SURGICAL DIRECTIVES: PEDIATRIC SURGERY

SURGICAL DIRECTIVES: PEDIATRIC SURGERY

Editor

PETER MATTEI, M.D.

Assistant Professor
Department of Surgery
Thomas Jefferson University
Philadelphia, Pennsylvania
Pediatric Surgeon
Department of Surgery
Alfred I. duPont Hospital for Children
Wilmington, Delaware

LIPPINCOTT WILLIAMS & WILKINS
A **Wolters Kluwer** Company
Philadelphia • Baltimore • New York • London
Buenos Aires • Hong Kong • Sydney • Tokyo

Acquisitions Editor: Lisa McAllister
Developmental Editor: Kerry Barrett
Production Editor: Thomas J. Foley
Manufacturing Manager: Benjamin Rivera
Cover Designer: Mark Lerner
Compositor: Lippincott Williams & Wilkins Desktop Division
Printer: Quebecor World, Dubuque

530 Walnut Street
Philadelphia, PA 19106 USA
LWW.com

Printed in the USA

Library of Congress Cataloging-in-Publication Data

Pediatric surgery / editor, Peter Mattei.
p. ; cm. — (Surgical directives)
Includes bibliographical references and index.
ISBN 0-7817-3000-7
1. Children—Surgery. 2. Pediatrics. I. Mattei, Peter, M.D. II. Series.
[DNLM: 1. Surgical Procedures, Operative—Child. 2. Pediatrics. WO 925 P3716 2003]
RD137 .P432 2003
617.9′8—dc21

2002141568

Care has been taken to confirm the accuracy of the information presented and to describe generally accepted practices. However, the authors, editor, and publisher are not responsible for errors or omissions or for any consequences from application of the information in this book and make no warranty, expressed or implied, with respect to the currency, completeness, or accuracy of the contents of the publication. Application of this information in a particular situation remains the professional responsibility of the practitioner.

The authors, editor, and publisher have exerted every effort to ensure that drug selection and dosage set forth in this text are in accordance with current recommendations and practice at the time of publication. However, in view of ongoing research, changes in government regulations, and the constant flow of information relating to drug therapy and drug reactions, the reader is urged to check the package insert for each drug for any change in indications and dosage and for added warnings and precautions. This is particularly important when the recommended agent is a new or infrequently employed drug.

Some drugs and medical devices presented in this publication have Food and Drug Administration (FDA) clearance for limited use in restricted research settings. It is the responsibility of the health care provider to ascertain the FDA status of each drug or device planned for use in their clinical practice.

10 9 8 7 6 5 4 3 2 1

To my son and my hero, Peter, whose daily triumph over autism, unfailing sense of humor, and fearless spirit are an example and an inspiration for me every day.

CONTENTS

CONTRIBUTING AUTHORS

Lisa P. Abramson, M.D. Resident, Department of Surgery, University of California, Davis, Sacramento, California; and Research Fellow, Department of Pediatric General Surgery, Children's Memorial Hospital, Chicago, Illinois

Robert D. Acton, M.D. Pediatric Surgery Fellow, Department of Pediatric General Surgery, Children's Memorial Hospital, Chicago, Illinois

Craig T. Albanese, M.D. Associate Professor and Attending Surgeon, Department of Surgery, Division of Pediatric Surgery, The University of California, San Francisco, and The University of California San Francisco Medical Center, San Francisco, California

Maria H. Alonso, M.D. Assistant Professor, Department of Surgery, Division of Pediatric Surgery, University of Cincinnati, and Cincinnati Children's Hospital Medical Center, Cincinnati, Ohio

Richard J. Andrassy, M.D. Denton A. Cooley Professor, Department of Surgery, University of Texas–Houston Medical School; and Surgeon-in-Chief and Chief, Department of Pediatric Surgical Oncology, Memorial-Hermann Hospital, M.D. Anderson Cancer Center, Houston, Texas

Harry Applebaum, M.D. Clinical Associate Professor, Department of Surgery, University of California at Los Angeles, School of Medicine; and Head, Division of Pediatric Surgery, Kaiser Permanente Medical Center, Los Angeles, California

Marjorie J. Arca, M.D. Assistant Professor, Departments of Clinical Surgery and Pediatric Surgery, Ohio State University College of Medicine and Public Health; and Director, Minimally Invasive Pediatric Surgery, Department of Pediatric Surgery, Children's Hospital, Columbus, Ohio

Robert M. Arensman, M.D. Professor, Departments of Surgery and Pediatrics, Northwestern University Medical School; and Chief, Department of Pediatric General Surgery, Children's Memorial Hospital, Chicago, Illinois

Keith W. Ashcraft, M.D. Professor, Emeritus, Department of Surgery, Children's Mercy Hospital, Kansas City, Missouri

Richard G. Azizkhan, M.D. Professor, Departments of Surgery and Pediatrics, University of Cincinnati; and Surgeon-in-Chief, Department of Pediatric Surgery, Cincinnati Children's Hospital Medical Center, Cincinnati, Ohio

William F. Balistreri, M.D. Professor, Department of Pediatrics, University of Cincinnati; and Chairman, Department of Pediatrics, Gastroenterology, Hepatology, and Nutrition, Cincinnati Children's Hospital Medical Center, Cincinnati, Ohio

Edward M. Barksdale, Jr., M.D. Associate Professor, UPP/Department of Surgery-PUH, University of Pittsburgh; and Co-director, Fetal Diagnosis and Treatment, Division of Pediatric Surgery, Children's Hospital of Pittsburgh, Pittsburgh, Pennsylvania

Julia S. Barthold, M.D. Associate Professor, Department of Urology, Thomas Jefferson University, Philadelphia, Pennsylvania; and Associate Chief, Division of Urology, Alfred I. duPont Hospital for Children, Wilmington, Delaware

Thomas L. Bauer, M.D. Cardiothoracic Surgery Resident, Department of Surgery, Jefferson Medical College and Thomas Jefferson University Hospital, Thomas Jefferson University, Philadelphia, Pennsylvania

Gail E. Besner, M.D. Associate Professor, Departments of Surgery and Pediatrics, The Ohio State University and Children's Hospital, Columbus, Ohio

Mary L. Brandt, M.D. Professor, Michael E. DeBakey Department of Surgery, Division of Pediatric Surgery, Baylor College of Medicine; and Clinic Chief, Department of Pediatric Surgery, Texas Children's Hospital, Houston, Texas

B. Randall Brenn, M.D. Assistant Professor, Department of Anesthesia and Critical Care, Thomas Jefferson University, Philadelphia, Pennsylvania; and Staff Anesthesiologist, Department of Anesthesia and Critical Care, Alfred I. duPont Hospital for Children, Wilmington, Delaware

Mary Brindle, M.D. Research Fellow, Department of General Surgery, Department of Pediatrics, Stanford University Medical School; and Research Fellow, Division of Pediatric Surgery, Lucile Packard Children's Hospital, Palo Alto, California

Steven W. Bruch, M.D. Pediatric Surgeon, Department of General Surgery, Division of Pediatric Surgery, Naval Medical Center, Portsmouth, Virginia

Donna A. Caniano, M.D. Professor, Departments of Clinical Surgery and Pediatrics, Ohio State University College of Medicine and Public Health; and Surgeon-in-Chief, Children's Hospital, Columbus, Ohio

Pat Casale, M.D. Senior Resident, Department of Urology, Thomas Jefferson University, Philadelphia, Pennsylvania

Adela T. Casas-Melley, M.D. Assistant Professor, Department of Surgery, Thomas Jefferson University, Philadelphia, Pennsylvania; and Surgeon, Division of Solid Organ Transplantation, Alfred I. duPont Hospital for Children, Wilmington, Delaware

John C. Chandler, M.D. Attending Surgeon, Departments of Surgery and Pediatrics, Greenville Hospital System, Greenville, South Carolina

Francisco G. Cigarroa, M.D. President, Offices of the President, The University of Texas Health Science Center at San Antonio; and Active, Department of Surgery, University Hospital, San Antonio, Texas

William S. Cobb, M.D. Chief Resident, Department of General Surgery, Greenville Hospital System, Greenville, South Carolina

Paul M. Colombani, M.D. Professor, Department of Surgery, Johns Hopkins University School of Medicine; and Children's Surgeon-in-Chief, Department of Pediatric Surgery, Johns Hopkins Hospital, Baltimore, Maryland

Steven P. Cook, M.D. Clinical Assistant Professor, Department of Otolaryngology, Thomas Jefferson University, Philadelphia, Pennsylvania; and Chief, Division of Pediatric Otolaryngology, Department of Surgery, Alfred I. duPont Hospital for Children, Wilmington, Delaware

Arnold G. Coran, M.D. Professor and Chief, Section of Pediatric Surgery, University of Michigan Medical School; and Surgeon-in-Chief, the C.S. Mott Children's Hospital, Ann Arbor, Michigan

Robin T. Cotton, M.D., F.A.C.S., F.R.C.S (C) Professor, Department of Otolaryngology—Head and Neck Surgery, University of Cincinnati; and Director, Department of Otolaryngology—Head and Neck Surgery, Cincinnati Children's Hospital Medical Center, Cincinnati, Ohio

Andrew M. Davidoff, M.D. Assistant Professor, Departments of Surgery and Pediatrics, University of Tennessee, Memphis, School of Medicine; and Assistant Member, Department of Surgery, St. Jude Children's Research Hospital, Memphis, Tennessee

Ellen S. Deutsch, M.D., F.A.C.S., F.A.A.P. Associate Professor, Departments of Otolaryngology—Head and Neck Surgery and Pediatrics, Thomas Jefferson University, Philadelphia, Pennsylvania; and Pediatric Otolaryngologist, Department of Surgery, Alfred I. duPont Hospital for Children, Wilmington, Delaware

Reed A. Dimmitt, M.D. Assistant Professor, Department of Pediatrics, University of Alabama at Birmingham; and Associate Director, Department of Pediatrics, NICK—Children's Hospital of Alabama, Birmingham, Alabama

Stephen E. Dolgin, M.D. Chief and Associate Professor, Departments of Surgery, Pediatrics, Anatomy, and Functional Morphology, Mt. Sinai School of Medicine and Mt. Sinai Hospital, New York, New York

Edward J. Doolin, M.D. Clinical Professor, Department of Surgery, University of Pennsylvania; and Department of Surgery, Children's Hospital of Philadelphia, Philadelphia, Pennsylvania

George T. Drugas, M.D. Assistant Professor, Departments of Surgery and Pediatrics, University of Rochester School of Medicine; and Pediatric Surgeon, Department of Surgery, Strong Memorial Hospital, Rochester, New York

Stephen P. Dunn, M.D. Professor, Departments of Surgery and Pediatrics, Thomas Jefferson University, Philadelphia, Pennsylvania; and Department of Surgery, Alfred I. duPont Hospital for Children, Wilmington, Delaware

Sigmund H. Ein, M.D., C.M., F.R.C.S.C., F.A.C.S., F.A.A.P. Associate Professor, Department of Surgery, Division of General Surgery, Faculty of Medicine, University of Toronto; and Staff Surgeon, Division of General Surgery, The Hospital for Sick Children, Toronto, Ontario, Canada

Ravindhra G. Elluru, M.D., Ph.D. Clinical Fellow, Department of Pediatric Otolaryngology, University of Cincinnati; and Clinical Fellow, Department of Pediatric Otolaryngology, Cincinnati Children's Hospital Medical Center, Cincinnati, Ohio

Sherif G.S. Emil, M.D., C.M., F.R.C.S.C. Assistant Clinical Professor, Division of Pediatric Surgery, University of California, Irvine College of Medicine, Irvine, California; and Attending Staff Surgeon, Department of Pediatric Surgery, Miller Children's Hospital, Long Beach, California

Mohammad A. Emran, M.D. Postdoctoral Fellow, Departments of Pediatric Surgery and Cancer Biology, Northwestern University Medical School, and Children's Memorial Hospital, Chicago, Illinois

Michael Erhard, M.D. Chief, Department of Pediatric Urology, Nemours Children's Clinic; and Assistant Professor, Department of Urology, Mayo Medical School, Jacksonville, Florida

Mary E. Fallat, M.D. Professor, Department of Surgery, Division of Pediatric Surgery, University of Louisville; and Trauma Chief, Kosair Children's Hospital, Louisville, Kentucky

Neil R. Feins, M.D. Senior Surgeon, Department of Surgery, The Children's Hospital, Harvard Medical School, Boston, Massachusetts

T. Ernesto Figueroa, M.D., F.A.A.P., F.A.C.S. Clinical Associate Professor, Department of Urology, Thomas Jefferson University, Philadelphia, Pennsylvania; and Chief, Division of Pediatric Urology, Alfred I. duPont Hospital for Children, Wilmington, Delaware

Christine M. Finck, M.D. Fellow, Department of Pediatric Surgery, Arkansas Children's Hospital, Little Rock, Arkansas

Anne C. Fischer, M.D., Ph.D. Assistant Professor, Department of Surgery, Division of Pediatric Surgery, Johns Hopkins Hospital, Baltimore, Maryland

Phoebe Fisher, M.D. Department of Anesthesiology and Critical Care, Alfred I. duPont Hospital for Children, Wilmington, Delaware

Steven J. Fishman, M.D. Assistant Professor, Department of Surgery, Harvard University Medical School; and Assistant in Surgery, Department of Surgery, Children's Hospital, Boston, Massachusetts

Hélène Flageole, M.D., M.Sc., F.R.C.S.(C), F.A.C.S. Assistant Professor, Department of Surgery, McGill University; and Department of Pediatric Surgical Services, Montreal Children's Hospital, Montreal, Quebec, Canada

Alan W. Flake, M.D. Professor, Department of Pediatric Surgery, University of Pennsylvania; and Department of Surgery, Children's Hospital of Philadelphia, Philadelphia, Pennsylvania

David S. Foley, M.D. Clinical Assistant Professor, Department of Surgery, Oklahoma University Medical Center; and Chief Resident, Department of Pediatric Surgery, Children's Hospital at Oklahoma University Medical Center, Oklahoma City, Oklahoma

Frazier W. Frantz, M.D., F.A.C.S. Staff Surgeon, Department of Surgery, and Head, Division of Pediatric Surgery, Naval Medical Center, Portsmouth, Virginia

Victor F. Garcia, M.D. Associate Professor, Department of Surgery, University of Cincinnati; and Director, Trauma Services Medical Center, Cincinnati Children's Hospital Medical Center, Cincinnati, Ohio

Michael W.L. Gauderer, M.D. Professor, Department of Pediatric Surgery, University of South Carolina, School of Medicine, Columbia, South Carolina; and Chief, Department of Pediatric Surgery, Children's Hospital, Greenville Hospital System, Greenville, South Carolina

Keith E. Georgeson, M.D. Professor, Department of Surgery, and Director, Division of Pediatric Surgery, University of Alabama School of Medicine; and Surgeon-in-Chief, Department of Pediatric Surgery, Children's Hospital of Alabama, Birmingham, Alabama

Frances T. Gill, M.S.N., R.N., C.S., C.P.N.P. Advanced Practice Nurse, Department of Pediatric General Surgery, Alfred I. duPont Hospital for Children, Wilmington, Delaware

Kim H. Giordano, M.S.N., R.N., C.S., C.P.N.P. Advanced Practice Nurse, Department of Pediatric General Surgery, Alfred I. duPont Hospital for Children, Wilmington, Delaware

Julie R. Glasson, M.D. Chief Fellow, Department of Pediatric Surgery, Children's Hospital of Michigan, Detroit, Michigan

Philip L. Glick, M.D. Chair (Interim) and Professor, Departments of Surgery, Pediatrics, and OBGYN, The State University of New York at Buffalo; and Surgeon-in-Chief, and Clinical Director, Department of Pediatric Surgery Services, The Children's Hospital of Buffalo, Buffalo, New York

Michael J. Goretsky, M.D. Assistant Professor, Department of Surgery, Eastern Virginia Medical School; and Pediatric Surgeon, Department of Surgery, Children's Hospital of the King's Daughters, Norfolk, Virginia

Kathleen Graziano, M.D. Department of General Surgery, University of Michigan Medical School and The C.S. Mott Children's Hospital, Ann Arbor, Michigan

Jeffrey H. Haynes, M.D. Associate Professor, Department of Surgery and Pediatrics, Medical College of Virginia, Virginia Commonwealth University, Richmond, Virginia

André Hebra, M.D. Director, Minimally Invasive Pediatric Surgery Program, Department of Surgery, University of South Florida, and All Children's Hospital, St. Petersburg, Florida

Michael A. Helmrath, M.D. Surgical Fellow, Department of Pediatric Surgery, Baylor College of Medicine; and Surgical Fellow, Department of Pediatric Surgery, Texas Children's Hospital, Houston, Texas

James H. Hertzog, M.D. Associate Professor, Department of Pediatrics, Thomas Jefferson University, Philadelphia, Pennsylvania; and Pediatric Intensivist, Department of Anesthesiology and Critical Care Medicine, Alfred I. duPont Hospital for Children, Wilmington, Delaware

Bruce A. Holm, Ph.D. Senior Vice Provost, Office of the Provost, The State University of New York at Buffalo; and Professor, Department of Pediatrics/OB GYN, The Children's Hospital of Buffalo, Buffalo, New York

Andrew R. Hong, M.D. Assistant Professor, Departments of Surgery and Pediatrics, Albert Einstein College of Medicine, Bronx, New York; and Assistant Attending in Surgery, and Director, Pediatric Trauma Center and Pediatric Minimally Invasive Surgery, Department of Pediatric Surgery, Schneider Children's Hospital, New Hyde Park, New York

J. David Hoover, M.D. Attending Surgeon, Departments of Surgery and Pediatrics, Northwestern Memorial Hospital; and Critical Care Surgeon, Department of Pediatric General Surgery, Children's Memorial Hospital, Chicago, Illinois

Thomas H. Inge, M.D., Ph.D. Assistant Professor, Department of Surgery, University of Cincinnati; and Pediatric Surgeon, Department of Pediatric Surgery, Cincinnati Children's Hospital Medical Center, Cincinnati, Ohio

Michael B. Ishitani, M.D. Associate Professor, Department of Surgery, Divisions of Pediatric Surgery and Transplantation, Mayo Clinic, Rochester, Minnesota

Joseph S. Janik, M.D., F.A.C.S. Assistant Professor, Department of Pediatric Surgery, University of Colorado Health Sciences Center, School of Medicine; and Pediatric Surgeon, and Director of Surgical Outreach, Department of Pediatric Surgery, The Children's Hospital Association, Denver, Colorado

Dale G. Johnson, M.D. Professor, Department of Surgery, Division of Pediatric Surgery, University of Utah School of Medicine; and Surgeon-in-Chief, Division of Pediatric Surgery, Primary Children's Medical Center, Salt Lake City, Utah

Mustafa Kabeer, M.D. Fellow, Department of Pediatric Surgery, Children's Hospital of Michigan, Detroit, Michigan

Timothy D. Kane, M.D. Assistant Professor, Department of Surgery, University of Pittsburgh School of Medicine; and Director, Pediatric Minimally Invasive Pediatric Surgery, Children's Hospital of Pittsburgh, Pittsburgh, Pennsylvania

Frederick M. Karrer, M.D. Associate Professor, Department of Surgery, University of Colorado, School of Medicine; and Chairman, Department of Pediatric Surgery, The Children's Hospital, Denver, Colorado

Aviva L. Katz, M.D. Assistant Professor, Departments of Surgery and Pediatrics, Thomas Jefferson University, Philadelphia, Pennsylvania, and Alfred I. duPont Hospital for Children, Wilmington, Delaware

Michael A. Keating, M.D. Clinical Professor, Department of Surgery, Division of Urology, University of South Florida, Tampa, Florida; and Chairman, Department of Children's Surgery, Arnold Palmer Hospital for Children, Orlando, Florida

Michael D. Klein, M.D. Arvin I. Philippart MD Endowed Chair, Department of Surgery, Wayne State University; and Surgeon-in-Chief, Department of Surgery, Children's Hospital of Michigan, Detroit, Michigan

Karen M. Kling, M.D. Department of Pediatric Surgery, Johns Hopkins University School of Medicine, and Johns Hopkins Hospital, Baltimore, Maryland

Rupa V. Kothandapani, M.D. Urology Resident, Department of Surgery, Division of Urology, University of Cincinnati; and Pediatric Urology Resident, Division of Pediatric Urology, Cincinnati Children's Hospital Medical Center, Cincinnati, Ohio

M. Ann Kuhn, M.D. Departments of Surgery and Pediatrics, The Ohio State University and Children's Hospital Columbus, Ohio

Jean-Martin Laberge, M.D., F.R.C.S. (C), F.A.C.S. Associate Professor, Department of Surgery, McGill University; and Director, Division of Pediatric General Surgery, Montreal Children's Hospital, Montreal, Quebec, Canada

Alan P. Ladd, M.D. Assistant Professor, Department of Surgery, Indiana University School of Medicine; and Deaprtment of Surgery, J.W. Riley Hospital for Children, Indianapolis, Indiana

Scott E. Langenburg, M.D., F.A.C.S. Assistant Professor, Department of Surgery, Wayne State University; and Surgeon, Department of Pediatric General and Thoracic Surgery, Children's Hospital of Michigan, Detroit, Michigan

Michael P. La Quaglia, M.D. Professor, Department of Surgery, Weill-Cornell University Medical School; and Chief, Department of Pediatric Surgery, Memorial Sloan-Kettering Cancer Center, New York, New York

Eric Lazar, M.D. Department of Pediatric Surgery, Columbia College of Physicians and Surgeons, New York, New York

Robert W. Letton, Jr., M.D., F.A.C.S., F.A.A.P. Assistant Professor, Departments of Surgery and Pediatrics, Wake Forest University School of Medicine, Winston-Salem, North Carolina

Fawn C. Lewis, M.D. Clinical Instructor, Department of Surgery, Northwestern University Medical School; and Surgical Critical Care Attending, Department of Pediatric General Surgery, Children's Memorial Hospital, Chicago, Illinois

Nicola A. Lewis, M.D., F.R.C.S. Research Fellow, Departments of Surgery and Pediatrics, The State University of New York at Buffalo; and Research Fellow, Department of Surgery, The Children's Hospital of Buffalo, Buffalo, New York

Thom E Lobe, M.D. Professor, Department of Pediatrics and Preventive Medicine, University of Tennessee, and LeBonheur Children's Medical Center, Memphis, Tennessee

Susan R. Luck, M.D. Professor, Departments of Surgery and Pediatrics, Northwestern University Medical School; and Attending Surgeon, Department of Pediatric General Surgery, Children's Memorial Hospital, Chicago, Illinois

François I. Luks, M.D., Ph.D. Associate Professor, Departments of Surgery and Pediatrics, Brown Medical School; and Attending Surgeon, Division of Pediatric Surgery, Hasbro Children's Hospital, Providence, Rhode Island

Dennis P. Lund, M.D. Associate Professor, and Chairman, Department of Surgery, Division of General Surgery, University of Wisconsin; and Surgeon-in-Chief, University of Wisconsin Children's Hospital, Madison, Wisconsin

Irene W.Y. Ma, M.D. Chief Medical Resident, Department of Medicine, University of British Columbia, Vancouver, British Columbia, Canada

Tippi C. MacKenzie, M.D. Fetal Surgery Fellow, Department of Surgery, Children's Hospital of Philadelphia, Philadelphia, Pennsylvania

Peter B. Manning, M.D. Associate Professor, Department of Surgery, University of Cincinnati School of Medicine; and Director, Department of Pediatric Cardiothoracic Surgery, Cincinnati Children's Hospital Medical Center, Cincinnati, Ohio

Peter Mattei, M.D. Assistant Professor, Department of Surgery, Thomas Jefferson University, Philadelphia, Pennsylvania; and Surgeon, Department of Pediatric Surgery, Alfred I. duPont Hospital for Children, Wilmington, Delaware

Mark McCollum, M.D. Chief Resident, General Surgery, University of Utah, Primary Children's Medical Center, Salt Lake City, Utah

Milissa A. McKee, M.D. Assistant Professor, Departments of Surgery and Pediatrics, Yale University School of Medicine, New Haven, Connecticut

Rebecka L. Meyers, M.D. Associate Professor, Adjunct Professor, and Division Chief of Pediatric Surgery, Department of Surgery, University of Utah School of Medicine; and Pediatric Surgical Director, Liver and Transplant Program, Division of Pediatric Surgery, Primary Children's Medical Center, Salt Lake City, Utah

R. Lawrence Moss, M.D. Associate Professor, Department of Surgery, Yale University School of Medicine; and Surgeon-in-Chief, Department of Surgery, Yale-New Haven Children's Hospital, New Haven, Connecticut

Stephen G. Murphy, M.D. Assistant Professor, Department of Surgery, Thomas Jefferson University, Philadelphia, Pennsylvania; and Department of Surgery, Alfred I. duPont Hospital for Children, Wilmington, Delaware

George B. Mychaliska, M.D. Pediatric Surgery Fellow, Department of Pediatric General Surgery, Children's Hospital of Michigan, Detroit, Michigan

Michael L. Nance, M.D. Assistant Professor, Department of Surgery, University of Pennsylvania; and Attending Surgeon, Department of Surgery, Children's Hospital of Philadelphia, Philadelphia, Pennsylvania

Deborah A. Neigut, M.D. Assistant Professor, Department of Pediatrics, The University of Texas Health Sciences Center at San Antonio, San Antonio, Texas

Holly L. Neville, M.D. Resident, Department of Surgery, University of Texas-Houston Medical School, Houston, Texas

Kurt D. Newman, M.D. Professor, Departments of Surgery and Pediatrics, The George Washington University School of Medicine; and Vice Chair, Department of Surgery, Children's Hospital, Washington, D.C.

Peter F. Nichol, M.D., Ph.D. Senior Resident, Department of Surgery, Division of General Surgery, University of Wisconsin Hospitals and Clinics, Madison, Wisconsin

James A. O'Neill, Jr., M.D. Professor of Surgery Emeritus and Surgeon-in-Chief Emeritus, Section of Surgical Sciences, Vanderbilt University Medical Center, Nashville, Tennessee

Charles N. Paidas, M.D. Associate Professor, Department of Pediatric Surgery, Johns Hopkins University School of Medicine and Johns Hopkins Hospital, Baltimore, Maryland

Konstantinos Papadakis, M.D. Department of Surgery, Children's Hospital, Harvard Medical School, Boston, Massachusetts

Walter Pegoli, Jr., M.D. Chief, Division of Pediatric Surgery, Department of Surgery, University of Rochester School of Medicine and University of Rochester Medical Center, Rochester, New York

Alberto Peña, M.D. Professor, Department of Surgery, Albert Einstein College of Medicine, Bronx, New York; and Chief, Department of Pediatric Surgery, Schneider Children's Hospital, New Hyde Park, New York

Scott Penfil, M.D. Clinical Assistant Professor, Department of Pediatrics, Thomas Jefferson University, Philadelphia, Pennsylvania; and Pediatric Intensivist, Department of Anesthesiology and Critical Care Medicine, Alfred I. duPont Hospital for Children, Wilmington, Delaware

J. Duncan Phillips, M.D. Associate Professor, Department of Surgery, University of North Carolina at Chapel Hill; and Attending Pediatric Surgeon, Department of Surgery, North Carolina Children's Hospital, Chapel Hill, North Carolina

John F. Pohl, M.D. Assistant Professor, Department of Pediatrics, Section of Pediatric Gastroenterology, Scott and White Hospital, Texas A&M Health Science Center, Temple, Texas

Todd A. Ponsky, M.D. Resident, Department of Surgery, The George Washington University School of Medicine, and The George Washington University Hospital, Washington, D.C.

Joseph Queenan, M.D. Chief, Division of Neurosurgery, Alfred I. duPont Hospital for Children, Wilmington, Delaware

Shawn J. Rangel, M.D. Post Doctoral Fellow, Division of Pediatric Surgery, Stanford University School of Medicine, Stanford, California

Marleta Reynolds, M.D. Associate Professor, Department of Surgery, Northwestern University Medical School; and Attending Surgeon, Department of Pediatric General Surgery, Children's Memorial Hospital, Chicago, Illinois

Mark A. Rich, M.D. Clinical Associate Professor, Department of Urology, University of South Florida, Tampa; and Director, Division of Pediatric Urology, Nemours Children's Clinic, Orlando, Florida

Catherine Richards, M. Chir., F.R.C.S. (Paed) Consultant Pediatric and Neonatal Surgeon, Department of Pediatrics, University Hospital, Lewisham, London, United Kingdom

Richard R. Ricketts, M.D. Professor, Departments of Surgery and Pediatrics, Emory Children's Center; and Chief, Department of Surgery, Division of Pediatrics, Children's Healthcare of Atlanta at Egleston, Atlanta, Georgia

Bradley M. Rodgers, M.D. Professor, Department of Surgery, and Chief, Division of Pediatric Surgery, University of Virginia Health System, Charlottesville, Virginia

Jonathan H. Ross, M.D. Head, Section of Pediatric Urology, The Urological Institute, Cleveland Clinic Foundation, Cleveland, Ohio

Stephen A. Rowe, M.D. 4th Year Surgical Resident, Department of General Surgery, University of Louisville, Louisville, Kentucky

Michael J. Rutter, B.H.B., M.B.C.L.B., F.R.A.C.S. Assistant Professor, Department of Pediatric Otolaryngology–Head and Neck Surgery, University of Cincinnati; and Pediatrict Otolaryngologist, Department of Otolaryngology–Head and Neck Surgery, Cincinnati Children's Hospital Medical Center, Cincinnati, Ohio

Frederick C. Ryckman, M.D. Professor, Department of Surgery, Division of Pediatric Surgery, University of Cincinnati, and Cincinnati Children's Hospital Medical Center, Cincinnati, Ohio

Eric R. Scaife, M.D. Assistant Professor, Department of Surgery, Division of Pediatric Surgery, University of Utah School of Medicine; and Medical Director, Trauma Program, Division of Pediatric Surgery, Primary Children's Medical Center, Salt Lake City, Utah

L.R. Scherer III, M.D. Department of Surgery, Section of Pediatric Surgery, Indiana University School of Medicine; and Department of Surgery, J.W. Riley Hospital for Children, Indianapolis, Indiana

Marshall Z. Schwartz, M.D. Professor, and Vice Chairman, Department of Surgery, Thomas Jefferson University, Philadelphia, Pennsylvania; and Vice Chairman, Department of Surgery, Alfred I. duPont Hospital for Children, Wilmington, Delaware

Curtis A. Sheldon, M.D., F.A.C.S., F.A.A.P. Professor, Department of Surgery, University of Cincinnati; and Director, Division of Pediatric Urology, Cincinnati Children's Hospital Medical Center, Cincinnati, Ohio

Nicholas A. Shorter, M.D. Department of Surgery, Weill-Cornell University Medical School; and Associate Attending Surgeon, Department of Pediatric Surgery, Memorial Sloan-Kettering Cancer Center, New York, New York

Samuel D. Smith, M.D. Professor, Department of Surgery, University of Arkansas for Medical Sciences; and Chief of Staff, and Chief, Department of Pediatric Surgery, Arkansas Children's Hospital, Little Rock, Arkansas

Samuel Z. Soffer, M.D. Resident, Division of Pediatric Surgery, Department of Surgery, Columbia University College of Physicians and Surgeons, and Children's Hospital of New York, New York, New York

Lewis Spitz, Ph.D., F.R.C.S. Nuffield Professor, Department of Pediatric Surgery, Institute of Child Health, University College London, Great Ormond Street Hospital, London, United Kingdom

Ala Stanford, M.D. Research Fellow, Department of Pediatric Surgery, Children's Hospital of Pittsburgh, Pittsburgh, Pennsylvania

Robert P. Stanton, M.D., F.A.C.S. Director, Musculoskeletal Tumor Program, Department of Surgery, Alfred I. duPont Hospital for Children, Wilmington, Delaware

Richard J. Stevenson, M.D. Associate Professor, Department of Clinical Surgery, Division of Pediatric Surgery, University of Cincinnati, and Cincinnati Children's Hospital Medical Center, Cincinnati, Ohio

Charles J.H. Stolar, M.D. Director, Division of Pediatric Surgery, Department of Surgery, Columbia University College of Physicians and Surgeons, and Children's Hospital of New York, New York, New York

Steven Stylianos, M.D. Associate Professor, Departments of Surgery and Pediatrics, Columbia University College of Physicians and Surgeons; and Director, Regional Pediatric Trauma Program, Children's Hospital of New York–Presbyterian, New York, New York

Riccardo A. Superina, M.D. Professor, Department of Surgery, Northwestern University Medical School; and Director, Department of Transplant Surgery, Children's Memorial Hospital, Chicago, Illinois

Roman M. Sydorak, M.D. Postgaduate Research Fellow, and Surgical Resident, Department of Surgery, Division of Pediatric Surgery, The University of California, San Francisco, and the University of California San Francisco Medical Center, San Francisco, California

Lesli Taylor, M.D. Associate Professor, Department of Pediatric Surgery, University of North Carolina at Chapel Hill, School of Medicine, Chapel Hill, North Carolina

Daniel H. Teitelbaum, M.D. Associate Professor, Department of Surgery, Section of Pediatric Surgery, University of Michigan Medical School, and C.S. Mott Children's Hospital, Ann Arbor, Michigan

John T. Tomicic, M.D. Fellow in Surgical Oncology, Boston University, Boston, Massachusetts; and Roger Williams Hospital, Providence, Rhode Island

David W. Tuggle, M.D. Paula Milburn Miller, CMRI, Chair, Department of Pediatric Surgery, Oklahoma University Medical Center; and Chief, Section of Pediatric Surgery, Children's Hospital at Oklahoma Medical Center, Oklahoma City, Oklahoma

Daniel von Allmen, M.D. Assistant Professor, Department of Surgery, Division of Pediatric Surgery, University of Pennsylvania School of Medicine; and Staff Surgeon, Department of General and Thoracic Surgery, Children's Hospital of Philadelphia, Philadelphia, Pennsylvania

Brad W. Warner, M.D. Professor, Department of Surgery, University of Cincinnati College of Medicine; and Attending Surgeon, Division of Pediatric Surgery, Cincinnati Children's Hospital Medical Center, Cincinnati, Ohio

H. Warner Webb, M.D. Professor of Surgery, Department of Pediatric Surgery, University of Florida; and Pediatric Surgeon, Department of Children's Surgical Services, Wolfson Children's Hospital, Jacksonville, Florida

Thomas V. Whalen, M.D., M.M.M. Professor, Departments of Surgery and Pediatrics, University of Medicine and Dentistry of New Jersey-Robert Wood Johnson Medical School, New Brunswick, New Jersey

Philip J. Wolfson, M.D. Professor, Department of Surgery, Thomas Jefferson University, Philadelphia, Pennsylvania; and Chief, Division of General Surgery, Alfred I. duPont Hospital for Children, Wilmington, Delaware

Mark L. Wulkan, M.D. Assistant Professor, Department of Surgery, Division of Pediatric Surgery, Emory Children's Center; and Surgical Director, PICU, Department of Pediatric Surgery, Children's Healthcare of Atlanta at Egleston, Atlanta, Georgia

Uzay Yasar, M.D. Chief Resident, Department of Surgery, Division of Urology, University of Cincinnati; and Division of Pediatric Urology, Cincinnati Children's Hospital Medical Center, Cincinnati, Ohio

Garrett Zallen, M.D. Pediatric Surgery Fellow, Department of Pediatric Surgery, Children's Hospital of Buffalo, Buffalo, New York

Moritz M. Ziegler, M.D. Professor, Department of Surgery, Harvard Medical School; and Chairman, and Surgeon-in-Chief, Department of Surgery, Children's Hospital, Boston, Massachusetts

FOREWORD

Surgical Directives: Pediatric Surgery continues a trend in textbooks that started with the *Current Therapy* series. This series, which includes textbooks in Surgery, Neurosurgery, Gastroenterology, etc., is meant to supplement the general textbooks in their fields. The general textbooks are marvelous reference texts that contain extensive descriptions of presentation, diagnosis, pathogenesis, pathophysiology, and a clinical course of diseases in each field. Due to the length of such textbooks, and the time and effort required to put such a text together, they generally are only revised every six to eight years. This often makes the discussions on therapy outdated. With the newer format of textbooks, as exemplified by *Surgical Directives: Pediatric Surgery*, the interval between new editions has been shortened substantially, often to a period of every three years. This allows the therapy section, the section that is most important to the experienced practitioner, to be kept up to date. This textbook edited by Dr. Peter Mattei, with multiple contributors, produces such a text for pediatric surgeons. If one wants to thoroughly investigate a disease process, learn about pathogenesis, pathophysiology, diagnosis, and have access to an extensive bibliography, Dr. Mattei's text will not substitute for the several superb general textbooks of pediatric surgery available. For the busy practitioner, however, who wants immediate access to the most up-to-date information concerning management of a disease, this text is superb.

Surgical Directives: Pediatric Surgery contains 139 chapters with over 150 contributors. Most of the contributors are from the United States, but there is some international participation as well. The contributors vary from nurse practitioners, residents and fellows, to Division Chiefs and Department Chairmen. All are experts with substantial experience in the field about which they write. The chapters do not necessarily contain all treatment options for a disease. They do, however, present a therapeutic option by an expert in the field who through his or her experience has developed a proven way of managing the disease entity about which they write. This book is not written for medical students. The text assumes basic knowledge of anatomy, pathophysiology, and diagnostic methods. The book is thus aimed at senior residents in general surgery, pediatric surgical fellows, and the experienced pediatric surgeon in both the academic and community setting. Each chapter contains a Suggested Readings Section at the end of the chapter, which includes several key articles or chapters on the topic dealt with in the chapter. Extensive bibliographies that are difficult to sort through for key publications, are not present. The Suggested Reading List allows the reader to go directly to the important key publications in that field.

I presume this will be the first in a series of editions of *Surgical Directives: Pediatric Surgery* over the years to come. If the authors of the chapters change in each new edition, each will be additive to the one that precedes it. With each new edition, the pediatric surgeon will have another expert's opinion on how to manage a clinical situation or a disease entity. The continuing editions of *Surgical Directives: Pediatric Surgery*, along with a standard general pediatric surgical textbook, will provide the pediatric surgical trainee, and the practicing pediatric surgeon with the broad overview of pediatric surgery and the most up-to-date information on therapy that are required to remain a current superb practitioner of their art.

John L. Cameron, M.D.
Baltimore, Maryland
June, 2002

PREFACE

There are several fine textbooks already available that discuss the scientific and clinical basis of pediatric surgery. These texts, written and revised by some of the most highly respected surgeons in the field, pass on a rich tradition of surgical techniques developed and refined by cumulative experience. Many of these techniques have become the standard approach to pediatric surgical problems for generations of pediatric surgery fellows. The purpose of *Surgical Directives: Pediatric Surgery* is to extend this tradition. It is intended to be a complement to these fine works, not a replacement.

Surgical textbooks generally provide detailed discussion of background, anatomy, pathophysiology, and standard approaches to management. They are understandably limited in their discussion of the more complex and sometimes controversial aspects of surgical management. This volume is a forum in which the subtleties of patient management are discussed in detail, and novel approaches to common problems are presented. It is my hope that residents, fellows, and attendings will find this work useful as a resource for keeping abreast of current management strategies, and for studying for certification and recertification examinations. Ideally this book will serve yet another purpose: to foster the progressive and enthusiastic attitude characteristic of pediatric surgeons since the days of William Ladd.

Each author was asked to produce an authoritative monograph on a very specific topic using direct, first-person perspective, as though they were trying to pass on their expertise on the subject to a fellow or chief resident. The chapters are not meant to be an expansive discussion of all possible ways to treat a particular problem, nor do they claim to represent the only correct approach. Rather, they are meant to present one reasonable approach that is based on the opinion and judgement of an experienced pediatric surgeon. Some authors were given the opportunity to elaborate on very narrow topics that are rarely covered in other texts, which are important in the care of pediatric surgical patients. Certain topics, such as Hirschsprung's disease and esophageal atresia, are divided into several chapters. This allows particular aspects of these conditions to be addressed specifically, without the usual constraints inherent in writing a comprehensive chapter on a much broader subject. The reader also benefits from what is effectively a collaboration of several experts presenting slightly different points of view.

Surgical Directives: Pediatric Surgery differs from other pediatric surgery texts in that it is designed for senior practitioners and senior surgery residents, pediatric surgery fellows, and attendings. The authors assume the reader has a grasp of the fundamental anatomy and physiology but would like to know how to approach a problem clinically. Each chapter discusses the aspects of real patient care that a chief resident is expected to understand by the end of fellowship. These aspects include the work up, preoperative preparation, operative technique, and postoperative care–with special emphasis on pitfalls, complications, and follow-up care. The chapters are first-hand descriptions of individualistic approaches to a wide variety of pediatric surgical problems presented by experts with real clinical experience.

Nearly every aspect of pediatric surgery relevant to a practitioner in a typical clinical practice is covered. Pediatric surgery is a field that is continually evolving, and engendering ever more focused subspecialties. This book tries to be true to the general surgery core of pediatric surgery, with in-depth coverage of specialized subjects that are still relevant to many practicing pediatric surgeons. There are chapters that cover aspects of alimentary tract surgery, thoracic surgery, surgical oncology, trauma, endocrine surgery, head and neck surgery, and skin and soft tissue surgery. In addition, topics related to perioperative care, transplantation, urology, and critical care are covered. There is also an emphasis on the innovative concepts being advanced by the current generation of pediatric surgical pioneers that are rapidly being incorporated into mainstream pediatric surgery, especially minimally invasive techniques and creative approaches to common surgical problems.

Above all, *Surgical Directives: Pediatric Surgery* is a text by pediatric surgeons for pediatric surgeons. It is meant to be a practical guide for the daily care of pediatric surgical patients that can be carried in a backpack or referred to late at night in a call room, rather than collecting dust on a library shelf to be referenced only on special occasions. It is also intended to represent the current state-of-the-art, rather than a review of basic concepts, and as such may help to stimulate new ideas and a further advancement of pediatric surgical science.

Peter Mattei, M.D.

ACKNOWLEDGMENTS

I am fortunate to have had several extraordinary mentors over the years to whom I will always be grateful, especially Dr. Richard M. Schultz at the University of Pennsylvania, Dr. John L. Cameron at The Johns Hopkins University School of Medicine, and Dr. Moritz M. Ziegler at the Cincinnati Children's Hospital Medical Center, now at Harvard Medical School.

I would also like to acknowledge the many pediatric surgeons and subspecialists who wrote each of the chapters of this book and whose hard work and skill certainly made my job as editor much easier.

I would like to thank my partners in the Division of Pediatric Surgery at Alfred I. duPont Hospital for Children for their support; Dr. Robert Brislin, Department of Anesthesia, for his expert editorial assistance at several key points in the project; and Jennifer Adams, my Administrative Assistant, for her help in keeping me organized throughout the process.

Most importantly, I am supremely grateful to my wife, Kimberly Keenen Mattei. Without her constant inspiration, understanding, and support I could accomplish nothing and without her sensibility, insight, and timely advice I could accomplish nothing of value.

SURGICAL DIRECTIVES: PEDIATRIC SURGERY

SECTION I

PREOPERATIVE AND POSTOPERATIVE CARE

1

PREOPERATIVE EVALUATION AND TESTING

B. RANDALL BRENN

Preoperative evaluation of pediatric surgical patients has undergone changes in the past 20 years due to altered financial dynamics as well as new medical knowledge. More patients and procedures are shifting from inpatient to outpatient status. Consequently, the preparation of patients has moved to surgeons' offices, presurgical clinics, and preoperative areas on the day of surgery. Parents' work schedules also limit the time available for preparation of patients. The time available to prepare patients is diminished, but the task is certainly no less important.

The goals of preoperative preparation are similar for adults and children: to identify and optimize coexisting diseases and introduce the patient to the perioperative process. The psychological preparation differs in that there are different psychological needs depending on the age of the patient. In addition, with pediatric patients, the whole family prepares for the surgery.

This chapter focuses on the preoperative preparation of pediatric patients and their families. It highlights common issues involving normal patients and children with certain pediatric diseases that require consideration prior to receiving anesthesia and surgery.

RISKS OF ANESTHESIA

One of the most common questions asked by parents is "what are the risks of anesthesia?" It is not uncommon for parents to ask this of the surgeons, nurses, and clerks, even though the pediatric anesthesiologist is probably the best one to answer the question. Unfortunately, this question has no simple answer—estimates from large series do not account for all anesthetics administered. The common minor complications of anesthesia are related to the specific techniques used such as sore throat, nausea, vomiting, croup, and minor oral trauma. More major problems are postoperative apnea, untoward drug reactions, aspiration pneumonia, arrhythmias and cardiac arrest. Usually the major complications are associated with a predisposing history, such as cardiac disease, pulmonary disease or apnea of prematurity.

Studies from Great Britain during the 1980s have estimated a mortality rate of 1 in 185,000 due to anesthesia alone. In the United States, since the implementation of monitoring standards, the incidence of mortality in healthy patients may be as high as 1 in 200,000. The Pediatric Perioperative Cardiac Arrest Study revealed a rate of 2.5 cardiac arrests (not deaths) in 10,000, with the incidence 0.6 per 10,000 (1 in 166,000) in healthy pediatric patients. Modern monitoring, specifically pulse-oximetry and capnography, combined with in-depth training of pediatric subspecialists has allowed safer surgical procedures on patients who are more compromised.

The American Society of Anesthesiologists (ASA) physical status score allows anesthesiologists to communicate the physical condition of the patient, independent of the planned operation. The physical status serves as a common language among different practitioners and institutions for subsequent analysis reporting of morbidity and mortality. The ASA status is not intended to give an estimation of risk, but it is a patient-centered classification to warn of potential morbidity related to the patient's preexisting disease processes (Table 1.1).

INFORMATION GATHERING

Once it has been decided that a patient needs elective surgery, it is necessary that the patient and his or her caregivers become oriented to the perioperative process. Patients can be seen prior to or on the day of surgery, depending on the health of the patient and the procedure. Although there is a tendency in modern medicine to speed

B. R. Brenn: Department of Anesthesia and Critical Care, Thomas Jefferson University, Philadelphia, Pennsylvania; and Department of Anesthesia and Critical Care, Alfred I. duPont Hospital for Children, Wilmington, Delaware.

TABLE 1.1. THE PHYSICAL STATUS CLASSIFICATION OF THE AMERICAN SOCIETY OF ANESTHESIOLOGISTS

Physical Status Classification	Description
PS-1	A normal healthy patient
PS-2	A patient with mild systemic disease that results in no functional limitations Examples: hypertension, diabetes mellitus, chronic bronchitis, morbid obesity, extremes of age
PS-3	A patient with severe systemic disease that results in functional limitations Examples: poorly controlled hypertension, diabetes mellitus with vascular complications, angina pectoris, prior myocardial infarction, pulmonary disease that limits activity
PS-4	A patient with severe systemic disease that is a constant threat to life Examples: congestive heart failure, unstable angina pectoris, advanced pulmonary, renal, or hepatic dysfunction
PS-5	A moribund patient who is not expected to survive without the operation Examples: ruptured abdominal aneurysm, pulmonary embolus, head injury with increased intracranial pressure
PS-6	A declared brain-dead patient whose organs are being removed for donor purposes
Emergency operation (E)	Any patient in whom an emergency operation is required Example: An otherwise healthy 39-year-old woman who requires dilation and curettage for moderate but persistent vaginal bleeding (PS-1E)

Reprinted from Smethan GW. Preoperative pulmonary evaluation. *N Engl J Med* 1999;340:937–944; with permission.

up the preoperative process, just having the patient show up on the day of surgery is not always the best strategy for pediatric patients, especially those new to the hospital and surgical milieu. Parents as well as their children all experience anxiety prior to the day of surgery. Young children can sense the anxiety in their parents, although they may not know what is happening. Reductions in anxiety of the whole family through preoperative teaching programs are felt to improve coping on the day of surgery.

Our institution encourages all participating surgeons to send their patients to our preoperative clinic to begin preparing for the upcoming surgery. Most patients come a few days prior to the surgery to have a screening history and physical examination performed by nurse practitioners specifically entrusted to gather the necessary information to ensure a safe anesthetic and surgery. Including the patient history and results of the physical examination on the chart allow for quick access and alert the anesthesiologists to potential problems prior to the day of surgery.

Preoperative nurses offer an educational program in addition to managing the paperwork. Many recent reviews of pediatric preoperative programs have concluded that the best programs have age-specific materials. These educational programs provide an opportunity for the family and patient to take some time to digest the often voluminous new information about the child's upcoming procedure. Usually the well-prepared parent will be able to translate for their child what is to occur and reduce anxiety. This preparation paves the way for a smooth perioperative course.

The family is encouraged to contact the department of anesthesia or the surgeon if there are any pressing questions, and an anesthesiologist is available if there are any issues that need resolution on the day of the preoperative visit. On the day of surgery the family and patient will meet the anesthesiologist, nurse anesthetists, residents, operating room nurses, and any other personnel involved with the case. This is the opportunity for the anesthesiologist to develop a relationship prior to going to the operating room.

AGE-RELATED PSYCHOLOGICAL CONCERNS

It is helpful to split the pediatric population into different age groups to be able to generalize about the kinds of problems that may occur. A typical grouping would include the young infant (0–6 months), the older infant/toddler (6 months to 3 years), the young child (3–7 years), the older child (7–12 years), and the adolescent (12 years and above). Note that these distinctions are arbitrary and many children may not fit perfectly into these groups because of accelerated or stunted development.

The young infant may be physiologically challenging to manage in the perioperative period, but is often psychologically easy to prepare. Usually the infant can be handled by anyone with a kind and caring manner and there is little risk for separation anxiety. The parents may have a more difficult time with the idea of their child going to the operating room where they do not control what is happening. The parents need to be reassured that the anesthetic agents are reversible and that their child will receive pain medication intraoperatively and postoperatively.

The older infant/young child is undergoing a tremendous amount of social and developmental change that can be derailed with the onset of an illness or the stress of surgery. Language is just being developed, and children this age cannot completely comprehend what is happening to them. Separation anxiety becomes firmly established as children learn how to interact with other children and adults. This group is most prone to regressive behaviors during the perioperative process. It is not uncommon to have the toddler stop sleeping through the night or suffer night terrors after a surgical procedure. Bedwetting could occur just when the child has started developing bladder control. It is necessary to assure parents that such behavioral changes will be temporary.

Young children are more able to converse and comprehend what is happening to them and know that they may be "sick." However, they may have magical ideation, and may view the hospitalization as punishment for being sick. These patients develop vivid and exaggerated memories of noxious events. Having an intravenous line is not simply a "little poke" or a "bee sting." It is considered being harpooned! Hearing that the anesthesiologist will "put them to sleep" can be misinterpreted to mean what happened when Rover got old. Separation from caregivers is a potentially traumatic event, especially in repeat patients, and parents are usually amazed when their child happily rolls to the operating room after a well-dosed and well-timed premedication.

Fortunately, this population also is extremely responsive to well-designed preoperative teaching programs. Role-playing and play-acting are a part of everyday life, and this group can usually be cajoled to play along. The media of choice vary as the technology of communication progresses. In the past, books were the staple, followed by movies and videotapes. Now parents are availing themselves of interactive Internet sites that have additional information.

Preadolescents usually become accustomed to separation from their caregivers because of attending school. They usually understand "if-then" scenarios and can be told more about their procedure and what is expected. They usually become actively involved with the preoperative process, and the operative plan should be explained to them. They also need to know about postoperative pain control techniques that are appropriate to their age and to the procedure. Care must be taken in that stressful situations may bring out the more dependent tendencies in these children. After all, they still are children and they still look to their parents for guidance and support. Their trust has to be earned. Woe to the anesthesiologist or surgeon who says "there won't be any pain when you wake up," and then pain does occur. The child may be forever frightened and suspicious, and the medical profession will have lost much of its credibility in the child's eyes.

Adolescent patients, despite their reputation for difficulty, are usually easy to communicate with in the perioperative period. Adolescents can understand the procedure and the consequences thereof, although they may not be happy about them. It is important to not circumvent these patients in conversations about the procedure with parents. Adolescents should be included in the decisions about induction techniques, intravenous lines, pain treatment options, and so forth—the parent may want the child to have a spinal block and the adolescent patient may object, making for an interesting preoperative debate. Because they may be able to hide many of their fears about the procedure and the potential disfigurement that might result, special care with adolescents is crucial.

NPO GUIDELINES

The strict "NPO after midnight" has never worked well in the younger pediatric population, and pediatric anesthesiologists have been parting from the fold for years. In addition, a controversy over whether or not breast milk should be considered a "clear liquid" has been debated. Unfortunately, NPO (nothing by mouth) guidelines vary from institution to institution based on differing interpretations of an incomplete body of literature on the subject. What is not debated is that if a patient aspirates a certain volume of gastric fluid of acidic pH, there is a high likelihood of developing severe aspiration pneumonia and the potential for respiratory failure requiring an intensive care stay. Most practitioners and parents understand that this is an unacceptable risk in an otherwise healthy patient undergoing elective surgery.

Our institution has arrived at the following guidelines that apply to healthy patients undergoing elective surgery:

1. All healthy patients may have *clear liquids until 2 hours* prior to arrival at the hospital. Clear liquids are considered those that are transparent, such as sugar water, Pedialyte, apple juice, white grape juice, flavored gelatin, and Gatorade. Obviously this list is not all-inclusive, and some parents may choose another sugar-based clear drink that is perfectly appropriate.
2. Infants under *one year of age* may have *breast milk 4 hours* prior to arrival at the hospital and solids and formula 6 hours prior to arrival at the hospital.

3. Children over *one year of age* must not have any *solids or milk for 8 hours* prior to arrival at the hospital.

It should be noted that we decided on "prior to arrival at the hospital" in an attempt to ensure that the guidelines are most successfully met. It is important that the surgical fellow is aware of the NPO guidelines of his or her hospital to avoid misunderstandings that result in delayed or canceled surgeries.

NEONATAL CONCERNS

The medical history of a child, especially a young infant, starts prior to birth. Knowledge of the maternal history, gestational complications, and birth history are essential because certain problems may extend into the newborn period and the childhood years. Table 1.2 lists some points in the patient's history that can have profound influences on the outcome.

TABLE 1.2. THE MEDICAL HISTORY AND REVIEW OF SYSTEMS WITH ANESTHETIC IMPLICATIONS

System	History	Possible Anesthetic Implication
Central nervous and neuromuscular systems	Seizures	Medications: drug interactions, possible inadequate serum levels, valproate-induced hepatitis
	Head trauma	Elevated intracranial pressure; anemia
	Hydrocephalus	Possible elevated intracranial pressure
	CNS tumor	Possible elevated intracranial pressure; chemotherapeutic drugs and interactions
	Developmental delay	Bulbar dysfunction and risk of aspiration
	Neuromuscular disease	Altered response to relaxants
	Muscle disease	Risk of malignant hyperthermia; hyperkalemia after succinylcholine
	Muscular dystrophy	Possible risk of malignant hyperthermia
Cardiovascular system	Heart murmur	Septal defect; avoid IV air bubbles; hemoconcentration; endocarditis prophylaxis
	Cyanosis	Right-to-left cardiac shunt: IV air bubbles; hemoconcentration; endocarditis prophylaxis
	History of squatting	Possible tetralogy of Fallot
	Diaphoresis with feedings	Congestive heart failure
	Hypertension	Possible coarctation of the aorta; renal disease; pheochromocytoma
	Transplant recipient	Fixed heart rate; insensitivity to anticholinergic drugs
Respiratory system	Prematurity	Increased risk of postoperative apnea; possible lower respiratory tract illness
	Bronchopulmonary dysplasia	Lower airway obstruction; reactive airways; possible subglottic stensosis; possible postoperative hypoxia and apnea; pulmonary hypertension
	Lower respiratory infection, cough	Reactive airways; bronchospasm; medication history; drug interactions
	Croup	Possible subglottic stenosis/anomaly
	Snoring, sleep apnea	Perioperative airway obstruction; hypoxia
	Asthma	β agonist or theophylline drugs; pulmonary hypertension or cor pulmonale; steroid use: adrenal insufficiency, postoperative hypoxia
	Cystic fibrosis	Drug interactions; pulmonary toilet; pulmonary dysfunction; reactive airways
	Recent cold	Possible lower respiratory tract infection: reactive airways
Gastrointestinal/ hepatic system	Vomiting, diarrhea	Electrolyte abnormality; dehydration; full stomach
	Growth failure	Possible anemia
	Gastroesophageal reflux	Risk of aspiration; reactive airways; hypoxia
	Jaundice	Altered drug metabolism; risk of hypoglycemia
	Liver transplant recipient	Altered drug metabolism; immunosuppression
	Frequency, nocturia	Unrecognized diabetes; urinary tract infection
	Renal failure/dialysis	Electrolyte abnormality; hyper- or hypovolemia; anemia; medication history
	Renal transplant recipient	Immunosuppression
Endocrine/metabolic system	Hypoglycemia	Hypoglycemia
	Diabetes	Insulin requirement; intraoperative hypoglycemia
	Steroid therapy	Adrenal insufficiency
	Pregnancy	Teratogenic effects of N_2O and other drugs; risk for spontaneous abortion
Hematologic system	Anemia	Transfusion requirements
	Bruising, excessive bleeding	Coagulopathy
	Sickle cell disease	Anemia; transfusion; hydration; oxygenation; orthopedic tourniquet use
	AIDS	Susceptibility to infection; infectious risk to medical personnel
Allergies	Medication history	Drug reactions; drug interactions
Dental	Loose teeth	Dental trauma; aspiration of tooth

Modified from Coté CJ, Todres ID, Ryan JF. In: Ryan JF, Todres ID, Coté CJ, Goudsouzian N, eds. *A practice of anesthesia in infants and children.* New York: Grune and Stratton, 1986; with permission.

Some major anomalies of the developing organs are detected on routine fetal ultrasonography, and clues can be gleaned from the amniotic fluid estimation. A history of polyhydramnios usually indicates gastrointestinal anomalies, such as tracheoesophageal fistula or gastroschisis, duodenal atresia, or diaphragmatic hernia. It also may be an indicator of central nervous system anomalies, chromosomal defects, and maternal diabetes. Oligohydramnios is associated with renal and lung hypoplasia (Potter's syndrome) or other urologic abnormalities. Oligohydramnios associated with premature rupture of membranes increases the risk for neonatal infections. Uncontrolled maternal diabetes causes fetal macrosomia, anomalies of the gastrointestinal tract, and neonatal hypoglycemia.

Knowledge of the gestational age of the newborn gives clues about the maturity of the major organ systems. The 24-week premature infant has a greater incidence of respiratory distress syndrome, intraventricular hemorrhage, and necrotizing enterocolitis than the term newborn. The size of the infant relative to the gestational age may indicate external problems such as placental insufficiency and infections, and may be associated with metabolic defects and malnutrition in the newborn period. The Apgar scores reveal much about the condition of the infant at birth, from transiently depressed to asphyxiated with the need for resuscitation. Low Apgar scores and a rocky early newborn course is associated with cerebral palsy.

RESPIRATORY CONCERNS

Upper respiratory tract infections (URIs) are extremely common in children. Children have an average of six acute URIs per year, more if they are in day care, and scheduling elective procedures around these events can become challenging. A viral URI causes increased upper airway secretions that predispose the patient to laryngospasm on induction of anesthesia, bronchospasm, endotracheal tube plugging, oxygen desaturation, and hypoventilation. However, the literature dealing with URIs and anesthesia presents a confusing array of recommendations. Pediatric anesthesiologists differ as much in their management as the patients differ in their presentation. The main decisions to be made are when to cancel an elective procedure, and if canceled, when to reschedule.

The ultimate course of action should be to achieve a patient-focused outcome that all parties can agree upon. In general, if the patient has a mild URI consisting of rhinorrhea but without a fever or cough, the procedure could proceed with few sequelae. If the child has a significant cough, wheezing, or fever and it is clear the child is not in his or her normal state of health, then a lower respiratory tract infection may be present and the surgery ought to be rescheduled. The effects of the illness, the respiratory irritability, and secretions can linger for a considerable period after the acute illness is over. The surgery should be rescheduled for at least 4 to 6 weeks later to give time for optimum recovery.

Patients with a history of reactive airway disease demand more concern because the viral URI may progress to significant bronchospastic episodes. The initial bronchospasm may be well treated with β agonists, but the inflammatory component of the disease may take 6 to 7 weeks to subside. The partially treated asthmatic can develop the most severe bronchospasm on intubation or with light anesthesia; therefore, it is always preferable that these patients be at their best prior to an elective procedure.

Apnea and associated bradycardia may occur in any premature infant and in term infants after general anesthesia. The literature contains case reports of prematurely delivered infants who at 44 to 60 weeks' postconceptual age (the sum of the gestational and postnatal ages) developed life-threatening apnea after surgical procedures with multiple types of anesthetics. Therefore, hospital admission with respiratory monitoring is required for infants at risk for apnea, which include infants with a history of apnea, premature infants who were mechanically ventilated as newborns, term infants who may have had asphyxial events (low Apgar scores) at birth, and infants with anemia at the time of surgery. Our institution has adopted 52 weeks as the cutoff for automatic postoperative admission.

The prematurely delivered infant also may have other pulmonary problems, such as subglottic stenosis or bronchopulmonary dysplasia (BPD). Subglottic stenosis results from prolonged intubation in the newborn period resulting in a scarred narrowing in the upper trachea. These infants have stridor, which may be of little consequence, or which during URIs can result in an increased work of breathing and even episodes of respiratory failure.

Bronchopulmonary dysplasia results from mechanical ventilation with high airway pressures and high concentrations of oxygen in the newborn period. Diseases that cause respiratory failure necessitating mechanical ventilation, such as severe respiratory distress syndrome and meconium aspiration syndrome, are the usual predisposing factors. The lungs develop peribronchiolar fibrosis with smooth muscle hypertrophy, as well as dilatation and distortion of the lung parenchyma. The result is a group of patients who are chronically oxygen dependent with marked hyperactive lungs, not unlike chronic asthmatics. The medications used for asthma are also effective for BPD, and should be continued through the perioperative period. Like asthmatics, these patients require preoperative pulmonary tuning to assure that they are in the best condition possible for even the most minor operative procedure. Even in asymptomatic patients, if there is a history of mechanical ventilation of greater than a week, the patients should be treated as if they have reactive airways disease.

CARDIOVASCULAR CONCERNS

Evaluation of the cardiovascular system is critical to the delivery of safe anesthesia and recovery of patients in the postoperative period. All anesthetic agents have effects on the cardiovascular system, and major surgery can result in changes in preload and afterload. Fortunately, most children have healthy hearts with significant reserve to handle the stresses of surgery.

Innocent heart murmurs are common because they can be heard in up to 80% of healthy children less than 4 years of age. The ability to hear subtle murmurs decreases with age due to the development and expansion of the chest wall, but may still be detectable in 20% of adolescents. Common pediatric problems such anemia, fever, and exercise can accentuate innocent murmurs by increasing cardiac output. The genesis of these types of murmurs can be from turbulent flow at the aortic and pulmonic roots or turbulent flow at the subclavian and pulmonary arteries.

It is important to obtain a full history and perform a physical examination that may uncover a history of diaphoresis or tachypnea with feedings, or failure to thrive in infants, which may indicate cardiac disease. Older children may have shortness of breath, inability to exercise, or syncope that might have a cardiac origin. Any historical evidence of cardiovascular disease associated with a murmur should be explored with radiography and electrocardiography, and usually referred to a pediatric cardiologist for further evaluation. Certainly this workup should proceed well in advance of an elective procedure to avoid any delay or cancellation on the day of surgery.

It is not uncommon to have children with previous heart surgery undergo other procedures. A full history and physical examination, as well as knowledge of the lesion, the repair, and the patient's current functional status, are required prior to undertaking elective surgery. Knowledge of the presence of any residual intracardiac shunts, either congenital or surgical, is of paramount importance because of the risk for paradoxic embolism of air or thrombi, as well as the need for endocarditis prophylaxis.

Subacute bacterial endocarditis is a risk in patients who have congenital heart lesions and who have had repairs of congenital heart lesions. Transient bacteremia caused by genitourinary, bowel, airway, sinus, and oral procedures may infect damaged heart valves or intracardiac shunts. Seemingly insignificant heart lesions such as mitral valve prolapse and bicuspid aortic valves also require prophylaxis. The full recommendations are available through American Heart Association (AHA) publications. Although the AHA recommends oral medications for adults up to 30 minutes prior to surgery, the recommendations are often altered for the pediatric population. Typically we will induce anesthesia first, then administer the antibiotics (ampicillin and gentamicin) intravenously during the surgical preparation time prior to the start of the operative procedure.

HEMATOLOGIC CONCERNS

The hemoglobin level varies throughout childhood. Term infants are born with hemoglobin values of 14.5 to 18 gram/dL. This value typically drops to its lowest levels at 1 to 2 months of age (the so-called physiologic nadir) with values of 9.4 to 11.2 gram/dL. Because much of the circulating blood volume is acquired during the third trimester, premature infants are born with a relative anemia that predisposes them to greater degrees of anemia within the first 2 months of life. The hemoglobin levels then increase throughout childhood to the normal adult levels. There are few data to suggest that an optimum hemoglobin level is required prior to surgery. A routine hemoglobin determination is not performed as part of the preoperative process if the history and physical do not suggest a problem. If a child is recognized to have anemia, it is important to know if the change is chronic or the result of an acute process.

Routine testing of the coagulation system is also not believed to be cost effective given the poor ability of the standard tests of hemostasis to predict the likelihood of intraoperative bleeding. However, if the history should suggest a problem of coagulation, frequent nosebleeds, bruising, and bleeding from prior incisions, it is necessary to have a full workup, perhaps under the direction of a hematologist. Occasionally Von Willebrand's disease, acquired thrombocytopenias, or hemophilia can be uncovered.

Sickle cell disease often is asymptomatic in early childhood, and screening is usually undertaken only in the older child. In the child with known sickle cell disease, hypoxia, acidosis, dehydration, hypothermia, and use of tourniquets can induce a sickle crisis. The optimum level of hemoglobin for patients with hemoglobin S and hemoglobin C is unknown, but the traditional aggressive transfusion regimens that required preoperative transfusions to ensure a hemoglobin S level below 30% have been challenged. A large multicenter trial comparing the aggressive versus conservative transfusion regimens recommends transfusing the patient to a hemoglobin level of 10 g/dL without regard to the hemoglobin S level.

Von Willebrand's disease is characterized by an inability of platelets to adhere appropriately to the sites of endothelial injury due to the lack of production of or the presence of atypical von Willebrand's factor. It has an incidence of 1% in the general population and is typically inherited in an autosomal-dominant fashion. The disorder manifests itself as mucocutaneous bleeding, or prolonged bleeding after circumcision or tonsillectomy. A specific assay is required to formally diagnose the disease because standard tests of coagulation such as the partial thromboplastin time and bleeding time may not reveal abnormalities in some patients with the disorder.

Desmopressin (DDAVP) increases the levels of von Willebrand's factor from the endothelium, which may be all the treatment necessary for mild von Willebrand's disease. More severe cases require hematology consultation and the administration of cryoprecipitate.

ONCOLOGIC CONCERNS

The success of oncology programs and bone marrow transplantation on the survival of children with neoplastic disorders has resulted in a population of patients that deserve special consideration when undergoing elective surgical procedures. These patients may have had traumatic experiences from early childhood, with vivid memories of needlesticks, surgical trauma, infections, intractable nausea and vomiting, and pain. Often a visit to the hospital was viewed as a major setback. The psychological preparation may be especially challenging. In addition, specific antineoplastic agents have long-term systemic effects that have anesthetic and perioperative implications. If a patient is known to have had a neoplasm as a child, it is extremely important to elucidate which agents and what dosages were used.

Pulmonary fibrosis can result from several agents, for example, bleomycin, BCNU (carmustine), busulfan, and rarely cyclophosphamide. Bleomycin, a plant alkaloid agent, is typically used in the induction chemotherapy for bone marrow transplantation. These agents, especially in combination with radiation therapy, can cause accelerated and progressive pulmonary fibrosis, leading to respiratory failure. Of concern to anesthesiologists is the potential for further lung scarring due to elevated levels of oxygen during anesthesia. The management of ventilation in these cases is to try to avoid high concentrations of oxygen and undue barotrauma if the patients are intubated.

Several agents are associated with myocardial dysfunction. The anthracyclines adriamycin and cerubidine (doxarubicin and daunorubicin, respectively) both can cause myocyte damage in a dose-dependent fashion. A high dose of greater than 400 mg/m^2 is associated with acute myocardial dropout and can result in acute cardiomyopathy. However, doses lower than this have been associated with myocardial damage in adults who had received 200 mg/m^2 as children. It is generally believed that although they received the drugs as children and were asymptomatic then, as they developed into teenagers and young adults the damaged myocardium may not have developed as well. It has recently been suggested that a prolonged QT interval (QTc $\geq$ 0.43) may be a marker for patients at risk for cardiac decompensation. Although arrhythmias are common after these drugs have been administered, there does not appear to be evidence for long-term arrhythmogenic potential.

Extra care physically and psychologically needs to be taken with patients with a known history of neoplasm, however remote. Although in remission and asymptomatic, some of these patients may still bear physical and mental scars from their ordeal.

CENTRAL NERVOUS SYSTEM DYSFUNCTION

Children with neurologic problems often require procedures throughout childhood. Cerebral palsy, hydrocephalus, neuromuscular disease, seizure activity, and developmental delay are concerns that can complicate the most trivial procedure. Children with developmental delay may have communication and behavioral problems that require patience and care. *Cerebral palsy* is a term used to describe a host of manifestations associated with an insult to the infant's developing brain. Although the hallmark of this disorder is its motor manifestations, these patients are prone to gastroesophageal reflux, aspiration pneumonia, restrictive and obstructive lung disease, hypothermia, seizures, and altered pharmacokinetics of medications. Often these patients have had a history of intracranial hemorrhage and may have ventriculoperitoneal shunts, which can become infected or obstructed. Vomiting in the postoperative period might not be due to ileus, and fever might not be due to atelectasis.

Children with a history of seizures are often being treated with multiple anticonvulsant medications that can alter the metabolism of other medications and alter liver function. Usually these medications are long acting, and it is not a problem to schedule the operative procedure or adjust the medication schedule to accommodate. It is important to emphasize that the stress of surgery, operations near the liver, and blood transfusions can alter the anticonvulsant levels that may predispose to seizure activity in the postoperative period.

Spina bifida is associated with latex allergy due to the chronic exposure of latex products associated with neurogenic bladder regimens. Some of these patients may have undergone testing for sensitivity to latex products, but regardless of their status, it is prudent to avoid contact with latex product in these patients to reduce the chances of future sensitization. Latex precautions are standard for these patients in our hospital and are not only confined to the operating room but also the inpatient floors.

RENAL CONCERNS

There are multiple concerns for the patients with renal insufficiency who present for operative procedures. Intravascular volume status must be assessed prior to surgery. These patients most often are at risk for volume overload, and attention to the patient's dialysis schedule is critical. They also may be at risk for hypovolemia if recently dialyzed, and are at risk for further renal dysfunction if the kidneys are hypoperfused. Likewise, hyper- and hypotension can complicate the perioperative period so that particular attention to antihypertensive medication regimens is key.

Electrolyte disturbances are common, and few chronic renal failure patients undergoing elective surgery make it into an operating room without a recent electrolyte panel. Specific attention to "kalemia," either hyper- or hypo-, is necessary because both have potential cardiac effects. If the patient is at risk to receive blood during the procedure, the blood may provide an additional potassium load. Along with electrolytes, the acid/base status of patients with renal disease should be assessed.

Patients with uremia and end-stage renal disease may have coagulopathies due to platelet dysfunction. It is also a concern in patients undergoing hemodialysis who may have residual heparin effect in the hours immediately postdialysis.

ENDOCRINOLOGIC CONCERNS

Adrenal insufficiency is not a common disease of childhood, but certain conditions such as panhypopituitarism, congenital adrenal hyperplasia, and rheumatic diseases require chronic replacement steroids, which may impair the hypophyseal–pituitary axis (HPA) during times of stress.

Glucocorticoids are required for the conversion of norepinephrine to epinephrine in the adrenal medulla, which is essential to maintain cardiovascular responsiveness to catecholamines. In addition, the adrenal cortex is critical in the stress response process because it causes gluconeogenesis and retention of sodium to preserve plasma volume. Patients with panhypopituitarism and congenital adrenal hyperplasia rely on exogenous steroids for survival, whereas patients with rheumatic disease use exogenous steroids as antiinflammatory agents. All of these patients are at risk for acute adrenal crisis in the perioperative period, because the stresses of surgery may outstrip the catecholamine response in the absence of corticosteroids.

The classic presentation of a patient with adrenal crisis is nausea and vomiting, fatigue, and hypotension, with the associated laboratory findings of hypoglycemia, hyponatremia, hyperkalemia, metabolic acidosis, and potential cardiovascular collapse. This syndrome is obviously difficult to detect in the immediate postoperative period; thus, treatment regimens focus on prevention of the crisis. For patients who have complete reliance on exogenous steroids it is accepted that replacement therapy will need to be supplemented by stress dose coverage. It is more problematic in patients who have recently been on a course of steroids. It is accepted that patients that have received greater than 15 mg/m^2 will develop HPA suppression. The problem is that the recovery of the HPA after steroid administration is highly variable, as little as 2 to 4 weeks in some children, but as long as 9 months in adults.

Migeon and Donohoe recently reviewed this issue and categorized patients who had received a course of steroids in the preceding year. In the first category, if patients had received glucocorticoids at less than replacement levels, there should be no HPA suppression and no need for supplemental steroids (e.g., a patient who received a pulse of steroid after an asthmatic attack). In the second category, if the patient had received glucocorticoids in excess of replacement dosages, then HPA suppression is assured. If the therapy was of short duration (2–4 weeks), then suppression usually had a prompt recovery (2–4 weeks) and no supplementation needed to be given. If the therapy was of longer duration (>4 weeks), then HPA suppression could last up to 6 months.

What does replacement therapy mean? For uncomplicated procedures, sedations, and diagnostic studies, a one-time dose of 50 mg/m^2 of hydrocortisone hemisuccinate is recommended. For more complicated procedures, an initial bolus of 25 to 50 mg/m^2 is followed by 100 mg/m^2 as a continuous infusion or divided into four daily doses. For major operations with significant blood loss, this regimen is continued for 1 to 3 days postoperatively, preferably under the management of an endocrinologist.

Thyroid dysfunction is also not a common finding in childhood. Hypothyroidism can be congenital or acquired and is associated with temperature instability, decreased cardiac output due to decreases in heart rate and stroke volume, and prolonged recovery from various medications (narcotics, muscle relaxants) used in the perioperative period. The elective patient should be euthyroid prior to surgery if possible, and usually a 2-week period is required to achieve this pharmacologically.

Hyperthyroidism also can be congenital or acquired (Graves' disease) and results from excess circulating thyroid hormone. Elective procedures should be postponed until the patient is euthyroid, and patients usually revert to having normal vital signs, temperature, and deep tendon reflexes. Once on therapy, the likelihood of an uncontrolled thyroid storm is diminished, although some patients who are pharmacologically euthyroid will still be on antihypertensive medications.

Insulin-dependent diabetes mellitus is relatively common in children (1 in 500) and is always a management challenge in patients undergoing elective surgery. The typical "brittle" diabetic can have his or her tightly controlled insulin regimen thrown completely out of whack from the stress of surgery. The goal of perioperative management is to ensure that life-threatening hypoglycemia and uncontrolled hyperglycemia are avoided. The typical management involves the patient observing the typical 8-hour solid food fast, with clear liquids up to 2 hours prior to surgery. It is best if the patient is scheduled as the first case of the day if possible. Half of the dose of regular insulin is given after an intravenous solution containing glucose (D5 0.45% normal saline typically) is administered. Glucose determination should be performed regularly during the course of the operative procedure. Hyperglycemia in excess of 250 mg/dL should be treated using subcutaneous or intravenous regular insulin. Uncontrolled hyperglycemia may result in undesirable diuresis and cerebral edema.

PHARMACOGENETIC SYNDROMES

Malignant hyperthermia (MH) and pseudocholinesterase deficiency are disorders that are of particular interest with surgeons and anesthesiologists because they typically manifest themselves only in the perioperative period.

Malignant hyperthermia is characterized by a fulminant hypermetabolic reaction of skeletal muscle triggered by the muscle relaxant succinylcholine, and volatile anesthetic agents. The primary defect is excessive intracellular calcium, which is primarily due to increased calcium release and inhibition of uptake by the sarcoplasmic reticulum. The resulting elevated intracellular calcium causes actin and myosin in the muscle to contract, resulting in hydrolysis of adenosine triphosphate, heat production, uncoupling of oxidative phosphorylation, and eventual cell breakdown with release of intracellular contents, potassium, creatine kinase, and myoglobin. The patients develop a rigor mortis-like muscle rigidity associated with arrhythmias, hypertension, and hypercarbia. Subsequently, elevation of temperature, metabolic acidosis, and myoglobinuria is followed by cardiovascular and renal collapse. Treatment consists of dantrolene and intensive supportive care.

Malignant hyperthermia is associated with central core disease, but is unlikely in Duchenne's muscular dystrophy. Its incidence among the general population is estimated at 1 in 40,000 adults and 1 in 14,000 children. A family history of problems with surgical procedures or anesthesia should warrant further investigation. It is important to have a member of the anesthesia department plan the anesthetic well in advance. If there is a suggestive history, it is optimal to have the patient scheduled as the first case of the day to allow for purging the anesthesia machine of traces of inhalation agents and of vaporizers, and to ensure than dantrolene is available in the event of an episode. In known MH-susceptible patients, prophylactic dantrolene may be warranted.

Pseudocholinesterase or plasma cholinesterase is a serine protease that has an obscure role in normal patients, and lack of the enzyme or production of atypical pseudocholinesterase is not associated with any abnormal growth or development. Various combinations of alleles exist in the general population with varying sensitivity to succinylcholine. However, certain patients in this population have potentially life-threatening prolongation of neuromuscular blockade after administration of succinylcholine. Typically the family describes the patient as being allergic to anesthesia, not "waking up" after anesthesia, or being "very weak" after anesthesia. Fortunately the use of succinylcholine in pediatric anesthesia is uncommon, but patients with a family history of this problem will undoubtedly have many questions at the time of surgery.

LABORATORY TESTING

The only routine laboratory test ordered preoperatively in our institution is a urine pregnancy test in females who have achieved menarche. The fear is that some adolescent girls may not discuss their sexual experiences with their parents, and it is hospital policy to perform the urine pregnancy test rather than risk the potential for adverse outcomes. In the state of Delaware, an adolescent 12 years of age or older is emancipated with regard to her reproductive health and is entitled to the same rights as an adult regarding issues of confidentiality. An adolescent girl who feels that she may be pregnant may give written consent for her own treatment without parental notification, except in issues regarding abortion.

Other than the urine pregnancy test, it has been recognized that routine preoperative laboratory testing in healthy children is not cost effective, wastes time, may lead to erroneous results, and is often traumatic for the child and family. Laboratory tests should be ordered when the history indicates a problem or when abnormalities are anticipated due to the surgery and the postoperative course. Hemoglobin determinations are indicated in those patients with a history of anemia, or those who may have significant blood loss during surgery. It is not uncommon for anesthesiologists to draw baseline samples after the child is anesthetized. Electrolyte determinations are essential in patients with pyloric stenosis or renal anomalies, and are necessary prior to the induction of anesthesia because potassium levels can influence myocardial function. Coagulation studies are indicated in children with known disorders as a guide to the management of the coagulation system intraoperatively. Routine coagulation screening for all patients has been challenged successfully and is no longer a part of standard batteries.

HOW TO KEEP THE PROCEDURE FROM BEING CANCELED

Procedures are canceled or postponed for a variety of reasons, at various steps in the process. In our institution the most common patient cause for delay or cancellation is violation of the NPO guidelines. It is amazing that after extensive education, reinforcement of the education, sending the family home with written instructions, and calling them on the phone the day prior to the procedure to tell them of the time of the procedure and the proper NPO time, some patients still arrive at the hospital for elective surgery after eating a full breakfast. Usually there is a simple mistake, or the child will have been caught sneaking something. We make every attempt to rearrange the schedule to accommodate the surgeon and the families, although this may not always be possible. If it is an emergency surgery, the patient is assumed to have a full stomach, appropriate steps are taken, and the surgery proceeds.

"Out of whack" laboratory values, especially electrolytes, are an occasional cause for delay. There are real risks to proceeding with potassium, sodium, calcium, and glucose abnormalities. Coagulation disorders are also seen, and pose a dilemma when the potential for blood loss is high. Proceeding in the face of such risks opens the door to unnecessary complications that are always best avoided.

When a child arrives with an acute illness or an acute exacerbation of an existing illness, it is customary to cancel the procedure so that the illness can be addressed. Consideration must be given to the urgency of the case and the severity of the illness, but all parties should be informed to make the best decision. Healthy debates often ensue with regard to children with URIs. The best policy is for all parties involved to agree on the course of action to be taken. If the family or the anesthesiologist is uncomfortable with the case, this should be communicated to the surgeon. Clearly the worst course of action is for one party to get their way with the other two dissenting. This goes for the anesthesiologist as well, who is not making any allies by canceling every child with a sniffle. The decision should be patient focused, with an open discussion of the risks and benefits of proceeding.

CONCLUSIONS

Surgery on pediatric patients is safer than ever due to the advances in knowledge of disease processes, improvements and standardization of monitoring techniques, and the skill of the practitioners involved. Despite these improvements, proper preparation of children includes meticulous attention to detail to anticipate and treat possible untoward problems in the perioperative period.

EDITOR'S NOTES

It is often tempting to allow the anesthetists to assume complete responsibility for the evaluation and testing of our patients prior to an operation. Indeed, except for the presence of certain obvious medical conditions (e.g., coagulopathy, obesity) that could impact the safe completion of the procedure, most of the risk associated with the operation is related to the administration of the anesthetic and management of the patients while under general anesthesia. Our anesthesia colleagues are also usually quite conscientious in their approach to the preoperative evaluation, making the whole process safer for the patients and certainly easier for us and our staff. However, I think most would agree that we as surgeons share in the responsibility for the care of the patient in the perioperative period and that we should, at minimum, facilitate the preoperative evaluation. This includes a thorough and well-documented history and physical examination and addressing any potential complicating factors well in advance of the scheduled date of surgery. This also includes working closely with the anesthesiologists in a collegial way, rather than as adversaries.

Fortunately, most children who require elective surgery have few potentially complicating health issues, making the preoperative evaluation relatively straightforward from the medical standpoint. It is nevertheless important to discuss the entire process in detail with the family, including some of the basics of the anesthesia component, which is often the greater source of anxiety for them. It is tempting to try to avoid giving "too much" information for fear that this might dissuade them from having the procedure or frighten them excessively. For most patients, however, providing an abundance of information actually serves to allay anxiety rather than worsen it and provides parents with a sense of control.

–P.M.

SUGGESTED READINGS

Cote CJ. Preoperative preparation and premedication. *Br J Anesth* 1999;83:16–28.

Eichhorn JH. Effect of monitoring standards on anesthesia outcome. *Int Anesthesiol Clin* 1993;31:181–196.

Evaluation and preparation of pediatric patients undergoing anesthesia. American Academy of Pediatrics Section on Anesthesiology. *Pediatrics* 1996;98(part 1):502–508.

Kain ZN, Caramico LA, Mayes LC, et al. Preoperative preparation programs in children: a comparative examination. *Anesth Analg* 1998;87:1249–1255.

Krane EJ, Davis PJ, Smith RM. Preoperative preparation. In: Motoyama EK, Davis PJ, ed. *Smith's anesthesia for infants and children, 6th ed.* St. Louis: CV Mosby, 1996:213–228.

Litman RS, Berger AA, Chibber A. An evaluation of preoperative anxiety in a population of parents of infants and children undergoing ambulatory surgery. *Paediatr Anaesth* 1996;6:443–447.

Means LJ. Preoperative evaluation. In: Badgewell JM, ed. *Clinical pediatric anesthesia.* Philadelphia: Lippincott-Raven, 1997:1–13.

Migeon CJ, Donohoe PA. Adrenal disorders. In: Kappy MS, Blizzard RM, Migeon CJ, eds. *The diagnosis and treatment of endocrine disorders in childhood and adolescence.* Springfield, IL. Charles C. Thomas, 1994.

Steward DJ, Screening tests before surgery in children. *Can J Anaesth* 1991;38:693–695.

2

PRENATAL DIAGNOSIS AND COUNSELING

NICOLA A. LEWIS
PHILIP L. GLICK

Antenatal screening for high-risk pregnancies has become extremely common over the past two decades, and many congenital anomalies are now being routinely detected *in utero*. Fetal imaging and certain invasive techniques aid in the diagnosis of specific anomalies. Advances in the prenatal diagnosis of fetal anomalies afford us the opportunity to educate and inform the expectant family regarding the natural history of the anomaly and to help them choose the management of the pregnancy and the place, time, and mode of delivery. Postnatal treatment options can be discussed in advance when emotions are relatively calm, and strategies aimed at minimizing maternal and fetal morbidity and mortality can be implemented.

At many medical centers, pediatric surgeons are involved in antenatal screening programs and participate in maternal-fetal medicine patient care conferences where antenatal diagnoses are discussed. In this chapter we provide an overview of some of the specific terms and techniques used in prenatal assessment followed by a discussion of some of the more common diagnoses that we are asked to discuss with families prior to delivery.

ANTENATAL SCREENING

Routine antenatal care can identify the at-risk fetus through careful assessment of the maternal history, family history, and maternal serum α-fetoprotein (AFP) levels. Pertinent factors in the maternal history include alcohol or drug history, obstetric history, family history, maternal and paternal ages, and medical history. A history of frequent miscarriages, stillbirths, or offspring with chromosomal abnormalities indicates the need for further assessment.

MATERNAL SERUM α-FETOPROTEIN

Alpha-fetoprotein is a fetal glycoprotein produced initially by the fetal yolk sac, and subsequently by the fetal liver. AFP is filtered by the kidneys and excreted into the amniotic fluid. Transudation of AFP across nonkeratinized fetal skin may contribute to amniotic AFP levels. Fetal production of AFP reaches its peak at the end of the second trimester. AFP enters the maternal circulation via the placenta or the amniotic membranes, and maternal serum AFP (MS-AFP) is solely synthesized by the fetus. MS-AFP increases throughout the second trimester and gradually decreases after 30 to 32 weeks. Variations in MS-AFP occur with gestational age, race, weight, and a history of insulin-dependent diabetes mellitus. Hence, levels must be corrected prior to the interpretation of results.

Maternal serum AFP was originally used to detect neural tube defects; however, it was soon discovered to be useful in the diagnosis of other anomalies. Screening is performed at 15 to 20 weeks of gestation, when less biologic variation occurs. Elevated levels of MS-AFP are seen with anencephaly, neural tube defects, sacrococcygeal teratoma, anterior abdominal wall defects, intestinal atresia, and cystic hygroma. Low MS-AFP levels are found in trisomies 21, 18, and 13, and in congenital diaphragmatic hernia (CDH).

Screening MS-AFP levels are associated with a 40% false-positive rate. Known causes of false-positive results include inaccurate gestational ages, multiple gestation pregnancies, fetal demise, and fetal-maternal transfusion. Following the verification of initial MS-AFP results, level II ultrasonography is performed to confirm gestational age and viability of the pregnancy, to rule out multiple pregnancies, to determine amniotic fluid volume and the posi-

N. A. Lewis and P. L. Glick: Departments of Surgery and Pediatrics, The State University of New York at Buffalo; and Department of Surgery, The Children's Hospital of Buffalo, Buffalo, New York.

tion of the placenta, and to detect structural anomalies known to be associated with abnormal MS-AFP levels. Amniocentesis, chorionic villus sampling (CVS), or cordocentesis are performed as indicated.

FETAL IMAGING

Various modalities are used for detailed imaging of the fetus: computed tomographic (CT) scanning, ultrafast fetal magnetic resonance imaging (MRI), and amniography. Ultrasonography is easily available, noninvasive, and cost effective, and therefore remains the gold standard for fetal imaging. With it, an experienced operator can accurately detect many fetal anomalies. Ultrasonographic imaging can be limited by maternal obesity, bad fetal lie, and oligohydramnios. Anatomic defects can be detected by visualization of the defect itself, the absence of normal anatomic structure, abnormal fetal biometry, or the consequences of the defect (e.g., hydronephrosis). The timing of the study is important, and repeated examination is required for full evaluation of dynamic anomalies. Detection rates for specific anomalies vary from 90% for lethal anomalies, 75% for anomalies requiring intensive care, and 30% for some minor anomalies.

Conventional classification of ultrasonographic examinations includes three levels. A level I examination is available in most obstetric offices. It is useful in the determination of fetal viability, estimation of gestational age, and detection of multiple pregnancies, and allows a limited examination of the fetus. A level II examination is performed by an experienced sonographer and in consultation with a perinatologist. Amniotic fluid volume is estimated and is a useful indicator of fetal anomalies. Polyhydramnios is associated with CDH and lesions that decrease fetal swallowing (e.g., tracheoesophageal fistula or cervical masses) and the absorption of fluid from the gastrointestinal tract (e.g., intestinal atresias). Oligohydramnios is seen in renal dysplasia and obstructive uropathy. The gross appearance and size of the fetus is used to confirm gestational age and appropriate growth, and to exclude gross structural anomalies. The placenta and umbilical cord insertion are examined, and the individual organ systems are systematically scrutinized for congenital anomalies. During a level III examination, previously identified anomalies and all other organ systems are surveyed to detect associated birth defects as well as secondary effects, and a more comprehensive examination is performed.

FURTHER INVESTIGATIONS

For the couple at risk for a fetus with a chromosomal disorder, chromosomal and genetic investigations are required. This involves invasive techniques to obtain amniotic fluid, fetal cells, or fetal blood samples.

Amniocentesis is indicated if the woman is of advanced maternal age, if the parents are known carriers of genetic disorders, if other children have chromosomal abnormalities or neural tube defects, or if the woman has an obstetric history of multiple first-trimester miscarriages or a previous stillbirth. Amniocentesis is usually performed in the second trimester between the 14th and 16th week. Under ultrasonographic guidance and using a sterile percutaneous technique, approximately 20 mL of amniotic fluid is aspirated for biochemical analysis, DNA analysis, and cytogenetic studies. Complications of amniocentesis include amnionitis, amniotic fluid leaks, vaginal spotting, and respiratory distress syndrome or pneumonia in the newborn. A fetal loss rate of 1% has been reported.

Amniotic fluid AFP (AF-AFP) and acetylcholinesterase levels are means of additional screening. AF-AFP levels are elevated in conditions known to be associated with elevated MS-AFP levels. There is a false-positive rate of approximately 0.7%, which is thought to be mainly due to contamination of amniotic fluid with fetal blood cells. Amniotic fluid acetylcholinesterase levels are markedly elevated in neural tube defects and are found to be normal in approximately 90% of cases in which the AF-AFP was falsely elevated. Amniotic fluid acetylcholinesterase is therefore important in decreasing the false-positive rate and in differentiating neural tube defects from other causes of an elevated AF-AFP level. Amniocytes obtained from the amniotic fluid sample can be cultured for 3 weeks prior to cytogenetic studies, DNA analysis, and fetal enzyme assays. Cytogenetic analysis is usually performed on samples from CVS and amniocentesis, and identifies major chromosomal abnormalities. Karyotyping is performed during metaphase, when changes in chromosomal numbers can be identified. By using special banding techniques and karyotyping and by comparing the chromosomes with known standards, major chromosomal abnormalities can be identified. These abnormalities can be due to deletion, duplication, or translocation of genetic material.

If the fetus is known to be at risk for specific genetic defects, DNA analysis is performed. Genetic defects range from alterations in single base pairs to major alterations in genes. This translates into the modification of the structure, function, and quantity of enzymes or proteins coded for by the gene. When the mutation and the site of the mutation are known, recombinant techniques can be used to identify these alterations in the fetus.

The indications for CVS are similar to those for amniocentesis, except when amniotic fluid biochemistry is required. The chorionic villus is derived from the zygote. Therefore, chromosomal, biochemical, and DNA analysis of these cells should yield results similar to that obtained from cultured amniocytes. One advantage of CVS is that it can be performed between the 9th and 12th weeks of gestation, allowing families more options. A transvaginal ultrasonographic examination is performed to confirm fetal viability and to determine the position of the fetus and placenta. Under ultrasonographic guidance, the catheter is passed transcervically (most common route), transvaginally, or transabdominally into the body of the placenta. Samples of trophoblastic tissue are obtained by the application of negative pressure to the catheter.

Cells obtained via CVS are more actively dividing than amniocytes retrieved via amniocentesis; hence, results from CVS are obtained more quickly from cell cultures (7–10 days) or on analysis of extracted cells (24–48 hours). However, diagnostic errors may result if mosaicism or maternal cell contamination occurs. CVS is associated with a 2% fetal loss rate.

Fetal umbilical blood sampling (FUBS) is performed by ultrasonographically guided transabdominal umbilical cord sampling. FUBS is performed between the 15th and 20th weeks of gestation and is useful for fetal karyotyping and hematologic analysis. Fluorescent *in situ* hybridization can be performed in 24 to 48 hours for rapid karyotyping or in 5 to 7 days for full-banded karyotyping. The indications for FUBS are suspected fetal infections and screening for inherited blood and metabolic disorders.

FREQUENTLY DIAGNOSED PEDIATRIC SURGERY PROBLEMS

There are several diagnoses for which antenatal consultation with a pediatric surgeon can be useful for parents. The goal is to help inform and educate the parents about the suspected anomaly, so that they might be able to discuss the treatment plan in a calmer environment and be better prepared to become involved in decision making.

FETAL OBSTRUCTIVE UROPATHY

Significant urinary tract dilatation is frequently detectable on ultrasonographic examination in the second trimester. Approximately 20% of urinary tract dilatations are due to urologic abnormalities, whereas 80% are due to functional pelviectasis. The most common cause of upper tract dilatation is ureteropelvic junction obstruction. Other common causes are vesicoureteral reflux, vesicoureteral obstruction, and posterior urethral valves. Lower urinary tract obstruction results from developmental abnormalities of the urethra, including posterior urethral valves, urethral atresia, urethral hypoplasia, and rarely meatal stenosis, hypospadias, or epispadias. Lower urinary tract obstruction is also associated with cloacal anomalies or as part of a urogenital sinus syndrome in females. Features of lower urinary tract obstruction are bladder distension ("keyhole" sign), bladder wall hypertrophy, bilateral hydronephrosis, and oligohydramnios.

In addition to hydronephrosis, *in utero* obstruction can lead to renal dysplasia, loss of bladder wall compliance, and bladder wall hypertrophy. Subsequent oligohydramnios can cause pulmonary hypoplasia, Potter facies (due to compression of the skull against the uterus), limb deformities, and prune belly syndrome. The degree of pulmonary hypoplasia is a major determinant of survival in the early neonatal period.

Prenatal diagnosis identifies patients requiring postnatal surveillance and intervention. Postnatal ultrasonography should be performed in the first week of life and again at 1 month if results of the initial scan are normal. If the results are abnormal, the initiation of prophylactic antibiotics should be followed by a complete radiologic evaluation, including voiding cystoureterography.

When lower urinary tract obstruction is associated with oligohydramnios, antenatal intervention should be considered. *In utero* relief of the obstruction and restoration of amniotic fluid volume can improve lung growth and development and prevent further renal injury. The selection of patients who would benefit from prenatal intervention is based on karyotype analysis, detailed ultrasonographic evaluation, and serial urine evaluation. Current indications include bilateral hydronephrosis with oligohydramnios and no evidence of irreversible renal failure. Serial urinalysis can help in decision making and involves repeated fine-needle bladder aspiration (vesicocentesis) at set intervals and measurement of urine osmolality, electrolytes, and β_2 microglobulin. A poor prognosis is associated with osmolality of greater than 210 mOsm, sodium greater than 100 mEq/mL and chloride greater than 90 mEq/mL. In patients under 32 weeks of age with oligohydramnios, isolated renal tract anomalies, a normal male karyotype, and improving urinary measurements, vesicoamniotic shunting can improve outcome. In fetuses over 32 weeks of age, early delivery and postnatal decompression should be considered

CONGENITAL DIAPHRAGMATIC HERNIA

High-resolution ultrasonography and routine prenatal screening have increased the *in utero* diagnosis of CDH. In a 1984 North American study, approximately 20% of cases were detected on routine obstetric evaluation. In 2001, this number was more than 90%. In two thirds of patients, mothers were found to be large for gestational stage, prompting more detailed prenatal study. Ultrasonographic findings were variable and included polyhydramnios (76% of cases), intrathoracic gastric bubbles, abnormal upper abdominal findings, and mediastinal shift.

The diagnosis of CDH is frequently made in the second trimester. Differential diagnosis includes cystic lung disease (cystic adenomatoid malformation, pulmonary sequestration) and mediastinal cystic processes (cystic teratoma, thymic cysts). In up to one half of patients, CDH is associ ated with other congenital anomalies, such as cardiac defects, ventricular hypoplasia, urogenital anomalies, or neural tube defects or chromosomal defects such as trisomy 21, 18, or 13. Prenatal detection of CDH necessitates a search for other anomalies. Karyotype analysis, fetal echocardiography and level III ultrasonography are typically recommended.

The pathophysiology of CDH remains incompletely understood. Pulmonary hypoplasia is associated with immature surfactant- and antioxidant-producing systems, left ventricular hypoplasia, pulmonary hypertension, and a tendency toward persistent fetal circulation. Pulmonary hypoplasia remains a major determinant of fetal outcome. Approximately 70% to 80% of liveborn patients with CDH survive the neonatal period. A poor prognosis is associated with a low left ventricular mass, coexisting cardiac defects, low lung-to-thoracic transverse ratio and a contralateral lung-to-head circumference ratio of less than 0.6.

Surgical techniques for *in utero* intervention have been developed in the fetal lamb model and small clinical trials. No single prenatal parameter has been shown to reliably predict the occurrence of lethal pulmonary hypoplasia; hence, selection criteria for antenatal intervention remains controversial. Primary repair during the fetal period is no longer recommended. Early studies suggested that the babies most likely to benefit from the operation are the ones with the mildest form of the defect, who are the ones most likely to do well with postnatal management. Tracheal occlusion during the fetal period is currently being studied as an alternative to primary repair.

Antenatal discussion with the family should include a frank discussion of the survival rate (50% to 70%) as well as what they can expect when the baby is born. They should be told that the baby might be intubated soon after birth and could develop pulmonary hypertension and remain critically ill for some time. They should be warned about the need for extracorporeal membrane oxygenation (ECMO) therapy and what that entails. They should be informed regarding the possibility of associated anomalies and what studies are likely to take place early on to exclude these anomalies. They should be educated as to the natural history of the disease and that, in many respects, the actual repair of the defect becomes a secondary concern until the baby's physiology stabilizes.

ABDOMINAL WALL DEFECTS

Elevated MS-AFP levels may be the first indicator of an anterior abdominal wall defect. Most defects can be identified in the second trimester (first-trimester "abdominal wall defects" are physiologic) by ultrasonography. The presence of an intact sac or herniated liver distinguishes an omphalocele from gastroschisis, in which loops of intestine float freely in the amniotic fluid.

In cases of omphalocele, karyotype analysis should be performed, as should serial sonograms to detect associated anomalies and to assess the size of the defect. Parents should be informed of the risk for associated anomalies and the need for echocardiography, renal ultrasonography, and glucose monitoring soon after delivery. The details of reduction and repair should be discussed in the context of how large the defect is expected to be. They should be aware that repair of an omphalocele with an intact membrane is semi-elective, usually within the first 2 days of life, allowing time to pursue screening studies.

For patients with gastroschisis, the timing and mode of delivery remains somewhat controversial. Some protocols suggest weekly ultrasonographic evaluation during late pregnancy to monitor fetal growth and the quality of the herniated bowel. Intrauterine growth retardation, bowel thickening and dilatation may indicate a need for early delivery because of concern about vascular compromise of the bowel. Most studies suggest that vaginal delivery is safe for babies with gastroschisis. The decision regarding cesarean section is therefore left to the obstetric team and should be based on the usual issues of maternal health and fetal distress.

Parents should be made aware that the baby with gastroschisis requires emergent operation within the first few hours of life, requiring in some cases separation of the baby from the mother. They should also understand the indications and implications of a staged approach using a silo. The second hurdle is weaning from the ventilator, which takes several days in some cases. Parents should be made aware that although babies with gastroschisis are at no higher risk for other anomalies than other babies, they often have a prolonged ileus requiring parenteral nutrition and some form of central access. Some babies develop a stricture or an atresia that requires further surgery. Lastly, parents should be made aware that the overall survival for babies with gastroschisis is approximately 90% (not 100%) and that their child is at risk for complications such as sepsis, bowel obstruction, thromboembolic disorders, and necrotizing enterocolitis.

CONGENITAL CYSTIC ADENOMATOID MALFORMATIONS

Congenital cystic adenomatoid malformations (CCAMs) of the lungs are believed to be due to the abnormal development of lung segments. The diagnosis is frequently made on prenatal ultrasonography. Two types of lesions can be distinguished on prenatal ultrasonography: microcystic and macrocystic lesions. Macrocystic lesions contain a single or multiple large cysts (>5 mm). Microcystic lesions contain smaller cysts (<5 mm) and tend to appear more solid and bulky. Microcystic lesions are more commonly associated with hydrops. The natural history of these lesions is variable; some lesions disappear *in utero,* others result in fetal or neonatal demise, most become symptomatic in the first month (respiratory difficulty or recurrent infections), and some patients remain asymptomatic. Congenital anomalies are associated with 10% to 20% of cases, including renal agenesis or dysgenesis, intestinal atresia, cardiac anomalies, and imperforate anus.

Large masses detected *in utero* may lead to pulmonary compression and subsequent lung hypoplasia. Esophageal compression leads to decreased fetal swallowing and polyhydramnios. The development of fetal hydrops secondary to mediastinal shift and compression of major cardiac vessels is almost always a marker for fetal demise. Hence, large masses should be monitored closely for early development of fetal hydrops (an indication for fetal intervention or early delivery). The insertion of a thoracoamniotic shunt *in utero* can lead to successful decompression of macrocystic lesions. Open fetal lobectomy is required for the microcystic variant. Fetal intervention is associated with the resolution of fetal hydrops and growth of the hypoplastic lung. Fetuses that do not develop hydrops may require serial amniocentesis for polyhydramnios or high-frequency oscillatory ventilation (HFVO) and ECMO in the early neonatal period. All CCAMs need to be removed postnatally to avoid recurrent infections and the risk for malignant degeneration.

Antenatal intervention should be discussed with parents with referral to a fetal intervention program should they desire to pursue such an option. They should be informed of the possibility that the CCAM may resolve spontaneously before birth but that they do not do so after delivery. They should also be made aware of the risk for hydrops and subsequent fetal demise. They should undergo frequent serial ultrasonographic examinations late in pregnancy in the hope that hydrops can be identified early enough for intervention to be considered. Surgical options should be discussed according to institutional practices. Most infants undergo thoracotomy in the first week of life; however, some stable infants can be discharged with plans for an elective thoracotomy. Newborns should undergo an imaging study, usually either a CT scan or an MRI, to allow proper planning for the surgical approach and to rule out the presence of multiple CCAMs or other pulmonary lesions, such as pulmonary sequestration.

SACROCOCCYGEAL TERATOMA

Sacrococcygeal teratoma (SCT) is the most common tumor of the newborn and usually occurs as an isolated anomaly. Nearly all of these lesions are benign. Fetal SCTs may present with polyhydramnios, elevated MSAFP levels, and a lesion detected on sonography. Fetal MRI can delineate pelvic extension and aids in the classification of the tumor: type I is predominantly external tumor with minimal presacral involvement; type II is predominantly external tumor with significant intrapelvic component; type III is partially exterior tumor with predominantly intrapelvic and abdominal extension; type IV is presacral, with no external extension.

Rapidly enlarging lesions demand a high blood flow, which may lead to cardiac failure and fetal hydrops. Polyhydramnios and the increased fetal mass may lead to increased uterine irritability and premature delivery. In the majority of cases, high-output cardiac failure does not occur, and most patients can be monitored by serial ultrasonography.

When cardiac failure and hydrops develop, emergency cesarean section should be offered. If the fetus is likely to have immature lungs, open fetal surgery and tumor resection may be considered. Few cases of successful open fetal surgery for SCT have been reported.

Parents should be informed of the likelihood of a premature delivery and an infant who is small for gestational age. All newborns with an SCT should have an imaging study, usually either a CT scan or an MRI, mainly to assess the size of the intrapelvic extension and to aid in planning the operative strategy. Most sacrococcygeal teratomas are type I or type II and are therefore amenable to safe resection. Technical difficulty and the risk for significant complications correlates directly with the size of the intraabdominal component of the mass. The biggest risk is that for hemorrhage, either because of rupture of the mass or during surgical resection. Lastly, parents should be warned of the cosmetic issues that can result after resection of such a large tumor, but they can be reassured that the functional results (bowel and bladder function, reproduction) are usually very good.

DUODENAL ATRESIA

The double bubble of duodenal atresia may be identified by antenatal ultrasonography. The results of duodenoduodenostomy in the newborn period are usually good, and the lesion is not currently an indication for antenatal intervention. Prenatal consultation with a pediatric surgeon can be helpful for the parents to anticipate the surgery and its implications.

One third of babies with duodenal atresia have trisomy 21. Karyotyping should be offered, especially in patients who are otherwise at high risk for trisomy 21, either due to maternal age, elevated MS-AFP, or additional suggestive sonographic findings. Duodenal atresia is also associated with congenital heart disease, genitourinary anomalies, esophageal atresia with tracheoesophageal fistula, and imperforate anus. Newborns should be screened with a thorough physical examination, passage of a nasogastric tube, echocardiography, and renal ultrasonography. Parents should be informed of the excellent results of surgery and the likelihood that, in most cases, the infant will be able to tolerate oral feedings within 2 to 3 weeks of surgery.

BOWEL OBSTRUCTION AND ATRESIA

Occasionally, ultrasonographic findings suggest the possibility of a bowel obstruction or intestinal atresia. Except for some cases of jejunal atresia in which polyhydramnios may develop, the majority are asymptomatic and progress to term. Newborns should be assessed carefully with a physical examination and plain radiographs. Although some will remain asymptomatic and even warrant a feeding trial, those with abdominal distension, bilious emesis, or dilated loops on radiography require further workup. In certain cases, the radiograph is diagnostic and plans are made for urgent laparotomy. In other cases, it may be more prudent to proceed with a diagnostic study. A contrast enema can diagnose and sometimes treat meconium plug syndrome or meconium ileus. It also can suggest the possibility of Hirschsprung's disease, which would alter the subsequent management considerably. Occasionally, an upper gastrointestinal contrast study may be considered, although in most cases of an obvious obstruction without evidence of a process that can be treated nonoperatively, the infant should be prepared for laparotomy. The differential diagnosis should be discussed with the parents, including the possibility that cystic fibrosis will need to be ruled out. The operative approach, including the possibility of bowel resection and temporizing stoma, and complications such as stricture and short bowel syndrome should all be discussed with the parents during the antenatal visit.

COUNSELING

Counseling should begin when a high-risk pregnancy is identified or as soon as the diagnosis is known. This should continue into the postnatal period. Adequate counseling brings the family up to date on current medical facts related to the disorder. It also allows them to select the best course of action suited to their situation, facilitates adjustment to the disorder, and equips them to understand the risk for recurrence. A multidisciplinary approach should be used involving a social worker, ethicist, clergy, geneticists, obstetricians, neonatologist, and a pediatric surgeon.

SUGGESTED READINGS

Adzick NS, Harrison MR, Glick PL, et al. Diaphragmatic hernia in the fetus: prenatal diagnosis and outcome in 94 cases. *J Pediatr Surg* 1985;20:357–361.

Glick PL, Harrison MR, Adzick SN, et al. Correction of congenital hydronephrosis in utero IV: in utero decompression prevents renal dysplasia. *J Pediatr Surg* 1984;19:649–655.

Glick PL, Irish MS, Holm B, eds. New insights into the pathophysiology of congenital diaphragmatic hernia. *Clin Perinatol* 1996;23 (4):625–653.

Glick PL, Pohlson EC, Resta R, et al. Maternal serum alpha-fetoprotein is a marker for fetal anomalies in pediatric surgery. *J Pediatr Surg* 1988;23:16–20.

Golbus MS, Filly RA, Callen PW, et al. Fetal urinary tract obstruction: management and selection for treatment. *Semin Perinatol* 1985;9:91–97.

Harrison MR, Golbus MS, Filly RA, eds. *The unborn patient: prenatal diagnosis and treatment, 2nd ed.* Philadelphia: WB Saunders, 1991.

Kapur P, Holm B, Sokolowski J, et al. Lung physiology and metabolic changes in lambs with congenital diaphragmatic hernia after administration of prenatal maternal corticosteroids. *J Pediatr Surg* 1999;34:354–356.

3

PREPARING CHILDREN WITH SPECIAL NEEDS FOR DISCHARGE: GASTROINTESTINAL TUBES AND STOMAS

FRANCES T. GILL
KIM H. GIORDANO

Nowhere is the statement "Discharge starts at admission" more accurate than in the case of the surgical patient with special needs. Frequently, the surgical therapy and the immediate postoperative management are discussed in detail and accomplished smoothly, whereas the discharge process is taken for granted. Because care of the patient does not end with discharge, a seamless transition process should be viewed as a critical element in the holistic care of the child and family. It is often underestimated to what degree hospitalization, a complicated diagnosis, and advanced technologic needs can change the daily life of the child as well as that of the entire family unit. A multidisciplinary approach to the total care needs is imperative during the transitional period prior to discharge.

ANCILLARY SUPPORT

A complicated diagnosis inherently brings intricate issues to light. Early intervention from a social worker affords parental support coupled with the savvy to intervene with complex insurance and home care issues. Providing written orders for necessary supplies (formula, feeding pumps, intravenous medications, central line equipment, ostomy supplies) help to ease the transition to home. Detailed prescriptions are needed for each item. It is most helpful to prescribe a 1-month supply, while documenting the diagnosis directly on the prescription. In this time of constant scrutiny from third-party payers, letters of medical necessity from the physician may be needed to ensure that the appropriate equipment is financially covered and readily available.

F. T. Gill and K. H. Giordano: Department of Pediatric General Surgery, Alfred I. duPont Hospital for Children, Wilmington, Delaware.

Skilled nursing home visits may be offered to the family and ordered based on individual needs. This opportunity for assistance and support should not be underestimated. This is also the avenue to take when initiating multiple services on an outpatient basis (physical therapy, occupational therapy, speech therapy). Many managed care companies will agree to compensate for home visits if the hospital care team documents the clinical need and specifies the number of visits requested per week. When an agency has been identified by the social worker, written detailed orders are again necessary. The orders need to include all medications, including dose, intervals, route, and flush instructions; feeding instructions, including volume, route, and flow rate; oxygen requirements and pulse oximetry parameters; bathing instructions; gastrostomy/jejunostomy orders, including flushing, cleansing, securing, venting, residual parameters, and troubleshooting; and activity restrictions, including return to physical therapy, occupational therapy, speech therapy, and school.

Intervention from a nutritionist is another important adjunct during the postoperative period. Analysis of the caloric and fluid needs for each child is imperative. Guidance regarding the individual child's needs based on level of activity, future goals, and degree of healing is invaluable. For children who depend on tube feedings, suggestions regarding the appropriate formula for age and disease process and the rate calculated as a particular volume per kilogram can help in preventing postoperative feeding complications.

Families often verbalize a need to speak with others who "have been through the same thing." Providing them with information on support groups for particular diagnosis can provide a beacon of hope during a very challenging time.

A collaborative relationship with an advanced practice nurse (APN) can help to streamline coordination of the discharge process coupled with attentive follow-up care. Skilled nurse practitioners can provide an element of continuity that is important to and appreciated by the patient and family forced to cope with a complicated treatment plan.

GASTROINTESTINAL TUBES

Gastrointestinal tubes include gastrostomy, jejunostomy, gastrojejunostomy, and cecostomy tubes. The tubes come in a staggering variety of shapes, sizes, materials, and brand names. Most institutions and home health-care companies develop preferences and patterns so that the list of devices used in your hospital and locality may be limited to a handful of products. Tables 3.1 and 3.2 list some of the more common tubes and their qualities used for gastrostomies and jejunostomies.

The type of tube used in a given patient is determined by the operation performed and the needs of the child and his or her family. Sometimes a surgeon places a Mallecot or Foley catheter at the time of surgery with the intention of converting the tube to a more standard feeding device such as a Silastic gastrostomy tube or button device when the tract has matured. Securing these temporary tubes to prevent accidental dislodgment before the tract has matured can be a challenge. Sutures placed in the operating room have a tendency to erode and pull through, leaving only the balloon or mushroom tip to keep the tube in place. In the immediate postoperative period the tube can be secured with cloth tape. For home use, we have found the Hollister drain tube attachment device (Hollister, Inc., Libertyville, IL, 1-800-323-4060, product No. 9782) to be reliable and easy to use. Hollister devices should be changed every 3 days and on an as-needed basis. Skin integrity needs to be assessed frequently as well.

Patients and families need to be instructed as to how to maintain the tube sites. Mild soap and water are all that is needed to cleanse the tube site. If clear exudate collects around the tube, a solution of half-strength peroxide can be used to lift crusts. Dressings or creams and lotions are usually not necessary.

Gastrostomy tubes should be opened and "vented" frequently. Parents need to be advised to vent the tube prior to bolus feedings and as needed for fussiness, retching, gagging, or abdominal distention. Children receiving continuous jejunal feedings often need to leave the gastrostomy to drainage. The drainage should exhibit gastric contents. If the gastrostomy tube drainage appears bilious or milky, a contrast study through the jejunal tube will document the placement of the jejunal tube. If this study is inconclusive, further evaluation is needed.

Complications of gastrointestinal tubes are frequent and numerous. The formation of an overgrowth of granulation tissue is a normal response to the new tube. This granulation tissue often oozes a yellowish fluid that can be mistaken for a sign of infection. If surrounding erythema, edema, and pain are not evident, infection is unlikely. Granulation tissue often resolves on its own as the tract matures and scar tissue forms. Topical treatment with silver nitrate (applied daily for 3–5 consecutive days) or 0.1% triamcinolone cream (applied three times daily for 2–4 weeks) may help it to resolve more quickly. In rare cases, granulation tissue that is exuberant or refractory to local therapy requires surgical excision under local or general anesthesia. Families need to be reassured that the formation of granulation tissue is to be expected and in most cases resolves without surgical intervention.

Cellulitis of a tube site is a relatively frequent occurrence, although it can be difficult to distinguish from the redness, edema, pain, and discharge associated with local foreign body reaction and inflammatory changes that result from exposure to leaking intestinal contents. When in doubt, an empiric course of an antibiotic such as cephalexin (25–50 mg/kg/day divided into four daily doses) or ampicillin/sulbactam (45 mg/kg/day divided into two daily doses) may be warranted. Rarely does a true tract infection or abscess develop that requires surgical intervention. Erythema associated with multiple tiny pustules suggests the presence of a

TABLE 3.1. GASTROSTOMY TUBES

Gastrostomy Tube	Manufacturer	Sizes Available	Comments
Mallecot catheter	Multiple vendors	12 F and higher	May contain latex
MIC gastrostomy	Ballard Medical	12–18 F (5-mL balloon) 14–26 F (20-mL balloon)	1-800-528-5591
Mic-Key gastrostomy button	Ballard Medical	14–28 F (5-mL balloon) 0.8–4.5 cm length	1-800-528-5591
BARD gastrostomy device	Bard Endoscopic Tech.	18–28 F rigid mushroom 1.2–4.3 cm length	1-800-826-2273
Hide-A-Port	Ross Products	14–24 F (6-mL balloon) 0.8–4.5 cm	1-800-231-3330
Mini gastrostomy button	Applied Medical Technology	12–24 F (5-mL balloon) 0.8–4.4 cm length	1-800-869-7382
Foley catheter	Multiple vendors	8–30 F	May contain latex

TABLE 3.2. JEJUNOSTOMY TUBES

Jejunostomy	Manufacturer	Sizes Available	Comments
Mic-Key jejunostomy button	Ballard Medical	14–18 F 0.8–4.5 cm length Inflate balloon with 2 mL	1-800-528-5591
Mic-Key G button (for roux-en-Y)	Ballard Medical	See sizes above	1-800-528-5591
GJ tubes		16–18 F/25 cm length (5 mL)	
Mic-Gastro-Enteric	Ballard Medical	16–18 F/56.5 cm length (28 mL) 22–30 F/56.5 cm length (28 mL)	1-800-528-5591

Candida infection. Treatment with nystatin powder or cream for 2 weeks usually results in prompt resolution.

Leakage of intestinal contents around a gastrointestinal tube can be a particularly frustrating problem and one that causes a great deal of anxiety for the family. The tube should be assessed for size and fit. Granulation tissue and local infections should be treated appropriately. A common cause of leakage is distal obstruction due to poor gastric emptying, partial small bowel obstruction, or overfeeding. Occasionally, a contrast study is necessary to rule out obstruction. One should consider the possibility that the balloon has migrated distally, resulting in obstruction of the pylorus or jejunum. Meanwhile, the skin should be protected with a barrier ointment and movement of the tube should be minimized. Replacing the tube with one of a larger diameter, while tempting, results in a larger opening and more leakage and should therefore be avoided. A better strategy is to remove the tube completely (only if the tract is well established) for a period of up to several hours to allow the opening to close slightly and then replace it with the same size tube. Overfilling the balloon slightly and applying gentle traction on the tube so as to pull the balloon tighter against the abdominal wall may help, but needs to be done carefully and for only a short period of time to prevent necrosis of the stomach or intestine.

When a gastrostomy tube is scheduled to be changed, it must be ascertained if this was a surgical or Percutaneous Endoscopic Gastrostomy (PEG) placement. If a PEG approach was used, 12 weeks must pass prior to a tube change. In all cases, the first PEG tube change must be performed under fluoroscopy. Scheduled changes for new surgically placed gastrostomy tubes should occur at 4 and 12 weeks, depending on the preference of the individual surgeon. If the tube is changed to a short button-type tube (Mickey, Ballard Medical Products, Draper, Utah; Ross Hide-a-Port, Columbus, Ohio), the depth of the track must be determined with an appropriate measuring device. The initial surgical tube should be removed with gentle traction. The tube size should be ascertained and the new tube quickly replaced. Auscultation of the abdomen and aspiration of stomach contents are helpful in evaluating the patient for successful placement. Balloons should be inflated with 5 mL of sterile water. It is prudent to check the specific product recommendations. If appropriate time for healing has taken place postoperatively, fluoroscopy should not be needed. If there are any concerns about tube placement, radiologic confirmation is imperative.

Jejunal tubes can be changed within 4 to 12 weeks under fluoroscopy. Using a MIC-KEY jejunostomy tube, cut to appropriate length, provides a more secure tube. If the surgeon used a Roux-en-Y approach, a button gastrostomy device can be placed. For jejunostomy tubes, the balloon should only be inflated with 2 mL water to avoid obstruction of the small bowel lumen.

If the child's tube has come out and there has been a delay in intervention, it is often difficult to replace. The surgeon should determine what size tube was in place and attempt to pass a tube that is one size smaller, continuing to decrease the diameter of the tube size until a tube can be easily passed. One must never force any tube into the tract. If a tube cannot be passed, the child may need surgical intervention for dilatation of the track under anesthesia. Prevention of this problem is important. The tube should be secured appropriately. The family should be provided with a replacement tube and instructed to replace the tube themselves or to proceed to the nearest emergency room as quickly as possible so that the tube can be replaced before it closes.

Many children return with the complaint of a clogged tube. The first attempt to unclog the tube should be made with warm water injected from a small-volume syringe. Other solutions that can be used include carbonated beverages and cranberry juice. If these do not work, a solution of a meat tenderizer that contains papain can be used (1 teaspoon in 2 ounces of warm water). Pancreatic enzyme preparations also can be used (one capsule with sodium bicarbonate 325 mg mixed in 5 mL of water). If the tube cannot be opened with these techniques, then replacement will be necessary. Prevention is effected by appropriate flushing after feedings and administration of medications (especially antiseizure drugs).

STOMA CARE

The type of ostomy appliance is dependent on the type of diversion that is created, type and volume of effluent, and the stoma location on the abdomen. A variety of ostomy products are available. A selection should be implemented as soon as bowel function resumes in the early postoperative period. A flexible one-piece system is usually optimal immediately after surgery. Based on the age, size, and individual preferences of the patient and family, a two-piece system also can be used. These products snap together to form one unit. Whatever is used, it is important to aim for a pouch-wearing time of more than 24 hours. If changes occur more frequently, the risk of peristomal skin irritation, family and patient frustration, and financial impact increases. Table 3.3 lists some of the more commonly used ostomy appliance devices and their qualities. Table 3.4 lists common ostomy care accessories.

The skin surrounding an ostomy is at risk for compromised integrity because of reaction to ostomy supplies, and because of contact with liquid effluent causing contact dermatitis or fungal infections. The size, shape, configuration and location of the stoma can be a challenge. An improperly fitted pouch can compound these problems. The opening on the wafer should be 3 mm (1/8 inch) wider than the stoma. This will allow a snug fit around the stoma, protecting the surrounding skin surfaces without compromising the mucosa. When skin irritation begins, it should be covered immediately with the ostomy product. It is a common mistake to make the opening wider, exposing more skin surface. Remeasuring the stoma opening, followed by applying a thin layer of paste to the barrier wafer, enhances coverage and adhesiveness. Allowing the paste to dry prior to application to the skin surface enhances evaporation of the alcohol in the product and decreases skin irritation. Stoma powder is an alternative adhesive material that does not contain alcohol. Warming the pouch with a hair dryer increases flexibility and adhesiveness. If irritation persists, the products in use should be reevaluated. Cleansing products, adhesive removers, or enhancers or the ostomy products may be the cause of skin irritation. Skin problems may include local irritation with evidence of bright red erythema with flat or raised vesicular lesions. Dermatitis is usually limited to the area of contact. Discontinuing the products and cleansing with mild soap and water followed by application of a warmed pouch should be initiated.

Fungal infections due to *Candida albicans* are a common problem. This migratory infection presents with a red, shiny, macular rash that causes itching. The peristomal area should be cleansed and dried, followed by application of a small amount of topical antifungal powder (nystatin) and the pouching device. If needed, antifungal and stoma adhesive powders can be mixed together (1:1) to assure a good seal.

Stomal management problems may arise from a variety of issues. Uneven skin surfaces or flattened stomas can make the use of an appropriate appliance a true challenge. Troubleshooting this problem includes the addition of convexity to the ostomy product. Manufactured pouches that incorporate convexity are available by major vendors (Hollister, Libertyville, Illinois; Convatec, Princeton, New Jersey). Convexity also can be accomplished by adding a skin barrier ring (Eakins seal by Convatec, Princeton, New Jersey) around the stoma prior to application of a standard pouch.

Stoma prolapse is more frequently seen in children with transverse or loop colostomies. Prolapse can be difficult to manage. If it is minimal and the circulation is not compromised, apply the ostomy pouch while the patient is supine. If the prolapse is significant, circulation may be at risk, requiring manual reduction of the bowel. It may be necessary to increase the opening size of the pouch or change the

TABLE 3.3. OSTOMY PRODUCTS

Patient Age	Vendor Information	Product Information
Premature/low-birth-weight infant	Hollister	Pouchkins two-piece system no. 3777 (16 mm) 15/box or no. 3778 (35 mm × 22 mm) 15/box
Infant/small child	Convatec	Little Ones Active Life no. 209–22 one-piece system, 2-inch drainable pouch, 15/box
	Hollister	Pouchkins nos. 9766, 9768 one-piece system, 2-inch drainable pouch, 15/box
Children	Convatec	Little Ones Sur-Fit no. 401925 1¼-inch wafer, 5/box no. 401927 1¼-inch drainable pouch, 10/box no. 401926 1¾-inch wafer, 5/box no. 401928 1¾-inch drainable pouch, 10/box
	Hollister	Softflex-Centerpoint~Lock Floating Flange no. 3770 1¼-inch no starter hole, 5/box
Adolescent	Convatec	Active Life no. 22771 one-piece drainable pouch, cuts to fit ¾ inch to 2½ inches, 10/box
	Hollister	Premier no. 8631 one-piece drainable pouch, cuts to fit up to 2½ inches, 10/box.

TABLE 3.4. OSTOMY ACCESSORIES

Ostomy Accessories	Vendor	Product Information
Paste	Convatec	Stomahesive paste no. 183910
	Hollister	Karaya paste no. 7919
Powder	Convatec	Stomahesive powder no. 25510
	Hollister	Karaya powder no. 7906
Tail closures (for bag)	Convatec	no. 175635 (10/box)
Odor eliminators	Hollister	M9 drop deodorizer no. 7717
		M9 odor eliminator spray no. 7733

product to accommodate prolapse or edema. Surgical revision of the stoma may be required.

Peristomal herniation causes an uneven abdominal surface with concomitant problems of adherence of the ostomy appliance. Application with the patient supine may help. Older children and adolescents may use an ostomy belt for further support. Stomal stenosis should be considered if there are changes in the volume and consistency of the effluent. Other obstructive symptoms, such as abdominal distention, vomiting, decreased appetite, cramping, or irritability may be present. Stool cultures testing for rotavirus and *Clostridium difficile* should be considered. The abdominal examination may reveal a palpable mass. This may represent a retained fecaloma, thus raising suspicion for a distal stricture. Evaluation of the stoma, including a digital examination, is imperative. If unable to complete the digital examination, a lubricated catheter or Hegar dilator can be gently passed into the stoma. A contrast enema may be necessary to confirm the diagnosis of stricture. Surgical revision of the stoma may be warranted.

Patient and family education should be initiated at the time of admission and reviewed throughout hospitalization. Families need to demonstrate the ability to care for their child's ostomy. Careful attention to the discharge process cannot be overemphasized.

Children who have undergone closure of a colostomy often suffer from complicated skin care issues. During the initial postoperative period, patients tend to pass many loose stools, often up to 10 or 15 per day. Severe skin breakdown can occur from the acidic nature of the stool. Although aggressive skin care is necessary, normal diaper rash remedies often are not sufficient. Skin barrier products are recommended to decrease stool–skin contact. In many cases, a standard over-the-counter zinc oxide preparation, applied after every bowel movement, is sufficient. The product should be used prophylactically, before any signs of skin irritation are present. Other barrier creams and ointments are also useful and are made by a variety of manufacturers. Again, frequent application and prophylactic use are essential. In severe cases, a prescription product may be necessary. We have had success with ILEX barrier cream (MedCon Technologies, Tel Aviv, Israel). This rubbery paste forms an excellent barrier to moisture and needs to be applied three to four times daily. It is also important to instruct families not to scrub it off, which worsens the skin irritation. SensiCare Protective Barrier (Convatec) can be applied with each diaper change and also works well for some families. Helpful adjuncts include instructing the family to refrain from using diaper wipes of any kind due to the multiple additives in these products. The skin should be washed with mild soap and water only. Soothing tub baths are comforting. Exposing the buttocks to air, or blowing air from the "cool" setting of a blow dryer may hasten the healing process. Fungal skin infection is a common postoperative complication. Treatment must address the underlying cause while providing protection for the skin.

SUPPORT GROUPS

Finally, support groups can provide a great deal of comfort and emotional support for families trying to cope with a new or complicated diagnosis. They can also provide a great deal of useful information via their literature, websites, and meetings. The following is a brief list of commonly used support groups for our patients:

International Foundation for Functional Gastrointestinal Disorders (IFFGD)
Pediatric Division
P.O. Box 170864
Milwaukee, WI 53217-8076
1-414-964-1799
E-mail: *IFFGD@IFFGD.org*

Biliary Atresia & Liver Transplant Network (BALT)
3835 Richmond Avenue, Box 190
Staten Island, NY 10312-3828
Website: *livertx.org*

Cherubs (Association of Congenital Diaphragmatic Hernia Research Advocacy and Support)
P.O. Box 1150
Oxford, NC 27522
E-mail:*cherubs@gloryroad.net*
Website: *www.gloryroad.net/~cherubs*

EA/TEF Child & Family Support Connection Inc.
111 W. Jackson Blvd. Suite 1145
Chicago, IL 60604-3502
312-987-9085
E-mail: *eatef2@aol.com*

Crohn's, Colitis Foundation of America
386 Park Avenue South, 17th Floor
New York, NY 10016-8804
800-932-2423
E-mail: *info@ccfa.org*
Website: *www.ccfa.org*

Pediatric Crohn's, Colitis and Ileitis Association
Box 188
Newton, MA 02168
617-489-5854 (Colitis/Crohn's)
508-358-5147 (Ileitis)

The Pull-Thru Network (Anorectal Malformations)
316 Thomas Street
Bessemer, AL 34020
205-428-5953
E-mail: *pullthru@bellsouth.net*
Website: *www.pullthrough.org*

TEF/Vater International Support Network
c/o Jeff and Terri Burke
15301 Grey Fox Road
Upper Marlboro, MD 20772
301-952-6837

United Ostomy Association
19772 MacArthur Blvd., Suite 200
Irvine, CA 92612-2405
800-826-0826

4

ENTERAL NUTRITION

FRAZIER W. FRANTZ

Providing optimal nutrition to pediatric patients is essential, not only to meet metabolic and physiologic needs, but to support growth and development. In surgical patients, good nutrition decreases morbidity, shortens hospital stays, and improves outcome. Unfortunately, many children who present for surgery suffer from malnutrition, either due to an underlying feeding disorder or because of the nature of the disease process for which they require surgery. Moreover, the high nutrient requirements associated with surgical stress and wound healing in the postoperative period place the pediatric surgical patient at significant risk for becoming malnourished.

Pediatric nutritional support is designed to prevent and correct nutrient deficiencies associated with malnutrition and to provide adequate nutrition to meet the patient's needs. Enteral nutrition refers to nourishment provided through the gastrointestinal (GI) tract, either by oral feeding or through a feeding tube. In comparison with parenteral nutrition, enteral support is more physiologic, more economic, easier to administer, and results in fewer complications. In patients with a functional or even a partially functioning GI tract, enteral nutrition should be initiated as soon as the child is clinically stable, because even small volumes of enteral feedings facilitate preservation of normal intestinal villus and microvillus structure and may help to prevent bacterial translocation and septicemia. The single most important stimulus for intestinal mucosal growth and function is the presence of food in the gut.

Most healthy full-term infants tolerate oral feedings without difficulty. In other children, either because of severe prematurity (<32 to 34 weeks' gestation with uncoordinated suck/swallow) or due to underlying medical or surgical conditions, oral feedings are not tolerated or are inadequate in meeting nutritional requirements. Included in these conditions are functional problems, such as neurologic disorders and diseases associated with increased metabolic needs or altered absorption/metabolism, as well as anatomic abnormalities, encompassing congenital anomalies, obstruction or injury to the aerodigestive tract, and intestinal surgery. It is this population of children that requires enteral nutritional support.

It is important as a pediatric surgeon to master the principles of enteral nutrition because we treat patients of all ages and with many different diseases that directly or indirectly impact the body's ability to consume and absorb adequate nutrients to heal and grow. In no group of patients is nutrition more important or challenging than in neonates, particularly those delivered prematurely. For this reason, the majority of this chapter focuses on guidelines for enteral nutrition in full-term and preterm infants. Attention is directed toward nutritional assessment, determination of nutritional requirements, feeding access, formula selection and initiation/administration, monitoring and complications of tube feedings, and transitional feedings.

NUTRITIONAL ASSESSMENT

The assessment of a child's nutritional status requires consideration of the medical history, anthropometric data, laboratory data, physical findings, and dietary history. Many hospitals use some form of nutritional screening, such as the subjective global assessment (SGA), to identify patients with varying degrees of malnutrition. The SGA includes a history and physical examination focused on identifying underlying nutrition-related disease processes and potential signs or risk factors for malnutrition, such as weight loss, anorexia, diarrhea, emesis, or other feeding problems.

The most commonly used anthropometric data are height, weight, and head circumference. These measurements are plotted on a standardized growth curve such as that of the National Center for Health Statistics (NCHS). From this information, the expected weight-for-height index can be calculated. These data help determine if the child is within the 5th and 95th percentiles of growth and will serve as data points for subsequent comparison in time to assess the child's growth trends. For newborns, these parameters are checked frequently with length and head

F. W. Frantz: Department of Surgery, Division of Pediatric Surgery, Naval Medical Center, Portsmouth, Virginia.

circumference measured weekly and weight checked daily. The anticipated increments in these parameters in preterm newborns receiving adequate nutrition are weight 15 to 18 g/kg/day, length 0.8 to 1.1 cm/week, and head circumference 0.5 to 0.8 cm/week. For full-term infants the anticipated increments are weight 20 to 30 g/kg/day, length 0.69 to 0.75 cm/week, and head circumference 0.33 cm/week. After 3 months of age, these growth rates gradually slow. It is important to remember that all newborns lose weight during the first 1 to 2 weeks of life as a result of postnatal diuresis. This weight loss varies from 10% of birth weight in full-term babies to as much as 20% in micropremies (<1,000 g). For this reason, weight gain reflecting growth may not be present for 2 weeks after birth. As this anthropometric data is followed for growth trends, deviations from the child's usual growth pattern, especially an increase or decrease across two major percentiles or measurements below the 5th percentile for weight or height, should be noted.

The most commonly used biochemical markers to monitor nutritional status are serum albumin and prealbumin. Although the serum albumin level is affected by hydration status and may be a relatively late indicator of nutritional depletion because of its long half-life (20 days), it is an inexpensive and readily available test, and levels do correlate with the degree of malnutrition. Prealbumin has a much shorter half-life (2–3 days) and is a sensitive correlate of visceral protein status. These values can be checked weekly with the initiation of enteral support. During the first week of life in infants requiring enteral support, serum electrolytes, glucose, creatinine, and blood urea nitrogen are usually monitored daily. Serum calcium, phosphorus, and magnesium levels are checked biweekly. In many premature infants, hemoglobin/hematocrit and alkaline phosphatase levels also should be assessed every 2 weeks.

NUTRITIONAL REQUIREMENTS

Many factors affect the nutritional requirements of infants. Caloric and protein requirement estimates based on recommended dietary allowances (RDAs) serve only as starting points, and nutrient delivery should be adjusted based on the individual child's nutritional parameters after initiation of enteral feeding. Typical caloric requirements for healthy full-term infants are approximately 110 to 120 kcal/kg/day, whereas preterm infants require 120 to 130 kcal/kg/day. Protein requirements for full-term infants are estimated to be 2.0 to 2.5 g/kg/day, whereas preterm infants need 3.0 to 4.0 g/kg/day. Increased energy requirements should be anticipated during recovery from surgery, sepsis, and respiratory distress. Postoperative neonates usually require 120 to 140 kcal/kg/day and 2.5 to 4.0 g protein/kg/day to account for the increased energy demands of stress and healing.

Once calorie and protein requirements have been determined, the final diet should provide 35% to 65% of calories as carbohydrates, 7% to 16% as protein, and 30% to 55% as fat. A disproportionate amount of any of these elements may lead to unwanted metabolic or clinical sequelae. If more that 55% of calories are fat, ketosis may develop. Excess carbohydrates may overwhelm absorption capacity and cause diarrhea. Protein intakes exceeding 5 g/kg/day can cause azotemia.

In addition to calories and protein, vitamins and minerals are important requirements that must be included in nutritional support to ensure adequate growth and development. This is particularly true in preterm infants, who require higher intake of calcium, phosphorus, and magnesium (the primary components of skeletal tissue) than do full-term infants. The special vitamin and mineral requirements of the preterm infant are usually met by fortified human milk or premature infant formula. Iron supplementation is important for both full-term and preterm infants, and needs usually can be met with iron-fortified formula. For iron supplementation, the American Academy of Pediatrics recommends 1 mg/kg/day for the full-term infant by 4 months of age and 2 mg/kg/day for preterm infants starting at no later than 2 months of age. In infants who have undergone bowel resection and ileostomy, particular attention should be directed to zinc levels, because excessive ostomy losses may result in deficiency of this important trace mineral.

As a general rule, RDAs for calories and protein requirements in the pediatric population decrease with age. From 6 months to 3 years of age, calorie and protein requirements are estimated at 100 kcal/kg/day and 1.2 to 1.6 g/kg/day, respectively. By 7 to 10 years of age, these requirements decrease to 70 kcal/kg/day and 1.0 g/kg/day for protein. Beyond this age, values stabilize between 40 to 50 kcal/kg/day and 0.8 to 1.0 g/kg/day for protein.

FEEDING ACCESS

Feeding routes for enteral nutrition include oral intake, nasogastric (NG) or orogastric (OG) tubes, nasoduodenal tubes, gastrostomy tubes, and jejunostomy tubes. For infants who have an abnormal suck or swallow or those that are not alert enough to swallow, feeding tube placement is required to serve as the primary access for enteral nutrition. In infants who can tolerate oral intake but do not consume adequate calories to maintain growth, despite maximizing formula concentration, feeding tube placement can be used to supplement oral intake.

When tube feeding is required, direct gastric feeding is preferable to intestinal feeding because it allows for a more natural digestive process. Gastric feedings are associated with a larger osmotic and volume tolerance, a more flexible feeding schedule, easier tube insertion, a lower frequency of diarrhea and dumping syndrome, and beneficial bactericidal effects of gastric acid. NG feeding tubes can be used for short-term (6–8 weeks) therapy. A variety of soft, small-bore (5–8 French) NG tubes are available. In neonates, who are obligate nose breathers, OG tube placement may be preferable to prevent airway occlusion. After NG/OG tube placement, confirmation of position must be obtained by either aspiration of gastric contents or by radiography. One disadvantage of these tubes, especially when used for supplemental feedings, is that they may interfere with oral intake.

For children expected to require tube feeding for longer than 6 to 8 weeks, consideration should be given to gastrostomy tube placement. The tube can be placed using an open or endoscopic approach, depending on the size of the child. For the open route, I prefer the Stamm technique through a small midline incision. With either placement technique, feedings can usually be safely started within 24 hours. In many cases, the decision to place a gastrostomy tube requires an evaluation of the patient for the presence of gastroesophageal reflux (GER). This is particularly true for children who present with neurologic or developmental disorders and failure to thrive. The rationale for this investigation is that if GER is present, it is usually made worse by the placement of a gastrostomy tube. This workup usually entails some combination of an upper GI series, esophageal pH monitoring, and a gastric emptying scan. If significant GER is detected, fundoplication with gastrostomy tube placement or enterostomy tube placement is likely indicated.

To present a different approach, if I am consulted for gastrostomy tube placement in an infant—especially if the child is preterm, under 6 months of age, and tolerating NG/OG feedings without emesis, aspiration, or "spells" that could be attributed to GER—I usually proceed to gastrostomy placement without a GER workup. NG/OG feeding tolerance has proven a good litmus test and may avoid unnecessary fundoplication in a child who, even if mild GER is present, may outgrow it with age. As with gastrostomy tube placement under any scenario, it is important to explain to the parents that GER may occur afterwards and could require further medical or surgical therapy.

One often underappreciated advantage of gastrostomy feedings in patients who require enteral support is that the need for a tube through the patient's oropharyngeal cavity is obviated. In infants, this often results in less feeding aversion and facilitates development and maintenance of oral feeding skills. In older patients, particularly for long-term management, it results in better compliance with supplemental feedings.

Transpyloric feeding tube placement is desirable for patients who are at high risk for aspiration by virtue of diminished gag reflex, delayed gastric emptying, frequent vomiting, or severe GER. Placement of transpyloric nasoduodenal or nasojejunal tubes is more complicated than NG tube placement and requires confirmation of position by radiography or pH analysis of aspirates. Placement of nasojejunal tubes can be facilitated by fluoroscopy and metoclopramide.

With regard to feeding jejunostomies, those that are placed endoscopically or radiographically through existing gastrostomies or those placed surgically via the transgastric route are probably the easiest to maintain. This can be accomplished using an available combination device, or separate tubes (standard gastrostomy tube and adjacent small-bore enterostomy tube) can be placed. "Straight" jejunostomy tubes can be difficult to place and maintain in small children and should probably be reserved for exceptional cases. A general dictum regarding all of the transpyloric feeding tubes is that although they are desirable for short-term bypass of the stomach in "aspiration-risk" children, they inherently commit the child to continuous feedings and may lead to significant, though reversible, compromise in gastric capacity for eventual oral or direct gastric feeding.

ENTERAL FORMULA SELECTION

Many commercially available formulas can be used for pediatric patients. Proper product selection depends on several patient-specific factors, including age, intestinal function, underlying disease, nutrient requirements, and feeding route. Table 4.1 lists the different formula compositions and their indications for use. The preferred enteral diet for the full-term newborn is human milk, providing sufficient energy, macronutrients, minerals, and water for normal growth. The preterm infant may not grow as fast on human milk alone because of considerably higher nutritional requirements. Milk from mothers of preterm infants has more calories, protein, and sodium than milk obtained at term and occasionally provides for adequate growth in larger and healthier preterm infants. Most of the time, however, fortification with one of the commercially available supplements is necessary to provide additional energy, protein, vitamins, and minerals. Using these human milk fortifiers (HMFs), such as Enfamil HMF (Mead Johnson, Evansville, IN) and Similac HMF (Ross), an additional 4 kcal/oz can be added to provide 24 kcal/oz fortified breast milk.

Infant enteral formulas generally mimic breast milk in caloric density (20 kcal/oz) but provide more protein, calcium, phosphorus, and iron. They are adequate to meet the needs of full-term and larger preterm infants (>1,800 g) with an intact GI tract and normal fluid requirements. Products designed for premature infants contain even higher concentrations of these constituents, and many include a substantial portion of fat substrate as medium-chain triglycerides (MCTs). MCTs do not require bile salts for absorption and can be directly absorbed into the portal

TABLE 4.1. INFANT AND PEDIATRIC FORMULA SELECTION

Formula Classification	Possible Indications for Use	Infant Formula (Manufacturer)	Pediatric Formula (Manufacturer)
Standard milk-based	Normally functioning GI tract	Human milk Similac (Ross) Enfamil (Mead Johnson) Carnation Good Start (Nestle)	Carnation Follow-Up Formula (Nestle)
Preterm formulation, milk-based	Infants <34 weeks' gestation and/or weight <2 kg	Special Care 24 (Similac) Enfamil Premature 24 (Mead Johnson)	
Standard milk-based, lactose-free	Term infant with acute lactase deficiency (i.e., acute gastroenteritis) Standard product ages 1–10 yr	LactoFree (Mead Johnson) Lactose Free (Similac)	Resource Just for Kids (Novartis) Pediasure and Pediasure with fiber (Ross) Kindercal (Mead Johnson)
Standard soy-based, lactose-free	Infants >1,800 g with primary or secondary lactase deficiency	Isomil (Ross) Prosobee (Mead Johnson) Carnation Alsoy (Nestle)	
Semi-elemental (casein hydrolysates)	Malabsorption (i.e., intestinal resection, short gut syndrome) Liver disease Cystic fibrosis Allergy to cow's milk and soy proteins	Pregestimil (Mead Johnson) Alimentum (Ross) Nutramigen (Mead Johnson)	
Elemental	Allergy to cow's milk or multiple food protein intolerance Short gut syndrome	Neocate (SHS) Ele-Care (Ross)	Neocate One+ (SHS) Vivonex Pediatric (Novartis) Peptamen Junior (Nestle)
Follow-up/discharge formulas	Premature infants for 1st year of life, especially if birthweight <1,250 g	Similac Neosure (Ross) EnfaCare (Mead Johnson)	
Special needs: lactose-free, modified fat	Chylothorax, severe steatorrhea, liver disease	Portagen (Mead Johnson)	
Standard milk-based, added rice starch	Mild reflux	Enfamil AR (Mead Johnson)	

venous circulation. Preterm formulas also contain less lactose and substitute glucose polymers to provide half of the calories derived from carbohydrates. These formulas are available in 20, 22, and 24 kcal/oz preparations and can be used until the infant reaches 2.5 to 3.6 kg.

Soy protein formulas should be reserved for infants with a strong family history of cow's milk protein allergy who are not being fed human milk. These formulas have lower protein, vitamin, and mineral content and are not indicated for premature infants under 1,800 g. Lactose-free formulas, intended for the full-term infant with acute lactase deficiency, do not meet the nutritional requirements of premature infants either. Semielemental (contain protein hydrolysates) and elemental formulas are used in infants with malabsorption, abnormal GI tracts, or severe protein allergy. Most of these formulas contain MCTs, Pregestimil having the most, with 55% of total fat content. Occasionally these formulas are useful after a severe episode of infectious gastroenteritis with mucosal injury and resulting protein or lactose intolerance. The nutrient content of protein hydrolysate formulas is inadequate for the preterm infant, and calcium and phosphorus need to be supplemented. Depending on the infant's feeding history and the indications for using a semielemental or elemental formula, consideration should be given, when appropriate, to switching to a premature formula to improve nutrient intake.

Children with increased caloric requirements and those who are subject to volume restriction may benefit from a more concentrated formula than is typically used. Concentration of a base infant formula by adding less water is generally recommended up to 24 or 26 kcal/oz. When concentrating formulas, it is safest to advance caloric density gradually by 2 kcal/oz every 24 hours. When higher energy densities are required, use of modular components should be considered for further caloric enhancement (maximum 30 kcal/oz). Available modular additives to increase caloric density include glucose polymers (Polycose, Ross) or fats such as vegetable oil or MCTs. Each teaspoon of Polycose powder provides 8 kcal. Corn oil provides 8.3 kcal/mL, whereas MCT oil provides 7.7 kcal/mL. Additional protein can be added using Resource (Novartis) instant protein powder, which provides 1.5 g of protein per teaspoon. Soluble dietary fiber is an additional supplement that is added to formulas to enhance feeding tolerance, particularly in children with altered GI function. A good source for this is Resource Benefiber powder, which provides 1.5 g of fiber and approximately 5 kcal per teaspoon. When concentrating formulas, particular attention should be directed to (a) adequacy of fluid intake, because excessively concentrated formula may have a high renal solute load; (b) the final osmolarity of the formula feeding, because hyperosmolar feedings may not be tolerated by some infants; and (c) maintenance of normal carbohydrate, fat, and protein ratios, particularly if modular components are used.

TIMING OF INITIATION OF ENTERAL FEEDING

Prior to initiating enteral feeding, the child should meet certain clinical criteria to optimize safety and to maximize the chances for feeding tolerance. Overall, the child should be stable from a respiratory and cardiovascular standpoint. Oral feedings can be started safely when the respiratory rate is below 60 breaths/min. For gavage feedings, a rate below 80 breaths/min is usually recommended. Clinical signs of acute sepsis, hypotension, and significant apnea and bradycardia should be absent. No signs of intestinal obstruction should be present, including emesis or bilious gastric drainage. Evidence of intact intestinal function should be confirmed as active bowel sounds or passage of meconium, stool, or flatus. No evidence of GI tract hemorrhage should be present. On physical examination, the abdomen should be nondistended and nontender to palpation.

Contraindications for the initiation of enteral nutrition in pediatric patients include necrotizing enterocolitis (NEC), bowel obstruction, intestinal atresia, severe inflammatory bowel disease, severe intestinal side effects of cancer therapy, and acute pancreatitis. In addition to these, there are certain clinical scenarios that occur predominantly in neonates and which may warrant withholding of enteral nutrition, for example, the infant who is recovering from shock or asphyxia. In this setting, enteral feedings should probably be discontinued for 24 to 72 hours to allow recovery of the bowel from the ischemic injury and to decrease the risk for NEC. Other scenarios where withholding of enteral feedings is appropriate because of a higher risk of bowel ischemia include the neonate with an umbilical artery catheter in place or one who has a patent ductus arteriosus that is symptomatic or being treated with indomethacin.

After an abdominal operation, enteral feedings are often withheld for 3 or more days awaiting return of intestinal motility and function. Otherwise healthy postoperative pediatric patients can usually withstand a period of 5 to 7 days without nutritional intake while they recover. Infants and patients who were malnourished preoperatively will require prompt initiation of nutritional support after surgery. These patients may be managed via enteral or parenteral nutrition, or a combination of these, depending on the extent of surgery, the affected portion of the GI tract, and the child's general medical condition. Early initiation of small bowel feedings can be safe and effective if monitored closely. Aside from their nutritive role, enteral feedings are trophic for the gut and, even at low rates, may help to preserve intestinal structure and function. Because motility of the small bowel returns before that of the stomach after GI surgery, feeding tubes advanced beyond the pylorus or past a proximal small bowel anastomosis can be used to initiate and advance enteral feedings while the stomach recovers and anastomoses heal.

ADMINISTRATION OF ENTERAL FEEDING

Tube feedings can be administered as intermittent boluses, continuous infusion, or a combination of the two, depending on the child's condition, site of enteral access, status or gastric function and capacity, and the needs of the family. Bolus feedings can mimic or supplement meals and are easier to administer. A feeding pump is not usually required, and the child is free to move about without restrictions between feedings.

Bolus feedings are typically administered over 15 to 20 minutes. Once total formula volume has been calculated, feedings should begin with 25% of the volume goal on the first day and increase by 25% daily as tolerated with total volume equally divided between five and eight feedings. Bolus feedings may not be well tolerated in children with conditions associated with poor volume tolerance, such as GER or delayed gastric emptying. Continuous feedings require a pump, and the child remains attached to feeding equipment through the duration of feeding. Battery-powered portable pumps can improve mobility in ambulatory children who are on continuous feedings. Continuous administration is the preferred method for patients with altered GI function and those receiving transpyloric feedings. Supplemental tube feedings can be given via continuous infusion nocturnally to avoid disruption of the daytime schedule and oral intake. In children on total enteral nutritional support, continuous feedings can be administered over 24 hours or can be cycled over shorter time periods depending on the age and medical condition of the patient. Older children usually tolerate a "window" period of 12 hours, whereas infants may tolerate a period of only 4 to 6 hours before hypoglycemia develops.

Although the decision between bolus and continuous tube feedings can appear somewhat arbitrary at times, continuous feedings have been shown to be advantageous in several settings. In preterm infants, continuous feedings are associated with lower energy expenditure and better growth compared with bolus feedings. In hypermetabolic burn patients, they have been associated with fewer stools and reduced time to reach nutritional goals. They are particularly beneficial in children with impaired absorption, such as short gut syndrome.

Regardless of which feeding route is selected, non-nutritive sucking during tube feedings should be encouraged because it accelerates maturation of the sucking reflex, decreases intestinal transit time, and has been reported to facilitate more rapid weight gain with decreased hospital stay.

There is no single "right" answer for initiating and advancing enteral nutrition in pediatric patients. Many different recommendations exist based on institutional practices and modifications of adult regimens. Table 4.2 contains reasonable guidelines for several different age ranges. In general, the rate of feeding advancement is contingent on the structure and function of the patient's GI tract. Children who are malnourished or those being weaned from parenteral nutrition require a more conservative feeding progression than what is typically administered to children with normal GI function.

Enteral feedings should be initiated with isotonic formulas (300 mOsm/L), breast milk, or 20 kcal/oz formula. An exception to this is very-low-birth-weight (<1,500 g) premature infants, who should be started on half-strength breast milk or quarter-strength formula. Initial dilute feedings also may be beneficial in patients with altered GI function or those beginning transitional feeding following prolonged parenteral feeding. For full-term infants and older children, a 2- to 5-day plan to reach nutritional goals is appropriate. Preterm infants will require more time. During advancement, simultaneous changes in volume and concentration should not be made. Volume should be increased before concentration with transpyloric feedings, and concentration should be advanced before volume with gastric feedings. If evidence of feeding intolerance develops, feedings should be returned to the previously tolerated concentration and volume, from which they can subsequently be advanced more slowly. For preterm infants, once feeding volumes reach 100 to 120 mL/kg/day, fortifier should be added to human milk, and preterm formula should be increased to 24 kcal/oz.

MONITORING OF TUBE FEEDINGS

Successful enteral nutrition must be carefully planned and monitored. In the early stages of tube feeding, monitoring is focused on assessing the patient's tolerance of the feeding plan. Daily weight, total fluid and caloric intake (all intravenous and enteral solutions), total output (all drains, stomas, emesis, stools, and urine), and appropriate biochemical parameters must be closely followed when enteral feedings are initiated and during advancement. Although monitoring is important in all children receiving enteral support, it is even more so in neonates because of their unique risk factors. Routine monitoring should include measurement of gastric residuals, measurement of abdominal girth, and stool testing. The goal of this detailed surveillance is to detect early signs of feeding intolerance, sepsis, or NEC. When abnormal parameters are detected or clinical signs of illness, such as apnea and bradycardia or temperature instability, are present, feedings may need to be decreased, diluted, or discontinued.

For infants receiving bolus feedings, gastric residuals should be checked before all feedings (every 2–3 hours) initially and then every 6 to 8 hours. Residual volumes greater than 50% of the previous feeding or progressive increases in serial measurements may warrant, at a minimum, a reduction in feeding volume or temporary withholding of feed-

TABLE 4.2. PEDIATRIC ENTERAL FEEDING GUIDELINES

Patient Age	Initial Volume	Advancement Rate	Goal Feedings
Bolus feedings			
Preterm <1,500 g	1–2 mL/kg every 1–2 h	1 mL every other feeding, maximum 10–15 mL/kg/day advance	150–175 mL/kg/day divided every 2–3 h
Preterm >1,500 g	2–4 mL/kg every 2–3 h	2 mL every other feeding, maximum 20–30 mL/kg/day advance	120–175 mL/kg/day divided every 2–3 h
0–12 mo	5–10 mL/kg every 2–3 h	15–30 mL/feeding	15–30 mL/kg every 3–5 h
1–6 yr	5–10 mL/kg every 3 h	30–45 mL/feeding	15–20 mL/kg every 4–5 h
7–10 yr	90–120 mL every 3–4 h	60–90 mL/feeding	360–480 mL every 4–5 h
Continuous feedings			
Preterm	1–2 mL/kg/h	10–15 mL/kg/day	120–175 mL/kg/day
0–12 mo	1–2 mL/kg/h	1–2 mL/kg every 12 h	5–6 mL/kg/h
1–6 yr	1–2 mL/kg/h	1–2 mL/kg every 12 h	4–5 mL/kg/h
7–10 yr	20–30 mL/h	10–30 mL every 12 h	75–120 mL/h

ings. For continuous gastric feedings, residuals should be checked at least every 4 hours during initiation and feeding advancement. If the residual volume is greater than the volume infused over the previous 2 hours, the infusion can be interrupted for an hour or two, restarted, and rechecked at the next interval. Unless they are mostly mucous, gastric aspirates should be returned to the stomach after checking residuals. In addition to the quantity of aspirate obtained, attention should be directed to the consistency of the fluid when checking residuals. Bile in the aspirate may be a sign of significant ileus or obstruction.

Abdominal girth should be measured every 4 to 8 hours during feeding initiation and advancement. Increases of greater than 1.5 to 2.0 cm on serial measurements are significant and should prompt withholding of feedings and a search for other signs of feeding intolerance. Routine stool testing should be performed daily during feeding advancement to detect the presence of blood or evidence of malabsorption (presence of reducing substance, pH <6.0).

Overt signs of feeding intolerance are emesis, abdominal distension, and high stool output or diarrhea. Any of these should prompt a temporary withholding or decrease in feeding volume until the source of the problem has been identified and addressed. A good starting point for infants with emesis or abdominal distension is plain abdominal films to check feeding tube position and to look for evidence of intestinal obstruction or NEC. Stool output of greater than 40 mL/kg/day or diarrhea may indicate underlying malabsorption. The stool should be tested for undigested carbohydrate and fat, and stool cultures should be obtained.

COMPLICATIONS

Complications of enteral feeding are generally classified into mechanical (tube-related), GI, and metabolic categories. Some complications may be a function of the enteral access route. Mechanical complications include tube clogging, tube displacement, and, occasionally, intestinal perforation associated with tube placement or migration. Tube clogging can generally be prevented by regular flushing of the tube, particularly before and after feedings and residual checks, and by infusing liquid formulations or completely dissolved crushed tablets when administering medications. Any suspicion of tube displacement based on clinical findings (coughing or vomiting) or inadvertent dislodgment should result in withholding of feedings and confirmation of tube position.

A wide spectrum of GI complications can be encountered, including reflux with aspiration pneumonia, gas bloating, diarrhea, dumping syndrome, and vomiting. Although aspiration pneumonia may be due to feeding tube malposition or mechanical impairment of the lower esophageal sphincter by an NG tube, most of the time it is a complication of underlying GER or delayed gastric emptying. Diarrhea in tube-fed patients can result from antibiotics, malabsorption, feedings that are too high in volume or concentration, low fiber intake, or food allergies. Diarrhea caused by bacterial contamination of formula can be minimized by limiting hang times to 8 to 12 hours for commercially manufactured formulas and 4 hours for breast milk. Dumping syndrome will usually respond to lowering of the feeding rate. The importance of enteral feeding as a risk factor in NEC has been well described. Techniques that may minimize the incidence of NEC include avoidance of rapid escalation of feeding volumes and hyperosmolar feedings and postponement of initiation of enteral feedings in "sick" newborns who have experienced respiratory or hemodynamic compromise.

Although less common that those associated with parenteral nutrition, metabolic complications can occur with enteral feeding. Dehydration is not uncommon, particularly in children on concentrated feedings. In severely malnourished children, refeeding must be approached cautiously. Starting at too high an initial nutrient level/rate or advancing too rapidly can lead to hyperglycemia, hypophosphatemia, hypokalemia, and hypomagnesemia. Clinically, volume overload with signs of cardiac or respiratory failure can occur. To avoid this, refeeding should begin at no more than 25% of goal with gradual advancement over 7 to 10 days. Failure to demonstrate consistent weight gain on enteral support should prompt reevaluation of the adequacy of nutrient intake and, if deemed appropriate, an investigation for potential malabsorption.

TRANSITIONAL FEEDINGS

Transitional feeding refers to a change from one feeding modality to another. This is typically a sign of progress toward providing optimal nutritional intake for the patient based on the child's medical condition, structure and function of the GI tract, and desired quality of life for the child and family. Transitional feedings should not be considered until the patient has achieved a satisfactory nutritional status because weight loss can occur during the transition. Although the needs of each child need to be considered individually, the most commonly used transitions in pediatric patients involve parenteral to enteral, parenteral to oral, continuous enteral to intermittent enteral, and enteral to oral feedings.

The transition from parenteral to enteral or oral nutrition is fairly straightforward. Caloric requirements of enterally fed patients are generally 10% higher than for parenterally fed patients. For enteral transitioning, small-volume continuous feedings (either gastric or transpyloric) are tolerated best after prolonged parenteral feeding.

For patients who have impaired absorption and those who have had no enteral nutrition for more than 5 to 7 days, feedings should be initiated with a semielemental formula. Most other patients will tolerate an isotonic, full-strength, lactose-free formula for initial feeding. Once tolerance is established at 15% to 20% of the desired volume, children receiving semielemental formula can be switched to a polymeric (intact nutrients) formula, and those already receiving polymeric formula can begin formula concentration. As enteral feedings reach 35% to 50% of calculated enteral requirements, total parenteral nutrition (TPN) may be tapered milliliter per milliliter for further increases in enteral feeding. When enteral feedings reach 75% to 100% of calculated requirements, TPN can be discontinued. For fluid-restricted patients, the lipid infusion can be continued until the enteral nutrition goal rate is achieved, at which point formula concentration can increase as the lipids are tapered. The transition from parenteral to enteral nutrition must be gradual and usually requires at least a week.

For oral transitioning, oral feedings should begin with small, frequent volumes of full-strength formula or breast milk for infants and clear liquids for children. Feedings are advanced in volume for infants and to full liquids and, eventually, solid foods in children. When full liquids are tolerated, parenteral feedings can be decreased by 10% to 25% daily. Daily adequate oral intake to meet all nutrient needs is required before TPN can be discontinued. Because appetite suppression is not uncommon after long-term parenteral feedings, commercial enteral liquid supplements may be helpful in the final stages of weaning to help maintain caloric intake. The time required for transition from parenteral to oral nutrition correlates well with the length of parenteral infusion.

Transition from continuous enteral to intermittent (gastric) enteral feedings can usually be accomplished by gradually increasing the rate of feeding and lengthening the time between feedings or by progressing to a combination of daytime bolus feedings and nighttime continuous feedings. Using the first method, the total daily feeding volume can be divided by the desired number of daily feedings, so that for feedings given every 3 hours, eight daily feedings would be required. This feeding volume, one eighth of the daily total, is then given at higher rates over progressively shorter times, and the feeding pump is shut off between feedings. For "target" 3-hour feeding intervals, a reasonable progression would be: 2-hour infusion/1 hour off (day 1), 1-hour infusion/2 hours off (day 3), and bolus over 15 to 30 minutes/pump off (day 5). The rapidity of weaning is based on patient tolerance and acceptable gastric residual volumes. In the second method, the total feeding volume is divided between daytime and nighttime feedings. Once a desirable feeding schedule is determined, bolus feedings can be started at one half to two thirds of the total volume that would have been given over the designated time period via continuous infusion. The daily formula volume remaining after daytime boluses can then be infused continuously over an 8- to 12-hour nighttime cycle. Gradual advancement of bolus feeding volumes will be dictated, again, by patient tolerance.

The transition from enteral to oral feedings can be an arduous one, primarily due to underdeveloped oral motor skills and swallowing capabilities and the multitude of behavioral problems that are common in tube-fed children. To minimize these problems, oral feedings by nipple- or breast-feeding should be instituted as soon as medically possible. Although the transition to oral feedings can be made from continuous or bolus feedings, it is easier from the latter. In older children, the bolus feeding schedule can be adjusted further to approximate three meals and two to three snacks per day to facilitate the transition. Introducing the sensation of hunger is a tool that is helpful when transitioning to oral feedings. Tube feeding is usually reduced by 25% initially to promote hunger. Using the bolus schedule as a baseline, oral feedings can be offered first when the child is hungry, and any remaining feeding volume can be given as a bolus through the feeding tube. Alternatively, inadequate oral intake during daytime feedings can be compensated for using nighttime feedings. When oral intake is consistent, growth is acceptable, and feeding problems are decreasing, tube feedings can be decreased further in 25% increments. When 75% of calories required are from oral intake, tube feedings can be discontinued. In infants who are transitioning to oral feedings from continuous enteral feedings, allowing the child to nipple-feed the hourly volume with the pump off every 8 to 12 hours is a good starting point. The continuous rate over subsequent hours can be adjusted to compensate for any feeding volume discrepancies. This process can be gradually accelerated with nipple-feeding every 3 to 4 hours and progressive increases in oral feeding volumes and intervals with tube feedings held. When transitioning from tube feedings to oral feedings in infants, it is important to limit nipple feeding to 20 minutes per feeding to prevent fatigue and excess energy expenditure. Because it is more difficult to quantitate feeding volumes and requires more energy of the infant, breast-feeding is slowly introduced during oral transitioning with careful monitoring of weight gain and nutritional parameters.

SUGGESTED READINGS

Anderson DM. Nutrition for premature infants. In: Samour PQ, Helm KK, Lang CE, eds. *Handbook of pediatric nutrition, 2nd ed.* Gaithersburg, MD: Aspen, 1999:43–63.

Corrales KM, Bechard LJ, Kanek A, et al. Enteral nutrition. In: Hendricks KM, Duggan C, Walker WA, eds. *Manual of pediatric nutrition, 3rd ed.* Hamilton, Ontario, Canada: BC Decker, 2000: 186–241.

Davis A. Transitional and combination feeds. In: Baker SB, Baker RD, Davis A, eds. *Pediatric enteral nutrition.* New York: Chapman & Hall, 1994:139–156.

Fletcher AB. Nutrition. In: Avery GB, Fletcher MA, MacDonald MG, eds. *Neonatology: pathophysiology and management of the newborn, 4th ed.* Philadelphia: JB Lippincott, 1994:330–342.

Marchand V, Baker SS, Baker RD. Enteral nutrition in the pediatric population. *Gastrointest Endosc Clin North Am* 1998;8: 669–703.

Nevin-Folino N, Miller M. Enteral nutrition. In: Samour PQ, Helm KK, Lang CE, eds. *Handbook of pediatric nutrition, 2nd ed.* Gaithersburg, MD: Aspen, 1999:513–545.

Teitelbaum DH, Coran AG. Perioperative nutritional support in pediatrics. *Nutrition* 1998;14:130–142.

5

COMPLICATIONS

JEFFREY H. HAYNES

The accurate and honest analysis of all surgical complications is one of the major cornerstones of surgical practice. The basis for this has always been clearly understood: to make sure the correct operation is being performed and is being performed correctly, including postoperative care. It is only through a forthright discussion of adverse events, along with their proper reconciliation, that similar events may then be prevented. The evaluation and management of specific complications in pediatric surgery is beyond the scope of this chapter and will be addressed on a topic-by-topic basis within this book. Rather, the intent is to reinforce the importance of evaluating complications and to provide a brief framework for their evaluation through which improved patient care may be assured.

ORIGINS OF EVIDENCE BASED MEDICINE

The systematic evaluation of complications is just one part of what today is known as evidence-based medicine. The origins of this practice extend back to the beginning of the 20th century in Boston. Ernest A. Codman, a surgeon, realized that both short- and long-term follow-up was necessary to assess the efficacy of his surgical interventions. He put forth the "end result idea" as well as other measures to modify care if patient outcomes were undesirable. To that end, he opened his own 10-bed hospital in Boston in 1911, routinely following his patients for 1 year postoperatively. He gathered his own data to be able to speak accurately and convincingly of his results. Although his contemporaries belittled his systematic approach to these issues, he clearly had in mind the approaches held as standards today by most hospitals and carried forth under various monikers such as quality assurance, continuous quality improvement, and evidence-based medicine. Again, the stringent evaluation of short- and long-term complications is an integral component of all the above systems, whose purpose is to assure delivery of first-rate health care.

J. H. Haynes: Department of Surgery and Pediatrics, Medical College of Virginia, Virginia Commonwealth University, Richmond, Virginia.

COMPLICATIONS AND MANAGED CARE

In this era of managed care, despite public discontent with the overall system, there is ever-increasing pressure to deliver high-quality, cost-efficient health care. Measures of this performance include length of stay, cost basis, and mortality and morbidity (or complications). Costs in particular are closely monitored and are probably the easiest parameter to measure. Today it is unusual not to receive periodic statements from health maintenance organizations, as well as hospitals, comparing physicians' individual costs with those of their peer group, often in striking detail. It is presumably only a matter of time before equivalent complication and outcome data are included in such reports based on reporting of adverse events. The move for such data to be part of a national database is well underway in order to help patients make an informed decision. Thus, it will become even more critical that we as surgeons track our own morbidities and mortalities, as well as the associated costs. We must see that they are reported with accuracy and interpreted correctly with respect to patient comorbidity, as well as use them as the critical basis to improve the art and science of pediatric surgery. Clearly, if we are not proactive in this arena, outside interests will gather and interpret such data for us. Undoubtedly, erroneous interpretation and subsequent conclusion will follow.

REVIEW OF COMPLICATIONS

As encouragement for internal review, departmental discussions of complications are considered privileged from a legal standpoint. As mentioned, however, more and more hospitals are tracking these data institutionally rather than leaving such discussions entirely within the confines of a department of surgery. Again, while still legally privileged, hospital quality assurance programs tracking this data must be able to interpret it appropriately.

The critical review of complications is an extremely valuable teaching tool at all levels of surgical education. Therefore, it should be conducted with formality and in an ordered fashion. Pediatric surgeons in the United States, being mostly trained in the Halstedian tradition as general surgeons prior to pediatric surgical residency, all have a similar grasp of the conduct of a morbidity and mortality conference. There are many other formats, of course, but certain characteristics transcend all types of these conferences.

Conferences should be held on a regular basis; service volume will dictate the frequency. The conference should be held at a time when other commitments are minimized and attendance should be mandatory. If possible, both the attending surgeon as well as the operating resident or intern should be present. There is little value in trying to develop the nuances of a case if one or the other is absent. An appropriate peer group should be present to provide insight or a larger experience to the problem at hand; the vision of someone one step removed from the problem is often extraordinary. The presenting resident should have a firm grasp of the literature regarding the surgical therapy of a given case; this is a learning experience for all present. This also allows determination of whether the observed complication is at significant variation with the published experience. The atmosphere in which the presentation occurs deserves comment. An austere, punitive environment is most certainly counterproductive. Rather, discussions should occur in a positive fashion, in which case an equivalent if not greater lesson will be learned. Individual mistakes will occur and must be tracked, but there is little point in a belittling approach to them. After presentation, an open discussion should follow as to further questions and interpretation of events. It is surprising how often new light is shed on a seemingly simple clinical problem.

After final assessment, it is useful and often required to categorize the complication as follows:

1. Error in surgical technique
2. Error in surgical judgment or patient selection
3. Known risk of procedure
4. Known risk due to patient disease or comorbidity

Such a categorization permits category assignment of "preventable" or "not preventable" to the adverse event. Trends may then be analyzed, which might suggest corrective actions in patient selection, surgical techniques, or physician education.

On a proactive note, it will be important to closely assess ongoing attempts at instituting clinical pathways. Many such pathways are effective in cutting costs without affecting quality of care. Because these efforts are clearly cost driven, it must be ensured that they are supported by evidence-based medicine prior to their routine use.

SUMMARY

Complications in pediatric surgery are part of everyday practice and are taken into account each time the risk:benefit ratio for a surgical operation is considered. It is essential, however, that any adverse event be discussed in a systematic fashion to ultimately determine if it may have been preventable. This is a crucial component of evidence-based medicine and assures that therapeutic interventions will continue to be appropriate as well as beneficial to the patient. In an era of ever-increasing cost control as well as clinical scrutiny, we must remain proactive in leading these discussions. Failure to systematically follow and learn from our own complications will result in third party involvement and possible erroneous interpretation of any adverse event. Such a sequence would clearly not be in the best interest of the surgeon or patient.

SUGGESTED READINGS

Badger TG. Quality management within a cost-constrained service. *J Nurs Manag* 1999;7:323–329.

Dudley RA, Bowers LV, Luft HS. Reconciling quality measurement with financial risk adjustment in health plans. *Jt Comm J Qual Improv* 2000;26:137–146.

Kaska SC, Weinstein JN. Historical perspective: Ernest Amory Codman, 1869–1940. A pioneer of evidence-based medicine: the end result idea. *Spine* 1998;23:629–633.

6

EPIDURAL AND REGIONAL ANESTHESIA

PHOEBE FISHER

Regional anesthesia in children has become a valuable tool in perioperative care. The benefits include a decrease in the hormonal stress response and lower intraoperative requirements of potent agents, allowing a more rapid return to alertness, decrease in postoperative parenteral narcotic use, and a high level of patient and family satisfaction. In addition, an interesting report by Taddio et al. in 1997 found that pain in the neonatal period may have significant long-term consequences. This study looked at circumcised infants, comparing those who were given analgesics and those who were not, and then how they responded to later painful stimuli (vaccinations). Those given analgesics at the time of circumcision were significantly calmer months later for their vaccinations. The most common blocks used for general surgical procedures are the epidural block via the caudal, lumbar, or thoracic approach, the ilioinguinal/iliohypogastric block, and the penile block.

In adults, these blocks are generally placed while the patient is awake and can be used frequently in lieu of a general anesthetic. Children are unable to cooperate with the positioning and sensations involved with block placement, and thus the block is almost always placed after the induction of general anesthesia. This adds a greater element of risk to block placement. An awake patient can describe paresthesias associated with accidental intraneuronal needle placement, as well as identify the early signs of local anesthetic toxicity. Nonetheless, large studies have shown that these blocks can be done by trained anesthesiologists in relative safety, with the benefits considerably outweighing the risks.

EPIDURAL BLOCKS

The epidural space is a potential space located just outside the dura. The spinal cord is a solid structure down to L3 in neonates and does not reach the adult position of L1 until 1 year of age. The dural sack extends to S2/S3.

P. Fisher: Department of Anesthesiology and Critical Care, Alfred I. duPont Hospital for Children, Wilmington, Delaware.

Access to the epidural space in the lumbar and thoracic regions is generally done for placement of an epidural catheter for continuous infusion. For this purpose, the epidural space is most often identified by a loss-of-resistance technique, as a needle is advanced in the midline anteriorly and cephalad between two spinous processes. The epidural space is 2 to 5 mm across. Once it is identified, a test dose of an epinephrine-containing solution is injected through the needle to rule out intravascular placement. Intrathecal placement is usually obvious, with the free flow of cerebrospinal fluid back through the large-bore needle. A catheter is then threaded approximately 5 cm into the space. The catheter can be difficult to pass for several reasons. These include false identification of the space, the catheter tip passing into a neural foramen, or a kinked catheter. There are several manipulations of the needle and catheter that can be used to salvage the attempt, although once the catheter has passed the tip of the needle, it should be withdrawn with great care, or not at all, because the tip can be sheared off. If these manipulations fail, the needle and catheter must be withdrawn as a unit and the procedure attempted again. Once the catheter does pass, it is gently aspirated to look for intravascular or intrathecal positioning. A negative aspiration, however, does not rule out improper placement, and a second test dose must then be given. The therapeutic dose should be given incrementally, each time with prior aspiration, because there have been incidences of catheter "migration" into the intravascular or intrathecal space.

Complications of continuous catheter use can be divided into those related to needle and catheter placement, and those that are drug related. Placement complications include backache, total spinal, postdural puncture headache (PDPH), and nerve injury. Backache is probably related to direct needle trauma to the tissues of the back, and generally resolve within a few weeks. A total spinal is caused by intrathecal injection of an epidural dose or a portion of an epidural dose of local anesthetic. In an already anesthetized and intubated patient, the blood pressure may need some support; otherwise, the effect should wear off in 1 to 3 hours, usually without sequelae. If the dura is punctured, there is a risk of PDPH. This can be treated conservatively with fluids, bed rest, and caffeine, but the most effective treatment is an epidural blood patch. The epidural space is accessed again in the same area, and 10 to 15 mL of the patient's own blood is injected with sterile precautions; this can result in immediate relief of symptoms. Nerve injury is fortunately rare. It can be caused by direct trauma to a single nerve root, causing paresthesias, pain, and numbness, all of which generally resolve in a period of weeks, or by direct cord trauma by the needle at the thoracic level. This can result in a significant injury. Nerve injury also can be caused by cord compression due to a mass effect from hematoma or abscess. Hematoma formation in the absence of a coagulopathy is almost unheard of, and an abscess is also rare. Such a mass lesion presents with back pain and neurologic changes. This presentation mandates an urgent imaging study and surgical decompression.

Complications related to drugs primarily relate to central nervous system toxicity and cardiotoxicity of local anesthetics and side effects of neuroaxial narcotics. Local anesthetics are sodium channel blockers. They function by blocking conduction along the neural pathways. Peak systemic concentration of local anesthetics is dependent on dose, site of injection, and the speed of injection. Signs of early toxicity include tinnitus, headache, circumoral numbness, and a change in mental status. As the serum level increases, the patient may develop seizures or cardiac toxicity. Lidocaine is a class 1 antiarrhythmic drug. It impairs myocardial contractility, but does not facilitate reentrant ventricular arrhythmia. Bupivacaine, however, is far more cardiotoxic, causing malignant arrhythmias that can be difficult to treat. Treatment includes bretylium 5 mg/kg (up to 30 mg/kg), and some success has been shown with phenytoin 5 mg/kg (up to 15 mg/kg). Resuscitation should be continued for a prolonged period of time because bupivacaine takes a long time to clear from the myocardium.

The early signs of local anesthetic toxicity are, of course, not recognized during general anesthesia. To replace this warning, epinephrine is added to the local anesthetic as a marker to indicate intravascular absorption. During injection, the electrocardiogram tracing is watched closely for epinephrine-induced changes. The first sign is peaked T waves. This is normally followed by tachycardia, but in the presence of bupivacaine there often is a decrease in the heart rate, followed by ST-wave elevation and hypertension. If these occur, the injection needs to be stopped, and the needle or catheter repositioned or the block abandoned.

Neuroaxial opioids can be a good adjunct or alternative to local anesthetics. The side effects of pruritis and nausea are treatable, but might be sufficiently annoying to the patient that the opioid needs to be removed from the continuous infusion. Neuroaxial opioids work in synergy with parenteral narcotics and can cause significant respiratory depression. Some studies have shown that the risk of respiratory depression lasts no more than 12 hours after the last dose.

In young children, the epidural space is most frequently accessed from the sacral hiatus either as a single-shot technique or with a catheter for continuous infusion. A caudal epidural block works well for almost any procedure of the abdomen and can even be used to cover a thoracotomy, such as ligation of a patent arterial ductus. A single-shot technique works very well for outpatients. A block with bupivacaine can provide good pain relief for 3 to 6 hours. This may allow the child to get dressed and travel home in relative comfort. The parents should be instructed to start oral analgesics before the block wears off. A continuous caudal catheter also can be used, although care must be taken to keep the entry site clean. Studies have showed varying degrees of success in placing the tip of the catheter at a desired level, but it can be imaged postoperatively to confirm location and dose requirements.

The caudal block is a safe block. A survey published in 1991 from 119 hospitals showed an incidence of catastrophic complications of 1:40,000. Less serious complications include intravascular or intraosseous injection, hematoma, and infection, but these are also uncommon. Although unusual with the one-shot technique, urinary retention is a common sequela with continuous infusion through an epidural catheter, necessitating placement of an indwelling urinary catheter in all patients.

Contraindications to neuroaxial blocks include sepsis, coagulopathy, local infection, and anatomic abnormalities at the lower spine. They are also contraindicated in patients with increased intracranial pressure.

SPINAL BLOCKS

Spinal anesthesia is less commonly used in children. However, it can be a valuable tool in selected cases. It can be used in former premature infants with lung disease of prematurity. It is safe enough to be used before an intravenous catheter is placed. Once the block is established, the intravenous line can be started in a lower extremity without distressing the infant. The procedure can then be performed with the infant awake and gently restrained. Spinal blocks also can be used as an adjunct to general anesthesia for postoperative pain control, but can be complicated by urinary retention and postdural puncture headache.

ILIOINGUINAL/ILIOHYPOGASTRIC BLOCK

This is a simple block to perform and is most useful for inguinal hernia repair. The ilioinguinal and iliohypogastric nerves originate from the lumbar plexus and provide cutaneous sensory innervation to the area above the inguinal ligament, the scrotum, and the inner thigh. Placement of the block prior to incision gives the advantages of preemptive analgesia, and lower intraoperative anesthesia requirements.

The block is placed one fingerbreadth medial and inferior to the anterior superior iliac spine, where the nerves pass in a plane between the transversus abdominus and the internal oblique muscles. A generous dose of a long-acting anesthetic such as bupivacaine should be given, with frequent checks to avoid intravascular injection. Because the block is placed well out of the surgical field, it will not distort the anatomy. Complications are rare and include inadvertent intravenous injection, intraperitoneal injection, and hematoma.

PENILE BLOCK

The penile block works well for circumcision or distal hypospadius repair. It can be performed by one of several techniques. A ring block can be performed at the base of the penis by injecting the local anesthetic subcutaneously and circumferentially, taking care not to puncture the subcutaneous veins. Of course, the anesthetic solution should never contain epinephrine. Another technique is to block the two dorsal penile nerves as they pass below the pubic symphysis. Here it is critical to avoid injury to the blood vessels that travel in close proximity to the nerves, because ischemia of the penis can result.

INTRAOPERATIVE BLOCKS

The intercostal block is useful for thoracotomies. Bupivacaine 0.25% with epinephrine 1:200,000 is injected from the pleural side, 0.25 to 3 mL per level, posterior to the thoracotomy incision. The block should be placed two interspaces above and two interspaces below the incision to cover the required dermatomes. Of note, intercostal blocks have the highest rate of systemic absorption; therefore, the maximum allowable dose must not be exceeded.

The penile ring block also can be performed by the surgeon after skin preparation and draping, but is best placed prior to the procedure to allow preemptive analgesia and the advantages of lower anesthetic requirements. Bupivacaine 0.25% *without* epinephrine 1 mL per year of age (maximum dose 5 mL) should be used.

Infiltration of the skin prior to incision can be helpful, but is also valuable when it is placed at the conclusion of surgery. The earlier infiltration is done, the earlier emergence from general anesthesia can be initiated. If the local anesthetic cannot be given until the last moment, mixing bupivacaine and lidocaine can induce a more rapid onset, without sacrificing the duration of the block. It is best to be generous with the local anesthetic. The maximum dose of bupivacaine is 3 mg/kg, or approximately 1 mL/kg of the 0.25% solution, with or without epinephrine, up to 20 mL. For lidocaine, the maximum dose is 5 mg/kg without epinephrine (1 mL/kg of the 0.5% solution) and 10 mg/kg with epinephrine.

SUGGESTED READINGS

Broadman LM. Complications of pediatric regional anesthesia. *Reg Anesth Pain Med* 1996;21(suppl):64–70.

Longnecker DE, Tinker JH, Morgan GE Jr, eds. *Principles and practice of anesthesiology, 2nd ed.* St. Louis: Mosby-Yearbook, 1997: 1306–1308.

Markakis DA. Regional anesthesia in pediatrics. *Anesthesiol Clin North Am* 2000;18:355–381, vii.

Taddio A, Katz J, Ilersich AL, et al. Effect of neonatal circumcision on pain response during subsequent routine vaccination. *Lancet* 1997;349:599–603.

SECTION

II

CRITICAL CARE

7

SHOCK

SCOTT PENFIL

Shock has been defined in many ways over the years. These definitions have included criteria for blood pressure, heart rate, peripheral perfusion, and presence of a metabolic acidosis. However, the best definition of shock is "an acute, complex state of circulatory dysfunction that results in failure to deliver sufficient amounts of oxygen and other nutrients to meet tissue metabolic demand" (1).

Note that this definition does not include any of the parameters listed above, including blood pressure. It is important to note that a patient may be in shock with a blood pressure that is high, low, or normal. For example, a patient with severe peripheral vasoconstriction may be hypertensive, but may still be in shock due to inadequate delivery of oxygen and other nutrients to end organs. The body's response to the shock state is to vasoconstrict to improve blood pressure and to maintain perfusion to the brain, heart, and adrenal glands. However, delivery to other organ systems may be compromised.

In order to properly evaluate and treat the patient in shock, there are some simple general principles that must be understood. First, the shock state is usually associated with an attempt by the body to increase cardiac output:

$$CO = HR \times SV$$

where CO = cardiac output, HR = heart rate, and SV = stroke volume. Thus, as SV becomes decreased due to hypovolemia, poor cardiac contractility, or increased afterload, the patient develops tachycardia to try to maintain CO.

In addition, oxygen delivery is described by the following equation:

$$DO_2 = CO \times CaO_2 \times 10$$

where DO_2 = oxygen delivery and CaO_2 = arterial O_2 content.

S. Penfil: Department of Pediatrics, Thomas Jefferson University, Philadelphia, Pennsylvania; and Department of Anesthesiology and Critical Care Medicine, Alfred I. duPont Hospital for Children, Wilmington, Delaware.

Arterial O_2 content is described by:

$$CaO_2 = (Hgb \times \%\ saturation \times 1.34) + (PaO_2 \times 0.003)$$

where PaO_2 = partial pressure of arterial oxygen.

The first part of the equation above refers to bound oxygen that is readily available to tissues. The number 1.34 is a constant that represents the amount of oxygen that 1 g of hemoglobin can carry. The second part of the equation refers to dissolved oxygen, which must diffuse across a concentration gradient to enter the cell. This is an inefficient process, because less than 1% of this oxygen is available to tissues (represented by the constant 0.003). In most situations, the second part of the equation is negligible and can be ignored. The exception to this is when there has been significant acute blood loss and the hemoglobin is extremely low. In this situation, dissolved oxygen may be a significant contributor to oxygen delivery.

From the above equation, it is easy to see that the quickest, most efficient way to improve a patient's oxygen delivery is to transfuse packed red blood cells. This almost immediately increases the amount of bound oxygen, which is readily available to tissues, and should improve the shock state.

TYPES OF SHOCK

Shock can be classified in many ways. In general, there are five main types of shock: anaphylactic, neurogenic, cardiogenic, septic, and hypovolemic. Anaphylactic shock results from the generation and release of a variety of potent endogenous chemical mediators in response to an allergic stimulus. Respiratory failure, shock, and death can occur within minutes. Neurogenic shock occurs when there is depressed activity of the higher vasomotor centers in the brainstem, such as a vasovagal response. Blood pressure drops acutely, and the patient can lose consciousness. The effect is generally brief, and spontaneous recovery is the rule. High cervical spine injuries also can lead to neurogenic shock. Cardiogenic shock occurs when there is significantly decreased cardiac output as a result of myocardial dysfunction. Viral myocarditis is a common cause of cardiogenic shock in children. In addition, a pericardial effusion or tension pneumothorax can significantly decrease cardiac output by not allowing the heart to fill and thus decreasing preload. Septic shock occurs as a result of the body's response to the presence of an infection, most commonly bacterial. A systemic inflammatory response syndrome (SIRS) may develop, and there is generation and release of endogenous chemical mediators that result in a shock state. Hypovolemic shock occurs when there has been a sudden decrease in the circulating intravascular blood volume that is beyond the body's ability to compensate by vasoconstriction and increases in heart rate. Shock associated with trauma is usually due to hypovolemia from blood loss. Hypovolemia from dehydration is the most common cause of shock in young children. For our purposes, this chapter will concentrate on the evaluation and treatment of septic and hypovolemic shock.

EVALUATION AND ASSESSMENT

When approaching a patient who may be in shock, the history is extremely important. Often it will give significant clues as to the underlying cause of the shock. For example, a child who presents with a several day history of diarrhea and emesis is likely to be hypovolemic; a child who presents after a motor vehicle accident may have significant blood loss; a child who presents with a high fever and petechial rash is likely to be septic.

Once the history is obtained, a rapid evaluation of the patient should take place. This evaluation should take only a few minutes, or even less, and give you all the information you need to initially proceed and begin to treat the shock state. As usual, the ABCs (airway, breathing, circulation) must be evaluated. If the patient does not have a patent airway and spontaneous respirations, then he or she must be ventilated with a bag-mask apparatus until an endotracheal tube can be placed. If there is no spontaneous circulation, then chest compressions must be immediately begun as the evaluation and treatment continues. Once it has been determined that the patient has a patent airway, and has a spontaneous respiratory effort and spontaneous circulation, then attention should be turned to an evaluation of the shock state. This must include an evaluation of cerebral perfusion, peripheral perfusion, and respiratory effort.

The first thing that must be evaluated is the patient's mental status. A patient who is lethargic, difficult to arouse, or has slurred speech (in the absence of a head injury) has evidence of inadequate cerebral perfusion. Because we know that the body does all it can to preserve cerebral perfusion, a change in mental status generally indicates an advanced shock state in which the patient is no longer able to compensate. In this situation, you must take action quickly to avoid further deterioration.

The second thing that must be evaluated is the peripheral perfusion. Are the extremities warm or cold? If they are cold, where do they become warm—at the ankle, midshin, or knee? Is the capillary refill brisk, normal, or delayed? Are peripheral pulses bounding, normal, weak, or nonpalpable? The answers to these questions will help determine if the patient is in "warm" shock versus "cold" shock. "Warm" shock is associated with bounding pulses, brisk capillary refill, warm extremities, and a widened pulse pressure. These findings are the result of significant peripheral vasodilatation related to loss of vasomotor tone. Diastolic pressure may be low in this situation. "Cold" shock is associated with cool or cold extremities, delayed capillary refill, weak or absent peripheral pulses, and a narrow pulse pressure. Traditionally, it was believed that there was a progression from warm to cold shock, and that the patient in cold shock likely had a more advanced state of shock. We now know that this is not true. The body's response to shock may vary, and "cold" versus "warm" does not indicate the degree of advancement or severity of shock.

Finally, one must evaluate the patient's respiratory status. Specifically, the work of breathing must be assessed. In the absence of pulmonary or neurologic pathology, the only reason for a patient to have increased work of breathing (tachypnea, intercostal or subcostal retractions with use of accessory muscles, nasal flaring) is to compensate for a metabolic acidosis by "blowing off" CO_2 and increasing blood pH. Therefore, if the patient is in respiratory distress without obvious underlying pulmonary pathology, it should be assumed that the patient has a significant metabolic acidosis. Action must be taken quickly to prevent further deterioration.

Note that this initial evaluation of cerebral perfusion, peripheral perfusion, and respiratory effort does not require any laboratory or radiographic studies. Once again, this evaluation should be completed quickly so that appropriate treatment can begin promptly.

TREATMENT

The treatment of the shock state is similar regardless of the underlying cause, unless there is active blood loss. If there is active blood loss, then this must be controlled with direct pressure if possible. If not possible due to internal bleeding, the patient may need urgent surgical intervention. In addition, packed red blood cells should be transfused as soon as possible. In the absence of active blood loss, there are four parameters that we may manipulate to increase cardiac output and improve end organ perfusion: heart rate, preload, contractility, and afterload.

The first approach is to increase preload by the rapid infusion of large amounts of fluids. It is extremely important to ensure that intravascular volume is adequate. Chronotropes, inotropes, and pressors will not have optimal effect if preload is inadequate. Although boluses of fluids in 10 to 20 mL/kg aliquots is appropriate, there is no real limit to the total volume that must be given. Total circulating volume in a normal child is approximately 75 to 80 mL/kg. However, it may sometimes be necessary to give 80 to 100 mL/kg of fluid or more to adequately increase preload. This is because only 25% to 35% of the fluid will stay in the intravascular space. The majority of the fluid is lost through leaky capillary beds and will accumulate in interstitial tissue. This effect seems to be more dramatic in septic shock as compared with hypovolemic shock associated with trauma, probably as a result of the SIRS reaction. Finally, fluid boluses should be given as rapidly as possible. Fluid that is ordered to infuse over 1 hour should not be considered a "bolus" and will likely have minimal effect.

The optimal type of fluid to use for resuscitation remains an area of controversy. Traditionally, it was taught that colloid infusion was more efficient in repleting the vascular space and maintaining a normal serum osmotic pressure. Due to the protein contained in colloid mixtures, it was believed that less fluid would third space and more would stay in the intravascular space. In addition, this would result in less interstitial pulmonary fluid and help minimize pulmonary dysfunction, a common complication of the shock state. However, the results of recent clinical and laboratory studies dispute this. In fact, several studies indicate a tendency toward a worse outcome in trauma patients resuscitated with colloid as compared with crystalloid solutions. As a result of the increased cost and increased risk of transmitted infection with colloid solutions, in conjunction with the lack of proven benefit over crystalloid solutions, it is currently recommended that crystalloid solutions be used in fluid resuscitation. However, the fluid used must be at least isotonic. Hypotonic solutions will contribute to increased third spacing, and much more fluid will be required. Either normal saline solution or Ringers lactate solution should be the fluid of choice.

Recently, the use of hypertonic saline solutions, most commonly 3% saline, have been studied as a resuscitation fluid, especially in shock associated with trauma. The early results appear promising. Hypertonic saline has been associated with rapid improvement of blood pressure, less total fluid requirements, and a tendency toward improved outcomes. Hypertonic saline also has been shown to be beneficial for patients with traumatic brain injuries by decreasing intracranial pressure and cerebral edema and increasing cerebral perfusion pressure. Aliquots of 1 to 5 mL/kg tend to be effective, and they should be infused over 10 to 20 minutes to avoid rapid changes in serum osmolarity. Although this is a promising area of research, the current recommendation is to use isotonic solutions.

In a trauma patient who does not respond to the first 20 to 40 mL/kg of fluid, transfusion of packed red blood cells should be considered. For pediatric patients, volumes of 10-20 ml/kg are appropriate.

To ensure that fluid resuscitation has been adequate, central venous pressure (CVP) or pulmonary capillary wedge pressure (PCWP) should be measured. In order to measure PCWP, a pulmonary artery (PA) catheter must be placed. However, PA catheters are rarely used in children. The recent results of an adult study indicating a worse outcome in patients who had PA catheters, in combination with the morbidity and increased difficulty placing PA catheters in small children, has led to this practice. In addition, a good clinical examination, possibly in conjunction with an echocardiogram, should provide similar information. If a PA catheter is placed, then fluids should be given to maintain the PCWP between 15 and 18 mm Hg. All patients in shock will require adequate intravenous access, so virtually all patients in shock should have a central venous catheter. Regardless of the placement of the tip of the catheter (iliac vein, subclavian vein, etc.), as long as there is a continuous fluid column between the tip of the catheter and the right atrium, then CVP measurement should be accurate. When using CVP to assess intravascular volume, fluids should be given until the CVP is maintained at 10 to 15 mm Hg.

Once adequate preload has been established, the shock state may resolve. If the patient remains in a shock state, we must then augment contractility, heart rate, and afterload by the use of inotropes and pressors. Not all inotropes are pressors. For example, dobutamine is a synthetic β agonist, which is a potent chronotrope and inotrope. It will increase cardiac contractility. However, it is also a peripheral vasodilator and decreases afterload. Although this combination should increase cardiac output, it may not affect blood pressure, or may even cause a decrease in blood pressure, due to the afterload effects. In addition, if there is enough peripheral vasodilatation, blood may pool in the peripheral vascular system and decrease preload. Therefore, it is important to understand the effects of the various agents so that they can be chosen wisely. For our purposes, I will limit this discussion mainly to the use of epinephrine, dopamine, dobutamine and norepinephrine.

In general, patients in "warm" shock are peripherally vasodilated. These patients require a medication that will cause vasoconstriction and improve vasomotor tone. In this situation, the best agents to use are dopamine (5–20 μg/kg/min) and epinephrine (0.05–1.00 μg/kg/min). Both of these drugs increase heart rate, contractility, and blood pressure. If doses of epinephrine higher than 0.2 to 0.3 μg/kg/min are required, there is an associated vasoconstriction of the splanchnic bed, and renal perfusion may be compromised. Therefore, the use of epinephrine with "renal-dose" dopamine (2–5 μg/kg/min) to help maintain renal perfusion is an effective combination. If a patient is in "cold" shock, then they have significant peripheral vasoconstriction and increased afterload. The agent of choice must cause some degree of vasodilatation to ensure adequate end organ perfusion. The vasoconstriction we can appreciate by examining the extremities is also occurring internally. In this situation, the use of low-dose epinephrine (0.2 μg/kg/min) or dobutamine (5–20 μg/kg/min) should be the agent of choice. At low doses, the β effects of epinephrine predominate over the α effects, and the result is afterload reduction. As afterload is reduced, more blood may pool in the periphery and preload may decrease. If this occurs, fluid should be given to maintain CVP or PCWP as noted above.

Other agents that can be used include norepinephrine, milrinone, amrinone, and isoproterenol. Norepinephrine is an α agonist. It increases afterload and blood pressure, but does not support myocardial function. It is generally not considered a first-line agent in children and is used less commonly than in the adult population. In some situations, however, norepinephrine can be very useful. Patients with significant tachycardia, hypotension, and vasodilation may do well with norepinephrine, because it has no significant chronotropic effect and will not worsen the tachycardia. Also, in shock refractory to dopamine, dobutamine, and epinephrine, the addition of norepinephrine may help stabilize the hemodynamics. Milrinone and amrinone have effects similar to those of dobutamine: increasing heart rate and contractility while decreasing afterload. However, they are more difficult to titrate to effect due to their long half-lives, and they are associated with several adverse effects. Isoproterenol may be useful in third-degree heart block to increase ventricular rate, but otherwise has no advantages over the other agents. The vast majority of patients are stabilized with the right combination of dopamine, epinephrine, and dobutamine.

One of the most common errors made when treating a patient in shock is the failure to consider early endotracheal intubation. In the normal state, the respiratory muscles use approximately 8% to 10% of cardiac output. In shock states, when the work of breathing is increased to compensate for metabolic acidosis, this can increase to over 30%. Early endotracheal intubation and use of mechanical ventilation can divert the cardiac output to more vital organs, such as the brain, heart, and adrenal glands. In addition, as long as preload is maintained, positive pressure ventilation increases cardiac output by decreasing afterload on the left ventricle. Even in the absence of airway, pulmonary, or neurologic pathology, early intubation must be considered for any patient in shock, especially those that do not respond to initial fluid resuscitation. Finally, if the patient has an abnormal mental status that does not improve with initial fluid resuscitation, the patient must be intubated.

Both septic shock and shock related to trauma may be associated with coagulation defects. In septic shock, this is usually the result of disseminated intravascular coagulation. In shock related to trauma, this may be the result of loss of circulating clotting factors due to hemorrhage. In either case, laboratory studies should include measurement of prothrombin time (PT), partial thromboplastin time (PTT), and fibrinogen. If PT or PTT are significantly elevated and there is ongoing blood loss or "oozing" from puncture sites, then the infusion of 10 to 20 mL/kg of plasma should be considered. Plasma is available as either fresh frozen plasma or solvent detergent plasma. Similarly, if the fibrinogen level is under 100 mg/dL, coagulation will be significantly impaired. In this case, the use of cryoprecipitate provides a good source of fibrinogen. The usual dose is 1 to 2 units per 10 kg of body weight.

In some severe cases, despite maximal aggressive therapy, the patient does not respond and remains in shock. In these situations, two additional therapies may be useful. One is the infusion of calcium. All inotropes and pressors ultimately work by increasing intracellular calcium concentrations, albeit by different mechanisms. If serum calcium is low, their effect may be limited. If serum ionized calcium is low, then supplemental calcium should be given. Calcium may be given as calcium gluconate (50–200 mg/kg, maximum dose 2 g) or calcium chloride (10–20 mg/kg, maximum dose 500 mg, infused over 15–30 minutes). If calcium chloride is used, it must be given via a central venous catheter due to the risk of infiltration into the skin if a peripheral vein is used. Also, supplemental calcium should not be used if the serum-ionized calcium is normal, because high levels of calcium can theoretically hasten cell death. The use of stress doses of steroids also may be helpful in improving blood pressure and cardiac output. Hydrocortisone at a dose of 50 mg/m^2/day is most commonly used, although any steroid with equivalent glucocorticoid effect may be used. This dose should be continued for 1 to 3 days, and then tapered to a maintenance dose of 12.5 mg/m^2/day.

If there is any concern that the cause of the shock may be related to infection, antibiotics must be given as early as possible. Community-acquired infections, intestinal perforation, and intraabdominal trauma are the most common causes of septic shock in previously healthy patients. For cases of community-acquired infection, the empiric antibiotic regimen must include vancomycin due to the emergence of resistant strains of *Pneumococcus.* In addition to vancomycin, a third-generation cephalosporin, meropenem, or ticarcillin/clavulanate should be included until culture results are known. In the case of intestinal perforation with or without trauma, the patient must be covered for enteric bacteria, including anaerobes. Many combinations of antibiotics provide adequate coverage. Traditionally, triple antibiotic coverage with ampicillin, gentamicin, and clindamycin or metronidazole has been used. Alternatives include ticarcillin/clavulanate and meropenem.

Once the patient has stabilized, it is important to document that oxygen delivery is adequate. This can be accomplished in one of two ways. First, serum lactate levels can be measured. If oxygen delivery is adequate, the serum lactate level should be stabilized or decreasing. If it is increasing, the patient should be re-evaluated. Additional fluid, transfusion of packed red blood cells, or changes in inotropes may be necessary. The second method is to compare arterial oxygen saturation to mixed venous oxygen saturation, termed $AVDO_2$. This difference should be 20% to 30%. If it is higher than 30%, it is indicative of increased oxygen extraction. The tissues are increasing their ability to extract oxygen because oxygen delivery is low or inadequate.

Once stabilized, or even during the efforts to stabilize, the patient in shock should be admitted to an intensive care unit setting for close monitoring and ongoing care to prevent further deterioration.

MORBIDITY AND MORTALITY

The overall mortality rate for shock in pediatric patients is approximately 25% to 30%. Appropriate and aggressive care can affect the outcome of these patients, especially those related to trauma. The care in the first few hours may make the difference between survival and death, as well as decrease the morbidity for survivors. Unfortunately, not all survivors are left unscathed. Adverse outcomes for survivors may include limb loss, chronic renal failure, chronic lung disease, prolonged muscular weakness, or central nervous system injury.

EDITOR'S NOTES

The treatment of all forms of shock should have the same goal: to optimize tissue oxygen delivery. This entails diligent clinical assessment and careful analysis of available data, but ultimately "treating the patient, not the numbers." This is especially true for very young patients, in whom a seemingly minor error in management can have dire consequences. The elegance of the simple approach detailed in this chapter lies in its broad applicability to shock regardless of the cause or the age of the patient.

The cause of shock in pediatric surgical patients is not always obvious, but a careful assessment usually results in a treatment plan that is appropriately individualized as well as therapeutic. Unlike many adults, most children have intact and robust organ systems that can compensate for the physiologic stresses of the shock state and withstand the adverse effects of treatment. Two notable exceptions are complex trauma patients and newborns. Trauma patients who develop shock are best treated according to the acute trauma life-support protocols established by the American College of Surgeons. The treating physician needs to be cognizant of the fact that several mechanisms may be at work to produce shock in these complex patients. Although the presumption should be that hypovolemia due to hemorrhage is the major factor, it is not uncommon for the same patient to have a neurogenic component (e.g., spinal cord injury) or a cardiogenic component (e.g., cardiac contusion or pericardial tamponade). Similarly, the response to treatment may be altered by the reflex bradycardia and hypertension seen with associated severe head injury. Again, constantly assessing tissue perfusion and oxygen delivery will allow proper management in most patients despite the sometimes confusing clinical picture.

Although the treatment of newborns in shock can be challenging, the general approach to diagnosis and treatment still applies. "Poor perfusion" (listlessness, dusky coloration, cool extremities, low urine output) is commonly seen in infants, especially in the premature, and is essentially a euphemism for the shock state. It is often easily reversible with intravenous hydration but sometimes requires a diagnostic workup if the cause cannot be attributed to simple dehydration. One needs to consider other sources of fluid loss that might seem insignificant but can be important in a tiny infant. For example, increased insensible water loss from mechanical ventilation, phototherapy, or high ambient temperature may be the cause. Anemia can be caused by sepsis, intraventricular hemorrhage, or hemolytic processes and needs to be considered. Infants who do not respond appropriately to adequate hydration or transfusion therapy should have an echocardiogram to rule out an otherwise occult cardiac anomaly or a patent ductus arteriosus. There should also be a low threshold to treat newborns with signs of shock empirically for sepsis (after blood cultures and lumbar puncture) until infection can be ruled out with some degree of certainty. Similarly, premature infants often develop apnea or bradycardia and, as in older patients in shock, there should be a low threshold to intubate and mechanically ventilate these patients until the shock state can be fully reversed. Lastly, one needs to consider the possibility that refractory shock in a newborn may be due to adrenal insufficiency, with or without evidence of adrenal hemorrhage on imaging studies. Empiric corticosteroid therapy may be indicated in these situations.

–P.M.

REFERENCE

1. Perkin RM, Levin DL. Shock in the pediatric patient. *J Pediatr* 1982;101:163.

SUGGESTED READINGS

Rogers MC, ed. *Textbook of pediatric intensive care, 3rd ed.* Baltimore: Williams & Wilkins, 1996.

Fuhrman BP, Zimmerman JJ, eds. *Pediatric critical care, 2nd ed.* St. Louis: Mosby-Year Book, 1998.

8

ELECTROLYTE DISORDERS

ROBERT W. LETTON, JR.

Despite the advances that have been made in caring for critically ill infants, the mismanagement of fluid and electrolyte therapy remains a potential cause of morbidity and mortality in this patient population. Managing fluids in the critically ill pediatric population requires dynamic monitoring and frequent adjustment of fluids and electrolytes. Subtle differences in the perioperative management of these patients can be amplified more so than in the adult population. Fluid and electrolyte balance should be viewed from the three perspectives: total amount of water and solute in the body, distribution of water and solute in the various body compartments, and the osmolar concentration of each in these various compartments.

The most abundant component of the human body is water. Total body water (TBW) can be calculated from the patient's body weight, with adults having $0.6 \times$ kg, infants $0.7 \times$ kg, and neonates $0.8 \times$ kg. TBW can be divided into extracellular fluid (ECF) and intracellular fluid (ICF) compartments. The major components of the ECF compartment are an intravascular component (plasma volume) and an interstitial component. The principal cation of the ECF compartment is sodium; the principal anions are chloride and bicarbonate. In the ICF compartment, potassium is the principal cation, whereas phosphates and nondiffusible proteins are the principal anions. The ICF compartment consists of the fluid found inside the cells of the body. It is separated from the ECF compartment by the cell membrane. ICF volume is estimated as the difference between TBW and ECF volumes. Because cell membranes are freely permeable to water, the osmolality values of the ICF and ECF are always equal.

During the course of gestation, there is a decrease in the percentage of body weight represented by TBW and a relative decrease in the ECF to ICF compartment ratio. At 20 weeks' gestation, TBW accounts for 85% of total weight, three fourths of which is in the ECF (60% of body weight) versus only one fourth in the ICF (25% of body weight). At full term, TBW is equal to roughly 80% of total body weight, with nearly equal distribution between the ECF and ICF compartments (45% and 35% of body weight, respectively). By 18 months of age, fluid and electrolyte distribution reaches adult proportions, with the TBW compartment representing 60% of total body weight, two thirds of which is now intracellular (40% body weight), and one third extracellular (20% body weight). The plasma compartment in newborn infants represents approximately 8% of total body weight and decreases to the adult volume of 6% of total body weight by 12 to 18 months of age.

Water expenditure in the neonatal and infant populations can be divided into insensible water loss, excretion of renal solute, water loss in stool, and water and electrolytes lost during normal homeostasis. Insensible losses are free water losses that occur through the skin and respiratory tract. The rate of loss via the respiratory tract is dependent on tidal volume, respiratory rate, temperature, and the humidity of inspired/expired air. In all infants, regardless of age, transepithelial water loss (TEWL) makes up the majority of insensible losses. The degree of TEWL varies inversely with body weight and age, since younger infants have a higher ratio of body surface area to body weight. Using radiant warmers and phototherapy can increase temperature and decrease humidity, exacerbating evaporative losses. TEWL can be reduced significantly during transport by the use of an impermeable plastic cover. Fever can increase insensible losses by approximately 7 mL/kg/day for each degree above 99°F. Because hyperosmolality can lead to an increased risk of intracerebral hemorrhage, free water should be used to replace insensible losses. The simplest estimate of TEWL is 30 to 60 mL/kg/day for neonates weighing less than 1,500 g, and 15 to 35 mL/kg/day in neonates weighing more than 1,500 g.

SODIUM

Sodium balance plays a major role in the maintenance of the ECF volume. It is the total amount of sodium present in the whole body, not just the serum concentration of

R.W. Letton, Jr.: Departments of Surgery and Pediatrics, Wake Forest University School of Medicine, Winston–Salem, North Carolina.

sodium that determines the ECF volume. A decrease, an increase, or no change in the sodium concentration can accompany changes in the ECF volume. The total amount of sodium in an adult is approximately 60 mEq/kg. The sodium content of the fetus is much higher, approximately 85 to 90 mEq/kg, due to the proportionally increased ECF compartment as compared with the adult. Serum osmolality is, in large part (approximately 80%), dependent on the sodium concentration, but also on blood urea nitrogen (BUN) and glucose concentrations, and can be estimated with the following formula:

$$2[Na^+] + BUN/2.8 + glucose/18.$$

Hyponatremia

Hyponatremia is defined as a serum concentration of sodium of less than 135 mEq/L and may occur with hypovolemia, euvolemia, or hypervolemia. Symptoms usually do not become apparent until the level decreases to below 120 mEg/L. Because water can easily cross the blood–brain barrier into the central nervous system, symptoms arise due to cerebral overhydration and include apathy, nausea, vomiting, headache, seizures, and coma. The rate and magnitude of the shift determines the degree of symptoms. Acute hyponatremia, which occurs over a period of 24 hours or less, is associated with the most rapid onset of symptoms. Rapid movement of water into the brain initiates protective mechanisms in the central nervous system, and intracellular amino acids and potassium are lost in order to reduce cellular swelling. Because of these changes, the brain is particularly susceptible to dehydration during the fluid and electrolyte correction phase. Rapid correction of the low plasma sodium increases the plasma osmolality in advance of correction in the cerebral intracellular compartment, and a net shift of fluid out of the brain may occur, leading to central pontine myelinolysis. Therapeutic correction of hyponatremia should occur over 24 to 48 hours in order to avoid secondary injury from this mechanism.

The renal response to hyponatremia is to produce dilute urine; however, this can be complicated by release of antidiuretic hormone (ADH). Urine sodium concentration is a useful measure because it may provide clues to the underlying condition causing the hyponatremia. Urine sodium concentrations of less than 10 mEq/L indicate that renal sodium handling is intact and that effective blood volume is decreased. A sodium concentration of greater than 20 mEq/L indicates intrinsic renal tubular damage or a natriuretic response to a state of hypervolemia. Pseudohyponatremia can develop in states of hyperlipidemia and hyperproteinemia due to a decreased percentage of plasma water in the sample. Factitious hyponatremia is due to hyperglycemia or the presence of mannitol, and is associated with a true hyponatremia secondary to redistribution of water from the intracellular to extracellular space. This occurs in the face of an abnormally high serum osmolality. The serum sodium should be reduced by 1.6 mEq/L for every 100 mg/dL increase in glucose concentration above normal. As the underlying condition is corrected, the sodium concentration returns to normal.

Hypovolemic hyponatremia occurs with losses of sodium in relative excess to water and is associated with total body sodium depletion and ECF volume contraction. The most common cause is secondary to increased gastrointestinal losses from vomiting, diarrhea, or fistula output. Increased losses through perspiration can occur, especially in infants with cystic fibrosis and adrenal insufficiency. Intake of hypotonic solutions then leads to a hyponatremic hypovolemic ECF volume, and the hyponatremia is maintained by the kidney's inability to excrete free water. The excessive renal loss of sodium induced by diuretics can lead to a hypovolemic hyponatremia. Adrenal insufficiency should be suspected when hypovolemic hyponatremia exists in conjunction with hyperkalemia and renal sodium wasting (urinary sodium >20 mEq/L) despite normal renal function. Intrinsic renal disease can lead to an impaired ability to conserve sodium, resulting in hyponatremia.

Euvolemic hyponatremia is rarely euvolemic, and usually exists in a state of increased ECF volume, often associated with a normal amount of total body sodium. The syndrome of inappropriate secretion of ADH (SIADH) is the most common cause in children. It is diagnosed by exclusion and is found in certain malignancies, pulmonary diseases, and disorders of the central nervous system. SIADH is a problem of water retention, not decreased sodium, and should be managed with fluid restriction. Attempts to correct this condition with the administration of saline solutions usually causes an increase in renal sodium excretion with little change in serum sodium. Increased levels of ADH postoperatively, combined with the infusion of hypotonic fluids, can place the infant at risk for iatrogenic hyponatremia. Acute water intoxication is rare but can occur in infants due to their inability to effectively excrete a water load.

Cerebral salt wasting syndrome is another cause of hyponatremia associated with central nervous system injury that is similar to SIADH. Rather than euvolemic or hypervolemic hyponatremia, this syndrome results in a hypovolemic hyponatremia, and is best treated by hydration and salt replacement, not fluid restriction. It is most likely secondary to increased levels of atrial natriuretic factor, and clinically is distinguished from SIADH by the fact that the patients have urine salt wasting and volume depletion.

Patients with hypervolemic hyponatremia present with peripheral and pulmonary edema. Despite the low serum concentration of sodium, they usually have elevated total body sodium and body water. This condition can occur in infants with congestive heart failure, cirrhosis of the liver, nephrotic syndrome, and renal failure. The hyponatremia is a result of a decreased effective blood volume, which leads to an increased release of ADH, resulting in water retention. A decreased glomerular filtration rate leads to increased water reabsorption, and, with active sodium reabsorption, urine sodium is usually less than 20 mEq/L.

Any patient with significant symptoms of hyponatremia and a serum sodium of less than 120 mEq/L should receive hypertonic saline in order to rapidly (over 4 hours) increase the sodium to 125 mEq/L. Further correction toward normal should then occur more slowly over the next 24 to 48 hours, and subsequent therapy will be based on the patient's volume status. Hypovolemic patients should receive isotonic saline or isooncotic colloid solutions. An estimate of sodium necessary for adequate correction can be obtained with the following formula:

$$\text{mEq Na required} = (\text{desired } [Na^+] - \text{actual } [Na^+]) \times 0.6 \times \text{kg}$$

Euvolemic patients with SIADH require fluid restriction, and if symptoms persist with little change in serum sodium, furosemide followed by hypertonic saline may be effective. In chronic SIADH, lithium and demeclocycline can inhibit the renal response to ADH. Hypervolemic patients require both salt and water restriction. The amount of fluid excess can be calculated from the following formula:

$$\text{Liters } H_2O \text{ excess} = \text{TBW} \times (1 - Na^+]/140)$$

Acute hyponatremia can be corrected at a rate of 12 to 14 mEq/L/day, and chronic hyponatremia should be corrected no faster than 12 mEq/L/day. In instances of renal failure, diuretics and dialysis will also help correct the hyponatremia.

Hypernatremia

Hypernatremia is defined as a serum sodium concentration greater than 145 mEq/L and is most often a disorder of water balance as opposed to sodium balance. Total body sodium content may be high, normal, or low in relation to TBW content, depending on the cause of the hypernatremia. The most common cause of hypernatremia in the pediatric population is the loss of hypotonic fluid without adequate water intake. Although diarrhea most often leads to isonatremic or hyponatremic dehydration, when it is additionally associated with decreased fluid intake or prolonged vomiting, hypernatremic dehydration may occur. Excess sodium intake is unusual, but can occur iatrogenically if infants are fed an inappropriately concentrated formula. The loss of pure water, which occurs in diabetes insipidus, is characterized by decreased secretion of ADH (primary) or end organ unresponsiveness (secondary). Excessive sweating or increased insensible losses, especially in the premature infant, result in increased free water loss.

Hypernatremic dehydration is associated with extremely dry mucous membranes and "doughy" skin. Periods of lethargy and irritability, increased muscle tone, seizures, and coma also can occur. In the central nervous system, the shrinkage of brain matter associated with intracellular fluid losses can result in intracerebral hemorrhage from the tearing of cerebral vessels. In response to persistent hypernatremia, the accumulation of intracellular taurine occurs in an attempt to increase the osmotic gradient for the intracellular return of water. Hypernatremic dehydration should first be treated with volume expansion using isotonic crystalloid solutions to promote volume expansion. When urine output has been reestablished, hypotonic solutions should be used to correct the hypernatremia in no less than 48 hours. Free water deficit can be calculated from the following formula:

$$\text{Free } H_2O \text{ deficit} = \text{TBW} \times ([Na^+]/140 - 1)$$

Rapid rehydration leads to cellular swelling and cerebral edema, thus increasing the likelihood of permanent neurologic deficit. Hypocalcemia is commonly associated with hypernatremia and also may require correction. In cases of central diabetes insipidus, the administration of vasopressin can be used cautiously as an adjunct to volume expansion to help correct the hypernatremia.

POTASSIUM

The most important function of the potassium ion is the role it plays in regulating the electrical activity of biologic systems. Disorders of potassium homeostasis occur frequently in the hospitalized pediatric population and can lead to signs and symptoms ranging from muscle weakness to cardiac arrhythmias. Potassium is the principal intracellular cation, remaining primarily unbound and osmotically active. Although it is not freely diffusible through the cytoplasmic membrane, it is more easily diffusible than sodium or calcium.

Hypokalemia

Relatively common in the pediatric surgical population, hypokalemia is often iatrogenic, for example, when diuretics are administered without appropriate potassium replacement. Loop diuretics promote potassium secretion and trigger the release of aldosterone, which further aggravates the hypokalemia. In addition to renal loss, extrarenal potassium losses are also common in the pediatric population, and the urine concentration of potassium can be helpful in distinguishing between the two. A urine concentration of potassium that is less than 15 mEq/L indicates renal conservation of potassium, suggesting loss from an extrarenal source. Increased gastrointestinal losses through vomiting and diarrhea lead to a dehydrated, contracted physiologic state, which can be associated with significant potassium losses. Increased secretion of insulin and catecholamines cause a significant shift of potassium into the cells, leading to a loss of extracellular potassium, even though total body potassium remains constant.

Treatment of mild hypokalemia in asymptomatic patients may not be necessary, except in patients receiving digitalis preparations (to whom supplements should be given). In severe depletion, potassium replacement should be given parenterally. Doses of 0.5 to 1 mEq/kg KCl are given with frequent electrocardiographic monitoring and measurement of serum values. Concentrations of 40 to 60 mEq/L can be tolerated in peripheral veins, but concentrations of 1 mEq/3 mL can be given via central access with continuous heart monitoring required. Because potassium is located intracellularly, it is difficult to calculate the exact deficit; therefore, frequent monitoring of the plasma potassium level should be performed as repletion is continued. Generally, a 1 mEq/L decrease in serum potassium (due to actual decrease in total body potassium) represents a loss of approximately 5% to 10% of body potassium. In patients with a significant hypochloremic alkalosis, such as infants with pyloric stenosis, potassium is difficult to replace until the chloride is corrected. This is also true for patients who have a significant hypomagnesemia.

Hyperkalemia

Hyperkalemia is most often present in patients who have impaired renal excretion. Children with congenital urologic abnormalities, such as reflux nephropathy and prune belly syndrome associated with bilateral hydronephrosis, have an associated dysfunction of the tubular epithelium. If this involves the epithelium responsible for potassium secretion, an associated hyperkalemic, hyperchloremic metabolic acidosis may ensue. Adrenal insufficiency causes hyperkalemia due to impaired secretion of potassium in the kidney and colon (secondary to decreased mineralocorticoid production). Insulin-dependent diabetes mellitus limits the ability of muscle and liver to take up potassium. Severe crush injuries associated with trauma or the lysis of tumor cells associated with chemotherapy can lead to acute life-threatening hyperkalemia. Excess hydrogen ion decreases the membrane electrical gradient, allowing potassium to follow its chemical gradient out of the cell into the extracellular fluid. In adults, for every decrease in pH of 0.1 units, a shift of 1.5 mEq of potassium occurs.

Hyperkalemia causes clinical sequelae by depolarizing electrically excitable cells. Early electrocardiograms show peaked T waves, which progress to a lengthening of the PR interval and a widening of the QRS complex. If hyperkalemia persists, the infant is at risk for life-threatening arrhythmias, including asystole. When the QRS complex is widened or asystole is present, immediate intravenous infusion of 10% calcium gluconate (1 mL/kg/dose) increases the threshold potential, allowing cells to repolarize and once again generate action potentials. The hyperkalemia itself should be treated with an infusion of insulin (0.1 U/kg) and glucose ($D_{50}W$ 1 mL/kg), which will transiently shift potassium into the intracellular compartment. If a metabolic acidosis also exists, the administration of bicarbonate ($NaHCO_3$ 1 mEq/kg) will shift potassium into the intracellular compartment. These maneuvers will transiently lower the extracellular potassium concentration for a few hours, allowing time to more definitively reduce total body potassium. Loop diuretics are effective at removing potassium in patients with adequate renal function. In patients without adequate renal function and with severe hyperkalemia, the administration of sodium polystyrene sulfanate powder (Kayexalate, Sanofi Winthrop, New York, New York; 1 g/kg orally for 6 hours), a cation-exchange resin, into the gastrointestinal tract will bond potassium and remove it from the system. Kayexalate is usually administered with sorbitol to enhance its removal from the gastrointestinal tract and avoid obstruction due to concretion formation. Hemodialysis or peritoneal dialysis is effective at correcting the hyperkalemia as well as the associated metabolic acidosis.

OTHER ELECTROLYTES

Hypocalcemia is relatively common in the neonate. An exaggerated primary parathyroid response often persists into adulthood, but with a relatively benign course. The immunologic compromise associated with DiGeorge's syndrome results in a hypoparathyroid hypocalcemia that requires aggressive management. A decreased parathyroid hormone response leads to neonatal hypocalcemia in infants of mothers with maternal diabetes, and may be related to hypomagnesemia. In this condition, a postprandial decrease in ionized calcium fails to elicit an appropriate parathyroid response when compared with normal newborns. States of maternal hypocalcemia, hypercalcemia, hypomagnesemia, and hypermagnesemia predispose the neonate to calcium abnormalities. Hypoalbuminemia leads to a factitious hypocalcemia and can be corrected using the following formula:

$$\text{Corrected Ca}^{2+} = [\text{Ca}^{2+}] + [0.8 \times (\text{normal albumin} - \text{current albumin})]$$

Diminished cardiac function results from decreased ionized calcium levels. Rate, rhythm, contractility, and afterload are all dependent on the maintenance of ionized calcium within a physiologic range. The range at which ionized calcium remains physiologic is also dependent on other variables such as adrenergic activity, preload, and oxygen delivery. Left ventricular contractility increases with calcium administration in hypocalcemic state, but when given to a normocalcemic individual, blood pressure elevations are more likely due to increased peripheral resistance. Calcium chloride boluses can be dangerous, resulting in acute cardiac decompensation in digitalized or hypokalemic individuals. Calcium only benefits a cardiac arrest associated with hyperkalemia or arrest due to hypoglycemia-induced arrhythmias. When calcium therapy is required, calcium gluconate should be administered slowly, preferably by continuous infusion into high flow veins. The repletion dose is 20 mg/kg/dose of calcium, with 10% calcium gluconate equal to 9 mg/mL of calcium, and 10% calcium chloride equal to 27 mg/mL of calcium.

Although hypocalcemia is more common in the neonatal population, many disease states in neonates can result in hypercalcemia. The clinical expression of familial hypercalcemic hypocalciuria is variable and is related to a neonatal state of hyperparathyroidism, which requires initial aggressive resuscitation and may potentially necessitate parathyroidectomy. Patients receiving hyperalimentation or vitamin supplements can develop hypercalcemia secondary to hypervitaminosis A. Those receiving hyperalimentation are also susceptible to hypercalcemia resulting from hypophosphatemia. Primary and tertiary hyperparathyroidism can cause hypercalcemia. Hyperthyroid individuals, during periods of immobilization, are subject to hypercalcemia, and hypothyroidism can cause hypercalcemia secondary to associated calcitonin insufficiency. Solid tumors, which can cause hypercalcemia secondary to paraneoplastic syndromes, are not as common in infants and children as in adults, but tumors with metastases to bone and multiple myeloma may cause hypercalcemia in children. Hypercalcemia can predispose patients to pancreatitis due to increased pancreatic duct permeability.

Chloride is the major anion of the extracellular fluid and its intake and output parallel that of sodium. It follows electrochemical gradients created largely by movement of sodium via passive diffusion. Active transport occurs in the ascending limb of the loop of Henle. Although chloride is not directly involved in the regulation of acid-base homeostasis, as adjustments are made in the levels of bicarbonate, chloride often shifts in a reciprocal fashion. Chloride must be given in addition to potassium in order to correct hypokalemia, and chloride administration is necessary to correct most forms of metabolic alkalosis. Prompt administration of potassium and sodium chloride results in excretion of bicarbonate into the urine and correction of the alkalosis. Renal correction of metabolic alkalosis results in reabsorption of chloride in excess of sodium and potassium. The measurement of chloride is necessary for calculation of the anion gap. The concentration of sodium is greater than the sum of chloride and potassium, thus resulting in an anion gap of 8 to 16 mEq/L under normal conditions. This is due to the presence of unmeasured anions, which exceed the concentration of unmeasured cations.

Magnesium plays a major role in intracellular enzymatic activity and is the fourth most abundant cation in the body. It is a crucial cofactor in glycolysis and in the stimulation of ATPases. Sixty percent of the body's total magnesium is bound in bone, with only one third of this freely exchangeable. The remaining magnesium is intracellular, the majority in muscle and liver, and is bound to proteins, RNA, and ATP. Extracellular magnesium is maintained at a low level within a narrow physiologic range and is freely interchangeable with the bone pool. Absorption of magnesium occurs in the upper gastrointestinal tract by a mechanism that is enhanced by vitamin D, parathyroid hormone, and increased sodium absorption. It remains incomplete, however, with only one third being absorbed. Repletion of magnesium can be given enterally or parenterally at doses of 0.5 mEq/kg/dose two to three times a day.

SUMMARY

Fluid and electrolyte management requires continuous monitoring in the infant and child and remains a potential cause of morbidity and mortality. Despite aggressive titration and monitoring to prevent electrolyte imbalance, these disorders still often occur. With a few common formulas (Table 8.1), most of these can usually be safely corrected without permanent injury to the child. It is imperative that physicians caring for sick infants be familiar with these basic concepts.

TABLE 8.1. COMMON FLUID AND ELECTROLYTE FORMULAS

Serum osmolality	2[Na] + BUN/2.8 + Glucose/18	
Total body water (TBW)	Neonate:	0.8 × kg
	Infant:	0.7 × kg
	Adult:	0.6 × kg
Electrolyte deficit (d)	d × kg × (desired [mEq/L] – actual [mEq/L])	
	Sodium	d = 0.6
	Bicarbonate	d = 0.4
	Chloride	d = 0.2
Free water deficit	TBW × ([Na]/140 – 1)	
Free water excess	TBW × (1 – [Na]/140)	
Corrected calcium (hypoalbuminemia)	[Ca] + [0.8 × (normal – current albumin)]	
Corrected sodium (hyperglycemia)	Serum [Na] + [1.8 × (glucose – 100)]	

d, distribution factor.

EDITOR'S NOTES

Most of the electrolyte disorders that we as pediatric surgeons are required to manage involve the sometimes large perturbations of fluid status that affect our patients before, during, and after operation. Dehydration is often accompanied by gastrointestinal losses from vomiting or diarrhea, so that water, sodium, potassium and acid-base balance all need to be addressed simultaneously. Additional fluid losses from "third-spacing" contribute to the problem in the postoperative period. Anticipation of these changes and adherence to standard principles of fluid management prevent serious electrolyte disturbances in the majority of cases, so that clinical acumen can be an adequate substitute for frequent blood draws. Nevertheless, infants still present a significant challenge in some cases and require diligent assessment of electrolyte status.

Some minor electrolyte disorders result from the inappropriate use of so-called "maintenance fluids." Maintenance fluid requirements are calculated for patients based on body weight and are supposed to represent the minimum fluid and electrolytes that a patient needs to avoid dehydration. Roughly half of the calculated amount represents insensible loss of free water while the other half represents mandatory renal losses for excretion of solutes. In children and adults, this is usually best managed with half normal saline and 10 to 20 mEq of potassium per liter, while in neonates the fluid composition should be calculated on a per-kilogram basis. This typically ends up being very close to quarter normal saline with 5 to 10 mEq of potassium per liter. This becomes a reasonable approximation for basic fluid needs in the postoperative period, except in the patient who has had significant blood loss or who has become relatively depleted of intravascular fluid due to a third space shift of fluid. These patients need boluses of isotonic fluid (10–20 mL/kg of normal saline or lactated Ringer's solution) rather than half normal saline or increasing to "maintenance-and-a-half" rates of fluid administration. This practice tends to give patients too much free water, worsens postoperative edema, and contributes to the tendency for postoperative hyponatremia caused by secretion of antidiuretic hormone.

Hyperkalemia in infants and children who have normal renal function is nearly always factitious, caused by hemolysis of the blood specimen due to a difficult blood draw or improper handling of the specimen. If this cannot be confirmed, the test needs to be repeated to document a normal potassium level. True hypokalemia is more common but is well tolerated and rarely requires replacement therapy. Replacement of potassium requires careful calculation, good venous access, and proper monitoring to avoid complications. In general, mild hypokalemia (>2.9 mEq/L) requires no specific therapy beyond standard hydration measures. This is also true in infants with pyloric stenosis, who are usually deficient in total body potassium (although the laboratory nearly always reports hyperkalemia due to hemolysis of the specimen) but who generally recover normal levels with isotonic fluid resuscitation and rarely require potassium administration.

Management of electrolyte disorders in infants and children can be challenging and sometimes requires intervention that at first seems counterintuitive, but with an understanding of the physiology of fluid balance and a thoughtful approach to management, most patients are treated safely even in an unmonitored setting.

–P.M.

SUGGESTED READINGS

Coran AG, Drongowski RA. Body fluid compartment changes following neonatal surgery. *J Pediatr Surg* 1989;24:829–832.

Filston HC. Fluid and electrolyte management in the pediatric surgical patient. *Surg Clin North Am* 1992;72:1189–1205.

Friis-Hanse B. Body water compartments in children: changes during growth and related changes in body composition. *Pediatrics* 1961; 28:169.

Pestana C. *Fluids and electrolytes in the surgical patient.* Baltimore: Williams & Wilkins, 1985.

Winthrop AL, Jones PJH, Schoeller DA, et al. Changes in the body composition of the surgical infant in the early post-operative period. *J Pediatr Surg* 1987;22:546–549.

9

VASCULAR ACCESS

PETER MATTEI

Central venous access is one of the most common reasons for pediatric surgical consultation. Common indications for venous access procedures include infections requiring long-term antibiotics, parenteral nutrition, and malignancy. Premature neonates also frequently require central access, and occasionally we are asked to establish venous access when attempts to gain standard peripheral venous access have been unsuccessful.

The type of catheter used, the route of access, and the placement technique are determined by the needs of the patient. The most commonly used devices include temporary central venous catheters, permanent (tunneled) central venous catheters, and implantable devices (subcutaneous ports). Using the Seldinger technique, catheters can be placed into the subclavian vein, the femoral vein, or the internal jugular vein. Catheters also may be placed by cutdown using the external jugular vein, the facial vein, the internal jugular vein, the saphenous vein, or any other vein that can be accessed safely through a small incision.

The first step for a surgeon when consulted for intravenous access is to determine whether placement of a peripheral IV would be adequate, even as a temporary measure, and to personally assess the child for a suitable peripheral vein. Few clinical scenarios are more gratifying for a surgeon than to resolve an intravenous access "crisis" by starting an IV in a child after "everyone in the hospital" has tried but failed. Starting peripheral IVs should be part of the practical education for surgical residents and fellows, and it is a skill that as attending pediatric surgeons we should try to maintain over time.

In difficult cases, a useful site to consider is the saphenous vein at the ankle. Often considered a "blind stick" just above and slightly medial to the medial malleolus, with experience the clinician can learn to detect the vein. The technique is most useful in infants and toddlers, and the vein will usually accommodate a slightly larger cannula than a typical upper extremity vein.

P. Mattei: Department of Surgery, Thomas Jefferson University, Philadelphia, Pennsylvania; and Department of Pediatric Surgery, Alfred I. duPont Hospital for Children, Wilmington, Delaware.

Although placement of an intravenous cannula by venous cutdown has been promoted in the past as the first alternative when conventional percutaneous techniques fail, it has been replaced in most centers by percutaneous central venous access and intraosseous infusions. Nevertheless, it is a valuable technique and can be useful in certain situations. The most common site for peripheral venous cutdown is probably the saphenous vein at the ankle. Using a sterile technique, the vein can be identified rapidly through a transverse incision just above and slightly anterior to the medial malleolus. The vein is secured between ligatures and ligated distally. The vein can then be accessed directly or by venotomy. The cannula is then secured with a ligature around the vein and with sutures to the skin. The incision is partially closed if the cannula was placed directly or can be completely closed if the cannula was placed through a separate puncture site. Removal of the catheter does not usually require another procedure, and hemostasis is achieved by direct pressure over the site. Complications are rare but include cellulitis, phlebitis, and thrombosis. There are no sequelae except for scarring and inability to use the site again.

PERCUTANEOUS CENTRAL LINES

Percutaneous or "temporary" central lines are placed using the Seldinger technique and are not designed for long-term access. Indications include a short, defined course of intravenous antibiotics, short-term parenteral nutrition, central access for the critically ill patient, and perioperative access for the patient with limited peripheral access. These catheters are usually made of plastic and are produced by various manufacturers. They should not be used for more than 2 or 3 weeks. Beyond 4 weeks, the risks for infection, thrombosis, and catheter decay and malfunction are high. Advantages include ease and safety of placement, the availability of multiple lumens and ports, and ease of removal with minimal discomfort in the office or at the bedside. Disadvantages include the need for conscious sedation or general anesthesia for placement in children and a slightly higher risk for infection and thrombosis when compared with tunneled Silastic catheters. Nevertheless these appliances have a good overall safety record.

Placement of percutaneous catheters in children requires general anesthesia or deep conscious sedation so that the child is comfortable and motionless. I do not feel that placement with mild sedation and local anesthetic, as is often done in adults, is prudent, except when a patient is critically ill or obtunded. The two most useful sites for percutaneous central access are the subclavian vein and the femoral vein. The internal jugular vein can be used in older children but only with extreme caution: the carotid artery is at significant risk for injury, and lines emerging from the neck are not tolerated well by most children.

Subclavian vein access is generally straightforward and safe. In experienced hands, the risk of pneumothorax or hemothorax is negligible. Placement of a subclavian catheter is immensely simplified by the use of fluoroscopy. It ensures access to the superior vena cava (SVC), helps to confirm intavenous placement of the device, reduces the incidence of injury to the SVC, and confirms the final position of the catheter so that the need for repositioning of the catheter is eliminated. The technique is similar to that used for adults. The patient should be placed in a gentle head-down position, and a roll may be placed behind the shoulders. I find that a small rolled towel placed between the scapulae works best. The roll should gently exaggerate the posterior angulation of the clavicles without raising the patient's shoulders off the table. The vein is usually easier to access (and the artery more easily avoided) when the puncture is made more medial than is commonly used for adults, at or just lateral to the medial angle of the clavicle. Placement of the catheter between the head of the clavicle and the first rib should be avoided to prevent catheter shearing and embolization. The vein in small children is superficial and small, so good flow must be appreciated and the needle must be secured extremely well before the syringe is removed and the guide wire is placed. Central positioning of the wire is confirmed by the stimulation of ectopic electrical activity on the electrocardiogram or by visualization under fluoroscopy. It is common for the guide wire to find its way into the internal jugular vein or opposite subclavian vein. When manipulation of the wire under fluoroscopy is necessary, the access needle should be replaced with a small-gauge intravenous cannula; this makes wire manipulation easier and ensures venous access if the wire is pulled back too far. When the wire is confirmed to be in the right atrium or SVC, the tract is dilated gently and the catheter is placed using the Seldinger technique. To avoid the potentially life-threatening complication of traumatic injury to the SVC, placement of dilators and catheters over guide wires is ideally done under "live" fluoroscopy.

The optimal location of the tip of the subclavian catheter is considered to be in the SVC at the SVC–right atrial junction. However, the catheter tip must point straight down to avoid SVC injury either by catheter erosion or by hyperosmolar solutions. In most children, placing the tip in the SVC or at the SVC–right atrial junction causes the tip of the catheter to point toward the wall of the SVC. For this reason, I usually place the catheter so that the tip resides in the superior aspect of the right atrium (the "proximal" right atrium). However, placing catheters deep in the atrium should be avoided because this can result in atrial perforation or bothersome arrhythmias.

Given that the difference between optimal line position and poor line position is so small, choosing the appropriate size of catheter is important. Neonates can tolerate the smallest catheters, which are 3 French (single lumen) or 4 French (double lumen). A 5-cm catheter can be used on the right side and an 8-cm catheter on the left side. In larger patients it is best to use a measuring tape and the standard landmarks on the chest wall to estimate the appropriate length of the catheter. Standard catheter lengths are 8, 10, 12, and 15 cm. Most patients in this age group are best served by a double-lumen catheter in the 4 to 5.5 French range. Larger patients occasionally require a larger diameter catheter or a triple-lumen catheter.

Central catheters also can be placed in the femoral vein using a percutaneous approach. Exposure to urine and stool in young patients and limitation of mobility in older patients make it less than optimal in most cases, but it can be a useful access in the operating room and in the critical care setting when more traditional sites are not available. The size varies from a 3 or 4 French in neonates to a 5 or 6 French in larger patients. The appropriate length also varies from approximately 8 cm in neonates to 16 cm in older patients. The length should be individualized so that the tip lies in a central location in the distal inferior vena cava (IVC; just below the level of the umbilicus). The location should be confirmed by plain radiographs or fluoroscopy.

Safe placement of a percutaneous femoral venous line depends on clear anatomic landmarks, especially a distinctly palpable femoral artery. In children the neurovascular bundle is usually more lateral than in adults. The vein is also quite close to the artery and sometimes seems to be somewhat posterior to it. I approach the femoral vein at least a fingerbreadth below the inguinal crease. The vein is medial to the artery and in young children is often quite superficial. If good blood flow is established, a guide wire can usually be passed and the catheter placed using the Seldinger technique. Prior to passing a dilator or large catheter, one must be absolutely certain that the artery has not been entered inadvertently. Femoral arterial catheters in children under 12 years of age can result in severe ischemia and should be used only with extreme caution, if ever. Immediately after placement of a femoral venous catheter, infants often demonstrate a bluish discoloration or mottling of the lower extremity due to transient poor venous drainage. This typically resolves within 4 hours; however, the limb should be monitored carefully by the surgeon to be certain that it resolves completely. Persistent discoloration or edema mandates immediate removal of the catheter and careful attention to return of good perfusion.

Percutaneous catheters should be secured to the skin with two sutures and covered with a sterile dressing. In younger patients, creative dressing techniques may be required to prevent inadvertent removal of the catheter. The catheters are usually periodically flushed with a heparin-saline solution and require scheduled sterile dressing changes according to the established practices of the institution.

Removal of percutaneous catheters can be performed at the bedside or in the office. The sutures are removed, the catheter is gently withdrawn, and hemostasis is achieved with gentle pressure at the puncture site. A dressing is placed, and the family is instructed in standard wound care. The catheter itself should be inspected carefully upon removal to be certain that it has been removed in its entirety. The tip of a line that is removed for infection should be sent for culture, but this is not done routinely.

TUNNELED CENTRAL VENOUS LINES

Catheters placed for long-term use (e.g., Hickman, Broviac) are made of silicone elastomer, are placed in such a way that a portion of the catheter is tunneled in the subcutaneous space, and have a felt cuff that allows tissue ingrowth and prevents dislodgment. These catheters are placed under general anesthesia and, in the absence of infection or thrombosis, may last for many months or even years.

My preferred approach is to access the subclavian vein percutaneously and place the catheter using a peel-away sheath system. This technique can be used in patients weighing as little as 1,500 g and has the advantage of avoiding a cutdown in the neck. The patient is under general anesthesia with, at minimum, electrocardiographic, oxygen saturation, and blood pressure monitoring. Fluoroscopy should be available, although this may not be feasible when the catheter is being placed in the neonatal intensive care unit (NICU). A small roll is placed between the scapulae, and in infants the arms should be taped to the diaper to apply gentle downward traction on the shoulders. The neck is gently extended with the head in a midline position, and the neck and chest are sterilely prepared and draped bilaterally. The patient is placed in a slight head-down position, and the subclavian vein is accessed with a needle using the standard approach. The anesthetist should suspend positive pressure ventilation during needle insertion. A guide wire is inserted and the needle is removed. At this point, confirming a central location of the wire is essential. This is most easily done by using fluoroscopy to confirm that the wire tip is in the right atrium. If fluoroscopy is not available, the generation of ectopic electrocardiographic activity is a reasonably accurate way to confirm that the wire is in the atrium. If the wire has found its way into the opposite subclavian vein or the jugular vein, manipulation and redirection of the wire into the atrium is best achieved using a standard IV cannula, the smallest one that will pass easily over the guide wire, as a sheath to maintain intavenous access in case the wire is dislodged and to prevent trauma to the vessel itself. Once the wire is confirmed to be in a central location, an incision is made on the anterior chest wall. I prefer to place the incision just lateral to the sternum at approximately the level of the third or fourth intercostal space, regardless of the size of the patient. The subclavian puncture site is enlarged slightly, and the catheter is tunneled between the two incisions. Although this can be done with commercially available "tunnelers," it also can be done easily using a Fraser suction tip, a tendon passer, or, in neonates, a silver probe that has a slit at one end. The cuff should be placed at least 1 cm from the entry site. I prefer to leave it no more than 2 or 3 cm from the site, making it easier to remove without a second incision. Others place the cuff much deeper to prevent dislodgment.

Catheters come in many sizes, and in single-, double- or triple-lumen varieties. In neonates, 3 French catheters are used. In children weighing less than 10 kg, 4 to 6 French catheters are used, whereas in children weighing over 10 kg, a 6.5 French single-lumen or 7 French double-lumen catheter can be used. In rare cases, a catheter larger than 7 French or one with more than two lumens is required. Once the catheter has been tunneled, it should be cut to size. The tip should come to lie in the proximal right atrium and can be estimated by draping the catheter across the chest in a way that corresponds to the anatomy of the central venous system and cutting it just above the nipple line. I prefer to cut the catheter on a slight angle. The catheter is then placed in the vein using a peel-away sheath system. The tip is confirmed to be central by fluoroscopy or plain radiography and flushed with heparinized saline according to standard protocol. It is important to confirm that blood can be withdrawn easily into a syringe prior to flushing. If the catheter is found to be in a location other than the proximal right atrium, it can be withdrawn carefully through the subclavian incision and manipulated under fluoroscopy into the correct location. Catheters that are too long or too short need to be replaced. Catheters that are in the jugular vein or opposite subclavian vein can sometimes be manipulated by a forceful jet of saline injected through a small-volume syringe, which can flip the catheter tip into position. The catheter should be secured to the chest wall with a permanent monofilament suture and the subclavian incision is closed with a single fine absorbable suture and sterile strips. A dry sterile dressing is applied, and the catheter is further secured with tape.

If the subclavian vein is not accessible by percutaneous puncture, the opposite subclavian vein should be attempted. If neither is accessible, the neck is available for cutdown. My preference is to use the right facial vein. Although in most patients the external jugular vein is the most superficial large neck vein and is preferred by some pediatric surgeons, I have found it to be unreliable, in that it is often difficult to maneuver a catheter into the SVC. The facial vein, on the other hand, provides direct access to the internal jugular vein and is relatively constant in location. The vein can be approached from either side of the neck, but the right side is preferred. The patient is under anesthesia, positioned with a small roll behind the shoulders, and in a slight head-down position. The head is turned slightly away from the surgical site, and the anterior neck and chest are sterilely prepared and draped. A small incision is made in the superior aspect of the anterior triangle of the neck, between the sternocleidomastoid muscle and the carotid pulse. A natural skin crease may be used if present in this location. The incision is continued by blunt dissection through the platysma. The facial vein is usually easily visualized and controlled with fine sutures. If not, then the internal jugular vein should be controlled and a search made for an appropriate branch. After the vein is isolated and deemed to be of appropriate size, a small incision is made on the anterior chest wall and a catheter is tunneled between the two incisions. The catheter is cut to size on an angle, and the vein is ligated distally. A venotomy is performed, and the catheter is fed gently into the vein in a proximal direction. The catheter is secured in the vein with the proximal suture and the incision is closed with absorbable sutures and sterile strips. The catheter is flushed with heparinized saline and secured to the skin. The proper location of the catheter tip (proximal right atrium) is confirmed by radiography.

When the facial vein is not suitable, the internal jugular vein may be used. Although in infants the vein may be safely sacrificed, this should be avoided whenever possible by placing the catheter through a small lateral venotomy. In older patients, a monofilament purse-string suture can be placed in the wall of the vein to control bleeding at the site. In neonates, a venotomy made with a 23-gauge needle will allow a 3 French catheter to be placed securely and with good hemostasis.

Catheters also can be placed via the femoral vein and then tunneled either up onto the abdomen or to a more distal site on the thigh. The femoral vein can be accessed percutaneously or by cutdown. When a cutdown is used, the saphenous vein should be used. I try to avoid using the femoral vein proper because of the potential for thrombosis. A small transverse incision is made over the neurovascular bundle one to two fingerbreadths below the inguinal crease. Careful dissection will reveal the saphenous vein at the saphenofemoral junction. The vein is controlled proximally and ligated distally. The catheter is flushed, tunneled, and cut to size. The catheter is placed through a small venotomy and fed into the femoral vein. The proximal location of the tip should be confirmed radiographically and should be located in the distal IVC below the level of the renal veins (L2–3). The catheter is then secured and dressed in the usual fashion. The patient should be examined periodically by the surgeon to be sure that the typical mottling of the lower extremity that occurs after femoral venous catheter placement resolves.

IMPLANTABLE DEVICES

Another option for patients who require long-term central venous access is an implantable device. These have the advantages of being completely subcutaneous, allowing the patient greater freedom in activities, no need for dressing changes, and no risk of accidental dislodgment. Disadvantages include the need for more dissection at operation and thus more postoperative discomfort, higher risk for wound complications, and less likelihood of salvaging a catheter that has become infected or colonized. Another disadvantage is that the ports are accessed with a needle through intact skin; however, this has been less of a problem since effective topical anesthetics have become available.

Placement of the catheter is the same as for the tunneled devices, and can be done percutaneously or by cutdown. The port chamber is placed subcutaneously at least a few centimeters from the vein puncture site. Optimal placement is over a relatively flat and immobile area of the chest wall, where the subcutaneous fat is neither too thin nor too thick. I prefer to place it on the upper chest just lateral to the sternum. After access to the vein has been secured either with a guide wire or by cutdown, a transverse incision is made and a subcutaneous pocket is developed bluntly in a plane just above the pectoralis fascia. Hemostasis must be excellent to prevent a hematoma. The port should be fixed to the fascia with at least three permanent monofilament sutures. The catheter is then tunneled, cut to size, and placed intravascularly. The line position is confirmed radiographically, and the port is flushed with heparinized saline (typically 100 U/mL). Scarpa's fascia should be closed as a separate layer with interrupted absorbable suture. I prefer to close the skin with interrupted deep-dermal absorbable stitches, given that the skin closure is typically under slight tension and these patients are often at higher risk for wound complications. Initially the ports are difficult and painful to localize and access. If the port is to be used within a week, it is best to leave it accessed with a 90° Huber needle.

LINE REMOVAL

Removal of percutaneous lines is usually straightforward. The sutures are divided, the line is removed, hemostasis is achieved with gentle pressure, and a light sterile dressing is applied. In most cases, this can be done in the office or at the bedside without anesthetic or sedation. One must examine the tip carefully to be certain that the entire catheter has been removed.

Tunneled catheters require sharp dissection of the cuff from the subcutaneous tissues. This should be done under general anesthesia in nearly all patients, with possible exceptions being neonates still in the NICU and the rare teenager who can tolerate the procedure with local anesthetic. If the cuff is less than 3 cm away, the cuff can be excised through the skin entry site after it has been enlarged slightly; otherwise a small incision needs to be made directly over the cuff. With gentle traction on the catheter itself, and with a combination of blunt and sharp dissection, most cuffs can be excised with only a small pair of scissors. The catheter tip should be inspected to be certain that it was removed in its entirety. A sterile technique should be used, but because the site is assumed to be colonized with bacteria, the wound is best left open to heal by second intention. Gaping wounds may benefit from a loose approximation, and certainly an incision placed over the cuff should be closed in standard fashion. Some catheters are designed to break away from the cuff, leading some to remove only the catheter, leaving the cuff in the patient. I recommend against this. The cuffs can become infected, albeit rarely, but more importantly, it is typical for families to regard this as a retained foreign body or a technical error.

Removal of implantable ports always requires a general anesthetic but can usually be done on an outpatient basis. The approach is through the old incision, and all foreign material must be removed. The port is encased in a fibrous pseudocapsule, which does not need to be completely excised. The wound is closed in layers after meticulous hemostasis is achieved.

COMPLICATIONS

Central lines are associated with numerous potential complications. Catheter dislodgment is a constant risk and requires that the catheter be carefully secured, typically with skin sutures, tape, and a sturdy dressing. Cuffed catheters do not usually require resuturing if they have been in place for more than 2 weeks and the cuff itself is securely embedded. An exposed cuff portends further catheter extrusion and a high likelihood of infection. If the tip is still intravascular, the catheter can be used for a short period of time, but will need to be replaced if needed long-term. Tunneled catheters are made of a resilient Silastic material but are prone to breaks and cracks. Repair kits are available and are relatively easy to use. If the break occurs close to the skin, the catheter will need to be replaced.

Catheters are prone to infections, which can be endovascular or subcutaneous. Endovascular infections are confirmed by blood cultures drawn through the line. Infected temporary catheters should be removed. Tunneled catheters and ports can sometimes be sterilized with antibiotic therapy, but often need to be removed. The likelihood of salvage depends somewhat on the organism involved: roughly 50% for *Staphylococcus epidermidis*, 20% for gram-negative organisms, and zero for fungal line infections. Infections that involve the subcutaneous portion of the catheter take the form of cellulitis or an abscess. Cellulitis can occasionally be treated with antibiotics alone, whereas an abscess requires drainage and usually removal of the line. In the presence of bacteremia, the line should be removed and the patient treated with appropriate antibiotics for at least 24 hours. The line is replaced only if the patient is afebrile and blood cultures are negative.

Catheters can become occluded by clot or crystallization of infusate. A plain radiograph should be obtained to exclude a kink or mechanical obstruction. Tissue plasminogen activator (tPA) is approved for use in thrombosed catheters. Clinicians should always refer to their institutional protocols and policies regarding its use, but the standard concentration is 1 mg/mL. The solution is infused into the catheter (up to 2 mL) and allowed to dwell for 2 to 4 hours. It is then aspirated from the line (not flushed). If crystallized parenteral nutrition solution is the likely cause, a small volume of sterile 0.1 N HCl can be used instead. A particularly frustrating problem is a catheter that flushes easily but does not allow blood to be drawn back. This can be due either to a flap of fibrin that creates a valve effect at the tip of the catheter or by the tip of the catheter being drawn up against the wall of the vessel by negative pressure. A trial of tPA is occasionally successful, but usually the catheter needs to be replaced. Some have suggested that not cutting the catheter at an angle or cutting the tip twice to create a double bevel can prevent this problem.

Deep venous thrombosis can be induced by central venous lines. Fortunately, they appear to be uncommon and are typically well tolerated by infants and children. Reports of pulmonary embolism, for example, are exceptionally rare. Nevertheless, edema or mottling of an extremity mandates prompt removal of the catheter. Symptoms typically resolve quickly, and sequelae are unusual, even though the vein may never regain patency. Thrombosis of the SVC or IVC, on the other hand, can have severe repercussions. Although symptoms may improve after immediate line removal, intravenous heparinization should be administered in most cases. In the case of thrombosis without occlusion, we have used subcutaneous enoxaparin with good results.

Catheters in the atrium or ventricle of the heart can cause bothersome arrhythmias, such as supraventricular tachycardia and ventricular tachycardia, or heart block and should be repositioned or replaced. Catheter tips also can erode through the wall of the SVC or right atrium, especially in infants and those receiving hyperosmolar infusions (parenteral nutrition). The result is a right hydrothorax or pericardial effusion, both of which can cause severe hemodynamic compromise. These potentially lethal complications must be recognized and treated without delay. The key is a high index of suspicion–it should be considered when a child with a central line unexpectedly develops hypoxia or shock. Physical examination findings may suggest the cause, while a chest radiograph should confirm it. Treatment is by thoracentesis or pericardiocentesis and removal of the line. Fortunately (and inexplicably), the perforations nearly always seal spontaneously and rarely require operative repair.

In summary, a large component of the practice of the typical pediatric surgeon is the placement of central venous lines and the management of their numerous potential complications. It is an important service that we provide and contributes greatly to the care and well–being of our patients.

SUGGESTED READINGS

Andropoulos DB, Bent ST, Skjonsby B, et al. The optimal length of insertion of central venous catheters for pediatric patients. *Anesth Analg* 2001;93:883–886.

Choi M, Massicotte MP, Marzinotto V, et al. The use of alteplase to restore patency of central venous lines in pediatric patients: a cohort study. *J Pediatr* 2001;139:152–156.

Kurekci E, Kaye R, Koehler M. Chylothorax and chylopericardium: a complication of a central venous catheter. *J Pediatr* 1998;132: 1064–1066.

Shaul DB, Scheer B, Rokhsar S, et al. Risk factors for early infection of central venous catheters in pediatric patients. *J Am Coll Surg* 1998;186:654–658.

Somme S, Gedalia U, Caceres M, et al. Wireless replacement of the "lost" central venous line in children. *Am Surg* 2001;67:817–820.

Taylor L, O'Neill JA Jr. Total parenteral nutrition in the pediatric patient. *Surg Clin North Am* 1991;71:477–491.

van Engelenburg KC, Festen C. Cardiac tamponade: a rare but life-threatening complication of central venous catheters in children. *J Pediatr Surg* 1998;33:1822–1824.

Warner BW, Ryckman FC. A simple technique to redirect malpositioned Silastic central venous catheters. *J Parenter Enter Nutr* 1992; 16:473–476.

Wesley JR. Permanent central venous access devices. *Semin Pediatr Surg* 1992;1:188–201.

10

NONTRADITIONAL CENTRAL VENOUS ACCESS

THOMAS L. BAUER
PHILIP J. WOLFSON

The ability to gain reliable access to the central venous system in infants and children is extremely important when peripheral veins are scarce, long-term infusions of total parenteral nutrition or chemotherapy are necessary, and hemodynamic monitoring is needed. In many instances, central venous catheters (CVCs) are literally "lifelines," and the ultimate survival of the child is dependent on the ability to maintain continued intravenous infusion.

As premature infants, critically ill patients, and children with malignancies have ever higher survival rates, central venous catheterization has become increasingly common in the pediatric population. Although catheter insertion in children and especially infants can be far more formidable than in adults and is usually regarded as a surgical procedure to be performed by a highly qualified individual, the current armamentarium of techniques and equipment available provides for a high success rate with an acceptably low incidence of complications. However, as more children require these lines for longer periods of time, their veins increasingly become thrombosed and traditional cannulation sites become unavailable for use.

Central venous catheterization is usually performed with relatively nonthrombogenic silicone catheters, which have a subcutaneously tunneled cuff to resist ascending infection and prevent dislodgment. Catheters may be inserted by "cutdown" or percutaneously, using a peel-away sheath system. Veins are more often cut down in infants and commonly include the external jugular vein (EJV), facial vein (FCV), internal jugular vein (IJV), and saphenous vein (SAV) at the groin. We usually reserve percutaneous cannulations for older children (>1 year of age) and most often use the subclavian vein (SBV), with the IJV and femoral vein (FMV) as less frequent alternatives. Others have demonstrated the feasibility of percutaneous cannulation in infants weighing as little as 1,000 g. Recently there has been increased usage of extremely thin silicone, peripherally inserted, centrally placed catheters (PICC lines). They may be used in both infants and older children and are often placed by neonatologists, intensivists, or nurses. However, the narrow caliber of these lines allows for only a limited infusion rate, and blood cannot be drawn or infused.

The following is a description of some of the more innovative central catheterization techniques that have been used in children when the more traditional routes are precluded from usage.

Careful preoperative assessment of the patient with a potentially difficult access problem is essential. If a child has had several previous CVCs, a known thrombotic complication of a prior cannulation, or any clinical evidence of venous thrombosis (unexplained peripheral edema or visible dilatation of superficial veins), duplex Doppler ultrasonography or venography should be performed to assess the patency of the central venous system and its tributaries in order to plan the operative strategy.

REUSE OF EXISTING VENOTOMY SITE

Traditionally, veins that have already been ligated and cannulated by cutdown are considered no longer available. Brevetti et al. described a technique whereby a vein that still contains a malfunctioning catheter can be reused, so long as the catheter is not infected and the central veins are not thrombosed.

An incision is made at the previous cutdown site, and the fibrous tunnel that has formed around the catheter before it enters the vein is circumferentially dissected and divided. Stay sutures are placed on the proximal fibrous tunnel segment, the catheter is removed, and a new line is inserted between the stay sutures to the same measured distance as the previous catheter. It is estimated that a sufficient fibrous tunnel will have developed by 4 weeks after a CVC has been in place.

T. L. Bauer: Department of Surgery, Jefferson Medical College and Thomas Jefferson University Hospital, Thomas Jefferson University, Philadelphia, Pennsylvania.

P. J. Wolfson: Department of Surgery, Thomas Jefferson University, Philadelphia, Pennsylvania; and Divsion of General Surgery, Alfred I. duPont Children's Hospital, Wilmington, Delaware.

CEPHALIC VEIN

The cephalic vein is small in tiny neonates but may be a viable cannulation site in larger infants and children with a patent SVC in whom the EJV, FCV, IJV, and SAVs are unavailable, and as an alternative to percutaneous cannulation of the SBV.

The cephalic vein is located in the deltopectoral triangle and drains directly into the SBV. It is approached through an incision in the deltopectoral groove, medial to the coracoid process and just below the lateral third of the clavicle (Fig. 10.1). The deltoid and pectoralis muscles are separated and the interposed adipose tissue is dissected to reveal the cephalic vein. The floor of the deltopectoral triangle is formed by the pectoralis minor muscle (whose fibers run at right angles to the other muscles) and indicates the lower limit of the dissection. If necessary, the junction of the cephalic vein and SCV can be exposed by dividing a few fibers of the pectoralis major. If the cephalic vein proves unavailable, tributaries may be found in the chest wall at this level that also drain into the SBV and can be used.

AXILLARY VEIN

The axillary vein may be cut down and cannulated even in neonates, in many of the same situations for which the cephalic vein would be used (patent SVC, unavailability of or preference not to use other veins). It is relatively large and does not need to be ligated, and its utilization will not block jugular flow.

The arm is extended and abducted, with the face straight up or directed ipsilaterally. A transverse incision is made in the midaxillary line in the deepest skin fold of the axilla (Fig. 10.2). The axillary vein is the most superficial and inferior structure encountered in the axillary sheath. The ulnar

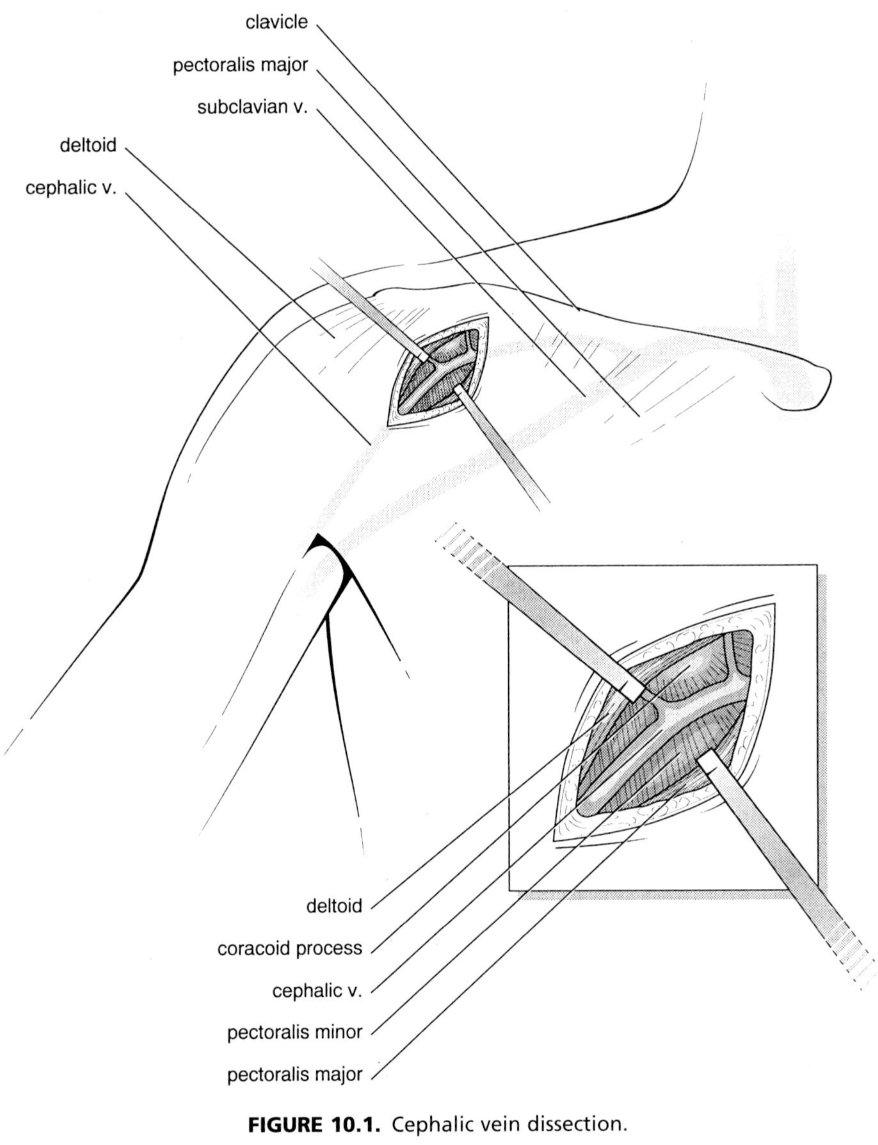

FIGURE 10.1. Cephalic vein dissection.

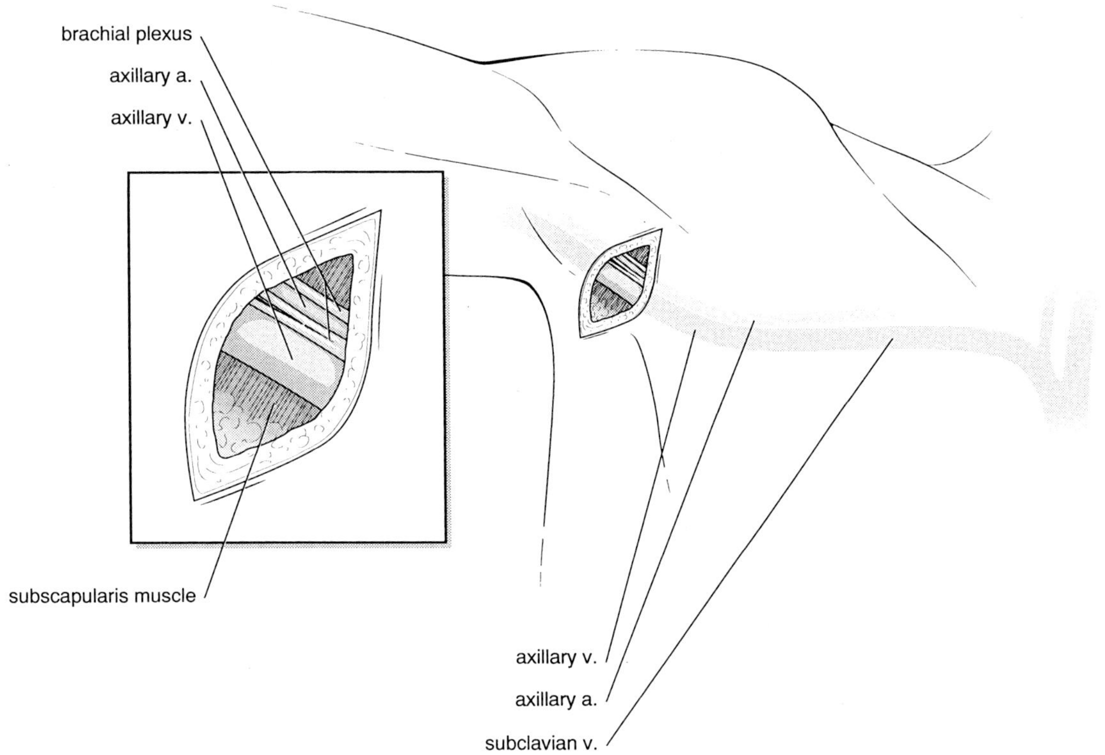

FIGURE 10.2. Axillary vein dissection.

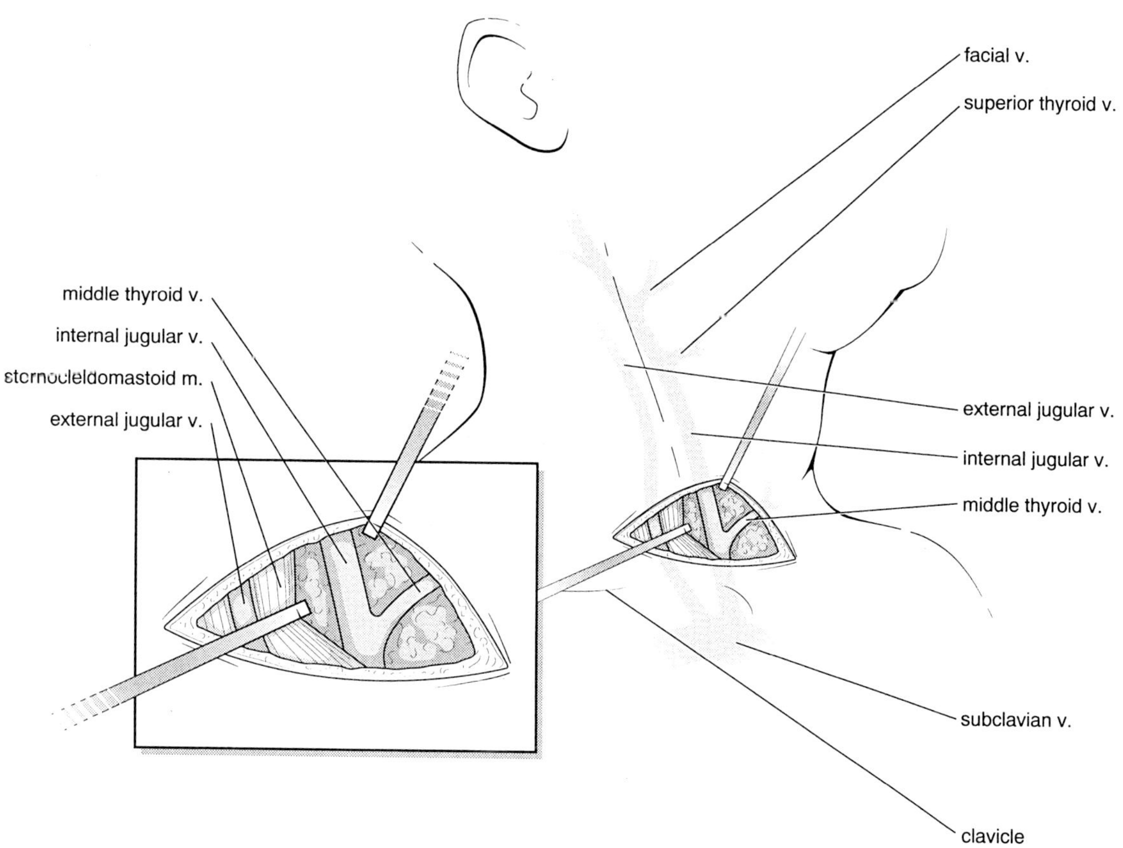

FIGURE 10.3. Middle thyroid vein dissection.

branch of the brachial plexus is found adjacent to the vein. Although the axillary artery is not usually directly visualized, its pulsations can serve as a landmark. Dissection into muscle or deep fat indicates that the vein has been missed. The axillary vein does not need to be ligated, but the venotomy is closed around the catheter with a fine suture.

MIDDLE THYROID VEIN

The middle thyroid vein enters the IJV medially in the lower neck, below the FCV branch of the IJV. Although the middle thyroid vein is not as large or constant as the FCV, it may be cannulated when an attempt at EJV cutdown fails, because this incision is usually placed too low for its medial extension to expose the FCV. The middle thyroid vein also may be used in patients in whom the FCVs and EJVs have all been used.

If an incision has already been made to cannulate the EJV, it is extended medially; otherwise, a transverse incision is placed 2 cm above the clavicle. The IJV is exposed, and the middle thyroid vein is identified where it enters the medial aspect of the IJV (Fig. 10.3).

INTERNAL MAMMARY VEIN

The internal mammary vein is the first tributary of the innominate vein, and on the right side has an angle favorable to catheter insertion into the SVC. Although the SVC and right innominate vein must be patent, the internal mammary vein may be used when the SBVs, IJVs, and inferior caval system are no longer available due to prior use or thrombosis. It does not require a thoracotomy.

A transverse incision is performed in the second right intercostal space. The intercostal muscles are dissected from the sternal border laterally, taking care not to injure the artery, until the internal mammary vein is identified (Fig. 10.4). The catheter tends to thread up and into the SVC.

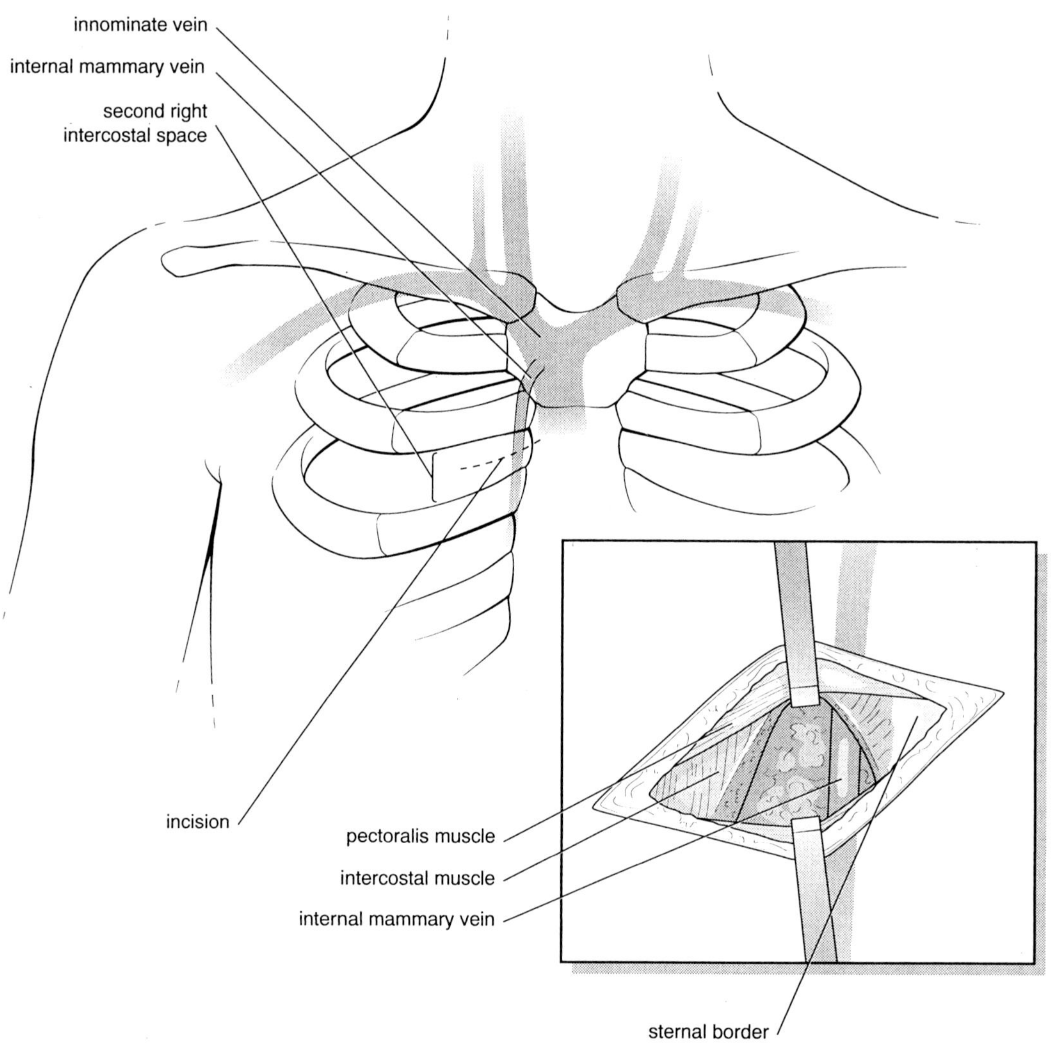

FIGURE 10.4. Internal mammary vein dissection.

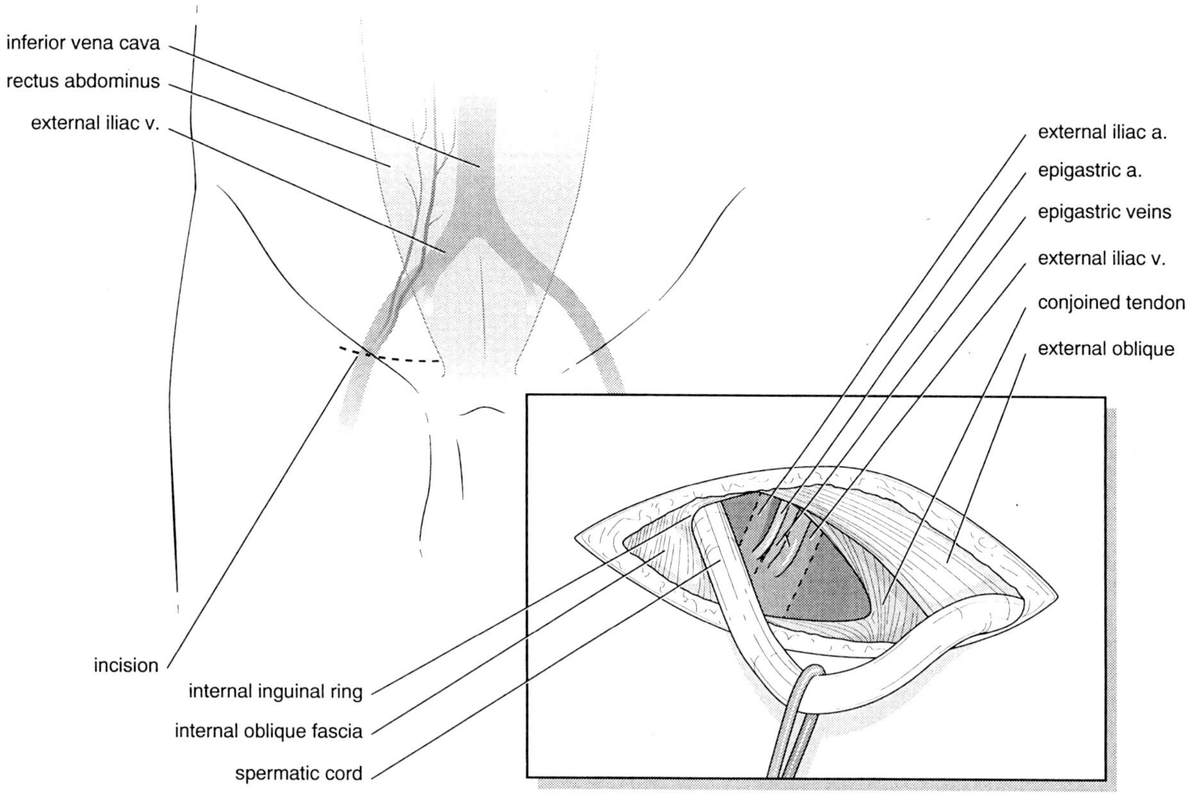

FIGURE 10.5. Inferior epigastric vein dissection.

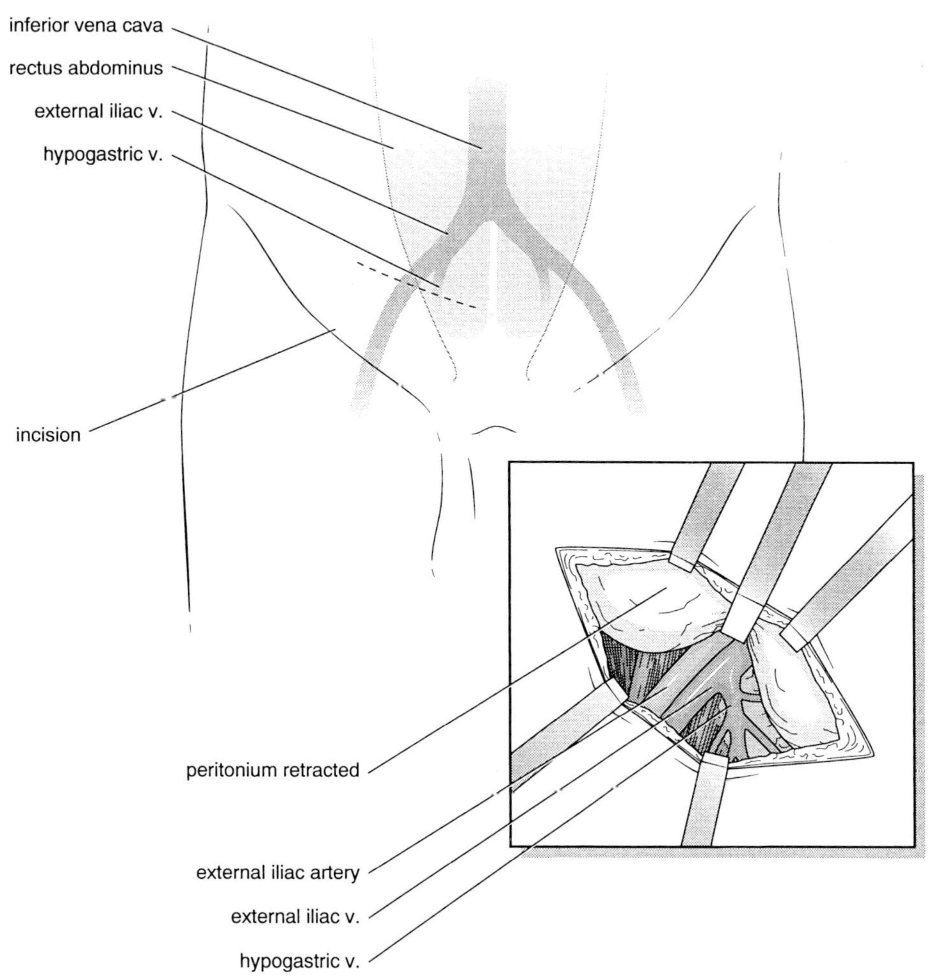

FIGURE 10.6. Hypogastric vein dissection.

INFERIOR EPIGASTRIC VEIN

The inferior epigastric vein courses inferiorly, deep to the rectus abdominis muscle, before turning cephalad and medially at the internal inguinal ring to enter the external iliac vein. It is useful if the patient has no access sites above the diaphragm and a patent IVC.

The inferior epigastric vein is exposed through the same incision as for an inguinal hernia repair (Fig. 10.5). After the external oblique has been opened, the inferior epigastric vessels (usually two veins and one artery) are located just medial to the internal ring. The larger vein is cannulated cephalad to the IVC.

HYPOGASTRIC VEIN

The hypogastric vein, like the inferior epigastric vein, can be cannulated in patients with a patent IVC but no access sites above the diaphragm. A right or left lower quadrant muscle-splitting McBurney type of incision is carried down to the peritoneum (Fig. 10.6). Retroperitoneal dissection exposes the iliac vessels; the hypogastric vein is identified and cannulated.

PERCUTANEOUS TRANSLUMBAR IVC CATHETERIZATION

In a child with SVC thrombosis, in whom the lower extremity veins are also not available, the IVC may be cannulated directly through a percutaneous approach, analogous to that used for translumbar aortograms in adults.

The patient is placed prone and a small needle (21 gauge) is directed under ultrasonographic or fluoroscopic guidance into the IVC (Fig. 10.7). The puncture site is several centimeters lateral to the transverse process of L3, and the needle is directed 45 degrees medially until it touches the body of L3. The needle is then directed slightly anteriorly until blood is aspirated from the IVC, which is confirmed with a contrast injection. Using the Seldinger technique, a guide wire and dilators are passed, followed by a peel-away sheath and the silicone catheter. The catheter tip is placed at the right atrium–IVC junction.

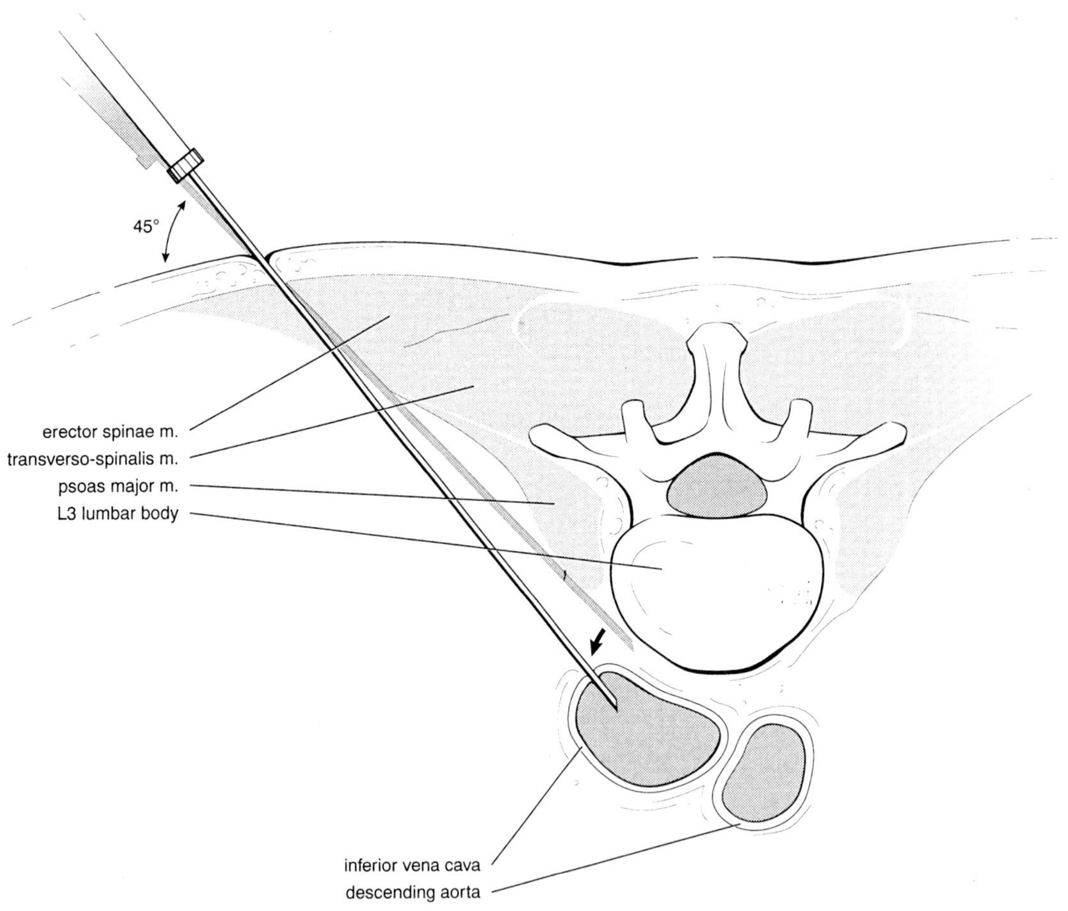

FIGURE 10.7. Percutaneous translumbar catheterization of the inferior vena cava.

AZYGOS VEIN

In children with both SVC and IVC thrombosis, the azygous system represents an alternative route for central venous access. Although the intercostal veins at the level of the ribs are usually small, and using them to access the azygous system may be difficult, the azygos vein can be more readily cannulated centrally.

The azygos vein is readily exposed through a right posterolateral, extrapleural thoracotomy in the fourth intercostal space, similar to the approach used for esophageal atresia repair. The azygos vein can be catheterized directly or via one of its high intercostal branches. The catheter tip is threaded to the right atrium, and the other end tunneled outside through the chest wall.

An intriguing thoracoscopic approach to the azygos vein in children also has been described (Fig. 10.8). The child is placed in a left lateral decubitus position, with the arm abducted over the head. A 5-mm port is inserted just below the tip of the scapula for the camera, and another port is placed in the midaxillary line at the second or third intercostal space to retract the lung. Using external pressure on the child's back to select the optimal intercostal space, a needle is introduced percutaneously and extrapleurally between the medial edge of the scapula and the spine. The needle is advanced extrapleurally, and into a suitable intercostal vein or directly into the azygos vein. A guide wire is inserted, the needle is withdrawn, and a dilator with a peelaway sheath is placed over the wire. The wire is removed and a tunneled catheter inserted.

INTERCOSTAL VEIN

The intercostal vein at the level of the ribs has been cannulated in children weighing as little as 5.5 kg using a very

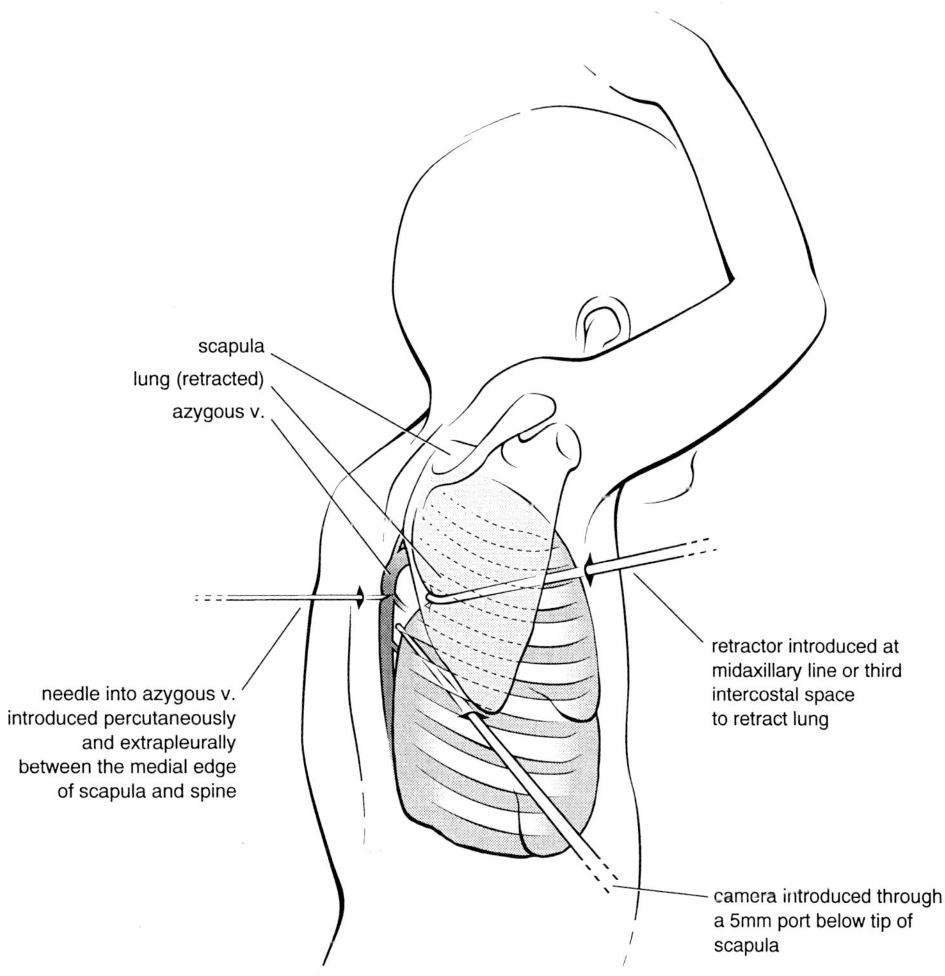

FIGURE 10.8. Thoracoscopic cannulation of the azygos vein.

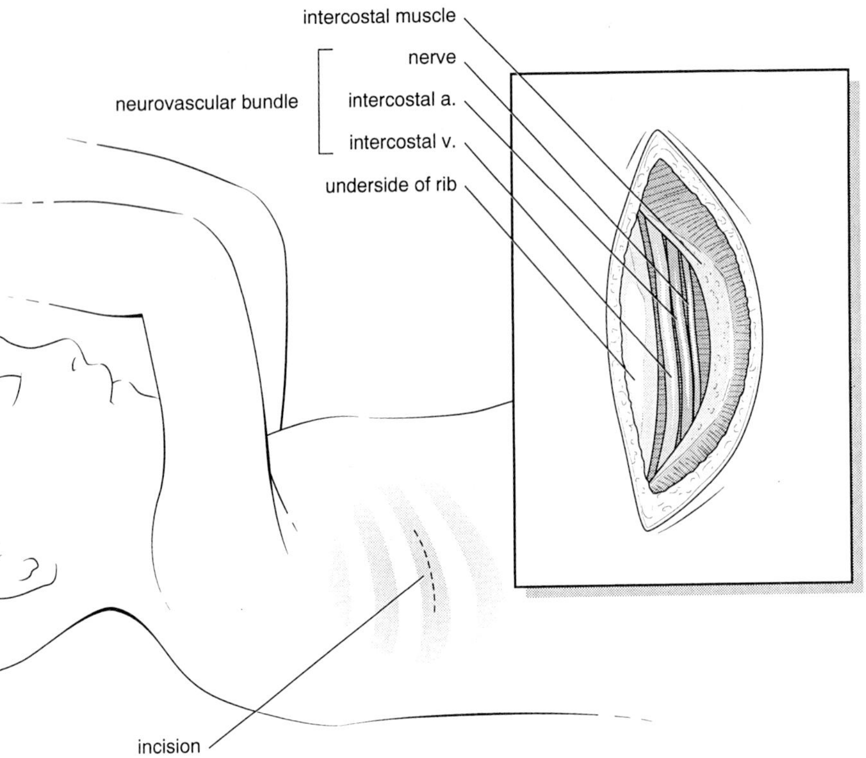

FIGURE 10.9. Intercostal vein dissection.

narrow silicone catheter on a blunt-tip needle, which is subsequently cemented to a Broviac catheter with a silicone strut slid over the connection.

With the patient in the lateral decubitus position, an incision is made over the chosen interspace and carried down to the intercostal muscles. These are dissected from the undersurface of the rib until the intercostal neurovascular bundle is identified (Fig. 10.9). A thin silicone catheter is threaded into the intercostal vein through a venotomy until the azygos vein is entered and blood can be aspirated. This catheter is then joined to the larger one, which is tunneled externally.

PERCUTANEOUS HEPATIC VEIN CANNULATION

A hepatic vein can be cannulated as an alternative to the azygos vein and direct right atrium cannulation in individuals with SVC and IVC thrombosis, and has been successful even in infants.

The technique is similar to that of translumbar IVC cannulation (Fig. 10.10). The patient is supine, and under ultrasonographic guidance, a 20- or 21-gauge spinal needle is introduced percutaneously at the lowermost right costal margin, inserted through the hepatic parenchyma, and into the right or middle hepatic vein. Using the Seldinger technique, a catheter is placed with its tip at the right

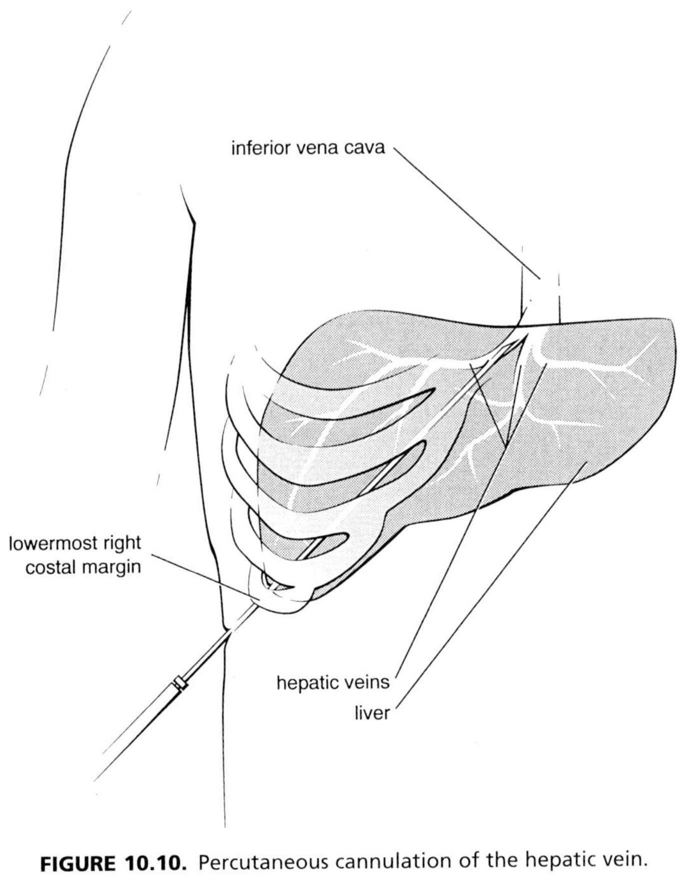

FIGURE 10.10. Percutaneous cannulation of the hepatic vein.

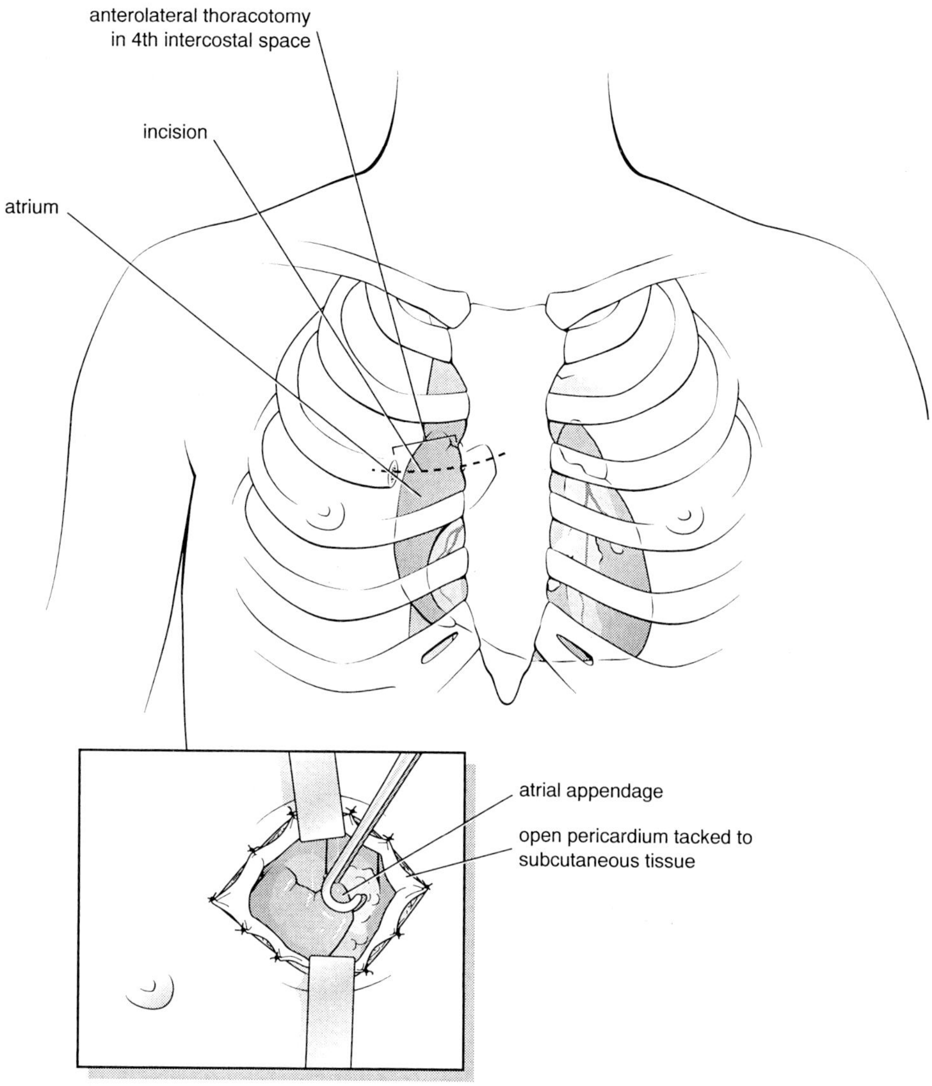

FIGURE 10.11. Direct catheterization of the right atrium.

atrium–SVC junction, allowing sufficient catheter length for respiratory movement of the liver and growth of the child.

DIRECT RIGHT ATRIUM CATHETERIZATION

Finally, if both the SVC and IVC are thrombosed, the right atrium may be cannulated directly.

The pericardium may be exposed through an anterolateral thoracotomy in the fourth intercostal space, or via the mediastinum in the bed of the excised right third costal cartilage (Fig. 10.11). The opened pericardium may be tacked to the subcutaneous tissue with traction sutures to enhance exposure. The atrial appendage is grasped with a small vascular clamp, a nonabsorbable purse-string suture is placed, and the catheter is inserted directly into the atrium.

SUGGESTED READINGS

Azizkhan RG, Taylor LA, Jaques PF, et al. Pecutaneous translumbar and transhepatic inferior vena caval catheters for prolonged vascular access in children. *J Pediatr Surg* 1992;2:165–169.

Bax NMA, van der Zee DC. Thoracoscopic guided percutaneous cannulation of the azygos vein in children. *Surg Endosc* 1996;10: 862–864.

Brevetti LS, Kalliainen L, Kimura K. A surgical technique that allows reuse of an existing venotomy site for multiple central venous catheterizations. *J Pediatr Surg* 1996;31:939–940.

Core GB, Chaudhry SS, Egozi L, et al. Use of the internal mammary vein for central venous access. *Surg Gynecol Obstet* 1990;171: 343–344.

Donahoe PK, Kim SH. The inferior epigastric vein as an alternate site for central venous hyperalimentation. *J Pediatr Surg* 1980;15: 737–738.

Eichelberger MR, Rous PG, Hoelzer DJ, et al. Percutaneous subclavian venous catheters in neonates and children. *J Pediatr Surg* 1981;16:547–553.

Gorman RC, Buzby GP. Difficult access problems. *Surg Oncol Clin North Am* 1995;4:453–447.

Hogan L, Pulito AR. Broviac central venous catheters inserted via the saphenous or femoral vein in the NICU under local anesthesia. *J Pediatr Surg* 1992;27:1185–1188.

Kanter RK, Zimmerman JJ, Strauss RH, et al. Central venous catheter insertion by femoral vein: safety and effectiveness for the pediatric patient. *Pediatrics* 1986;77:842–847.

Kosloske AM, Klein MD. Techniques of central venous access for long term parenteral nutrition in infants. *Surg Gynecol Obstet* 1982;154:395–399.

Krausz MM, Berlatzky Y, Ayalon A, et al. Percutaneous cannulation of the internal jugular vein in infants and children. *Surg Gynecol Obstet* 1979;148:591–594.

Lobe TE, Schropp KP, Rogers DA, et al. A "smart needle" to facilitate vascular access in pediatric patients. *J Pediatr Surg* 1993;10: 1401–1402.

Mulvihill SJ, Fonkalsrud EW. Complications of superior versus inferior vena cava occlusion in infants receiving central total parenteral nutrition. *J Pediatr Surg* 1984;19:752–757.

Newman BM, Cooney DR, Karp MP, et al. The intercostal vein: an alternate route for central venous alimentation. *J Pediatr Surg* 1983;18:732–733.

Pokorny WJ, McGill CW, Harberg FJ. Use of azygos vein for central catheter insertion. *Surgery* 1985;97:362.

Robards JB, Jaques PF, Mauro MA, et al. Percutaneous translumbar inferior vena cava central line placement in a critically ill child. *Pediatr Radiol* 1989;19:140–141.

Robertson LJ, Jaques PF, Mauro MA, et al. Percutaneous inferior vena cava placement of tunneled Silastic catheters for prolonged vascular access in infants. *J Pediatr Surg* 1990;25:596–598.

Silverman SH, Stringel G. Two techniques for central catheter placement in the hypogastric and azygos veins. *Pediatr Surg Int* 1988; 3:62–63.

Stephens BL, Lelli JL, Allen D, et al. Silastic catheterization of the axillary vein in neonates: an alternative to the internal jugular vein. *J Pediatr Surg* 1993;28:31–35.

Toufanian A, Knight P. The middle thyroid vein: an alternative route for central venous catheter insertion. *J Pediatr Surg* 1983;18: 156–157.

11

ACUTE RENAL FAILURE

MUSTAFA KABEER
MICHAEL D. KLEIN

Acute renal failure (ARF) contributes significantly to morbidity and mortality in pediatric surgical patients. The neonatal mortality rate for ARF is 60%, and the overall mortality rate for ARF in children and neonates is 30%. If patients are to survive, there must be a high index of suspicion, a rapid diagnosis, and early recognition of reversibility, so that treatment can be instituted expeditiously.

Acute renal failure is an abrupt decrease in glomerular filtration rate (GFR), with associated tubular dysfunction resulting in retention of nitrogenous and other metabolic waste. This prevents the kidneys from regulating volume and electrolyte composition and may be associated with diminished urine output and elevated levels of blood urea nitrogen (BUN) and creatinine. Oliguric renal failure is easier to detect due to insufficient urine output, clinically defined in neonates and children as less than 1 mL/kg/h. Renal failure can occur despite excellent urine output. Nonoliguric renal failure is most often detected by an increase in creatinine of at least 0.3 mg/dL/day.

PATHOPHYSIOLOGY

The fetal kidney has a high vascular resistance that decreases over the first 48 hours after birth, but lack of autoregulation persists in premature neonates and leaves them susceptible to prerenal ARF. Newborns are additionally susceptible to renal failure due to diminished tubular glucose reabsorption leading to glycosuria, with resultant osmotic diuresis and dehydration. GFR is also low due to high vascular resistance. GFR in the fetal kidney is less than 1 mL/min until 34 weeks of gestational age and only 4 mL/min at term. There is a gradual increase after birth to about 20 mL/min by 3 days of age, and after that it slowly increases until plateauing at 1 year of age.

Prerenal ARF accounts for roughly half of all cases of renal insufficiency in neonates. Autoregulation attempts to maintain GFR over a wide range of perfusion pressure by regulating renal blood flow. This is usually done by afferent glomerular capillary dilation (mediated by prostaglandin) and may also require efferent glomerular capillary constriction (mediated by angiotensin II). Autoregulation in newborns is often immature and easily impaired by maternal factors and drugs. Angiotensin-converting enzyme inhibitors that block production of angiotensin II and nonsteroidal antiinflammatory drugs that block prostaglandin synthesis can lead to failure of the autoregulation mechanism. Cortical nephrons mature from the inner to outer cortex, and blood flow is greater to the inner cortex in newborns. During hypovolemia, autoregulation is impaired and newborns lose more renal function than do older children and adults because the inner cortex, with more functioning nephrons, is affected to a greater extent.

Prerenal failure occurs when autoregulation fails to maintain normal GFR and leads to increases in water and solute reabsorption. This is accomplished by elevated renin and aldosterone, with resultant increased sodium reabsorption by cortical and medullary collecting tubules. Release of antidiuretic hormone in response to insufficient intravascular volume leads to increased water reabsorption in the collecting tubules. This leads to the overall picture of decreased urine output and increased urine osmolality.

Hypoxic injury accounts for 70% of prerenal ARF in the neonate. Hypoxia can lead to changes in autoregulation and shunting of blood from the kidney to improve oxygenation of the brain. Hypoxia also can cause intrinsic renal injury. Volume depletion without hypoxia is responsible for the remaining cases. Emesis and diarrhea due to gastroenteritis are a common cause.

Intrinsic renal failure is due to malfunction within the kidney parenchyma and leads to decreased ability to concentrate urine. Isosthenuria due to tubular cell damage is a hallmark of intrinsic renal failure. Severity ranges from mild

M. Kabeer: Department of Pediatric Surgery, Children's Hospital of Michigan, Detroit, Michigan.

M.D. Klein: Department of Surgery, Wayne State University; and Department of Surgery, Children's Hospital of Michigan, Detroit, Michigan.

tubular dysfunction to acute tubular necrosis with or without oliguria/anuria to renal infarction and cortical necrosis. Such damage leads to changes in ultrastructure with decreased permeability of glomerular capillaries and intratubular obstruction due to tubular flow by cellular debris. The most common cause of intrinsic renal failure in neonates is perinatal asphyxia and hypoxia. Increased production of uric acid occurs after tissue hypoxia, and due to partial deficiencies in purine metabolism, increased urinary uric acid excretion is observed. This leads to precipitation of uric acid or monosodium urate crystals within the tubules of the nephron. Neonates are especially vulnerable to this because of the increased fractional excretion of uric acid and an increased urinary burden, increasing the risk of precipitation of urate crystals. Other causes of intrinsic renal failure are noted in Table 11.1.

Postrenal failure is due to obstructive uropathy. It accounts for about 10% of cases of neonatal ARF, predominantly in boys with posterior urethral valves. Obstruction due to nonpatency of an existing Foley catheter should initially be ruled out. Other causes are listed in Table 11.1.

DIAGNOSIS

History and Physical Examination

The history may reveal risk factors for dehydration such as emesis, diarrhea, decreased oral intake, or fever. Clinical findings may include decreased urine output, anemia, or lethargy. Physical examination can demonstrate hypertension, edema, a flank mass, or even posterior pharynx erythema or a rash that can be related to glomerulonephritis.

TABLE 11.1. CAUSES OF ACUTE RENAL FAILURE

- Prerenal failure
  - Hypovolemia
    - Hemorrhage
      - Adrenal hemorrhage
      - Intraventricular hemorrhage
      - Trauma
      - Twin-twin transfusion
    - Dehydration
    - "3rd spacing"
      - Postoperative
      - Sepsis
      - ECMO
      - NEC
      - Ascites
      - Pancreatitis
      - Peritonitis
    - Burns
    - Osmotic diuresis: diabetes mellitus
    - Insensible losses: bilirubin lights, fever
  - Hypoperfusion
    - Cardiac failure
    - Hypotension
    - Ineffective circulating volume
  - Hypoxia
- Renal failure (intrinsic)
  - Allergic/collagen vascular disease
    - SLE
    - Polyarteritis nodosa
    - Henoch-Schonlein purpura
    - Acute interstitial nephritis
  - ATN
    - Postoperative (abdominal, cardiac)
    - Nephrotoxins
  - Congenital
    - Renal agenesis
    - Renal dysplasia
    - Polycystic kidney disease
  - Infectious
    - Poststreptococcal glomerulonephritis
    - Bacterial endocarditis
    - Congital syphilis, CMV
    - Sepsis
  - Metabolic
    - Uric acid, oxalic acid nephropathy
    - Pigment: hemoglobinuria, myoglobinuria
  - Heavy metals
  - Neoplasia
    - Tumor infiltration
    - Uric acid nephropathy
  - Pharmacologic
    - Radiocontrast agents
    - Indomethacin
  - Trauma
  - Vascular
    - HUS
    - TTP
    - Drug-induced vasculitis
    - Renal artery thrombosis
    - Renal vein thrombosis
    - Aortic thrombosis
  - Hypoxia
  - Uric acid nephropathy
- After renal failure (obstructive)
  - Congenital
  - Extrinsic obstruction
    - Tumor compression
  - Intrinsic obstruction
    - Bilateral ureteropelvic junction obstruction
    - Posterior urethral valves
  - Neurogenic
    - Myelomeningocele

ECMO, extracorporeal membrane oxygenation; NEC, necrotizing enterocolitis; SLE, systemic lupus erythematosus; ATN, acute tubular necrosis; CMV, cytomegalovirus; HUS, hemolytic uremic syndrome; TTP, thrombotic thrombocytopenic purpura.

Laboratory Evaluation

Laboratory findings are important in determining the type and degree of renal failure (Table 11.2). Urinalysis with microscopic evaluation should be obtained. Glomerular disease is suspected if the urine tests positive for blood and albumin. If red blood cell casts are present, glomerulonephritis, hemolytic uremic syndrome or vasculitis are possible diagnoses. The presence of hemoglobin without red blood cells suggests hemolysis or rhabdomyolysis. Interstitial nephritis is discovered by leukocyte casts and eosinophils. Tumor lysis syndrome is associated with uric acid crystals on urinalysis.

Urine output of less than 1 mL/kg/h requires investigation, but oliguria can be unreliable due to either inaccurate documentation or incorrect as occurs in cases of watery diarrhea. It is only present in 50% of patients with ARF.

Elevated serum BUN and creatinine are hallmarks of ARF. Elevated BUN can also be due to a high-protein diet, starvation, gastrointestinal bleeding, dehydration, steroid use, and sepsis with hypercatabolism. As a result, other findings are used in conjunction, such as an elevated creatinine, which directly reflects tubular function.

Electrolyte and water abnormalities are clinically crucial aspects of renal failure. Potassium excess and metabolic acidosis often occur and are detected by routine serum measurements. If a patient has urine output, urinary electrolytes and creatinine as well as osmolality should be assessed at the same time as serum studies. These values may not be reliable if a patient has recently received diuretics. These results will allow for calculation of the fractional excretion of sodium (FE_{Na}).

$$FE_{Na} = \frac{Ur_{Na} \times Se_{Cr}}{Se_{Na} \times Ur_{Cr}} \times 100$$

FE_{Na} of less than 1% in full-term infants and children or less than 2.5% in neonates suggests prerenal azotemia. FE_{Na} of 1% to 3% may indicate obstructive renal failure. FE_{Na} of greater than 2.5% suggests intrinsic renal failure.

The FE_{Na} is complicated by maturational change in sodium handling with poor specificity for prerenal failure in the very-low-birth-weight infant because values for prerenal failure overlap with those for intrinsic renal failure. In fact, infants delivered before 32 weeks' gestation have a normal FE_{Na} of greater than 5%.

Urine specific gravity should be less than 1.030 to show adequate hydration. In general, urine osmolality is a more reliable indicator of concentrating ability than is specific gravity.

Serum electrolytes and especially BUN and creatinine are the best indicators of glomerular and tubular function. An increase in creatinine by 0.3 to 0.5 mg/dL/day can sig-

TABLE 11.2. INDICES OF RENAL FAILURE

	Prerenal	Renal (Intrinsic)
Important (main indices)		
Fractional excretion sodium (FE_{Na})	<1 (<2.5 neonate)	>2 (>2.5 neonate)
Serum Creatinine (Cr)	Normal	Elevated
Serum BUN	Increased	Increased
Urine osmolality (osm)	>500 (>400 neonate)	<350 (<400 neonate)
Other indices		
Urine sodium (Na)	<10	>20
Urine urea/serum urea	>8	<3
Urine Cr/serum Cr	>40 (>30 neonate)	<20 (<10 neonate)
Urine osm/serum osm	>1.3	<1.1 (<1 neonate)
Renal failure index (RFI)	<1 (<3 neonate)	>1 (>3 neonate)
Fractional excretion urea (FE_{urea})	0.2–0.3	0.4–0.7

Formulas:

$$\textit{Creatinine clearance} = (140 - \textit{age in years}) \times \frac{\textit{wt in kg}}{72} \times Se_{Cr}\ (mg/dL)$$

$$= \frac{Ur_{Cr}\ (mg/dL) \times \text{Urine volume (mL/day)}}{Se_{Cr}\ (mg/dL) \times 1440\ \text{min/day}}$$

$$= \frac{0.48 \times \textit{length (cm)}}{Se_{Cr}}\ \text{(for children)}$$

Fractional excretion of sodium:

$$FE_{Na} = \frac{Ur_{Na} \times Se_{Cr}}{Se_{Na} \times Ur_{Cr}} \times 100$$

$$\textit{Renal failure index (RFI)} = \frac{Ur_{Na} \times Se_{Cr}}{Ur_{Cr}}$$

$$\textit{Bicarbonate deficit} = 0.5 \times wt\ (kg) \times (\textit{desired } HCO_3 - \textit{measured } HCO_3)$$

nify an acute decrease in GFR. A newborn can have a higher creatinine level, which reflects maternal creatinine levels, but should decrease to 0.3 to 0.4 mg/dL within the first 3 to 4 days of life. A diagnosis of ARF should be considered if serum creatinine fails to decrease in the first week. It should be noted that creatinine can be falsely elevated by chromogens such as ketones and cephalosporins. A BUN/creatinine ratio of greater than 20 suggests that there is increased urea production or increased tubular reabsorption of urea and not renal failure. Monitoring serum electrolytes is important because grave imbalances can cause life-threatening arrythmia or sudden cardiac arrest.

Imaging

The size of the kidneys, collecting system, and bladder should be evaluated by ultrasonography. The renal vessels should be assessed for patency and resistive indices.

Radionuclide imaging can provide more information about renal perfusion and function. Radiotracers such as technetium 99 diethylenetriamine pentacetic acid (^{99}Tc-DTPA) and technetium 99 disodium N-mercaptoacetylglycylglycyl-glycinate 2-N-S-oxotechnetate (^{99}Tc-MAG_3) demonstrate renal function and parenchymal uptake. DTPA is less effective in neonates and patients with impaired renal function because of its dependence on GFR. MAG_3 is currently the best choice for neonates because it approximates effective renal plasma flow (its excretion is by glomerular filtration and active renal tubular transport). This agent has excellent specificity for the kidney, gives high kidney:background ratios and allows measurement of split renal function. In evaluating for obstruction, MAG_3 can be used for diuretic renography. This allows for tracer to be eliminated from the dilated collecting system in cases not involving obstruction and slow clearance or increased activity in the collecting system with obstruction.

Voiding cystourethrography is also used to evaluate lower urinary tract abnormalities such as vesicoureteral reflux, posterior urethral valves, or bladder diverticuli.

When the diagnosis remains in doubt and a treatment plan is uncertain, renal biopsy can be performed percutaneously with ultrasonographic guidance.

COMPLICATIONS

Complications of ARF include fluid overload, hyperkalemia, and acidosis. Fluid overload can lead to substantial edema and may cause hypertension and pulmonary compromise. Increasing oxygen requirements in a patient with renal failure suggest impending respiratory compromise due to pulmonary edema. Fluid restriction and pharmacologic diuresis may not be sufficient, and dialysis or hemofiltration may be required. Unfortunately, malnutrition often follows fluid restriction because total parenteral nutrition is often the only source of fluid that may be discarded in favor of other medications. Hyperkalemia and acidosis can lead to diminished cardiac function and fatal arrhythmias. Other electrolyte imbalances such as hyponatremia, hyperphosphatemia, and hypocalcemia also can be seen and should be monitored so that corrective measures can be taken as needed.

Long-term consequences from ARF include chronic renal insufficiency with or without dependence on renal replacement therapy. Patients also may experience persistence of hypertension and renal tubular dysfunction. Forty percent of patients surviving ARF will have abnormal creatinine clearance and a decreased ability to concentrate urine. Ten percent will have small kidneys by ultrasonographic analysis up to 15 years later.

TREATMENT

In cases of acute oliguria, attention should first be directed to correcting hypoxemia and hypotension by addressing their underlying causes. A Foley catheter should be placed or flushed if present. If oliguria persists, a fluid challenge of 10 to 20 mL/kg of 0.45% normal saline can be administered as a diagnostic and therapeutic strategy. Up to 70% of neonates and infants with oliguria respond favorably to a fluid challenge. Return of adequate urine production with fluid administration suggests a prerenal cause. Central venous pressure (CVP) monitoring is sometimes useful and should exceed 10 mm Hg to suggest adequate volume resuscitation. Assessing fluid intake and output, body weight, and vital signs is also useful in determining fluid status. After 1 to 2 hours of monitoring for hourly urine output, urine electrolytes, creatinine, osmolality, and urinalysis should be analyzed concurrently with serum electrolytes, BUN, and creatinine. If the CVP or clinical judgment suggests adequate resuscitation, a trial of furosemide at 3 to 5 mg/kg should be administered intravenously over 20 to 30 minutes and a furosemide drip at 0.1 to 0.3 mg/kg/h for 3 to 4 hours can be considered. A dopamine drip at 3 to 5 μg/kg/min also can be used to augment renal flow. If there is still no response, intrinsic renal failure is suspected.

The next clinical strategy is the management of intrinsic renal failure. This can be achieved by adjusting medications (Table 11.3), restricting use of nephrotoxic agents, restricting fluid intake to insensible losses, and obtaining frequent electrolyte measurements.

Anecdotally, we examined two premature infants (gestational age of 28–32 weeks and weight of 800–1,100 g) who presented with hypotension, respiratory distress, and anuric renal failure. Both neonates required ventilator support, had adequate fluid resuscitation, and received pressor support with dopamine, dobutamine, and epinephrine. Despite a systolic blood pressure of more than 50 mm Hg, no urine output was noted. A single dose of furosemide at 4 to 6 mg/kg was administered without any effect. In both infants, one dose of dexamethasone at 2 mg/kg was administered after no results from other measures. Both infants

TABLE 11.3. COMMONLY USED MEDICATIONS IN ICU PATIENTS REQUIRING DRUG ADJUSTMENTS FOR RENAL FAILURE

Aminoglycosides
Amphotericin B
Cephalosporins
Chloral hydrate
Digoxin
Penicillins
Phenobarbital
Ranitidine
Spironolactone
Vancomycin

Every patient with renal failure should have a pharmacy and nephrology consult.
Most medications use the same dosage but vary the dosing interval depending on creatinine clearance or glomerular filtration rate.
Drugs removed by dialysis: penicillin, sulfonamide, cephalosporin, aminoglycoside.
Drugs not removed by dialysis: amphotericin B, steroids, coumadin, digoxin, furosemide.

began to have a brisk diuresis 6 to 8 hours after the steroid dose. Patent ductus arteriosus and congenital heart disease should be ruled out with an echocardiogram as these can also lead to renal insufficiency.

Control of hyperkalemia begins with eliminating any administration of exogenous potassium. In emergent situations, such as markedly elevated serum potassium or electrocardiographic changes, the administration of sodium bicarbonate, calcium gluconate, and combinations of glucose and insulin have been used. However, these measures only redistribute potassium rather than eliminate it. Kayexalate (Sanofi Winthrop, New York), an ion exchange resin that permanently binds potassium, can be administered orally or as an enema and will lower serum potassium 1mEq/L in 4 to 6 hours. Dialysis may be required on an urgent basis to control hyperkalemia.

In nonoliguric renal failure, detected by an increasing creatinine level, treatment is easier because fluid restriction is not as critical, and the prognosis is usually excellent. Figure 11.1 shows a treatment algorithm.

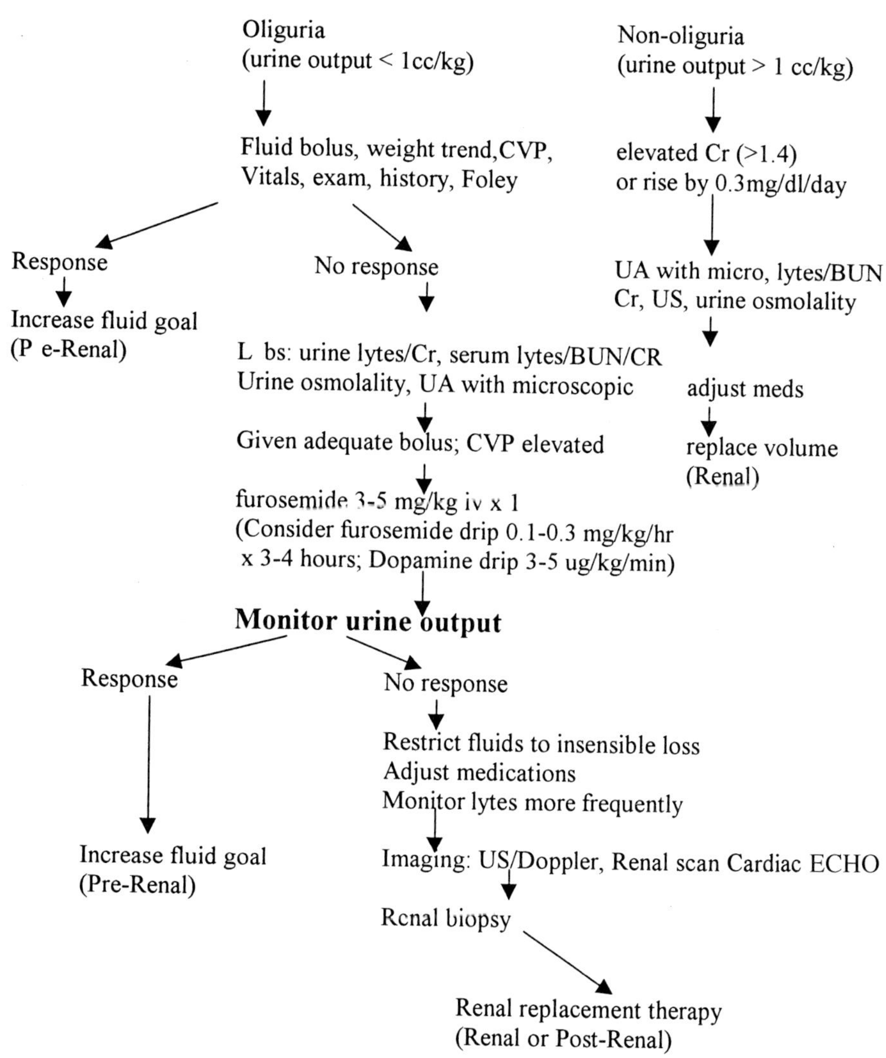

FIGURE 11.1. Algorithm for renal failure.

RENAL REPLACEMENT THERAPY

When management of volume and electrolytes with less invasive means begins to fail, renal replacement therapy can maintain homeostasis for months to years. In ARF it is instituted with the expectation of recovery in 2 to 6 weeks. Included in renal replacement therapies are peritoneal dialysis (PD), hemodialysis, or hemofiltration. Indications for considering these therapeutic measures are excessive fluid retention, electrolyte imbalance, compromised respiratory function, and inability for adequate nutritional or medicinal infusions. Hyperkalemia refractory to medical management may require urgent dialysis.

Peritoneal dialysis is most commonly used in neonates and infants. Patients requiring renal replacement therapy are quite ill (1-year mortality rate of 35%). Only 26% undergo complete recovery. A Tenckhoff catheter is placed into the peritoneal cavity and dialysate is chosen based on the patient's hydration status using a more concentrated dialysate (3.86%) in hypervolemic patients and a more dilute solution (1.36%) in hypovolemic patients. Infusion volumes of 20 to 50 mL/kg are used per exchange, and dwell time varies depending on peritoneal membrane permeability. Peritoneal dialysis can remove urea, creatinine, PO_4, and many drugs, in addition to electrolytes. Careful monitoring is required to prevent dehydration and hypernatremia from hyperosmolar dialysate. Complications of PD include fluid balance error, catheter malfunction and loss of peritoneal domain, bowel perforation, peritonitis, and protein losses.

Hemodialysis is used routinely in children and adults but requires special consideration in infants. Extracorporeal blood volume needs to be minimized and careful monitoring of vital signs must be accomplished. Vascular access that is dependable and functional is a major challenge in neonates, especially in those weighing less than 2 to 3 kg. Comorbid conditions make these neonates more prone to hypotension with initiation of hemodialysis.

Hemofiltration is not as efficient at removing solute as it is at removing fluid, while minimizing hypotensive episodes. The process allows for aggressive management of fluid overload. The inefficiency at solute removal requires the removal of much more fluid in order to remove the same amount of solute. When a patient on extracorporeal membrane oxygenation is receiving hemofiltration for both volume removal and solute removal, it is necessary to remove much more fluid and then subsequently return some of the volume without the unwanted solutes. For example, if the goal is to remove 30 mL/h and also some potassium, one has to hemofilter at 100mL/h and replace it with 70 mL/h of 0.45 normal saline to achieve both goals of eliminating volume and solutes.

SUGGESTED READINGS

Ronco C, Ronconi M, Bellomo R. Acute renal failure in infants and children. In: Grenvik A, Ayres SM, Holbrook PR, et al., eds. *Textbook of critical care, 4th ed.* Philadelphia: WB Saunders. 2000: 1690–1702.

Seri I, Jacquelyn E, Tulassay T. Renal insufficiency and acute renal failure. In: Taeusch HW, Ballard RA, eds. *Avery's disease of the newborn, 7th ed.* Philadelphia: WB Saunders. 1998:1158–1164.

Stapleton FB, Jones DP, Green RS. Acute renal failure in neonates: incidence, etiology and outcome. *Pediatric Nephrology* 1987;1: 314–320.

Stewart CL, Barnett R. Acute renal failure in infants, children, and adults. *Crit Care Clin* 1997;13:575–590.

12

RESPIRATORY FAILURE AND SUPPORT

JAMES H. HERTZOG

Respiratory failure is the most common reason for admission to the pediatric intensive care unit. Respiratory failure may be preexistent in children requiring surgical treatment, may be a direct result of the surgical condition, or may be the sequela of surgical intervention. Therefore, an appreciation for both the causes of respiratory failure in children and the methods of respiratory management is vital for pediatric surgeons.

I ask myself five questions when I am evaluating the etiology of respiratory failure in a child. First, *does the child have the drive to breathe?* Premature infants are at risk for the development of apnea at any time due to the immaturity of their respiratory drive system. Electrolyte imbalance, hypothermia, or intercurrent infection may accentuate this risk. Furthermore, full-term infants who are less than 48 to 52 weeks' conceptual age have an increased risk of apnea associated with anesthetics, narcotics, and sedatives. Metabolic derangements, central sleep apnea, intoxication, primary central nervous system disease, infection, or traumatic brain injury also may contribute to an inadequate respiratory drive in children. Second, *does the child have the strength to breathe?* Higher airway resistance due to smaller airway caliber, greater chest wall compliance, the relative weakness of the intercostal muscles, and the greater fatigability of the diaphragm in infants and children increases the risk of respiratory failure due to inadequate strength. Preexisting thoracic dystrophy or surgical alterations of the thoracic cage, increased abdominal size with impingement on the diaphragm, phrenic or intercostal nerve injury, splinting secondary to inadequate analgesia, and inadequate nutritional reserve may further exacerbate these problems. Together, inadequate respiratory drive and strength can be considered a failure of the "respiratory pump."

Third, I ask, *is there a problem with the extrathoracic airway?* Obstruction of the airway from precedent infection, intrinsic masses or malacia, extrinsic compression, or postoperative edema may necessitate respiratory support. Functional obstruction also may need to be addressed in those children with obstructive sleep apnea or pharyngeal hypotonia who require postoperative narcotic analgesia or pharmacologic restraint. Fourth, I ask, *is dysfunction of the intrathoracic airways or gas-exchanging units present?* Smaller airway caliber and alveolar size, the lack of collateral alveolar ventilation, and the similarity between closing capacity and functional residual capacity in infants and small children increases the possibility of atelectasis. Primary lung disease or direct surgical lung injury, as well as secondary lung injury from the inflammatory response elicited by the underlying disease process and surgery, also may result in respiratory failure. Extrathoracic airway abnormalities and intrathoracic pulmonary dysfunction can be grouped together as a failure in the "lung."

Lastly, I consider, *is there an abnormality in another organ system or a special therapeutic need that might require the implementation of respiratory support, even though a problem has not been identified by the preceding four questions?* For example, children who have inadequate oxygen delivery secondary to cardiac failure, have evolving neurologic failure, or need to be kept motionless postoperatively will require respiratory support.

BASIC RESPIRATORY SUPPORT

The support of children with impending or existing respiratory failure varies in complexity and invasiveness. The first step, however, is to provide supplemental oxygen. Oxygen is a cheap and readily available drug that no patient should be denied. As with any drug, care must be used when administering oxygen. The toxic effects of high concentrations of inspired oxygen to the lung and the immature retina is demonstrated within hours, and children with parallel pulmonary and systemic circulations may develop excessive pulmonary blood flow at the expense of systemic blood flow because oxygen lowers the pulmonary vascular resistance. Oxygen may be delivered in a variety of ways. Nasal cannula oxygen provides modest levels of supplemen-

J. H. Hertzog: Department of Pediatrics, Thomas Jefferson University, Philadelphia, Pennsylvania; and Department of Anesthesiology and Critical Care Medicine, Alfred I. duPont Hospital for Children, Wilmington, Delaware.

tal oxygen and may be relatively more effective than other devices in infants who are obligate nose breathers. Cannulas are generally well tolerated and allow easy access to the child. Oxygen flow rates should generally not exceed 4 L/min, because higher flows are more likely to cause mucosal irritation. The amount of oxygen delivered to the gas-exchanging units is difficult to quantify and dependent on the oxygen flow rate, anatomic dead space, minute ventilation, and amount of room air entrained by the child. Oxygen masks in general deliver higher concentrations of oxygen. Options for masks include the simple mask, partial rebreather mask, Venturi mask, and nonrebreather mask, each providing higher concentrations of supplemental oxygen, respectively. Maintaining the placement of a mask may be difficult in infants and young children. The use of oxygen hoods and tents avoids this difficulty, but oxygen concentrations are diminished whenever the hood or tent is entered, and visual monitoring of the child becomes more difficult.

INTERMEDIATE RESPIRATORY SUPPORT

Therapies aimed at enhancing the clearance of tracheobronchial secretions and recruiting atelectatic lung units are often used. Chest physiotherapy and postural drainage has a long tradition of use in children who require assistance in the mobilization of secretions, but any advantage that this procedure may provide must be weighed against the effect of transferred kinetic energy on suture lines and the concurrent increase in oxygen consumption. Incentive spirometry devices, or simpler methods such as blowing bubbles, are also used in an effort to reverse atelectasis and have few side effects except for the possibility of gastric distension from swallowed air. Mechanical devices also may be used to help promote cough and the reversal of atelectasis. Intermittent positive pressure breathing provides short periods of positive pressure to the tracheobronchial tree via a mouthpiece, a facemask, or an artificial airway. A "cough-o-lator" also adds active exhalation (i.e., a negative pressure), while intrapulmonary ventilation (IPV) provides high-frequency oscillatory breaths for short periods, again via a mouthpiece, facemask, or artificial airway. Despite their extensive use, there are no studies that demonstrate conclusively the effectiveness of these therapies in children. If the potential risks of these therapies are acceptable, then it may be worth trying these therapies and monitoring for effectiveness. In my experience, timely postoperative mobilization, along with effective analgesia to prevent splinting and hypoventilation, are often the most effective strategies. Bronchodilators, in addition to their effect on airway smooth muscle, also may enhance mucociliary motility and the clearance of secretions. Although this effect may not be dramatic, it may be worth a trial of bronchodilator therapy if there are no contraindications to their use.

When caring for an infant who may be at risk for postoperative apnea secondary to an immature central respiratory drive, the administration of central respiratory stimulants may be considered. Both caffeine and theophylline are used for this purpose.

Noninvasive forms of administering positive airway pressure or ventilatory support for more than just brief periods are the next level of respiratory support complexity to be considered. Continuous positive airway pressure (CPAP) may reverse atelectasis and restore functional residual capacity, improving oxygenation and abolishing apnea. In infants, a simple nasal cannula with a 2- to 4-L gas flow may provide some level of CPAP. This level is likely to be low, and CPAP is probably only effectively delivered by this method in small infants. In larger infants or in those infants who require a higher level of CPAP, nasal prongs or tubes that extend to the posterior pharynx may be effective, whereas older children and adolescents may receive CPAP via a nasal or full facemask. Initial CPAP levels of 3 to 5 cm water may be used and subsequently increased based on clinical response. Likewise, supplemental oxygen provided through the CPAP system can be titrated to effect based on pulse oximetry measurements. CPAP levels above 10 to 12 cm water are difficult to maintain and suggests that another strategy be considered if the desired clinical results have not been obtained. Infants and children commonly tolerate CPAP quite well. The drawbacks to this technique include the risk of gastric distension, although this is uncommon for the levels of CPAP outlined above, the relative contraindication to oral or nasogastric feeding, and the risk of skin breakdown from a tightly applied facemask. The possibility of aspiration is often discussed but is not reported in pediatric series. Likewise, the development of subcutaneous emphysema, especially after airway or facial surgery, is possible but has not been reported.

When ventilatory support is needed, it can be delivered noninvasively by using mask bilevel positive airway pressure (BiPAP). Although less efficient than positive pressure ventilation delivered via a tracheal tube, BiPAP can be effective either as a primary support modality or as a "bridge" between ventilation via a tracheal tube and spontaneous ventilation. BiPAP can be delivered in a spontaneous mode, where each spontaneous patient breath is supported; a timed mode, where a set number of breaths is delivered independent of patient effort; or a timed/spontaneous mode, where the attributes of both modes are combined. I generally avoid the timed mode because of the potential patient–ventilator dissynchrony. Settings to be determined include an inspiratory positive airway pressure (IPAP, analogous to peak inspiratory pressure, or PIP), an expiratory positive airway pressure (EPAP, analogous to positive end-expiratory pressure, or PEEP), and an inspiratory time and mechanical breath rate when a timed mode is used. Supplemental oxygen is typically added by a separate oxygen flow connected directly to the mask. I begin with low settings, such as an IPAP of 4 to 6 cm water and an EPAP of 2 to 3 cm water, to allow the child time to adjust to the sensation of pressure being introduced into the pharynx and larynx. As tolerated, the settings are increased until clinical goals are met. I generally do not exceed an IPAP of 20 cm water or an EPAP of 12 cm water, because higher pressures are difficult to achieve with BiPAP, the risk of gastric distension increases, and it is likely that another strategy needs to be considered. As with CPAP, BiPAP is generally well tolerated, although in some cases judicious use of sedation may be required. The major advantage of BiPAP is that it avoids tracheal intubation and provides support that can be intermittently discontinued as tolerated. The risks of BiPAP are as outlined for CPAP.

Another form of noninvasive ventilation is negative pressure ventilation. With negative pressure ventilation, the child is placed in a tank device or body suit. A negative pressure is generated around the thorax at a specified rate interval such that gas flow from the atmosphere into the lung is augmented. Negative pressures up to −30 cm water are often used, delivered at rates titrated to clinical effect. Supplemental oxygen can be introduced at the nose and mouth as needed. Negative pressure ventilation is advantageous for the same reasons as for BiPAP. In addition, patients with "passive" pulmonary circulation may benefit from the augmented pulmonary blood flow created by the negative intrathoracic pressure. The disadvantages of negative pressure ventilation include the relative inaccessibility of the child, the limitations in positioning, and the risk of skin breakdown on the neck where a tight seal must be maintained. These problems and the increased use of other ventilatory modalities have made negative pressure ventilation uncommon.

ADVANCED RESPIRATORY SUPPORT

Positive pressure ventilation via a tracheal tube remains the most common form of ventilatory support. "Conventional" modes of ventilation include volume control and pressure control. With volume control, a tidal volume is selected, whereas with pressure control a peak inspiratory pressure (PIP) is selected. The advantage of volume control is that a known minute ventilation is delivered and changes in pulmonary compliance can be detected by changes in the PIP. The disadvantage is that high PIPs may be achieved with excessive tidal volumes or markedly diminished pulmonary compliance. These advantages and disadvantages are inverted for pressure control ventilation, in that dangerously high PIPs can be avoided but minute ventilation varies with compliance changes. I generally select volume control ventilation, but if the resultant PIPs generated by a tidal volume necessary for adequate gas exchange exceed 35 to 40 cm water, I convert to pressure control ventilation. I also choose pressure control ventilation in situations where excessive airway pressures may endanger suture lines in the airway or for the ventilation of premature infants who are at greater risk for barotrauma.

A second decision that must be made when using either of these modes is the manner in which breaths are to be delivered. I use synchronized intermittent mandatory ventilation (SIMV). With SIMV, a preselected number of breaths are delivered but synchronized to the child's respiratory effort. In addition, a continuous gas flow through the breathing circuit is available for spontaneous breathing between machine breaths. This results in less patient/ventilator dissynchrony. Also, as the mechanical ventilator rate is decreased during weaning, the child still receives the benefit of a fully supported mechanical breath, decreasing the risk of atelectasis development. Another option sometimes used in pediatric patients is assist-control ventilation, where every patient-initiated breath receives full mechanical support. The disadvantage to this method is that weaning requires a decrease in tidal volume or PIP, potentially increasing the risk for atelectasis as these parameters are minimized.

I select an initial tidal volume of 7 to 10 mL/kg when using volume control or an initial PIP of 20 to 25 cm water (and lower in premature infants) when using pressure control ventilation. Subsequently I evaluate for good chest rise and air movement and evidence of adequate gas exchange, adjusting the tidal volume or PIP as appropriate. Other ventilatory parameters that must be set include a PEEP, respiratory rate, inspiratory time, and fraction of inspired oxygen (FiO_2). I initially choose a PEEP of 3 to 5 cm water for children with minimally diseased or normal lungs. If oxygenation is suboptimal or atelectasis is present, increasing levels of PEEP are used. Generally PEEP levels of up to 15 cm water can be well tolerated, but if higher levels are needed it may be reasonable to consider a high-frequency ventilatory strategy. Mechanical respiratory rates are based on age-appropriate rates, with rates of 10 to 15, 15 to 25, and 25 to 40 breaths per minute being appropriate for adolescents, children, and infants, respectively. Subsequent adjustments are made based on the adequacy of ventilation and patient comfort. Inspiratory times are also age based, with a common range from 0.5 to 1 second from infancy to adolescence, resulting in an inspiratory to expiratory (I:E) ratio of roughly 1:4. Under certain circumstances, such as with acute lung injury, extending the inspiratory time and equalizing or inversing the I:E ratio may be helpful in alveolar recruitment and oxygenation. With the initiation of mechanical ventilation, I use an FiO_2 of 100%, but as the situation stabilizes, an immediate priority is to decrease the FiO_2 based on pulse oximetry measurements. An FiO_2 of less than 60% is generally considered to be a nontoxic level, although further reduction is warranted if oxygenation is acceptable, because any level of supplemental oxygen is potentially toxic.

Another consideration is the use of pressure support ventilation. Pressure support ventilation delivers a preset level of pressure to the airway when the child initiates a breath. This pressure is continued through the majority of the inspiratory cycle, then discontinued so that expiration is not impeded. There is no control component to this form of ventilation, so no mechanical breaths are guaranteed. Although I do not generally use pressure support as a primary mode of ventilatory support in children, I often use low levels of pressure support in conjunction with SIMV. Pressure support levels of 5 to 10 cm water assist the child in overcoming the resistance to spontaneous breathing resulting from the ventilator and the circuit while adding little to no true ventilatory support.

ALTERNATIVE RESPIRATORY SUPPORT MEASURES

Although the majority of children with respiratory failure can be adequately managed with the above-outlined respiratory supports, acceptable gas exchange may not be achieved with these methods in some children with severe pulmonary processes. "Acceptable" gas exchange includes maintaining the arterial pH above 7.25 either through ventilation or the provision of exogenous buffers (an approach termed permissive hypercarbia) and maintaining adequate arterial oxygenation such that lactic acidosis does not develop secondary to inadequate oxygen delivery. I consider the use of "alternative" respiratory therapies when the PIP exceeds 35 to 40 cm water, when the FiO_2 cannot be decreased to 60% or less, or when a PEEP exceeding 12 to 15 cm water is needed. When oxygenation is the issue, prone positioning may be extremely effective and is relatively simple to perform in infants and children. This may not be possible, however, in patients who have undergone abdominal surgery. As mentioned above, equalizing or inverting the I:E ratio also may improve oxygenation, but ventilation may suffer. Surfactant administration by tracheal instillation is a well-proven therapy in premature infants with respiratory distress syndrome secondary to surfactant deficiency. Success with this therapy also has been demonstrated in older infants and children and may be considered.

If there is still no improvement in the child's status, high-frequency oscillatory ventilation (HFOV) should be considered. The advantage to HFOV is that high mean airway pressures to recruit atelectatic alveoli can be achieved without overstretching the gas-exchanging units, as occurs with high levels of volume or pressure control ventilation. Thus, the risks for barotrauma (or more precisely volutrauma) are minimized. In addition, HFOV can be used in the management of pulmonary air leak syndromes. The disadvantage of HFOV is that with every disconnection of the ventilator, alveolar derecruitment occurs and it may take 1 or 2 hours to regain this lost volume. Therefore, children who need frequent tracheal suctioning are not good candidates for HFOV. In addition, the intrathoracic pressure produced by HFOV diminishes preload and may decrease cardiac output in intravascularly depleted children. Furthermore, children with heterogeneous lung disease may not do well with HFOV, because relatively healthy areas of the lung may be overdistended as efforts are made to reexpand affected lung spaces.

To initiate HFOV, the following settings must be determined. A mean airway pressure (MAP) must be selected, and commonly is set at 4 to 8 cm water above the MAP that is being used for conventional ventilation. The frequency of oscillations is measured in hertz, and this setting is determined by patient age. The available range of hertz is 15 (used in infants) to 3 (used in adolescents and adults). The power or "Δ P" refers to the extent of piston displacement and is qualitatively determined by the "wiggle factor." The optimal wiggle factor is achieved when oscillations are visualized between the child's clavicles and pelvis. Inspiratory time is routinely set at 33%, a bias flow of 20 L/min or greater is used, and the initial FiO_2 is set at 100%. As the child is started on HFOV, the pulse oximeter is monitored so that the oxygen saturation (SpO_2) is maintained above 90%. If the SpO_2 decreases below this level, the MAP may be increased by 1 or 2 cm water until the desired saturations are achieved. After about an hour of ventilation, a chest roentgenogram is obtained, and lung expansion to nine posterior ribs in the midclavicular line suggests ideal lung recruitment. Subsequently, decreasing the FiO_2 to 60% or less is the first priority. As the child improves, support is diminished by decreasing the FiO_2 and MAP as long as oxygenation is adequate and by decreasing the Δ P as long as ventilation is adequate. The hertz, inspiratory time, and bias flow are generally not manipulated. When HFOV is being used to manage an air leak syndrome, lower MAP and higher FiO_2 are used in an effort to allow the air leak to seal.

Nitric oxide is another therapy that may be considered in children with severe oxygenation deficits or pulmonary hypertension. When used as an inhaled gas through the ventilator circuit, it selectively produces pulmonary vasodilation in ventilated lung units, thus improving ventilation/perfusion matching. Although initial trials have demonstrated that nitric oxide decreases pulmonary artery pressures and improves oxygenation in many children with respiratory failure, no change in mortality rates with its use has been demonstrated, although a decreased need for extracorporeal membrane oxygenation has been shown. Currently, nitric oxide is only approved for patients with documented pulmonary hypertension.

Extracorporeal supports for respiratory failure, such as extracorporeal membrane oxygenation and extracorporeal carbon dioxide removal, have been successfully used as a "rescue" therapy when other therapies have failed, and they are discussed in other chapters. Liquid ventilation, where gas exchange is achieved by the use of oxygenated perfluorocarbon, has shown promise in animal studies and small clinical trials but has not been approved for routine clinical use.

EDITOR'S NOTES

Although we are often amazed by the resilience of children who endure huge operations and tolerate significant physiologic challenges, we realize quickly how fragile they are when they demonstrate airway compromise or significant respiratory embarrassment. Dealing effectively with a patient with respiratory compromise requires not only skill and experience, but also a "cool head" and a systematic approach that is both logical and flexible. In addition, the primary surgical team's active participation in the care of the patients and help in balancing postoperative factors and primary respiratory issues cannot be overemphasized.

The goals for postoperative patients who require respiratory support are to get the patient back to his or her baseline respiratory status (or better) as soon as possible and to avoid complications of the support mechanisms we use. This includes using the least invasive and lowest level of support that the patient requires without avoiding more aggressive therapy (intubation and mechanical ventilation) when clearly indicated.

In infants, a simple nasal cannula often can deliver significant "ventilatory support" by providing some degree of positive pressure and a stimulus to breathe. On the other hand, without flow the nasal cannula apparatus obstructs air flow and can result in hypoxia and distress if the oxygen is merely turned off and the cannula is left in place. Newborns who have general anesthesia even for relatively minor surgical procedures often require intubation and ventilation in a monitored setting. This is attributable to central apnea that can be exaggerated during the first 12 to 24 hours due to a lingering effect of anesthetic agents and narcotics. A discussion regarding this routine and generally safe practice with the parents prior to the operation goes a long way to help ease their apprehension and avoid the perception that there has been a complication of the surgery.

Drug-induced paralysis (pancuronium) was commonly used in the past, especially for infants; however, it is no longer used routinely in most centers. There are several well-known disadvantages, including tachycardia, excessive edema from capillary leak, the potential for paralysis without adequate sedation, and muscular atrophy with prolonged use, and few specific advantages except in certain circumstances.

When weaning a patient from ventilatory support, it is a common error to focus on the CO_2 measurement alone, without considering the patient's overall acid-base status. For example, in a patient with a significant metabolic alkalosis, an elevated CO_2 represents normal physiology, not hypoventilation. Similarly, a patient compensates for a metabolic acidosis with hyperventilation and a low CO_2 so that weaning support prematurely in this situation results in increased work of breathing and worsening patient anxiety.

–P.M.

SUGGESTED READINGS

Arnold JH, Hanson JH, Toro-Figuero LO, et al. Prospective, randomized comparison of high-frequency oscillatory ventilation and conventional mechanical ventilation in pediatric respiratory failure. *Crit Care Med* 1994;22:1530–1539.

Dreyfuss D, Saumon G. Ventilator-induced lung injury. *Am J Respir Crit Care Med* 1998;157:294–323.

Padman R, Lawless ST, Kettrick RG. Noninvasive ventilation via bilevel positive airway pressure support in pediatric practice. *Crit Care Med* 1998;26:169–173.

Rodgers MC ed. *Textbook of pediatric intensive care, 3rd ed.* Baltimore: Williams & Wilkins, 1996.

Willson DF, Zaritsky A, Bauman LA, et al. Instillation of calf lung surfactant extract (calfactant) is beneficial in pediatric acute hypoxemic respiratory failure. *Crit Care Med* 1999;27:188–195.

13

EXTRACORPOREAL MEMBRANE OXYGENATION

FAWN C. LEWIS
MARLETA REYNOLDS
ROBERT M. ARENSMAN

Extracorporeal membrane oxygenation (ECMO) or extracorporeal life support describes a method of partial bedside cardiopulmonary support derived from the cardiopulmonary bypass experience in open-heart surgery. When conventional methods of pulmonary support are inadequate or when short-term mechanical cardiac assistance is indicated, ECMO therapy should be considered.

Diagnoses most often associated with referral for possible ECMO include meconium aspiration, persistent pulmonary hypertension of the newborn (PPHN), sepsis, pneumonia, congenital diaphragmatic hernia (CDH), and respiratory distress syndrome. In general terms, ECMO is considered when adequate ventilatory or circulatory support cannot be achieved with conventional therapy. ECMO is a means of providing temporary cardiopulmonary support and is not in and of itself a therapeutic process. Therefore, patients are only considered for ECMO support if the disease process being treated is transient, self-limited, or generally responsive to therapy. The inclusion criteria for ECMO are listed in Table 13.1. Intractable hypotension, hypercarbia, or hypotension form the basic criteria. Infants with treatable congenital pulmonary or cardiac anomalies or severe but transient pulmonary compromise (meconium aspiration, pulmonary hypertension) represent the majority of patients treated with ECMO, although occasionally older children or adolescents are candidates for ECMO therapy.

The contraindications to ECMO therapy are listed in Table 13.2. Because full systemic anticoagulation is mandatory, those with a contraindication to heparin therapy constitute the majority of patients who are not considered candidates. Infants with grade 1 intraventricular hemorrhage are considered for therapy in some ECMO programs; however, precautions are usually taken, such as allowing slightly longer activated clotting times and performing daily head ultrasonography. There is also an understanding that if the hemorrhage worsens, ECMO will be discontinued. Those with otherwise fatal conditions or irreversible disease processes are also generally excluded. This includes patients who have been exposed to prolonged high levels of support and in whom the effects of barotrauma on the lung parenchyma are irreversible (remodeling, fibrosis).

F. C. Lewis, M. Reynolds, and R. M. Arensman: Departments of Surgery and Pediatrics, Northwestern University Medical School; and Department of Pediatric General Surgery, Children's Memorial Hospital, Chicago, Illinois.

MODES OF ECMO

Venovenous ECMO is instituted via a double-lumen cannula placed from the right internal jugular vein into the right atrium of the heart. Side holes in the cannula allow blood returning to the right atrium to be directed through the catheter to the ECMO circuit (Fig. 13.1) where it passes through a countercurrent membrane oxygenator and a pumping mechanism. Blood is then returned via the tip of the double-lumen catheter into the right atrium toward the tricuspid valve where it continues its normal course through the cardiopulmonary circulation. Venovenous ECMO provides little cardiovascular support and is typically used only in patients who require only respiratory support and who have relatively normal cardiac function.

The advantages of venovenous ECMO include preservation of the carotid artery, relative ease of cannulation and decannulation, excellent CO_2 removal, maintenance of pulsatile systemic blood flow, and relative ease of weaning. The disadvantages include reliance on native cardiac function for cardiac output, flow that is sometimes limited by venous return to heart and by flow through the smaller venous side of the double-lumen cannula, and oxygen delivery that is limited because oxygenated blood is mixed with venous blood within the right atrium.

Venoarterial ECMO is instituted via single-lumen catheters placed into the right internal jugular vein and the right carotid artery. Blood is withdrawn from the right atrium, and after passing through the membrane oxygena-

TABLE 13.1. INCLUSION CRITERIA FOR ECMO SUPPORT

Inability to maintain Pa_{O_2} > 50 despite optimal conventional or oscillating ventilator therapy
Intractable respiratory acidosis
Barotrauma resulting in pneumothoraces and limiting conventional therapy
Respiratory insufficiency with expected short-term treatment response (<3–4 wk)
Bridge to cardiac transplantation
Postoperative cardiac dysfunction
Absence of absolute exclusion criteria

ECMO, extracorporeal membrane oxygenation.

TABLE 13.2. EXCLUSION CRITERIA FOR ECMO THERAPY

Weight <2.0 kg
Prolonged severe hypoxia
Multiple system disease
Prolonged mechanical ventilation (>7 days in neonates, longer in children and adults)
Contraindications to anticoagulation
Intraventricular hemorrhage (IVH)
Prematurity (neonates <35 weeks' gestation have a very high incidence of IVH)
Menstruation (patients at risk for menstruation can be hormonally controlled)
Head trauma
Fatal genetic condition or other unrelated fatal diagnosis
Lack of parental consent

ECMO, extracorporeal membrane oxygenation.

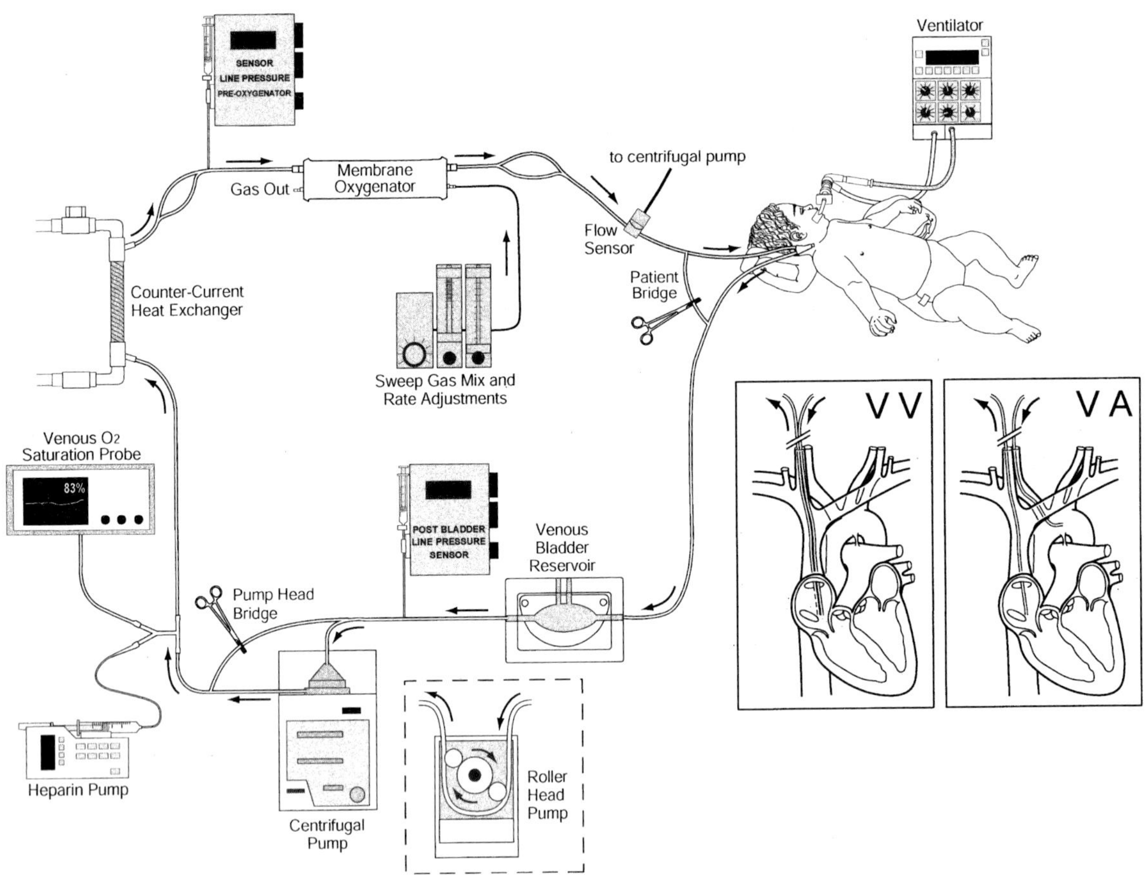

FIGURE 13.1. ECMO circuit. ECLS for Respiratory Dx.

tor is delivered directly into the aortic arch. Oxygen delivery is therefore superior to that achieved with venovenous ECMO, although the oxygenated blood may be diluted somewhat by blood shunted through a patent ductus arteriosus (PDA). Other advantages of venoarterial ECMO include excellent CO_2 removal, little dependence on native cardiac output, and ability to minimize ventilator settings and pressor requirements.

The decision whether to use venovenous or venoarterial ECMO depends partly on institutional and surgeon preference. In general, venovenous ECMO is preferred when there is primary respiratory failure and stable hemodynamics. Venoarterial ECMO is more appropriate when the primary indication is cardiac insufficiency or when respiratory disease is accompanied by significant cardiac dysfunction.

PREPARATION FOR ECMO

Candidates for ECMO need ultrasonography of the brain to rule out intraventricular hemorrhage and echocardiography to exclude significant cardiac anomalies. The history and all available laboratory and radiographic data are reviewed. If the disease process is felt to be reversible, conventional therapy has been optimized, and there are no contraindications, ECMO therapy should be discussed with the parents. Informed consent should be obtained for cannulation, ECMO therapy, anticoagulation, and decannulation after the indications, alternatives, anticipated benefits, and potential risks have been carefully explained to the parents. Mortality and morbidity statistics are plainly given, specifically for the patient's age and particular disease. Hemorrhagic, infectious, developmental, and hearing complications should be explained. Parents must understand that ECMO is not a specific therapy to cure the patient's disease, but a method to provide pulmonary and cardiac support while allowing the patient's respiratory and cardiac status to improve. At our center, this includes discussion of our ECMO nonresponder end point of 3 weeks: infants who show no improvement and no success at weaning after 3 weeks have a low chance of ever weaning and higher risk for all complications. After 3 weeks, our practice is to withdraw ECMO support and resume conventional medical therapy. The data regarding longer ECMO support, survival, and complications are not as clear in older patients; thus, ECMO runs for older patients might be allowed to continue longer depending on the patient's age and overall status.

Extracorporeal membrane oxygenation centers have specialists on call who prime the circuit in preparation for cannulation. Priming also involves removing oxygen from the circuit, which can produce emboli, and allowing the tubing to be coated with plasma proteins in order to minimize loss of serum proteins. Priming the circuit with blood to avoid a dilutional anemia is the final step, especially in infants. The circuit volume is usually two to three times greater than an infant's blood volume. In large children it may not be critical, but in our center we use a blood prime for all children. In filling the circuit tubing, CO_2, lactated Ringer's solution, fresh frozen plasma, and packed red blood cells are sequentially circulated. Before cannulation, medications are added to the circuit: heparin, calcium gluconate, and sodium bicarbonate.

While the circuit is being primed, a right radial artery catheter (preductal) is placed if desired. If a cutdown is performed, the site is well dressed in anticipation of anticoagulation. If an umbilical artery catheter is present and functioning well, we often omit the radial catheter. Some centers recommend removal of umbilical venous catheters and other central venous lines to prevent air embolus. The patient is placed in a radiant-warming, radiographically transparent bed on a lambswool pad to facilitate cannulation, to avoid movement of the patient for radiographs, and to protect from pressure necrosis. A first-generation cephalosporin is given for prophylaxis.

CANNULATION

Cannulation occurs in the intensive care unit with the assistance of a circulating nurse and a scrub nurse. An operating room back table, trays of instruments and supplies, drapes, suction, electrocautery, and a headlamp are available. Cannulation is usually via right neck cutdown with a horizontal shoulder roll behind the patient's shoulders and with the head midline or turned slightly to the left. The incision is made in a skin crease in the lower neck over the sternocleidomastoid muscle. The vessels can be approached between the two heads of the muscle or just medial to it. Dissection is done with electrocautery to avoid subsequent bleeding while on heparin. The internal jugular vein (IJ) is isolated first and encircled with suture, then the carotid artery. The IJ is isolated first because it can be used for venovenous ECMO if the patient rapidly deteriorates. Even in cases of cannulation for venovenous ECMO, the carotid artery is isolated and encircled so that it can be easily found should the need arise to convert to venoarterial ECMO. Conversion from venovenous to venoarterial ECMO becomes technically more difficult as time passes and edema progresses; if conversion is necessary, it is better to do so within the first 24 hours of ECMO.

When the vessels have been isolated, the patient is given 100 U/kg heparin. The venous cannula is placed first. The IJ is ligated high in the neck and the catheter is placed via venotomy. Some surgeons place stay sutures of fine monofilament suture at each side of the venotomy to retract the vessel and aid in cannulation. The cannula can be coated with sterile water-soluble lubricant. With great care the largest venous cannula that will fit into the vein without causing a tear is placed. In most infants, a 12 or 14

French catheter is preferred, but in smaller neonates, a 10 French catheter may be adequate. If the vein tears, the vein should be ligated and a venotomy made more proximal. Placement of a smaller cannula should also be considered. Tearing the vessel at the clavicle can be catastrophic and may require division of the clavicle or a thoracotomy to control the bleeding and allow cannulation. For venovenous ECMO, a 14 or 16 French cannula is preferred. The double-lumen catheter is measured externally to the xiphoid, and placed so that the multiple venous side holes are oriented posterolaterally to the right to maximize exposure to the superior and inferior vena cavae as they enter the atrium. If the heart is shifted, it is usually also rotated, and the ideal cannula insertion angle and rotational position may need to be altered. Venous cannula position is very important. It is confirmed immediately in most centers on a plain radiograph, while some centers have advocated concurrent echocardiography to confirm tip position within the right atrium. The venous catheter should be well into the right atrium but not touching the tricuspid valve. The cannula is secured with heavy permanent suture over a Silastic bumper.

The arterial cannula is usually 10 or 12 French and is placed via arterotomy after ligation of the common carotid artery. The catheter is inserted to the 2- or 3-cm mark, so that the tip resides within the artery or the aortic arch. Placement of the arterial cannula too far into the arch can cause a jet effect that decreases blood flow to the left carotid artery. The cannula is secured with heavy suture, usually over a Silastic bumper. Confirmation of arterial catheter position is not usually necessary.

After the cannulas are in place, the circuit tubing is connected. The tubing is lightly attached at first and the line inspected for air bubbles before the connections are joined more securely. Clamps are removed from the lines, a clamp is placed on the bridge in the circuit, and pump flow is begun. Full bypass is estimated at 120 mL/kg/min, which for a 3- to 4-kg infant is approximately 300 to 400 mL/min. Pump flow is sometimes limited by the maximum flow allowed by the venous cannula. The sweep gas is usually begun near 0.5 L/min with a fraction of inspired oxygen (FiO_2) of 100%. The catheters are secured to the skin over the mastoid process with heavy braided suture, and the wound is loosely approximated with a running monofilament suture. Some centers routinely use fibrin glue to prevent bleeding, although most find it unnecessary and expensive.

ECMO THERAPY

After initiation and establishment of good flow, we use standardized orders. Full sets of blood gases (pump arterial, pump venous, and right radial or umbilical artery) are obtained immediately and every 4 hours for the first 24 hours. The frequency then decreases to every 8 hours. An activated clotting time (ACT), complete blood count (CBC) with platelets, and potassium level are obtained soon after cannulation. ACTs are obtained every 30 minutes until the ACT is below 300s, at which time a heparin drip is begun at 10 U/kg/h. ACTs are taken at half-hour intervals until values are within the therapeutic range (180–200s or 200–220s). The heparin drip is titrated to maintain the ACTs within range (measured hourly).

Monitoring is based on protocol and includes many routine data measurements. We use the following regimen. At 4 A.M. daily, CBC with differential white blood cell count, platelet count, electrolyte panel, blood urea nitrogen level, creatinine level, protime, prothrombin time, fibrinogen level, fibrin split product analysis, plasma free hemoglobin, and portable chest radiography are performed. At 4 A.M. every 48 hours, albumin, magnesium, phosphate, and total and direct bilirubin levels are determined. Every 6 hours, potassium level and platelet count are checked. CBC is determined every 12 hours. Blood cultures are drawn every evening. Head ultrasonography is performed daily for 5 days because the majority of intraventricular hemorrhage occurs in the first 5 days. An endotracheal tube culture is taken every 3 days. Throughout the ECMO run, stagnant parts of the circuit (the patient bridge and the pump bridge) are unclamped to allow flow every 15 to 20 minutes in order to prevent thrombus formation.

Ventilator weaning (to reach rest settings) may be achieved rapidly on venoarterial ECMO but may take 2 to 3 days on venovenous ECMO. The minimum settings for the ventilator should provide little pressure to the lungs and minimize barotrauma, while maintaining a positive end-expiratory pressure (PEEP) that prevents atelectasis. We use a rate of 10 breaths/min, a peak inspiratory pressure (PIP) of 20, PEEP of 10, and FiO_2 of 21% as standard neonatal rest settings. Pediatric rest settings may have a slightly larger PIP. Weaning off of vasoactive drips also may be achieved rapidly on venoarterial ECMO but may take several days on venovenous ECMO.

In using the ECMO pump for oxygenation and ventilation, the sweep gas flowing through the oxygenator acts as a regulator of ventilation. Increasing the sweep flow increases CO_2 clearance. Regulation of oxygenation, however, is generally managed by changes in the pump blood flow; at a constant sweep gas FiO_2, increasing the pump blood flow increases the patient's partial pressure of arterial oxygen (PaO_2). Some centers blend CO_2 into the sweep gas as a regulatory mechanism for CO_2 diffusion. Others just blend O_2 and air to achieve the desired FiO_2 and use the sweep velocity to regulate ventilation.

The mixed venous oxygen saturation (SvO_2) of the blood returning to the pump in the venous cannula is continually monitored. In venoarterial ECMO, the SvO_2 is interpreted normally as an indication of peripheral extraction and adequacy of oxygen delivery. In venovenous ECMO, high SvO_2

in the pump venous system usually represents recirculation. The oxygenated blood delivered from the pump to the heart is sucked back into the venous cannula and returned to the pump. This can be addressed by repositioning the cannula, adding volume to the patient to improve venous return, or most often by decreasing the pump flow a small amount.

On venovenous ECMO, continuing PPHN can be a cause of continued systemic hypotension because oxygenated blood returned to the right atrium still has resistance to flow through the pulmonary vasculature and is shunted through the ductus arteriosus. Most of these patients now receive nitric oxide therapy when ECMO begins, and it may be beneficial to delay weaning the nitric oxide to promote pulmonary vasodilation.

During the first hours a new circuit is used, the patient's blood equilibrates with the inner surface of the tubing. Blood proteins deposit on the inner surface of the circuit, acute-phase reactants are increased, and platelets are activated to a certain degree. Clinically this process results in the appearance of a systemic inflammatory response syndrome (SIRS) with pulmonary "whiteout" on the chest radiograph and capillary leak with peripheral edema. Relative hypotension and increased cardiac output are difficult to identify with the ECMO circuit in series or in parallel with the native circulation. The signs of SIRS usually clear in about 2 days. As the circuit ages, there is a window of quiescence lasting approximately 3 to 9 days during which the patient's blood is in relative equilibrium with the circuit surfaces. After this interval, the patient's platelet counts begin to drop faster, fibrinogen levels decrease, fibrin split products increase, blood clots in the circuit increase in size, and there is the appearance of diffuse intravascular coagulation. Before there is a problem large enough to compromise circuit flow, the circuit is changed for a new circuit. The SIRS-like clinical picture again occurs. Those centers using centrifugal pumps also see hemolysis with increased plasma-free hemoglobin and hematuria as indicators of turbulence, high pump flows, or an aging circuit. The centrifugal pump head also begins to sound gritty or rough instead of smooth as the circuit ages.

At the onset of ECMO therapy, patients are commonly on continuous drips of vasoactive pressors as well as narcotics, benzodiazepines, and paralytics. It is our practice to eliminate the paralytics after the patient has stabilized on ECMO; this is almost always successful in neonates, and occasionally in older children. Paralytics are restarted if patient motion jeopardizes circuit flow or cannula position. Phenobarbitol is ordered as seizure prophylaxis for the duration of paralytic therapy, and unexplained hypertension or tachycardia is considered possible evidence of occult seizure activity and investigated. In neonates, cranial ultrasonography is performed to best evaluate for intraventricular hemorrhage. In addition, unexplained hypertension, tachycardia, agitation, or shunting through the PDA could be tachyphylaxis to the narcotic and sedative drips; increased doses should be considered.

As part of the daily evaluation, the patient is hand-ventilated with an inline manometer to judge pulmonary compliance. Breath sounds and airway pressure achieved with normal hand ventilation are noted, as is the presence or absence of visible chest rise with 30 to 40 cm H_2O airway pressure. As the lungs begin to heal, there will be a noticeable increase in compliance and chest rise with less airway pressure. On venoarterial ECMO, the arterial saturation may decrease as pulmonary hypertension decreases, allowing increased pulmonary blood flow and increased flow through the minimally ventilated lungs instead of through the circuit. On venovenous ECMO, the sweep gas requirement decreases as native pulmonary flow improves. With a centrifugal pump, the specialists often note a concomitant decrease in circuit blood flow with unchanged pump revolutions per minute.

When a patient is placed on venoarterial ECMO, it is not uncommon that urine output is poor for one to several days. Nonpulsatile flow to the kidneys may be responsible for this phenomenon. Patients with frank renal failure at the onset of ECMO or marginal renal function, increasing creatinine levels, and anuria are treated with continuous venovenous hemofiltration, the tubing for which can be spliced directly into the ECMO circuit. There are recent advances in the development of a hepatic cartridge that can be spliced into the ECMO circuit as therapy for patients with transiently poor liver function (e.g., shock liver caused by the process that triggered the initial requirement for ECMO) or as a bridge to liver transplantation.

WITHDRAWAL OF SUPPORT

There are situations when it becomes clear that continuation of therapy is futile or contraindicated. These include children with severe (grade 3 or 4) intraventricular hemorrhage, severe congenital cardiac malformations in which the heart fails after surgical correction (if deemed unacceptable candidates for transplantation), overwhelming sepsis, uncontrollable hemorrhage, brain death, or cardiac death. Lack of improvement, the onset of new diseases, or new organ system dysfunction are compelling reasons for prolonged ECMO therapy to be terminated and for a return to mechanical ventilatory support. If immediate death is expected on withdrawal of ECMO or if complete withdrawal of life support is planned, the parents should be prepared for this eventuality. The cannulas are clamped and divided at the neck, and a plunger from a disposable syringe is inserted into the end of each cannula so that the awkward clamps can be removed for the benefit of the parents. With neonates or small children, the parents can sit at the bedside and hold their child.

WEANING

When pulmonary compliance and function improve, the patient is diuresing, and general improvement is evident, ECMO weaning is attempted. The ventilator support is increased to moderate settings: PIP = 25 or so, FiO_2 = 30% to 35% (if the pump cannot be weaned with the ventilator $FiO_2 \leq 40\%$, it is probably too early to wean), the PEEP is turned down to 6 to 7 cm H_2O, and the rate is increased to approximately 40 breaths/min for a neonate. There must be sufficient room to increase the ventilatory support significantly if needed via conventional means after decannulation.

On venovenous ECMO, removal of support is accomplished by increasing the ventilator support as above, then gradually decreasing the sweep gas flow and sweep FiO_2. This gradually decreases the effect the oxygenator has on the blood and allows the native lungs, in series with the oxygenator, to resume function. The circuit blood flow is not decreased below about 200 mL/min in order to prevent coagulation within the circuit. If the patient tolerates decrease of sweep FiO_2 to 21% and gradual removal of the sweep gas flow as monitored by frequent arterial blood gases, then the oxygenator is capped off. This entails disconnecting the sweep gas tubing from its source and connecting the sweep inlet to the sweep outlet to prevent any ventilation effect via the circuit. If the patient tolerates this maneuver, he or she is truly already removed from ECMO support, and the venovenous cannula is only functioning as a large central venous catheter.

After increasing the ventilator on venoarterial ECMO, the sweep FiO_2 cannot be weaned because the blood passing through the pump is delivered directly into the aortic arch. The blood fraction diverted through the circuit is diminished, but it cannot be left unoxygenated and unventilated. Pump blood flow is gradually decreased, allowing a greater fraction to proceed normally through the cardiopulmonary system. The patient's blood oxygenation and arterial CO_2 are monitored closely. When the pump flow is at the minimum safe rate to prevent thrombosis within the circuit (200 mL/min), a "trial off" is performed. The arterial and venous cannulas are clamped at the baby's head, and the bridge is opened to allow the pump to maintain flow. Blood gases are obtained immediately, at 20 to 30 minutes, and again at an hour. If all is well, the patient is ready for decannulation. The catheters are unclamped every 10 minutes or so to prevent thrombosis in case the patient is not yet ready for decannulation.

DECANNULATION

The decannulation procedure requires a surgeon and assistant, a sterile field, suction, headlamp, instrument tray, and a single- or double-lumen Broviac catheter. The wound is reopened and the vessels are identified and exposed in the wound. If the carotid artery was cannulated, that cannula is removed and the vessel ligated proximally. In the case of venovenous ECMO, the isolating suture around the carotid artery is simply removed. Some surgeons prefer to repair the carotid artery. The risks of repair include embolism, stenosis, aneurysm formation and rupture from repair in a contaminated field. The reported stenosis rate is 2% to 4% after repair, and the infection rate is not different from that in patients with ligated vessels. Cerebral blood flow studies and neurodevelopmental evaluations show no compelling evidence in favor of either ligation or repair. The internal jugular vein is surrounded proximally with nonabsorbable sutures, and the previous ties around the cannula are removed. The vein is decannulated and an appropriate sized Broviac catheter is placed into the lumen. The sutures are tied around the catheter in the vein, taking care not to obstruct the small, pliable catheter. Some centers feel that the ECMO cannula wound is contaminated, and that the catheter should be tunneled and brought out through a separate incision. We habitually bring the Broviac straight through the operative wound without any increase in infectious catheter complications. After the catheter is in place, the wound is reapproximated at the skin level with several widely spaced interrupted sutures. The arterial and venous umbilical artery catheters are not removed for 24 hours after decannulation to allow resolution of the coagulopathy. After that time, an effort is made to remove all umbilical lines and arterial lines as soon as possible.

FOLLOW-UP

After decannulation, treatment returns to normal medical therapy for the given diagnosis. Physical therapy, often begun gently during ECMO, is continued after decannulation and after discharge as indicated. Before discharge from the hospital, all patients undergo a developmental evaluation, computed tomography of the brain, and audiology screening in the form of an auditory brainstem response (ABR) test. Patients are seen 1 week after hospital discharge in the ECMO clinic to continue treatment of any ongoing medical issues and to coordinate follow-up care. Follow-up also consists of developmental evaluations at 4, 8, 12, 18, and 24 months after discharge. If results of these evaluations are normal, screening continues annually for 7 to 8 years. Hearing tests are performed at 6-month intervals for 6 years. Some centers also do cerebral blood flow scanning, repeated vision screening, and electroencephalography. These additional tests may not be cost effective or yield clinically significant data.

OUTCOMES

Morbidity attributable to ECMO independent of illness and other medical therapies is difficult to identify. Many

TABLE 13.3. ACCUMULATED DATA FROM THE ELSO REGISTRY, 1987–2000: NEONATAL RESPIRATORY ECMO RUNS BY DIAGNOSIS

Diagnosis	Total Runs	Average Run Time (h)	Longest Run Time (h)	Survived	% Survived
CDH	3,422	219	1,072	1,861	54
Meconium aspiration	5,509	128	936	5,172	94
PPHN	2,227	139	1,176	1,759	79
RDS	1,301	132	1,093	1,094	84
Sepsis	2,107	137	1,200	1,601	76
Pneumonia	187	207	936	103	55
Air leak syndrome	78	153	490	55	71
Other	868	165	1,131	584	67

ECMO, extracorporeal membrane oxygenation; CDH, congenital diaphragmatic hernia; PPHN, persistent pulmonary hypertension of the newborn; RDS, respiratory distress syndrome.

reviews report no difference in morbidity for ECMO patients compared with near-miss ECMO patients, whereas others show an increase in developmental delay and sensorineural hearing loss (SNHL) in ECMO patients with CDH as compared to those with other diagnoses. Overall, severe neurodevelopmental impairment is seen in 12% of ECMO survivors, and up to one third have been identified as being "at risk" for an inability to progress through school in the usual manner. SNHL has been reported in 15% to 25% of ECMO survivors, equivalent to the incidence reported in non-ECMO ventilated babies. Many patients are discharged from the hospital with normal ABR screens but develop progressive deficits months or years later. Similar results are reported between ECMO and near-miss ECMO patients. The variables found to correlate most consistently with the presence of a developmental deficit or SNHL were number of hospital days, number of ECMO days, and number of ventilated days.

Data from the Extracorporeal Life Support Organization Registry show that survival varies by diagnosis (Table 13.3). Neonates with meconium aspiration have a 94% survival rate compared with 54% for CDH. Survival also varies by age: neonates have a better outcome than do children or adults. Figure 13.2 shows the data for patients on ECMO for all respiratory diagnoses: although neonates have a 78% survival rate, only 55% of children and 49% of adults survive to discharge. The results equalize, however, for patients placed on ECMO for cardiac reasons: adult survival was 32%, whereas survival for children and neonates was 39% (Fig. 13.3).

New therapies such as high-frequency oscillatory ventilation (HFOV) and inhaled nitric oxide (iNO) have been successful in treating babies with neonatal respiratory distress and PPHN, and the number of ECMO cases in the United States has fallen dramatically over the past 4 years (Fig. 13.4). The concern is that the present success with therapies such as HFOV and iNO will lead to a delay in ECMO referral for refractory patients. There is concern that neonates with longer courses of maximum ventilation and marginal oxygenation before cannulation will have

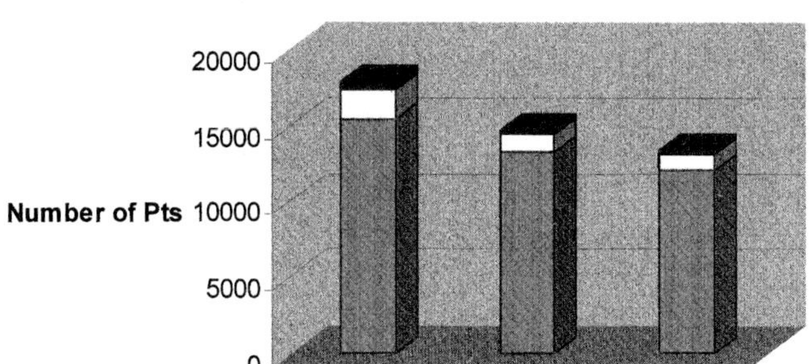

	Total	Off ECLS	Dischg
■ Adult	554	297	273
□ Pediatric	1912	1191	1052
▨ Neonatal	15525	13319	12158

Survival

FIGURE 13.2. ECLS for Cardiac Dx. Accumulated data from the Extracorporeal Life Support Organization Registry, 1987-2000.

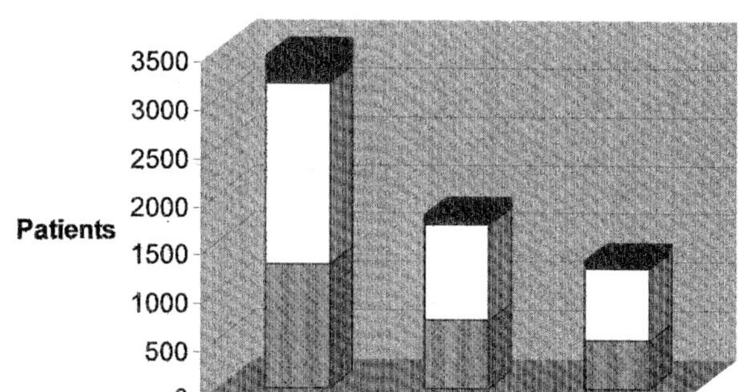

	Total	Off ECLS	Dischg
■ Adult	285	111	91
□ Pediatric	1880	992	744
▨ Neonatal	1279	704	498

Survival

FIGURE 13.3. Accumulated data from the Extracorporeal Life Support Organization Registry, 1987-2000.

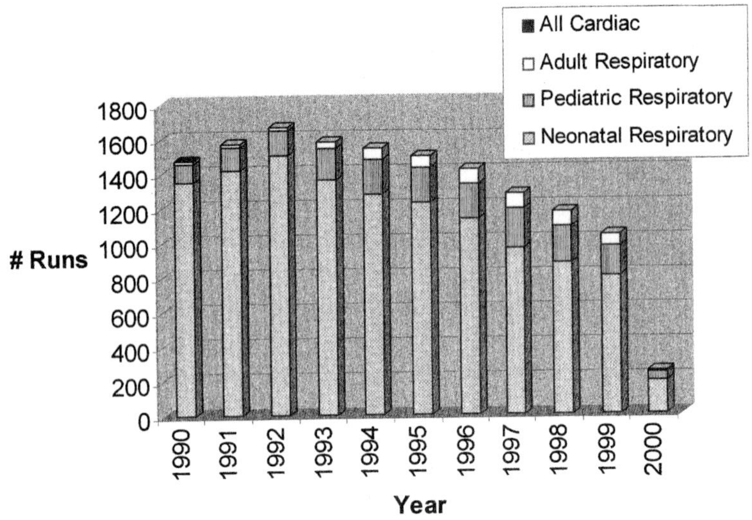

FIGURE 13.4. Accumulated data from the Extracorporeal Life Support Organization Registry, 1987–2000.

longer ECMO runs, as well as higher rates of morbidity and mortality, and that survivors may have increased pulmonary and neurologic sequelae. Careful evaluation of outcomes during the next few years will assist in guiding the combined use of HFOV, iNO, and ECMO to achieve maximal benefit.

In the interest of further improvement, work is being performed to develop improvements in ECMO technology such as pulsatile flow and more efficient oxygenator cartridges. An experimental therapy now in the trial stage is liquid ventilation. Results from this modality alone and combined with other methods of therapy are eagerly awaited. There is particular interest in liquid ventilation with regard to support of premature or low-birth-weight infants, and those who do not otherwise qualify for ECMO. Experimentation is also being performed on possible intravascular oxygenation and CO_2 removal devices designed for adults.

EDITOR'S NOTE

Extracorporeal membrane oxygenation is essentially a method of cardiopulmonary bypass that is used primarily for support of infants with severe but reversible respiratory compromise and older children with correctable cardiac dysfunction. It requires that an institutional program be in place that includes a large team of specialists: surgeons, nurses, pump specialists, biomedical engineers, equipment maintenance personnel, and physicians and nurses who coordinate team activities. Patient care is typically protocol driven but relies heavily on the collective experience, expertise, and good judgment of the team members. In most programs, surgeons continue to play a prominent role—not only as technicians who cannulate and decannulate patients, but also as members of the primary care team that is involved in daily patient care and major decisions.

The management of the patient on ECMO involves an intricate balance of data analysis and patient assessment. The goal from the very beginning should be to get the patient off ECMO. Ventilator settings are minimized to "rest" the lungs, and treatment of the primary disease process should continue. During the initial 2 to 3 days of the run, patients experience a huge cytokine release with capillary leak syndrome and pulmonary edema that results in a "white-out" of the lung fields on radiography. This is accompanied by large fluid requirements and extremely stiff, poorly compliant lungs. When this picture resolves, steps should be taken in anticipation of coming off ECMO. This includes decreasing fluid intake and using diuretics to initiate negative fluid balance. Insensible losses are huge while on ECMO, and when measured intake and output are equal, the infant is actually losing fluid overall. Electrolytes need to be monitored carefully during this stage as well. Hand-bagging to test compliance and to recruit collapsed airways should be performed daily. Vent settings might be increased gradually for the same reasons. Likewise, pump flow should be decreased gradually to the minimum rate needed by the child to maintain adequate preductal oxygen saturation, good systemic perfusion (pink with warm extremities and good urine output), and a normal SvO_2.

An infant on venovenous ECMO will usually maintain cardiovascular function at pre-ECMO levels, including the need for pressor support. Maintaining volume status becomes important and should be monitored closely. When venoarterial ECMO is initiated, there will be an immediate dampening of the arterial pressure tracing, although the mean blood pressure should remain relatively unchanged. This is thought to be due to the effect of having blood flow generated by the ECMO circuit in parallel to the normal circulation. In fact, overdampening (a flat tracing) can be a sign of hypovolemia that will improve with fluid administration. Others have suggested that this is a physiologic "cardiac stun" that correlates with the cytokine release and edema one sees in these patients. Despite the difference in philosophy and approach, the treatment is essentially the same (fluid and pressors, as needed). Impending hypovolemia also can sometimes be predicted by the presence of "chatter" in the circuit or an exaggerated sway of the portion of the venous drainage tubing that is draped between the patient and the circuit.

Some controversy exists as to the appropriate way to measure the effects of the therapy. Some propose that postductal oxygen saturation should be kept within a normal range, whereas others feel that the only important measurement is preductal oxygenation (oxygen delivery to the brain and heart). A reasonable compromise adopted by many programs is to have two different thresholds of concern for the preductal and postductal saturation measurements, so that a lower level is accepted in a postductal organ system but never in the preductal system. Oxygen levels should be maintained above 60 mm Hg as measured by preductal arterial blood gases. Oxygen levels in excess of 100 mm Hg suggest that less flow may be tolerated or that the patient is hypovolemic. The two parallel circuits result in mixing of highly oxygenated blood from the ECMO circuit with relatively poorly oxygenated blood from the native circulation. Hypovolemia decreases the relative contribution of the native circuit allowing for greater oxygen levels. Whether or not lowering flows should be considered depends on the Svo_2. An Svo_2 measurement of less than 65% suggests that oxygen extraction by the tissues is maximal and that flows may actually need to be increased. High Svo_2 (>85%) suggests that oxygen delivery is very high and that lower flows may be tolerated. Rarely does it suggest the presence of a hyperdynamic state as is traditionally described for sepsis. The oxygenator is extremely efficient at removing CO_2, even at very low pump flows, so CO_2 levels do not reflect flow dynamics. Carbon dioxide elimination is therefore regulated by altering the concentration of CO_2 in the sweep gas.

Besides these physiologic effects and elevated oxygen levels, hypovolemia can have detrimental effects on pump function. Venous drainage is essentially passive and reliant on gravity. Hypovolemia can cause poor venous drainage and tripping of the low pressure alarm ("bladder box") that is part of all ECMO circuits. If the alarm continues to sound frequently despite the administration of fluid or blood products, one can consider physically raising the patient relative to the circuit to increase the gradient produced by gravity; however, persistently poor venous drainage despite these maneuvers is usually due to improper venous cannula position (too high or up against the tricuspid valve). After chest radiographic or echocardiographic confirmation, reoperation to reposition the cannula is often necessary.

Hemorrhage is one of the most important potential complications while on ECMO. The ACT is kept within a defined narrow range, depending on the perceived risk in a given patient. For the patient felt to be at average risk, a range of 200 to 220s may be acceptable, whereas patients at high risk for bleeding may need to have ACTs between 180 and 200s or even lower. The potential downside with tolerating lower ACTs is that clot will accumulate within the circuit more quickly than usual and may require that the circuit be exchanged before the run is completed. Patients who need to undergo surgery while on ECMO present a unique challenge. Some advocate lowering the ACT levels to 160 to 180 and increasing the platelet transfusions. Others routinely use aminocaproic acid (Amicar, Immunex, Seattle, Washington) to inhibit fibrinolysis. In cases of ongoing bleeding, the options are to stop heparin therapy altogether (with sacrifice of the circuit), aborting the ECMO run altogether, or delaying the surgery until the patient can come off ECMO as originally planned.

–P.M.

SUGGESTED READINGS

Bartlett RH, Burns NE, Fong SW, et al. Prolonged partial venoarterial bypass: physiologic, biochemical and hematologic responses. *Surg Forum* 1972;23:178–180.

Bartlett RH, Roloff DW, Custer JR, et al. Extracorporeal life support: the University of Michigan Experience. *JAMA* 2000;283: 904–908.

Desai SA, Stanley C, Gringlas M, et al. Five-year follow-up of neonates with reconstructed right common carotid arteries after extracorporeal membrane oxygenation. *J Pediatr* 1999;134: 428–433.

Garber SJ, Stewart DL, Cook LN, et al. Evaluation of post extracorporeal membrane oxygenation follow-up testing. *ASAIO J* 1998; 44:171–174.

History of the development of extracorporeal circulation. In: Arensman RM, Cornish JD, eds. *Extracorporeal life support.* Boston: Blackwell Scientific, 1993.

Nield TA, Langenbacher D, Poulsen MK, et al. Neurodevelopmental outcome at 3.5 years of age in children treated with extracorporeal life support: relationship to primary diagnosis. *J Pediatr* 2000;136: 338–344.

Rais-Bahrami K, Wagner AE, Coffman C, et al. Neurodevelopmental outcome in ECMO vs. near-miss ECMO patients at 5 years of age. *Clin Pediatr (Phila)* 2000;39:145–152.

Southgate WM, Annibale DJ, Hulsey TC, et al. International experience with trisomy 21 infants placed on extracorporeal membrane oxygenation. *Pediatrics* 2001;107:549–552.

Zahraa JN, Moler FW, Annich GM, et al. Venovenous versus venoarterial extracorporeal life support for pediatric respiratory failure: are there differences in survival and acute complications? *Crit Care Med* 2000;28:521–525.

Zwischenberger JB, Steinhorn RH, Bartlett RH. *ECMO extracorporeal cardiopulmonary support in critical care, 2nd ed.* Extracorporeal Life Support Organization, 2000.

SECTION III

TRAUMA

14

PEDIATRIC TRAUMA RESUSCITATION

VICTOR F. GARCIA

An understanding of the epidemiology of pediatric trauma, the most common causes of death, and the most immediate life-threatening conditions is essential in pediatric trauma resuscitation. Unintentional blunt injuries are the most common form of childhood injury and are usually motor vehicle related. Head injury is the major cause of death in these instances. Half of the deaths attributed to head injury are complicated by inappropriate treatment of hypovolemia or hypoxia. Loss of the airway results in death in 3 to 4 minutes. Inability to breathe results in death in 5 to 7 minutes, and severe hemorrhage results in death in about 10 to 12 minutes.

TRAUMA TEAM

The attributes of highly effective trauma teams have been well studied and should be cultivated in every trauma center. The essential characteristic is a well-orchestrated, multidisciplinary, self-directed team that evaluates, diagnoses, and treats virtually concurrently. Each member of the team must be highly trained and self-sufficient. Team members must not only know their role but also how their role impacts on the role of other team members. To a large extent, individual team members must be goal directed but responsive to the team leader's redirection of effort. The team leader actively and continuously prioritizes, monitors, assesses, and, as dictated by the patient's clinical response, reprioritizes individual and collective efforts.

Information regarding the mechanism of injury and the child's response during the prehospital phase of resuscitation is invaluable. It enables the team to postulate the child's pattern of injury, anticipate needed radiologic and laboratory tests, and prioritize their initial focus and interventions.

V. F. Garcia: Department of Surgery, University of Cincinnati; and Trauma Services Medical Center, Cincinnati Children's Hospital Medical Center, Cincinnati, Ohio.

EVIDENCE-BASED PATHWAYS

The more severely injured the child, the less time should be spent in the trauma bay. In this regard, evidence-based pathways for the initial phase of resuscitation are very useful. Pathways should specify and prioritize which laboratory tests should be obtained (tailored to the severity of injury), which drugs should be used for intubation (based on the patient's hemodynamic status), the appropriateness and sequence of radiologic tests, and the criteria for clinically clearing the cervical spine. Such provisions expedite care, minimize provider-generated variations in treatment, and reduce health-care costs without increasing morbidity or mortality.

TRIAGE

Most severely injured children have multisystem injuries. Early morbidity and mortality are usually related to the severity of the brain injury, degree of airway compromise, and presence of hypovolemic shock. The majority of injured children who experience cardiac arrest before they reach the hospital die despite resuscitation. Severe brain injury and pulseless electrical activity are a fatal combination, and prolonged efforts at resuscitation are unwarranted. Aggressive resuscitation of children with signs of life (nondilated pupils, spontaneous respiratory efforts, response to pain, cardiac activity associated with peripheral pulses) may return cardiopulmonary function without neurologic recovery. Solid organ donation is possible in up to 9% of such patients.

AIRWAY MANAGEMENT

Early and appropriate management of the airway is especially important in patients with severe brain injury. The examining physician should always assume that the cervical spine is injured and immobilize the head and neck to prevent unintentional manipulation of the spinal cord. How the airway is managed depends on the likelihood of airway compromise and the patient's breathing. Oxygen should always be administered. Although hypercarbia is generally tolerated well, hypoxia is potentially catastrophic.

Altered level of consciousness, impending or actual upper airway obstruction, and hemodynamic instability are indications for intubation. A rapid-sequence intubation technique minimizes the risk of aspiration of gastric contents. All equipment for intubation must be readily available. Laryngoscopy blades of varying lengths, an assortment of airway forceps, a ventilation bag, suction, and proper sized endotracheal tubes should be within easy reach. The appropriate size of an endotracheal tube can be estimated by gauging the size of the child's fifth finger or diameter of the naris, or by using Cole's formula: tube size (millimeters internal diameter) = (years of age/4) + 4. The tube should pass easily and allow gas to leak around it at about 15 to 30 cm H_2O pressure. Cuffed tubes are recommended for children over 8 to 10 years of age because their cricoid ring is no longer restrictive. A severely compromised airway requires that expertise with flexible bronchoscopy, needle cricoid-thyroidotomy, surgical cricoid-thyroidotomy, and surgical tracheostomy be immediately available.

Laryngoscopy and intubation are noxious stimuli and increase intracranial pressure. Intubation under the protection of profound sedation with the assistance of neuromuscular blockade attenuates this phenomenon. It is extremely important to perform a reliable mini-neurologic examination prior to sedating or paralyzing the patient.

Anticholinergic agents such as atropine are recommended in order to decrease oral secretions and prevent the bradycardia associated with laryngoscopy. The choice of a sedative agent depends on the patient's hemodynamic status. Thiopental is short acting, decreases cerebral oxygen consumption, and lowers intracranial pressure. However, it is also a potent myocardial depressant and decreases peripheral vascular resistance. This can result in cardiovascular collapse in patients with hypovolemia. Etomidate is another short-acting agent that decreases cerebral oxygen consumption and intracranial pressure but without the adverse effects on cardiovascular function. It is the preferred agent in the setting of circulatory dysfunction.

Depolarizing agents or nondepolarizing agents can be used for muscle paralysis. The only depolarizing relaxant in clinical use is succinylcholine. It has a rapid onset and short duration of action, but the disadvantages associated with its use (Table 14.1) have kindled interest in newer short-acting agents. Most agents in use are nondepolarizing relaxants with similar actions, although there are differences in their hemodynamic effects. Pancuronium, vecuronium, atracurium, and rocuronium all have little hemodynamic effect and have a short onset of action.

Intubation of the injured child is a multiperson task. All other activities, especially those that are likely to agitate or stimulate the patient (insertion of urinary and gastric tubes), should be deferred until the airway is secured. To improve exposure, the anterior portion of the cervical collar can be removed. One person immobilizes the cervical spine. Preoxygenation is critical. The team member with the most experience with intubation places the oral endotracheal tube. A third person applies cricoid pressure to protect against aspiration of gastric contents and to minimize gastric distention during bag mask ventilation. After the intubating drugs take effect, the pharynx is suctioned. Prolonged periods of apnea may be avoided if the person performing the intubation holds his or her breath during the procedure.

There is a tendency to insert the tube too deep. Placing the tip of the tube just below the true vocal cords guards against this common occurrence. Observation of moisture condensation in the tube, symmetric chest expansion, equal breath sounds, and adequate oxygenation confirms proper placement of the tube. The most reliable means of ensuring correct tube placement is documentation of CO_2 in the expired gas. Hyperventilation and resulting hypocarbia reduces cerebral blood flow and should be avoided.

Patients with closed head injury are at greater risk for increased intracranial pressure and require a modification of the usual intubation protocol in order to avoid increasing intracranial pressure further. Preoxygenation should be accomplished with 100% oxygen and assisted ventilation. Atropine sulfate (0.1–0.5 mg) is administered, followed by sedation and neuromuscular blockade. In the absence of circulatory dysfunction or hypovolemia, thiopental (4–6 mg/kg), lidocaine (1 mg/kg), and vecuronium (0.1 mg/kg) can be administered intravenously in rapid succession. In the presence of hypovolemia or circulatory compromise, etomidate or midazolam (0.1 mg/kg) is used instead of thiopental. The patient should be mask ventilated until the drugs take effect, then the patient is intubated in a way that minimizes coughing and retching.

Complex craniofacial injury or laryngeal trauma may require tracheostomy, needle cricothyroidotomy, or surgical cricothyroidotomy. Surgical cricothyroidotomy is not recommended in infants or young children because of the risk to the small and relatively soft trachea.

TABLE 14.1. DISADVANTAGES OF SUCCINYLCHOLINE

Muscle fasciculation in patients over 4 years of age
Increased intracranial, intraocular, and intragastric pressure
Hyperkalemia in certain circumstances
Risk of malignant hyperthermia and myoglobinuria

BREATHING

Thoracic injury occurs in 4.5% of injured children. Immediately life-threatening chest injuries include tension pneumothorax, massive hemothorax, pericardial tamponade, flail chest, and massive pulmonary contusion. The quality and symmetry of breath sounds are best assessed by auscultation in the axilla. Diminished breath sounds, in the presence of appropriate end-tidal CO_2 readings, usually occur because the endotracheal tube is placed too far distally and are less likely a result of a tension pneumothorax. Nonetheless, diminished breath sounds and hypotension may be due to a tension pneumothorax given the compliant nature of a child's mediastinum. A tension pneumothorax should be rapidly decompressed by placing a large-bore catheter into the second intercostal space along the midclavicular line. Once the tension is relieved, a chest tube should be placed in a deliberate and sterile manner.

The presence of a pneumothorax or hemothorax requires placement of a thoracostomy tube. Rib fractures suggest the transfer of a significant degree of energy and are a reliable indicator of other associated injuries. Physiologically significant pulmonary contusion is uncommon. If it results in significant ventilation-perfusion mismatch, the patient may benefit from differential lung ventilation with a double-lumen endotracheal tube or prone positioning.

CIRCULATION

The ability to compensate for large losses in blood volume by an increase in heart rate and peripheral vascular resistance is one of the most remarkable aspects of a child's physiology. Tachycardia is the most immediate and easily measured response to the loss of blood volume. It may not be present in a well-conditioned athlete who has suffered a major blood loss. Despite progressive hypovolemia and decrease in cardiac output, a concomitant increase in peripheral vascular resistance maintains the blood pressure at a relatively normal level. A child may maintain a near normal blood pressure until about 40% blood volume loss, when vascular constrictive ability is totally lost and blood pressure rapidly decreases. Consequently, hypotension is a notoriously late sign of bleeding.

Earlier signs of significant blood loss are found in the quality of central and peripheral pulses, heart rate, capillary refill, skin color, and a subjective sense of the adequacy of perfusion. Large-bore intravenous catheters or intraosseous needles should be inserted peripherally. Commercially available catheter exchange kits permit placement of a larger, more appropriately sized catheter through an existing intravenous site. Blood samples are drawn for cross-matching and other appropriate tests that should include lactate and blood gas determinations to monitor the adequacy of volume resuscitation.

The initial infusion should be a 20 mL/kg rapid bolus of warmed crystalloid solution. The child's clinical response, as evidenced by an improvement in heart rate, blood pressure, and capillary refill, determines whether a second 20 mL/kg bolus is needed. If there is a fleeting or insignificant improvement after the second bolus, then as a third bolus of crystalloid is administered, 10 mL/kg of packed red blood cells is prepared. Children who require blood transfusions are likely to require operative intervention to stop ongoing hemorrhage. There is some evidence to suggest that patients who have suffered severe brain injury (Glasgow Coma Scale score <8) and are hypotensive may have better outcomes if resuscitated with hypertonic saline.

NEUROLOGIC ASSESSMENT

Brain injury is adversely affected by hypotension and hypoxia. Hypotension on admission in patients with severe head injury is associated with more than double the mortality as compared with patients with no hypotension. The presence of hypoxia in addition to hypotension is associated with a mortality of approximately 75%. Avoiding secondary brain injury from hypoxia and hypotension is an obvious and immediate priority during resuscitation. Eucapnia should be maintained and hypocapnia avoided. Hyperventilation-mediated cerebral vasoconstriction further compromises an already ischemic injured brain.

The initial neurologic assessment consists of determining the level of consciousness and the equality and responsiveness of the pupils and is a prelude to determining the Glasgow Coma Scale score. During the secondary survey, the Glasgow Coma Scale score (modified for children under 4 years of age) is determined and used throughout the hospital course to follow and communicate changes in the patient's level of consciousness and neurologic function. The best motor response elicited is the most accurate prognostic indicator. As stated previously, it is extremely important to obtain a reliable mini-neurologic examination prior to sedating or paralyzing the patient.

EXPOSURE AND ENVIRONMENT

Complete and adequate evaluation requires that the child's clothing be completely removed to expose the entire front and back for thorough evaluation. Keep in mind that an exposed and severely injured child is especially susceptible to hypothermia. Adjuncts in maintaining core body temperatures include increasing the ambient temperature, warming infused fluids, and using body warming devices, such as the Bair Hugger (Augustine Medical, Eden Prairie, Minnesota). Crystalloid solutions (but not blood) may be warmed in a microwave oven. Efforts to rewarm the patient and to prevent hypothermia should be considered to be as important as any other component of the resuscitation phase.

IMAGING STUDIES

Radiography should not delay the resuscitation of the patient. Three radiographs should be considered as part of the initial resuscitation: a lateral cervical spine, an anteroposterior (AP) chest film, and an AP pelvis film. The cervical spine should be clinically cleared if the child is alert and communicative with no distracting injuries, no tenderness to palpation of the cervical spine, and no pain with active full range of motion of the neck. Similarly, a radiograph of the pelvis may not be necessary if the patient is alert and there is no evidence of pain or instability of the pelvis on examination.

SECONDARY SURVEY

The secondary survey is the final phase of the initial resuscitation and begins when the primary survey is completed, resuscitative efforts are well established, and the patient has normal vital functions. It entails a complete history and head-to-toe physical examination and is intended to identify concurrent injuries that are not immediately life threatening. Each region of the body is carefully examined. The potential for missing an injury in an unresponsive child is great and argues for a routine tertiary survey within 12 to 24 hours following admission.

HISTORY

The mechanism of the injury greatly influences the patient's pattern of injury. The child who is in a motor vehicle–pedestrian crash and experiences respiratory arrest at the scene is likely to have severe brain injury or atlantooccipital dislocation of the cervical spine. The child restrained with only a lap belt, involved in a frontal motor vehicle collision, and who complains of abdominal and back pain may have cervical spine and brain injury as well as intraabdominal and lumbar spine injuries. Children who are injured by a discharged air bag should be evaluated for chest, eye, neck, and head injuries.

SPECIAL STUDIES

Ultrasonography does not have the same reliability in children as it has in adults. As many as 30% of children with solid organ injuries demonstrated by computed tomography (CT) will not have free fluid demonstrated on ultrasonography performed in the trauma bay. Its sensitivity in detecting free fluid is useful in determining whether hypotension in an unresponsive child with a severe closed head injury is due to intraabdominal hemorrhage. Absence of massive amounts of peritoneal fluid on ultrasonography may be helpful in determining whether the child should be stabilized with fluids and vasopressors and taken for CT scan of the head or taken directly to the operating room for abdominal exploration.

Contrast-enhanced CT is the most useful tool to identify the scope and magnitude of multisystem injuries. Although there is debate whether oral contrast is necessary, we have found its use invaluable in delineating the retroperitoneal structures as well as elucidating the possibility of hollow viscus injury. Interestingly, we have found water to be as effective as traditional oral contrast agents.

In summary, the resuscitation of the acutely injured child is one of the most challenging responsibilities of the surgeon or team leader. Appreciation of the mechanism of injury, the vagaries of the child's physiologic response, and the limitations and advantages of the available diagnostic modalities available are essential.

SUGGESTED READINGS

Battistella FD, Nugent W, Owings JT, et al. Field triage of the pulseless trauma patient. *Arch Surg* 1999;134:742–745.

Brain Trauma Foundation. American Association of Neurological Surgeons. Joint Section on Neurotrauma and Critical Care. Resuscitation of blood pressure and oxygenation. *J Neurotrauma* 2000; 17:471–478.

Corbett SW, Andrews HG, Baker EM, et al. ED evaluation of the pediatric trauma patient by ultrasonography. *Am J Emerg Med* 2000;18:244–249.

Fisher B, Worthen M. Cardiac arrest induced by blunt trauma in children. *Pediatr Emerg Care* 1999;15:274–276.

Harris BH, Butler LJ. Teamwork in pediatric trauma centers. *Semin Pediatr Surg* 2001;10:35–37.

Kochanek PM, Clark RS, Ruppel RA, et al. Cerebral resuscitation after traumatic brain injury and cardiopulmonary arrest in infants and children in the new millennium. *Pediatr Clin North Am* 2001; 48:661–681.

Levy RJ, Helfaer MA. Pediatric airway issues. *Crit Care Clin* 2000;16: 489–504.

Sanchez JI, Paidas CN. Childhood trauma. Now and in the new millennium. *Surg Clin North Am* 1999;79:1503–1535.

Simma B, Burger R, Falk M, et al. A prospective, randomized, and controlled study of fluid management in children with severe head injury: lactated Ringer's solution versus hypertonic saline. *Crit Care Med* 1998;26:1265–1270.

Thomas NJ, Carcillo JA. Hypovolemic shock in pediatric patients. *New Horiz* 1998;6:120–129.

Surgical Directives: Pediatric Surgery, edited by Peter Mattei. Lippincott Williams & Wilkins, Philadelphia

15

HEAD TRAUMA

JOSEPH QUEENAN
PETER MATTEI

Surgeons are usually the first responders to the trauma victim. Children are more likely to suffer a head injury than an adult for any given mechanism of trauma. This is probably due to the disproportionate size of their head when compared with the adult population as well as the relative weakness of their neck musculature. Moreover, severe head injuries are responsible for the vast majority of deaths and long-term disability in children who sustain traumatic injuries. Although definitive therapy is typically managed by the pediatric neurosurgeon, resuscitation and initial management of the head-injured child demands attention to detail, knowledge of current therapeutic guidelines, and an efficient, systematic approach.

The most common mechanisms of head injury in children include motor vehicle accidents and falls, although nonaccidental injury such as child abuse and other forms of violence are also common. In adolescents, penetrating injuries due to gunshot wounds and impalement injuries become more significant as well. The severity of the mechanism does not always correlate with the degree of injury in children, so that a seemingly minor traffic accident, for example, may easily result in a lethal head injury in an infant or small child. A high index of suspicion is therefore imperative. It is also important to realize that the skull provides little protection to penetrating injury in infants, even in blunt-force impacts. A small child with a laceration or puncture wound of the face or scalp after a fall or crash should be assessed for the possibility of intracranial injury or open skull fracture. The usual historical points should be elicited such as loss of consciousness, amnesia, or a reported change in mental status, although these are often difficult to assess in the small child. Likewise, lethargy or irritability or both are typical in the injured child, as is the characteristic sleepiness seen in toddlers and young children who sustain even minor head injuries, so that, again, a high index of suspicion, often erring on the side of caution, is important.

J. Queenan: Division of Neurosurgery, Alfred I. duPont Hospital for Children, Wilmington, Delaware.

P. Mattei: Department of Surgery, Thomas Jefferson University, Philadelphia, Pennsylvania; and Department of Pediatric Surgery, Alfred I. duPont Hospital for Children, Wilmington, Delaware.

RESUSCITATION AND INITIAL MANAGEMENT

The initial protocol emphasizes stabilization of the spine and the ABCs (airway, breathing, circulation) of trauma resuscitation. Usually, a cervical collar is applied in the field. It is important to realize that all head-injured patients are considered at risk for cervical spine injury. This includes both penetrating and blunt trauma. Once in the trauma bay, inline stabilization of the spine is imperative and should be assigned to an experienced individual who has no other potentially distracting duties. Often the collar placed on the child in the field is of an inappropriate size. A broad range of sizes of stiff collars should be available, and a poorly fitted collar should be removed and replaced. Assessment of the airway, with emphasis on respiratory and circulatory issues, is always the highest priority in any injured patient, even in the setting of an isolated head injury. Concerns related to whether the resuscitation fluids should contain dextrose or whether the solute load is adequate are less important than maintaining oxygenation and an adequate blood pressure. Nevertheless, these are certainly relevant issues, and protocols should be in place ahead of time so that the discussion of these concerns does not delay or otherwise compromise the care of the patient.

The initial evaluation of the child should include a rapid assessment of the scalp. If there is a laceration, immediate attention should be directed at stopping the blood loss, which in a small child can result in exsanguination. Collars and other stabilizing devices need to be carefully removed to allow full assessment of the entire scalp. Direct pressure is applied initially, although hemostatic clips, skin staples, or sutures should be applied as soon as possible in the trauma bay. This will avoid the possibility of exsanguination, although definitive wound management, including irrigation and formal repair, needs to be performed later when the patient is more stable.

The pupils should be inspected. Care should be taken to ensure that they are equal and reactive to light. Although anisocoria of less than 1 mm is considered to be within normal limits, a detailed history should be sought for confirmation, and the pupils should be assessed at frequent intervals to detect any progression in the size discrepancy. In the event of a fixed and dilated pupil without obvious signs of direct trauma to the orbit, a mass lesion should be suspected and treatment for elevated intracranial pressure (ICP) should immediately ensue. Disconjugate gaze should be documented; however, it is normal to have disconjugate pupils during sleep, and this state may not have the same implications when observed as an isolated finding.

The cervical spine should be evaluated clinically and radiographically, because both are required to rule out an injury. Examination is by inspection and palpation of the neck, looking for step-offs and point tenderness, in addition to a complete neurologic examination. In the cooperative patient, active movements (never performed by the examiner) of the neck might elicit pain and suggest the need for further studies. The minimum radiologic investigation includes visualization of the cervical spine from the base of the occiput to the top of the body of the first thoracic vertebra. Further evaluation with CT or magnetic resonance imaging (MRI) is sometimes required when an injury cannot be ruled out on the basis of physical examination and plain radiographs, especially at the level of C1–C2. Thoracic and lumbar spinal films should be obtained in all patients with a cervical spine injury. Patients with suspected spinal cord injuries are given corticosteroids according to standard protocol.

The remainder of the physical examination should be directed at obtaining a Glasgow Coma Scale (GCS) score. In children, the GCS can be difficult to assess, because the examination must be directed to the appropriate age level (Table 15.1). The GCS provides a way of relating information to consultants with some interobserver reliability. It also helps to provide some prognostic information, although making predictions based on the initial GCS score are notoriously unreliable. When performed in serial fashion it can also provide a somewhat objective measure of clinical progress. Patients with a GCS score of less than 8 are considered to be in a coma.

TABLE 15.1. GLASGOW COMA SCALE, MODIFIED FOR CHILDREN

Score	Eyes Open	Verbal	Motor
6	—	—	Spontaneous
5	—	Age appropriate	Localizes
4	Spontaneous	Cries/consolable	Withdraws
3	To voice	Irritable	Flexion posture
2	To pain	Restless	Extension posture
1	None	None	None

Other important findings on physical examination include the respiratory rate and whether there is evidence of the Cushing reflex (bradycardia and hypertension), which suggests the presence of elevated ICP. The respiratory rate can be severely depressed or erratic. In the comatose patient, it is important to assess cranial nerve and extremity reflexes prior to the administration of sedating or paralyzing drugs. This includes documentation of gag and corneal reflexes, which can have important prognostic significance and provides data points in the event that a brain death evaluation becomes necessary. Lastly, examination of the ears for evidence of hemotympanum or cerebrospinal fluid (CSF) leak should be performed as part of the initial survey.

When managing a head-injured patient, the goal should be to complete the initial assessment and resuscitation so that the child can undergo a CT scan of the brain as quickly as possible, ideally within 30 to 45 minutes. There is rarely a reason for exploratory burr holes or other invasive measures. One should be able to obtain appropriate radiographic studies in a timely fashion at all facilities involved with trauma. Further intervention will be planned based on the results of the CT scan, and time is critical.

Intravenous (i.v.) or intraosseous access should be obtained immediately, as should fluid resuscitation instituted with normal saline solution or lactated Ringer solution according to institutional protocol. It is important to avoid the use of hypotonic fluids and to prevent overhydration, both of which can contribute to increased ICP. Hyperglycemia has been shown to worsen brain injury in patients with head injury; therefore, the initial resuscitation fluid should not contain dextrose. Boluses of 10 to 20 mL/kg are given rapidly but should be titrated to the blood pressure and overall signs of peripheral perfusion. If pressor support is needed, a carefully titrated i.v. epinephrine drip is the preferred drug in the head-injured patient. Midazolam should be considered for the anxious child, especially in anticipation of the CT scan, but only after a complete neurologic assessment has been performed.

Endotracheal intubation should be considered in comatose patients, in patients with signs of elevated ICP, and in patients who would ordinarily satisfy criteria for intubation in the trauma setting. Any patient who cannot protect his airway or is expected to deteriorate en route to or during the CT scan should be considered for intubation as well. Intubation should be performed with inline stabilization of the cervical spine and minimal, if any, extension of the neck. Protocols vary according to the standards of the institution, but some common principles apply. Rapid-sequence intubation with cricoid pressure to reduce gastric insufflation is usually practiced. Lidocaine (2 mg/kg i.v.) can be given to suppress cough and the incidence of arrhythmia. In children less than one year of age, atropine (20 μg/kg i.v., minimum 100 μg) may be given to prevent bradycardia and minimize secretions. Sodium pentothal (1–5 mg/kg i.v.) or etomidate (0.3 mg/kg i.v.) can be given for sedation and amnesia. Lastly, succinyl choline (1–2 mg/kg i.v.) can be given safely prior to intubation in most head-injured patients. Most patients should be ventilated according to the usual protocols, unless a hyperventilation strategy is adopted for elevated ICP. An orogastric tube should be inserted to prevent gastric distension. Nasogastric and nasotracheal tubes are generally avoided in the event of a cribriform plate fracture.

TREATMENT OF ELEVATED INTRACRANIAL PRESSURE

If after the initial assessment the patient is felt to have elevated ICP, then some treatment should be instituted immediately. Elevated ICP may be suspected on the basis of systemic signs, such as hypertension, bradycardia, and respiratory changes, or due to localizing signs, such as fixed dilated pupil, hemiparesis, or flexion or extension posturing. Treatment for increased ICP includes hyperventilation and mannitol, if the patient's blood pressure can tolerate it. Remember that approximately 10% of patients with a severe isolated head injury present with profound hypotension. Also, although it is somewhat routine to place a Foley catheter at the time of the initial assessment and stabilization, it is imperative that a catheter be placed whenever an obtunded or unconscious patient is administered a diuretic.

The principal goal is to relieve ICP and support cerebral perfusion pressure. Cerebral perfusion pressure (CPP) is the difference between mean arterial pressure (MAP) and ICP (CPP = MAP – ICP). To optimize CPP, MAP is supported by maintaining adequate hydration and pressor support. Hyperventilation lowers the partial pressure of CO_2 (P_{CO_2}), which results in reflex cerebral vasoconstriction. This decreases cerebral blood volume and thus ICP. Severe and prolonged hyperventilation can result in cerebral ischemia and should therefore be avoided. Hyperventilation therapy should only be used for acutely elevated ICP and should be limited to as short a period of time as possible.

Mannitol presumably works by increasing the osmotic gradient in favor of loss of interstital fluid from the brain. The typical dose in children is 0.5 mg/kg i.v. The dose can be repeated every 4 to 6 hours and is titrated to keep serum osmolarity between 300 and 320 mOsm/L.

In the event that the patient must be taken immediately to the operating room and cannot be evaluated with a CT scan, then placement of an ICP monitor must be considered. This is usually in the form of a ventriculostomy catheter. If the patient has high ICP or lateralizing signs, then the need for exploratory burr holes also must be considered. Patients requiring neurosurgical intervention are those with symptomatic mass lesions, mass lesions felt to be at too high risk for further expansion if left alone, and some patients with penetrating trauma.

After the patient has undergone placement of an ICP monitor, ventriculostomy, or craniotomy, he or she will be placed in the intensive care unit (ICU) setting. It is often best to follow CPP, but absolute numbers in children are difficult to assess because they have varied MAPs. In general we try to keep the ICP below 20 and the CPP above 50. In older children, a CPP closer to 70 may be preferable. Monitoring a patient with elevated ICP requires central venous and peripheral arterial catheters in addition to the usual monitoring equipment.

Treatment of ICP can be done with a combination of CSF drainage, administration of diuretics, sedation, paralyzation, and, in severe cases, pharmacologic coma. Pentobarbital (3 mg/kg every 20 minutes three times, followed by 1 mg/kg/h by i.v. drip) is the most commonly used agent for inducing coma for treatment of elevated ICP. There is currently no indication for the use of steroids in the head-injured patient. It is our preference to reserve hyperventilation for acute increases in ICP unresponsive to other measures. This is because of the deleterious effects on cerebral blood flow mentioned above.

In addition to the management of ICP per se, care in the ICU should also emphasize optimization of other physiologic parameters that are important to minimizing brain injury and maximizing the potential for meaningful recovery. Core body temperature should be monitored closely and maintained between 36° and 37°C. The head of the bed is typically elevated to about 30 degrees. Cervical spine injury must be ruled out as quickly as possible, by CT or MRI if necessary, to avoid prolonged immobilization in a collar and so that steroid therapy can be instituted early. Unless a hyperventilation strategy is in effect, P_{CO_2} should be maintained between 35 and 40 mm Hg. In children over 5 years of age, i.v. hydration is performed using normal saline solution supplemented with potassium at a rate between two thirds and the full "maintenance" rate. Pain and anxiety should be treated with fentanyl (1–2 μg/kg/h as an i.v. drip) or midazolam (0.1–0.2 mg/kg/h). Of course, sedating drugs should be used with caution in a patient whose neurologic status is being observed closely for anticipated changes. In severely injured patients, an i.v. phenylephrine drip can be used to increase MAP in favor of a higher CPP. Seizures should be treated aggressively with fosphenytoin (15–20 phosphenytoin equivalents/kg followed by 2.5–4 phosphenytoin equivalents/kg every 12 hours). Nutrition should not be neglected, and enteral feeds should be instituted as early in the ICU course as is feasible. This is usually in the form of continuous nasogastric tube feedings.

Follow-up CT scans should be reserved for those patients with clinical deterioration or an unexplained increase in ICP. It is important to involve physical, occupational, and speech therapists as early as clinically feasible. This will help to make the patient's transition to rehabilitation more seamless.

COMPLICATIONS

Delayed complications of head injury include the development of hydrocephalus, seizure disorders, learning difficulties, behavioral problems, and persistent neurologic deficits. About 13% of children suffering a head injury will leave the hospital in a vegetative state. If no improvement is seen in the first 6 months, patients are unlikely to make any significant gains.

As in any trauma, the most important time is the acute period. The cervical spine should be immobilized until cleared. The patient needs to be rapidly assessed for areas of scalp laceration or open skull fracture. A quick assessment of the neurologic function to determine if there are lateralizing signs or systemic signs consistent with elevated ICP should be performed. Thereafter, CT of the head should be performed as quickly as possible. Once an assessment of the CT has been made, a decision about ICP monitoring and the need for craniotomy can be made. The postoperative patient should be monitored closely until he or she has stabilized neurologically and the ICP is controlled. Involving rehabilitation services early on and keeping lines of communication open with the parents, including repeating realistic goals for the patient, can facilitate transfer to rehabilitation when the patient is stable.

SUGGESTED READINGS

Bruce DA. Imaging after head trauma: why, when and which. *Childs Nerv Syst* 2000;16:755–759.

Bruce DA, Raphaely RC, Goldberg AI, et al. Pathophysiology, treatment and outcome following severe head injury in children. *Childs Brain* 1979;5:174–191.

Harpold TL, McComb JG, Levy ML. Neonatal neurosurgical trauma. *Neurosurg Clin North Am* 1998;9:141–154.

Kochanek PM, Clark RS, Ruppel RA, et al. Cerebral resuscitation after traumatic brain injury and cardiopulmonary arrest in infants and children in the new millennium. *Pediatr Clin North Am* 2001; 48:661–681.

Schenarts PJ, Diaz J, Kaiser C, et al. Prospective comparison of admission computed tomographic scan and plain films of the upper cervical spine in trauma patients with altered mental status. *J Trauma* 2001;51:663–668.

Schutzman SA, Barnes P, Duhaime AC, et al. Evaluation and management of children younger than two years old with apparently minor head trauma: proposed guidelines. *Pediatrics* 2001;107: 983–993.

Teasdale G, Jennett B. Assessment of coma and impaired consciousness. A practical scale. *Lancet* 1974;13:81–84.

Surgical Directives: Pediatric Surgery, edited by Peter Mattei. Lippincott Williams & Wilkins, Philadelphia © 2002

16

PENETRATING NECK INJURIES

VICTOR F. GARCIA

Penetrating injuries of the neck are uncommon but challenging conditions to evaluate and manage. Missiles wounds (gunshot and BB) and stab wounds are the two most common types of injury. Vascular and aerodigestive injuries are indications for immediate operative management. Selective management has replaced mandatory exploration of the neck of an asymptomatic patient with a wound that penetrates the platysma but without evidence of vascular or aerodigestive injury.

Details of the event and an examination of the wound can suggest the direction of the missile and how much energy has been transferred to the surrounding tissues. In turn, this information may suggest organs at risk for injury and the extent of damage. A round entrance wound indicates a straight impact. An oval entrance wound suggests an angular impact. The spin of a high-velocity missile abrades the skin edges. If the missile passes at an angle, the side with the most abrasions is the side from which the bullet was traveling. Flame burns on the skin suggest that the muzzle was within 10 cm of the skin. Smoke particles on the skin suggest that the weapon was within 20 cm. Exit wounds tend to be stellate and do not have burns or abrasions as seen in entrance wounds. The anatomic structures at risk may be surmised by lining up entrance and exit wounds, although it should be kept in mind that missiles passing through tissue do not always travel in a straight line. Similarly, cavitation effects from high-velocity missiles and injury to structures that are adjacent to the missile tract can be more extensive than that suggested by the trajectory itself.

DIAGNOSIS

Indicators of injury to major vessels or the aerodigestive tract are noted in Tables 16.1 and 16.2. Signs of vascular injury are noted on careful serial physical examinations and include active hemorrhage, expanding hematoma, the presence of a bruit, and diminished pulses in the upper extremity. Shock that does not respond to the administration of intravenous fluids and has no other obvious etiology should be assumed to be due to an occult vascular injury and ongoing blood loss.

Signs of injury to the esophagus or trachea also may be evident by history or physical examination and include hoarseness, stridor, hemoptysis, dysphagia, painful swallowing, midline neck swelling, subcutaneous emphysema, or tracheal deviation. The examination is supplemented with a plain lateral radiograph, which may reveal retropharyngeal emphysema.

Neurologic deficits can be central, due to cerebral ischemia from a disrupted carotid or vertebral artery, or peripheral, due to an injury to the brachial plexus. The possibility of airway penetration or external hematoma compressing the airway is the first consideration during the evaluation of a patient with a penetrating injury of the neck. Penetration of the airway may require that the airway be secured by passing the endotracheal tube through the defect in the skin and into the trachea. A lateral or posterior injury tract requires that the endotracheal tube be inserted orally, preferably over a bronchoscope, to provide direct visualization of the trachea. Attempts at blind intubation often result in additional injury to the airway or placement of the tube through the defect and outside of the trachea. An injury tract close to the major vessels increases the risk of airway compression by an expanding hematoma and lowers the threshold for intubation. Additional indications for

TABLE 16.1. SIGNS OF VASCULAR INJURY

Active hemorrhage
Expanding hematoma
Shock not responding to fluid resuscitation
Bruit
Diminished radial pulse

V.F. Garcia: Department of Surgery, University of Cincinnati; and Trauma Services Medical Center, Cincinnati Children's Hospital Medical Center, Cincinnati, Ohio.

TABLE 16.2. SIGNS OF INJURY TO THE AERODIGESTIVE TRACT

Hoarseness
Hemoptysis
Dysphagia
Odynophagia
Midline swelling of the neck.
Subcutaneous emphysema
Retropharyngeal air on radiograph
Tracheal deviation

intubation include the presence of a large or expanding hematoma, decreasing level of consciousness, pharyngeal hemorrhage, significant mandibular injury, and tracheal injury.

Evidence of vascular or aerodigestive injury such as those listed above are indications for immediate operation. Penetration of the platysma is no longer considered an absolute indication for neck exploration. Selective management of patients who are asymptomatic or have minor symptoms has been shown to be safe and effective. The need for operation is determined by the results of barium swallow, esophagoscopy, fiberoptic laryngoscopy, arteriography, and color flow Doppler imaging. The initial study of the digestive tract should be a barium swallow with cineradiography in anterior and posterior views. No further evaluation of the esophagus is necessary if results of the barium swallow are normal. If results are inconclusive, rigid esophagoscopy should be performed under general anesthesia.

Arteriography is nearly 100% accurate in detecting a vascular injury. Color flow Doppler imaging closely parallels the specificity and sensitivity of arteriography in detecting clinically significant vascular injury. If the patient is asymptomatic, there is no evidence of vascular injury on physical examination, and the chest radiograph is normal, further testing of the vascular system may not be necessary. Some centers suggest that careful physical examination and color flow Doppler imaging provide a reliable, less morbid, and more cost-effective way to assess the major vessels of the neck following penetrating neck trauma. However, reducing the interval to definitive treatment reduces morbidity and mortality. Consequently, the decision to pursue diagnostic evaluation and the testing itself must be made with a sense of utmost urgency.

CLASSIFICATION OF INJURIES

The neck is arbitrarily divided into three zones. This classification is used in determining the likelihood of major vascular injury, need for arteriography, and mortality risk. Zone I extends from the thoracic inlet to the cricoid cartilage. Zone II begins at the cricoid cartilage and ends at the level of the angle of the mandible. Zone III extends from the angle of the mandible to the base of the skull. Traditionally, arteriography is recommended in patients with injuries in zones I and III because of the difficulty encountered in obtaining vascular control.

AIRWAY MANAGEMENT

A secure airway is the first priority in the management of a patient with a penetrating neck injury. Given the difficulty posed by anatomy distorted by hematoma, subcutaneous air, and active hemorrhage, securing the airway should be approached methodically and expeditiously. Facility with establishing a surgical airway and use of flexible bronchoscopy should be immediately available.

If intubation is necessary, the airway should be secured with an orotracheal tube preceded by preoxygenation. To protect against prolonged periods of hypoxia, the individual intubating the patient should hold their breath to appropriately gauge the duration of individual attempts at intubation. If intubation is unsuccessful, needle cricothyroidotomy, surgical cricothyroidotomy, or tracheostomy should be performed. Needle cricothyroidotomy can provide adequate oxygenation for approximately 30 to 45 minutes. Surgical cricothyroidotomy should not be performed in children under 12 years of age and in patients with evidence of laryngeal injury on physical examination.

SURGICAL APPROACH

Incision along the anterior border of the sternocleidomastoid muscle provides excellent exposure to the hypopharynx, esophagus, trachea, and vasculature of the neck. Alternatively, a generous collar incision can be used or, in the case of a stab wound, the laceration may be extended along the course of the anterior border of the sternocleidomastoid muscle.

AIRWAY INJURIES

Laryngeal injuries are best managed by a team consisting of a trauma surgeon, otolaryngologist, and anesthesiologist. Submucosal hematomas, minor lacerations, and mucosal disruptions can be managed with endotracheal intubation until airway edema resolves. More extensive mucosal disruptions and lacerations, major fractures of the larynx, or disruption of the cricoarytenoids are best managed with the timely support of an otolaryngologist familiar with anterior approaches to the larynx.

ESOPHAGEAL INJURIES

Barium cineradiography in two views (anterior and posterior) is the most accurate imaging study to establish the presence of esophageal injury. Penetrating injuries of the esophagus are repaired with a two-layer closure, consisting of an inner layer of absorbable suture and the surgeon's preference for an outer layer. Large wounds may require mobilization of the esophagus to permit a tension-free closure. Care must be taken to avoid injury to the recurrent laryngeal nerves. Extensive wounds may preclude primary repair and require lateral cervical esophagostomy. Regardless of the approach, all esophageal injuries should be actively drained. If there is a concomitant airway or vascular injury, a tissue flap, usually consisting of one of the strap muscles, should be interposed between the repair sites.

VASCULAR INJURIES

The vessels in zone I are the innominate, subclavian, and axillary arteries. If the patient is stable and the clinical picture suggests a vascular injury, arteriographic identification of the site of injury confirms the need for surgery and improves operative planning and exposure.

The innominate and proximal subclavian arteries are best approached through a median sternotomy incision, rather than a trapdoor incision of the upper chest. The second and third portions of the subclavian artery are best exposed with a supraclavicular cervical incision. Resecting the medial head of the clavicle facilitates dissection and proximal control of the subclavian vessels. The axillary artery is approached with an incision along the deltopectoral groove. Dividing the pectoralis major muscle 1 cm from its insertion on the humerus and the pectoralis minor muscle from the coracoid process can expose nearly the entire extent of the axillary artery.

Arterial vessels can be repaired either by simple arteriorrhaphy or end-to-end anastomosis using a fine monofilament suture. Resection of more than 2 cm of artery usually requires interposition of a saphenous vein or prosthetic graft. Given the generous collateral supply of the subclavian and axillary arteries, ligation is an option in the unstable patient with extensive injuries.

The vessels at risk in zones II and III are the common, internal, and external carotid arteries. These vessels are best approached through an incision along the anterior border of the sternocleidomastoid muscle. Exposure of the distal internal carotid artery can be problematic. Dislocating the temperomandibular joint anteriorly may improve access to this aspect of the internal carotid artery.

The external carotid artery may be ligated with impunity. Management of injuries to the common and internal carotid arteries is controversial. Concern over converting a "dry" infarct into a "hemorrhagic" infarct prompts some surgeons to favor ligation over primary repair in patients who present in coma or with a dense neurologic deficit. Patients who do not have a neurologic deficit on admission will in all likelihood do well regardless of whether ligation or repair is performed. Patients who have neurologic deficits and are revascularized are at risk for developing cerebral edema and may benefit from monitoring and management of increased intracranial pressure.

Vertebral artery injuries are rare. Most injuries result from a posterior neck wound and are recognized in the course of four-vessel arteriography in anticipation of selective nonoperative management. If the patient is stable, the disrupted vertebral artery can be embolized. If the injury is noted during neck exploration, proximal and distal ligation is acceptable.

Venous injuries in any zone can result in exsanguinating hemorrhage, tracheal deviation, and airway obstruction. Venous injuries are rarely isolated and usually are noted while addressing injuries to juxtaposed arteries. Fortunately, injuries to these veins can be ligated without significant morbidity.

SUMMARY

Penetrating neck injuries in children are uncommon but are a challenge to expeditiously diagnose and manage. Clinical guidelines based on available evidence facilitate decision making and management. Overt bleeding, an enlarging hematoma, or airway compromise are indications for immediate exploration of the neck. The asymptomatic patient with normal chest radiographs may be observed and the patient with minor symptoms may be selectively evaluated.

SUGGESTED READINGS

Atteberry LR, Dennis JW, Menawat SS, et al. Physical examination alone is safe and accurate for evaluation of vascular injuries in penetrating zone II neck trauma. *J Am Coll Surg* 1994;179:657–662.

Biffl WL, Moore EE, Rehse DH, et al. Selective management of penetrating neck trauma based on cervical level of injury. *Am J Surg* 1997;174:678–682.

Demetriades D, Theodorou D, Cornwell E III, et al. Penetrating injuries of the neck in patients in stable condition. Physical examination, angiography, or color flow Doppler imaging. *Arch Surg* 1995;130:971–975.

Demetriades D, Theodorou D, Cornwell E, et al. Evaluation of penetrating injuries of the neck: prospective study of 223 patients. *World J Surg* 1997;21:41–47.

Desjardins G, Varon AJ. Airway management for penetrating neck injuries: the Miami experience. *Resuscitation* 2001;48:71–75.

Ginzburg E, Montalvo B, LeBlang S, et al. The use of duplex ultrasonography in penetrating neck trauma. *Arch Surg* 1996;131: 691–693.

Kim MK, Buckman R, Szeremeta W. Penetrating neck trauma in children: an urban hospital's experience. *Otolaryngol Head Neck Surg* 2000;123:439–443.

Montalvo BM, LeBlang SD, Nunez DB Jr, et al. Color Doppler sonography in penetrating injuries of the neck. *AJNR* 1996;17: 943–951.

Mutabagani KH, Beaver BL, Cooney DR, et al. Penetrating neck trauma in children: a reappraisal. *J Pediatr Surg* 1995;30:341–344.

Shott SR. Penetrating trauma to the face, neck, and oral cavity in children. *Facial Plast Surg* 1999;7:153–160, viii.

17

BURNS

DAVID W. TUGGLE
DAVID S. FOLEY

More than 2 million burn injuries occur every year, resulting in 150,000 hospitalized patients. It has been estimated that 50% of all burned children will require up to 1 month of hospitalization. Deaths caused by thermal injuries occur most commonly in residential fires, especially in multifamily dwellings and low-income areas, and are the leading cause of death in the home for children under the age of 14. Ten percent of these deaths are the result of children playing with matches and cigarette lighters. It has been estimated that 12 people die in residential fires every day, and young children are among the most frequent victims. Burns are also a substantial form of child abuse. However, over the past 5 years, deaths associated with residential fires and thermal injuries have declined. This is most likely due to increased burn prevention education and awareness, which has resulted in decreased water heater temperature, more smoke alarms, improved building design, flame-resistant clothing, and the safer use of appliances. Improved burn care also has helped to decrease mortality rates.

RESUSCITATION

As with any injury, the initial resuscitation of a burned child consists of first managing the airway. Endotracheal intubation should be considered in any child with significant facial burns or inhalation injury. The burn wound edema that typically results from fluid resuscitation often causes obstruction of the airway in the presence of significant neck and facial burns. In addition, if significant chest wall burns are present, the edema that develops within a few hours can cause a restrictive lung defect, which can severely impair ventilation. If a child was in a closed space where a significant amount of smoke was present, such as a residential or vehicular fire, then an inhalation injury should be suspected. An inhalation injury is the most common factor in the cause of death in burned children. A carboxyhemoglobin value determined from an arterial blood gas taken as early as possible after extraction from the fire will give a good estimate of the degree of inhalation injury; however, the administration of supplemental oxygen during transport can decrease the detectable level of carboxyhemoglobin. Acute respiratory distress can develop up to 36 to 48 hours after smoke exposure; therefore, a high index of suspicion must be maintained. Examination of the child's airway with a fiberoptic bronchoscope will identify patients with oropharyngeal and tracheobronchial injuries. The typical bronchoscopic picture of airway edema, mucosal necrosis, hemorrhage, ulceration, or the presence of bronchial casts confirms the diagnosis.

Care should be taken to secure the airway because the topical treatment of the burn wound often makes securing the endotracheal tube problematic. If the mechanism of the injury suggests the possibility of traumatic injuries other than burns, a careful evaluation of the patient's ventilation and oxygenation is required. If the child sustained burns in a motor vehicle collision, the usual evaluation for traumatic injuries takes precedence over the burn wound management. Chest radiography and placement of chest tubes when appropriate should be considered early in resuscitation.

The fluid resuscitation of the burned child is extremely important. There is an obligatory increase in capillary permeability that occurs in the first 24 hours after burn injury and is most pronounced in burns involving more than 20% of the total body surface area. This creates a loss of isotonic intravascular fluid, most notably into the burned tissue but also into unburned soft tissue. A significant burn wound injury is a systemic injury; therefore, aggressive fluid resuscitation is associated with improved survival. It has been suggested that the earlier fluid resuscitation is begun, the better survival is. Several burn resuscitation formulas are advocated for use in children (Table 17.1).

The Parkland burn formula consists of giving 4 mL of lactated Ringer's solution per kilogram of body weight per

D.W. Tuggle and **D.S. Foley:** Department of Surgery, University of Oklahoma Medical Center; and Section of Pediatric Surgery, Children's Hospital at Oklahoma University Medical Center, Oklahoma City, Oklahoma.

TABLE 17.1. COMMONLY USED BURN RESUSCITATION FORMULAS

Formula	First 24 Hours	Subsequent Treatment
Parkland	Lactated Ringer solution 4 mL/kg/TBSA ½ in first 8 h; ½ in next 16 h Add maintenance fluids to calculated resuscitation to find total 24-h volume	D5 ¼ NS or D5 ½ NS at maintenance rate or greater Add potassium as needed
Shriners	Lactated Ringer solution 5,000 mL per m^2 burn area 2,000 mL per m^2 body surface area ½ total in first 8 h; ½ in next 16 h	3,750 mL per m^2 burn area + 1,500 mL per m^2 body surface area
Brookes	Lactated Ringer solution 3 mL/kg/TBSA ½ in first 8 h; ½ in next 16 h Plus maintenance fluids	Maintenance fluids to maintain urine output at 0.5–1 mL/h
Hypertonic	Hypertonic sodium lactate 2 mL/kg/TBSA	0.6 mL/kg/TBSA + maintenance fluids

TBSA, total body surface area; NS, normal saline.

the percentage of total body surface area burned. Half of the total volume is given within the first 8 hours after injury, and the remaining half is given over the next 16 hours. When infants and small children are being resuscitated, the standard calculation for maintenance fluid should be added to the 24-hour resuscitation volume, and the total should be given as noted above. This combination of resuscitation fluid and maintenance fluid is necessary for smaller children because their fluid requirements are much greater on a per-kilogram basis than are those of older children and adults. For example, a 10-kg infant with a 40% surface area burn would receive 1,600 mL of fluid in 24 hours based on the Parkland formula. This amount of fluid would result in a child with inadequate resuscitation. The addition of the usual 1,000 mL daily maintenance volume for this child would result in a total 24-hour fluid volume of 2,600 mL, which would more adequately resuscitate the child and provide for the expected insensible water losses.

Another widely used formula is the Shriners burn resuscitation formula. This formula provides for fluid resuscitation for the burn based on a surface area calculation and fluid resuscitation for maintenance on a surface area basis. Half of the calculated fluid volume is given during the first 8 hours, and the remaining half is given over the next 16 hours. Although some burn surgeons have advocated hypertonic saline resuscitation of burned children, the majority of burn centers use either the Parkland or the Shriners burn formulas.

All fluid resuscitation calculations are based on starting the resuscitation at the time of the burn. In many circumstances, the child may need to be transported to a regional burn center and often is under-resuscitated during transport. It has been shown that the first 8-hour resuscitation volume can be safely compressed into 4 hours without adverse effect to the child. Albumin is often added to the resuscitation at 12 to 24 hours after the injury. This is given in an effort to prevent hypoalbuminemia with a goal of maintaining the serum albumin concentration at greater than 2.0 g/dL. The best monitor of adequate fluid resuscitation is urine output, which should be maintained at a rate of 0.5 to 2 mL/kg/h. Serum electrolytes and osmolality should be maintained at normal levels. After 24 hours, the increased capillary permeability starts to decrease toward normal. At this point the maintenance fluid requirements are typically reduced to more normal rates, with an effort directed toward maintaining a normal volume status, normal electrolytes, and replacing insensible water loss. Glucose is an important early component of fluid resuscitation in children due to their relatively low glycogen stores. Approximately 3,750 mL of water is evaporated from each square meter of burns surface per 24 hours. Because of this volume loss of free water, the typical solution after the first 24-hour resuscitation should consist of 5% dextrose with 0.25% to 0.5% normal saline.

An accurate estimate of the burn size is essential in calculating the initial fluid resuscitation. The "rule of nines" is commonly used in adult patients and is appropriate for teenagers as well. However, the percentage of skin surface area represented by various anatomic regions is significantly different from infancy to the teen years (Table 17.2). For example, the head of an infant comprises 19% of the total body surface area (TBSA) and only 9% in a teenager or adult. Therefore, the burn wound size should be calculated from a nomogram or a table that takes into account the age, weight, height, or surface area of a child.

As the child is resuscitated, burn wound edema develops. If a child has a full-thickness circumferential burn to an extremity or the trunk, circulation or ventilation may be impaired. This burn wound edema is most prominent at 6 to 24 hours postburn. The peripheral arteries at the wrist or ankle should be monitored with a Doppler device on a regular basis during the first 24 to 36 hours of resuscitation. If

TABLE 17.2. CALCULATIONS OF BURN WOUND SIZE IN CHILDREN USED AT CHILDREN'S HOSPITAL OF OKLAHOMA

Area	Infant	1–4 yr	5–9 yr	10–14 yr	15 yr	Adult
Head	19	17	13	11	9	7
Neck	2	2	2	2	2	2
Anterior trunk	13	13	13	13	13	13
Posterior trunk	13	13	13	13	13	13
Right buttock	2.5	2.5	2.5	2.5	2.5	2.5
Left buttock	2.5	2.5	2.5	2.5	2.5	2.5
Genitalia	1	1	1	1	1	1
Right upper arm	4	4	4	4	4	4
Left upper arm	4	4	4	4	4	4
Right lower arm	3	3	3	3	3	3
Left lower arm	3	3	3	3	3	3
Right hand	2.5	2.5	2.5	2.5	2.5	2.5
Left hand	2.5	2.5	2.5	2.5	2.5	2.5
Right thigh	5.5	6.5	8	8.5	9	9.5
Left thigh	5.5	6.5	8	8.5	9	9.5
Right leg	5	5	5.5	6	6.5	7
Left leg	5	5	5.5	6	6.5	7
Right foot	3.5	3.5	3.5	3.5	3.5	3.5
Left foot	3.5	3.5	3.5	3.5	3.5	3.5

the peripheral artery Doppler signal becomes noticeably diminished or absent, burn wound escharotomy is indicated to relieve the constrictive effect of the edema. An escharotomy of an extremity is usually undertaken in a longitudinal fashion and can be extended onto involved digits. An escharotomy of the trunk is most often undertaken in a W or M pattern to allow expansion of the chest wall and improved ventilation.

Intravenous access can be a difficult problem, especially in burned infants. Peripheral intravenous access is often used early in resuscitation, but central venous access often becomes necessary soon after resuscitation is begun. A cutdown for intravenous access may be necessary, but should be avoided if possible. Central venous access by way of the femoral vein, subclavian vein, or internal jugular vein is a more reliable technique. An intraosseous technique also can be used initially for children under 6 years of age.

BURN WOUND CARE

After the initial assessment and resuscitation of the child is begun, attention is turned to care of the burn wound. The skin prevents the invasion of bacteria to deeper structures and controls insensible water loss. Burned tissue is nonviable and provides an excellent medium for the colonization of bacteria and fungi. The most common bacteria seen on burns come from the patient's own skin or intestinal tract. The most common topical agent used initially on burn wounds is silver sulfadiazine (Table 17.3). It has a broad spectrum of antibacterial effect, but does not penetrate the burn wound eschar. The most common side effect of silver sulfadiazine use is leukopenia. Children who are treated with silver sulfadiazine should have white blood cell monitoring on a daily basis. If the white blood cell count decreases to less than 4,000 cells/mm^3, another topical agent should be selected. Silver sulfadiazine can be used in combination with other topical agents, especially nystatin, which has the effect of reducing the incidence of *Candida* colonization or infection. Mafenide acetate is the next most commonly used topical agent. Its antibacterial effect has been shown to penetrate through full-thickness burn wounds to the unburned tissue underneath. Mafenide acetate is a significant carbonic anhydrase inhibitor and can create a metabolic acidosis when used over an extensive area of burn wound. Patients usually compensate for this metabolic acidosis by an increased respiratory rate and a compensatory respiratory alkalosis. Typically only 20% of the total burn surface area should be treated with mafenide acetate at any time to decrease the risk of this complication. Other topical agents can be used if silver sulfadiazine and mafenide treatments are contraindicated.

TABLE 17.3. TOPICAL ANTIMICROBIAL AGENTS USED TO TREAT BURNS

Silver sulfadiazine
Mafenide acetate
Silver sulfadiazine–cerium nitrate
Nystatin
Bacitracin
Polysporin/bacitracin
Silver nitrate
Povidone-iodine
Gentamicin

In addition to the use of topical antimicrobial agents, burn wound dressing changes are typically instituted. Dressing changes are performed every 8 to 24 hours depending on the burn size and risk of infection. The wounds should be cleaned and gently debrided with every dressing change. Dressing changes should be performed in as sterile an environment as possible. Burn wounds are typically cleaned with an antimicrobial soap. Occasionally a dilute hypochlorite solution might be used for selected bacterial colonization, such as with *Pseudomonas.* The goal of treatment is to maintain the bacterial colonization at less than 10^2 organisms per gram of tissue. Burn wound colonization is monitored by quantitative burn wound cultures, typically taken three times per week. Any bacterial wound count of 10^5 or greater indicates a probable burn wound infection, and a change in topical treatment is recommended.

Partial-thickness burns that are minimally colonized can be covered with a variety of biologic, bioengineered, or manufactured surfaces. This has been shown to decrease pain and increase healing, decrease inpatient days, and possibly improve cosmetic outcome. Pigskin (xenograft) or cadaver skin (allograft) has been used extensively but can result in tissue reactions due to genetic mismatches. The use of bilaminar nylon sheeting (Biobrane, Bertek Pharmaceuticals, Inc., Pittsburgh, PA) or cultured neonatal fibroblasts on nylon sheeting (TransCyte, Advanced Tissue Sciences, LaJolla, CA) is gaining popularity with respect to treatment of partial-thickness burns in children.

Intravenous antibiotics are not typically indicated during the initial treatment of an extensive burn wound. Systemic antibiotics are indicated when clinical sepsis is present. Examples of infection that would require systemic treatment include burn wound cellulitis, burn wound biopsy with greater than 10^5 organisms per gram of tissue, positive blood culture, urinary tract infection, or pulmonary infection. Even in the absence of positive cultures, empiric systemic antibiotic therapy should be instituted in the presence of fever, hypothermia, tachypnea, tachycardia, ileus, central nervous system changes, thrombocytopenia, leukocytosis, hyperglycemia, a large base deficit, or unexplained acidosis. In addition, intravenous antibiotics are indicated prior to burn wound excision and grafting, and are continued for 2 to 3 days postoperatively.

Early burn wound excision and grafting for deep partial-thickness and full-thickness burns have been shown to decrease mortality rates, burn wound infections, and hospital length of stay. Typically, burn wound excision is undertaken within 2 to 5 days following a thermal injury. In a young child, the surgical excision of a deep partial-thickness or full-thickness burn is most often down to fascia. This results in a more disfiguring burn wound, but has an associated lower blood loss. In older children, tangential excision of the partial-thickness burn with preservation of the unburned deep dermal layer or subcutaneous fat can be used with a better cosmetic result, but with more blood loss during surgery. Harvesting unburned skin by tangential excision with autografting provides the most efficient wound coverage. In most circumstances the skin is meshed to provide coverage of the wound in excess of the size of the donor site. Donor skin meshing can be 2:1, 3:1, 4:1, or as much as 9:1 when limited donor sites are available. The hands, face, and neck should be covered with unmeshed skin if possible. Meshing also allows for exudative fluid and blood to escape the donor graft–wound interface without interfering with graft adhesion and ingrowth. Skin grafts are usually secured to the wound bed with stainless steel staples. Smaller grafts can be secured with absorbable sutures. If there is insufficient unburned skin to provide adequate donor skin grafts, alternative coverage of the burn wound is available through a variety of sources. Cadaver skin, pigskin, and bioengineered burn wound coverage are all reasonable alternatives. Cultured epidermal autografts can be grown from small skin biopsy samples and applied to clean, previously excised burn wounds. The donor site can be covered with a variety of techniques and most often is chosen based on the preference of the surgeon.

The treatment of burn wounds can cause significant pain and anxiety, and the use of analgesics and anxiolytics is essential in the treatment of burned children. An intravenous narcotic in combination with amnestics or mood-altering drugs is most appropriate for patients with large surface area burns. Smaller burns can be treated with oral medications given enough in advance of treatment to be absorbed from the intestines.

NUTRITION

Patients with burns greater than 20% TBSA have an increased metabolic rate that requires nutritional supplementation. Children with a 40% or greater burn area may have increases in the metabolic rate up to 100% above basal levels. Maintenance of a child's weight during the postburn period can be accomplished by enteral or parenteral alimentation. A rough approximation of the required calories is 25 kcal/kg plus 40 kcal per the percentage of TBSA burned. The Shriners Burn Institute uses a formula based on the age and surface area of the patient and the burn. Children under 1 year of age receive 2,100 kcal/m^2 surface area plus 1,000 kcal/m^2 of burn surface area. Children 1 to 11 years of age receive 1,800 kcal/m^2 surface area and 1,300 kcal/m^2 burn surface area. Both of these formulas are calculated to provide adequate nutrition so that maintenance of body fat and muscle mass can be maintained. Nutritional support is best provided enterally and can be instituted as early as 3 hours after the burn injury. Enteral feedings instituted within hours of a burn injury decrease bacterial translocation, metabolic rate, mucosal atrophy, and the incidence of sepsis. Total parenteral nutrition has been shown to increase the mortality rate after burn injury when compared with enteral feedings. The early administration of parenteral nutrition also has detrimental effects on the immune system. Intravenous nutrition is only recommended in burn patients with prolonged gastrointestinal dysfunction or other contraindications to enteral feedings.

CHEMICAL INJURY

When a chemical burn injury occurs, the speed at which care is rendered is of prime importance. In general, all clothing should be removed, and the injured area liberally irrigated with large amounts of water. The effluent should be carefully removed so that a secondary injury does not occur. Alkali injuries often involve chemicals such as potassium hydroxide and sodium hydroxide and most commonly occur in children under 6 years of age. Alkaline agents bind with proteins to produce compounds with hydroxyl ions. These free radicals can cause deep secondary injury if not treated aggressively. No attempt should be made to neutralize the alkali with acid, because the heat generated by this exothermic reaction can worsen tissue injury.

Acid burns require more selective management. As with all chemical burns, copious irrigation with water is of prime importance. Burns caused by acids such as formic acid or hydrofluoric acid may require additional treatment to the wound, along with careful observation for electrolyte abnormalities in the case of formic acid exposure, and hypocalcemia for hydrofluoric acid burns.

ELECTRICAL INJURY

High-voltage electrical injuries in children are uncommon, and typically present with distinctive entry and exit wounds. Electrical burns have fewer cutaneous manifestations, but often cause deep muscle necrosis, along with bone and nerve damage. The resuscitation of children with severe electrical burns typically requires more fluid than would be calculated using standard burn resuscitation formulas.

The electrical current near the heart can give rise to dysrhythmias for up to 48 hours postinjury. A fasciotomy of an involved limb may be required if extensive muscular destruction results in a compartment syndrome. Some patients require debridement of necrotic muscle and fascia in an extremity, or even amputation in severe cases. Extensive muscular injury is associated with the early appearance of myoglobinuria. Myoglobinuria must be treated aggressively with large volumes of intravenous fluid to maintain a brisk diuresis. Mannitol can be used to assist with the maintenance of high urine output, but not at the expense of intravascular volume. Sodium bicarbonate is administered to alkalinize the urine and reduce precipitation of myoglobin in the renal tubules. Biting an electrical cord causes the electrical injury most commonly seen in small children. This manifests as a burn wound at the corners of the mouth involving the vermilion border. These burns cause limited disability and rarely have cardiac effects from the electrical shock. The most common problem associated with the mouth burns from cord bites occurs when the eschar separates, and bleeding occurs.

REHABILITATION AND PSYCHOLOGIC SUPPORT

Rehabilitation of the burned child should begin shortly after admission. The physical therapy team should be involved in the early stages of the burn care of all children with extensive burns, or burns involving the hands, feet, or face. Extremity splints are created to maintain joint mobility and prevent joint complications or contractures. The addition of constant pressure to a burn wound decreases the incidence of hypertrophic scarring. This pressure is applied in the form of measured elastic garments and should be maintained 24 hours a day for a year or more. If reconstructive procedures are planned, they should be undertaken when the burn wound healing is completed.

In a similar fashion, the psychologic aspects of burn care should be addressed early during hospitalization. The psychologist or psychiatrist can be instrumental in helping the child develop strategies to cope with the pain associated with daily wound care treatments. Children tend to adjust better to disfiguring injuries than do adults. The psychologic support for the child also should be extended to the entire family.

BURNS AND CHILD ABUSE

Approximately 20% of burn injuries in children are caused by child abuse. These burns are typically seen in children less than 5 years of age, and most are scald burns. In children of this age, this is also the type of burn most likely to be accidental. Other clues to the possibility of abuse are the reactions of the parents. The abusing parent or parents often show a relative lack of concern about the wound. The burn is often reported days after it was sustained. Other indications of abuse are the existence of wound symmetry, full-thickness wound, and occasionally wounds from struggle or flight. The treating physician should maintain a high index of suspicion, and in all 50 states, medical personnel are required to report their suspicions of abuse to governmental authorities.

EDITOR'S NOTES

Outside the setting of a tertiary burn center, the typical pediatric general surgeon manages burns either as part of a trauma resuscitation or as a relatively minor outpatient or emergency room referral. Two important issues become resuscitation of the severely burned child and the criteria for referral of smaller burn injuries to a burn center.

Resuscitation is outlined nicely in the chapter. Airway, breathing, and circulation, including intravenous access and aggressive hydration are, of course, paramount. Secondary but equally important issues include temperature regulation, exclusion of associated injuries, and patient comfort. In the absence of a true medical contraindication, it is inexcusable to withhold narcotic pain relief and anxiolytics from a child who has suffered significant burns. The assessment and resuscitation should be humane, efficient, and rapid, with transport to a burn unit within an hour of arrival, if possible. It is often advisable to establish telephone contact with the burn unit early in the resuscitation to ensure a smooth transition.

Deciding when a burn patient should be hospitalized or referred to a tertiary burn center can be difficult. Criteria vary depending on the services and expertise available at your institution and the comfort level of the staff and the family. General guidelines for hospitalization include second- or third-degree burns involving 10% or more body surface area (5% in children under 2 years of age); burns that involve the hands, feet, face, or genitalia; severe chemical burns; and high-voltage electrical burns. Children also should be admitted when there is any suspicion that the burns were the result of child abuse. Referral to a burn center is indicated whenever the primary facilities are felt to be inadequate for the acute care of the burn itself, or if there is a likelihood of significant long-term sequelae that would best be managed by the extended services provided by a burn center, for example, extensive reconstructive procedures, physical rehabilitation, or psychiatric support. In general, burns involving 25% or more body surface area, those associated with inhalation injury, or burns likely to result in significant functional or cosmetic concerns, for example, those involving joints or the female breast, should be referred to a specialty burn center either acutely or for follow-up.

Burns are often a form of child abuse, and a high index of suspicion should be maintained. Burns involving the palm of the hand (e.g., after touching an iron) or the sole of the foot are usually relatively superficial. The extent of injury is limited by the thickness of the skin and the reflex withdrawal caused by a painful stimulus. Deep second- or third-degree burns of the palm or sole raise the suspicion that the child was purposely held against the hot surface. Similarly, scald burns with sharply demarcated borders can be the result of a dipping injury and strongly suggest child abuse. When any suspicion of child abuse is raised, the child should be hospitalized and appropriate social services should be consulted.

–P.M.

SUGGESTED READINGS

Beushausen T, Mucke K. Anesthesia and pain management in pediatric burn patients. *Pediatr Surg Int* 1997;12:327–333.

Carvajal HF. Fluid resuscitation of pediatric burn victims: a critical appraisal. *Pediatr Nephrol* 1994;8:357–366.

Hansbrough JF, Hansbrough W. Pediatric burns. *Pediatr Rev* 1999; 20:117–123.

Rodriguez DJ. Nutrition in patients with severe burns: state of the art. *J Burn Care Rehabil* 1996;17:62–70.

Wolf SE, Debroy M, Herndon DN. The cornerstones and directions of pediatric burn care. *Pediatr Surg Int* 1997;12:312–320.

18

BLUNT ABDOMINAL TRAUMA

ROBERT W. LETTON, JR

Blunt abdominal trauma accounts for the vast majority of abdominal injuries occurring in childhood and infancy. Significant intraabdominal injuries are found in almost 25% of children sustaining multisystem trauma. Many of the injuries can be managed with minimal morbidity to the child. However, unrecognized injuries can lead to shock, multisystem organ failure, and ultimately death. It is important that individuals managing pediatric trauma always keep the "black box" known as the abdominal compartment in mind as a source of shock in the injured child.

The very nature of pediatric trauma often makes clinical assessment of the abdominal compartment very difficult. Anxiety and developmental immaturity may preclude an accurate physical examination of the abdomen. Often there are distracting injuries, which can result in shock themselves, and determining whether an aggravating abdominal injury needs to be addressed first can be difficult. This chapter will outline basic principles of management that when applied to the blunt pediatric trauma patient should allow rapid and accurate assessment of the abdominal compartment. Then will follow a brief discussion of the operative management in the stable and unstable child. With rapid and accurate assessment, appropriate intervention, and proper critical care, the child with abdominal trauma can and should have an excellent outcome.

ANATOMY AND PATHOPHYSIOLOGY

Compared with an adult, any impact in a child is absorbed over a smaller surface area and mass, making the energy delivered comparatively higher. The rib cage, which protects the upper abdominal viscera, is less calcified and more pliable. It is less likely to protect the liver and spleen and rarely shows visible signs of injury despite a significant impact. The spleen is only partially protected by this pliable rib cage, and is the most commonly injured organ. The liver is less often injured than the spleen, but more likely to lead to significant blood loss. Injury to the liver is the most common abdominal injury in pediatric trauma that leads to death.

Pediatric abdominal musculature is less well developed than in the adult and provides less protection to the colon and small intestine. In small children the dome of the bladder is located in the abdomen and is also less well protected. Even retroperitoneal structures such as the kidneys, pancreas, duodenum, aorta, and inferior vena cava are more vulnerable to injury than in the adult. The pancreas and duodenum are injured less often than other organs, but have serious consequences when they are.

The thin pediatric abdominal wall should make physical examination of the abdomen much easier than in the adult. However, anxiety, fear, and pain cause the child to cry, distending the stomach, and causing muscles to tighten, which makes assessment very difficult. Gastric distension also can cause respiratory compromise. Children who have received bag valve ventilation in the field can experience significant distension of their stomachs, and early decompression with an orogastric (OG) or nasogastric (NG) tube should be performed.

PRIMARY SURVEY

Rapid assessment of the child's airway, breathing, and circulation comes first in all injured patients. Most children with significant abdominal trauma remain hemodynamically stable, allowing their abdominal workup to be part of the secondary survey. However, it is not uncommon to have a child with an intraabdominal injury causing hemodynamic instability that must be addressed as part of the primary survey. As the anxious child continues to cry, the stomach becomes distended such that it might compromise ventilation. During resuscitation and stabilization, an NG or OG tube should be placed to decompress the stomach. Often the quickest way to identify the abdomen as the source of hypotension is to rule out the other most likely sources. Hypotension in a child with a normal chest radi-

R.W. Letton, Jr.: Departments of Surgery and Pediatrics, Wake Forest University School of Medicine, Winston–Salem, North Carolina.

ograph, normal pelvic film, and without significant lacerations or long bone fractures is due to abdominal hemorrhage until proven otherwise. The child *in extremis* who is in shock without a life-threatening cause identified in the primary survey deserves a trip to the operating room to stop the bleeding prior to continuing with the secondary survey.

The focused abdominal sonography for trauma (FAST) examination has become popular in the management of adult trauma, and its role in pediatric trauma is being defined as well. In the past the quickest method for assessing the abdomen for significant hemoperitoneum was with diagnostic peritoneal lavage. In the hands of an experienced surgeon it is an effective means for identifying patients with abdominal injury requiring laparotomy from bleeding or bowel injury, but not very good at looking for injury to retroperitoneal structures. With FAST, one now has a quick method to determine if there is a significant amount of fluid in the abdomen. Identifying the source of the fluid may be difficult, but in the face of hemodynamic instability and multisystem trauma, it can determine the likelihood of an abdominal source of significant hemorrhage.

SECONDARY SURVEY

After stabilization the child should be exposed and a complete head-to-toe examination performed. The abdominal wall should be inspected for bruises, abrasions, and other marks such as a seat belt stripe, bicycle handlebar bruise, or flank ecchymosis. Is the abdomen scaphoid or markedly distended? Auscultation of bowel sounds is difficult in a noisy examination room and will rarely lead to a significant alteration in plan. Palpation of the abdomen should then be performed. Placing an NG/OG tube will help to ensure that any tenderness or peritoneal signs are not due to gastric distension. If a seat belt stripe is present, the clinician should attempt to elicit peritoneal signs away from the area of bruising. It can be difficult to tell tenderness from the abdominal wall bruise from peritoneal irritation. If there is any suspicion of an occult bowel injury, serial abdominal examination is necessary. The clinician should check for signs of chest trauma, as well as for stability of the pelvic ring. A rectal examination should be performed in all trauma patients to assess for blood, sphincter tone, or a high riding prostate in boys with pelvic fracture prior to placing a Foley catheter. Long bone fractures and large lacerations, which could result in significant blood loss, should quickly be identified as well. Absence of other injury and persistent fluid requirements by the patient suggest significant hemoperitoneum.

LABORATORY

Blood work is occasionally useful in identifying those patients at increased risk for abdominal injury. The trauma panel usually consists of a complete blood count with differential, electrolytes with liver function tests, amylase, lipase, type and screen or crossmatch, urinalysis, and in some centers a lactic acid and arterial blood gas analysis. In the acute trauma setting, normal laboratory values are not very sensitive for ruling out injury, because equilibration after hemorrhage may not have occurred yet. However, values that are inappropriately high or low should raise suspicion for injury. A low hematocrit and hemoglobin should cause alarm for bleeding; elevation of liver transaminases (>200U/L) in an otherwise healthy child should cause concern for a liver laceration. Elevated amylase in the absence of facial trauma or elevated lipase should raise concern for pancreatic injury. Hematuria is a hallmark for genitourinary trauma, but is also often associated with other organ injury, and is used as an indication for further abdominal imaging in many trauma centers. Gross hematuria requires a cystogram to rule out a bladder injury, in addition to abdominal imaging to rule out an injury to the kidneys or collecting systems.

RADIOLOGIC STUDIES

Plain abdominal films are useful for evaluating bony structures, but unless pneumoperitoneum is noted, they are not of much use for identifying abdominal injury. FAST includes ultrasonography of the abdomen that specifically looks for free fluid. Four cardinal areas are examined: subxiphoid, right subcostal, left subcostal, and the pelvis. The sensitivity of the examination is exquisitely operator dependent. In a hemodynamically unstable patient with multiple injuries that could be the source of hypotension (e.g., pelvic or femur fracture), FAST can be an effective adjunct early in the trauma resuscitation to determine whether or not there is significant fluid in the abdomen. It does not identify the type of fluid and is not useful for identifying bowel injuries or grading solid organ injuries. The sensitivity of FAST has ranged from only 50% to 70%, with a negative predictive value in the same range. At present it would appear to have insufficient sensitivity and negative predictive value to be used as a screening test in hemodynamically stable children with blunt trauma.

Computed tomography (CT) of the abdomen is the most effective means of evaluating the abdomen in the blunt trauma patient. Nevertheless, it has limitations that are important to recognize. A limitation in the past has been the time required to obtain and process the CT scan. Slow scanners located far from the trauma bay were not safe places to take potentially unstable trauma patients. With the newer, faster scanners, the process has become less time consuming. Furthermore, most trauma centers now have a CT scanner in or near the emergency department dedicated for trauma and emergency scans. Most pediatric trauma victims remain stable enough to undergo abdominal CT. Controversy exists as to the necessity of oral contrast for scanning. Oral contrast is rarely essential for diagnosis of intraabdominal injury. Although it improves the sensitivity for identifying pancreatic injuries, it does not improve the diagnosis of those requiring surgery. Even with oral contrast, CT is just as insensitive for bowel injuries, and many centers have gone to immediate CT of the abdomen without oral contrast (but with intravenous contrast) to prevent the risk for aspiration.

Computed tomography is an excellent diagnostic study for solid organ injury, as well as retroperitoneal injury. Grading systems for solid organs have been developed based on CT criteria, and our management of these patients has become progressively more refined based on the CT appearance. The Achilles heel of CT scanning remains the poor sensitivity and specificity for hollow viscus injuries: the duodenum, small bowel, colon, and bladder. The presence of secondary signs of injury, such as free fluid, pneumoperitoneum, and bowel wall thickening, is currently the only way to identify individuals at risk for bowel injury. Isolated intraperitoneal fluid without solid organ injury is noted in approximately 10% of pediatric blunt trauma patients. Intraabdominal injury requiring surgery occurs in 15% to 25% of these patients; thus, operating based on the presence of fluid alone would result in a significant number of nontherapeutic laparotomies. The diagnosis is best made with a high index of suspicion, and signs of peritoneal irritation on serial examination. Because bowel perforation can present up to 3 days after injury, these patients should be observed closely for several days.

INJURY MANAGEMENT: THE UNSTABLE CHILD

Any child with hemodynamic instability, a negative primary survey for life-threatening injuries, negative chest and pelvic films, and absence of long bone fractures or external bleeding needs immediate laparotomy for presumed intraabdominal bleeding. Taking the unstable child with absence of other injury to the CT scanner will delay diagnosis and increase morbidity by extending the period of uncompensated hemorrhagic shock. Fortunately, this scenario is uncommon in the pediatric trauma victim. Regardless of the indication for surgery, a thorough exploration of the abdomen should be performed, including the retroperitoneum and lesser sac. Usually this is best accomplished with a midline incision, although infants under 2 years of age can usually be adequately exposed through a transverse incision. The chest should be prepared as well because sternotomy or thoracic extension may be required for severe liver or retroperitoneal aortocaval injuries.

If hemoperitoneum is encountered, the falciform ligament should be taken down, followed by four-quadrant packing and a systematic search for the source of bleeding. Severe liver lacerations can be extremely difficult to manage. The liver laceration should be approximated and compressed in order to give the anesthesia team time to catch up with the blood loss. With the help of a competent assistant, suture ligation of bleeding vessels in the liver parenchyma is often successful with a Pringle maneuver applied. If this does not control the bleeding, a retrohepatic caval or hepatic vein injury should be sought. Sternotomy and hepatic exclusion is often necessary to repair these injuries. If the child becomes cold, acidotic, and coagulopathic, a salvage operation should be performed. The liver should be packed, and the child should be brought to the pediatric intensive care unit (PICU) for aggressive resuscitation. This is followed in 12 to 24 hours by reexploration when the patient is warm and no longer coagulopathic. There are reports in the literature of hepatectomy for trauma followed by liver transplantation, but this would not appear to be a viable option in most centers.

Splenectomy is performed for unstable patients with spleen lacerations; splenorrhaphy should be attempted only if the patient is stable. Repair of associated hollow viscus injuries depends on the hemodynamic stability and temperature of the child. The concept of a "damage control laparotomy" currently practiced in the adult trauma patient should be similarly practiced in children. In the unstable patient, once the bleeding is controlled, if other injuries are present, they should be stapled off or packed, the abdomen temporarily closed, and the child resuscitated in the PICU until such time that reconstruction can be safely performed. Our institution uses a "vac-pac" closure similar to others described elsewhere. A bowel bag is pie-crusted with a no. 11 blade to allow drainage, placed over the bowel, and tucked under the fascia. A moist towel or cotton gauze is placed over this, followed by two closed suction drains connected to wall suction, and a large sterile drape to cover the abdomen. Peritoneal fluid losses can be monitored and replaced, and the child can be aggressively fluid resuscitated without fear of abdominal compartment syndrome. After reconstruction has been performed, it is our practice to pass a nasoduodenal tube, although some clinicians prefer placement of a feeding jejunostomy tube.

INJURY MANAGEMENT: THE STABLE CHILD

Solid organ injury to the spleen and liver will be discussed further in another chapter. Blunt injury to the kidney is more common in children than in adults due to increased mobility of the retroperitoneal structures. Any child with hematuria greater than 10 red blood cells per high-power field should have a CT scan with intravenous contrast not only to evaluate the kidneys, but also to rule out associated injuries that occur commonly with significant hematuria. Most kidney lacerations can be managed conservatively, although delayed nephrectomy for hypertension, persistent fever, or pain may be necessary in high-grade injuries. In the acute setting, controversy exists as to whether to repair a renal artery dissection or perform a primary nephrectomy due to prolonged warm ischemia. Gross hematuria in a boy with a pelvic fracture mandates urethrography followed by cystography to rule out intraperitoneal bladder rupture. A Foley catheter can be inserted in the urethra and the balloon slightly inflated. Contrast is injected and the catheter passed into the bladder if no urethral tear is noted. An abdominopelvic film with the bladder full of contrast followed by a postevacuation film should be obtained. Intraperitoneal rupture requires operative repair in two layers with Foley catheter drainage for 1 to 2 weeks; extraperitoneal rupture can be treated with Foley drainage alone for 7 to 10 days.

Pancreatic injuries are uncommon in children. They most frequently occur with seat belt, handlebar, or abuse injuries. The initial serum amylase level does not correlate well with the severity of pancreatic injury. Double-contrast CT scan is a more sensitive test than noncontrast CT or ultrasonography in diagnosing pancreatic injury; however, it does not increase the sensitivity for operative pancreatic trauma. The constellation of abdominal pain, an elevated serum amylase level, and a handlebar or "abdominal blow" mechanism of injury warrants hospitalization and investigation for injury. The majority of pancreatic injuries can be managed nonoperatively; however, distal duct injuries are best managed by prompt spleen-sparing distal pancreatectomy. As long as distal pancreatic injury presents within a few days of the traumatic event, distal pancreatectomy can usually be performed with some reports of successful spleen-sparing pancreatectomy up to 1 week after injury. Initial nonoperative management of injuries of the proximal pancreatic duct result in the formation of pancreatic pseudocyst. Often these can be managed by delayed percutaneous drainage. Despite weeks of hyperalimentation and possibly needing to perform an open cyst gastrostomy, this is often a better course for the child than early radical Whipple resection for proximal pancreatic duct injury. Controversy exists as to the benefit of closed drainage for management of minor pancreatic injuries discovered at laparotomy

Small bowel injuries are rarely life threatening, but their potential morbidity, combined with difficulty in diagnosis, gives them significant importance. Although the overall incidence of bowel injury from trauma in children is approximately 1%, in many studies looking at severely injured children the rate approached 8% to 10%, with reports of 15% to 25% of children with a lap belt stripe having small bowel injury. A discreet point of contact such as a lap belt, bicycle handlebar, or blow causes most hollow viscus injuries. Diagnosis can be difficult early in the course of evaluation. Reports of up to a 10% incidence of free intraperitoneal fluid on abdominal CT of all children is noted, and only 15% to 20% of these will have a surgical injury. The presence of free intraperitoneal fluid in more than one location increases the sensitivity to approximately 50%. Clearly, operating on the presence of fluid alone results in a number of nontherapeutic laparotomies. Furthermore, abdominal examination can frequently be misleading. It is this author's experience that many children with hemoperitoneum will react with significant abdominal tenderness, despite the absence of true peritonitis. This rapidly improves over time, and if persistent peritoneal irritation is present 12 to 24 hours after injury, exploration, or perhaps a repeat CT scan, is warranted to rule out an associated bowel injury.

In the absence of significant shock and contamination, primary repair of colon injuries is frequently possible, with diversion being used only in the face of severe shock and contamination, or to divert a rectal injury below the peritoneal reflection. In children with severe head injury and isolated peritoneal fluid on CT scan, a diagnostic peritoneal lavage can frequently help establish the presence or absence of bowel injury without formal laparotomy.

Duodenal hematomas are usually self-limited, and do not warrant exploration. Transpyloric feeding can be accomplished safely for a few weeks until the hematoma resorbs and duodenal obstruction resolves. Duodenal perforation is often delayed in presentation. Due to the retroperitoneal position of the duodenum and the relative absence of bacteria in the gastrointestinal tract at this level, development of peritonitis is delayed. Simple lacerations can be repaired and patched with serosa or omentum. Complex repair should be diverted with temporary pyloric exclusion, gastrostomy, suture closure of the pylorus from within the stomach, and side-to-side gastrojejunostomy.

Diaphragmatic rupture may be suggested on chest radiography by visualizing the NG tube coiled in the stomach above the diaphragm, or on CT scan, but the sensitivity is low. Left-sided rupture is often associated with splenic injury; therefore, laparoscopy may not be as useful in the diagnosis of blunt diaphragmatic rupture as it may be in cases of penetrating trauma to the lower chest. Gastric rupture occurs infrequently and is usually easily repaired in two layers, with consideration for placing a gastrostomy tube in severe injury.

CONCLUSION

Blunt abdominal trauma occurs in a significant number of children. Early management principles are aimed at recognizing and treating shock, followed by definitive diagnosis of injury and subsequent repair. The trauma physician should approach the care of the child with adherence to the common principles of adult trauma, along with the knowledge that different anatomic, physiologic, and mechanistic patterns exist in the pediatric trauma patient.

SUGGESTED READINGS

Albanese CT, Meza MP, Gardner MJ, et al. Is computed tomography a useful adjunct to physical examination for diagnosis of pediatric gastrointestinal perforation from blunt trauma in children. *J Trauma* 1996;40:417–421.

Bond SJ, Eichelberger MR, Gotschall CS, et al. Non-operative management of blunt hepatic trauma and splenic injury in children. *Ann Surg* 1996;223:286–289.

Coley BD, Mutabagani KH, Martin LC, et al. Focused abdominal sonography for trauma (FAST) in children with blunt abdominal trauma. *J Trauma* 2000;48:902–906.

Haller JA, Papa P, Drugas G, et al. Non-operative management of solid organ injury—is it safe? *Ann Surg* 1994;219:625–628.

Keller MS, Stafford PW, Vane DW. Conservative management of pancreatic trauma in children. *J Trauma* 1997;42:1097–1100.

Newman KD, Bowman LM, Eichelberger MR, et al. The lap belt complex: intestinal and lumbar spine injury in children. *J Trauma* 1990;30:1133–1138.

Sivit CJ, Taylor GA, Newman KD, et al. Safety belt injuries in children with lap belt ecchymosis: computed tomography findings in 61 patients. *Am J Radiol* 1991;57:111–114.

Taylor GA, Eichelberger MR, O'Donnell R, et al. Indications for computed tomography in children with blunt abdominal trauma. *Ann Surg* 1991;213:212–218.

Surgical Directives: Pediatric Surgery, edited by Peter Mattei. Lippincott Williams & Wilkins, Philadelphia © 2002

19

PENETRATING ABDOMINAL TRAUMA

MICHAEL L. NANCE

Trauma is the leading cause of death and disability in the pediatric age group. Penetrating injuries represent 8% to 12% of the trauma population at most major institutions. Despite declining national trends in firearm-related injury, gunshot wounds are the most common cause of penetrating wounds in the pediatric age group and represent the leading cause of death in the male African-American population 15 to 24 years of age. In the urban setting, firearm injuries are usually related to violence, whereas in nonurban regions they tend to be unintentional. In children with gunshot wounds, approximately 25% sustain an intraabdominal injury, including 14% who are fatally injured. Other causes of penetrating injuries include stab wounds, impalements, animal bites, and machinery related accidents (Table 19.1).

Initial evaluation of the child with a penetrating abdominal injury should follow the well-established guidelines developed by the American College of Surgeons Committee on Trauma and taught through the advanced trauma life support course. The evaluation begins with an assessment of the airway, breathing, and circulation. Large-bore intravenous access should be established for volume resuscitation and to address the potential for blood loss and transfusion requirements. Uncrossmatched blood should be immediately available for transfusion if needed and a specimen sent to prepare type-specific and crossmatched blood components. Because the vast majority of penetrating injuries to the abdomen will require surgical intervention, preparation of an operating room for laparotomy should occur simultaneously with patient assessment. As part of the secondary survey during the trauma assessment, the abdomen is evaluated. It is imperative that the patient be completely exposed to help identify all wounds of entrance and exit. Consideration of the trajectory is important, because many patients with intraabdominal injuries will have remote entrance wounds such as the thigh, buttock, or chest. It should be kept in mind that 15% of children with an intraabdominal injury also have injuries to other body regions. Wound location provides a general idea as to possible intraabdominal injuries and may help determine operative strategy. Physical findings are also helpful in determining possible intraabdominal pathology. Distention may develop from hemorrhage or hollow visceral injury with free air. Percussion of the abdomen may help distinguish the dullness of fluid from the tympany of free air. Tenderness may be present as a result of diffuse peritoneal inflammation from blood or enteric contents, or locally as a result of soft tissue destruction.

Radiologic evaluation (abdominal plain film) is usually indicated to help determine bullet trajectory and search for possible retained missiles, fragments, or bony injury. It is useful to place radiopaque markers on the skin to mark wounds of entrance and exit. Wounds and identified bullets need to match up to minimize the risk for missed injuries. A decubitus or upright view is rarely necessary, but may demonstrate free air in the abdomen. It may be necessary to obtain chest films, pelvis films, or femur films to locate foreign bodies.

If violation of the peritoneum is in doubt based on physical examination or the suspected trajectory of the missile, adjunctive measures may be useful to evaluate the patient. CT scan has been advocated for evaluating tangential abdominal wounds or wounds in the hepatic region that may not require celiotomy. If an extraperitoneal path can be verified, laparotomy may be avoided. In addition, injuries that clearly involve the liver, in the absence of other indications for surgical intervention, may be managed expectantly. Data supporting this approach in the child is anecdotal and should be considered on a case-by-case basis. CT

TABLE 19.1. PENETRATING ABDOMINAL INJURY MECHANISM

Mechanism	Frequency
Gunshot wound	60%
Stab wound	24%
Animal bite	8%
Machinery related	8%

M.L. Nance: Department of Surgery, University of Pennsylvania; and Department of Surgery, Children's Hospital of Philadelphia, Philadelphia, Pennsylvania.

scan may be of benefit in the evaluation of injuries to the gluteal region to help detect a possible rectal injury. CT scans obtained to evaluate transpelvic gunshot wounds should include intravenous, oral, and rectal contrast. Although experience with this modality for evaluation of transpelvic injuries in the adult population is promising, information is limited in the pediatric population.

Diagnostic peritoneal lavage (DPL) has been advocated as a tool to determine the need for laparotomy in the penetrating trauma setting. Detection of blood, white blood cells, or fecal matter in the lavage effluent is an indication of intraabdominal injury and necessitates operative intervention. Other clinicians have found this technique less reliable and nonspecific. The decision to perform DPL should be that of the operating surgeon because the interpretation of the results will determine the need for laparotomy.

Laparoscopy also may be useful to help determine whether peritoneal violation has occurred. If peritoneal penetration were identified, most would advocate converting to formal laparotomy for thorough exploration. The laparoscope also may be valuable in assessing the diaphragm in those cases in which the trajectory suggests a possible thoracoabdominal path.

In selected patients, nonoperative management of stab wounds or gunshot wounds may be indicated. This decision must be individualized and the patient examined at frequent intervals to detect peritoneal signs. Deterioration of the physical examination or vital signs mandates urgent laparotomy.

Intraabdominal injuries from a gunshot wound are variable and unpredictable; therefore, one must prepare for the worst (Table 19.2). The chest, abdomen, and groin should be prepared and draped into the operative field. The left arm is extended above the head to provide access to the chest in case thoracotomy is necessary. Maintaining the patient's core body temperature is a priority during the laparotomy. The operating room should be warmed, and all fluids and blood products should be run through a warming device. Broad-spectrum antibiotics are administered preoperatively. Immediately upon entering the abdomen, all four quadrants should be packed with laparotomy sponges to control hemorrhage. Each quadrant is then inspected for ongoing hemorrhage and repacked if necessary. Control of hemorrhage is of primary importance. After control of hemorrhage, attention turns to identification of injuries. The bowel should be inspected meticulously from diaphragm to rectum. In general, an even number of enterotomies should be identified because bowel injuries are typically through and through. Retroperitoneal hematomas should be explored to identify potential major vascular injuries.

TABLE 19.2. ORGAN INJURIES ENCOUNTERED IN PENETRATING ABDOMINAL TRAUMA

Organ Injured	Frequency
Liver	22%
Small bowel	18%
Colon	16%
Vascular	10%
Stomach	10%
Spleen	9%
Kidney	9%
Pancreas	6%
Duodenum	4%
Other	9%

The management of hollow organ injuries is based on the extent of injury. Focal injuries with minimal blast effect can be managed with debridement and primary repair if adequate caliber can be assured. Extensive injury or tissue devitalization usually requires resection and reconstruction. Multiple injuries in close proximity (as often occur in the small bowel) are best managed by limited bowel resection incorporating all holes with a primary anastomosis rather than repair of individual wounds. The management of colonic injuries remains controversial. Most adult studies suggest that primary repair or resection with repair is appropriate for the majority of colonic injuries. Colostomy is reserved for complex injuries or the unstable patient. Such an approach is likely safe in children but is as yet unproven.

Solid organ injuries such as those involving the liver or spleen are typically amenable to packing or local maneuvers. In the minority of cases, resection may be required for hemostasis. Attempts at splenic salvage are warranted in the stable pediatric patient to avoid the potential for overwhelming postsplenectomy sepsis.

Abdominal vascular injuries, although somewhat uncommon, are associated with a high mortality rate. Hemodynamic instability in the setting of an abdominal gunshot wound is likely the result of a vascular injury. Consideration should be given to thoracotomy and cross-clamping of the aorta prior to entering the abdomen because decompression of abdominal tamponade effect may prove rapidly fatal. Additional maneuvers to control exsanguinating hemorrhage include cross-clamping of the aorta at the suprahepatic level or compression of the aorta with an instrument. Once the vascular injury is identified, local control should be established and aortic occlusion released. Management of the injured vessel should be individualized. Most injuries are amenable to debridement with primary repair. Ligation may be necessary in some cases. If vascular reconstruction is necessary, native internal jugular vein or hypogastric artery are potential conduits.

Damage control has been applied to the pediatric trauma population. The approach is appropriate for the most severely injured subset of patients with life-threatening hemorrhage. The initial laparotomy is abbreviated and involves expeditious tamponade of active bleeding with packing and control of contamination by closure of enterotomies. No attempts are made to definitively manage injuries that can safely be delayed until the patient is more stable. A temporary abdominal closure of skin only is performed to prevent intraabdominal hypertension. In the second phase, aggressive resuscitation continues in the intensive care unit with a focus on rewarming and correction of acidosis and coagulopathy. The resuscitation phase typically lasts 12 to 24 hours. The third phase involves definitive management of injuries and fascial closure and should be undertaken when adequate resuscitation has been achieved. This approach, which is very resource intensive, may salvage patients with an otherwise high risk for death.

Impalements represent a truly unique subset of penetrating injuries. These injuries are best managed in the operating room, where complete assessment of injuries can be performed and a treatment strategy developed. The management is highly individualized based on the nature and trajectory of the impaling instrument. Management of these injuries is frequently a team effort involving surgery, neurosurgery, and orthopedic surgery.

SUGGESTED READINGS

Nance ML, Stafford PW, Schwab CW. Firearm injury among urban youth during the last decade: an escalation in violence. *J Pediatr Surg* 1997;32:949–952.

Stylianos S, Templeton JM Jr. Abdomen. In: Ivatury RR, Cayten CG, eds. *The textbook of penetrating trauma, 1st ed.* Media, PA: Williams & Wilkins, 1996:813–816.

Cooper A, Barlow B, DiScala C, et al. Mortality and thoracoabdominal injury: the pediatric perspective. *J Pediatr Surg* 1994;29:33–38.

Surgical Directives: Pediatric Surgery, edited by Peter Mattei. Lippincott Williams & Wilkins, Philadelphia

20

GUIDELINES FOR THE TREATMENT OF CHILDREN WITH BLUNT SPLEEN OR LIVER INJURY

STEVEN STYLIANOS

Evidence-based medicine involves integrating current best evidence (medical literature) with clinical expertise and patient preferences in making decisions about the care of individual patients. Evidence-based methodology is the emerging cornerstone of the clinical practice guideline process. Recently, several trauma societies have used evidence-based methodology to develop practice guidelines for adult patients with cervical spine injuries, blunt cardiac injury, intraperitoneal colon injury, and for venous thromboembolism prophylaxis, antibiotic use, and other conditions.

There are no randomized, controlled trials (class I evidence) regarding optimal resource utilization in children with isolated spleen or liver injury. Therefore, using evidence-based methodology, standards of care cannot be proposed in the absence of class I data. Formal consensus development techniques using expert opinion is required to develop practice guidelines whenever adequate evidence is lacking (Table 20.1). A recently completed study by the American Pediatric Surgical Association (APSA) Trauma Committee regarding children with isolated spleen or liver injury used evidence from multiple sources, including published, nonrandomized trials (class II evidence), historical controls, and expert clinical experience and consensus (class II and III). Thus, the term *guidelines* is appropriate for the proposed recommendations.

Although nonoperative treatment of children with isolated, blunt spleen or liver injury has been universally accepted, there is great variation in the management algorithms used by pediatric surgeons. Review of the National Pediatric Trauma Registry and two recent surveys of the APSA membership confirm the wide disparity in care acknowledging the limitations of trauma registry and survey reviews. The evolution and refinement of nonoperative treatment in children with isolated spleen or liver injury have been well documented at individual centers. However, guidelines for intensive care unit (ICU) admission, number of hospital days, the need for predischarge or postdischarge imaging, or the appropriate interval of restricted physical activity remain undefined.

To define evidence-based guidelines for children with spleen or liver injury assuring efficient, cost-effective utilization of resources while maximizing patient safety, it was essential to determine current practice. Data from the case records of 856 children with isolated spleen or liver injury treated at 32 pediatric surgical centers from July 1995 to June 1997 were collected. The patients were grouped by severity of injury as classified by computed tomography (CT) grade, and patients with grade V injuries were excluded from analysis or recommendation. These data and the available literature were analyzed for consensus. Clinical parameters in the 832 patients are described in Table 20.2. Five guidelines are proposed for all *hemodynamically stable* patients (Table 20.3). Admission to the ICU is reserved for patients with grade IV injuries only. Children with grade I to III injuries had transfusion rates of only 2% to 10% and operation rates of under 3%, supporting the omission of

TABLE 20.1. EVIDENCE-BASED GUIDELINE DEVELOPMENT

1. Topic selection (area of variability)
2. Selection of "expert" panel
3. Clarification of proposed guideline purpose and scope
4. Listing specific goals and questions
5. Grading scientific evidence
6. Establishing recommendations
7. Presentation
8. Dissemination and Implementation
9. Evaluation and Revision

S. Stylianos: Departments of Surgery and Pediatrics, Columbia University College of Physicians and Surgeons; and Regional Pediatric Trauma Program, Children's Hospital of NewYork–Presbyterian, New York, New York.

TABLE 20.2. RESOURCE UTILIZATION AND ACTIVITY RESTRICTION IN 832 CHILDREN WITH ISOLATED SPLEEN OR LIVER INJURY

	Computed Tomography Grade			
	I	II	III	IV
Admitted to ICU	55.0%	54.3%	72.3%	85.4%
No. of hospital days (mean)	4.3 days	5.3 days	7.1 days	7.6 days
No. of hospital days (range)	1–7 days	2–9 days	3–9 days	4–10 days
Transfused	1.8%	5.2%	10.1%[a]	26.6%[a]
Laparotomy	None	1.0%	2.7%[b]	12.6%[b]
Predischarge imaging	13.9%	32.4%	34.8%	37.9%
Postdischarge imaging	29.8%	33.7%	44.0%	43.2%
Activity restriction (mean)	5.1 wk	6.2 wk	7.5 wk	9.2 wk
Activity restriction (range)	2–6 wk	2–8 wk	4–12 wk	6–12 wk

[a]Grade III vs. grade IV, $p < 0.014$.
[b]Grade III vs. grade IV, $p < 0.0001$.

ICU stay. The proposed number of hospital days and weeks of physical activity restriction were chosen by determining what was done safely in at least 25% of the patients entered in the study. Fewer than half of the patients had pre- or postdischarge follow-up imaging studies, thus supporting our recommendation of no follow-up imaging in routine cases. Based on the data analysis, literature search, and consensus conference, we propose the guidelines in Table 20.2 for the safe and optimal utilization of resources in routine cases. *It is important to emphasize that no recommendation falls outside the 25th percentile of current practice at participating centers.*

Despite the diversity, clear patterns emerged, showing a continued decrease in the resources used without a compromise in safety or outcome. Several descriptive studies have recommended shorter ICU and hospital stays in children with stable spleen or liver injury. Gandhi et al. showed significant reduction of hospital stay in children with spleen injury after adopting a clinical pathway. Their recommendations for hospital stay and interval of activity restriction did not stratify for injury severity. The evidence in our study for eliminating ICU admission in stable patients with grades I through III injury is current transfusion rates of only 2% to 10% and operation rates of under 3% in this cohort. Intensive care unit admission for patients with grade IV injuries is supported by the significant increase in the rate of transfusion and operation than in children with less severe injuries. *It is imperative to emphasize that these proposed guidelines assume hemodynamic stability.* The extremely low rates of transfusion and operation document the stability in the study cohort of patients.

The safe interval of restricted physical activity after solid organ injury has been debated for nearly 30 years. Many clinicians have used radiologic "healing" as criteria for allowing children to return to normal physical activity. Controversy exists over the need for follow-up imaging before and after discharge in children with successful nonoperative treatment of spleen or liver injury and the potential significance of these studies on limitation of physical activity. Attempts to define the time required for healing of the injured spleen by imaging studies have been inconclusive. Multiple studies from pediatric trauma centers evaluating the use of routine follow-up ultrasonography or CT after successful nonoperative treatment showed that interval

TABLE 20.3. PROPOSED GUIDELINES FOR RESOURCE UTILIZATION IN CHILDREN WITH ISOLATED SPLEEN OR LIVER INJURY

	CT Grade			
	I	II	III	IV
ICU days	None	None	None	1 day
Hospital stay	2 days	3 days	4 days	5 days
Predischarge imaging	None	None	None	None
Postdischarge imaging	None	None	None	None
Activity restriction*	3 wk	4 wk	5 wk	6 wk

*Return to **full-contact, competitive sports** (e.g., football, wrestling, hockey, lacrosse, mountain climbing, etc.) should be at the discretion of the individual pediatric trauma surgeon. The proposed guidelines for return to unrestricted activity include "normal" age-appropriate activities.

to radiologic "healing" correlated roughly with CT grade of injury. However, the appearance of the spleen or liver on imaging studies may not necessarily correlate with the integrity of the organ and, therefore, offers little help to the clinician in advising the period of restricted physical activity after injury. Many clinicians believe that assessment of healing by imaging studies can be misleading and unreliable in defining a safe interval for restriction of physical activity. Our data show that less than 50% of patients currently undergo follow-up imaging in the 32 participating centers without sequelae. Our recommendation is that no routine follow-up imaging be obtained. Rather, focused imaging based on clinical symptoms is encouraged.

This detailed review of 832 patients confirmed the diversity of treatment, with attendant variation in resource utilization, in children with isolated spleen and liver injury of comparable severity. A unique aspect of our study is strict stratification of patients by injury severity (CT grade). This allowed for a more rational analysis of resource utilization. Our findings stimulated a prospective study with the objective of validating the five proposed evidence-based guidelines. These guidelines were applied prospectively in 312 children at 16 centers from 1998 to 2000. Specific guideline compliance was 81% for ICU stay, 82% for hospital stay, 87% for follow-up imaging, and 78% for interval of activity restriction. There was a significant improvement in compliance from year 1 to year 2 for ICU stay (77% vs. 88%, $p < 0.02$) and interval of activity restriction (73% vs. 87%, $p < 0.01$). There were no differences in compliance by age or organ injured. Deviation from the guidelines was the surgeon's choice in 90% of cases, and patient related in 10%. Six patients (1.9%) were readmitted. None of the six required operation.

Prospective application of specific treatment guidelines has resulted in conformity in patient management, improved utilization of resources, and validation of guideline safety. Reduction of ICU stay, hospital stay, follow-up imaging, and length of activity restriction was achieved without adverse sequelae when compared with a historical database. The impact of developing clinical guidelines on costs can be significant. Once validated, guidelines should have direct economic relevance by eliminating unnecessary ICU days, hospital days, and imaging studies while enhancing patient satisfaction in safely returning to normal activities. This evidence-based study design can bring order and conformity to patient management, resulting in optimal utilization of resources while maximizing patient safety. The rapidly changing health-care environment has put new pressures of accountability on physicians. There is a great need and opportunity to apply evidence-based methodology in pediatric surgery to enhance the care for our patients. Evidence-based studies such as this will allow pediatric surgeons to proactively define optimal care rather than to be reactive, responding after the fact to the concerns of others with less expertise and differing motivations.

IMMEDIATE SURGERY FOR BLUNT ABDOMINAL INJURIES

Surgeons treating children with abdominal injuries have refined nonoperative management over the past three decades. Review of the National Pediatric Trauma Registry from 1995 through 1999 shows that only 11% of 1,177 children with spleen injuries and only 6% of 1,179 children with liver injuries required surgery. In a recent report from the APSA Trauma Committee, only 28 (2.5%) of 1,144 children with *isolated* spleen or liver injury underwent surgery. These data indicate that few surgeons will have extensive experience with massive abdominal solid organ injury requiring immediate surgery. It is imperative that surgeons familiarize themselves with current treatment algorithms for life-threatening abdominal trauma.

The indications for immediate surgery following abdominal trauma in children include hemodynamic instability, evidence of persistent hemorrhage, suspicion of hollow viscus perforation, and major pancreatic ductal disruption. Maintenance of physiologic stability during the struggle for surgical control of severe bleeding is a formidable challenge even for the most experienced surgeon, particularly when hypothermia, coagulopathy, and acidosis occur. This triad creates a vicious cycle whereby each derangement augments and exacerbates the others and the physiologic and metabolic consequences of the triad often preclude completion of the procedure. Increased emphasis on physiologic and metabolic stability in emergency abdominal operations has led to the development of staged, multidisciplinary treatment plans, including abbreviated laparotomy, perihepatic packing, temporary abdominal closure, angiographic embolization, and endoscopic biliary stenting. Asensio et al. reported on 22 patients with grade IV or V injuries treated between 1992 and 1997. Mean blood loss was estimated at 4.6 L and mean packed red cell transfusion requirement was 15 units. Ten patients were packed at the first operation. Fifteen patients underwent postoperative angiographic embolization in an attempt to control hemorrhage. Survival was 92% in 13 grade IV patients and 78% in 9 grade V patients.

Abbreviated laparotomy with packing for hemostasis allowing resuscitation prior to planned reoperation is an alternative in unstable patients where further blood loss would be untenable. Once hypothermia is reversed, coagulation factors are replaced, and oxygen delivery optimized, the patients can be returned to the operating room for pack removal and definitive repair of injuries. Although abdominal packing (PACKS) with planned reoperation has been used with increasing frequency in adults during the past two decades, little experience in children has been reported. A recent review reported 22 patients with refractory hemorrhage (ages 6 days to 20 years) who were treated with PACKS. The anatomic site of hemorrhage was the liver and/or hepatic veins in 14, retroperitoneum and/or pelvis in

7, and the pancreatic bed in 1. Fifteen patients (68%) had PACKS inserted during a primary operative procedure. Insertion of abdominal packing was accomplished in a mean of 2.5 hours (1–5 hours) after the start of the primary procedure. Seven patients (32%) had PACKS inserted during a reexploration for persistent hemorrhage in a mean of 1 hour (1–2 hours) after the start of the reexploration. Twenty patients (91%) were coagulopathic (mean prothrombin time >16 seconds), hypothermic (mean temperature <35°C), and acidotic (mean pH <7.2) at the time of packing. The mean volume of intraoperative blood product transfusion prior to PACKS was 190 mL/kg (50–600 mL/kg). Primary fascial closure was accomplished in 12 patients (55%), whereas temporary skin closure or prosthetic material was used in the other 10. PACKS controlled hemorrhage in 21 of 22 (95%) patients. Removal of PACKS was possible within 72 hours in 18 patients (82%). No patient rebled after PACKS removal, but 2 patients died with PACKS in place. Seven patients (32%) developed an abdominal or pelvic abscess. All were successfully drained by laparotomy (6 patients) or percutaneous (1 patient) approach. Six of these seven patients with abdominal sepsis survived. Eighteen patients (82%) survived. Two deaths were due to multisystem organ failure, one succumbed to cardiac failure from complex cardiac anomalies, and one death was from exsanguination after blunt traumatic liver injury. There were no differences in volume of intraoperative blood product transfusion, time to initiate PACKS, physiologic status, or type of abdominal closure between survivors and nonsurvivors.

The consequences of prolonged operations with massive blood product replacement include hypothermia, coagulopathy, and acidosis. Although the surgical team may keep pace with blood loss, life-threatening physiologic and metabolic consequences are inevitable, and many of these critically ill patients are unlikely to survive once their physiologic reserves have been exceeded. Review of nearly 700 patients with abdominal packing from several institutions demonstrated hemostasis in 80%, survival of 32% to 73%, and abdominal abscess rates of 10% to 40%. It is essential to emphasize that the success of the abbreviated laparotomy and planned reoperation depends on an early decision to employ this strategy prior to irreversible shock. A staged operative strategy for unstable patients represents advanced surgical care and requires sound surgical judgment and expertise. Abdominal packing, when employed as a desperate, last-ditch resort after prolonged attempts at hemostasis have failed, has been uniformly unsuccessful.

The optimal time for reexploration is controversial because neither the physiologic end points of resuscitation nor the increased risk of infection with prolonged packing are well defined. The obvious benefits of hemostasis provided by packing are also balanced against the potential detrimental effects of increased intraabdominal pressure on ventilation, cardiac output, renal function, mesenteric circulation, and intracranial pressure. Timely alleviation of the secondary "abdominal compartment syndrome" may be a critical salvage maneuver for patients. Temporary abdominal wall closure at the time of packing can prevent the abdominal compartment syndrome. We recommend temporary abdominal wall expansion in all patients requiring packing until the hemostasis is obtained and visceral edema subsides.

A staged operative strategy for unstable trauma patients represents *advanced* surgical care and requires sound judgment and technical expertise. Intraabdominal packing for control of exsanguinating hemorrhage is a life-saving maneuver in highly selected patients in whom coagulopathy, hypothermia, and acidosis render further surgical procedures unduly hazardous. Early identification of patients likely to benefit from abbreviated laparotomy techniques is crucial for success.

EDITOR'S NOTES

The concepts of an evidence-based approach to surgical therapy and the establishment of practice guidelines for some of the more common pediatric surgical problems are gradually becoming accepted within the pediatric surgical community. Surgeons are now being placed in the unfamiliar position of having to justify their treatment plans and management schemes based on available evidence and consensus opinion, and the sometimes uncomfortable position of having to submit to analysis of their own outcomes. Although some of the pressure to conform certainly comes from hospitals and insurance companies, I would hope that most of us could see that these are ideas that make sense and that our patients are the ones who benefit directly. A beneficial side effect is that as more prospective data are gathered and analyzed, we are unlikely to be practicing in exactly the same way late in our careers as we did at the beginning, which is a relatively new concept for general and pediatric surgeons.

On the other hand, few would argue that there should be a wholesale acceptance or universal application of every practice guideline that is suggested, even if supported by the evidence. There is still an important role for healthy skepticism, clinical judgment, and "experience-based medicine" when applied rationally and thoughtfully. This is borne out in many of the recent prospective studies, in which compliance with the protocol is typically only 80% to 90%.

What we have learned about blunt solid organ injuries in children is that the previous protocols were unnecessarily restrictive and resulted in tremendous costs and wasteful utilization of resources with little demonstrable benefit to the patients. We now individualize the treatment plans based on severity of injury and established guidelines. This is elegantly demonstrated by the studies of Dr. Stylianos and others in the field, and validated by the experience of those of us who have applied the guidelines in our own practices.

It can be said that the only indication for operation in blunt solid organ is bleeding, although concomitant injury and unexplained hemodynamic instability are also clear indications. The apparent extent of injury by CT appearance and, more specifically, the grade of injury are not in and of themselves indications for operation in the absence of bleeding for hemodynamic instability. In fact, it has been suggested that the grading system of solid organ injuries does not correlate with need for operation or clinical outcome. Nevertheless, it serves as an empiric marker of extent of injury to the organ in question and is still used to help stratify patients for appropriate management. A more sophisticated and clinically useful grading system, one that incorporates injury severity score, concomitant injury, and other factors, is likely to be developed soon as a result of the prospective analysis of outcomes data that are currently being done.

The outcomes data for salvage procedures (abdominal packing with planned reoperation for exsanguinating hemorrhage) are compelling and should hopefully allow their successful application in a higher number of clinically appropriate situations. The complication rate is high, but given the alternative end result, this is certainly acceptable. Clinical judgment and experience play a big role in the decision-making process; therefore, the formulation of a simple algorithm or a list of criteria is not possible. Again, further analysis of outcomes data will help to better define the indications and the optimal application of this potentially life-saving strategy.

–P.M.

ACKNOWLEDGMENT

This work was supported in part by the APSA Foundation and the Arnold P. Gold Foundation.

SUGGESTED READINGS

Asensio JA, Demetriades D, Chahwan S, et al. Approach to the management of complex hepatic injuries. *J Trauma* 2000;48: 66–69.

Denton JR, Moore EE, Codwell DM. Multimodality treatment for grade V hepatic injuries: perihepatic packing, arterial embolization, and venous stenting. *J Trauma* 1997;42:964–968.

Ellrodt G, Cook DJ, Lee J, et al. Evidence-based disease management. *JAMA* 1997;278:1687–1692.

Fabian TC. Evidence-based medicine in trauma care: whither goest thou? *J Trauma* 1999;47:225–232.

Hoyt DB. Clinical practice guidelines. *Am J Surg* 1997;173:32–34.

Rotondo MF, Schwab CW, McGonigal MD, et al. Damage control: an approach for improved survival in exsanguinating penetrating abdominal injury. *J Trauma* 1993;35:375–383.

Stylianos S. Abdominal packing for severe hemorrhage. *J Pediatr Surg* 1998;33:339–342.

Stylianos S, and the APSA Trauma Committee. Evidence-based guidelines for resource utilization in children with isolated spleen or liver injury. *J Pediatr Surg* 2000;35:164–169.

Stylianos S, and the APSA Liver/Spleen Trauma Study Group. Compliance with evidence–based guidelines in children with isolated spleen or liver injury: a prospective study. *J Pediatr Surg* 2002; 37:453–456.

21

CHILD ABUSE

LESLI TAYLOR

> We see what we look for,
> We look for what we know.
> —Goethe

K.L. is a 2-year-old girl who was brought to the emergency room after reportedly falling from the back of a parked truck. She had multiple bruises on her back and blisters on one foot. She had diffuse abdominal tenderness. Head computed tomography (CT) showed old and new subdural hematomas. Abdominal CT scan showed thickened bowel loops, and mesenteric and intraabdominal fluid. There was no free air.

She underwent urgent abdominal exploration and was found to have a 40-cm segment of bowel that had been stripped of its mesentery and devascularized (Fig. 21.1). There was evidence of chronic bruising and foreshortening of the mesentery. A resection of the injured bowel and primary anastomosis was performed. Skeletal survey showed fractures of the left second, third, fourth, and fifth metatarsals that were approximately 2 weeks old as judged by the degree of calcification. She recovered from her surgery uneventfully and was discharged in the care of her grandmother.

PRESENTATION OF CHILD ABUSE

Physicians who care for children are mandated by law to report suspected child abuse. Abused children comprise about 10% of all children under the age of 6 years who present to the emergency room. There are over 1 million cases of child abuse in the United States each year, with about 5,000 deaths per year resulting from child abuse. It is the leading cause of death in children 6 to 12 months of age. Infants under 6 months of age are at highest risk for lethal injury. This chapter details common and uncommon presentations of child abuse, evaluation of injuries, and immediate and short-term management.

Children who are born prematurely or with disabilities or abnormalities are at increased risk, as are stepchildren. Parents at risk for committing child abuse include those involved with other domestic violence, or alcohol or substance abuse; those experiencing social isolation or high life stress; or those physically or emotionally abused themselves.

The recognition and reporting of child abuse in its earliest stages can prevent the predictable progression to more serious injury or death. Most inflicted injuries in children are not life threatening and do not require surgery. Bruises, lacerations, bites, dental and ocular trauma, and fractures are common early abusive injuries.

Fractures are present in about 25% of abuse victims. Inflicted fractures can be typical spiral or greenstick frac-

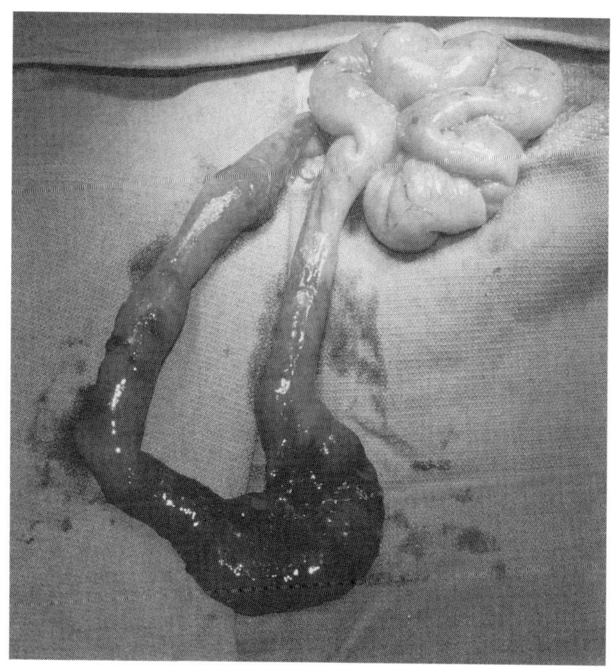

FIGURE 21.1. Blows to the abdomen caused stripping of the mesentery of a 40-cm loop of the middle of the small bowel with subsequent devascularization.

L. Taylor: Department of Pediatric Surgery, University of North Carolina School of Medicine, Chapel Hill, North Carolina.

tures. The age of the victim can be used to determine the suspiciousness of the injury. A spiral fracture in a child under 9 months of age and a femur fracture in a child under 2 years of age are particularly suspicious, especially if attributed to a fall. Bucket handle fracture, the chip fracture, and subperiosteal hematoma due to pulling or twisting the child's limb are occult bone injuries that are pathognomonic for child abuse. Fractures of the acromion process of the scapula or the proximal humerus are also suspect. Because children have very flexible ribs, rib fractures are rare in children unless significant force has been used. Bilateral rib fractures are especially worrisome. Callus formation may be the only evidence of an inflicted fracture.

Burn injuries occur in 10% to 20% of documented cases of child abuse. The median age of children suffering burns as part of their abuse is 18 months. Inflicted burns range from brandings with hot objects or cigarettes to life-threatening immersion burns. Any scald burn with a sharp border, especially of the hands, feet, or buttocks is suspicious for child abuse, as is dorsal location of contact burns of the hand. Porcelain contact sparing, flexor sparing, and a deep scald burn of uniform depth are highly suspicious for abuse. Regardless of burn size, any child with a suspected inflicted burn should be admitted to the hospital for protection and evaluation.

Head injuries are a late manifestation in the progression of child abuse and occur predominantly in infants. They are the third most common type of abuse, but are the most common cause of death in abused children. One third of abused children have head injuries. The most common mechanism is a blow to the head from a hand. Other mechanisms include violent shaking or being thrown against a wall. Injuries include blunt head trauma, skull fractures, and subdural hematoma from shaken baby syndrome. Children present with lethargy or coma with few external signs of abuse. Skull fractures attributed to a fall of less than 4 feet or in a "shattered eggshell" pattern are suspicious. Abuse injuries are more severe and diffuse compared with accidental head injuries, with much more severe long-term sequelae.

Although abdominal abuse is rare compared with other forms of child abuse, it can be life threatening or lethal. The mortality rate is about 50%, and is related to late presentation and recognition. Inflicted abdominal injuries are the second most common cause of death in child abuse and occur in approximately 2% of abused children. Many victims do not survive to reach the hospital. Toddlers are the most likely victims of abdominal abuse.

Children are particularly susceptible to severe internal injury from abdominal trauma because of several anatomic factors. They have a thin abdominal wall with poorly developed musculature. Widely splayed ribs provide little protection to viscera. The younger the child, the larger the liver is in proportion to the abdominal cavity, and the more at risk it is for injury from blows to the abdomen. The anteroposterior diameter of the abdomen in children is short compared with adults and predisposes to organs being crushed against the spine by a blow to the abdomen.

Blows or kicks to the abdomen cause predictable injuries of the hollow and solid viscera. Blunt abdominal injuries that should always be considered suspicious for child abuse include gastric rupture, duodenal hematoma, or duodenal perforation. The intestinal shearing injury with mesenteric hematoma and disruption, intestinal hematoma, or bowel perforation is pathognomonic for abuse. The most common site of intestinal shearing injury is at the duodenojejunal junction, with isolated duodenal injuries being next most common. Chylous ascites, although rare, may arise from mesenteric injury. Pancreatic contusion or transection from a blow to the epigastrium should arouse suspicion. Pancreatic pseudocysts have been reported as a late presentation of abdominal abuse. Colonic rupture and avulsion of the common bile duct also have been reported.

The majority of inflicted injuries of the abdomen and thorax are blunt rather than penetrating, following the pattern of accidental trauma. Boys are twice as likely to be abused as girls. Inflicted injuries differ from noninflicted injuries in other ways. Abused children are younger (average age 2.5 years) than children suffering accidental trauma. The typical perpetrator in abdominal abuse is male, either the child's father or the mother's boyfriend. There is a delay in presentation either because the perpetrator fails to realize the severity of the injury or has tried to conceal the injury until the child is *in extremis*. A story inconsistent with the injury is frequently given, such as the child fell from a couch, bed, or swing, or the injury was inflicted by a sibling or from a fall onto furniture. Because the most common victims of abdominal abuse are toddlers, it is rare that the child can contribute to the history. Significant intraabdominal injury can occur with no abdominal wall bruising. Child abuse should be considered in any child with unexplained shock, cardiac arrest or unconsciousness, with or without a suspected inflicted head injury.

The most common abdominal injury in abused children is a perforation of a hollow viscus from a blow to the upper abdomen. Children injured accidentally tend to have lower abdominal injuries or injury to a single solid organ. The liver is the organ most commonly injured in inflicted trauma, and the child may die from exsanguination. In accidental trauma, the spleen is the most commonly injured organ. The spleen is less likely to be injured in child abuse because the blows tend to be midline. Renal contusion and laceration are less common solid organ injuries. Bladder rupture also can occur from abdominal blows.

The mechanism of injury is usually a direct blow from a fist, knee, or foot. If an adult kneels on a child's abdomen, a severe shearing injury of the bowel, from being compressed against the spine, can occur. The surgeon should suspect child abuse when a hollow viscus injury is found and similarly should suspect the presence of a hollow viscus injury in a child presenting with abdominal findings and other evidence of child abuse. The cause of death in children with abdominal abuse is hemorrhagic shock from solid organ disruption, or septic shock from viscus perforation and peritonitis.

Thoracic injuries include rib fractures and lung contusion. Rib fractures in infancy should be considered highly suspicious for inflicted trauma, especially if posterior. Because an infant's ribs are so flexible and supple, an excessive amount of force is required to break an infant's rib. The mechanism may be due to direct blows or from striking the child against furniture. An abusive "bear hug" or severe shaking with anteroposterior squeezing of the chest also can cause multiple rib fractures. A pattern of bilateral thumbprint bruising on the front of the torso and multiple bilateral fingerprints on the back (trunk encirclement bruising) should lead one to suspect fractures. Pneumothorax, hemothorax, and traumatic chylous ascites have been described from abusive injuries.

Rectal injuries in children are always suspicious for child abuse, especially if there is associated anal or genital condylomata. All children presenting with vaginal tears, straddle injuries, and rectal trauma should be evaluated for abuse. Rectal abuse unrelated to sexual activity can occur when blunt objects are inserted into the rectum and cause laceration and perforation. Most accidental genital injuries in girls are asymmetric and do not transect the hymen. Sexual assault must be suspected for symmetric wounds that transect the hymen. These also have the highest likelihood for penetrating the peritoneal cavity. Examination under anesthesia is usually necessary to properly evaluate the injury. If sexual penetration is suspected, the wound should be irrigated and the specimen sent for examination for sperm. Girls who are 10 years of age and older are at greatest risk for sexual abuse, but it should be suspected in younger girls and even infants if there are perineal findings.

All surgeons must be aware of Munchausen syndrome by proxy (MSBP). Serious disease entities or symptoms are fabricated or induced in the child by the parent, almost always the mother, to gain attention of medical professionals. The triad of apnea, seizures, and cyanosis is the pattern of presentation most commonly seen in infants. Induced vomiting may lead to the involvement of the surgeon for surgical management of gastroesophageal reflux. Central venous catheter placement may be requested for management of the fabricated illnesses before the diagnosis of abuse with the risk of creating a portal for contamination of the blood stream and further fabrication. In a recent large study, approximately 17% of children who were victims of MSBP had central lines, and about 1% of children with central lines were victims of MSBP.

Initial MSBP behavior by the mother usually starts in the first year of the child's life. Resolution of symptoms when the child is separated from the parent is the key to diagnosis. Video telemetry in the case of smothering and toxin screens for cases of poisoning can aid in diagnosis.

EVALUATION

A full evaluation must be undertaken immediately when a child presents with injuries inconsistent with the stated mechanism or time frame. The child should be admitted to the hospital for protection and observation during this workup. Substantiation of inflicted injury is critical to successful prosecution in child abuse cases, and documentation must be graphic and impeccable.

Meticulous documentation of all physical findings as well as immediate photographs of the injuries, especially bruising, are imperative. Bruises should be measured and their color and location described in detail. A magnifying glass may help distinguish a pattern to the bruise, such as from carpet or the stitching or weave pattern of a belt. Fresh bruises will have a bluish-red color, while bruises older than 3 to 4 days will have brown, green, or yellow color. Bruises can take up to 14 days to fade. A child presenting with a single explanation for bruises of multiple colors should be considered abused. Bruises on the cheeks, trunk, buttocks, upper legs and genitalia are suspicious for abuse.

A standard evaluation for child abuse includes a radiologic survey for fractures. Radiographs should include skull, frontal and lateral cervical spine, thoracolumbar spine, frontal view of the chest, shoulders, hands, pelvis, and feet. Symmetric fractures or fractures in different stages of healing are suspicious, as are fractures of the ribs, clavicle, sternum, or spine in a very young child.

Symptoms of abdominal trauma include abdominal distension, tenderness, vomiting, and anemia. The child may present with septic or hypovolemic shock if there is a delay in seeking medical care. Peritonitis usually develops within 12 hours of an intestinal perforation. A crush injury of the small bowel may take 3 to 4 days to evolve, as tissue necrosis progresses to perforation and peritoneal contamination progresses to peritonitis. Duodenal and pancreatic injuries may remain occult for days and are sometimes difficult to diagnose with CT.

A patulous anus and blood in the rectal vault are suggestive of abusive rectal injury. If a rectal perforation extends to the level of the peritoneal reflection, the child may present with pelvic or lower abdominal pain. Photographs of the perineum should be obtained at the time of sigmoidoscopy, cystoscopy, or vaginoscopy.

If chest radiography and abdominal radiography are nondiagnostic, an urgent CT scan should be obtained to look for liver, splenic, and renal laceration and pancreatic injuries. Mesenteric and intestinal hematomas also may be recognized. Bowel perforation may be detected by free air or leak of contrast. A goal of CT evaluation is to document all injuries, although they may be clinically insignificant, because the pattern and spectrum of injuries can be critical in substantiating them as inflicted. Other contrast studies may be indicated in individual cases.

The surgical management of abusive injuries is similar to nonabusive injuries. Stable liver, splenic, and renal lacerations can be managed nonoperatively with supervision by a surgeon. Duodenal hematoma and pancreatic contusion can be managed with total parenteral nutrition and bowel rest. There is currently debate about the appropriate management of pancreatic lacerations and pancreatic transection, and each case should be assessed individually. Bowel perforation and intestinal shearing injury require emergency laparotomy and appropriate bowel resection as indicated by the findings. The decision for primary anastomosis or ostomy depends on the age of the injury and the amount of peritoneal contamination. If abdominal abuse has been chronic, scarring of the mesentery may cause it to be foreshortened. Rarely, the bowel injury may be so extensive that short bowel syndrome may be anticipated. The need for placement of a gastrostomy and central venous catheter at the time of abdominal exploration should be assessed. Penetrating abdominal trauma is a rare form of abdominal abuse and would be managed with standard trauma techniques.

Until child abuse can be eradicated by prevention, we must remain vigilant in the early recognition of abuse. Immediate intervention will prevent subsequent injury and death. A high level of suspicion and comprehensive radiologic evaluation will assure prompt recognition and management with the best chance for favorable outcome in abuse cases.

ACKNOWLEDGMENT

I would like to thank Dr. Tim Weiner for the use of the case report and photograph in Fig. 21.1.

SUGGESTED READINGS

Chadwick DL, Chin S, Salerno C, et al. Deaths from falls in children: how far is fatal? *J Trauma* 1991;31:1353–1355.

Feldman KW, Hickman RO. The central venous catheter as a source of medical chaos in Munchausen syndrome by proxy. *J Pediatr Surg* 1998;33:623–627.

Jenny C, Hymel KP, Ritzen A, et al. Analysis of missed cases of abusive head trauma. *JAMA* 1999;81:621–626.

Lacey SR, Cooper C, Runyan DK, et al. Munchausen syndrome by proxy: patterns of presentation to pediatric surgeons. *J Pediatr Surg* 1993;28:827–832.

Tarantino CA, Dowd MD, Murdock TC. Short vertical falls in infants. *Pediatr Emerg Care* 1999;15:5–8.

SECTION IV

AIRWAY AND HEAD AND NECK

22

MANAGEMENT OF THE EMERGENT AIRWAY AND TRACHEOTOMY

RAVINDHRA G. ELLURU
ROBIN T. COTTON

Care of the pediatric patient with an obstructed airway is technically and intellectually challenging. Management of these often acute situations demands preparation and decisive action. Infants have a small airway, and minimal change in the diameter of the airway leads to a significant percentage decrease in the cross-sectional area. This, in addition to having minimal energy stores and pulmonary reserve, can cause these patients to progress quickly to respiratory distress. The etiology of airway obstruction is varied, ranging from congenital anomalies such as laryngeal agenesis and aberrant innominate artery compression of the trachea, to iatrogenic causes such as subglottic stenosis from prolonged intubation or bilateral vocal cord paralysis from birth trauma. We will highlight the different options available for controlling the airway in an acute situation, how to perform a proper tracheotomy for long-term airway management, postoperative care of the tracheotomized patient, and the pitfalls or complications of tracheotomy.

MANAGEMENT OF THE EMERGENT AIRWAY

The key to successful management of the acutely obstructed airway is preparation and anticipation of potential problems. At our facility, any child with a suspected airway obstruction is evaluated by one of the staff otolaryngologists. However, this assessment could be performed by any experienced clinician who understands the anatomy and pathophysiology of the upper airway and is comfortable in managing potentially difficult airways. After careful assessment of the patient, the first decision we make is whether the patient can be simply observed or whether some method of airway intervention is necessary.

R. G. Elluru and R. T. Cotton: Department of Otolaryngology–Head and Neck Surgery, University of Cincinnati; and Department of Pediatric Otolaryngology, Cincinnati Children's Hospital Medical Center, Cincinnati, Ohio.

Certain disease states such as croup and epiglottitis can cause marked airway symptoms, but can often be managed with a combination of cool mist, antibiotics, steroids and careful observation. This is a viable option if the airway symptoms are not progressive, the child appears stable, and close monitoring by experienced ancillary staff in an intensive care setting is available. A physician must be readily available at all times, however, to manage the airway if symptoms progress and the patient decompensates. If airway intervention is thought to be even remotely necessary, we recommend securing a stable airway during the day when staff resources are abundant, as opposed to the middle of the night.

In a patient with emergent airway obstruction, heliox can be used to maintain oxygenation until a more stable solution can be found to resolve or bypass the obstruction. Helium has one of the lowest specific gravities of any gas, and when combined with oxygen, the overall density of the gas is lowered relative to that of room air or 100% oxygen. This lower density gas creates less turbulence and therefore has less resistance as it moves through the airway. Administering heliox to a patient with a partially obstructed airway decreases the work of breathing and stabilizes blood oxygenation until the obstructed airway can be definitively managed.

When the etiology of the obstruction is proximal, the patient can often be managed with an oral or nasal airway. For example, airway obstruction caused by large tonsils and adenoids can often be overcome with a nasal airway. The nasal airway should be long enough to stent the velopharynx open, but not too long that it induces gagging. Oral airways can be used in situations where a large or proptotic tongue obstructs the oropharynx, such as in a child with Down's syndrome. However, oral and nasal airways are poorly tolerated, and other methods of controlling the airway should be sought as required.

Another temporizing measure is the use of masked ventilation with continuous positive airway pressure. Small children can be effectively ventilated using a facemask, a combination of an oral airway or jaw thrust maneuver, and an ambu-bag to provide the positive airway pressure. This option is dependent on patient cooperation, airway anatomy, and the degree of airway obstruction. Although gentle sedation can be used to facilitate facemask ventilation, it is important to preserve spontaneous respirations until a stable airway is achieved.

When a more definitive method of obtaining a secure airway and bypassing obstructions of the upper airway is required, endotracheal intubation should be considered. In children, the subglottis is the narrowest region of the airway and dictates the size of the endotracheal tube used, as opposed to the adult, in whom the narrowest level is the glottis. Uncuffed endotracheal tubes are used, and the size of tube chosen is based on the patient's age, which roughly correlates with the size of the subglottis. Gentle sedation can be used, but it is important to preserve spontaneous respiration. An intubating laryngoscope is used to visualize the larynx, and the appropriate size of endotracheal tube is placed past the vocal cords and into the trachea. It is important to have suction equipment available to remove secretions or blood that interferes with visualization of the larynx. To confirm the appropriateness of endotracheal tube size, an applied positive airway pressure of less than 30 cm H_2O should cause a leak around the endotracheal tube. Intubations can be performed either transorally or transnasally. If the situation permits, we prefer the transnasal route both for patient comfort and because it is a more secure airway. The relative contraindications to endotracheal intubation are cervical spine instability, nasal or oral trauma, or situations where the integrity of the airway is in question.

The difficulty with endotracheal intubation arises when the larynx cannot be readily visualized using a laryngoscope, the case with many children with acute airway obstruction. Several options are available under these circumstances, including intubation using a flexible or rigid bronchoscope. With the patient awake or gently sedated, a flexible bronchoscope sheathed with an appropriate size of endotracheal tube is passed through the patient's nose and into the trachea. Local anesthetics such as lidocaine jelly or spray can be used before the procedure to anesthetize the nose and upper airway. Once the trachea is visualized, the endotracheal tube is slid over the bronchoscope and into the trachea. Once placement of the endotracheal tube in the trachea is confirmed, the bronchoscope is removed. A rigid bronchoscope can be used in the same way to intubate a patient transorally. The advantage of the rigid bronchoscope is that the patient can be ventilated directly through the bronchoscope, if necessary.

The laryngeal mask airway (LMA) provides another option for airway maintenance in patients with a poorly visualized larynx. We have found that the use of the LMA is particularly effective in patients with Pierre Robin sequence, where the cause of airway obstruction is micrognathia and a large, proptotic tongue. The LMA can be placed into the hypopharynx without specific visualization of the larynx. Additionally, some LMAs are designed to allow endotracheal intubation through the device once it is positioned in the hypopharynx. LMAs allow temporary management of the airway in an acute situation, creating time for long-term airway management options to be used.

Management of an acute airway obstruction requires preparation, anticipation, careful assessment of the patient, and an understanding of the patient's underlying pathophysiology. This requires a well-rehearsed algorithm for employing the various airway interventions discussed above, and being able to transition smoothly from one intervention to another as needed. Furthermore, it requires immediate access to all the equipment and ancillary staff necessary to employ any of the above airway interventions. At our facility, carts are available that have clearly labeled drawers containing all the essential equipment to handle a difficult airway. Furthermore, we prefer to evaluate and stabilize obstructed airways in the operating room, if the patient can be safely transported. This allows the benefit of having equipment close at hand, trained ancillary staff in the room, and the assistance of an anesthesia team. If a tracheotomy has to be performed, we can proceed in a controlled and sterile fashion.

TRACHEOTOMY

In theory, intubation may be maintained for prolonged periods without complications, provided that the endotracheal tube causes no mucosal injury. In practice, however, it is difficult to assess whether the endotracheal tube required to provide an adequate airway is injuring the underlying mucosa. Even if direct mucosal injury could be prevented, the presence of the endotracheal tube would eventually elicit a localized inflammatory reaction. Granulation tissue then forms in these areas, and eventually leads to scarring and stenosis. Portions of the airway at risk include the vocal processes, the posterior glottis, and the subglottis. Additionally, pressure necrosis from endotracheal tubes that are too large can lead to tracheomalacia and eventual tracheal collapse.

Although pediatric patients can be kept intubated longer than adults with careful monitoring, a tracheotomy should be considered for long-term airway management. The advantages of a tracheotomy are that the incidence of injury to the airway is decreased, the patient's comfort and mobility are markedly increased, and deglutition is enhanced. There are three major indications for long-term tracheotomy in children: airway obstruction, prolonged ventilatory support, and pulmonary toilet. The morbidity of a tracheotomy is minimal when proper technique and meticulous postoperative care is applied.

We perform all pediatric tracheotomies in the operating room after a careful airway evaluation by laryngoscopy and bronchoscopy to evaluate the nature of the obstruction. If the patient is not already intubated, we either intubate the patient or ventilate the patient through a bronchoscope. In rare situations, with difficult to intubate patients, we may use a facemask or laryngeal mask to provide ventilation. The patient is positioned supine on the operating room table. A shoulder roll is used to extend the neck and bring the trachea anteriorly. Neck extension should be minimized in patients with suspected cervical spine injuries or patients with congenital instability of the cervical spine, such as children with Down's syndrome. The anterior neck anatomy is palpated, and the level of the hyoid, thyroid, and cricoid cartilages are determined.

A 2-cm horizontal incision is marked out over the anterior neck, directly over the trachea and half way between the cricoid cartilage and the sternal notch. The skin is infiltrated with 1% lidocaine with 1:100,000 epinephrine. The patient is then prepared and draped, taking care to allow the anesthesiologist plenty of access to the airway. The skin incision is made sharply with a knife, and the subcutaneous fat is removed down to the anterior cervical fascia covering the strap muscles using electrocautery. Removal of the subcutaneous fat allows maturation of the tracheal stoma and allows better seating of the tracheotomy tube. The anterior cervical fascia is divided vertically with electrocautery, and the strap muscles are bluntly divided down the midline. With the strap muscles retracted laterally, the trachea and attached thyroid gland become visible. The isthmus of the thyroid gland can be retracted out of the way or divided with electrocautery to provide access to the trachea. If the thyroid isthmus is to be divided, it should be bluntly separated from the anterior tracheal wall with a curved hemostat and held away from the tracheal wall to avoid damage to the tracheal cartilage. Throughout the procedure, palpation of the cartilaginous airway allows the surgeon to maintain anatomic orientation.

Once the anterior tracheal wall is isolated, it is imperative to definitely determine the level of the cricoid cartilage and the first, second, and third tracheal rings. Vertical stitches using 4-0 nonabsorbable suture are then placed through the tracheal cartilage at the level of the second to third tracheal rings, on either side of midline (Fig. 22.1). These sutures are later taped to the chest wall and act as retaining sutures to pull the trachea anteriorly and the trachea-stoma open if the patient is accidentally decannulated in the perioperative period. They should be labeled (left and right) and kept in place until after the first tracheotomy tube change.

After informing the anesthesiologist, the tracheal lumen is entered using a knife to make a vertical incision between the retaining sutures, through tracheal ring 2 and, if necessary, tracheal ring 3. The first tracheal ring should be preserved, if possible. The size of the tracheal incision depends on the size of the tracheotomy tube to be placed. The edges of the skin incision are sewn directly to the cut edges of the tracheal cartilage using 4-0 chromic sutures (Fig. 22.2). The endotracheal tube or bronchoscope is then pulled back to the superior margin of the tracheotomy, and an appropriate size of tracheotomy tube is inserted into the trachea via the tracheotomy. As a rough rule, the formula of (age/4+4) can be used to estimate tracheotomy tube size for children over 10 months of age. On the other hand, one can just use a tracheotomy tube a half a size smaller than the endotracheal tube used to intubate the patient. Regardless, it is important to have the appropriate tracheotomy tube, as well as several size options, available before the tracheotomy is executed. Once inserted, ventilation is initiated via the tracheotomy tube and placement within the trachea is confirmed by return of CO_2, auscultation of breath sounds, and the ease of passing a suction catheter through the tracheotomy tube. In patients with thick, short necks and difficult to visualize tracheotomies, it is possible to create a false passage between the skin and the trachea during insertion of the tracheotomy tube. Therefore, it is crucial to visualize the tracheotomy during tube insertion and to confirm proper placement within the tracheal lumen. In addition, a flexible or rigid bronchoscopy is used to assess the level and position of the distal tip of the tracheotomy tube within the tracheal lumen. Finally, the endotracheal tube or bronchoscope is

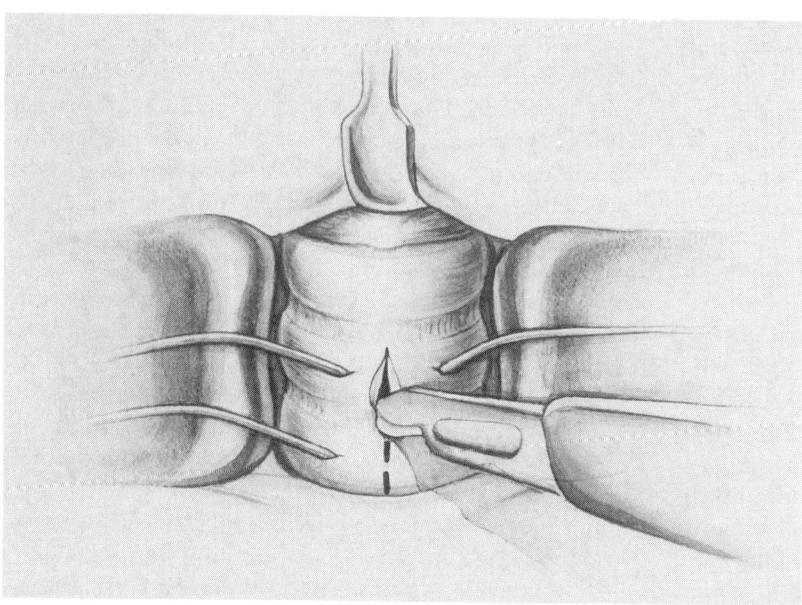

FIGURE 22.1. Retraction sutures are placed vertically around the planned midline tracheotomy incision. These sutures are clearly labeled as left and right, and are taped to the chest wall. In the case of accidental decannulation, these sutures are used to retract the stoma up to the skin and open. This aids in the proper replacement of the tracheotomy tube. These sutures are removed on postoperative day 5, after the first tracheotomy tube change. A midline tracheotomy incision is made in the anterior tracheal wall, mirroring the outer diameter of the tracheotomy tube.

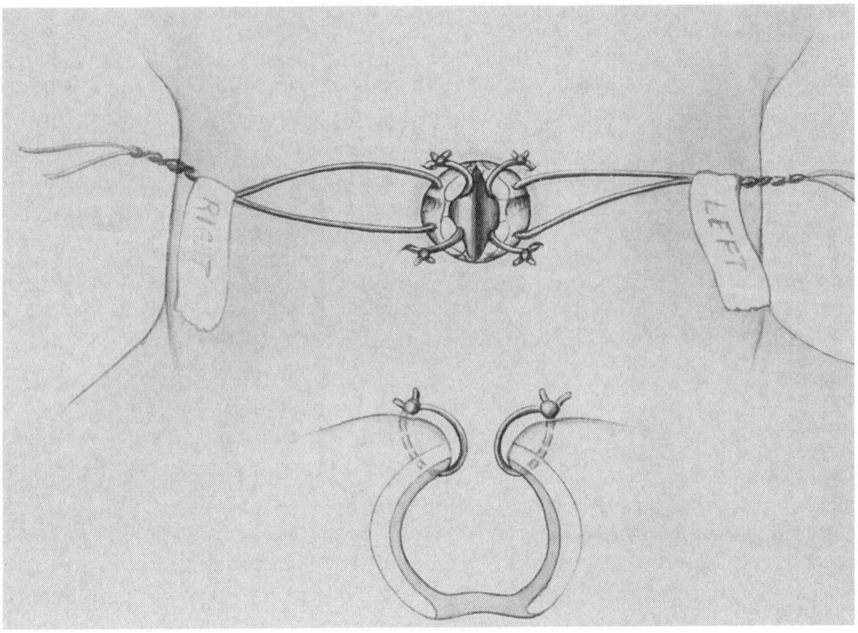

FIGURE 22.2. The skin edges are secured to the tracheal wall to form a matured stoma. This is important in case of accidental dislodgment. Tacking the skin to the trachea will help to guide the tracheotomy tube through the tracheotomy. This will help prevent the formation of a false passage anterior to the trachea during reinsertion.

completely removed. With the neck in the neutral position, tracheotomy ties are placed around the patient's neck and tied, allowing only one finger of slack between the tie and the neck. A postoperative chest radiograph is obtained to again check the position of the tracheotomy tube and to rule out a pneumothorax.

Once a proper tracheotomy is performed, meticulous postoperative care is initiated to avoid any of the early complications of tracheotomy discussed below. Ancillary staff is instructed not to change tracheotomy ties or tubes until after the first tube change by the otolaryngology staff on postoperative day 5. Routine wound care and tracheotomy tube suctioning is performed two to three times a day and as needed. Care is taken to never suction beyond the length of the tracheotomy tube. Supplemental humidified air or a humi-vent is kept on the patient at all times. Patients are kept in the hospital until after the first tracheotomy tube change.

During the patient's stay in the hospital, the parent (or at least two adult members of the immediate family) are instructed in tracheotomy care including suctioning and changing the tracheotomy tube. Additionally, family members are trained in basic life support techniques. The family members must demonstrate a proficiency in all of these skills before they can take the patient home. To facilitate this educational process, our facility has dedicated airway nurses for patient teaching, coordinating home care, and facilitating communication with the family after they have left the hospital. The patient and the family are sent home with a portable suction machine and tubing, and additional tracheotomy tubes of the same size and one size smaller. The smaller tracheotomy tube facilitates rapid replacement of a dislodged tracheotomy tube if difficulty is encountered replacing the original tube. A home health-care nurse is also arranged to stay with the patient about 8 hours a day, usually at night. This helps continue the educational process for the family, frees the family to tend to other matters, and continues careful monitoring of the patient.

COMPLICATIONS OF TRACHEOTOMY

Tracheotomy when properly performed and managed is associated with a low rate of morbidity and mortality. Early and late complications of tracheotomy are outlined in Table 22.1. In a large metanalysis of tracheotomy-associated complications, early complications ranged in frequency from 14% to 31% and late complications ranged in frequency from 14% to 50%. The most common long-term complication was formation of a suprastomal granuloma and persistent tracheocutaneous fistula after decannulation. Tracheotomy-related mortality was less than 2%.

Many of the complications listed in Table 22.1 can be avoided with proper surgical technique and postoperative care. Adhering to strict anatomic boundaries and fascial planes during the tracheotomy allows for a relatively bloodless procedure and a minimal chance of postoperative hemorrhage. Furthermore, careful anatomic orientation during the procedure will avoid such errors as inadvertently violating the pleural space at the root of the neck and causing a pneumothorax. If a pneumothorax does occur, expedient diagnosis and treatment consisting of chest tube placement, leads to a quick resolution. Avoiding tight neck wraps after a tracheotomy minimize the chance of air dissecting between the tracheal stoma and the skin into the mediastinum, leading to a pneumomediastinum. Stringent wound care and suctioning of secretions will decrease tracheotomy tube plugging and local wound infection. Cellulitis localized to the tracheotomy

TABLE 22.1. COMPLICATIONS OF PEDIATRIC TRACHEOSTOMY

Early or late
Accidental decannulation
Tracheotomy tube obstruction
Early
Pneumothorax
Pneumomediastinum
Hemorrhage
Local infection
Late
Local infection
Suprastomal collapse
Tracheal stenosis
Subglottic stenosis
Tracheoesophageal fistula
Tracheoinnominate fistula
Tracheal granuloma
Persistent tracheocutaneous fistula

site usually responds well to oral antibiotics. Each of these complications can be treated easily if detected early.

Accidental decannulation can occur early or late postoperatively. For this reason, we prefer to mature our tracheal stomas by suturing the edges of the skin incision directly to the trachea stoma. A mature tracheal stoma will not collapse or bleed when the tracheotomy tube is displaced, allowing easy replacement. Until the tracheal stoma heals and matures, we place retaining sutures, which can be used to open the tracheal stoma and provide access for replacing accidentally displaced tracheotomy tubes.

Subglottic stenosis is a rare complication of tracheotomy and is usually secondary to a high tracheotomy. It is imperative to clearly identify the cartilagenous landmarks of the upper airway before performing the tracheotomy. The tracheotomy should be below the second tracheal ring. If a high tracheotomy or cricothryoidotomy is performed, for example, in an emergent situation, it should be revised as soon as possible.

Suprastomal granulomas can be a recurrent problem. We examine all our tracheotomized patients at frequent intervals to evaluate for tracheotomy tube fit and positioning of the tracheotomy tube within the tracheal lumen. This is especially important in light of the fact that children are continually growing, their airways are getting larger and longer, and the tracheotomy tubes may no longer be of the appropriate size. During these examinations we also remove any granulation tissue bronchoscopically or via the tracheal stoma.

Tracheal stenosis, tracheoinnominate, and tracheoesophageal fistulas are rare complications of a tracheotomy. These complications arise from tracheotomy tubes that are not of the appropriate size or fit for the patient. Tracheotomy tubes are available in a variety of sizes, lengths, and shapes, allowing a nearly custom fit for any patient. The distal tip of the tracheotomy tube should fit within the tracheal lumen without placing pressure on the anterior or posterior tracheal wall. We confirm tracheotomy tube fit by performing a rigid or flexible bronchoscopic examination at the end of the procedure.

After decannulation, most tracheal stomas close without further intervention. In the rare case of a persistent tracheocutaneous fistula, we excise the epithelialized fistula tract, close the tracheotomy by suturing the edges together with 4-0 absorbable suture, sewing the strap muscles together over a rubber band drain, and then closing the skin. We observe the patient overnight for airway distress or accumulation of subcutaneous air. The drain is removed after 24 hours. If there is a sizable defect in the anterior tracheal wall, another option is to allow the tracheal stoma to heal by secondary intention after excising the epithelialized tract. In this situation, a tracheotomy tube is left in place until the patient is completely awake and is then removed. We have had equally good success with both of these options.

CONCLUSION

Management of the patient with an acutely obstructed airway requires preparation, and clear and decisive thinking. Surgeons may choose from many options for stabilizing a patient's airway. The choice of these options depends on the patient's disease process and airway anatomy. Tracheotomy for long-term airway management is a safe and effective option. Both proper technique and meticulous postoperative care are necessary to minimize complications.

SUGGESTED READING

Fitton CM, Myer CM III. Home care of the child with a tracheotomy. In: Myer CM III, Cotton RT, Shott SR, eds. *The pediatric airway: an interdisciplinary approach.* Philadelphia: JB Lippincott; 1995:171–177.

Lloyd-Thomas AR. Anesthesia. In: Cotton RT, Meyer CM III, eds. *Practical pediatric otolaryngology.* Philadelphia: Lippincott-Raven, 1999:153–174.

McMurray JS, Prescott CAJ. Tracheotomy in the pediatric patient. In: Cotton RT, Meyer CM III, eds. *Practical pediatric otolaryngology.* Philadelphia: Lippincott-Raven, 1999:575–593.

Sherman JM, Davis S, Albamonte-Petrick S, et al. Care of the child with a chronic tracheotomy. *Am J Respir Crit Care Med* 2000;161:297–308.

Wetmore RF. Management of acute airway obstruction. In: Wetmore RF, Muntz HR, McGill TJ, eds. *Pediatric otolaryngology: principles and practice pathways.* New York: Thieme, 2000:845–862.

23

AIRWAY ENDOSCOPY

ELLEN S. DEUTSCH

> Endoscopic ability cannot be bought with the instruments. As with all mechanical procedures, facility can be obtained only by educating the eye and the fingers in repeated exercise of a particular series of maneuvers. As with learning to play a musical instrument, a fundamental knowledge of technic, positions, and landmarks is necessary, after which only continued manual practice makes for proficiency.
>
> —Chevalier Jackson

Airway endoscopy provides a privileged view of intraluminal airway anatomy, not obtainable by any other method of evaluation. Endoscopy provides precise anatomic information, as well as details about mucosal characteristics and dynamic airway processes. Airway endoscopy can be a treacherous procedure because of the innate risks associated with manipulating an airway that may already be compromised. The availability of modern telescopes, ventilating bronchoscopes, advances in anesthesia, and the lessons learned from our predecessors contribute to the safety of modern endoscopy.

DIAGNOSTIC APPROACH

The airway endoscopist must make many complex choices concerning instruments, techniques, anesthesia and patient care settings to be used during airway endoscopy. Using information gathered from a patient's history, physical examination, and basic radiographs will help to refine the differential diagnosis and focus these decisions, thereby facilitating safe, purposeful, and effective endoscopy.

Stridor is probably the most common indication for diagnostic airway endoscopy in children, and is caused by turbulent airflow within a narrowed or distorted airway. Airway caliber can be compromised by lesions within the airway lumen, abnormalities of the walls of the airway, or extrinsic processes causing a mass effect. Abnormalities of the airway can be structural or dynamic. Lesions of the extrathoracic portion of the airway tend to cause inspiratory noises, whereas lesions of the intrathoracic airways tend to cause expiratory sounds. An exception is the severe lesion in any location, which can cause biphasic sounds (Fig. 23.1). Proximal lesions involving either the supraglottis or the vocal folds generally produce high-pitched noises, lesions in the trachea tend to cause low-pitched noises, and further distally, high-pitched noises come from the very small airways. An exception is laryngomalacia, which in older children produces a lower pitched sound. Wheezing is a classic example of a high-pitched expiratory noise originating in the distal intrathoracic airways. Bilateral vocal fold paralysis and laryngomalacia both cause high-pitched inspiratory stridor, but the stridor of laryngomalacia is more "choppy" and the stridor of vocal fold paralysis is increased with agitation, whereas the stridor of laryngomalacia is usually more evident in quiet states. Wet sounds suggest anatomic or neuromuscular difficulties with the clearance of secretions. Hoarseness suggests that the abnormality involves, but is not necessarily limited to, the true vocal folds.

Endoscopy is indicated if there is a history suggestive of foreign body aspiration despite lack of radiographic find-

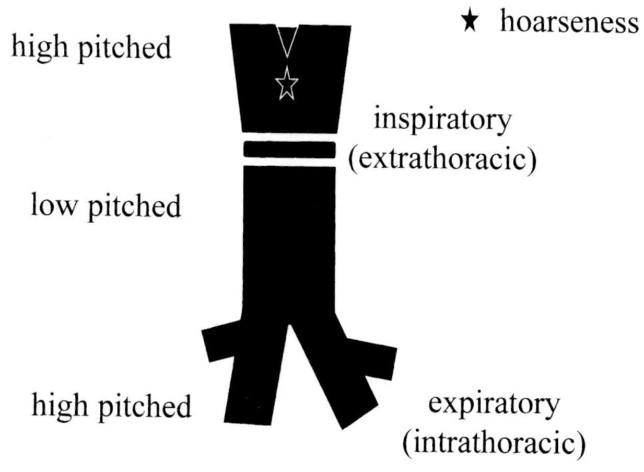

FIGURE 23.1. General topographic localizing characteristics for stridor.

F. S. Deutsch: Departments of Otolaryngology–Head and Neck Surgery, and Pediatrics, Thomas Jefferson University, Philadelphia, Pennsylvania; and Department of Surgery, Alfred I. duPont Hospital for Children, Wilmington, Delaware.

TABLE 23.1. INDICATIONS FOR URGENT AIRWAY ENDOSCOPY

- Significant respiratory distress
  - Child appears uncomfortable or fatigued
  - Child is newly cyanotic or has a new supplemental oxygen requirement
  - Child's condition is not explainable solely by other organ system problems
- Acute onset of stridor
  - Foreign body aspiration
  - Suspicion of certain infections, such as epiglottitis
  - Mechanical, thermal, or chemical airway trauma
- Significant dysphonia
  - Papilloma
  - Exudative infections, such as staphylococcal tracheitis
  - Foreign bodies

ings, or a suggestive radiograph despite lack of supportive history. Endoscopy is also indicated for any airway disease that does not respond to treatment as expected. For example, recurrent "croup" may be due to underlying subglottic stenosis, or persistent atelectasis may not be a result of pneumonia, but may be caused by an aspirated foreign body.

Endoscopy also may be indicated as a therapeutic procedure, to establish and maintain control of a patient's airway, or to manipulate or remove an endogenous or exogenous lesion that obstructs the airway. Superimposed on the question of how to proceed with airway endoscopy is the question of how urgently the endoscopy should be performed (Table 23.1). Certain airway lesions can progress to complete obstruction or cause respiratory collapse from exhaustion. Maintaining satisfactory oxygen saturation measured by pulse oximetry does not preclude imminent respiratory collapse.

Plain radiographs of the chest and lateral neck often provide useful preoperative information (Fig. 23.2). Lack of normal clarity, distorted shape, inappropriate masses or decreased caliber of the lumen are suggestive of an abnormality. Although the "steeple sign" suggests narrowing of the subglottis, it may also be seen if the child is phonating at the moment the radiograph is obtained.

Although sometimes a foreign body is visualized in a radiograph, more often only its sequelae are evident (Fig. 23.3). Air trapping may be demonstrated by comparing lung inflation on inspiratory and expiratory radiographs (Fig. 23.4), or on decubitus images. Airway fluoroscopy may be useful when a child is uncooperative or when the findings are subtle.

Information obtained by endoscopy may suggest the need for subsequent specialized radiographic examinations such as barium swallow, computed tomography (CT), magnetic resonance imaging (MRI), or tracheobronchography to further define airflow dynamics, distal anatomy, or the relationship between the airway and adjacent structures or masses.

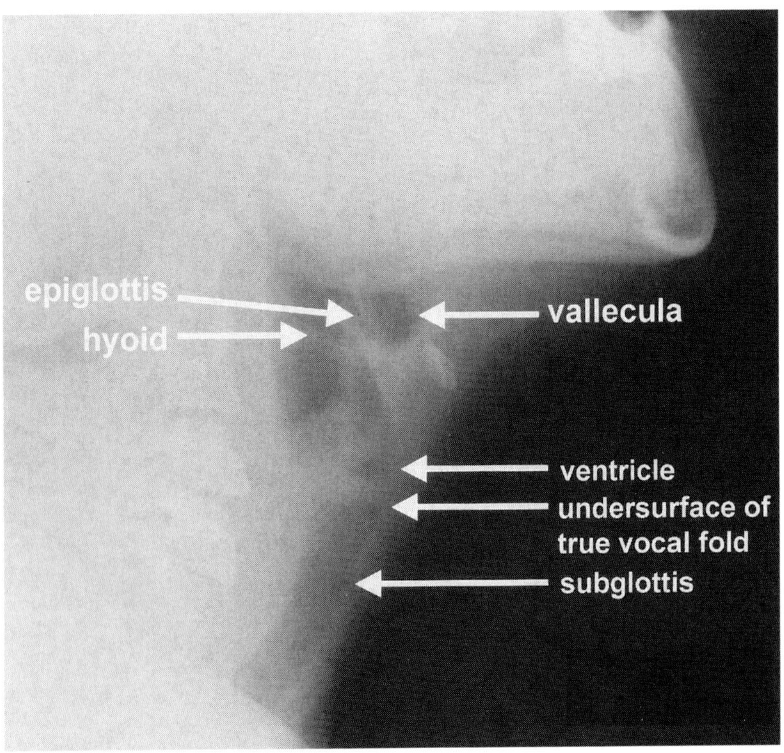

FIGURE 23.2. On good quality, inspiratory, lateral neck and chest radiographs, the laryngeal ventricle, the epiglottis, the aryepiglottic folds, much of the trachea, and often the undersurface of the vocal folds can be visualized.

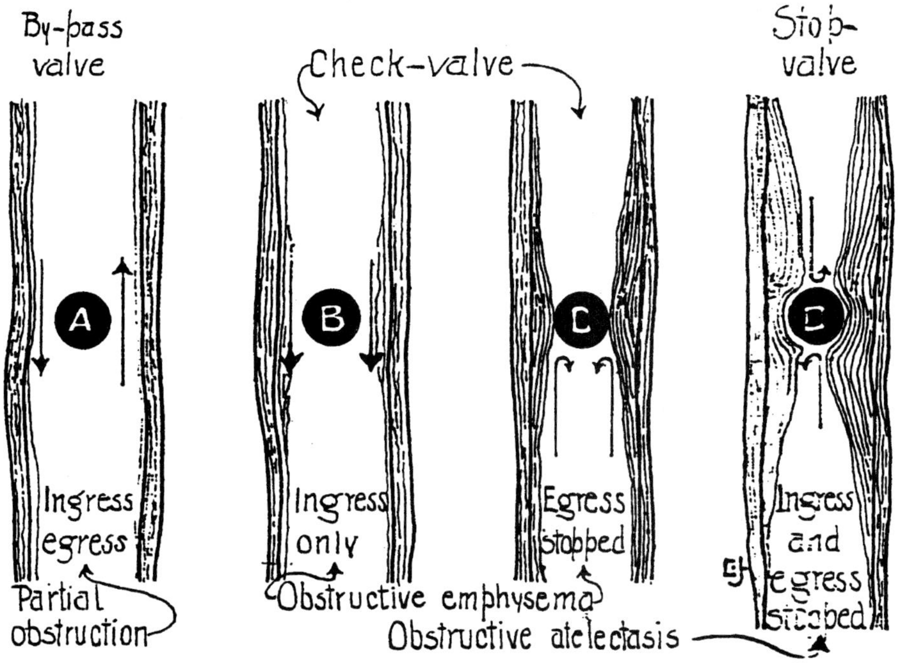

FIGURE 23.3. Airway foreign bodies that have a stop valve effect, with complete obstruction of airflow, can result in atelectasis of the lung distal to the obstruction. Foreign bodies that have a check valve effect, letting air flow distally with inspiration but not allowing egress with expiration, can result in air trapping or hyperinflation. Reprinted from Jackson C. *Bronchoscopy and esophagoscopy. A manual of peroral endoscopy and laryngeal surgery,* 2nd ed. Philadelphia: WB Saunders, 1927; with permission.

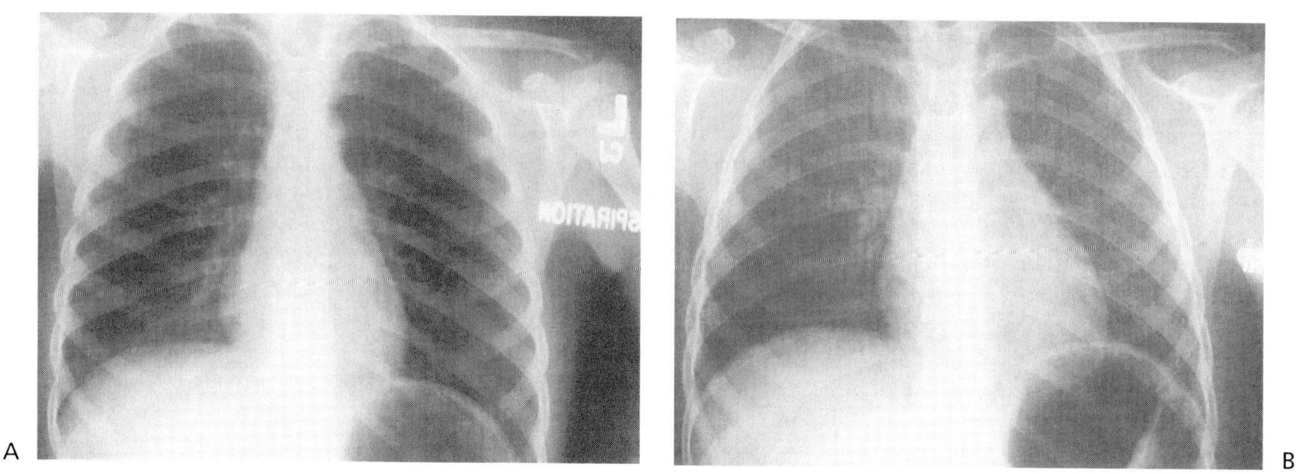

FIGURE 23.4. Inspiratory **(A)** and expiratory **(B)** chest radiographs demonstrating lack of deflation of the right lung during expiration, caused by a foreign body in the bronchus intermedius functioning as a check valve.

ENDOSCOPIC EQUIPMENT

Fiberoptic telescopes are valuable for evaluating dynamic lesions, such as hoarseness, laryngomalacia, tracheo- or bronchomalacia, or vocal fold paralysis, and for examination of distal airway lesions, as a wedge for broncheoalveolar lavage or as a conduit for fiberoptic lasers. Fiberoptic bronchoscopy may reveal significant airway collapse not evident during rigid bronchoscopy using general anesthesia. However, care must be taken to avoid overdiagnosis of airway dynamics, because the presence of the fiberoptic bronchoscope may increase airway resistance to the point that normal dynamics are exaggerated, particularly in infants whose airways are small and compliant. Fiberoptic telescopes are also useful in examining or securing the airway of patients with morbid obesity, micrognathia, cervical spine rigidity or instability, or temporomandibular joint immobility. Use of simultaneous fluoroscopic guidance may facilitate intralesional placement of brushes, biopsy forceps, or catheters. Fiberoptic telescopes are generally passed through the nose, allowing visualization of the nasopharynx and larynx without interfering with the position of oral cavity structures. If the fiberoptic telescope is passed through the mouth, bite blocks should be used to protect the telescope.

The selection of local anesthesia, sedation, or general anesthesia depends on the purpose and circumstances of the endoscopy. Passing a fiberoptic scope through and beyond the glottis is facilitated by the use of local or general anesthesia, to provide patient comfort and prevent laryngospasm. Maintaining spontaneous ventilation is also helpful, especially for the assessment of dynamic lesions, to prevent "stenting" of the airway by positive pressure ventilation. Alternately, a conduit such as an endotracheal tube can used. Adapters are available to minimize air leak and maintain mechanical ventilation and oxygen delivery, if necessary.

Standard pediatric fiberoptic bronchoscopes have a 3.5-mm outer diameter and an operating channel of 1.2 mm. Adult scopes are available with outer diameters up to 6.2 mm and side channel diameters up to 3.2 mm. The smallest of the ultrathin fiberoptic instruments with distal angulation (2.2 mm outer diameter, Olympus PF22, Olympus America Inc., Melville, NY) will pass through 2.5- to 4-mm (inner diameter) endotracheal tubes, a 3.5-mm scope can be used in 4.5- to 6-mm tubes, and a 4.0-mm scope (standard adult size) can be used in endotracheal tubes larger than 6 mm. Side channels can be used for suctioning, application of topical anesthetics or liquid radiographic contrast material, or for passage of instruments such as biopsy forceps, balloon catheters, laser fibers, and wire brushes. Side channels are not available in the smaller scopes.

Rigid Hopkins rod-lens telescopes are the workhorses of airway evaluation in the operating room. When combined with rigid bronchoscopes, they are the instruments of choice for removing tracheobronchial foreign bodies, controlling massive pulmonary hemorrhage, dilating stenoses, excising granulation tissue, debulking large tumors, evaluating tracheoesophageal fistulas or laryngeal clefts, and for performing laser therapy or inserting airway stents. The optics and image quality are superior to those of fiberoptic telescopes of comparable size.

A Hopkins rod telescope with an outer diameter of 4 mm and a length of 20 cm (such as the Storz 7200A telescope, Karl Storz Endoscopy–America, Culver City, CA) is particularly useful and should pass easily through the vocal folds and subglottis of a typical neonate. It is short enough to be handled easily, yet long enough to visualize beyond the carina in most children through school age. It is also large enough to provide a good quality image, sturdy enough to be used without being sheathed by a bronchoscope, and is of a convenient diameter for measuring lesions in infants and toddlers. Narrower telescopes are useful for evaluating stenotic airways, but provide lesser quality images and are more fragile. For pediatric endoscopy, a variety of telescopes are necessary to fit a variety of sizes of ventilating bronchoscopes, optical forceps, and other components. In general, straight (0 degree) telescopes are used, but occasionally telescopes able to view at 30, 45, or 70 degree angles are useful. Rigid telescopes are less flexible than fiberoptic telescopes, but this is rarely a practical limitation.

Ventilating bronchoscopes should be available during rigid airway endoscopy. They allow control of the airway, manipulation and instrumentation of the airway, and the capability for ventilation and oxygenation. They can be used to shield, protect, and guide fragile instruments, and provide a stable, protective conduit for manipulation and instrumentation. Rigid equipment provides tactile information and is compatible with both CO_2 and fiberoptic laser applications.

A variety of cameras that can be attached to rigid or fiberoptic telescopes or to microscopes (e.g., during suspension microlaryngoscopy) are available, allowing multiple observers, as well as documentation with still photography, video recordings, and digital recordings.

ADDITIONAL EQUIPMENT

Miller intubating laryngoscope blades are often used to facilitate laryngeal instrumentation or intubation, because their straight, open backs facilitate the passage of instruments. Other laryngoscopes are designed for specific purposes: Holinger anterior commissure laryngoscopes facilitate exposure of the anterior larynx, Lindholm laryngoscopes allow binocular vision and exposure of the supraglottis, Dedo laryngoscopes are modified for laser surgery, and Jackson sliding laryngoscopes facilitate instrumentation and intubation. Light clips can be attached to the proximal end of a laryngoscope, and suction catheters, ventilation, or light carriers may be inserted directly or through side channels.

Suctioning is usually necessary to remove secretions that interfere with visualization. After exposing the larynx with a laryngoscope, a flexible suction catheter is insinuated between the vocal folds (as if intubating the patient) to allow distal suctioning, and promptly withdrawn. Rigid suction catheters with thumb controls allow precise suctioning, and large-bore catheters may be used to suction thick material, but each can cause significant trauma if not inserted gently. Precise distal placement is guided by feel and by listening for the tip of the catheter to make contact with secretions. Small-caliber flexible catheters can be inserted via the side channel of ventilating bronchoscopes, which allows simultaneous visualization during suctioning. It may be necessary to use a smaller diameter telescope or a larger bronchoscope to allow room for the suction catheter to pass adjacent to the telescope within the lumen of the bronchoscope.

Optical forceps are useful for manipulating or removing airway lesions. They consist of peanut, biopsy, or cup forceps with double action jaws and a telescope for distal illumination and visualization with magnification (Fig. 23.5). Although optical forceps can be inserted unsheathed, they are fragile and therefore should be passed through a ventilating bronchoscope. They allow only a limited peripheral view, so visualization of the bronchoscope's sidewall ventilation ports indicates proximity to the distal opening of the bronchoscope. A longer instrument or a shorter bronchoscope will permit the expandable tip of the optical forcep to pass beyond the tip of the bronchoscope before the jaws are opened.

A variety of microlaryngeal instruments are available, including angled and straight scissors, cup forceps, alligator forceps, knife blades, retractors, and reflectors. Some also incorporate aspiration tubes. Older styles of forceps are available in a greater variety of configurations, but their lack of distal lighting and the limitations of proximal magnification restrict their use. Ring rotation forceps and rat-toothed forceps allow a grasped object to swivel into the plane of least resistance. A safety pin closer can be used to sheath the point of a pin within its keeper before it is removed (Fig. 23.6). In larger children, it is sometimes possible to pass a traditional instrument alongside a Hopkins rod telescope, but this can be very cumbersome and is usually not possible in small children.

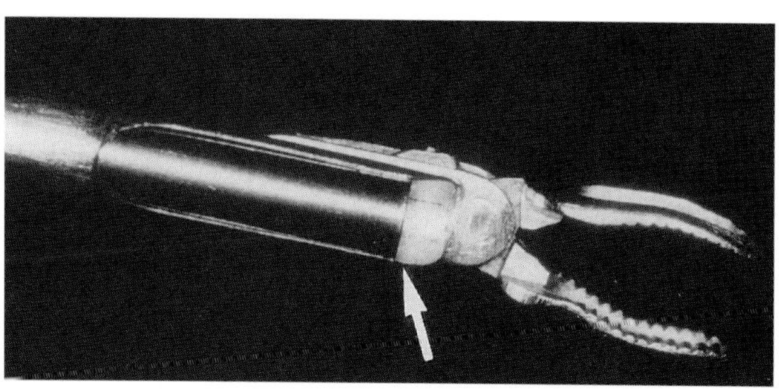

FIGURE 23.5. Optical forceps with peanut grasping jaws. Note tip of telescope (*arrow*).

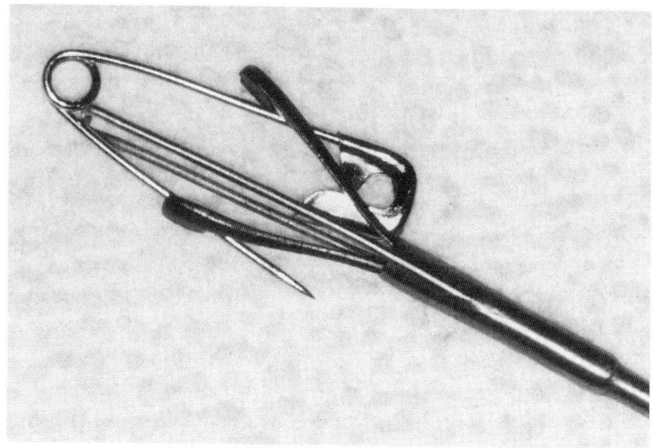

FIGURE 23.6. Safety pin closer.

PREOPERATIVE PREPARATION

Awake laryngoscopy can be performed in the office using a fiberoptic laryngoscope, a 70 or 90 degree rigid telescope, or a laryngeal mirror, and is useful if the findings would be likely to obviate the need for direct laryngoscopy and bronchoscopy under general anesthesia. Examples of lesions for which adequate evaluation may be obtained in awake office settings include laryngomalacia in a child with a classic history and typical endoscopic findings, vocal fold nodules, and vocal fold paralysis for which the etiology is suggested by the child's medical history, such as following ligation of a patent ductus arteriosus. The evaluation should be performed in the operating room if there is a need to visualize the airway below the level of the vocal folds, if there is significant airway distress, or if the child is significantly ill or uncooperative.

Establishing a routine, organized approach and reviewing the anticipated sequence of events with other members of the operating room team will facilitate efficient and directed patient management if any component of the procedure suddenly becomes urgent. The operating room should be arranged to optimize safety and ergonomic relationships between the patient, anesthesiologist, endoscopist and nurse. The arrangement should facilitate the ability of both the endoscopist and the anesthesiologist to access the patient's airway emergently, as well as allowing each person access to relevant equipment and supplies. The cephalad portion of the operating room table should protrude over the base, so that the endoscopist can sit comfortably at the head of the table. Ideally, instruments are passed over the right shoulder of a right-handed endoscopist. The assistant guides the distal tip of the instrument to the proximal opening of the laryngoscope.

Commercial defogging agents, soap, warm water, or touching adjacent mucosa to warm the tip of the telescope will minimize fogging of the lens. Lubricant or a moist gauze sponge applied to the upper lip allows instruments to glide gently; otherwise, the resistance of the instrument rubbing across the lip can be misinterpreted as resistance from the airway, giving a false impression of narrowing.

ANESTHESIA

For the child who requires examination of a dynamic laryngeal lesion in the operating room, limited sedation can be useful to achieve patient comfort, but oversedation or muscle paralysis will interfere with the endoscopist's ability to discriminate subtle dynamic findings. Selecting a safe and effective method of ventilation and oxygenation, while allowing adequate surgical exposure and access, requires planning and cooperation between endoscopist and anesthetist. Standard endotracheal tubes provide good airway control but interfere with the surgeon's ability to evaluate the posterior larynx or subglottis, and risk ignition during laser procedures. Supraglottic jet ventilation requires adequate laryngeal exposure and precise positioning of the tube. Laryngeal mask airways may be useful in patients with abnormal anatomy or as a conduit for fiberoptic-assisted intubation of a difficult airway, but they are contraindicated in patients with airway obstruction at or below the larynx, pharyngeal masses or edema, or high airway resistance, and they do not protect against aspiration. Intermittent apnea allows airway work without the presence of tubes obstructing surgical access or distorting laryngeal anatomy, but airway control and monitoring is limited. Spontaneous respiration allows evaluation of airway dynamics as well as anatomy, but requires a careful balance of adequate general anesthesia and sufficient spontaneous respiration. Risks include arrhythmias and inadequate ventilation as well as exposure of operating room personnel to anesthetic gases. Adjunctive topical anesthesia may be useful. Mask ventilation can often be used to temporize but may not be effective in patients with severe subglottic stenosis or obstructing lesions.

For transnasal examinations of awake patients, application of a topical decongestant and topical anesthetic to the nose may improve patient comfort. Because vasoconstricting agents can have systemic or cardiac effects, the anesthesiologist should always be informed of any medications administered.

Anesthetizing the supraglottis and glottis prior to awake endoscopy improves patient comfort and helps prevent coughing and laryngospasm. It also can be useful for procedures performed under general anesthesia. Anesthesia of portions of the hypopharynx and supraglottic larynx supplied by the internal branch of the superior laryngeal nerve can be accomplished by application of topical solutions or percutaneous superior laryngeal nerve block. Anesthesia of the trachea and subglottis, which are supplied by the recurrent laryngeal nerve, can be accomplished endoscopically or by transtracheal injection of lidocaine. Application of an anesthetic may interfere with assessments of sensation and neurologic integrity, and doses must be carefully calculated in children. The maximum dose of lidocaine with epinephrine is 7 mg/kg, not to exceed 500 mg; the maximum dose of lidocaine without epinephrine is 3 to 4 mg/kg, not to exceed 300 mg.

Steroids are often given preoperatively or intraoperatively to minimize edema, which may be an intrinsic component of the airway lesion, or may occur following airway manipulation. Edema generally occurs at the expense of the lumen, contributing to airway obstruction.

TECHNIQUE

The patient is placed in a supine position, with the head reaching the proximal edge of the table. The "sniffer" or Boyce-Jackson position provides the best visualization of the larynx, with the neck flexed on the shoulders and the head extended on the neck (Fig. 23.7). A gelatin pad, folded

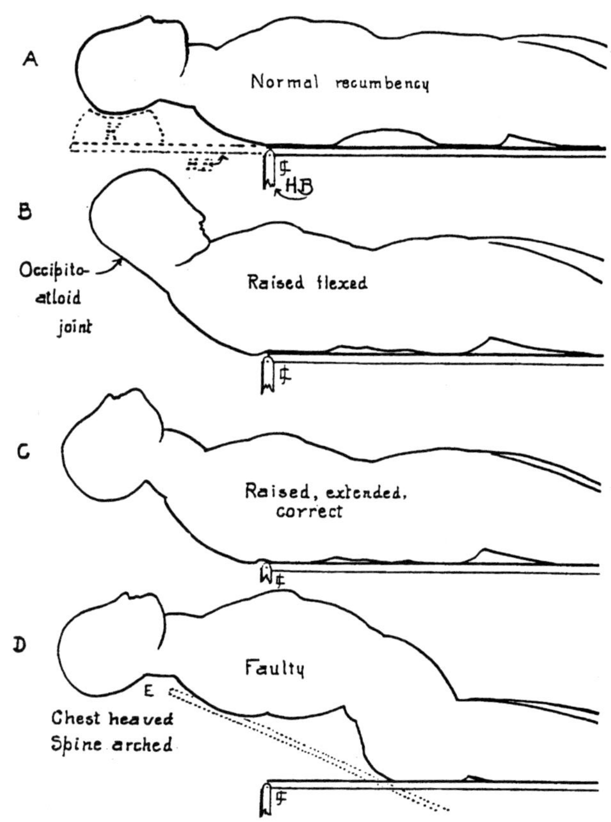

FIGURE 23.7. Optimum patient position for airway endoscopy. Reprinted from Jackson C. *Bronchoscopy and esophagoscopy. A manual of peroral endoscopy and laryngeal surgery.* Philadelphia: WB Saunders, 1922:78; with permission.

towel, or other support can be used to extend the head. A shoulder roll is useful in small children in whom the relatively large occiput may cause excessive neck flexion. Optimal patient positioning may entail the help of an assistant. Intubation prior to endoscopy is generally avoided because it may affect the findings, convert partial airway obstruction from a foreign body to full obstruction, or cause trauma. However, intubation may be indicated in selected patients for safe management of the airway.

During fiberoptic laryngoscopy and bronchoscopy, the control unit and proximal lens of the bronchoscope are held in the left hand, leaving the right hand free to manipulate the scope or insert instruments. The left thumb operates the angulation lever, which controls the angle of the distal tip, while the index finger is used to occlude the suction port as needed.

Rigid ("direct") laryngoscopy consists of two stages: initial exposure of the epiglottis and then elevation of the epiglottis and the tissues attached to the hyoid bone to expose the larynx. The blade of an intubation laryngoscope is passed along the right side of the tongue, sweeping the tongue to the left, and then the tip of the laryngoscope is placed in the vallecula (rather than under the epiglottis). The tip of the blade is lifted forward and upward (toward the corner of the room, where the wall in front of you meets the ceiling), exposing the epiglottis and vocal folds. The vocal folds should be well seen before the telescope or bronchoscope is inserted. External pressure on the thyroid cartilage can improve visualization of the anterior commissure.

Direct laryngoscopy and bronchoscopy are best accomplished, if possible, using an unsheathed telescope (i.e., without a bronchoscope) in order to optimize the size of the telescope and image quality, while minimizing the outer diameter of the instruments required. Once the telescope is advanced beyond the vocal folds, the laryngoscope blade can be withdrawn with a curved motion. At this point, increased neck extension may be required and can be accomplished by repositioning the patient's head and neck. Head position can sometimes be controlled by positioning a finger of the endoscopist's left hand on the maxilla. If necessary, a few extra centimeters of the airway may be viewed by rotating the telescope so that the light cable projects horizontally, along the oral commissure.

If a ventilating bronchoscope is used, it is positioned with the ventilation port accessible to the anesthesiologist and the long bevel parallel to the long axis of the vocal folds so that the light cable will be at a right angle to the camera cable. The bronchoscope is passed through the glottis with the long bevel in the center of the glottic opening, and the short bevel passing along the ipsilateral vocal fold. For example, if the bronchoscope is positioned so that the long bevel is on the right side, it is aimed slightly to the left of center as it is passed through the glottis. Once beyond the glottis, the ventilation port can be used, and the bronchoscope can be rotated in any desired direction, rotating the camera in a compensatory fashion to maintain an upright view on the monitor.

To visualize into the right main-stem bronchus and its branches with a rigid telescope, the child's head is rotated to the left and lowered, if necessary, as the instrument is advanced through the distal trachea. Turning the head to the right facilitates exposure of the left bronchial branches. Endoscopic tracheobronchial anatomy is illustrated in Fig. 23.8.

Suspension microlaryngoscopy frees the surgeon's hands and provides stable airway access during manipulation of supraglottic and glottic lesions, as well as selected subglottic or tracheal lesions. Visualization can be accomplished with a telescope, or a microscope with a 400-mm focal length lens. Procedures using lasers, microdebriders, or microlaryngeal instruments can be performed during intermittent periods of apnea, with intervening ventilation by jet ventilation or intubation. The laryngeal mucosa often becomes rather dry, and application of lubricant to the endotracheal tube facilitates passage.

POSTOPERATIVE CARE

Emergence from general anesthesia can be accomplished using mask ventilation or intubation, depending on both the condition of the airway and the anesthesiologist's preference, however minimizing airway manipulation is preferred when feasible. The level of care required after airway endoscopy is related to the severity of the airway lesion, and the type of anesthesia used. If the airway is marginal or if the patient remains intubated after the procedure, then a critical care setting may be most appropriate. Systemic steroids, and racemic epinephrine, with or without nebulized decadron, also may be indicated.

Patients should not eat or drink until they are awake and able to protect their airway, usually after the effects of topical anesthesia have worn off. Discomfort from the endoscopy itself is usually minor. Follow-up is based on the nature of the airway abnormality.

PITFALLS

To paraphrase a quotation historically attributed to Chevalier Jackson: "two minutes of preparation, two hours of surgery; two hours of preparation, two minutes of surgery." Before beginning the procedure, one must select, assemble, and test any equipment that is likely to be used, and locate any additional equipment that might be needed in an emergency. The surgeon should confirm that the set-up of the room is appropriate and anticipate management options if an adverse event should occur.

Airway structures should be handled in a gentle, atraumatic manner. Trauma can contribute to postoperative edema, and the long-term consequence of scarring. Scars

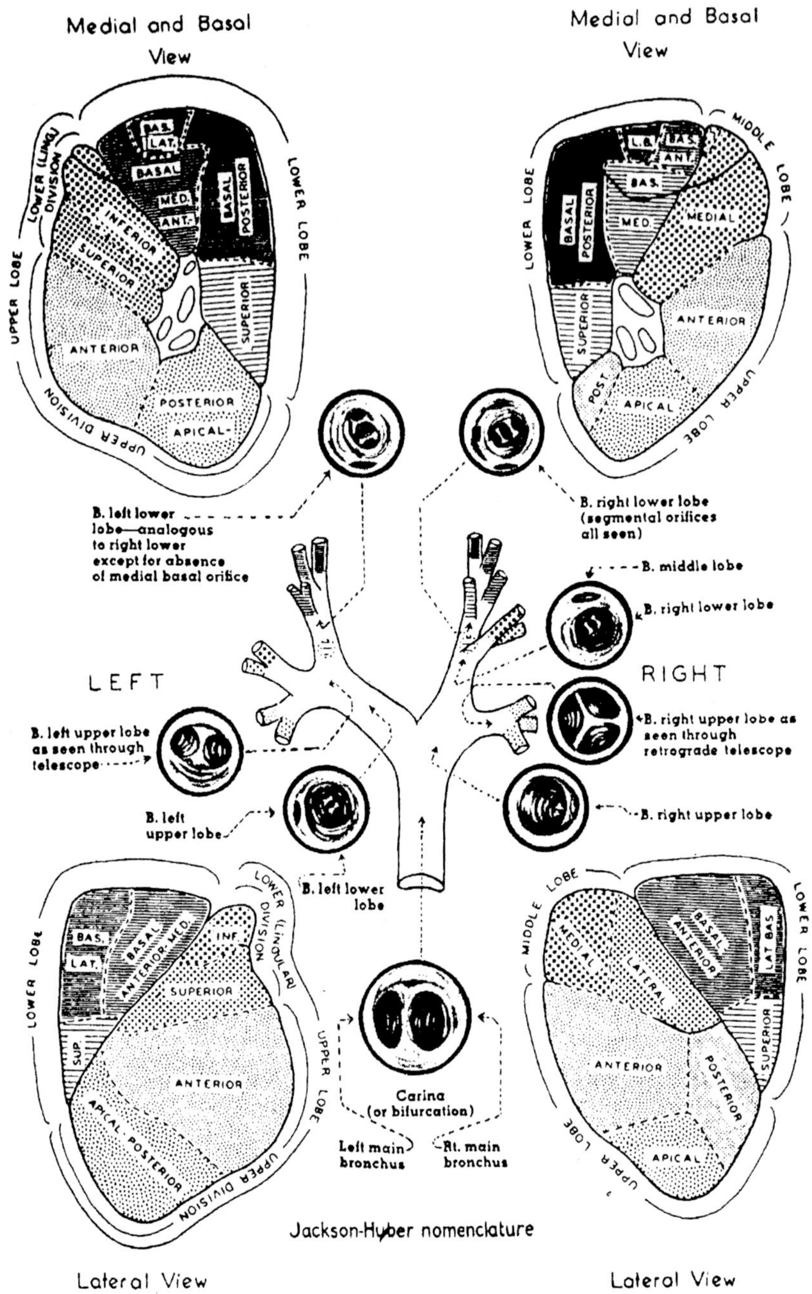

FIGURE 23.8. Tracheobronchial anatomy from the endoscopist's perspective. Reprinted from Ballenger JJ. *Diseases of the nose, throat, ear, head, and neck,* 14th ed. Philadelphia: Lea & Febiger, 1991:1280; with permission.

contract over time and may become stenoses. Evaluation of dynamic lesions, such as vocal fold paralysis or laryngomalacia, is more difficult if sedation is too deep, or if evaluation is attempted during emergence from general anesthesia.

Viewing the subglottis with a fiberoptic telescope from above the vocal folds can give the false impression of subglottic stenosis because of the angle of visualization. The subglottis is a difficult area to manipulate endoscopically. Securing the airway often involves passing a conduit for ventilation through the subglottis, which obstructs access to the subglottis itself. Placing the ventilation apparatus just above the subglottis can be precarious, and may not be feasible in small children. Lesions proximal to the subglottis may be visualized using suspension microlaryngoscopy techniques. The subglottic portion of the airway is particularly at risk for injury and complications because it is the narrowest portion of the airway in an infant and small child. In addition, the cricoid ring within the subglottis is a complete ring and is nondistensible, whereas the rest of the larynx and trachea contain a membranous posterior component, so the subglottis cannot expand to accommodate the passage of instruments.

Foods, particularly nuts, comprise the most common foreign bodies aspirated by children. Some foreign bodies (especially nuts) stimulate the growth of granulation tissue, exacerbating the airway obstruction. Airway foreign bodies must be grasped in a secure manner as loss of control of the foreign body may convert partial airway obstruction to total obstruction with an inability to ventilate the patient. This risk is increased in the subglottis, because of its intrinsic relative narrowness. If control over a foreign body is lost within the trachea or subglottis, risking complete airway obstruction, the foreign body can sometimes be pushed into a main bronchus, allowing ventilation of at least one lung. During removal of foreign bodies, "advancing points perforate, trailing points do not." Sharp points should be turned so that they trail during withdrawal, or sheathed by advancing the bronchoscope over them or withdrawing them into the lumen of the bronchoscope.

For selected foreign bodies with a lumen, such as beads, a Fogarty catheter can be passed through the lumen of the object, the balloon inflated, and the catheter withdrawn so that the foreign body is controlled between the balloon and the bronchoscope. Using a balloon catheter to dislodge a foreign body without proper visualization and control is not recommended. Application of cricoid pressure is sometimes advocated in the management of the patient with a full stomach who requires urgent endoscopy because of foreign body aspiration; however, application of pressure can also compress the larynx and interfere with the atraumatic extraction of a foreign body.

Fiberoptic bronchoscopy can cause partial or complete airway obstruction because the portion of the airway lumen occupied by the scope is not available for ventilation. A side-channel cup forceps can be used to obtain a mucosal biopsy, such as for assessment of ciliary motility. The specimen is grasped within the forceps and then the forceps are abruptly twisted and withdrawn. Aspirates or biopsy specimens obtained for culture should be placed in nonbacteriostatic saline; specimens that are obtained for evaluation of ciliary motility abnormalities that are not immediately evaluated are preserved in gluteraldehyde.

Granulation tissue, papillomas, or other mass lesions may be prudently removed, particularly if obstructing and pedunculated. Removal of large sessile masses, particularly if present in a circumferential distribution, may contribute to subsequent stenosis.

Visualization of distal structures or foreign bodies may be temporarily enhanced by having the anesthesiologist apply positive pressure ventilation, similar to a Valsalva maneuver. Before manipulating a distal lesion with the potential for airway obstruction, have a plan for how ventilation will be accomplished if the lesion becomes dislodged or if the airway becomes swollen or bloody. It may be best to use a smaller telescope, or to use alternative methods of investigation, such as medical imaging, to obtain additional information; however, this must be balanced against the risk of not proceeding. In very unusual circumstances, tracheotomy may be necessary to control the airway, and may allow removal of a foreign body via the stoma.

The American Heart Association recommends bacterial endocarditis prophylaxis for individuals with underlying structural cardiac defects undergoing surgical operations involving the respiratory mucosa, including bronchoscopy with rigid telescopes.

COMPLICATIONS

Edema may already be present, or may be caused or exacerbated by manipulation of an inflamed or narrowed portion of the airway. Steroids, racemic epinephrine, nebulized decadron, and intubation may be helpful.

Bleeding can interfere with visualization as well as ventilation. Techniques to control bleeding include irrigation, application of epinephrine using a catheter or neurosurgical sponges, dependent positioning of the bleeding hemithorax, bronchial tamponade with balloon catheters, bronchial artery embolization, laser coagulation, or open surgical procedures. Compensatory strategies include selective intubation of the nonbleeding lung.

Patients who struggle to breathe spontaneously against a partially or totally obstructed airway may develop postobstructive (noncardiogenic) pulmonary edema. Mechanical ventilation with positive end-expiratory pressures may be indicated.

SUGGESTED READINGS

Cordasco EM, Mehta AC, Ahmad M. Bronchoscopically induced bleeding. A summary of nine years' Cleveland clinic experience and review of the literature. *Chest* 1991;100:1141–1147.

de Blic J, Scheinmann P. Fibreoptic bronchoscopy in infants. *Arch Dis Child* 1992;67:159–161.

Deutsch ES, Smergel E, Crisci K, et al. Tracheobronchography in children. *Laryngoscope* 1996;106:1248–1254.

Good GM, Deutsch ES. Method for removing endobronchial beads. *Ann Otol Rhinol Laryngol* 1998;107:291–292.

Gotta AW, Sullivan CA. Anaesthesia of the upper airway using topical anaesthetic and superior laryngeal nerve block. *Br J Anaesth* 1981;53:1055–1058.

Hunsaker DH. Anesthesia for microlaryngeal surgery: the case for subglottic jet ventilation. *Laryngoscope* 1994;104:1–30.

Jackson C. *Bronchoscopy and esophagoscopy. A manual of peroral endoscopy and laryngeal surgery.* Philadelphia: WB Saunders, 1922.

Maze A, Bloch E. Stridor in pediatric patients. *Anesthesiology* 1979;50:132–145.

Prakash UB. Advances in bronchoscopic procedures [Review]. *Chest* 1999;116:1403–1408.

Wood RE. Pitfalls in the use of the flexible bronchoscope in pediatric patients. *Chest* 1990;97:199–203.

24

TRACHEAL STENOSIS AND RECONSTRUCTION

MICHAEL J. RUTTER
ROBIN T. COTTON

Tracheal stenosis is a relatively rare disorder in the pediatric population, and in contrast with the more common subglottic stenosis, is more often congenital than acquired. Subglottic stenosis is most commonly seen as an acquired lesion occurring as a consequence of prolonged intubation of a premature infant. Our unit currently manages at least 10 cases of subglottic stenosis for every case of tracheal stenosis. The predilection for acquired airway stenosis to occur at the subglottic level exists because the narrowest portion of the infant or child's airway is the cricoid ring, normally the only complete cartilaginous ring in the airway.

Congenital tracheal stenosis is usually due to complete tracheal rings, with or without associated vascular compression of the airway. Tracheal stenosis is sometimes seen as a component of certain syndromes such as Pfeiffer syndrome. If not severe, congenital tracheal stenosis may be a late presentation or an incidental finding.

Acquired tracheal stenosis is traumatic in origin in most cases, either as the result of direct injury (e.g., clothesline injury), or more commonly as a result of trauma from the tip of an endotracheal tube, particularly cuffed endotracheal tubes. Tracheal stenosis also may occur at the site of a tracheotomy, with either an A-frame deformity or a suprastomal collapse.

Although tracheal stenosis may coexist with tracheomalacia or vascular compression of the airway, it should not be confused with malacia or compression. The management of tracheomalacia or vascular compression of the airway is different from the management of tracheal stenosis.

A rare cause of congenital tracheal stenosis is a tracheal web, usually thin and amenable to endoscopic treatment. It is our belief that severe tracheal webs are often inadvertently treated at birth by emergent intubation, causing disruption of the web.

M.J. Rutter and R.T. Cotton: Department of Otolaryngology–Head and Neck Surgery, University of Cincinnati; and Department of Otolaryngology–Head and Neck Surgery, Cincinnati Children's Hospital Medical Center, Cincinnati, Ohio.

PRESENTATION

Congenital tracheal stenosis usually presents in the neonatal period with increasing respiratory distress, stridor, retraction, apnea, cyanosis, and occasionally dying spells. Some children will present with a very "wet" sounding airway due to tracheal secretions hanging up on an area of stenosis ("washing machine respiration"). Symptoms are most notable when the infant is agitated or upset, or when the infant is feeding.

In the first few weeks of life the infant tends to grow at a far greater rate than the stenotic airway, resulting in a deterioration of the airway from suboptimal to critical. An infant presenting with symptomatic tracheal stenosis in the neonatal period is therefore likely to require aggressive intervention.

A proportion of children with complete tracheal rings do not present during the neonatal period. This is due to the narrowest segment of the airway still being large enough to permit continued growth. Tracheal rings do spontaneously grow with time, and in these children it may be many years before their growth significantly exceeds the growth of the airway. Children usually present with exercise intolerance. Because of the insidious nature of the presentation, a child may have comparatively few symptoms despite a significantly narrowed airway. A further group of children may only be mildly symptomatic or asymptomatic despite complete tracheal rings, and in these children it is appropriate to observe because no definitive therapy may be needed. Often the airway stenosis is an incidental finding, for example, following a difficult intubation for an unrelated surgical procedure. Our unit follows several children with asymptomatic or minimally symptomatic complete tracheal rings, and our policy is to intervene only if the airway compromises the quality of life, such as limiting sporting activities. We have followed two of these children for over 15 years without intervention.

PREOPERATIVE PREPARATION

Most children with complete tracheal rings require operative repair. Optimal management requires a comprehensive preoperative evaluation. Imaging studies and endoscopic evaluation are essential. To minimize the risk to the patient during these procedures, a high index of suspicion is strongly recommended. If the child is stable, initial evaluation with high-kilovolt airway films may provide a warning of significant airway stenosis. Although airway films are an excellent screening tool for tracheal stenosis, more information is gained by spiral computed tomography or magnetic resonance imaging with contrast. This may provide information not only on the dimensions of the trachea, but also whether the bronchi are involved, and whether there are associated anomalies. The most common associated anomalies are hypoplasia of the right lung and cardiac defects, particularly pulmonary artery sling. Cardiac defects may be present in up to 50%, and echocardiography is a useful adjunctive investigation.

Although imaging studies may be useful, they also may be potentially misleading, and definitive assessment is undertaken via endoscopy. This should be performed with extreme care, because rough instrumentation in an area of stenosis may cause enough swelling to convert a narrow airway to a critical airway demanding abrupt intervention. Because of this, we routinely administer dexamethasone (0.5 mg/kg) on induction, and would prefer to note a tracheal stenosis, and not fully evaluate the distal airway, rather than force a telescope through a narrow stenosis.

The ideal aims of endoscopic evaluation are to confirm the diagnosis of tracheal stenosis, establish whether it is due to complete tracheal rings, estimate the size of the smallest ring, estimate the percentage of the airway involved with complete tracheal rings as well as the position of the rings within the trachea, and evaluate the bronchial anatomy. This is a situation where rigid endoscopy and flexible bronchoscopy are truly complimentary. Rigid bronchoscopy provides a superb optic evaluation of the trachea but carries a higher risk of compromising the airway during evaluation of the airway distal to the complete tracheal rings. Meanwhile, flexible bronchoscopy may permit a better evaluation of the distal trachea and main stem bronchi, particularly in an effort to exclude complete bronchial rings, while minimizing trauma to the narrowest segment of the airway. With a small airway, adequate evaluation is not undertaken with a ventilating bronchoscope, but rather with the Hopkins rod telescope (removed from the bronchoscope), which should be introduced independently into the airway to evaluate the stenosis.

An estimate of the size of the airway is valuable. In a normal full-term neonate, the narrowest point of the airway is at the cricoid and should measure 4.5 to 5.5 mm. Subglottic stenosis is defined as an airway diameter of less than 4 mm. Although the trachea should be of greater capacity than the cricoid, with complete tracheal rings the airway may be so small as to not easily permit safe passage of any form of instrumentation. For comparative purposes, the smallest Stortz 2.5 ventilating bronchoscope has an outer diameter of 3.7 mm. The smallest available endotracheal tube with a 2.0-mm inner diameter has an outer diameter of 3.1 mm. The smallest 20017 Hopkins rod telescope (as found in the Stortz 2.5 ventilating bronchoscope) has an outer diameter of 1.9 mm. It is remarkable how small an airway can be tolerated by a neonate with comparatively few symptoms.

Endoscopic evaluation of a critical airway carries risks and therefore should not be undertaken unless facilities exist to intervene should the child deteriorate during or after the evaluation. Although the council of perfection is to proceed straight to definitive repair should the child deteriorate, there are often practical and logistical problems that may prevent this. If the airway will permit, intubation with a 2.0-mm endotracheal tube may allow the child to be stabilized. However, complete tracheal rings presenting in the neonatal period may not permit passage of a 2.0-mm endotracheal tube, and even if this is possible, the smallest rings are often the most distal, close to the carina, and may cause significant problems with tube placement and stabilization. However, in a child where the complete tracheal rings cone down towards the carina, a 2.0-mm endotracheal tube may be wedged in the more capacious proximal rings, and still permit positive pressure ventilation, allowing time for more definitive intervention to be arranged. In a child where airway stabilization by intubation is not possible, extracorporeal membrane oxygenation (ECMO) is advisable if the facility is available. Tracheotomy is rarely helpful because the smallest complete tracheal rings tend to be more distal, and the smallest available tracheotomy tube is a Bivona 2.5-mm inner diameter, with an outer diameter of 3.9 mm. Attempted tracheotomy also may compromise the options of subsequent operative repair.

Certain patterns of complete tracheal rings may be recognized. The most common are (a) complete rings that are of reasonable size proximally, but cone down to a very small distal ring close to the carina; (b) the "stovepipe" airway with a long segment of complete tracheal rings of similar diameter; (c) "a short segment stenosis," often in the midtrachea; and (d) complete tracheal rings associated with a high "pig" bronchus.

Careful preoperative evaluation optimizes subsequent decision making. If the child has concomitant cardiac anomalies that require repair, particularly a pulmonary artery sling, then the complete tracheal rings are best tackled as a combined procedure through an anterior sternotomy under cardiopulmonary bypass. If the lower third of the trachea is involved, repair through an anterior sternotomy under cardiopulmonary bypass is also recommended. If only the upper or midtrachea is involved, then repair may be performed with routine anesthesia through a cervical approach. Hyperextension of an infant's neck over a shoulder roll will allow good access to the upper two thirds of the trachea through a cervical approach. Exposure can be further enhanced through a limited upper sternotomy if required.

TECHNICAL APPROACH

Although standard anesthetic techniques or jet ventilation techniques may allow access to the distal trachea without relying on cardiopulmonary bypass, we preferentially use cardiopulmonary bypass because it allows the heart and lungs to be decompressed, which enhances exposure of the distal airway. Even in a child already on ECMO, we prefer to convert to cardiopulmonary bypass for these reasons, and return to ECMO at the end of the procedure if required. It is often advantageous to resect the small pad of lymphatic tissue found in the region of the carina because this also facilitates airway exposure.

There are several methods for repair of complete tracheal rings. Our approach to the management of complete tracheal rings has evolved over the past 25 years, and our current recommendations are as follows.

Tracheal Resection

This is excellent for treating short-segment, complete tracheal rings (involving less than one third of the trachea). It is also excellent for treating acquired stenosis of the trachea. However, two precautions should be heeded. First, there are often more complete tracheal rings noted when the airway is actually opened than were noted during the endoscopic evaluation. Second, we are more cautious with resections involving the distal third of the trachea, because we try to avoid having an anastomosis close to the carina. This is because any anastomotic problems may ultimately require placement of a tracheotomy tube, and the tip of the tracheotomy tube must lie between the anastomosis and the carina, which may be very problematic if there is only 2 to 3 mm between the anastomosis and carina.

Tracheoplasty Using the Slide Technique

This involves estimating the center point of the complete tracheal rings, and transecting the airway at this level. The proximal segment of the trachea then has the back wall of the complete tracheal rings incised, while the distal segment of the trachea has the front wall of the complete tracheal rings incised. The transected ends of both segments are beveled, and the trachea is then overlapped upon itself, and the anastomosis completed with either running or interrupted 5.0 monocryl sutures. This is an excellent technique in that it greatly increases the size of the diameter of the airway while avoiding a transverse anastomosis. With this technique it is important to accurately estimate the midpoint of the complete tracheal rings, and intraoperative endoscopic evaluation may facilitate this. It is also technically more difficult to perform in infants whose complete tracheal rings are widely divergent in diameter in different segments of the airway (Fig. 24.1).

Tracheoplasty Using an Anterior Tracheal Patch

This is an excellent technique for long-segment, complete tracheal rings. One third to one half of the complete tracheal rings are removed, and the distal and proximal segments of the trachea anastomosed. The remaining complete

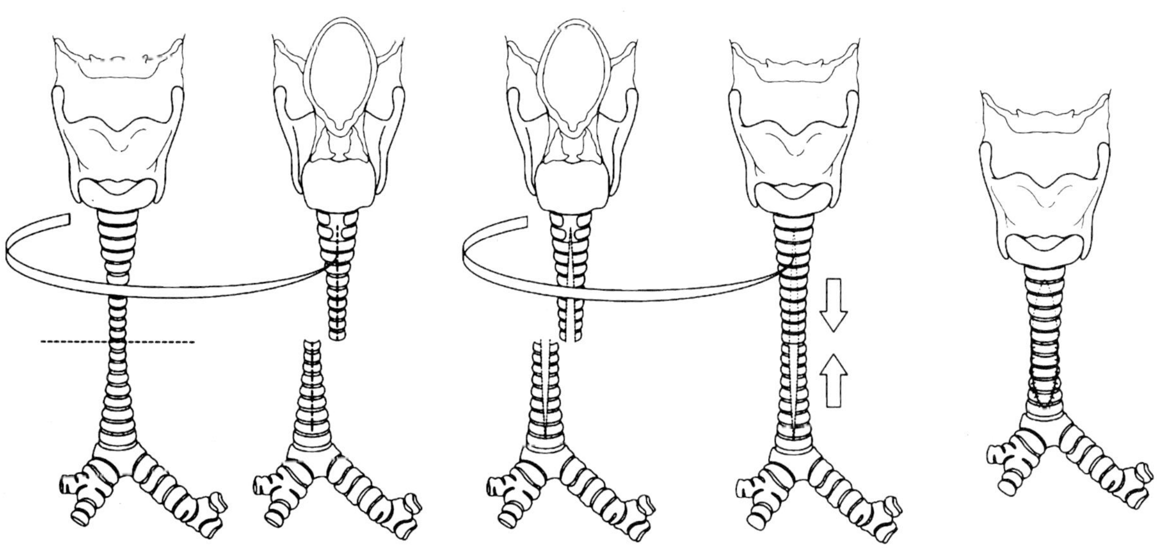

FIGURE 24.1. Tracheal slide technique.

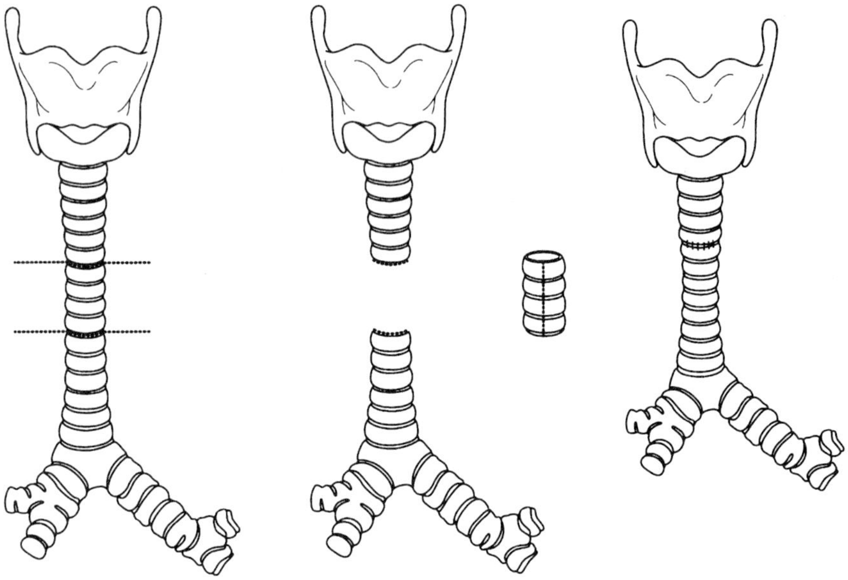

FIGURE 24.2. Tracheal slide technique.

tracheal rings are then split anteriorly, and the resected piece of trachea is split longitudinally, flattened out, and used as an anterior graft over the remaining anteriorly split complete rings. This technique can significantly expand the airway, although not as much as a slide tracheoplasty can do. The resected piece of trachea used as an anterior graft has far greater integral support than pericardium or perichondrium. It is helpful if the resected segment of the trachea includes the smallest complete tracheal rings, and the proximal and distal segments of the trachea need not have an equal number of complete tracheal rings on either side of the anastomosis. However, we still recommend trying to avoid an anastomosis of the proximal and distal segments of the trachea that lies close to carina (Figs. 24.2 and 24.3).

Pericardial Patch/Perichondrial Patch Tracheoplasty

We rarely perform this procedure. It is an excellent technique for children with mild to moderate tracheal stenosis due to complete tracheal rings. In such children any technique will have a good outcome. However, in children with very small diameter complete tracheal rings, especially when close to the carina, splitting the rings anteriorly and placing a patch will only allow a moderate gain in lumen size, and if too large a patch is placed, anterior tracheomalacia will result. There may be granulation tissue formation at the suture line, and this may require repeat visits to the operating room for management.

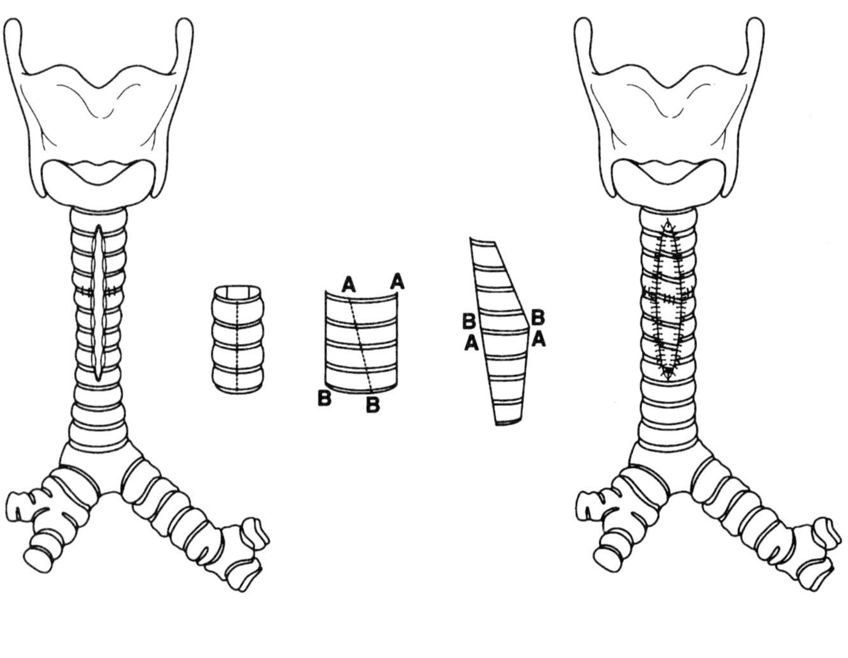

FIGURE 24.3. Tracheoplasty using an anterior tracheal patch technique.

Tracheoplasty Using Costal Cartilage Grafts

We do not perform this procedure for the same reasons that we rarely perform pericardial/perichondrial patch tracheoplasty. Although there is less of a risk for anterior tracheomalacia, this is replaced with the risk that the graft will prolapse into the airway. The survival of costal cartilage grafts in the upper trachea is dependent on revascularization from the overlying strap muscles. Muscle is not present over the lower trachea, and this decreases the survival rate of grafts placed in the distal trachea.

Tracheal Homograft

This is a technically challenging procedure in a young child, and a stormy postoperative course is expected. We reserve this procedure for children who have had failure of previous tracheal reconstructive attempts.

PITFALLS

1. A tracheotomy is rarely helpful in the management of complete tracheal rings prior to tracheal reconstruction.
2. Airway imaging may be hard to interpret.
3. Initial endoscopic evaluation should be performed carefully and gently, with an intervention plan available should the child decompensate postoperatively.
4. There are always more tracheal rings present than were appreciated during endoscopic evaluation.
5. The cardiovascular status of the child should be carefully evaluated, particularly with regard to a pulmonary artery sling.
6. Complete bronchial rings are a poor prognostic indicator.
7. Complete tracheal rings need not mandate intervention. In mild cases, growth of complete tracheal rings can be expected, and intervention may not be required.

CONTROVERSIES

Is it acceptable for complete tracheal rings to be managed conservatively? We have followed several children with complete tracheal rings for up to 15 years. We have documented the potential for spontaneous growth of complete tracheal rings. In some children the growth of complete tracheal rings is such that the child remains asymptomatic and intervention is not required. In other cases, the growth of the child is faster than the growth of the complete tracheal rings, with the child becoming more symptomatic with time. Under these circumstances, intervention is ultimately required, but operative management is more forgiving in an older child with a larger airway.

For decades the pericardial patch has been the standard of care for management of complete tracheal rings. Are we now advocating that this procedure be abandoned? For many years pericardial patch tracheoplasty was our standard of care as well. And as all physicians who have performed a significant number of pericardial patches know, children with more severe forms of tracheal stenosis tend to have a stormy postoperative course following pericardial patch tracheoplasty, usually due to granulation tissue in an airway that remains small despite the tracheoplasty. We have found that tracheal resection, slide tracheoplasty, and tracheoplasty using an anterior tracheal patch have provided us with satisfactory outcomes, both in the perioperative phase and long term.

POSTOPERATIVE CARE

Following tracheal repair we aim to extubate a child within 24 to 96 hours. During this time we try to avoid positive pressure ventilation so as not to threaten the anastomosis. Chest drains are ideally left in place until after the extubation. Preoperative presentation may be with an extremely unstable ventilated child, or a child already requiring ECMO. In this circumstance, postoperative ECMO may be required. The aim is to establish endotracheal ventilation and remove the child from ECMO as rapidly as possible.

COMPLICATIONS

In the early postoperative phase complications are most commonly seen that reflect the underlying health status of the child. These infants may be critically ill prior to tracheal repair, and often remain critically ill following tracheal repair. If postoperative ECMO is required, there are well-recognized short-term and long-term consequences of prolonged use, especially in the neonatal population.

The tracheal repair also may cause problems, including granulation tissue along suture lines, and restenosis or collapse at the anastomosis site. Failure of extubation usually results from one of these issues. Rarely, the anastomosis may dehisce. During the tracheal repair local soft tissue should be placed between the tracheal suture line and the innominate artery to minimize the risk of innominate artery fistula formation.

Granulation tissue is usually amenable to serial bronchoscopic management. Stenosis or collapse at the anastomosis site may require either regular dilation of the trachea, or placement of a tracheotomy tube, with the tip of the tracheotomy tube bypassing the area of concern.

FOLLOW-UP

We recommend that the tracheal repair be endoscopically evaluated within 7 to 10 days of the operation. It should then be reevaluated at increasing intervals if no problems are encountered, or on an as-required basis if there are any problems with granulation tissue, restenosis, or collapse. We would normally reevaluate an infant's airway at 1, 3, and 9 months following trachea repair. If the child required ECMO during management, follow-up neurologic and audiologic evaluation are recommended.

SUGGESTED READINGS

Andrews TM, Cotton RT, Bailey WW, et al. Tracheoplasty for congenital complete tracheal rings. *Arch Otolaryngol Head Neck Surg* 1994;120:1363–1369.

Backer CL, Mavroudis C, Gerber ME, et al. Tracheal surgery in children: an 18 year review of 4 techniques. *Eur J Cardiothorac Surg* 2001;19:777–784.

Cosentino CM, Backer CL, Idriss FS, et al. Pericardial patch tracheoplasty for severe tracheal stenosis in children: intermediate results. *J Pediatr Surg* 1991;26:879–884.

Cunningham MJ, Eavey RD, Vlahakes GJ, et al. Slide tracheoplasty for long-segment tracheal stenosis. *Arch Otolaryngol Head Neck Surg* 1998;124:98–103.

Jaquiss RD, Lusk RP, Spray TL, et al. Repair of long-segment tracheal stenosis in infancy. *J Thorac Cardiovasc Surg* 1995;110: 1504–1511; discussion 1511–1512.

Molter DW, Cotton RT. Management of tracheal stenosis in children. *Arta Otorhinolaryngol Belg* 1995;49:383–387.

25

TRACHEOMALACIA

EDWARD J. DOOLIN

Tracheomalacia is a dynamic problem of the usually passive trachea, in which opposing forces cause it to collapse and obstruct. This can occur at any age, although it is most common in the younger infant and newborn period. It has multiple and complementary causes. Because of the obscure nature of the disorder, different procedures are recommended depending on the clinical circumstances.

ETIOLOGY

There are multiple causes of tracheomalacia. Many of these are complementary and contribute to the ultimate symptoms and problems. The term *tracheomalacia* implies that the otherwise rigid airway is now too soft to maintain its tubular shape in the face of changes in the pressure gradient across its wall during respiration. Specifically, when the pressure within the lumen of the cervical trachea is less than atmospheric pressure during inspiration, the tube collapses and becomes occluded. During the expiratory phase, the extraluminal pressure in the thoracic portion of the trachea is higher than that within the lumen, again causing the tube to collapse and become occluded.

The trachea can usually withstand these normal forces by virtue of its cartilaginous ring structure. The most obvious cause of tracheomalacia is when the tracheal rings do not have the rigidity or resilience to support the organ during its dynamic functioning. In addition to providing intrinsic support, the shape of the tracheal ring is also critical. Typically omega shaped, the tracheal rings also supports the membranous posterior wall of the airway. If the rings are misshapen, the function of the posterior wall will be abnormal. When the tracheal rings are too broad or shallow, the anteroposterior diameter of the trachea is reduced and the support of the posterior tracheal wall is lost. This allows the soft posterior wall to collapse during inspiration to a great extent, further obstructing the airway. This leads us to the final factor that contributes to tracheomalacia, and that is the additional support of the posterior wall. The tracheal rings are not solely responsible for the support of the membranous portion of the tracheal wall. This area of the trachea is securely attached to the esophagus and posterior mediastinum. Disease processes in this area will cause the tracheal wall to be more mobile and hence render it more susceptible to collapse.

With these intrinsic malfunctions in mind, the clinical settings in which tracheomalacia is seen make a great deal of sense. Premature infants often have an incompletely developed trachea. The trachea also can be damaged or misshaped due to the long-term presence of an endotracheal tube. Mediastinal masses of any type, including tumors, bronchogenic cysts, an enlarged thymus, or compression from vascular rings can all put pressure on the trachea, resulting in a malformed trachea and a dysfunctional airway.

One of the most common causes of severe tracheomalacia is esophageal atresia. Because the airway develops in the face of compression by an enlarged proximal esophagus, it is at risk for malformation. In addition, the procedure needed to repair esophageal atresia entails mobilization of the esophagus from the trachea and renders the posterior membranous wall of the trachea unstable. This undoubtedly contributes to the severe tracheomalacia often seen in these children.

Finally, because the trachea is dependent on adjacent mediastinal structures to maintain its shape and posture, a distorted mediastinum can contribute to the malfunction of the trachea. This is particularly seen in children with severe spinal deformities, especially with high thoracic kyphoscoliosis.

DIAGNOSIS

Tracheomalacia produces symptoms related to airway compromise, the severity of which generally correlates with the degree of tracheomalacia. Stridor is the most common symptom. In its mildest form, the stridor may only be evident when the child is crying. The sound is characteristic

E.J. Doolin: Department of Surgery, University of Pennsylvania; and Department of Surgery, Children's Hospital of Philadelphia, Philadelphia, Pennsylvania.

and often allows the identification of the "tracheoesophageal fistula (TEF) baby" by experienced nurses from across the room. In cases of moderate tracheomalacia, the infant has stridor when tachypneic or sometimes at rest. The stridor is most pronounced on inspiration but can have an expiratory component as well. Severe cases present with prominent retractions, hypoxia, and signs of severe respiratory embarrassment. Intubation and ventilatory support is mandatory in these infants. With isolated tracheomalacia without pulmonary disease, minimal support with positive pressure ventilation is all that is required and results in a well-appearing infant who seems otherwise "extubatable."

The efforts to confirm the diagnosis of tracheomalacia generally follow two lines of pursuit. The first is to try to identify an anomaly that may be causing the tracheomalacia. A plain radiograph of the neck and chest occasionally demonstrate an alteration in the usual shape of the tracheal air column, but is often nonspecific. A barium swallow is sometimes used to look for compression of the esophageal lumen by a mediastinal cyst or a vascular ring. More commonly, a computed tomography scan of the chest is helpful to rule out the presence of a mediastinal tumor or a pulmonary or bronchial anomaly that could result in tracheomalacia.

The second approach is to assess the dynamic functioning of the airway. Although many efforts at using fluoroscopy or ultrasonography have been pursued, these usually fail to provide the appropriate dynamic image that is required to confirm this diagnosis. Studies such as pulmonary function tests can indeed isolate certain parameters, such as inspiratory volume and flow rate, which will support the diagnosis of the tracheomalacia, but are not useful in the small child.

The mainstay of diagnosis is endoscopic evaluation. Endoscopy allows not only an anatomic assessment of the trachea lumen and wall, which is key to the diagnosis, but also allows the surgeon to observe the trachea in a dynamic way during the respiratory cycle. With this in mind, it is important to allow the child to function as normally as possible during the assessment. This means that the child needs to be breathing spontaneously, without the intrinsic support provided by positive pressure ventilation. Rigid bronchoscopic evaluation is standard in many centers, but flexible fiberoptic bronchoscopy is a reasonable alternative, depending on the experience of the surgeon.

With the bronchoscope in the upper trachea, the trachea should be observed during spontaneous breathing and through several respiratory cycles. The membranous portion of the trachea normally moves in and out, but the anterior and posterior walls should not approximate. In the child with tracheomalacia, the walls of the trachea come together, and obstruction of the airway is evident. One should observe carefully whether the thoracic or cervical portions of the trachea, or both, are involved. Also, it should be noted whether the occlusion only occurs where the pulsatile anterior indentation of the aorta is visible. These factors may help decide whether surgical intervention is likely to be successful.

TREATMENT

In the majority of cases, the tracheomalacia is not severe enough to cause complete obstruction. Inspiratory stridor that is worse on exertion can be tolerated for a period of time if it is not causing undue duress and is not causing acute life-threatening events, such as apnea or cyanosis. As the child grows, several things will happen to the trachea that will help this condition improve. The first is that the trachea will enlarge in size. The second is that the soft cartilaginous tracheal rings will become more rigid with age. Finally, the mediastinum will enlarge, which will help support the trachea. These changes may take many months or, in some cases, even years before significant clinical improvement occurs.

If an extrinsic force, such as a mediastinal mass or vascular ring, is contributing to the tracheal weakness, this should be surgically corrected. Often, after surgical correction of the abnormality compressing the trachea, tracheomalacia will persist. At that point, the child is treated as outlined below. The surgical approach to the trachea should be considered for patients who have failed to improve for a period of nonoperative management and cannot be removed from positive pressure ventilatory support.

There are two basic techniques for the surgical correction of tracheomalacia. The first is to improve the mediastinal support, and the second is to support the trachea intrinsically. The tracheal obstruction in this disease is a complex result of soft tracheal rings, abnormal shapes, and a compressed airway. Although the aorta may not be the actual cause of the obstruction, it is an effective tool in reestablishing the airway. Aortic suspension can be performed to increase the anterior/posterior diameter of the trachea and reduce compression of the trachea by the weight of anterior mediastinal structures such as the great vessels. This involves securing the anterior aorta to the posterior aspect of the sternum. This can be done with or without a Dacron patch on the aorta, but the use of a patch is recommended. In a newborn baby, the distance between the aorta and the sternum is small and the structure is quite compliant. This allows the aorta to be adjacent to the sternum without surgery. As the child grows, the distance in the front of the aorta becomes larger and the aorta becomes more fixed in the mediastinum. Endoscopic assessment of the airway during the aortic suspension is useful in showing how much displacement of the aorta is required and tolerated by the child. Some surgeons describe preoperative endoscopic findings such as distinct impingement of the aorta as it crosses anterior to the trachea and a single defined area of tracheal occlusion ("fish mouth" deformity) as predictive of success of the aortic suspension procedure, suggesting that a diffuse involvement of the trachea is less likely to be ameliorated by the operation.

There are children in whom, because of the clinical situation, associated medical conditions or unfavorable mediastinal anatomy (such as severe kyphosis) the aortic suspension will not work. For these children, endoscopic placement of expansion stents can sometimes be useful in improving the tracheomalacia. My preference is to use the balloon-expanding Palmatz stent because of its ease of placement. Other stents, such as the Dumont stent, also have a role. It must be remembered that stenting is a palliative procedure. The devices that are put in place are fraught with short- and long-term complications. Operative complications include tracheal injury, misplacement of the stent, and missizing. Long-term complications include erosion through the airway, migration, bleeding, and obstructive granulation tissue.

Finally, if neither surgical technique is feasible, then a tracheostomy can always be used to palliate tracheomalacia. This not only fixes the trachea to the skin of the neck, which may or may not improve the functioning of the trachea, but it also allows a prosthesis to be put into the trachea, which will resolve the symptoms. Over time, the condition is expected to improve so that eventually the majority of these children can be decannulated.

SUGGESTED READINGS

Backer CL, Holinger LD, Mavroudis C. Innominate artery compression—division and reimplantation versus suspension. *J Thorac Cardiovasc Surg* 1992;103:817–820.

Benjamin B. *Diagnostic laryngology: adults and children.* Philadelphia: WB Saunders, 1990.

Blair GK, Cohen R, Filler RM. Treatment of tracheomalacia: eight years' experience. *J Pediatr Surg* 1986;21:781–785.

Nashef S, Dromer C, Velly JF, et al. Expanding wire stents in benign tracheobronchial disease: indications and complications. *Soc Thorac Surgeons* 1992;54:937–940.

Schild JA. Congenital malformation of the trachea and bronchi. In: Bluestone CD, Stool SE, Kenna MA, eds. *Pediatric otolaryngology,* 2nd ed., vol. 2. Philadelphia: WB Saunders, 1990:1129–1133.

Wiatrak BJ, Myer CM III, Cotton RT. Atypical tracheobronchial vascular compression. *Am J Otolaryngol* 1991;12:347–356.

26

POSTERIOR LARYNGEAL CLEFTS

MICHAEL J. RUTTER
ROBIN T. COTTON

A posterior laryngeal cleft is an abnormal communication between the trachea and esophagus that extends superiorly into the pharynx, and results from an embryologic failure of the laryngotracheal groove to fuse. The degree of clefting may vary considerably, from a deep interarytenoid notch that does not progress below the level of the true vocal cord, to a cleft that extends down the complete length of the trachea and into a bronchus. Posterior laryngeal clefts that progress below the level of the cricoid cartilage also may be termed laryngotracheoesophageal clefts.

A delay in diagnosis is commonplace and may adversely affect the long-term prognosis for the patient, because the risk of irreversible lung pathology due to chronic aspiration steadily increases with time. Although rare, increasing awareness of the condition and more successful techniques of repair have resulted in an improvement in survival rates from less than 60% 20 years ago to over 90% currently.

The severity of the posterior laryngeal cleft influences not only the ultimate survival rates, but also the rate of morbidity, the choice of operative procedure, and the likelihood that the surgical repair will be successful. Laryngeal clefts are best classified anatomically, as in the following modification of Benjamin and Inglis' excellent classification system (Fig. 26.1):

Type I. A supraglottic interarytenoid cleft extending to, but not below, the level of the true vocal cords. This could be considered a deep interarytenoid notch.

Type II. A partial cricoid cleft that extends below the level of the vocal cords, and into, but not through, the posterior cricoid cartilage.

Type III. A total cricoid cleft with or without extension of the cleft into the cervical trachea. This also may be termed a laryngotracheoesophageal cleft.

Type IV. A cleft extending to the thoracic trachea.

Type V. A cleft extending to the carina or into the mainstem bronchi.

M. J. Rutter and **R. T. Cotton:** Department of Otolaryngology-Head and Neck Surgery, University of Cincinnati; and Department of Otolaryngology-Head and Neck Surgery, Cincinnati Children's Hospital Medical Center, Cincinnati, Ohio.

DIAGNOSIS

The key to diagnosis is a high index of suspicion. Presenting symptoms are often nonspecific and may include choking on feeds, chronic cough, and repeated chest infections. Children with posterior laryngeal clefting have a high incidence of other congenital anomalies. Subtle airway symptoms (which often mimic other more common disorders) may be further disguised by more overt associated anomalies. In more severe cases, presentation may be early, with feeding problems, choking, wheezing, stridor, cyanotic spells, apnea, and aspiration pneumonia. Even with less impressive presentation, symptoms and signs are usually consistent with chronic aspiration.

Children with a posterior laryngeal cleft frequently present with airway compromise. Although this may be due to aspiration, in infants it is more commonly due to anatomic obstruction of the airway. Tracheomalacia and bronchomalacia are usually present to some degree, and severe cases may present with marked airway distress. Stridor is also common, usually due to excessive redundant mucosa on either edge of the posterior laryngeal cleft occluding the airway. It is also seen with subglottic stenosis and vocal cord paralysis, both of which may be associated with posterior laryngeal clefting. An abnormal cry can result from redundant mucosa impeding full glottic closure, or a unilateral vocal cord paralysis.

If there is clinical suspicion of a posterior laryngeal cleft, several supportive investigations may help aid in the diagnosis. A modified barium swallow or video swallow study may show evidence of aspiration, although in some cases redundant mucosa on the edges of the cleft may make this an intermittent phenomenon that is therefore difficult to diagnose radiologically. A functional endoscopic evaluation of swallowing (the glottis is inspected with a flexible nasopharyngoscope while the child feeds) also may be useful.

The definitive diagnosis of laryngotracheal cleft requires rigid endoscopic evaluation under general anesthesia. A high index of suspicion is still required, and to definitively

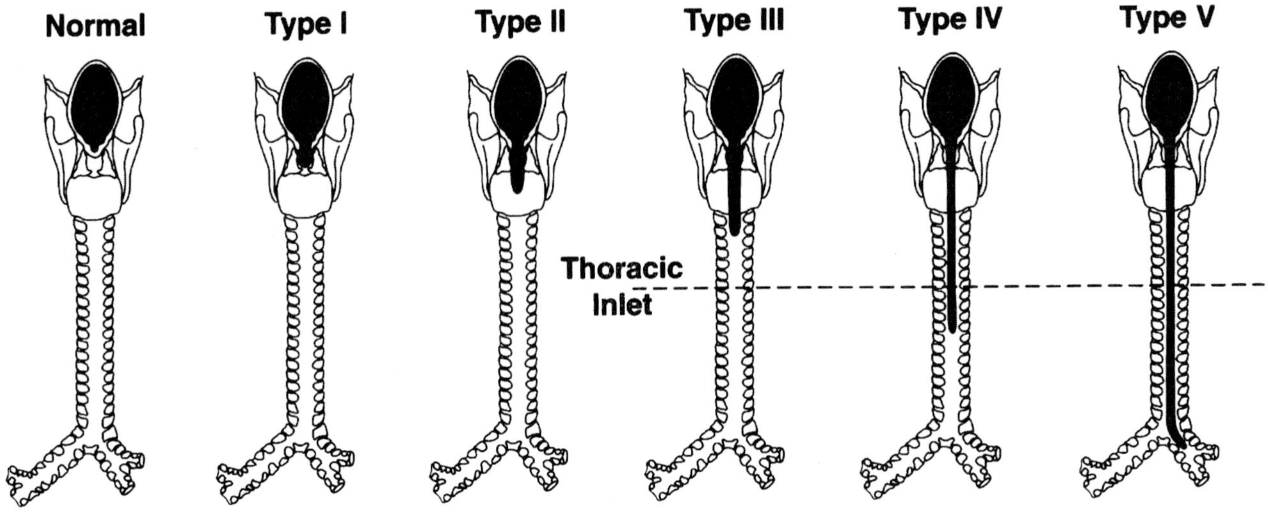

FIGURE 26.1. Classification of posterior laryngeal clefts (modified from Benjamin and Inglis). Posterior view of larynx and trachea is shown.

exclude a cleft, the interarytenoid notch should be probed with a right-angled hook while the vocal cords are splayed apart. This can be achieved by intubating the larynx, or by placing an esophagoscope. Endoscopic findings of excessive mucosa in the interarytenoid area are very suggestive of a posterior laryngeal cleft, as is a patulous upper esophageal sphincter. Although it is possible to establish the diagnosis with flexible bronchoscopy, this instrument does not provide a good view of the posterior glottis, and there is significant risk of missing the diagnosis and falsely reassuring the family and the physicians who are caring for the child.

During the endoscopic evaluation, the opportunity should be taken to carefully examine the rest of the airway and the esophagus to exclude other congenital anomalies. Bronchoscopy will confirm tracheomalacia and might show bronchomalacia, subglottic stenosis, innominate artery compression, or vocal cord paralysis. Esophagoscopy may show evidence of gastroesophageal reflux disease, or a retroesophageal subclavian artery. Twenty to 40% of children with a posterior laryngeal cleft have an associated tracheoesophageal fistula (whereas 10% of children with a tracheoesophageal fistula have a posterior laryngeal cleft), which is usually diagnosed prior to the diagnosis of a posterior laryngeal cleft.

Other congenital anomalies associated with a posterior laryngeal cleft include congenital heart defects, hypospadias, and imperforate anus. These may be seen in association with other syndromic congenital anomalies, with Opitz-Friaz syndrome commonly having an associated laryngotracheal esophageal cleft. A small number of children with the rarer Pallister-Hall syndrome also may have a posterior laryngeal cleft, and the presence of a posterior laryngeal cleft or bifid epiglottis may be the first anomaly noted in this syndrome.

PREOPERATIVE PREPARATION

Once the diagnosis of a posterior laryngeal cleft has been established, and any other more pressing congenital anomalies addressed (congenital heart defects, tracheoesophageal fistula), then consideration should be given to repair of the cleft. The patient should be optimized for surgery, and the repair performed as early as is practicable if there is no other reason to delay. There is considerable risk of pulmonary compromise from prolonged aspiration if cleft repair is delayed.

Three questions should be explored preoperatively: Does the child need a tracheotomy? Does the child need a gastrostomy? Does the child need a fundoplication? Most children with laryngeal clefting have significant gastroesophageal reflux disease. Gastroesophageal reflux adversely affects the outcome of laryngeal cleft repair. Although H_2 antagonists or proton pump inhibitors may provide adequate acid suppression in some children, most require more definitive intervention. Fundoplication is frequently required with simultaneous gastrostomy tube placement. An alternative is placement of a gastrojejunostomy tube or a jejunostomy tube, with concurrent acid suppression. The obvious benefit of gastrostomy or jejunostomy placement is the reduced potential for aspiration.

Consideration should be given to placement of a tracheotomy tube. This is mandatory if the child is in respiratory distress. Tracheotomy may be performed at the time of laryngeal cleft repair if desired. In selected circumstances it is appropriate to perform a laryngeal cleft repair as a single stage procedure without the requirement for a tracheotomy tube. The advantage of a single stage procedure is that a tracheotomy tube is avoided, and this is most relevant in children with moderate tracheomalacia. A child with moderate tracheomalacia may have few respiratory symptoms, but if a tracheotomy is placed, it may be difficult to remove for 2 or 3 years following the laryngeal cleft repair because the tracheotomy site produces anterior tracheal malacia. The disadvantage of a single stage procedure is that an endotracheal tube will lie against the suture line of the repair in the early postoperative period, and this may be further compounded by the presence of a nasogastric tube pressing against the other side of the repair if a gastrostomy was not placed. In most circumstances, the tracheotomy tube may be removed within weeks or months following a successful laryngeal cleft repair.

The next consideration is whether the cleft requires repair at all. If the child has other major congenital anomalies, particularly of the central nervous system, it may not be appropriate to repair the cleft. It is also noteworthy that not all type I posterior laryngeal clefts require repair. Type I laryngeal clefts are not common, yet have the potential to be overdiagnosed. Not all children with a type I laryngeal cleft are symptomatic, and if there is no clinical, radiologic, or pulmonary evidence of aspiration, then cleft repair is not required.

Finally, consideration should be given to the type of operative repair that is suited to the child. The three primary options are endoscopic cleft repair, open repair through a lateral pharyngotomy, and open repair through a transtracheal/translaryngeal approach.

TECHNICAL APPROACH

Endoscopic Repair

Endoscopic cleft repair should only be attempted for selected type I or type II laryngeal clefts. The technique involves using a laser to raise uneven flaps of arytenoid mucosa, and then performing a two-layer closure with endoscopically placed sutures. We have been disappointed with our results using this technique and rarely perform this procedure currently.

Open Repair via a Lateral Pharyngotomy Approach

A repair via a lateral pharyngotomy provides good access, particularly to the upper aspect of the cleft. However, the recurrent laryngeal nerve is highly vulnerable, and we have now abandoned this approach.

Open Repair via an Anterior Transtracheal/Translaryngeal Approach

We currently perform all of our open repairs via the anterior transtracheal/translaryngeal approach, which provides unparalleled access to the cleft without placing the recurrent laryngeal nerves at risk. The keys to this approach are that adequate access requires a complete laryngofissure, and an adequate repair requires a two-layer closure. All types of laryngeal clefting may be repaired using this approach.

Anesthesia is provided through a shortened oral RAE endotracheal tube placed through the tracheostomy. If a single-stage procedure is planned, then a temporary low tracheotomy may be placed. An esophageal bougie is then placed, and with the neck well extended over a shoulder roll, a transverse neck incision is made in the skin crease just below the level of the cricoid cartilage. Subplatysmal skin flaps are raised, and the strap muscles and thyroid isthmus are divided and carried laterally to expose the anterior trachea. A Beaver blade is used to enter the airway, staying strictly in the midline, with the initial incision passing from the second or third tracheal ring superiorly up through the cricoid cartilage and the cricothyroid membrane. Care must be taken performing the laryngofissure to prevent iatrogenic damage to the vocal cords. We strongly advise endoscopic guidance from above while the larynx is split, to aid the surgeon in staying exactly in the midline, especially at the anterior commissure. The airway is then held distracted with polypropylene sutures. The posterior cleft should now be clearly visible, with the esophageal bougie displayed lying in the esophagus.

The inferior aspect of the cleft needs to be determined, and the degree of redundant mucosa estimated. Excessive redundant mucosa is now removed from the edges of the cleft, and using sharp and blunt dissection a plane is developed between the tracheal mucosa and esophageal mucosa at the edges of the cleft. Infiltrating 1% lidocaine with 1/1,000 epinephrine prior to the excision of the edges of the cleft facilitates hemostasis. Mucosa should be incised or excised to a level at least 3 to 4 mm above the level of the true vocal cords. Monofilament stay sutures are then used to retract the tracheal layer of the cleft repair. The esophageal mucosa is then closed over the bougie with interrupted 4-0 or 5-0 absorbable sutures, with the knots lying in the lumen of the esophagus. The tracheal mucosa is then closed from the distal end to the proximal with interrupted 5-0 absorbable sutures, with the knots lying in the tracheal lumen. With both layers of the repair, particular attention should be directed to the most distal and most proximal sutures (Fig. 26.2).

If a tracheotomy is already present, the anterior airway can now be closed with interrupted 4-0 or 5-0 polypropylene sutures. Particular care is needed when reconstructing the anterior commissure so the vocal cords do not overlap. In a single-stage procedure, the patient should be nasally intubated prior to closure of the anterior trachea.

This technique may require modification in a child with a type IV laryngotracheoesophageal cleft that approaches the carina. To maintain anesthesia while allowing uninhibited access to the posterior tracheal wall, consideration should be given to performing the repair under cardiopulmonary bypass or extracorporeal membrane oxygenation.

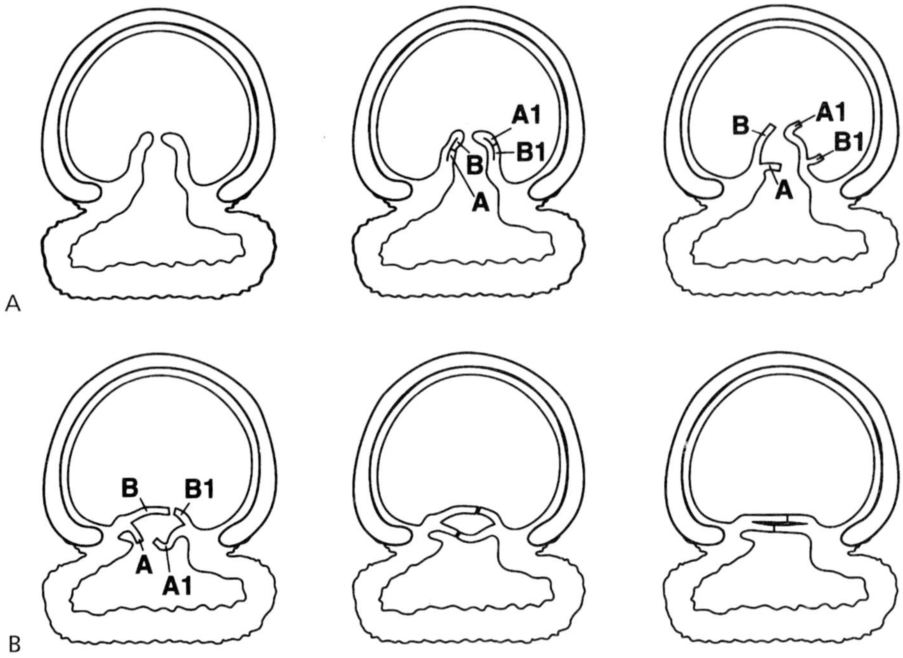

FIGURE 26.2. A and B: Posterior laryngeal cleft repair in two layers.

POSTOPERATIVE CARE

If the laryngeal cleft is being repaired as a single-stage procedure (without a tracheotomy tube), then extubation should be planned 3 to 5 days postoperatively. With either a single-stage or double-stage procedure, follow-up endoscopy of the repair should be planned in about 2 weeks, and if the repair is healthy, a barium swallow or video fluoroscopy is administered prior to the commencement of feeding. If the child has a tracheotomy tube, then this may be removed once he or she is able to feed without aspiration, and if the infant has an otherwise adequate airway.

COMPLICATIONS

The most likely short-term complication following cleft repair is breakdown of the repair. This is more likely to occur in the presence of gastroesophageal reflux disease, and is presumably more frequent when the suture lines lie between a nasogastric tube and an endotracheal tube. Breakdown of a repair is most likely to occur at the most distal aspect of the cleft, resulting in an "H" type tracheoesophageal fistula. Late breakdown is more common in the presence of chronic gastroesophageal reflux disease.

If inadequate redundant mucosa is excised at the time of repair, then there may still be prominent redundant mucosa present along the posterior tracheal wall following the repair. This may compromise the airway or contribute to tracheomalacia. If significant redundant mucosa remains at the vocal cord level, this may compromise the ability of the vocal cords to close, predisposing to aspiration. If the anterior commissure is not painstakingly repaired at the closure of the larynx, then the vocal folds will lie at different levels, resulting in a poor voice postoperatively.

With a single-stage procedure, complications may be encountered upon extubation of the patient. This may be due to redundant mucosa at the repair site, distal tracheomalacia, or glottic granulation tissue and edema resulting from the intubation. Reintubation of the patient may be required, and this should be done with extreme care so as not to disrupt the repair. It is recommended that the patient be reintubated with the bevel of the endotracheal tube lying anteriorly. If the patient repeatedly fails extubation, tracheotomy should be performed.

PITFALLS

1. The most important diagnostic tool is a high index of suspicion. If a cleft is suspected, the interarytenoid area should be carefully probed with a right-angled hook.
2. During open repair, uneven flaps should be created in the tracheal and esophageal mucosa to allow noncontiguous suture lines to be formed during two-layer closure of the cleft.
3. Every effort should be made to ensure a successful primary repair, because subsequent repairs of a laryngeal cleft are significantly more challenging.
4. A coexistent tracheoesophageal fistula is a poor prognostic indicator for the success of a laryngeal cleft repair.

CONTROVERSIES

The pediatric surgical literature has advocated the lateral pharyngotomy approach for repair of a posterior laryngeal cleft, while the otolaryngology literature advocates transtracheal repair of a posterior laryngeal cleft. Are there significant advantages of one approach over the other, and can we explain this disparity in operative approaches? The lateral pharyngotomy approach to the posterior larynx is familiar to both pediatric otolaryngologists and pediatric surgeons. However, this approach has limitations when dealing with long clefts, and there is a significant risk of damage to the recurrent laryngeal nerve with this procedure. Because pediatric otolaryngologists are more likely to have to live with the consequences of a paralyzed vocal cord, a viable alternative to a lateral pharyngotomy is very attractive. The transtracheal approach provides excellent exposure to the posterior cleft and carries no risk to the recurrent laryngeal nerve. However, it does involve entering the airway, as well as splitting the larynx, and having to take great care while reconstructing the larynx. It also involves having to share the airway with the anesthetic team, and although airway surgery is familiar territory to many pediatric otolaryngologists, it is often unfamiliar to many pediatric surgeons.

Repairing a laryngeal cleft without placing a tracheotomy tube carries significant risks. When is this technique justified? Some children present comparatively late, often without a tracheotomy. In a child who is already several months old and who does not have a tracheotomy, it is obviously attractive to try to avoid placing a tracheotomy. These children, almost by definition, have fewer symptoms than the more severe neonatal presentations. The other group of children in whom it is desirable to avoid tracheotomy if possible are those children who have moderate tracheomalacia, but who are relatively asymptomatic with it. Although it may seem illogical to try to avoid placing a tracheotomy in a child with potential airway obstruction, the rationale is that placement of a tracheotomy will usually obligate the child to be tracheotomy dependent for a number of years, because decannulating a child with significant tracheomalacia is often a difficult process. Under these circumstances a single-stage procedure carries a higher risk of ultimately requiring placement of a tracheotomy, but also carries a better chance of not being tracheotomy dependent 1 year following the repair.

SUGGESTED READINGS

Benjamin B, Inglis A. Minor congenital laryngeal clefts: diagnosis and classification. *Ann Otol Rhinol Laryngol* 1989;98:417–420.

Bent JP 3rd, Bauman NM, Smith RJ. Endoscopic repair of type 1A laryngeal clefts. *Laryngoscope* 1997;107:282–286.

Berkovits RN, Bax NM, van der Schans EJ. Surgical treatment of congenital laryngotracheo-oesophageal cleft. *Prog Pediatr Surg* 1987;21:36–46.

Donahoe PK, Gee PE. Complete laryngotracheoesophageal cleft: management and repair. *J Pediatr Surg* 1984;19:143–148.

Ryan DP, Muehrcke DD, Doody DP, et al. Laryngotracheoesophageal cleft (type IV): management and repair of lesions beyond the carina. *J Pediatr Surg* 1991;26:962–969; discussion 969–970.

Walner DL, Stern Y, Collins M, et al. Does the presence of a tracheoesophageal fistula predict the outcome of laryngeal cleft repair? *Arch Otolaryngol Head Neck Surg* 1999;125:782–784.

27

PARATHYROID DISORDERS

STEVEN W. BRUCH

The parathyroid glands develop from the third and fourth pharyngeal pouches. The two inferior parathyroid glands begin as the third pharyngeal pouch and descend to their normal position posterolaterally on the inferior portion of the thyroid gland. The two superior parathyroid glands begin their descent from the fourth pharyngeal pouch and come to lie on the posterolateral aspect of the superior portion of the thyroid gland. Abnormal migration occurs allowing the parathyroid glands to migrate anywhere from the superior neck to the anterior mediastinum. They can be found along the carotid sheath or the tracheoesophageal groove, within the thyroid gland, or in the substance of the thymus, which also originates from the third pharyngeal pouch.

DIAGNOSIS

Primary hyperparathyroidism is rare in children and requires parathyroidectomy as definitive treatment. Three clinical scenarios occur in children: neonatal hyperparathyroidism, which is usually due to diffuse hyperplasia; familial disorders, such as multiple endocrine neoplasia (MEN) types 1 and 2A, which result in diffuse hyperplasia; and sporadic cases, usually in older adolescents, usually caused by a single adenoma. Parathyroid cancer is extremely rare in children and presents similar to a solitary adenoma. The hallmark of primary hyperparathyroidism is hypercalcemia associated with an elevated parathyroid hormone level. Children may develop hypercalcemia for a number of other reasons, but the parathyroid hormone level will be normal or low in these children. Familial hypocalcuric hypercalcemia must be excluded in children with hypercalcemia using the calcium/creatinine excretion ratio on a 24-hour urine collection. Although a relatively common cause of hypercalcemia in adults, cancer rarely causes hypercalcemia in children. It can occur with the following childhood tumors: malignant rhabdoid tumors, mesoblastic nephroma, rhabdomyosarcoma, neuroblastoma, and lymphoma. Other causes of hypercalcemia in childhood include hypervitaminosis A and D, sarcoidosis, subcutaneous fat necrosis, prolonged immobilization, thiazide diuretics, Williams syndrome, thyrotoxicosis, hypophosphatemia, and hyperalimentation.

OPERATIVE APPROACH

The operative approach for hyperparathyroidism varies depending on the findings at exploration. Hyperparathyroidism develops from diffuse four-gland hyperplasia, or from a single adenoma. Classically, no preoperative localizing studies are performed, and the etiology of the hyperparathyroidism is uncovered in the operating room. A low transverse neck incision provides exposure. The thyroid gland is mobilized medially and the parathyroid glands are identified. Identification of one large gland and three normal-sized glands indicates a parathyroid adenoma. The adenoma is removed and the remaining three glands are left *in situ*. When the etiology of the hypercalcemia is diffuse hypertrophy, all four glands are enlarged. In this case, three and one half glands should be resected and the remaining parathyroid tissue should be marked and left in the neck. Alternatively, the remaining parathyroid tissue is removed, minced up, and placed in a pocket of muscle in the sternocleidomastoid or the nondominant forearm. If all four glands cannot be found, the appearance of the verified parathyroid glands determines the next step. If one large gland and two small or normal-sized glands are found, the large gland usually represents an adenoma and is removed. When fewer than four equally sized glands are found, the search for the remaining parathyroid gland or glands must continue. The carotid sheaths are opened bilaterally, and the tracheoesophageal grooves are explored. If the remaining parathyroid tissue is not found there, the thymus is brought up into the neck and explored. If the remaining parathyroid tissue still remains hidden, the thyroid lobe on the side of the missing parathyroid gland should be excised. The parathyroid gland is located within the substance of the thyroid 1% of the time.

S.W. Bruch: Department of General Surgery, Division of Pediatric Surgery, Naval Medical Center, Portsmouth, Virginia.

POSTOPERATIVE CARE

Postoperative hypercalcemia results from a missed adenoma or from leaving behind too much hypertrophied parathyroid tissue. These children require a thorough radiologic search for the missing parathyroid tissue. This workup includes ultrasonography, computed tomography, and radionucleotide studies, with the technetium Sestimibi scintiscan being the preferred nuclear medicine test. The results of these studies, in conjunction with a thorough review of the previous operative report, should direct the search for the remaining parathyroid tissue.

Recently, parathyroid surgeons have used these localizing tests to evaluate hyperparathyroid patients prior to the original exploration. When a well-defined single adenoma is found, the operation is limited to a local resection of the adenoma without the remainder of the parathyroid exploration. Published results of this technique reveal success in up to 98% of unilateral explorations with 3% temporary hypocalcemia rate. This technique may be useful in the older adolescent population whose hyperparathyroidism often stems from an adenoma. Children with familial hyperparathyroidism from diffuse hyperplasia should not be treated in this fashion.

Postoperative complications include bleeding with airway compromise, injury to the recurrent laryngeal nerve, hypocalcemia that is usually transient, and recurrent hypercalcemia. Careful dissection during the operation should avert the first two problems. The hypocalcemia may be transient or permanent. The usual cause is devascularization of the remaining parathyroid glands during dissection, or bone hunger due to suppressed normal glands following resection of an adenoma. The hypocalcemia is treated with intravenous calcium gluconate if necessary, then oral calcium and vitamin D supplements.

Although rare, neonatal primary hyperparathyroidism may be life threatening. The underlying abnormality is chief cell hyperplasia in all four parathyroid glands. Symptoms are nonspecific and consist of lethargy, hypotonicity, irritability, respiratory distress, polyuria, anorexia, constipation, and failure to thrive. Hypercalcemia often presents within the first few days of life, and generally develops by 3 months of age. Elevated serum calcium and parathyroid hormone levels make the diagnosis. The diffuse parathyroid hypertrophy requires total parathyroidectomy with heterotopic autotransplantation of a portion of one gland into the nondominant forearm or sternocleidomastoid muscle. Early diagnosis and treatment results in normal growth and development of the neonate.

Familial hyperparathyroidism occurs more commonly in children than adults. MEN 1 and 2A syndromes manifest chief cell hyperplasia of all four parathyroid glands. Hyperparathyroidism occurs in more than 90% of children with MEN 1 and 30% of children with MEN 2A syndrome. MEN 1 syndrome consists of hyperplasia or neoplasia of pancreatic islets (secreting gastrin, insulin, pancreatic polypeptide, or glucagon), the anterior pituitary (secreting prolactin), and the parathyroid glands. Children with the MEN 1 syndrome develop asymptomatic hypercalcemia around age 10. This is often the first detectable sign of the syndrome. The first clinical manifestations are those of pancreatic islet cell secretion. Kidney stones, hypertension, malaise, fatigue, and weakness develop later as a result of excessive parathyroid hormone release. The parathyroid glands are hyperplastic, but this hyperplasia may not be uniform. Exploration may show one or two large glands, with the remaining glands being of normal size. The normal-appearing glands often harbor hyperplastic chief cells and should be treated as diffuse hypertrophy.

Multiple endocrine neoplasia type 2A syndrome presents with medullary thyroid cancer in all cases, pheochromocytoma in 50% of cases, and hyperparathyroidism in 30% of cases. The hypercalcemia generally develops in the second or third decade of life. These children are now undergoing thyroidectomy at a young age after screening with the RET protooncogene. Few if any demonstrate hypercalcemia before age 5, when thyroidectomy should be undertaken. Current recommendations are to follow these children long term looking for hypercalcemia. When and if hypercalcemia develops, parathyroid tissue should be removed from the neck or the forearm if it was autotransplanted at the time of the original operation.

In older adolescents, a single adenoma is the most common cause of primary hyperparathyroidism. Symptoms, including irritability, weakness, and anorexia, are nonspecific and often not recognized until the calcium level returns to normal and the symptoms abate after treatment. Renal colic and hypertension are common in symptomatic children. In these older children with sporadic cases of primary hyperparathyroidism, the workup should include ultrasonography and a Sestimibi radionucleotide scan in addition to serum calcium and parathyroid hormone levels. If a solitary adenoma is confirmed on both the scintiscan and ultrasonography, a local exploration with intraoperative ultrasonographic guidance could be considered.

Secondary hyperparathyroidism results from a chronically decreased calcium level stimulating increased parathyroid hormone production. This occurs in children with renal insufficiency and malabsorption. Rarely, this results in severe renal osteodystrophy with fractures and metastatic calcifications. Most children respond to medical management, with the goal being decreased intestinal phosphate absorption. Severe cases may require parathyroidectomy with autotransplantation.

Tertiary hyperparathyroidism occurs when there is persistent hyperfunction of the parathyroid glands in a child with secondary hyperparathyroidism who has had the original stimulus for parathyroid hypersecretion removed. This commonly occurs in children with chronic renal failure after renal transplantation. Total parathyroidectomy with autotransplantation treats the resulting four-gland hyperplasia of tertiary hyperparathyroidism.

SUGGESTED READINGS

DiGeorge AM, LaFranchi S. Disorders of the parathyroid glands. In: Behrman RE, Kliegman RM, Arvin AM, eds. *Nelson textbook of pediatrics, 15th ed.* Philadelphia: WB Saunders, 1996:1605–1612.

Harman CR, vanHeerden JA, Farley DR, et al. Sporadic primary hyperparathyroidism in young patients: a separate disease entity? *Arch Surg* 1999;134:651–656.

Loh KC, Duh QY, Shoback D, et al. Clinical profile of primary hyperparathyroidism in adolescents and young adults. *Clin Endocrinol* 1998;48:435–443.

Skinner MA. Thyroid and parathyroid. In: Oldham KT, Colombani PM, Foglia RP, eds. *Surgery of infants and children. Scientific principles and practice.* Philadelphia: Lippincott-Raven, 1997: 857–868.

Skinner MA, Mayforth RD. Endocrine disorders and tumors. In: Ashcraft KW, Murphy JP, Sharp RJ, et al., eds. *Pediatric Surgery, 3rd ed.* Philadelphia: WB Saunders, 2000:1025–1032.

Smit PC, Rinkes IH, vanDalen A, et al. Direct, minimally invasive adenomectomy for primary hyperparathyroidism: an alternative to conventional neck exploration? *Ann Surg* 2000;231:559–565.

Thompson NW, Geiger JD. Thyroid/parathyroid. In: O'Neill JA Jr, Rowe MI, Grosfeld JL, et al., eds. *Pediatric surgery, 5th ed.* St. Louis: CV Mosby, 1998:743–755.

28

THYROID DISORDERS

STEVEN W. BRUCH

Three thyroid conditions require surgical intervention in the pediatric age group: congenital thyroglossal duct abnormalities, nonmalignant thyroid enlargement or hyperfunction, and thyroid cancer.

THYROGLOSSAL DUCT

The thyroglossal duct temporarily connects the thyroid gland to the foramen cecum at the base of the tongue, often passing through the hyoid bone. This duct normally obliterates after the thyroid completes its descent into the neck by the 7th week of gestation. Clinically, a thyroglossal duct cyst will present as a midline neck mass anywhere along its course from the base of the tongue to the thyroid gland. The cyst may become infected, resulting in spontaneous drainage or prompting surgical drainage through the skin. There is never a natural connection between a thyroglossal duct and the skin. The thyroglossal duct may harbor functioning thyroid tissue along the length of its tract. One should not be fooled by a lingual thyroid that may also present as a midline mass in the upper neck. The lingual thyroid results from failure of the thyroid gland to descend to its proper position in the neck and may harbor all of the child's functioning thyroid tissue.

The evaluation of a midline neck mass begins with an ultrasonographic examination to document the presence of a thyroglossal duct cyst, but more importantly, to identify the normal thyroid gland. If a thyroid gland is not found in its proper position, then a technetium 99 thyroid scan identifies the ectopic thyroid tissue.

Infected thyroglossal duct cysts require drainage, antibiotics, and time to reduce inflammation before attempting excision. A transverse neck incision over the mass allows adequate exposure. The cyst is separated from the surrounding structures, and the tract leading to the foramen cecum is located. This tract is followed and will pass just anterior, just posterior, or often through the middle of the hyoid bone. The midportion of the hyoid bone is resected to prevent recurrence. The remainder of the tract is dissected to the base of the tongue and suture ligated.

Complications include bleeding resulting in airway compromise, and recurrence. A recurrence presents as a mass in the neck, or a sinus tract draining through the wound. Failure to excise the entire tract leads to recurrences. This occurs more frequently when the thyroglossal duct cyst is inflamed at the time of operation. The recurrent tract must be followed back to the base of the tongue and completely reexcised.

GOITER

Congenital goiter and Graves' disease comprise the nonmalignant thyroid conditions requiring surgical management. Enlargement of the thyroid gland at birth may cause severe respiratory embarrassment and feeding difficulties due to pressure effects. Congenital goiter results from treatment of maternal thyrotoxicosis with antithyroid drugs or iodides. These and other goiterogenic drugs cross the placenta, interfere with fetal thyroid hormone synthesis, and result in goiter and hypothyroidism. Administration of thyroid hormone treats the hypothyroidism, speeds the disappearance of the goiter, and prevents brain damage. On rare occasion, the goiter causes severe respiratory obstruction and is best treated with partial thyroidectomy.

Graves' disease, an autoimmune disease manifested by immunoglobulins (IgG) directed against the thyroid-stimulating hormone (TSH) receptor, is the most common cause of hyperthyroidism in children. In children, Graves' disease presents with a goiter, exophthalmus, pretibial myxedema, and manifestation of thyrotoxicosis. The initial symptoms include emotional lability, nervousness, and worsening performance at school. Eventually, heat intolerance, sweating, palpitations, tremor, weight loss despite increased appetite, and general malaise follows. A goiter associated with elevated free tetraiodothyronine (T_4) and 3,5,5′-triiodothyronine (T_3) levels, a decreased TSH level, and presence of TSH

S.W. Bruch: Department of General Surgery, Division of Pediatric Surgery, Naval Medical Center, Portsmouth, Virginia.

receptor antibodies confirms the diagnosis. Although not necessary to diagnose Graves' disease, thyroid scintigraphy shows rapid, diffuse uptake that distinguishes it from Hashimoto's disease and toxic nodular goiter. The goal of the treatment of Graves' disease is to decrease the production and secretion of thyroid hormone. Three options exist at this time: antithyroid medication, radioactive iodine, and thyroidectomy. The choice of therapy should be individualized depending on the severity of the symptoms, the child's age, the family's preference, and the response to initial therapy.

Antithyroid medications constitute the first line of therapy for children with Graves' disease. Propylthiouracil and methimazole, both thionamide drugs, inhibit organification of iodide by the follicle cells, thus limiting thyroid hormone production. On average, it takes 8 weeks from the start of therapy to achieve euthyroidism. Beta-adrenergic blocking agents control acute symptoms more rapidly and are a useful adjunct in combination with the thionamides. These antithyroid medications result in a 25% remission rate at 2 years and a further 25% remission every 2-year period thereafter. Up to one third of children started on antithyroid drugs fail therapy due to drug reactions or noncompliance and require radioactive iodine treatment or thyroid surgery. Drug reactions range from minor side effects (nausea, skin rash, and pruritis), to serious complications, including granulocytopenia, thrombocytopenia, and hepatic dysfunction.

Although radioactive iodine is the treatment of choice in adults with Graves' disease, it has been used sparingly in children because of the risk of genetic mutation, cancer, and decreased fertility associated with ionizing radiation. Recent studies have followed children who received ablative doses of iodine 131 (^{131}I) and have shown no difference from the general population in the risk for teratogenic effects, cancer, or infertility. The benefits of radioactive iodine treatment include ease of administration, effectiveness, and low cost. Eighty-three percent of children require a single dose of radioactive iodine, and less than 5% have a recurrence after initial response to ^{131}I. The shortcomings of this treatment are its slow onset of action, up to 88% risk of developing hypothyroidism requiring lifelong thyroid hormone therapy, and abnormalities of parathyroid function. In preadolescent children, radioactive iodine is used selectively, but in older adolescents it has become the preferred treatment after antithyroid medication.

Thyroidectomy affords rapid and permanent treatment for Graves' disease. Controversy remains as to the optimum extent of thyroidectomy, subtotal versus total, for this disease. The disadvantages of thyroidectomy include risk of injury to the recurrent laryngeal nerve or the parathyroid glands, and the risk of recurrent hyperthyroidism with a subtotal thyroidectomy (14%). Hypothyroidism requiring long-term thyroid hormone replacement occurs in all children treated with a total thyroidectomy and in up to 54% of those treated with a subtotal thyroidectomy.

Hyperthyroid children require a period of preparation preoperatively to render them euthyroid, thus decreasing their risk of thyroid storm, and decreasing the vascularity of the gland, making the operation safer. Antithyroid medication requires 2 to 8 weeks to establish a euthyroid state, and then it is preferable to wait an additional 1 to 2 months prior to surgery. If the procedure must be performed before achieving euthyroidism, a β-adrenergic blocker controls the hyperthyroid physiology. Propranolol can safely prepare a child with Graves' disease for thyroidectomy in 10 to 14 days. The propranolol should be continued for 7 days postoperatively to prevent thyroid storm. All children receive Lugol's solution (5–10 drops one to three times daily) for 5 to 10 days before proceeding with surgery. This reduces the vascularity of the thyroid gland.

The extent of surgery for children with Graves' disease remains controversial. The factors to take into consideration when determining the extent of thyroidectomy should be the safety of the parathyroid glands and the recurrent laryngeal nerves, and the likelihood of recurrent Graves' disease postoperatively. Recurrent Graves' disease requires either a reoperation in the neck with a 10-fold increase in recurrent laryngeal nerve and parathyroid injury, or the need for ^{131}I therapy. The vast majority of children require thyroid hormone replacement therapy whether a total or subtotal thyroidectomy is performed. Therefore, a total thyroidectomy is the treatment of choice as long as at least one parathyroid gland is identified and preserved on each side of the neck and the recurrent laryngeal nerve is protected. If a rim of thyroid tissue must be left behind to protect the parathyroids and the nerve, this rim should be no more than 1 g of thyroid tissue on each side. If the parathyroid glands are devascularized, they should be minced and transplanted into a muscular pocket in the ipsilateral sternocleidomastoid, or the nondominant forearm.

Postoperative complications include thyroid storm, recurrent laryngeal nerve injury, hypocalcemia, and bleeding with airway compromise. Thyroid storm presents with symptoms similar to thyrotoxicosis. Fever is usually the earliest finding, followed by cardiovascular compromise (tachycardia, dysrhythmia, congestive failure, and even death), neurologic abnormalities (irritability, agitation, tremors, psychoses, and coma), and gastrointestinal symptoms (nausea, vomiting, diarrhea, and jaundice). Treatment involves general supportive care, blocking the peripheral effects of thyroid hormone with propranolol, and decreasing the production of thyroid hormone with antithyroid medications, supersaturated potassium iodide, and corticosteroids, which enhance the conversion of T_4 to the inactive form, reverse T_3.

Long-term follow-up is required for all children undergoing total or subtotal thyroidectomy. The majority will require thyroid hormone replacement, and those undergoing subtotal thyroidectomy also should be followed for the development of recurrent hyperthyroidism.

THYROID MALIGNANCY

Thyroid cancer occurs rarely in the pediatric population, making up 3% of all childhood malignancies. Girls are affected twice as often as boys, and the peak incidence occurs in adolescents between the ages of 10 and 18 years. The majority of childhood thyroid cancers are differentiated cancer, with papillary (80%) being more common than follicular (17%). Medullary cancer makes up 2% of the total, whereas undifferentiated anaplastic thyroid cancer is rare in children and is usually rapidly fatal.

The differentiated thyroid cancers–papillary, follicular, and follicular variants of papillary–usually present as a solitary thyroid nodule. Solitary thyroid nodules occur less frequently in children (1%) compared with adults (4%) but are more often malignant. Up to 20% of children with a solitary thyroid nodule harbor a malignancy. The risk of malignancy increases with a history of neck irradiation, either therapeutic or accidental, and in children treated for a previous malignancy. The Belarus population exposed to ionizing radiation from the Chernobyl accident has a 62-fold increase in thyroid cancer. In a series of second malignancies, thyroid cancer made up 9% of the cases. Children treated for Hodgkin's lymphoma comprised the group most likely to develop subsequent thyroid cancer. In addition to the radiation exposure, treatment with alkylating agents alone increases the risk of developing subsequent thyroid cancer.

Evaluation of a solitary thyroid nodule begins with a thorough history and physical examination looking for risk factors and additional neck masses, which may represent involved lymph nodes. Laboratory evaluation should include determination of T_4, T_3, and TSH levels to exclude subclinical thyrotoxicosis or hypothyroidism associated with Hashimoto disease. Radiologic evaluation should include chest radiography to look for pulmonary metastasis. Pulmonary spread often will not be appreciated on plain films but identified with the postoperative ^{131}I scan. Ultrasonography can be used to distinguish solid from cystic lesions. Both solid and cystic lesions may be malignant. Completely drained cystic lesions that do not recur on follow-up physical and ultrasonographic examination may be safely watched. If aspiration leaves a solid component, fine-needle aspiration (FNA) of the remaining solid portion is required. Thyroid scintigraphy classifies nodules as "hot" or "cold" depending on the ability to concentrate the isotope. Again, both hot and cold nodules may be malignant. Scintigraphy can be used to identify ectopic thyroid tissue and, along with thyroid function tests, to identify toxic nodules requiring preoperative preparation with antithyroid medication.

The role of FNA in children with thyroid nodules is evolving. An absolute must before using FNA is a group of pathologists comfortable evaluating thyroid cytology in this age group. Assuming the pathology department is on board, FNA is useful in adolescents over 13 years of age. This age group can cooperate without sedation, and the risk for their nodules being malignant is decreased—11% in one large series. Excisional biopsy with thyroid lobectomy is performed for malignant or indeterminate cytology, or if a cytologically benign nodule increases in size over time. All solitary thyroid nodules in children under 13 years of age should be sampled for biopsy via thyroid lobectomy. The use of exogenous thyroid hormone to cause regression of thyroid nodules in children is not recommended.

Treatment for differentiated thyroid cancer consists of surgical resection, followed by adjuvant ^{131}I treatment and thyroid hormone replacement. The extent of thyroidectomy remains a topic of controversy. Arguments in favor of subtotal thyroidectomy center around a decreased risk of permanent hypoparathyroidism and recurrent laryngeal nerve injury while maintaining the same overall mortality rate compared with total thyroidectomy. However, with proper identification of the parathyroid glands and the recurrent laryngeal nerves, a total thyroidectomy can be safely performed. A functioning recurrent laryngeal nerve should not be sacrificed even if surrounded by tumor. The tumor should be carefully dissected off the nerve, and any residual tumor can be controlled with postoperative ^{131}I treatment. If the parathyroids are devascularized during the dissection, they should be minced up and transplanted into the sternocleidomastoid or forearm muscle. Total thyroidectomy allows the use of ^{131}I scan to detect occult metastasis early. These are most commonly found in the lung. Although overall mortality does not change with total thyroidectomy, local and regional recurrence are decreased, thus minimizing the morbidity of a reexploration of the neck. Total thyroidectomy also allows follow-up with thyroglobulin levels to detect persistent or recurrent disease. For children with an FNA or frozen section biopsy that reveals differentiated thyroid cancer, a total thyroidectomy with central lymph node dissection should be performed. The lymph node dissection should extend from jugular vein to jugular vein and from the thyroid notch to the superior mediastinum. If suspicious nodes are found in the jugular chain, they are removed. Positive lymph nodes will be found in up to 75% of children with differentiated thyroid cancer, whereas pulmonary metastasis occurs in 6% at the time of initial treatment. Survival and recurrence are no different for children with and without cervical lymph node involvement.

Six weeks after total thyroidectomy, an ^{131}I scan is performed. If there is uptake in the lungs, around the recurrent laryngeal nerve, or in the lateral neck, a therapeutic dose of ^{131}I ablates the residual thyroid tissue. Thyroxin in doses sufficient to suppress TSH is required long term. Follow-up should consist of periodic physical examinations and thyroglobulin levels, and yearly ^{131}I scans. Recurrence rates range from 10% to 35%, with the most common site being the lateral neck followed by the thyroid bed and the lungs. Children under 10 years of age at diagnosis, and children with follicular or the follicular variant of papillary pathology have a higher recurrence rate. ^{131}I ablative treatment or reoperation are options for recurrent disease.

Children with differentiated thyroid cancer have a good prognosis, even with lymph node and pulmonary metastasis. In several large series with follow-up of 8 to 28 years, mortality was 0 to 3.5%. Those with poorer prognosis are younger children (<10 years of age) and children with extensive pulmonary metastatic disease with tracheal and laryngeal involvement.

Medullary thyroid cancer occurs sporadically or in association with multiple endocrine neoplasia (MEN) syndromes types 2A and 2B, or with the familial medullary thyroid cancer (FMTC) syndrome. The sporadic cases present similar to differentiated thyroid cancer with a thyroid nodule with or without cervical lymphadenopathy. The MEN and FMTC syndromes demonstrate autosomal-dominant inheritance and result in the development of medullary thyroid cancer at an early age. Mutations in the RET protooncogene on chromosome 10 identify children in the MEN and FMTC kindreds. All of these children will develop medullary thyroid carcinoma as part of their syndromes. Associated with the medullary thyroid carcinoma, children with MEN 2A develop pheochromocytomas (50%), and parathyroid hyperplasia (30%). Children with MEN 2B develop pheochromocytomas (50%), mucosal neuromas, and marfanoid habitus. Medullary thyroid carcinoma is the first tumor to develop in these children and is the most common cause of death. The treatment strategy now consists of early identification of children with the RET protooncogene mutation, and early thyroidectomy before the medullary thyroid cancer spreads beyond the thyroid gland. In children with MEN 2A syndrome thyroidectomy should be undertaken before age 5, whereas children with the more virulent MEN 2B syndrome require thyroidectomy prior to 1 year of age. Medullary thyroid cancer develops diffusely in the parafollicular C cells of the thyroid gland and therefore requires total thyroidectomy with central lymph node dissection as treatment. Eighty percent of children with MEN 2A syndrome who underwent prophylactic total thyroidectomy at a mean age of 10.5 years after the identification of the RET protooncogene mutation harbor foci of medullary thyroid carcinoma in their thyroid glands. Both before and after the operation, children with MEN 2A or 2B require screening for pheochromocytoma with plasma and urinary catecholamine levels, and those with MEN 2A require serum calcium levels to look for hyperparathyroidism.

SUGGESTED READINGS

DiGeorge AM, LaFranchi S. Disorders of the thyroid gland. In: Behrman RE, Kliegman RM, Arvin AM, ed. *Nelson textbook of pediatrics, 15th ed.* Philadelphia: WB Saunders, 1996:1587-1604.

Feimnesser R, Lubin E, Segal K, et al. Carcinoma of the thyroid in children—a review. *J Pediatr Endocrinol Metab*1997;10:561–568.

Geiger JD, Thompson NW. Thyroid tumors in children. *Otolaryngol Clin North Am* 1996;29:711–719.

Skinner MA. Thyroid and parathyroid. In: Oldham KT, Colombani PM, Foglia RP, eds. *Surgery of infants and children. Scientific principles and practice.* Philadelphia: Lippincott-Raven, 1997: 857–868.

Skinner MA, Mayforth RD. Endocrine disorders and tumors. In: Ashcraft KW, Murphy JP, Sharp RJ, et al., eds. *Pediatric surgery, 3rd ed.* Philadelphia: WB Saunders, 2000:1025–1032.

Skinner MA, Wells SA Jr. Medullary carcinoma of the thyroid gland and the MEN2 syndromes. *Semin Pediatr Surg* 1997;6:134–140.

Thompson NW, Geiger JD. Thyroid/parathyroid. In: O'Neill JA Jr, Rowe MI, Grosfeld JL, et al., eds. *Pediatric surgery, 5th ed.* St. Louis: CV Mosby, 1998:743–755.

Waldhausen JHT. Controversies related to the medical and surgical management of hyperthyroidism in children. *Semin Pediatr Surg* 1997;6:121–127.

Zimmerman D. Thyroid neoplasia in children. *Curr Opin Pediatr* 1997;9:413–418.

Surgical Directives: Pediatric Surgery, edited by Peter Mattei. Lippincott Williams & Wilkins, Philadelphia © 2002

29

THYROGLOSSAL DUCT CYSTS AND RELATED DISORDERS

STEVEN P. COOK

Most congenital neck masses present at birth or early childhood. The surgeon needs to be aware that they can manifest themselves at any age. Congenital defects must be considered in the differential diagnosis of a neck mass up until adulthood. The surgical management of congenital malformations is based on the embryologic development of the head and neck. This principle is particularly evident in the surgical treatment of thyroglossal duct cysts (TGDCs). Forty percent of all primary neck masses are TGDCs. They account for 70% of all congenital abnormalities of the neck.

Beginning in the third week of fetal development, the epithelium of the floor of the foregut begins to proliferate at the junction of the anterior two thirds and posterior third of the tongue. This is the area that will become the foramen cecum. The thyroid primordium migrates into the mesoderm and descends into the neck as a bilobed diverticulum. It passes between the first and second pharyngeal arches. By the seventh week it comes to lie in the lower neck anterior to the trachea. The thyroglossal duct is the tubular connection between the foramen cecum and the thyroid gland. It persists until the 8th to 10th week of fetal development.

As the thyroglossal duct passes from the foramen cecum, it runs anterior to the hyoid bone and hooks underneath the inferior border of the bone. It is closely approximated to the concave posterior surface of the hyoid. The duct then descends anterior to the thyrohyoid membrane. As we shall discover, the close relationship of the duct to the hyoid bone is of critical importance to effective surgical resection.

Faulty thyroid gland formation may lead to agenesis of the thyroid, abnormal thyroid gland position (ectopic gland), or cysts of the thyroglossal duct. Abnormalities of thyroid hormone can occur but will not be discussed here.

S. P. Cook: Department of Otolaryngology, Thomas Jefferson University, Philadelphia, Pennsylvania; and Department of Surgery, Division of Pediatric Otolaryngology, Alfred I. duPont Hospital for Children, Wilmington, Delaware.

PRESENTATION

Thyroglossal duct cysts are the most common of congenital head and neck masses. Typically, a TGDC appears as a nontender mass in the anterior neck in children of either sex, usually within the first 2 to 10 years of life (Fig. 29.1). Thirty percent of these lesions can appear as late as 20 years of age.

When embryologic rests of the thyroglossal duct fail to atrophy, they result in TGDCs. Classically, the patient presents with a cystic or fluctuant mass of variable size that is near the midportion of the hyoid bone. Because of the relationship of these cysts to the hyoid, they move with swallowing or tongue protrusion.

Thyroglossal ducts cysts can occur anywhere between the anterior borders of the sternocleidomastoid muscles laterally, and from the submental region above to the suprasternal notch below. In 25% of cases, the TGDC is superior to the hyoid in the submental region and may be confused with a palpable lymph node. The lesion is lower in the neck in fewer than 10% of cases. It is particularly unusual for TGDC to be located far from the midline. Multiple cysts are also possible.

Thyroglossal duct cysts may frequently present with the rapid onset of a tender inflamed anterior neck mass, particularly during an upper respiratory infection. The persistent connection between the foramen cecum and the thyroglossal duct may allow the entrance of infectious agents. Sudden swelling of duct remnants may cause dysphagia, dysarthria, or a sense of fullness in the neck.

If antibiotics do not resolve the acute infection, the inflamed cyst may require incision and drainage. Incision and drainage can result in a persistent sinus tract to the skin. With treatment the mass may decrease in size. Ward et al. reported that this might be accompanied by a foul taste as the cyst contents drain through the foramen cecum. Ideally, one should wait until the infection has resolved before attempting definitive surgical removal of the TGDC. Infections of the TGDC may recur.

The differential diagnosis should include an enlarged lymph node, particularly in masses above the hyoid bone. A

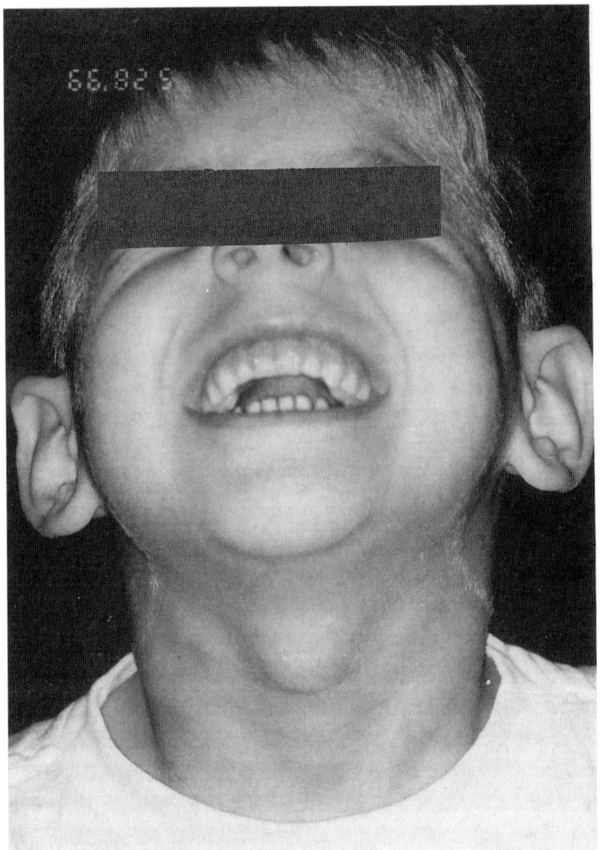

FIGURE 29.1. The typical presentation of a thyroglossal duct cyst as a midline mass related to the hyoid bone.

TGDC may mimic a branchial cleft cyst when it lies away from the midline toward the sternocleidomastoid muscle or in the lower neck. Other lesions to consider in the differential diagnosis are dermoid or sebaceous cysts, lipoma, hemangioma, and cystic hygroma. Cystic lesions may be difficult to distinguish from TGDC, even during surgery, so that the standard surgical approach, the Sistrunk procedure, should be undertaken in all instances.

Thyroid abnormalities such as a palpable pyramidal lobe or thyroid nodule must also be included in the differential diagnosis of an anterior neck mass in a child. Ectopic thyroid must be ruled out before any attempt at surgically removing a mass. Neoplastic lesions, either carcinoma of the thyroid or a metastasis, may rarely present in this fashion.

Laryngoceles and pharyngoceles may present like TGDCs. Intrusion of the TGDC into the larynx is unusual in children. In this case, the cyst may erode cartilage or pass through the thyrohyoid membrane and appear as a submucosal mass in the vallecula or supraglottis.

DIAGNOSTIC STUDIES

Given all the possible causes of an anterior neck mass, imaging becomes important. The extent of the mass and its relationship to adjacent structures may need to be defined. In most instances, the primary reason to image an anterior neck mass is to be sure the mass is not the only functioning thyroid tissue. Removing a functioning ectopic gland may result in hypothyroidism and lifelong consequences for the patient.

Computed tomography (CT) may be used to show the relationship of the mass to surrounding structures, demonstrate whether the thyroid gland is in its normal location, and differentiate a cyst from other pathologic entities. It is particularly useful when TGDCs are found away from their typical location. CT may be used to show the presence of an abscess that would require drainage. It is probably most helpful in the adult when one is concerned whether a lesion is solid, such as a metastatic node, or cystic. CT also may be used to define intralaryngeal cysts. The problem with CT in children is that it exposes the patient to ionizing radiation and may require sedation. Other studies may define an ectopic gland more simply.

Radioisotope scanning defines where functioning thyroid tissue resides in the neck. Radioisotope scanning is not specific for TGDC but may be used to show whether a lesion is an ectopic gland rather than a TGDC (Figs. 29.2 and 29.3).

Bimanual palpation of the pediatric thyroid gland is an unreliable indicator of whether a normally functioning gland is in its typical location. Since ectopic thyroid is not uncommon, preoperative radioisotope scanning is recommended. The majority of ectopic glands present in the tongue base. A thyroid scan would define whether this is functioning thyroid tissue. A normal scan does not eliminate the possibility of an ectopic gland. The presence of a TGDC implies that the thyroid gland itself must be distal to this lesion because the thyroid primordium is the leading structure that descends into the neck. Scanning certainly has value when the physician is concerned about thyroid agenesis.

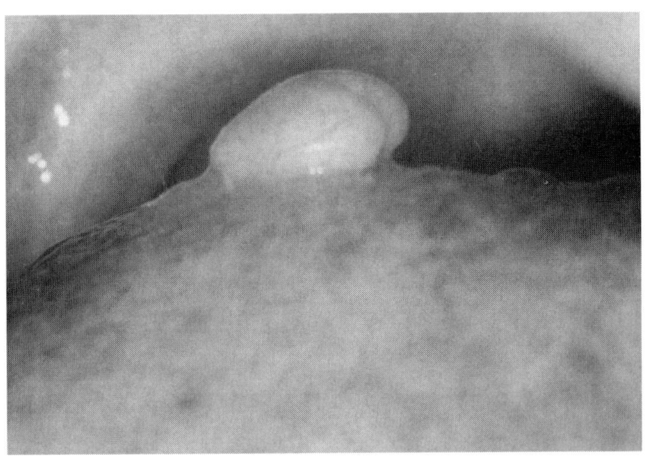

FIGURE 29.2. Ectopic thyroid presenting as a raised mass on the posterior tongue near the apex of the circumvallate papillae.

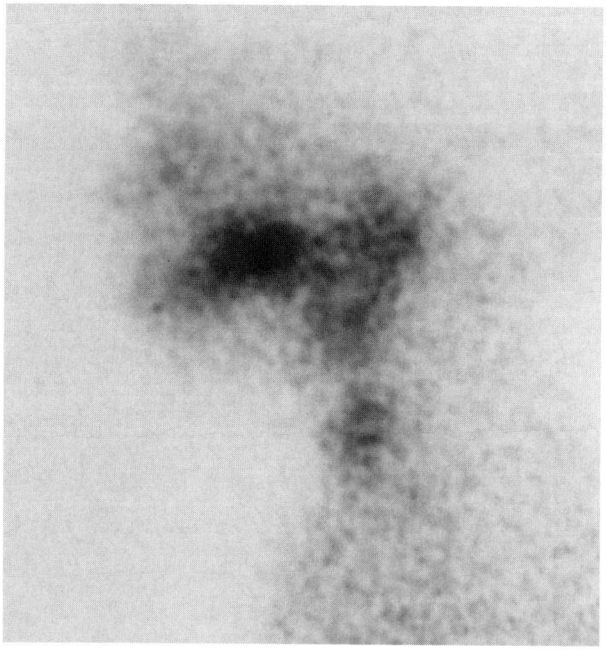

FIGURE 29.3. The same patient as in Fig. 29.2. Lateral thyroid scan demonstrating uptake within the tongue in a lingual or ectopic thyroid gland.

Ultrasonography is easy to perform and requires little patient cooperation. It may be used to demonstrate whether the thyroid gland resides in its normal location. Although ultrasonography should theoretically define whether the mass is solid or cystic, a false interpretation of a TGDC as being solid can occur. There is no exposure to ionizing radiation with ultrasonography. Should there be an absence of identifiable gland, or if an adequate ultrasonographic study cannot be completed, radioisotope scanning would then be of value.

Thyroid function studies have some limited value. Although there can be a wide range of thyroid function in ectopic thyroid, the ectopic gland is usually hypofunctional. In this case one would expect elevated thyroid-stimulating hormone levels.

SURGICAL CONSIDERATIONS

The major principle underlying TGDC surgery is prevention of recurrence. The historic treatment of TGDC consisted of incision and drainage or excision. This resulted in a draining sinus or recurrence in up to 50% of treated patients. In 1893, Schlange proposed removing the central portion of the hyoid bone with the cyst, reducing the recurrence rate to 20%. Sistrunk subsequently advocated removing the midportion of the hyoid bone without attempting to dissect the duct from the bone. He also stressed the importance of removing a core of the central tongue musculature from the hyoid bone up to the foramen cecum. His procedure reduced the rate of recurrence to 3% or less. Understanding the path of descent from the foramen cecum and the intimate relationship of the hyoid to the thyroglossal duct supports the rationale for the Sistrunk procedure. It is useful to assume that any anterior neck mass near the hyoid is likely to be a TGDC. The Sistrunk procedure should therefore be the procedure of choice. These principles should be followed every time the surgeon removes a suspected TGDC.

There are several reasons to remove a TGDC once it has been identified. Early surgical intervention provides the best chance of cure and reduces the risk of recurrence. TGDC excision alleviates the cosmetic deformity of an anterior neck mass and decreases the small, but distinct, risk for malignant degeneration.

The Sistrunk procedure involves a horizontal neck incision and raising subplatsyma skin flaps above and below the mass. If there is an opening to a sinus, an ellipse of skin around the opening should be included.

The thyroid cartilage and thyrohyoid membrane define the depth of dissection. Dissection is executed from the thyroid isthmus in a superior direction until the hyoid bone is encountered. Some sternohyoid muscle may be included. The cyst is typically located near the midportion of the bone. The superior and inferior portions of the hyoid, lateral to the cyst, are skeletonized to the level of the lesser cornua. The hyoid is elevated from the thyrohyoid membrane and divided at the lesser cornua. Intraoperative identification of the thyroid gland eliminates the possibility of removing a functioning ectopic gland.

A double-gloved finger is placed in the mouth to palpate the foramen cecum. A core of tongue musculature is dissected from the hyoid to this point. Care is taken not to enter the pharynx when the specimen is divided from the tongue mucosa. Hemostasis is achieved. The wound is irrigated and a small Penrose drain is placed. No attempt is made to approximate the hyoid remnants. The strap muscles are approximated, and the skin is closed in layers. Rapid absorbing sutures to close the skin will provide a good cosmetic result and obviates the need to remove sutures in the office. A fluffed gauze and mesh elastic tubular dressing provides gentle compression and is an easy dressing to remove on the first postoperative day. Odynophagia usually disappears by the first postoperative day. Excessive pain is unusual.

The surgeon should avoid those factors that may increase the risk for recurrence. Recurrences typically occur early, often within the first month of surgery. Avoiding prior incision and drainage will prevent draining sinuses and lessen the chance for recurrence. The hyoid must be resected to the lesser cornua, and no effort should be made to dissect the duct from the hyoid bone. The surgeon should try to prevent vertically fracturing the hyoid and removing the anterior portion of the bone while leaving the posterior aspect behind. Cyst rupture during excision is associated with an increase risk of recurrence.

Multiple tracts from the foramen cecum may be present and require removal of an adequate cuff of suprahyoid tissue. For this reason, recurrences can occur despite a seemingly adequate procedure. Removing infrahyoid tracts and the pyramidal lobe of the thyroid may be necessary. Multiple cysts are associated with an increased risk for recurrence.

Recurrence is more likely in the younger patient. Unfortunately, most TGDCs occur within the first few years of life.

Treatment of recurrence involves excision of the skin around a draining sinus. Removal of the contents of the anterior neck, which is superficial to the thyroid cartilage and thyrohyoid membrane, is executed from the thyroid isthmus to the level of the hyoid. The edges of the strap muscles should be included. The hyoid remnants are resected to the lesser cornua. An additional cuff of tongue muscle is removed.

Other complications are seroma or hematoma formation, suture abscess, and wound infection. Inadvertent entry into the oral cavity at the level of the foramen cecum is managed by closing the defect with a purse-string suture. The area must then be drained.

Intraoperative hemorrhage from lingual vessels or injury to the hypoglossal nerve is prevented by not dissecting lateral to the lesser cornua. Airway entry into the trachea or thyroid cartilage is possible, but unlikely if the surgeon recognizes all landmarks.

Hypothyroidism is avoided by preoperative imaging, as discussed earlier. Identifying the thyroid gland during the procedure should serve to obviate this problem.

Mention should be made regarding carcinoma in TGDCs. Papillary-follicular carcinoma is the cancer most often encountered in this situation. It can occur in ectopic rests of thyroid tissue. Treatment with a Sistrunk procedure may be adequate if surgical margins are negative. Some researchers argue that a thyroidectomy may be necessary as well.

EDITOR'S NOTES

Properly executed, excision of a thyroglossal duct cyst is very rewarding for the patient, their parents, and the surgeon. The "lump" is gone, patients usually recover quickly with little discomfort, and the incision is usually cosmetically quite acceptable. However, complications can develop and the cysts can recur, both of which occur less frequently when there is careful attention to detail before, during, and after the operation.

The differential diagnosis of a midline neck mass is broad, and this inherent diagnostic uncertainty should be shared with the family. Movement of the nodule with swallowing or protrusion of the tongue is somewhat overrated but is sometimes helpful. Laboratory and imaging studies of the nodule itself are unreliable and usually unnecessary. Despite the suggestion by some in the literature that it is expensive and unnecessary in most cases, I suspect most pediatric surgeons routinely perform an ultrasonographic examination to document the presence of a normal thyroid gland.

The patient should be in a modified Fowler position with the neck slightly hyperextended. Excessive hyperextension can distort the anatomy and tends to cause the hyoid bone to be pressed forcefully against the trachea, increasing the risk for injury to the airway. The incision should be placed in a skin crease. Once the nodule is exposed, a decision is made whether to proceed with a formal Sistrunk procedure or merely simple excision. It can be difficult to make this distinction, so unless the nodule is absolutely clearly identified as a dermoid cyst or lymph node, the patient should undergo formal excision including the central portion of the hyoid bone. The steps of the procedure are outlined nicely in this chapter. I would only emphasize that the trachea is sometimes surprisingly close to the plane of dissection and is at some risk for injury, especially when heavy instruments are introduced into the field to divide the hyoid bone.

Most patients can be treated as outpatients and recover rather quickly. They should be followed closely for the possibility of recurrence, for example at 2 weeks and again at 2 or 3 months after the operation. A simple wound infection is rare. The presence of redness, swelling, or drainage should raise the suspicion of a recurrent sinus tract. In contrast to the ease and elegance of the primary operation, operation for a recurrent thyroglossal duct remnant is often difficult and tedious. It is best to wait at least 4 to 6 weeks after the first operation before proceeding with the second. This allows local inflammatory changes to subside and should make the dissection easier and safer. In general, the steps of the Sistrunk procedure are repeated. The tract is typically embedded in thick scar and rarely visualized. The entire core of scar tissue should be excised, going through fresh tissue planes and excising more of the hyoid bone. The results of a second operation are generally good, but there are occasionally patients who require another attempt at resection.

–*P.M.*

SUGGESTED READINGS

Cunningham MJ. Congenital malformations of the head and neck. In: Cotton RT, Myer CM, eds. *Practical pediatric otolaryngology.* Philadelphia: Lippincott-Raven, 1999:663–680.

Ellis PDM, van Nostrand PAW. The applied anatomy of thyroglossal tract remnants. *Laryngoscope* 1977;87:765–770.

Pelausa EO, Forte V. Sistrunk revisited: a 10-year review of revision thyroglossal duct surgery at Toronto Hospital for Sick Children. *J Otolaryngol* 1989;18:325–333.

Sistrunk WE. The surgical treatment of cysts of the thyroglossal tract. *Ann Surg* 1920;71:121–124.

Sistrunk WE. Technique of removal of cysts and sinuses of the thyroglossal duct. *Surg Gynecol Obstet* 1928;46:109–112.

Ward PH, Strahan RW, Acqarelli M, et al. The many faces of the thyroglossal duct. *Trans Am Acad Ophthalmol Otolaryngol* 1970;74: 310–318.

30

LYMPHATIC MALFORMATIONS

PETER MATTEI

Lymphatic malformations occur mainly in the neck and axilla and usually present in infancy. They are composed of multiple large, thin-walled cysts that insinuate themselves between and around the normal structures of the neck and chest. They are usually asymptomatic but can be disfiguring and occasionally involve deeper structures, including the airway. Treatment of these benign lesions is surgical and involves a careful and sometimes tedious dissection in an effort to prevent recurrence but also preserve normal structures.

DIAGNOSIS

The typical presentation is that of an otherwise healthy and asymptomatic infant who is noted at birth or in the first few days of life to have a mass in the neck (Fig. 30.1). Some children present later, at the age of 1 or 2 years, with a slowly growing mass in the neck or axilla, although lymphatic malformations can develop anywhere in the body, including the abdomen or retroperitoneum. Parents and primary care physicians frequently describe the mass as "spongy" or "squishy," which, together with a typical location, leaves little doubt as to the diagnosis. A history of stridor or feeding difficulties suggests involvement of deeper structures, such as the airway or esophagus. The presence of fever, redness, and pain suggests that the lesion has become infected.

On physical examination, the mass is soft, fixed, fluid filled, and nontender. There are no overlying skin changes, except in the rare case of secondary infection, and the lesion can usually be transilluminated. Intralesional hemorrhage can occur and results in a rapidly expanding lesion or one that is firm to palpation. The child should be assessed clinically for evidence of stridor or drooling. The axilla should be examined, because lymphatic malformations of the neck are known to sometimes communicate with the axilla.

P. Mattei: Department of Surgery, Thomas Jefferson University, Philadelphia, Pennsylvania; and Department of Pediatric Surgery, Alfred I. duPont Hospital for Children, Wilmington, Delaware.

The diagnosis is usually obvious from physical examination, because there are few lesions with a similar appearance. Other diagnoses that should be considered include: hemangioma, lymphadenopathy, branchial cleft cyst, teratoma, and neoplasm. This is especially true of lesions that are symptomatic, infected, or firm to palpation.

The full extent of the lesion, particularly the involvement of deep structures, is impossible to determine on the basis of physical examination alone. All infants with lymphatic malformations should undergo an imaging study, and those with large neck lesions should be studied urgently because of the possibility of airway involvement. Ultrasonography will usually confirm the diagnosis and can provide some anatomic information, but it does not usually provide sufficient detail to plan properly for an operation. Computed

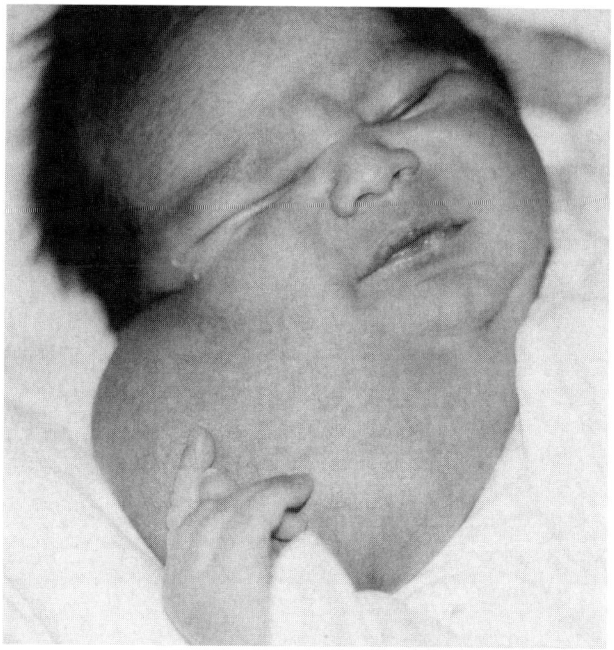

FIGURE 30.1. A large lymphatic malformation of the neck in a newborn infant. Note the extension of the mass onto the face. This is clearly a lesion in which airway involvement needs to be considered and ruled out with an imaging study.

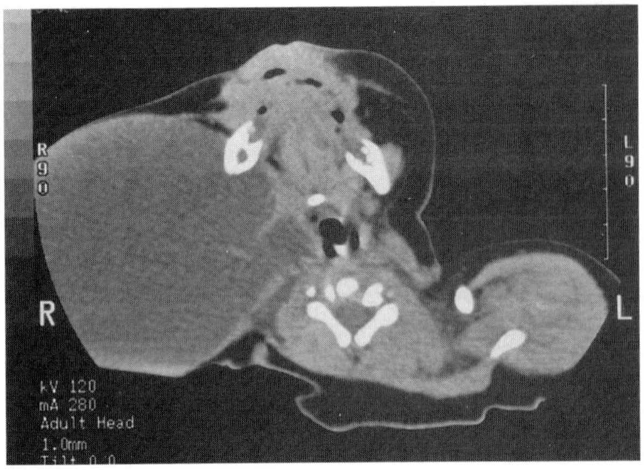

FIGURE 30.2. Computed tomography of the child pictured in Fig. 30.1. Note the proximity to the trachea with lack of true involvement or airway compromise. Careful inspection of the structures surrounding the upper airway by direct laryngoscopy prior to intubation is also useful to rule out airway compromise but does not obviate the imaging studies.

tomography (CT) provides much better images and is usually adequate for operative planning (Fig. 30.2). Magnetic resonance imaging is the preferred study for complex or extensive lesions. It produces images in multiple planes and provides information about adjacent structures that can be invaluable in planning the operative approach. The large fluid-filled cysts appear very intense on T2-weighted images and are usually easily distinguished from adjacent muscular and vascular structures (Fig. 30.3). The scanned area should always include the axilla and upper thorax, because these lesions are known to permeate deep into the mediastinum on occasion. Lymphatic malformations of the neck sometimes involve the parotid gland and the facial nerve.

TREATMENT

Treatment is primarily surgical. Simple aspiration of the cysts is followed by rapid reaccumulation of fluid and can result in infection or bleeding. There is a huge clinical experience with injection sclerotherapy in Japan that is being actively studied in this country, although the ideal sclerosing agent has yet to be identified. The utility of the technique is further compromised by the fact that lymphatic malformations are typically multilocular. The agents most often used include OK-432 (derived from a species of streptococci), sodium morrhuate, and bleomycin. Some clinicians also have used injection of triamcinolone with moderate success. Sclerotherapy might be considered in patients with extensive lesions, in those with recurrent fluid collections after surgical excision, and in those who are not otherwise good surgical candidates. However, it should probably be performed as part of a study protocol. Part of the problem with any form

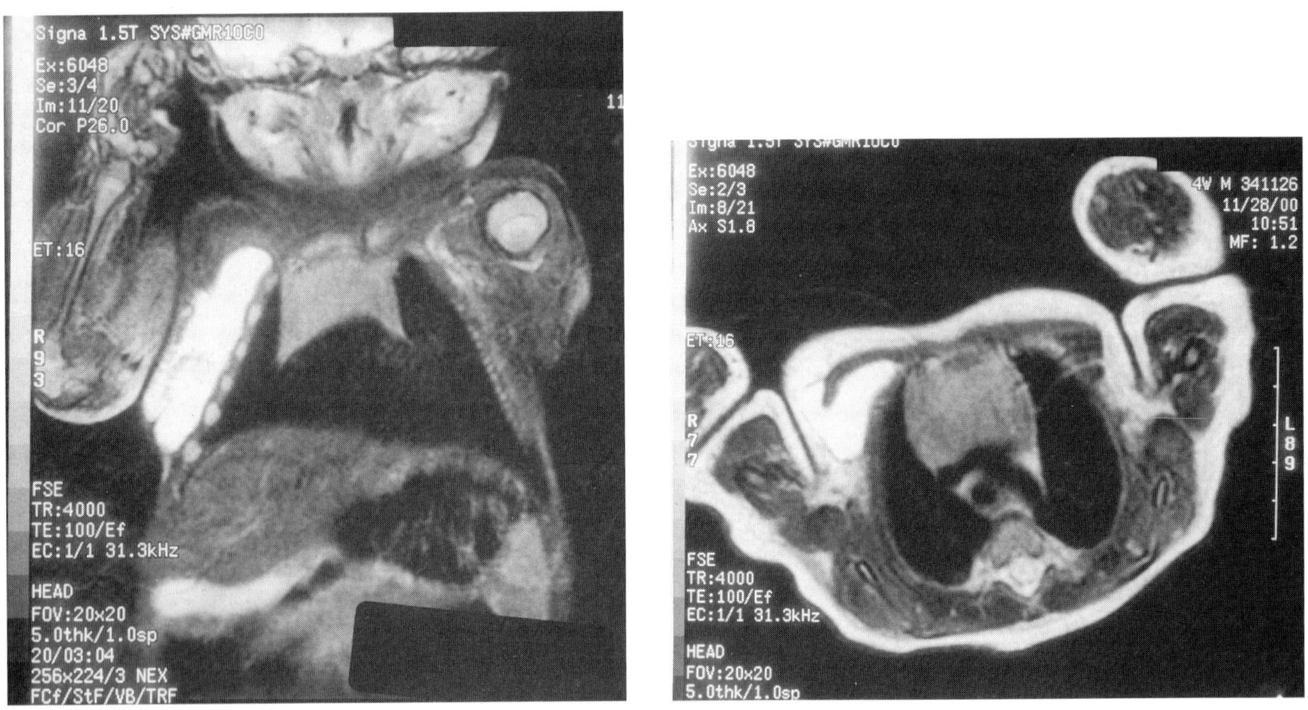

FIGURE 30.3. Magnetic resonance images (T2-weighted, with fat signal suppression) of a lymphatic malformation of the axilla and chest wall. Note the bright signal of the mass and the excellent detail provided of adjacent normal structures. The lesion involved the subareolar tissues and can be seen to extend deep to the pectoralis major muscle.

of injection therapy is that if it fails, subsequent surgical excision is often much more difficult because of hemorrhage and fibrosis. Expectant therapy is not a viable option in most cases, because these lesions rarely resolve spontaneously and when they do, it is often after the lesion has become infected, putting the infant at risk for sepsis.

The timing of surgery is variable. Large lesions that involve the airway require immediate attention. Infants with stridor should undergo laryngoscopy and, in rare cases, may require tracheotomy for safe airway management. In asymptomatic infants with lesions that do not involve the airway, the operation is delayed until 2 or 3 months of age. This allows for some somatic growth and adequate nutrition in anticipation of surgery. The family should be made aware of the risks of the procedure, including nerve injury, vocal cord paralysis, injury to other adjacent structures, and recurrence.

Surgical excision demands patience and meticulous attention to detail in order to achieve complete excision while protecting normal structures. The surgeon must anticipate that the anatomy may be severely distorted and that expected anatomic relationships will have been disrupted. This is especially true of nerves and their branches, which are frequently separated and isolated from their usual neighbors. The dissection should proceed as though any filamentous structure could represent an important nerve branch and should be preserved.

Lesions in the neck are approached through a transverse incision, preferably in a skin crease if one can be identified. If the lesion approaches the midline, direct laryngoscopy or bronchoscopy should be performed to assess the airway structures, which may be edematous or otherwise distorted. The infant is positioned with the head extended but the neck neutral or slightly flexed. The head is turned slightly away from the operative side. The skin preparation and draping should be wide, and if there is an axillary component, the arm may need to be included in the field. The presence of an orogastric tube helps with intraoperative identification of the esophagus.

The incision is continued down through the platysma, and subplatysmal flaps are raised widely, staying close to the wall of the lesion. The cyst wall is transparent and easily torn. Blunt dissection should be used as much as possible, and no structure should be divided unless it can be identified with certainty. Longitudinal structures appear to be completely surrounded by fluid-filled spaces but can usually be dissected free with careful blunt dissection. Often the cysts need to be opened in order to free the structure. In most cases, it is hopeless to expect that the lesion can be excised intact, without rupturing at least some of the cysts, and sometimes the extent of the lesion can be assessed better with access to the inside of the individual compartments. There is usually an adequate plane of dissection between the lesion and the normal structures, although it is acceptable to leave some of the cyst wall rather than sacrifice or compromise a critical structure. It is also acceptable to ligate and divide small vessels that are involved by the mass, including the middle thyroid vein and the facial vein.

Normal anatomic relationships are often distorted. The vagus nerve, for example, may be separated from the carotid artery and internal jugular vein by a pocket of fluid. More importantly, the recurrent laryngeal nerve may have been lifted out of the tracheoesophageal groove and its individual fibers may be separated, all of which puts it at high risk for not being easily identified and subsequently injured. The malformation should be separated from the esophagus and trachea along its entire length and superiorly to the insertion of the recurrent laryngeal nerve, where the nerve itself might look like a bundle of nonspecific connective tissue fibers. The marginal mandibular branch of the facial nerve is also at risk. Because the nerve is redundant in its course, looping down over the mass before it courses superiorly toward the mouth, it need not be sacrificed. It should be identified below the anterior mandible and carefully mobilized.

The spinal accessory nerve is also at significant risk of injury. This cranial nerve normally courses obliquely between the trapezius and the sternocleidomastoid muscles, but it can be very hard to identify. Again, meticulous technique should allow identification and protection of the nerve. Other nerves that may be injured and should therefore be sought out at operation include: the hypoglossal nerve, which is located at the bifurcation of the internal and external carotid arteries; the great auricular nerve, which is very superficial and can result in numbness of the ear lobe and face if injured; and the trunks and branches of the brachial plexus.

Lesions that involve the face put the branches of the facial nerve in danger of being injured. This dissection demands extraordinary patience and technical attention to detail. Lesions that communicate with the axilla will require a counterincision to allow mobilization of the inferior portion. Lesions that extend inferiorly and communicate with the axilla travel under the clavicle, placing the brachial plexus and subclavian vessels at risk. When the malformation extends into the mediastinum, a decision should be made whether it can be safely approached through the cervical incision or whether another approach is necessary. These lesions are sometimes treated in stages, with resection of the cervical portion first, and resection of the mediastinal portion after repeat imaging.

Lymphatic malformations are characterized by small finger-like extensions that taper off into tiny channels that might represent lymphatic channels. Failure to control these channels with ligation or sutures may be responsible for some recurrences and can also cause postoperative seromas. After the lesion has been completely excised, hemostasis must be meticulous. A closed suction drain should be placed through a separate incision, and the wound is closed in layers with absorbable sutures. The platysma should be closed as a separate layer. The skin will sometimes be quite redundant but usually need not be excised.

Lesions arising in other areas are treated according to the same principles of meticulous dissection and preservation of normal structures. Large cystic lymphangiomas that develop in the abdomen are often retroperitoneal and can develop within the mesentery or adjacent to other organs such as the pancreas. Retroperitoneal structures are dissected carefully, and the source of the fluid should be sought and controlled with suture techniques. Sacrifice of normal structures should be avoided. Recurrence can result in ascites or a recurrent cyst, which is often unilocular and therefore often more amenable to drainage or sclerosis. Lymphatic malformations can arise adjacent to segments of the small or large bowel and occasionally require bowel resection for complete control, but only if they cannot be separated safely from the bowel or mesentery.

POSTOPERATIVE CARE

Despite what is sometimes a long and extensive dissection, infants typically tolerate the procedure well. If edema or pain control are concerns, the patient may benefit from overnight intubation. If an extensive airway dissection was necessary, or if the soft tissues of the airway were edematous on laryngoscopy, extubation should be performed in a controlled setting so that the airway can be maintained safely. Administration of dexamethasone should be considered because it may help to reduce airway edema. Pain control is with morphine initially and can usually quickly be switched to acetaminophen.

After extubation, when the child is awake and alert, oral feedings can be started. Swallowing difficulties are uncommon, although inability to protect the airway can occur, sometimes with frank aspiration. Feedings are therefore started with water or an electrolyte solution and advanced to full-strength formula as tolerated. This is usually a transient phenomenon, but occasionally a formal assessment of swallowing becomes necessary if the problem persists.

Patients are discharged within 2 to 5 days, when they are tolerating full feedings and on oral pain management. Most are sent home with the drain in place, and the family is instructed to empty the collection device twice daily and record the volume. I prefer to see patients within 7 to 10 days after surgery, at which time the drain is usually draining minimal amounts of fluid and is ready to be discontinued. A seroma frequently occurs after the drain is removed. The parents should be warned that this is expected and does not necessarily mean that the malformation has recurred. Most seromas can be observed, although large ones may need to be drained. Drainage can be performed easily in the office with a small-gauge needle and syringe. The procedure is painless if the needle is inserted directly through the incision. Drainage may need to be repeated three or four times before the seroma resolves completely.

COMPLICATIONS

Besides the usual risks of cellulitis and bleeding, the principle complications seen after excision of a lymphatic malformation are related to injury to native structures. Nerve injuries predominate. The marginal mandibular branch of the facial nerve is at risk if there is dissection below the mandible anteriorly. This nerve is quite small and variable in location, making it somewhat difficult to protect. Patients present with a characteristic motor deficit of the lower lip in which the lower teeth on one side are not exposed when the patient smiles. Fortunately, this is often a transient deficit, presumably due to a neurapraxia rather than actually severing the nerve, although recovery may take up to a year and is not always complete.

Recurrent laryngeal nerve injury also may be transient and results in ipsilateral vocal cord paralysis. The deficit is normally well tolerated but can cause a persistent hoarse voice and occasionally more serious difficulties related to airway protection. The diagnosis is confirmed by direct laryngoscopy, which reveals a medial position of the true vocal cord and lack of normal movement during respiration. Bilateral vocal cord paralysis results in critical airway narrowing and usually necessitates tracheotomy. Patients should be followed closely by an experienced pediatric otolaryngologist and may eventually benefit from a cord lateralization procedure if the deficit does not resolve spontaneously.

The spinal accessory nerve is at high risk for being injured, given its superficial location. Patients should be evaluated for signs of injury; however, a drooping shoulder or winged scapula may be difficult to identify in an infant.

Recurrent lymphatic malformation can recur, albeit rarely. A period of observation is warranted because it may occasionally spontaneously resolve over the course of several weeks or months. Reoperation may be necessary and, as expected, is often fraught with considerable difficulty. These patients also can be considered for injection therapy, because recurrent cysts are often unilocular.

FOLLOW-UP

Patients are followed at 1- to 2-week intervals initially and then monthly, depending on their progress. After the first 3 months or so of follow-up, patients may be followed yearly or on an as-needed basis. Patients with neurologic injuries should be followed closely for evidence of recovery and to ensure appropriate referral for residual defects in 6 months to a year. Even patients with large lesions and excessive redundant skin eventually heal well, although occasionally patients may require scar revision.

In summary, lymphatic malformation is congenital and most commonly presents in the newborn period. Most are amenable to surgical excision, although all patients require

CT or magnetic resonance imaging to determine the true extent of the lesion and for proper operative planning. The operation can be tedious and requires meticulous technique to prevent recurrence and to avoid injury to adjacent native structures. Peripheral nerve injuries are common but are frequently transient. Most patients recover nicely from the operation and have an acceptable cosmetic result.

SUGGESTED READINGS

Charabi B, Bretlau P, Bille M, et al. Cystic hygroma of the head and neck—a long-term follow-up of 44 cases. *Acta Otolaryngol* 2000; 543(suppl):248–250.

Fonkalsrud EW. Congenital malformations of the lymphatic system. *Semin Pediatr Surg* 1994;3:62–69.

Fung K, Poenaru D, Soboleski DA, et al. Impact of magnetic resonance imaging on the surgical management of cystic hygromas. *J Pediatr Surg* 1998;33:839–841.

Lille ST, Rand RP, Tapper D, et al. The surgical management of giant cervicofacial lymphatic malformations. *J Pediatr Surg* 1996;31: 1648–1650.

Ogita S, Tsuto T, Nakamura K, et al. OK-432 therapy for lymphangioma in children: why and how does it work? *J Pediatr Surg* 1996;31:477–480.

Ricciardelli EJ, Richardson MA. Cervicofacial cystic hygroma. Patterns of recurrence and management of the difficult case. *Arch Otolaryngol Head Neck Surg* 1991;117:546–553.

Tran-Ngoc-Ninh, Tran-Xuan-Ninh. Cystic hygroma in children: a report of 126 cases. *J Pediatr Surg* 1974;9:191–195.

31

SALIVARY GLAND DISORDERS

STEVEN P. COOK

There is a broad spectrum of salivary gland diseases that may be either inflammatory or neoplastic. The task for the surgeon is to use the information gathered in the office history and examination, to determine the best diagnostic study, and to decide whether surgical or medical treatment is required.

In general, the same salivary gland conditions affect both children and adults. The treatment principles are essentially the same. The frequency varies between these problems. Mumps, congenital lesions, vascular tumors, recurrent parotitis, and sialorrhea are more common in children than in adults.

The typical complaints that bring the child to the physician are either a painful swelling or enlargement of the gland or a painless mass. Inflammatory disease is more common in children than in adults, but a nontender mass in a child is more likely to be malignant than it is in an adult.

The six major salivary glands and the numerous minor glands are all derived from ectoderm. The glands produce about 500 mL of saliva daily, primarily from the parotid and submandibular glands. At rest, the submandibular glands secrete most of the saliva.

Saliva acts to lubricate the oral cavity, and aids in mastication, deglutition, and digestion. Saliva is important in maintaining healthy dentition. Although hyposecretion may be seen in some disorders, such as Sjögren syndrome, true hypersecretory disorders are much more unusual.

PATIENT EVALUATION

The history should include inquiry about the duration and onset of symptoms. Inflammatory lesions tend to have a fairly rapid onset, usually with pain, tenderness, and possibly fever. Rapid onset of swelling with meals suggests obstruction to salivary outflow. Neoplasms generally present with the slow onset of a painless mass. In some less common instances, a malignancy may rapidly enlarge. A recurrent episode of parotid swelling is suggestive of recurrent parotitis of childhood. Usually only one gland is involved.

Age of the patient also will lead to the diagnosis. Acute suppurative parotitis of infancy is exclusively found in newborns, frequently in premature infants. Congenital cysts and vascular lesions also may present in infancy. Masses that increase in size with straining or crying suggest the latter.

Trauma to the duct orifice may be seen in older children. Cheek biting or irritation from dental appliances, such as braces, can cause outflow obstruction.

Skin changes such as discoloration, induration, erythema or firmness should be noted. Facial weakness or paralysis strongly suggests malignancy.

All histories should include a list of current medications, systemic illnesses, and recent infections or exposure to infected individuals. Mumps is the most common etiology of viral sialoadenitis and can only occur once in a patient's lifetime. To this end, one should ask about the patient's immunization status. Because catscratch disease can cause a necrotizing granulomatous infection of the parotid gland, exposure to pets should be noted.

The physical examination should include a good inspection of the entire oral cavity. The orifices of the ducts should be examined for inflammation (suggesting virus infection or irritation) or scarring from trauma. Attempts to milk saliva from each gland will show whether the saliva is clear or turbid. Obviously, one should note any intraoral mass, whether in the floor of mouth, buccal mucosa, or displacing the tonsil toward the midline.

Bimanual palpation is critical to reveal more subtle lesions. A dense fascia covers the parotid gland, and masses in this area may not otherwise be appreciated. Palpation of the ducts, particularly in the floor of the mouth, may reveal the presence of a stone. Palpation and inspection of the tail of the parotid gland in the infraauricular area should be included. The neck should be examined for palpable lymph nodes. Because the submandibular gland is confined to the

S. P. Cook: Department of Otolaryngology, Thomas Jefferson University, Philadelphia, Pennsylvania; and Department of Surgery, Division of Pediatric Otolaryngology, Alfred I. duPont Hospital for Children, Wilmington, Delaware.

anterior portion of the digastric triangle, any lesion here should not be palpable above the mandibular ramus.

The face should be visually inspected. Hemangiomas may have a slight bluish color from subcutaneous involvement or be frankly red when the skin becomes involved. Erythema and induration from bacterial infection should be obvious. The violaceous discoloration, with possible fluctuance or skin breakdown, may be seen in atypical *mycobacterial* infections. Because the facial nerve courses through the substance of the parotid gland, asymmetry from muscle weakness or paralysis should be noted because this strongly suggests malignancy.

Finally the mass itself should be examined. One should ask if the mass is firm, rock hard, fluctuant, or indurated. Is the mass ill defined and diffuse or discrete? Is it fixed or mobile, large or small, tender or nontender? Is this a single mass or is it multilobular or nodular?

DIAGNOSTIC STUDIES

Several imaging studies can be used to diagnose salivary diseases. The choice of the best procedure may be influenced by the ability of the child to cooperate for the study.

Sialography will demonstrate calculi, stricture, and ectasia of the duct. Recurrent parotitis has a typical sialographic picture of globular ductal ectasias. A sialogram may be difficult to accomplish in a child. It is contraindicated when the gland is acutely inflamed.

Radionucleotide scans generally are of little benefit in children. This study may be of some value in the evaluation of suspected congenital agenesis of major salivary glands, a rare condition. Technetium 99m–labeled red blood cell pool imaging is 100% specific for parotid hemangiomas if there is hypoperfusion in the early phase but with increased activity with the delayed image.

Plain radiography may show calculi, dystrophic calcification within the gland, or phleboliths, which can occur in hemangiomas. When it is clinically difficult to differentiate a parotid mass from a jaw lesion, a plain radiograph may demonstrate an erosive mandibular lesion. Dental occlusal films can demonstrate a radiopaque calculus of the anterior portion of the submandibular duct. Distal oblique occlusal views will demonstrate a calculus that is closer to the hilum. A panoramic view may show a parotid calculus. Because most submandibular stones are radiopaque, plain radiography can demonstrate a calculus 90% of the time.

Ultrasonography is rapid, noninvasive, and does not require sedation. In experienced hands, it can be used to demonstrate surrounding anatomic structures. High-resolution ultrasonography will identify hemangiomas, mixed parotid tumors, lymph nodes, or abscesses. Duct ectasia and hypoechoic areas, typical of recurrent parotitis, also can be identified.

Computed tomography (CT) can be used to demonstrate whether a mass is intrinsic or extrinsic to the gland and to define the relationship of the gland to adjacent bony and vascular structures. Tumors of the mandible or adjacent soft tissues may present as a parotid mass, and CT would show that these lesions are extrinsic to the gland. Contrast injection will demonstrate vascularity. Ring enhancement around a radiolucent area after contrast injection indicates abscess formation.

There are several disadvantages to CT, primarily exposure to ionizing radiation. As with many studies in children, sedation may be required. Allergic reactions to contrast medium also can occur.

Magnetic resonance imaging (MRI) is noninvasive, and imaging can be obtained in multiple planes. Excellent soft tissue detail permits localizing a mass to a specific space or anatomic structure. This improves diagnostic capability and helps to define the surgical approach. Because benign tumors remain confined to the tissue of origin, spread to adjacent compartments suggests malignancy. Imaging detail can identify the course of the facial nerve and whether there is perineural spread of disease. MRI can differentiate between hemangiomas and lymphangiomas. Cysts and abscesses are also identifiable. Although there is no radiation exposure or need to inject contrast material, the young child will likely require sedation or general anesthesia.

In the presence of suppurative sialoadenitis, a sample of saliva for culture and sensitivity may serve as a guide for antibiotic therapy. Unfortunately, cultures may yield only mouth flora. Cytopathologic diagnosis of saliva can reveal tumor cells. An experienced cytopathologist is necessary to provide a reliable diagnosis.

A tissue diagnosis is ultimately needed to determine definitive treatment of a salivary mass. Fine-needle aspiration will indicate whether a lesion is benign or malignant. This should help to define the extent of the surgical procedure. With an experienced cytopathologist, the sensitivity of diagnosing a malignancy is over 90%. Unfortunately, the ability of a child to cooperate for the procedure may limit its use in an office setting.

DIFFERENTIAL DIAGNOSIS AND MANAGEMENT

Congenital Diseases

Cysts or vascular lesions are the typical problems that present within the newborn period or early childhood. Two percent of all parotid masses are cystic. Dermoid cysts, retention cysts, or abnormalities of the first branchial arch may present within or adjacent to the parotid gland.

Initially, these masses are circumscribed and nontender unless secondarily infected. If untreated, an abscessed cyst may rupture and form a draining sinus tract.

W. P. Work had divided first branchial abnormalities by histologic elements into type I or type II cysts. Both types of first branchial abnormalities maintain a close and variable relationship to the facial nerve. Type I cysts are duplications of the external ear canal and present near to or within the substance of the parotid gland. Type I abnormalities are more common than type II abnormalities. Sinus tracts may present within the conchal bowl, pretragal area, or postauricular crease. It is not unusual to obtain a history of previous abscesses, often having required multiple incision and drainage procedures. The resultant scarring from previous infections may make surgical dissection difficult, particularly around the facial nerve.

Type II abnormalities are duplications of the external ear canal and the pinna. They contain ectodermal and mesodermal elements. They are generally infraparotid. They often have a sinus draining to the upper neck, near the hyoid. They frequently present with infections. Type II abnormalities may have a sinus tract that extends to the external canal, tympanic membrane, or middle ear. As with all cysts, fistulas, and sinus tracts, complete excision is required to prevent recurrence. Therefore, any preexisting inflammation must be completely resolved before definitive surgical removal.

Dermoids and congenital ductal cysts may become apparent in early childhood as unilateral swellings. As mentioned earlier, the dense fascia surrounding the parotid gland may hinder the diagnosis by physical examination.

Cysts are treated by excision. Unless frequent infections are a problem, it may be wise to defer surgical excision until the infant is older.

Vascular lesions, hemangiomas, and lymphangiomas are the most common benign salivary gland tumors of infancy. Hemangioma is the most common parotid tumor of childhood. Girls are more frequently affected than boys. A hemangioma may present initially with a tiny red skin component that can rapidly enlarge to involve adjacent structures, including the skin and soft tissues. Hemangiomas replace salivary parenchyma, unlike lymphangiomas. The masses are soft, compressible, and expand with crying or straining. They do not involve the facial nerve. The natural course of hemangiomas is of initial rapid growth. The lesion subsequently involutes by 2 to 5 years of age, and is replaced with fibrofatty tissue. In most instances, a conservative approach with observation is usually the best treatment. Surgery may place the child at risk for hemorrhagic complications or injury to the facial nerve. Given the dramatic and sometimes deforming appearance of hemangiomas, the child's family may exert pressure to "do something." True indications for surgery are ulceration, infection, hemorrhage, or functional impairment. Superficial parotidectomy and facial nerve dissection is the procedure of choice. There is a role for short courses of steroids when large lesions place vital organs, such as intraorbital structures, at risk.

Lymphangioma, or cystic hygroma, may occur by itself or in combination with a hemangioma. Lymphangioma is a cystic dilatation of the regional lymphatics. Most are present at birth, and 90% are present by the second year of life. They manifest as fluctuant, compressible masses. MRI should differentiate the lesion from hemangioma. Lymphangiomas rarely affect a salivary gland alone and usually involve other neck structures, particularly within the posterior triangle. Although they often enlarge slowly, trauma or upper respiratory infections can cause rapid expansion that may become secondarily infected. This can result in compression of the facial nerve or airway compromise. Airway obstruction is more common with lesions of the submandibular or sublingual gland areas.

Lymphangiomas are less likely to involute so that complete surgical excision is recommended. In the hope that the patient is one of the rare few that may experience spontaneous regression, deferring the procedure until the child is 3 to 5 years of age is a reasonable tactic. Lesions that become frequently infected or compromise the airway require earlier intervention. Aspiration of cysts carries a risk of infection or hemorrhage and is not recommended.

The cyst walls may be thin and easily ruptured during excision. Cysts tend to wrap around vital structures. There is a risk of nerve injury or recurrence due to retention of cyst walls. Staged resection may be required in some lesions. Recurrences may occur rapidly, usually within the first postoperative year. They are treated in the same manner. The risk of recurrence is higher with suprahyoid lesions.

Injection with sclerosing agents generally has met with little success. The exception may be current ongoing protocols using Picibanil [OK-432 (Chugai Pharmaceutical Co., Tokyo, Japan)].

Aplasia of major salivary glands is rare and is one of the few indications for a radionucleotide scan. Accessory glands, particularly anterior to the parotid capsule, have their own duct system. Aberrant glands do not have ducts but may fistulize to the pharynx, lateral neck, or middle ear. Imperforate submandibular ducts present as a swelling within the floor of the mouth (Fig. 31.1). Marsupialization or ductoplasty produces good long-term cure. Stenting is not needed.

Acute Inflammatory Disease

Numerous viruses may produce sialoadenitis. Mumps, coxsackie A virus, ECHO (enteric cytopathogenic human orphan) virus, and the virus of lymphocytic choriomeningitis can all cause parotid or submandibular gland involvement. Unless suppurative complications with abscess formation occur, treatment is supportive.

Acute suppurative parotitis can occur from duct obstruction secondary to a stone, stricture, or trauma to the orifice. Debility, dehydration, electrolyte imbalance, or salivary stasis are risk factors. The disease may be bilateral. It also can recur.

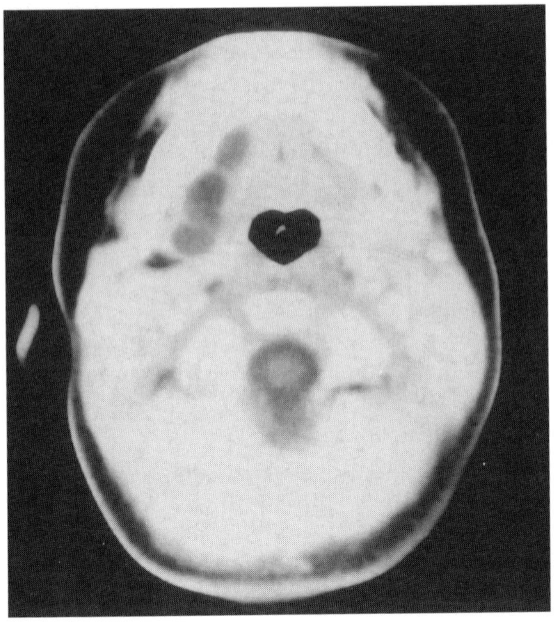

FIGURE 31.1. Computed tomography scan demonstrating congenital dilatation of the submandibular duct from failure of perforation of the duct orifice.

Staphylococcus aureus and *Streptococcus* species are common bacterial organisms for acute parotitis. *Escherichia coli* also has been identified, as has anaerobic organisms such as *Bacteroides* and *Peptostreptococcus*. Over 70% of species may be β-lactamase-producing organisms. Penicillinase-resistant penicillins or first-generation cephalosporins may be adequate. Clindamycin is another excellent choice, particularly because it is the only antibiotic secreted in saliva. Hydration, sialagogues, heat, and massage are also indicated.

Abscess is rare in children. When it occurs, it is more frequently in the parotid gland and in a younger age group. It requires incision and drainage. Because palpation of the parotid is not adequate to diagnose an abscess, CT with contrast will confirm the diagnosis. In the parotid area, a standard parotidectomy incision is made. A skin flap, superficial to the parotid fascia, is elevated. The fascia over the abscess should be incised parallel to the fibers of the facial nerve. Multiple drains may be needed. As with any neck abscess, extension to surrounding fascial spaces can occur.

Acute suppurative parotitis of infancy occurs exclusively in newborns, often in premature infants. The parotid gland is most frequently involved. Management follows the same principles outlined above.

Chronic Inflammatory Disease

Recurrent parotitis of childhood is a common cause of periodic parotid swelling. It is accompanied by the rapid onset of swelling, pain, and fever. It may last from several days to weeks. It usually affects only one gland. It occurs more frequently in boys. It usually starts between 5 to 7 years of age. Episodes may occur several times a year. The disease usually resolves by puberty. There is no effective prevention. Theoretically, the patient should avoid dehydration or medications that thicken or decrease salivary flow. Sialography, performed after resolution of the acute phase, will show a classic pattern of globular ductal ectasia. Ultrasonography will show small hypoechoic area. It may be necessary to rule out ductal calculi or possibly Sjögren syndrome.

The acute episode of recurrent parotitis is treated with antibiotics, heat, massage, and sialagogues. Dilatation of the ducts may be of some benefit in the acute phase. For long-term control, parotid duct ligation or tympanic neurectomy has been suggested. Rarely, superficial parotidectomy would need to be considered for extreme problems.

In addition to sialectasia, stricture from infections or duct trauma can lead to recurrent inflammation. Dilatation, possibly with incision of the duct and ductoplasty, may be helpful. Cystic fibrosis has been implicated in causing chronic enlargement of the submandibular glands.

Sjögren syndrome can occur in childhood as recurrent swelling. Steroids may be used as treatment. Biopsy of a minor salivary gland from the lip may aid in the diagnosis.

Granulomatous Disease

Tuberculosis (TB) or atypical mycobacterial infections can occur near both the parotid and submandibular glands. Atypical mycobacterial infections may be associated with a classic violaceous induration of the skin.

Mycobacterial infections produce painless masses that may mimic a neoplasm. A biopsy or fine-needle aspiration may be needed for accurate diagnosis. To rule out TB, analysis with a purified protein derivative and chest radiography is warranted. Culture results may take weeks or fail to show the growth of any organisms. Anti-TB antibiotics are warranted when results of cultures are positive.

Incision and drainage for a suspected abscess may cause a sinus tract (Fig. 31.2). Prolonged drainage would require serial curettage. Local superinfection with staphylococci can occur. When chronic infection produces a draining sinus of the submandibular area, gland excision may be the best way to promote healing. The surrounding inflammation of the skin places the marginal mandibular nerve at some risk of injury during gland resection. Clarithromycin and azithromycin may help to hasten resolution.

Catscratch disease, actinomycosis, brucellosis, and histoplasmosis can all produce granulomatous lesions of lymph nodes near the salivary glands or involving the glands themselves. Actinomycosis involves only one gland. It may lead to a sinus tract.

Sarcoidosis, particularly in patients of African descent, can cause a bilateral parotid swelling and involve the facial nerve. Chest radiography will demonstrate perihilar adenopathy. Treatment may require systemic steroids.

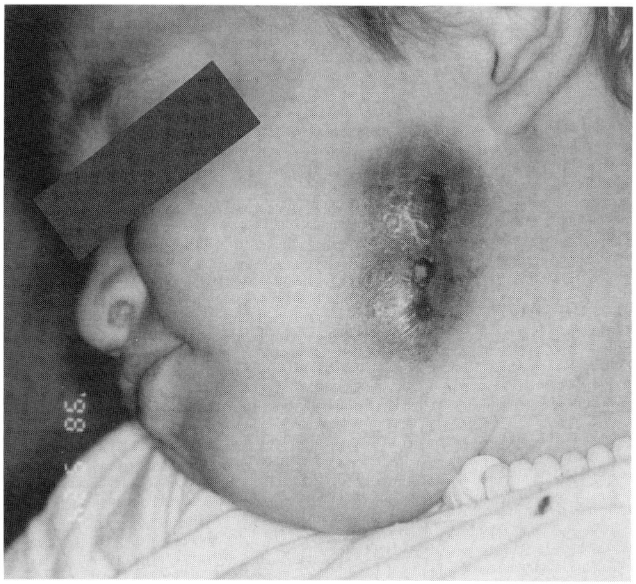

FIGURE 31.2. Draining sinuses from atypical mycobacterial infection.

Sialolithiasis

Calculi or stones in the salivary glands are uncommon in children. Classically, gland swelling occurs in conjunction with meals. The submandibular gland is most frequently involved for a number of reasons. The usual patient is a boy over 10 years of age. The stone is typically in a single gland. The need for bimanual palpation and dental occlusal films to aid in the diagnosis has already been mentioned. Most stones are near the duct orifice.

For stones near the orifice, stimulation of flow may allow passage of a small calculus from the duct. Dilatation may assist in this regard. Sialodochotomy, incising the duct over the stone, is the most common surgical treatment. During the procedure a ligature can be used to control the proximal portion of the duct. This prevents the stone from slipping in toward the gland. Stones near the hilum of the gland require submandibular gland excision.

Parotid duct stones may be managed by incision of the duct as well. Care must be taken to prevent injury to the buccal branch of the facial nerve. Because postoperative stricture is more likely in the parotid duct, stenting may be needed. If the stone cannot be removed intraorally, superficial parotidectomy may be needed.

Acquired Cysts

Parotid cysts can occur from recurrent sialoadenitis. Superficial parotidectomy may be needed. Polycystic disease is a rare condition from cysts arising from the intercalated ducts. The disease occurs in females, is bilateral, and is seen in the older child or young adult. Polycystic disease may be familial. Treatment is parotidectomy.

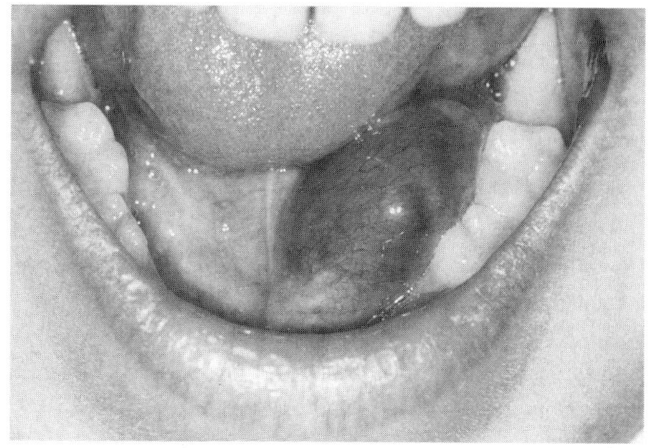

FIGURE 31.3. Ranula in the left floor of the mouth.

Parotid enlargement and lymphoepithelial cysts are features of infections involving human immunodeficiency virus in children. Uncomfortable or deforming cysts can be aspirated.

Ranulas are mucous retention cysts of the floor of the mouth arising in the sublingual glands (Fig. 31.3). They are thought to arise from ductal obstruction or trauma with salivary extravasation into the floor of the mouth. They may rupture spontaneously and recur. Ranulas appear as a painless, blue or translucent, unilateral swelling underneath the tongue. Plunging ranulas extend beyond the mylohyoid sling and appear in the neck. Plunging ranulas are thought to be pseudocysts from incomplete excision. For simple ranulas, marsupialization may be all that is needed. Excision requires removal of the adjacent sublingual gland to prevent recurrence. Meticulous hemostasis and protection of the lingual nerve and vessels as well as the submandibular duct will prevent complications. A plunging ranula may require a transcervical approach. Recurrent plunging ranulas may best be managed with transcervical excision, including the submandibular gland.

Mucoceles of the lower lip may be secondary to trauma to the minor salivary glands in this area. Because they can recur after removal, wide excision is needed to prevent this problem. Transient numbness on the same side of the lower lip is a common complication.

Trauma

A laceration of the parotid gland that is posterior to a vertical line drawn from the outer canthus of the eye and has associated facial weakness mandates nerve exploration. Epineural repair is required, possibly with nerve grafting to avoid tension on the nerve.

Involvement of the masseter muscle or saliva pooling in the wound indicates a laceration of the parotid duct. The duct can be ligated, rerouted, or repaired over a polyethylene tube stent. Stents should be used for at least 10 days. Failure to repair the duct leads to persistent salivary extravasation. Infection, obstructive cysts, abscess formation, or a draining sinus tract can be the result.

Drooling

Sialorrhea is rarely the result of excessive salivary production. Drooling is most common in those children with an underlying neurologic disease such as cerebral palsy or head injury. Medical therapy using agents like glycopyrrolate can help on a limited basis. The anticholinergic effects on bladder function limit their use. Correction of the causes of mouth breathing, such as adenotonsillar hypertrophy or chronic rhinitis, is the initial part of therapy.

If surgical therapy becomes warranted, several procedures can be considered. Wilkie and Brody described bilateral submandibular gland excision with parotid duct rerouting. Bilateral submandibular gland excision and parotid duct ligation has now become the procedure of choice. Bilateral parotid and submandibular duct ligation has recently been reported. Complications include facial swelling and pain, and parotitis.

There is a theoretical risk of ranula formation with submandibular duct ligation or rerouting. The sublingual ducts enter into the submandibular duct 1 cm from its orifice. If the sublingual ducts are injured, ranula will result.

Nerve injury and infection are risks associated with submandibular gland excision. Because only four of the major glands are addressed, a completely dry mouth is avoided. Some saliva is necessary for dental hygiene, comfort, and mastication and swallowing.

Benign Tumors

Most salivary gland neoplasms in children are located in the parotid gland. As previously discussed, tissue diagnosis is needed in the treatment of the solitary salivary mass. Fine-needle aspiration can be used to eliminate granulomatous diseases from the differential diagnosis. Knowing whether the mass is benign or malignant allows the surgeon, patient, and family to know ahead of time the extent of the proposed operation and whether the facial nerve can be preserved. CT and MRI will show whether the lesion is solely confined to the superficial lobe of the parotid gland. Frozen section diagnosis can be undertaken during surgery and may help with intraoperative decisions.

The most common nonvascular tumor of the salivary gland is pleomorphic adenoma. This presents as a slow-growing and freely mobile nodule. Patients typically present more than a year after the onset of the mass. The facial nerve is not involved. Because these tumors are encapsulated, superficial parotidectomy is the treatment of choice to avoid facial nerve injury and recurrence. Total parotidectomy is needed when the deep lobe is involved.

Less common benign lesions are Warthin's tumors, oncocytoma, and adenoma. Neurofibromas are rare but may involve the parotid or submandibular gland in those individuals with neurofibromatosis.

Malignant Tumors

Rapid growth of a firm salivary mass is highly suggestive of a malignancy. Malignancy also should be suspected in patients who present with pain, facial nerve involvement, or adenopathy. Thirty-five percent to 60% of pediatric salivary gland tumors are malignant.

Parotid neoplasms are less common in children than in adults but are more likely to be malignant. A firm parotid mass is 2.5 times as likely to be a malignancy in a child as in an adult. The parotid is the gland most frequently affected by malignancy. This is followed in frequency by the submandibular glands and the minor glands. These tumors tend to occur later in childhood, particularly mucoepidermoid carcinoma. The biologic behavior of salivary gland malignancies in children is similar to that in adults. Treatment recommendations are therefore similar. The guiding principle is that limited procedures increase the risk of recurrence.

As in adults, mucoepidermoid carcinoma is the most common salivary cancer in children. Acinic cell carcinomas, undifferentiated carcinomas, adenocarcinomas and adenoid cystic carcinomas follow in frequency. Squamous cell carcinoma is particularly rare.

Mucoepidermoid carcinoma is associated with slow growth and a risk of local recurrence. High-grade lesions are more locally aggressive and may recur or spread distantly. Total parotidectomy is indicated for high-grade and intermediate-grade tumors. Sacrifice of the facial nerve and radiation therapy may be indicated in the presence of perineural invasion. Low-grade mucoepidermoid and acinic cell tumors generally have a better prognosis than high-grade or histologically aggressive tumors.

Adenocarcinoma and adenoid cystic carcinoma are also best managed with total parotidectomy and facial nerve preservation. Radical neck dissection and radiation therapy should be considered with local cervical metastasis and in the face of recurrence.

Carcinomas involving the submandibular gland are treated by excision of the gland.

Radiation therapy in children carries the long-term risks of radiation-induced malignancies or effects on the growth of the child's face. These risks must be balanced by the benefits of preventing recurrence. Radiation therapy should be reserved for those children with facial nerve involvement, high-grade or histologically aggressive tumors, perineural invasion with adenoid cystic carcinoma, lymph node involvement, or with spread of disease to surrounding soft tissue.

Rhabdomyosarcoma and lymphoma are common pediatric head and neck tumors. They may present near the salivary glands. Detailed imaging studies should demonstrate that they are separate from the salivary glands so that appropriate biopsies and treatment can be initiated.

SURGICAL CONSIDERATIONS

Frank preoperative discussion with the patient's family about the risks and benefits of salivary surgery will allow realistic expectations about the results. The possibility of facial nerve injury, Frey's syndrome, scarring, or other cosmetic problems need to be brought to the attention of the family. Families need to be informed that there is a risk of recurrence when surgery is performed for tumors or on first branchial abnormalities.

Parotidectomy requires identification and protection of the facial nerve from surgical injury. The outer canthus of the eye and the commissure of the mouth should be visible in the surgical field. Intraoperative facial nerve monitoring is helpful and may be considered the standard of care in some localities. Monitors are available in most operating rooms. The surgeon should be familiar with the setup of the device and how to recognize recorded events. Monitors have electrodes to sense nerve stimulation and a probe to stimulate the nerve to confirm nerve integrity. One should avoid repeated intraoperative facial nerve stimulation that might fatigue the nerve.

The main trunk is located underneath the temporoparotid fascia, which runs from the tympanomastoid suture to the parotid gland. Once the nerve trunk is identified, the stimulator should be used to confirm the trunk. The branches of the pes anserinus can be followed until the lateral lobe is resected. At that point, the nerve stimulator should be used to confirm the integrity of each branch.

In some situations, such as after inflammation with subsequent scarring, the facial nerve trunk may be difficult to identify. Terminal nerve branches can be identified outside the gland and dissected back toward the trunk.

In infants and young children the mastoid may be underdeveloped and bony landmarks may be lacking. Additionally, in the very young patient the facial nerve is more superficial and the pes anserinus may be posterior to the mandible and outside the parotid gland.

Total parotidectomy may require sacrifice of some of the external carotid artery branches. The facial nerve can be gently retracted using vascular loops. The parotid duct is found during the procedure and should be ligated.

Frozen section diagnosis may help with intraoperative decision making, particularly if the facial nerve needs to be sacrificed. Preoperative discussion with the patient's family should be performed if nerve sacrifice is a consideration.

Meticulous hemostasis and gentle technique make nerve dissection easier and prevent postoperative hematoma or seroma. Bipolar cautery reduces the risk of injury to nerve branches. Active drains should be used at the end of the case. They are typically removed on the first postoperative day.

If there is facial nerve involvement, the nerve is cut at its trunk and at the terminal branches. The nerve ends are tagged to allow for identification and immediate microanastomosis of a graft. The sural nerve or the contralateral greater auricular nerve is used. Frozen section biopsies of the severed nerve endings are needed to assure that there is no residual tumor in the nerve stumps.

In the event of facial nerve injury or sacrifice there are several treatment options. Immediate nerve grafting or repair of nerve endings will give the best result in nerve regeneration. Protection of the cornea from drying may require patching, ophthalmic ointment, or lubricating eye drops. Nerve grafting, facial nerve–hypoglossal nerve hookup, fascial slings, and tarsorrhaphy are among the possible rehabilitative procedures that may be considered. Detailed discussion of the management of the paralyzed face is beyond the scope of this chapter.

The complications of parotidectomy include facial nerve injury, which is more likely to occur with total parotidectomy than with superficial parotidectomy. Temporary paresis from traction on the nerve should resolve. Gustatory sweating (Frey's syndrome) has been demonstrated in 50% of children who undergo parotidectomy. Cosmetic deformities such as hypertrophic scar, uneven ears, or facial asymmetry also have been reported.

Seromas or hematomas can be prevented with drains and pressure dressings. They may become infected or affect the viability of the skin flap. Temporary or permanent numbness to the ear lobe can occur from sacrifice of the greater auricular nerve. Salivary fistula is possible if the parotid duct was not ligated during the procedure.

Surgery to the submandibular gland may risk injury to the marginal mandibular nerve, lingual nerve, or hypoglossal nerve. A nerve monitor with electrode placement at the oral commissure can help with marginal mandibular nerve protection. Meticulous care to identify all vital structures will prevent injury to the lingual and hypoglossal nerves. Drains should prevent the complication from subcutaneous fluid collections. Hypertrophic scar is an additional possibility.

When serial curettage fails to resolve mycobacterial involvement of lymph nodes near salivary glands, gland removal may need to be considered. The friable, inflamed tissues cause poor definition of tissue planes. This results in a more difficult surgical dissection and increases the risk of nerve injury.

SUGGESTED READINGS

Cunningham MJ. Tumors of the head and neck. In: Bluestone CD, Stool SE, eds. *Atlas of pediatric otolaryngology.* Philadelphia: WB Saunders, 1995:529–571.

Myer C, Cotton RT. Salivary gland disease in children: a review. Part 1: Acquired non–neoplastic disease. *Pediatrics* 1986;25: 314–322.

Meyer C, Cotton RT. Salivary gland disease in children: a review. Part 2: Congenital lesions and neoplastic disease. *Pediatrics* 1986;25: 353–357.

Schuller DE, McCabe BF. Salivary gland neoplasms in children. *Otolaryngol Clin North Am* 1977;10:399–412.

Shikhani AH, Johns ME. Tumors of the major salivary glands in children. *Head Neck Surg* 1988;10:257–263.

Shott SR. Salivary disease in children. In: Cotton RT, Myer CM, eds. *Practical pediatric otolaryngology.* Philadelphia: Lippincott-Raven, 1999:693–710.

Siebert RW. Diseases of the salivary glands. In: Bluestone CD, Stool SE, Kenna MA, eds. *Pediatric otolaryngology, 3rd ed.* Philadelphia: WB Saunders, 1996:1093–1107.

Wilkie TF, Brody GS. The surgical treatment of drooling. *Plast Reconstr Surg* 1977;59:791–798.

Work WP. Cysts and congenital lesions of the parotid gland. *Otolaryngol Clin North Am* 1977;10:339–343.

32

TORTICOLLIS

PETER MATTEI

Torticollis is a term that refers to an unnatural tilted or turned position of the head. Although there are many potential causes, including adenitis, vertebral anomalies, and oculomotor abnormalities, the most common form is the result of unilateral shortening of the sternocleidomastoid muscle. It typically affects otherwise healthy newborns and the cause is unknown. Although once felt to be due primarily to birth trauma, it is now thought to rarely be the result of a traumatic injury to the muscle or its innervation. Pediatric surgeons are frequently consulted to aid in the diagnosis and treatment of the disorder, although therapy is primarily nonsurgical and the overall prognosis is quite good.

DIAGNOSIS

The typical newborn with torticollis is otherwise healthy and presents to the pediatric general surgeon in one of two ways. The classic presentation is that of a 1- to 2-month-old child who is noted by the mother or primary physician to preferentially turn his or her head to one side. The child may not be able to turn his head in the other direction despite all attempts to compel him to; in fact, there may be resistance to turning the head if an adult attempts to do so by force. The head is typically tilted to the side opposite the affected muscle, consistent with the expected function of the sternocleidomastoid muscle to bring the ipsilateral ear down toward the shoulder and forward toward the chest. On physical examination, the infant has limited range of motion of the head and neck to passive stretch. The degree of limitation should be documented for follow-up purposes. The sternocleidomastoid muscle often is foreshortened and taut, and there may a palpable thickening in the midportion of the muscle.

The second most common presentation is that of a newborn infant who is noted to have a cervical mass. The mass represents a fibrous "tumor" within the sternocleidomastoid muscle that is frequently associated with torticollis (*fibromatosis colli*). These infants may be too young to demonstrate true torticollis on casual observation. On physical examination, the mass is firm, nontender, and relatively fixed, although it may be slightly mobile in the anteroposterior plane. The differential diagnosis includes enlarged lymph node, branchial cleft cyst, and neoplasm. Although the location of the mass within the muscle is often evident on physical examination and essentially cinches the diagnosis, further studies may be necessary for more complete confirmation. An ultrasonographic examination performed by an experienced pediatric sonographer is the best study to rule out other diagnoses and establish the characteristic appearance of the fibrous mass associated with torticollis. Although the mass may be detectable by computed tomography and magnetic resonance imaging, these studies are unnecessary and expose the patient to the risks of radiation and anesthesia.

Some patients present to the pediatric neurosurgeon with plagiocephaly, or skull asymmetry caused by flattening of the posterior skull on one side. This is thought to be due to molding of the skull due to pressure placed on the one side during sleep. A child with torticollis who sleeps on his back will preferentially rest his head on the side opposite the torticollis. The flattening affects the entire skull, which assumes a rhomboid shape when viewed from above. Some patients respond to therapy with a custom-made plastic helmet that is worn during sleep. There is also a 10% incidence of congenital hip dysplasia in infants with torticollis.

TREATMENT

Once the diagnosis has been confirmed by physical examination or ultrasonography, a treatment plan is discussed with the parents. The parents should be reassured that the mass does not represent a malignant tumor, the long-term results of therapy are very good, and the babies usually develop otherwise normally. On the other hand, it needs to be emphasized to them that inadequate or delayed treatment can result in significant and irreversible deformity.

P. Mattei: Department of Surgery, Thomas Jefferson University, Philadelphia, Pennsylvania; and Department of Pediatric Surgery, Alfred I. duPont Hospital for Children, Wilmington, Delaware.

The mainstay of therapy is a passive stretch exercise regimen that the parents perform several times a day for several months. I prefer to refer the families to a qualified and experienced physical therapist who can demonstrate the proper techniques and assist in assuring vigilant follow-up. I follow patients in the surgery office initially at monthly intervals and then, if improvement is evident, at less frequent intervals. Most infants with motivated caregivers and close follow-up show definite signs of improvement within the first 2 months. It is important to remember, however, that some babies will probably improve without therapy, whereas others will progress despite the diligent and well-intentioned efforts of the family.

Surgical therapy is indicated for infants who develop facial hemihypoplasia. This is a curious phenomenon whereby the chronic and persistent tilting of the head to one side results in atrophy of the facial musculature and hypoplasia of the skeleton of the face. It can cause considerable facial asymmetry and distortion that may be irreversible. Although hemihypoplasia is felt by some clinicians to be the only indication for surgical intervention, persistent or worsening torticollis that does not improve after 9 months to a year of nonoperative therapy is also considered by some clinicians to be an indication for surgery.

SURGICAL TECHNIQUE

The surgical treatment of torticollis involves dividing the sternocleidomastoid muscle on the involved side. The patient is under general anesthesia and placed in a supine position. A small bump is placed under the shoulders, and the head is extended in the midline or turned slightly away from the operative site. A transverse incision is made directly over the inferior portion of the sternocleidomastoid muscle, preferably in a skin crease. The platysma is divided, and subplatysmal flaps are elevated to expose the sternocleidomastoid muscle. The muscle is then dissected circumferentially, with care to avoid injury to the carotid sheath structures. The muscle can be divided with electrocautery. It may be best to excise a portion of the muscle to prevent recurrence due to scarring. It is also important to adequately divide the external investing fascia within which the sternocleidomastoid muscle resides, because these fibers also may be fibrotic and foreshortened and contribute to the torticollis. The limits of the dissection are the anterior border of the trapezius muscle posteriorly and the midline anteriorly. In severe cases, the deeper fascia is involved and should also be carefully divided.

Hemostasis must be addressed meticulously. It is not necessary to excise the fibrotic tumor, if one is still present. The investing fascia is not approximated, but the platysma and skin should be closed as separate layers with absorbable suture. Placement of a drain is unnecessary.

Other treatments, including injection of botulinum toxin, sternocleidomastoid lengthening procedures, and endoscopic approaches to division of the muscle, have been described and may eventually prove to be superior to the standard approach. However, further intermediate- and long-range studies need to be conducted before these treatments can be recommended on a routine basis.

POSTOPERATIVE CARE AND FOLLOW-UP

Infants rarely have significant pain after the operation, and most can be treated on an outpatient basis. Diet is advanced as tolerated, and activity is not restricted. A less vigorous passive stretching exercise program can resume in 3 to 4 days and may prevent recurrence due to scarring. The risks of wound infection and bleeding are quite low. With meticulous technique and limited dissection, the risk of injury to the sensory nerves of the neck or the spinal accessory nerve should be negligible. The incision typically heals well with minimal scarring.

Division of the sternocleidomastoid muscle causes negligible functional impairment. The results are usually immediately apparent to the families, and the long-term results are quite good. Facial hemihypoplasia that was present before surgery might improve over time but may never resolve completely. In fact, the hemihypoplasia will sometimes become more apparent after surgery because the face, now being held in a more natural position, is better assessed for symmetry by the observer.

Patients are followed at 2 to 3 weeks after surgery for assessment of the wound, and then at 2 months and at 6 months for signs of recurrence.

In summary, torticollis is an uncommon problem that resolves without surgery in most cases. In fact, the operation should rarely be done and is reserved only for severe cases that result in facial hemihypoplasia.

SUGGESTED READINGS

Celayir AC. Congenital muscular torticollis: early and intensive treatment is critical. A prospective study. *Pediatr Int* 2000;42:504–507.

Cheng JC, Tang SP, Chen TM. Sternocleidomastoid pseudotumor and congenital muscular torticollis in infants: a prospective study of 510 cases. *J Pediatr* 1999;134:712–716.

Cheng JC, Wong MW, Tang SP, et al. Clinical determinants of the outcome of manual stretching in the treatment of congenital muscular torticollis in infants. A prospective study of eight hundred and twenty-one cases. *J Bone Joint Surg [Am]* 2001;83:679–687.

Golden KA, Beals SP, Littlefield TR, et al. Sternocleidomastoid imbalance versus congenital muscular torticollis: their relationship to positional plagiocephaly. *Cleft Palate Craniofac J* 1999;36:256–261.

Illingworth RS. Why blame the obstetrician? A review. *BMJ* 1979;1: 797–801.

Lawrence WT, Azizkhan RG. Congenital muscular torticollis: a spectrum of pathology. *Ann Plast Surg* 1989;23:523–530.

Porter SB, Blount BW. Pseudotumor of infancy and congenital muscular torticollis. *Am Fam Physician* 1995;52:1731–1736.

Stassen LF, Kerawala CJ. New surgical technique for the correction of congenital muscular torticollis (wry neck). *Br J Oral Maxillofac Surg* 2000;38:142–147.

Wei JL, Schwartz KM, Weaver AL, et al. Pseudotumor of infancy and congenital muscular torticollis: 170 cases. *Laryngoscope* 2001;111 (Part 1):688–695.

SECTION

V

ESOPHAGUS

33

ESOPHAGEAL ATRESIA AND TRACHEOESOPHAGEAL FISTULA

JEAN-MARTIN LABERGE

ESOPHAGEAL ATRESIA

Diagnosis

Esophageal atresia (EA) may be suspected on prenatal sonography by the absence of a gastric bubble, polyhydramnios, and distension of the upper esophagus during swallowing. After birth, a child with EA presents with excessive salivation, mucus coming out of the mouth or nose, and noisy breathing with episodes of choking or cyanosis. These symptoms worsen if oral feedings are attempted. Diagnosis is confirmed when a 10 French Replogle tube passed through the mouth or nose stops at about 10 cm. Smaller or more flexible catheters should be avoided because they can coil in the upper esophagus and give a false impression of esophageal patency. Anteroposterior and lateral radiographs that include the neck, chest, and abdomen (a "babygram") are then obtained while gentle pressure is maintained on the Replogle and 10 mL of air is injected through it. This delineates very well the location of the upper pouch in relation to the vertebral bodies. Contrast studies are not indicated and can lead to aspiration.

The radiograph is crucial in several ways:

1. The presence of abdominal gas confirms a distal fistula (~85% of cases), whereas its absence usually indicates a pure atresia.
2. The Replogle tip should project over C7 to T2; an abnormally high or low blockage may indicate pharyngeal or esophageal perforation rather than atresia, especially in a premature baby and when associated with blood-tinged return from the Replogle. In such circumstances, contrast studies are indicated, using 1 mL or less of a nonionic, isoosmotic, water-soluble agent.
3. Anomalies of vertebrae or ribs can be detected.
4. Cardiac malformations or a right aortic arch may be suspected.
5. The pattern of abdominal gas excludes a duodenal atresia.
6. The lungs are assessed for pneumonia, which usually occurs in the upper lobes and is related to a delay in diagnosis, and for respiratory distress syndrome (RDS) when the child is premature.

The initial diagnosis may have been made at another hospital before the neonate is transferred to a tertiary care pediatric center. During transfer, it is important to keep the baby warm, to keep the head elevated with the Replogle on continuous suction, to monitor O_2 saturation, and to give supplemental oxygen as required. On physical examination, one will assess the pulmonary status and look for signs of associated malformations such as cardiac, anal, limb, and chromosomal anomalies. A scaphoid abdomen suggests the diagnosis of a pure atresia. Thirty-five percent to 50% of infants with EA have other anomalies (Table 33.1). In about 10%, these occur in associations such as the VACTERL syndrome (abnormalities of vertebrae, anus, cardiovascular system, trachea, esophagus, renal system, and limb buds) or, less frequently, the CHARGE syndrome (coloboma of the eye, heart defects, atresia of the choanae, renal anomalies and retardation of growth or development, genital anomalies, and ear abnormalities or deafness).

Preoperative Preparation

We routinely obtain a complete blood count; assess levels of electrolytes, glucose, blood urea nitrogen, and creatinine; and send a specimen to be crossmatched for blood. Preoperative echocardiography and renal sonography are useful but can be performed postoperatively if the baby clinically demonstrates normal cardiac and renal function. Ampicillin and gentamicin are given preoperatively.

When life-threatening anomalies are suspected, it is wise to postpone surgery until appropriate investigations and consultations are obtained. Examples are trisomy 13 or 18, anuria, or suspicion of a complex cardiac malformation. In other cases, the operation should not be delayed because aspiration may occur from reflux of gastric secretions through the

J-M. Laberge: Department of Surgery, McGill University; and Department of Surgery, Division of Pediatric General Surgery, Montreal Children's Hospital, Montreal, Quebec, Canada.

TABLE 33.1. ASSOCIATED ANOMALIES

System	%
Cardiovascular	20–30
VSD, ASD, tetralogy of Fallot, PDA, coarctation	
Gastrointestinal	15–25
Imperforate anus, duodenal atresia, malrotation, Meckel's diverticulum, distal esophageal stenosis	
Genito-urinary	10–20
Hydronephrosis, renal agenesis, hypospadias, undescended testis	
Musculoskeletal	10–15
Extremity malformations, vertebral anomalies, hip dysplasia	
Craniofacial/CNS	5–10
Cleft lip/palate, dysmorphism, eye anomalies, spina bifida, hydrocephalus	
Chromosomal	3–5
Trisomy 21, 18, Turner's syndrome	
Respiratory tract (excluding tracheomalacia)	3–5
Lung hypoplasia/agenesis, choanal atresia, laryngeal web	
Miscellaneous	1
Omphalocele, CHARGE	

Only the most frequently associated anomalies are listed; many others have been described.

distal tracheoesophageal fistula (TEF). Even in premature babies with RDS, it is generally preferable to operate as soon as possible instead of waiting for the lungs to improve. These neonates usually get worse before they start to improve, with the risk that poor lung compliance will cause more of each tidal volume to escape through the fistula into the stomach. It then becomes impossible to maintain adequate ventilation, and gastric distension and perforation can occur. In such cases, a catheter may have to be placed at the bedside to decompress the pneumoperitoneum. Ideally, the distal TEF is controlled before one reaches that point.

Operative Approach

Intravenous access and monitoring devices are secured while hypothermia is prevented with heating lamps and a warming pad. We prefer to perform a rigid bronchoscopy before proceeding with the operation. We use a rigid ventilating bronchoscope with a Hopkins rod-lens telescope attached to a video camera, monitor, and videotape recorder. Once the child is asleep and intubated, and the anesthesiologist is ready, the surgeon places the bronchoscope to visualize the cords; the endotracheal tube is slowly removed, and the scope is advanced through the cords down to the level of the carina. The site of the distal fistula is clearly seen, and the presence of a proximal fistula can be eliminated. The side of the aortic arch can usually be appreciated from the pulsations transmitted through the tracheal wall. The scope is withdrawn slowly and then removed when the anesthesiologist is ready to reintubate. The whole procedure takes less than 5 minutes; everyone in the room can see, and the procedure is recorded for later review. We consider bronchoscopy essential in all patients suspected of a pure atresia, because these are treated with an initial feeding gastrostomy, followed by a delayed primary esophageal anastomosis 2 to 3 months later. There are reports that 10% or more of babies diagnosed with a pure EA by the absence of gastrointestinal gas have a *proximal* TEF; this results in recurrent aspirations and pneumonias during the 2- to 3-month waiting period. Furthermore, there have been reports of infants in whom small distal fistulas were obstructed by mucus.

After bronchoscopy, patients with pure EA undergo a gastrostomy through a midline epigastric incision. Because the stomach has not been distended by swallowed amniotic fluid, it is smaller and thinner than normal, making this operation more of a challenge than usual. The surgeon also has to decide which of the lesser or greater curvature he or she favors should esophageal replacement become necessary, although in our experience, a delayed primary esophageal anastomosis can be achieved in most cases.

In patients with EA–distal TEF, the bronchoscopy remains useful to (a) eliminate a proximal TEF, which could be missed during repair; (b) eliminate other malformations such as a laryngeal web, subglottic stenosis, or laryngotracheoesophageal cleft (LTEC); and (c) evaluate the site of the distal TEF. In the latter instance, if one sees a trifurcation fistula (a TEF at the carina) and the Replogle blocks at C7, the surgeon knows that it will be a "long-gap" atresia and will prepare for it accordingly. In such cases, we would position and prepare the baby with a free arm drape and include the neck in the sterile field; this allows mobilization of the upper pouch through a cervical incision and easier performance of circular or spiral esophageal myotomies.

The only situation where the risk of bronchoscopy may outweigh its benefits is in a premature baby with severe RDS. We prefer to perform a quick transpleural thoracotomy with control of the fistula; alternatively, if the baby does not even tolerate the lateral decubitus position, we have successfully occluded the fistula by passing a 6 or 8 French Foley catheter through a gastrostomy. Alternatively, some surgeons advocate placement of a Fogarty catheter in the fistula under bronchoscopic control as a method of blocking the fistula.

After bronchoscopy, the patient with EA-TEF is placed in the left lateral decubitus position with the right arm extended and a roll placed under the left chest. We use a limited posterolateral thoracotomy incision along the skin lines with the aim of entering the chest in the fourth intercostal space. The latissimus dorsi is divided, but the serratus anterior is simply reflected off the chest wall. The intercostal muscles are carefully divided to keep the pleura intact. We prefer an extrapleural dissection when possible; if a small postoperative anastomotic leak occurs (up to 5%–10% incidence), it can seal spontaneously without the risk of empyema. The dissection is begun posteriorly with a wet "peanut," then extended with a finger dissection or by gradually introducing a wet gauze into the extrapleural space. The areas where the pleura will most often tear during dissection are anteriorly, especially if the ribs are spread too rapidly before the dissection is completed, and posteriorly once the mediastinum is reached, in the area between the azygos vein and the distal esophagus.

The arch of the azygos vein is then divided between ties. The distal esophagus can usually be found just below this level, and it enters the trachea just above it in most instances. Identification of the vagus nerve and observation of air distending the esophagus confirms its position. Palpation is important to confirm the position of the trachea, mainstem bronchi, and aorta. A Silastic vessel loop is passed around the distal esophagus near its junction with the trachea after meticulous blunt dissection. Care is taken to avoid damage to the vascular and nervous supply to the lower esophagus. With a small amount of cephalad dissection and more fingertip palpation, the junction between the fistula and trachea becomes clear. The fistula is divided stepwise and closed with interrupted 5-0 synthetic resorbable sutures. This should be done close enough to the trachea to avoid leaving a diverticulum, while not causing tracheal stenosis. The area is then checked for air leaks before proceeding with identification of the proximal pouch.

The upper pouch is easy to see after the anesthesiologist is asked to gently push on the Replogle tube. A stay suture is then placed at the apex of the proximal pouch. With sharp and blunt dissection and gentle use of the cautery, the upper pouch is mobilized circumferentially. It often seems to share a common wall with the posterior part of the trachea in its lower portion. After the first 1 or 2 cm, the dissection usually becomes easier unless there is a proximal fistula. Because the upper pouch is thicker and better vascularized than the lower esophagus, it can be dissected as far as the pharynx if necessary.

The anastomosis is usually performed under some tension, yet heals adequately in most cases. If the two ends cannot be approximated after full mobilization of the upper pouch, available options include careful mobilization of the distal esophagus while maintaining its blood supply and upper pouch circular or spiral myotomy (allows a gain of 1–1.5 cm). If the two ends still do not meet after this, it is probably safer not to attempt an anastomosis, although some surgeons elect to mobilize the stomach through the hiatus or elongate the lower esophagus by creating a lesser curve gastric tube with the use of staplers (Collis-type). The more frequently used options are to close the lower esophagus and then: (a) tack it to the prevertebral fascia under some tension, (b) tack it to the upper pouch with the use of a heavy through-and-through silk suture, or (c) place pledgeted traction sutures on both upper and lower pouches, bring these out through the chest wall below and above the incision, and reapply traction daily. In the first case the child is fed by gastrostomy, allowing the lower esophagus to hypertrophy and elongate by the action of gastroesophageal reflux (GER), and perform an anastomosis 8 to 12 weeks later. The second option, called the suture-fistula technique, often results in a spontaneous fistula that can be dilated without the need for reoperation; otherwise a resection of the area and end-to-end anastomosis is required, usually under little tension. This technique should probably not be used in small premature babies because poor tissue healing may lead to fistulization to the mediastinum or pleural space with septic complications. The third option discussed, apparently allows a primary anastomosis to be achieved within one to two weeks.

Let us return to the "usual" anastomosis under mild or moderate tension. If the two ends can be brought in contact with the use of DeBakey forceps, then the distal esophagus is inspected and gently dilated with a fine hemostat to ensure an adequate lumen. There can be cartilage remnants in the wall of the lower esophagus close to the trachea, and occasionally one must resect a few millimeters of distal esophagus. A transverse opening is then made in the upper pouch. Two corner sutures of 4-0 or 5-0 synthetic resorbable sutures are placed in the full thickness of either end, so that the knots will be on the outside, but these are not yet tied. The posterior row of three or four sutures are placed with the knots inside the lumen to facilitate placement and tying. One must be careful during placement of the sutures, first because the mucosa tends to retract, and second to avoid trauma to the esophageal wall. With the posterior row in place, gradual tension is applied on all sutures, while the proximal and distal segments of the esophagus are brought in apposition with DeBakey forceps. The posterior and corner sutures are tied, the Replogle tube is gently advanced through the anastomosis and into the stomach to check distal esophageal patency, and the anastomosis is completed with four or five interrupted sutures with the knots on the outside. The tube is then withdrawn to 1 cm above the anastomosis and marked by the anesthesiologist. Air is injected through the tube after the anastomosis is placed under saline to detect leaks. Mediastinal tissue, pleura, or azygos vein are used to cover the tracheal side of the fistula. A small extrapleural chest tube is usually placed close to the anastomosis and tacked in the desired position with a catgut suture. This is connected to a sealed drainage system to prevent an extrapleural pneumothorax. The thoracotomy is closed in layers, avoiding excessively tight pericostal sutures that can lead to overlapping or fused ribs. It should be noted that some surgeons replace the Replogle tube during the anastomosis with a Silastic nasogastric tube, which is used for postoperative feeding; the chest tube is avoided by some surgeons in full-term babies with an "easy" anastomosis.

The patient is transferred intubated to the neonatal unit. Premature extubation with subsequent reintubation can lead to anastomotic disruption from neck hyperextension or inadvertent esophageal intubation. It should be noted that, throughout the operation, desaturations may occur, requiring the anesthesiologist to reexpand the right lung from time to time.

Postoperative Care and Complications

The patient is managed by a team approach that includes the surgeon, neonatologist, nurses, and respiratory therapists. In a near-term baby with an uncomplicated anastomosis, the anesthetic effects are allowed to wear off and extubation is achieved within 24 hours. Fentanyl is used for postoperative pain, either by boluses or a continuous drip. Some clinicians prefer to keep the child heavily sedated or even paralyzed for a few days, especially when the anastomosis has been performed under a lot of tension; extubation is then delayed for several days. Neck flexion also has been advocated to decrease tension on the anastomosis. We keep the Replogle tube above the anastomosis and under continuous suction. Parenteral nutrition is started as soon as possible.

The extrapleural chest tube is kept on underwater seal drainage, with gentle suction (5–10 cm H_2O) added for the first 24 hours. Usually only a minimal amount of serous drainage is noted. In a stable, extubated baby, we obtain a contrast esophagram and upper gastrointestinal series under fluoroscopy 5 to 7 days postoperatively. We usually start this study with a nonionic, isoosmolar, water-soluble agent, then switch to dilute barium if there is no aspiration or anastomotic leak. We observe the swallowing reflex, esophageal motility, anastomotic site, and distal esophagus. Then, if the baby is tolerating the procedure well, we fill the stomach enough to look for GER and assess gastric emptying and the position of the ligament of Treitz. It is normal for the esophageal anastomosis to appear narrowed and for the upper esophagus to appear dilated, but there should be no stasis. As long as there is no leak and good swallowing, feedings are initiated after this study, which help to gradually dilate the anastomosis and lower esophagus. The chest tube is removed the next day and the antibiotics are stopped. Feedings often progress slowly because of poor sucking or swallowing reflexes.

The infant is discharged when feeding well and gaining weight. Parents are warned about the signs of complications such as GER, tracheomalacia, anastomotic stricture, and recurrent fistula. Patients are followed up frequently in the first year of life, and then once or twice a year at least until school age, preferably until adulthood. It is important to explain to the parents that there will be some permanent scarring at the anastomosis, which prevents normal distensibility of the esophagus at this site. We therefore recommend pureed food up to 12 to 18 months, and then only minced food until 5 years of age when the child has learned to chew well before swallowing, and has adequate teeth to do so. All those caring for such children have seen patients admitted with an impacted foreign body at the anastomotic site despite normal appearance of the anastomosis. This may be food, often a piece of meat, or a foreign body.

Although most full-term babies do well after EA repair, some going home before 1 week of age, the potential complications are numerous. These can be related to associated problems such as prematurity and cardiac defects, or to the malformation itself and its treatment. Our discussion will focus on the latter. These may be divided roughly into early (<30 days), intermediate (1–3 months), and late complications (Table 33.2).

Anastomotic leaks occur in 5% to 10% of cases and can be suspected by the presence of frothy saliva in the chest tube drainage. Small extrapleural leaks that are well drained by the tube are treated with continued upper pouch suctioning and antibiotics because most seal spontaneously. Some surgeons even start feedings despite a leak, but we prefer to wait until radiologic evidence of resolution. A large pleural effusion or massive pneumothorax is usually caused by a large leak or a total anastomotic disruption; breakdown of the tracheal suture line also should be considered. The child may deteriorate rapidly and need more chest tubes and a thoracotomy. If the baby is not acutely ill, we perform a contrast study; extravasation of most of the contrast agent indicates the need for thoracotomy, whereas a smaller, well-drained leak can be treated nonoperatively. When thoracotomy is required, it is sometimes possible to simply repair the dehiscence, but only if the tissues appear healthy and if reanastomosis can be achieved with minimal tension; otherwise, it is safer to ligate the distal end and create a cervical esophagostomy and a gastrostomy, with repair delayed for some months. Surgeons should beware of anastomotic stenoses, which often develop within a few weeks after a leak.

TABLE 33.2. COMPLICATIONS OF ESOPHAGEAL ATRESIA REPAIR

Type	Timing	Rough Incidence of Significant/Symptomatic Complication
Anastomotic leak (+/– pneumothorax, empyema)	Early	5%
Anastomotic dehiscence	Early	1%
Recurrent fistula	Early	3–5%
Anastomotic stenosis	Early/intermediate	5–8%
Swallowing incoordination, aspiration, poor suck	Early/intermediate	5% + (higher in prematures)
Tracheomalacia	Early/intermediate	5–10%
Gastroesophageal reflux	Intermediate/late	30–50% (most treated medically)
Recurrent pneumonia/bronchitis/asthma	Intermediate/late	10–30%
Failure to thrive	Intermediate/late	10–20%
Scoliosis and chest wall deformities	Late	<5%

Patients who develop recurrent coughing, choking, apneic episodes, pneumonia, and vomiting or regurgitation present a diagnostic challenge. Choking during feedings may indicate a recurrent or missed fistula, tracheomalacia, esophageal stenosis, or swallowing incoordination with aspiration. Choking after feedings, with or without vomiting, is usually a manifestation of GER. The contrast esophagram with videofluoroscopy is the first and most important investigation. It is crucial for the surgeon and radiologist to cooperate on this study in order to evaluate swallowing coordination and esophageal motility. The patient is bottle fed initially to study the full progression of the contrast medium.

Tracheal narrowing may occur at the tracheal suture line or with *tracheomalacia*, most often at the level of the upper pouch. This often can be diagnosed on the lateral views. The tracheal diameter is evaluated during inspiration and expiration and with a bolus of swallowed contrast material.

A distal congenital stenosis may be difficult to differentiate from an acquired one due to reflux. If seen early and not responding to balloon dilations, it is more likely to be congenital and is likely to require resection. In order to evaluate the presence of GER, the rate of gastric emptying, and the position of the ligament of Treitz, more contrast may be required. If the baby is unable to swallow enough contrast material, a small feeding tube can be inserted gently under fluoroscopic control.

A recurrent TEF may be difficult to demonstrate. This study is best performed with the patient in the prone position, injecting the contrast through the feeding tube under pressure as it is gradually withdrawn from the lower esophagus.

Depending on the results of radiologic investigations, the precise symptoms, and their severity, further tests may be required. Bronchoscopy is the best procedure to evaluate fistula recurrence and the presence of a tracheal diverticulum at the fistula site. The bronchoscopy can be performed simply as a diagnostic procedure or as part of the definitive operation if the problem has been identified by the contrast study. When tracheomalacia is severe and is associated with "dying spells" (apnea and cyanosis during feeding or following a crying spell), aortopexy is indicated. Bronchoscopy is useful before, during, and after this procedure to assess the tracheal lumen. To confirm tracheomalacia, the tracheoscopy is performed with the patient breathing spontaneously under light general anesthesia, because the collapsed lumen is most obvious during expiration. Rare patients with diffuse tracheobronchomalacia may require more than a simple aortopexy. The reported incidence of severe tracheomalacia requiring aortopexy varies from 2.5% to more than 10%. This wide variation is explained in part by the fact that some patients in the past died without a diagnosis, or were treated by prolonged intubation or tracheostomy awaiting spontaneous improvement. Surgeons are now more aggressive with aortopexy, which is safe and effective. It is interesting to note that tracheomalacia is unusual in cases of pure EA, but there is no clear explanation for this observation. Another important point is that tracheomalacia may manifest itself early by the inability to extubate the child, with CO_2 retention as the child starts to breathe spontaneously, or it may become symptomatic much later, even a few weeks after discharge.

Fistula recurrence is a serious complication that can lead to death; aggressive investigation with fluoroscopy and bronchoscopy are essential. The identification and surgical repair of a recurrent fistula can be facilitated by the insertion of a ureteral catheter at bronchoscopy. The traditional approach is a repeat right thoracotomy, transpleural division of the fistula, and interposition of healthy tissue such as an intercostal pedicle or a pericardial flap. Some surgeons have approached this problem through a left thoracotomy or by means of a transtracheal repair. Less invasive ways to obliterate the fistula by bronchoscopy with laser, electrocoagulation, or synthetic glue and sclerosing agents are associated with a higher recurrence rate.

Gastroesophageal reflux may present with vomiting, recurrent pneumonia, asthma, failure to thrive, or stenosis of the lower esophagus or at the site of anastomosis. Evaluation should include an extended study performed with the tip of the pH probe in the midesophagus to pick up only the more significant refluxes, since nearly all EA patients have some degree of GER. Because of this, we liberally prescribe drugs to inhibit acid production and help motility in any patient presenting with symptoms suggestive of GER.

Fundoplication is required in 5% to 20% of patients after EA repair. The indications include life-threatening events, recurrent esophageal stenosis refractory to dilations, and failure of medical treatment. Fundoplication is more complicated in these patients. The esophagus is often short, the gastroesophageal junction having been pulled up into the chest at the time of esophageal repair. Because of abnormal esophageal peristalsis, the wrap is associated with a higher risk of causing a mechanical obstruction. Therefore, some clinicians suggest that a partial fundoplication (Thal, Toupet) is indicated because it may be less likely to result in significant dysphagia.

Symptomatic *anastomotic stenosis* often results from a leak; it also can be related to reflux or to an anastomosis constructed under extreme tension. Most stenoses can be treated with balloon dilation, which is the method preferred by most pediatric surgeons. It is thought to be safer, and is usually performed under fluoroscopy in the radiology suite, without general anesthesia. Failure to respond to repeated dilations over a period of several weeks despite appropriate treatment of associated reflux indicates the need for surgical correction. With proven GER, we usually perform a fundoplication first, then resect the anastomotic stricture if it recurs after two or three more dilatations.

Multiple simultaneous complications can occur in the same patient. The treatment sequence is based on a judgment of which is most life-threatening. Most infants after EA repair have abnormal esophageal peristalsis, some degree of GER, and tracheomalacia. When life-threatening symptoms are present, a careful history and appropriate investigation help decide what should be addressed first. In a child who had severe hypoxic spells associated with feeding or crying, and radiologic results showing both GER and tracheomalacia, we would perform a bronchoscopy to exclude a recurrent or missed fistula and would be prepared to perform an aortopexy during the same anesthesia if severe tracheomalacia was confirmed (i.e., apposition of the posterior and anterior tracheal walls during expiration).

Long-Term Results and Prognosis

Patients who are discharged from the hospital after successful restoration of esophageal continuity are often considered "cured." There is a general impression that feeding and respiratory problems completely disappear after a few years. Although it is true that most patients tend not to complain, and are reluctant to return for yearly follow-ups, one must be aware of the potential problems. Late mortality may occur from associated anomalies and from complications of the disease, or its treatment. In infants with a smooth initial course, unexpected death may result from tracheomalacia or food impaction in the esophagus. A surprisingly high incidence (>1%) of sudden infant death syndrome is noted in several large series, which gives some support to the theory of an immaturity of vagal reflexes in these patients. Tracheomalacia and GER also may contribute to these "crib deaths."

Late morbidity can be related to the esophageal anastomosis, to abnormal esophageal motility, to GER, and to respiratory problems. GER is probably the most troublesome because it can result in anastomotic or lower esophageal strictures, and may be accompanied by Barrett's esophagus. Esophageal adenocarcinoma has been reported 20 years after EA repair. Because most children grow up with their abnormally functioning esophagus, they tend not to realize that they have a problem. It was formerly thought that reflux improved with time, but several studies have shown that GER and esophagitis persist in a significant number of older children and adults. Closer follow-up and more aggressive treatment of GER are therefore required. Because reflux and esophagitis do not necessarily correlate with symptoms, surveillance esophagoscopy every 3 to 5 years has been recommended. The development of Barrett's esophagus calls for an antireflux procedure. Reflux also has been linked to respiratory problems such as recurrent pneumonia, bronchitis, and asthma.

The anastomotic scar and abnormal esophageal motility contribute to long-term dysphagia in about half the patients, although most do not complain about it. This frequently leads to swallowing difficulties and to food impaction requiring esophagoscopy for its removal.

Respiratory problems in the first year may be related to recurrent fistula, GER, tracheomalacia or associated anomalies such as an LTEC. Any of these may lead to serious morbidity and even mortality if not promptly recognized and treated. Later in life the respiratory symptoms tend to improve. In contrast to standard teachings, however, one study found that 40% of adults still had the typical barking cough of tracheomalacia, and 24% had intermittent respiratory problems such as asthma, pneumonia, and bronchitis. This finding was more common in patients who had these problems in early childhood. A daily cough was associated with symptoms of reflux and dysphagia.

Long-term growth and development have been considered within the normal range in most reviews, but in a large series of patients who underwent surgery at Great Ormond Street between 1980 and 1984, one third of them were below the third percentile for their age when assessed at 6 months to 5 years of age, including 21% in the good risk category.

Scoliosis may be secondary to vertebral or rib anomalies, anastomotic leak with pleural scarring, or an unnecessary long thoracotomy with rib excision. All patients should be followed closely for spine curvature, and that follow-up should include periodic radiography.

Overall, most adults who survive EA repair seem to enjoy a normal life and do not perceive their symptoms as significant. Several large series confirm the gradual improvement in survival in the past half century, despite the fact that smaller newborns with a higher frequency of associated anomalies are being treated. All investigators agree that associated anomalies are the most significant factor affecting the prognosis, but a small number of infants who "should" survive may continue to die of complications even in experienced centers. Waterston's classification has lost nearly all of its usefulness in the past two decades. The classification we have proposed (Table 33.3) highlights the fact that children with life-threatening anomalies and those with major anomalies combined with preoperative ventilator dependence (for example, extremely premature infants with severe hyaline membrane disease) are in a high-risk category, with an expected mortality rate of 40% or more, depending on the anomalies. The remainder have a good prognosis, with an expected survival of well over 90%.

TABLE 33.3. PROGNOSTIC CLASSIFICATION FOR ESOPHAGEAL ATRESIA

Class I (low risk)	All patients who do not satisfy Class II criteria
Class II (high risk)	Life-threatening associated anomalies (ex. bilateral renal agenesis, trisomy 13, hypoplastic left ventricle) Major associated anomalies with preoperative ventilator dependence

Modified from Poenaru D, Laberge J-M, Neilson IR, et al. A new prognostic classification for esophageal atresia. *Surgery* 1993;113:426.

ISOLATED TRACHEOESOPHAGEAL FISTULA

Diagnosis and Operative Approach

Choking and coughing in association with feedings, and repeated pneumonia (especially right upper lobe), suggest the possibility of an isolated congenital TEF. In some cases, asthma or impressive chronic abdominal distention are the predominant signs of the disorder. Excessive mucus or hypersalivation also may be noted. In most cases the symptoms start from birth, but the diagnosis is often delayed because of failure to investigate the problem, or as a result of falsely negative initial studies. The presence of other anomalies, such as laryngeal or tracheal atresia or stenosis may obscure the diagnosis. In distinction to the findings in babies with EA, a history of polyhydramnios is rare, and low birth weight is less common. Associated malformations may occur, but they are generally not as frequent and as severe as those associated with EA.

The next step in establishing diagnosis should be contrast esophagraphy with videofluoroscopy. Ideally this is performed in the prone or lateral decubitus position, injecting nonionic, water-soluble contrast material under pressure through a feeding tube, starting in the lower esophagus. The catheter is gradually withdrawn, and boluses of contrast are injected at various levels. This eliminates confusion with aspirated contrast from swallowing incoordination or an LTEC. This technique, by distending the esophagus, also facilitates opacification of the fistula because the tracheal opening is usually proximal to the esophageal opening.

In patients with persistent symptoms and negative esophagram results obtained under ideal conditions, rigid bronchoscopy should be performed. Special attention is directed to the posterior larynx to avoid missing an LTEC. This is followed by a thorough examination of the entire posterior tracheal wall to identify one or multiple TEFs if present. Even with positive contrast study results, bronchoscopy is an essential part of the operation. With the telescope just above the fistula and the operating room lights dimmed, one can visualize the bronchoscope light through the skin in the lower neck, confirming that the TEF can be approached through a cervical incision (as in 80%–90% of the cases). The fistula is then cannulated with a small Fogarty or ureteral catheter passed through the instrument channel. This step is essential to facilitate intraoperative identification of the fistula and minimize dissection, thereby decreasing the risk of recurrent laryngeal nerve (RLN) damage. I prefer to pass a 4 French Fogarty catheter, then inflate the balloon and pull it back. Esophagoscopy may be used to confirm that the balloon is up against the fistula. The ventilating bronchoscope is removed, and the patient is intubated. Since the Fogarty catheter is passed through the instrument channel of the scope, it should remain on the operating table next to the patient's head.

With the head kept in hyperextension, it is now turned to the left and the right neck is prepared and draped. Even with a fistula at the thoracic inlet, it is easier to pull it cephalad with the help of the Fogarty catheter than to work at the apex of the pleural cavity from a thoracic approach. Through a lower transverse incision along a skin fold, the sternomastoid and the carotid sheath are retracted laterally. Below the right lobe of the thyroid, the tracheoesophageal groove is exposed by blunt dissection. Palpation of the Fogarty catheter and balloon is facilitated when gentle traction is applied by the anesthesiologist. The right RLN is identified and preserved, avoiding traction to it. The fistula is carefully dissected and encircled with a vessel loop; it is always much thicker than is suggested by the contrast study. I prefer to put stay sutures of 5-0 synthetic resorbable sutures on the tracheal side at the cephalad and caudal ends of the TEF, then divide it close to the trachea as would be done in EA-TEF. Interrupted sutures are used to complete the tracheal closure, followed by esophageal closure. Ideally the tracheal suture line is then covered with healthy tissue such as the omohyoid muscle to prevent recurrence of the TEF. I usually leave a 5-mm Silastic drain connected to a low-pressure closed suction bulb, then close the wound in layers.

When a thoracic approach is required, a right transpleural exposure through the fourth interspace usually gives the best exposure. Again, the presence of the Fogarty catheter is invaluable. A thoracoscopic approach will undoubtedly be attempted in the future.

Postoperative Care and Complications

Immediate extubation is usually possible. The patient is usually maintained on parenteral nutrition until contrast esophagraphy is performed 3 to 5 days postoperatively. Others may choose to feed sooner and not perform a contrast study. In contrast to babies with EA, feeding difficulties are uncommon.

Intraoperative and early postoperative complications are common. They include accidental extubation, tracheal perforation, bradycardia and cardiac arrest, laryngeal edema, unilateral and even bilateral RLN damage with vocal cord palsy, missed or recurrent fistulas, mediastinitis, pneumothorax, and even phrenic palsy. Many of these complications can be avoided or minimized by identification and catheterization of the fistula preoperatively. Most of the reported complications were due to operations on patients who had only a clinical diagnosis, or those in whom the fistula was not catheterized. I would not perform a cervical exploration for presumed TEF if I could not visualize the fistula by bronchoscopy. Minimal dissection with preservation of the recurrent nerves, precise suturing of the trachea and esophagus, and verification of the cords at the end of the operation are important. Postoperative intubation may be required for vocal cord palsy or airway edema; in the latter situation, racemic epinephrine and steroids may be useful.

Late complications are uncommon, but a recurrent fistula may become apparent after several months. GER and abnormal esophageal peristalsis are uncommon.

The diagnosis and treatment of isolated TEF has improved over the years, and the prognosis is excellent. The satisfactory results obtained with cervical fistulas do not appear to warrant attempts at endoscopic occlusion.

SUGGESTED READINGS

Benjamin B, Phan T. Diagnosis of H-type tracheoesophageal fistula. *J Pediatr Surg* 1991;26:667–671.

Healy PJ, Sawin RS, Hall DG, et al. Delayed primary repair of esophageal atresia with tracheoesophageal fistula: is it worth the wait? *Arch Surg* 1998;133:552–556.

Kimura K, Nishijima E, Tsugawa C, et al. A new approach for the salvage of unsuccessful esophageal atresia repair: a spiral myotomy and delayed definitive operation. *J Pediatr Surg* 1987;22:981–983.

Laberge J-M, Guttman FM. Esophageal atresia and tracheoesophageal fistulas. In: Donnellan WL, ed. *Abdominal surgery of infancy and childhood.* Vol. I. Luxembourg: Harwood Academic, 1996:11/1–11/34.

Lindahl H, Rintala R. Sariola H. Chronic esophagitis and gastric metaplasia are frequent late complications of esophageal atresia. *J Pediatr Surg* 1993;28:1178–1180.

Myers NA, Beasley SW, Auldist AW. Oesophageal atresia and associated anomalies: a plea for uniform documentation: *Pediatr Surg Int* 1992;7:97–100.

Myers NA, Beasley SW, Auldist AW, et al. Oesophageal atresia without fistula—anastomosis or replacement? *Pediatr Surg Int* 1987; 2:216–222.

Ogita S, Tokiwa K, Takahaski T. Transabdominal closure of tracheoesophageal fistula: a new procedure for the management of poor-risk esophageal fistula. *J Pediatr Surg* 1986;21:812–814.

Schullinger JN, Vinocur C, Santulli TV. The suture fistula technique in the repair of selected cases of esophageal atresia. *J Pediatr Surg* 1982;17:234–236.

Spitz L, Kiely E, Brereton RJ. Esophageal atresia: five year experience with 148 cases. *J Pediatr Surg* 1987;22:103–108.

34

LONG GAP ESOPHAGEAL ATRESIA

PETER F. NICHOL
DENNIS P. LUND

The repair of long gap esophageal atresia (EA) represents one of the great technical challenges for the pediatric surgeon. Most surgeons would agree that the best repair uses the native esophagus whenever possible. This is not always feasible, and several esophageal substitution procedures have been developed.

Long gap EA is defined as an interruption of the esophageal lumen that exceeds a distance of 3.5 cm between the proximal and distal ends. This frequently occurs in the absence of a tracheoesophageal fistula (TEF), type A using the Gross classification. However, some cases of EA with distal TEF (type C) also involve a long gap between the ends of the esophagus. The term *extremely* or *ultra-long gap* EA typically refers to cases where the gap exceeds 5 cm. Gaps of this length require esophageal replacement in a large percentage of cases.

Esophageal atresia with or without TEF was at one time a uniformly fatal condition. The first successful primary repair of EA was performed by Dr. Cameron Haight in 1941 at the University of Michigan. Since that time, survival rates for these patients have increased from 15% in the 1950s to nearly 100% today. Outcome following repair of EA has been so successful that children who die with this anomaly in early childhood typically succumb to complications arising from other congenital defects that are associated with this lesion. Despite the improved survival with this condition, numerous difficulties, such as gastroesophageal reflux (GER), tracheomalacia, esophageal leak and stricture, and Barrett's esophagus, can affect children who undergo successful repair. These problems are more likely in children who have long gap EA.

Esophageal atresia occurs at a frequency of 2.4 per 10,000 births. The incidence of pure EA is reported to be about 7% of all TEF-EA in most series. There is a significant incidence of associated anomalies. Ein and Shandling reported a series of 69 infants with pure EA, seen over a 50-year period at their institution, and found that 52% were born prematurely. There was a 10% to 20% incidence of Down syndrome, and a 10% incidence of duodenal atresia. Polyhydramnios is frequently present, contributing to the likelihood of premature birth.

There are a number of risk factors associated with the development of EA. The incidence of EA is higher in white and male infants. There is a greater risk with the first pregnancy, with increased maternal age, in twins, and in siblings of children with EA. Other risk factors include diabetes mellitus, exposure to thalidomide, and prolonged exposure to oral contraceptives. Despite the known risk factors, the specific steps in embryogenesis that lead to EA remain unclear.

DIAGNOSIS

Antenatal diagnosis of this problem often can be made by ultrasonography. Typical findings include polyhydramnios and lack of a stomach bubble. Babies with EA-TEF, even if there is a long gap, are not usually diagnosed antenatally, and polyhydramnios is typically not present. The postnatal presentation and diagnosis of EA is well known. Neonates have excessive oral secretions and pooling of saliva in the posterior pharynx. Feedings are associated with choking or coughing and episodes of cyanosis. Definitive diagnosis is made by the failure to pass an orogastric (OG) tube into the stomach. Position of the OG tube in the proximal pouch is confirmed by fluoroscopy and can help delineate the length of the proximal pouch. If further confirmation is required, the surgeon may administer 1 mL of dilute barium into the upper pouch under fluoroscopy. An absolutely gasless abdomen on radiography is virtually pathognomonic of pure EA, whereas the baby who has EA with TEF will present with gas-filled loops of bowel.

PREOPERATIVE MANAGEMENT

Preoperative management of these patients begins immediately after birth. A sump tube is placed in the upper pouch

P. F. Nichol: Department of Surgery, University of Wisconsin Hospitals and Clinics, Madison, Wisconsin.

D. P. Lund: Department of Surgery, University of Wisconsin; and Department of Surgery, University of Wisconsin Children's Hospital, Madison, Wisconsin.

to remove secretions and minimize respiratory complications. The child is placed with the head of the bed elevated in order to minimize aspiration events. Intravenous lines are placed to maintain hydration. The baby should receive intravenous antibiotics, such as ampicillin and gentamicin. Other anomalies associated with the VACTERL syndrome (abnormalities of vertebrae, anus, cardiovascular tree, trachea, esophagus, renal system, and limb buds) should be sought. Echocardiography is routinely performed to establish the side of the aortic arch and to exclude cardiac anomalies. Renal and spinal ultrasonography should be performed at some point in the neonatal period to exclude renal anomalies and tethering of the spinal cord.

Pulmonary problems should be treated aggressively. If the baby has a TEF, intubation should be avoided, if possible. If intubation is necessary, the baby should be allowed to breathe spontaneously. Positive pressure ventilation will lead to distension of the stomach and intestine, which can lead to reflux of gastric contents into the lungs and subsequent pneumonitis. Abdominal distension in this setting can also severely limit ventilation and may necessitate emergency gastrostomy to decompress the stomach. In rare cases, the baby with TEF who requires positive pressure ventilation may need emergent thoracotomy and ligation of the fistula. Temporizing measures, such as occlusion of the fistula with a Fogarty balloon placed by bronchoscopy, are occasionally useful as well.

Typically, babies with EA-TEF should undergo surgery on the first day of life, after pulmonary stabilization and the initial evaluation are completed. A right posterolateral extrapleural thoracotomy is used. If the ends of the esophagus are found to be more than 3.5 vertebral bodies apart, we prefer to ligate and divide the fistula and to place a gastrostomy tube for feedings. If the distal fistula is divided, the end should be sutured to the periosteum of a rib as high in the mediastinum as possible so that the surgeon can go back later to try to perform primary repair. If this is not done, the fistula will retract, making primary repair much more difficult. If primary repair cannot be performed, a cervical esophagostomy should not be performed, but the baby is left on low intermittent sump suction via an OG tube.

In cases of pure EA, one should start first with gastrostomy tube placement. Intraoperatively, a small Bake's dilator can be passed up the distal esophagus through the gastrostomy, and fluoroscopy can be used to define the distance between the end of the distal pouch and the OG tube in the proximal pouch (Fig. 34.1). If the distance is greater than 3.5 vertebral bodies, it is wise not to attempt primary repair at this time. The baby can be fed by gastrostomy, and primary repair should be attempted at a later date.

After the initial procedure, the baby is allowed to recover from surgery and gastrostomy feedings are begun. These should be continued for 6 to 12 weeks, or until the baby is growing well. The distal pouch will elongate with time. The

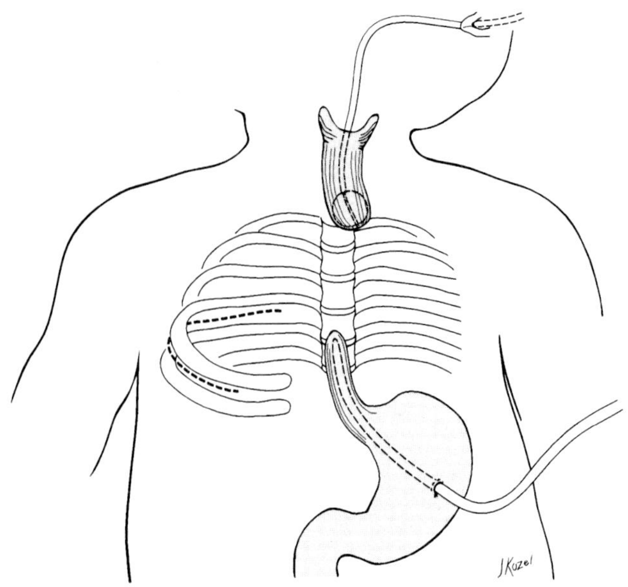

FIGURE 34.1. The two ends of the esophagus and the distance between them can be demonstrated by placing catheters from above (through the mouth) and below (through the stomach) and injecting contrast using fluoroscopy.

proximal pouch requires low intermittent suction to prevent aspiration events, but systems can be developed that allow this to be done at home with careful and competent parents. Some surgeons pass a small, blunt-tipped Maloney dilator once or twice a day by mouth to try to promote proximal pouch lengthening and thickening. The value of this practice has not been proven. Again, if desired, parents can be taught to do this safely on the child at home.

After a suitable period of time, both ends of the esophagus should be studied radiographically to assess the distance to be bridged. Contrast placed in the stomach via the gastrostomy will reflux into the distal esophagus, and the distance from the top of the distal pouch to the end of the OG tube is measured in vertebral bodies. Using esophageal mobilization and myotomies, gaps as large as five vertebral bodies can reliably be bridged. Regardless of the length of the gap to be bridged, we prefer not to consign a patient to esophageal substitution without an exploration and an attempt at primary repair.

PRIMARY REPAIR

Primary repair of long-segment EA requires extensive mobilization of the esophagus, a fair amount of tension, and often myotomies, all factors that can significantly impair the blood supply of this tenuous organ. It is essential that the surgeon understand the vascular anatomy of the esophagus as well as the important fact that the greatest strength layer of the esophagus is the mucosa. The proximal esophagus derives its blood supply longitudinally via the thyrocervical trunk through submucosal vessels. The distal esophagus has a segmental supply from the aorta as well as longitudinal supply from the left gastric artery. Despite the more redundant blood supply distally, it is thought that the proximal esophagus withstands extensive mobilization much better that the distal segment.

Proper positioning of the patient for operation is essential to successful repair. The patient is positioned for a posterolateral thoracotomy through the side opposite the aortic arch. A small axillary roll is placed to prevent brachial plexus injury, but the table should not be flexed, nor should any roll be placed under the chest to open up the intercostal spaces as one normally does for a thoracotomy. The reason for this is that bending the thoracic spine to open the intercostal spaces also moves the ends of the esophagus farther apart, creating more tension as one tries to perform the anastomosis. A relatively stiff OG tube or a Bake's dilator should be placed via the mouth into the proximal pouch so that it can be manipulated by the anesthesiologist intraoperatively. This will aid in dissection of the proximal pouch. The ipsilateral neck, chest, arm, and hand should be prepared into the field to allow access to the neck as well as the chest.

The operation begins with a posterolateral thoracotomy through the fourth or fifth interspace. If a previous thoracotomy was not performed, an extrapleural approach is best because a leak is less likely to result in empyema. However, a previous thoracotomy to ligate a fistula makes the extrapleural route nearly impossible; therefore, the surgeon should cross the pleura. In this case, a pleural flap can be developed later to wrap the anastomosis. The lung is gently retracted and the ends of the esophagus are sought. Previous suture of the distal esophagus with a long marking suture makes finding the distal pouch quite easy. If not, there is sometimes a small fibrous cord traversing the posterior mediastinum in the esophageal bed that leads to the distal esophagus near the diaphragm. The vagus and phrenic nerves should be identified and carefully preserved. If the distal pouch is hard to identify, inflating the stomach with air via the gastrostomy sometimes allows the distal pouch to be seen.

Identifying the proximal pouch is facilitated by applying gentle pressure on the catheter or dilator in the mouth. A bulge will be seen coming down from the posterior superior mediastinum when pressure is applied. With pressure on the catheter or dilator, the proximal pouch can be extensively dissected. It is important to stay immediately adjacent to the muscular layer of the esophagus as one dissects up into the neck so as not to damage the recurrent laryngeal nerves. There are usually somewhat dense adhesions to the back of the trachea that must be sharply divided. Some of these may contain small blood vessels from the bronchial circulation. They can be precisely cauterized using a Jacobsen hemostat. The surgeon must be on the lookout for the rare case of a fistula from the trachea to the upper pouch. If found, such a fistula should be closed carefully using the principles of repair of an H fistula.

Once the proximal pouch is mobilized thoroughly, attention is turned to the distal pouch. This can be mobilized carefully, but one should take care not to interrupt the segmental vessels that supply the esophagus. However, one can dissect the distal pouch all the way down to the diaphragmatic hiatus. Because there is no opportunity to place an instrument in the distal lumen to assist in dissection, an atraumatic suture can be placed in the end of the distal pouch for gentle traction. As with mobilization of the upper pouch, extensive handling with forceps should be avoided.

Once both ends of the esophagus have been mobilized in the chest, an assessment is made of the tension needed to bring both ends together in a successful anastomosis. The surgeon must judge at this point whether or not this can be safely accomplished. If the tension seems excessive, the anastomosis should not be undertaken.

If necessary, the surgeon can then proceed with techniques of lengthening the esophagus. It is important to realize that lengthening techniques can impair blood supply and make stricture or leak more likely. The oldest technique, and the one we prefer, is the use of the circular myotomy, first reported by Livaditis et al. in 1972. The technique is illustrated in Fig. 34.2. After mobilization of the esophagus, a 5 or 6 French Fogarty embolectomy catheter is placed through the mouth into the proximal pouch and inflated. This stretches out the muscle fibers, which are then circumferentially divided with a blade. Care should be taken to divide only the muscle fibers, not the submucosal blood vessels. Myotomies can be performed 1.5 cm apart, so that two myotomies can frequently be performed through the chest. The most distal myotomy should be no less than 1 cm from the end of the pouch. Each myotomy will lengthen the esophagus by about 1 cm. After one or two myotomies, the tension on an anastomosis must again be judged.

Mobilization of the proximal pouch can be even more extensive by use of a cervical incision. In this case, a transverse skin incision is used in a skin fold low in the neck. The sternocleidomastoid muscle is retracted, and the esophagus is identified behind the carotid and jugular vessels. Again the surgeon must stay directly on the esophagus to avoid the recurrent laryngeal nerves. Dissecting on the esophagus allows the surgeon to quickly develop a communication into the chest. This communication should be marked with a Penrose drain from the chest to the neck. Atraumatic traction sutures placed in the end of the proximal pouch are used to bring the pouch out of the neck incision. More extensive mobilization can be performed and another myotomy can be added high in the esophagus if needed. The proximal pouch is then placed back down in the chest along the track marked by the drain.

On occasion, the surgeon is confronted with a case of a very short proximal pouch and a fairly long distal pouch. If

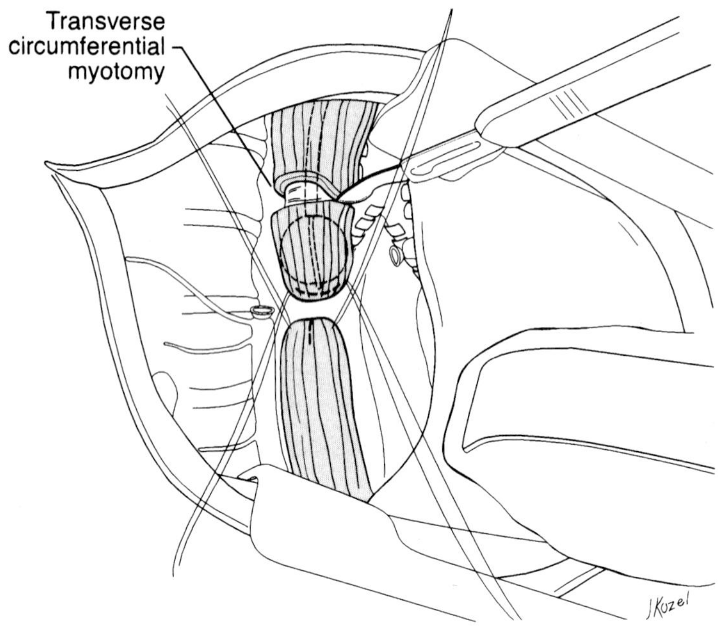

FIGURE 34.2. A circular myotomy is performed by distending the esophagus with a Fogarty embolectomy catheter and carefully incising the muscle down to the submucosa. Multiple myotomies can be performed in this way, and, if necessary, also can be executed on the distal pouch.

one takes care with the segmental blood supply, a distal pouch myotomy can be performed without interfering with the blood supply. The technique is the same as described above, but without opening the pouch one does not have the luxury of using a balloon catheter to distend the muscle fibers. Thus, an opening should be made in the end of the distal pouch, a Fogarty catheter inserted, and the myotomy completed as described above. We have used this technique successfully without subsequent leakage of the anastomosis.

After the esophagus has been mobilized and lengthened to the point where the ends meet without excessive tension, the anastomosis is undertaken (Fig. 34.3). This is accomplished with a single layer of interrupted monofilament sutures. We prefer using 5-0 polydioxanone suture material. The ends of the pouches are opened sharply in different planes, one sagittal and one coronal. A back wall of interrupted sutures is placed so that the knots are on the luminal side, taking great care that all sutures include sufficient mucosa. After the back wall sutures are tied, the anterior wall sutures are placed with the knots on the outside. These are then tied. The anastomosis should be buttressed with the azygos vein, which is ligated, divided, and mobilized, or with a flap of pleura that is mobilized and sutured over the esophagus. A chest tube should be placed and sutured to the

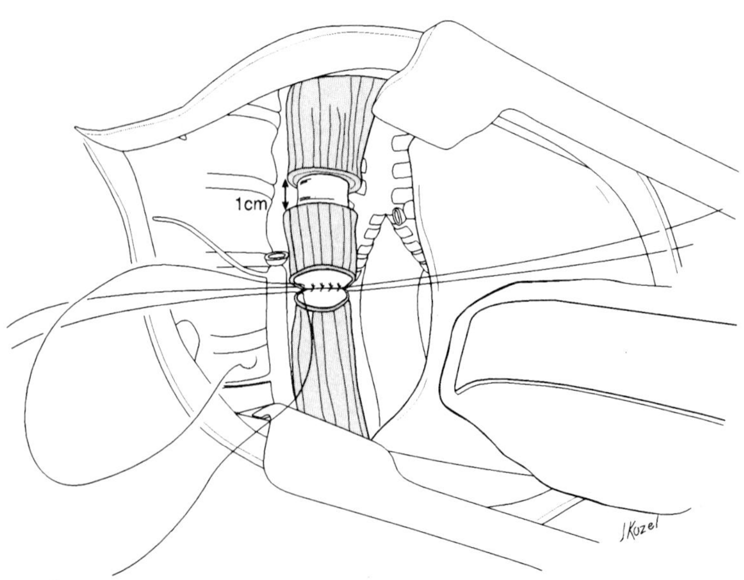

FIGURE 34.3. An end-to-end single-layer, interrupted anastomosis is performed with monofilament suture. Care must be taken to obtain good purchase on the mucosa with the sutures. The anastomosis can then be buttressed with an azygos vein flap or with a flap of pleura.

chest wall near, but not abutting, the esophagus. If a leak results, the contents will find their way out the tube, but the tube should not be allowed to press on or erode the anastomosis. The chest is then closed in standard fashion. Some surgeons prefer to pass a feeding tube across the anastomosis as it is performed, but this is not necessary in most cases because there is a gastrostomy present for feedings.

POSTOPERATIVE CARE

Placement of a thoracic epidural catheter by an experienced pediatric anesthesiologist makes postoperative management of these patients much simpler. We routinely use only bupivacaine in the epidural catheter, allowing us to use supplemental narcotics in much smaller doses. Use of ketorolac also helps to minimize narcotic use. The patient should be extubated only when one can be fairly certain that he or she will not require emergent reintubation. This most often occurs before the patient leaves the operating room. However, if there is any question about the airway, the patient should remain intubated until safely in the pediatric intensive care unit. Virtually all of these patients will have GER. Acid blockade with histamine2 (H_2) blockers or proton pump inhibitors is recommended. Care should be taken to be sure that the gastrostomy tube drains properly so that secretions do not build up in the stomach and reflux up against the fresh suture line.

A temporary central venous line is typically placed while the patient is in the operating room. This allows the use of intravenous hyperalimentation during the perioperative and postoperative periods, and until gastrointestinal feedings can commence. Perioperative antibiotics should be continued only for a short period as long as the patient is doing well.

The authors typically study these patients with an esophagram 7 to 10 days postoperatively to rule out an anastomotic leak prior to the initiation of feedings. If results of the study look normal, feeding can be begun using continuous gastrostomy feeding first and advancing gradually to bolus feeding as well as oral feeding. Because these children have not had oral feedings previously, it is usually necessary to use the services of the feeding team or speech therapy to assist with oral feeding.

COMPLICATIONS

Anastomotic Leak

Extensive mobilization of the esophagus, myotomies, and anastomotic tension all increase the likelihood of development of a postoperative leak after primary repair of long-segment EA. Although this is a great fear for surgeons who do these types of repairs, most can be managed conservatively. It is essential that a drainage tube is placed intraoperatively near but not abutting the anastomosis. This will allow drainage of esophageal contents promptly and prevent the development of empyema or mediastinitis. An anastomotic leak usually presents as a change in the character of the chest tube drainage and fever. Broad-spectrum antibiotics should be started. If there is a question of leakage, esophagraphy can be performed with water-soluble contrast. However, this is usually not necessary immediately because the drainage of salivary secretions out of the chest tube is diagnostic.

With antibiotics and good drainage, most leaks become controlled salivary fistulas. By giving the patient good nutrition and simply waiting, the majority of these fistulas heal. Rarely, if the patient becomes systemically ill, it may be necessary to operate. However, surgery in this circumstance almost always requires abandoning the primary repair and diverting the patient with a cervical esophagostomy. After the leak has stabilized, it should be assessed by esophagraphy using water-soluble contrast. Patience in the setting of good nutrition usually allows these leaks to seal. In order to use enteric nutrition, a transgastric jejunostomy tube can be placed under fluoroscopic guidance to allow weaning the patient from the intravenous nutrition.

Stricture

The same factors that can lead to an anastomotic leak—tension and ischemia—can also result in an anastomotic stricture. Stricture is more likely if there has been an anastomotic leak. Strictures manifest as increased oral secretions, unwillingness to swallow, or aspiration episodes. Patients also may present with food impacted in the esophagus requiring esophagoscopy and extraction. GER also promotes the formation of strictures. Because virtually all of these children develop reflux, it is best to begin aggressive antireflux therapy empirically after surgery.

Strictures usually respond to esophageal dilatation. Several techniques have been described. Direct esophagoscopy is helpful to assess the stricture and will help with passing a fiberglass filiform or wire across the stricture. Different types of followers or wire-guided dilators can then be used to dilate the stricture. We prefer not to use blind passage of Maloney dilators in these cases, because it is important to control the direction of the tip of the dilator. One must not be too aggressive with dilation since there is a significant risk of perforating the anastomosis of the esophagus. In the case of particularly recalcitrant strictures, it may be wise to leave a heavy suture across the stricture coming out the nares and the gastrostomy between dilations. Another helpful technique if one cannot get a wire or filiform to pass across the stricture from above is to try to pass one from the stomach side upward across the stricture. Finally, if the stricture is difficult, local injection of a small amount of triamcinolone may help to soften the stricture over time. However, data suggest that this form of steroid is systemically absorbed, so the doses should be kept small.

Persistent or nondilatable strictures require surgical therapy. Resection and primary reanastomosis is frequently possible, but other techniques that have been described may be necessary, such as use of a colonic or small bowel patch.

Gastroesophageal Reflux

Gastroesophageal reflux is virtually always present in children after esophageal repair. This GER is due to traction on the esophagus, which leads to less length of intraabdominal esophagus and straightening of the angle of His, as well as poor esophageal clearance due to impaired peristalsis. The child's GER should be treated aggressively with H_2 blockers or proton pump inhibitors, as well as properistaltic agents, such as metaclopramide. Severe, early postoperative GER should be treated with transgastric jejunostomy feedings because the GER may get better with time. Even with aggressive medical antireflux medications, the child's GER may not be well controlled. In these cases, surgical correction of the GER may be necessary. If fundoplication is undertaken, it is important not to make the wrap excessively tight because esophageal emptying is poor. If children have persistent GER, they should be followed long-term for development of the complications of GER such as respiratory problems, recurrent otitis, and even Barrett esophagus.

In summary, long-segment EA is a formidable challenge for the pediatric surgeon. Proper correction of the problem may take many months and multiple procedures. Every effort should be made to try to correct long-segment EA without resorting to esophageal substitution. Most often the native esophagus will empty better and have fewer long-term problems associated with it than with a substitute. The pediatric surgeon must form a close and understanding relationship with the patient and family. The surgeon must be persistent and the family must realize that complex problems such as EA often require complex solutions. Successful repair of long-segment EA not only is of great benefit to the child, but will also provide great satisfaction to the surgeon.

SUGGESTED READINGS

Chavin K, Field G, Chandler J, et al. Save the child's esophagus: management of major disruption after repair of esophageal atresia. *J Pediatr Surg* 1996;31:48–51.

Ein SH, Shandling B. Pure esophageal atresia: a 50-year review. *J Pediatr Surg* 1994;29:1208–1211.

Giacomoni MA, Tresoldi M, Zamana C, et al. Circular myotomy of the distal esophageal stump for long gap esophageal atresia. *J Pediatr Surg* 2001;36:855–857.

Hollands CM, Lankau CA Jr, Burnweit CA. Preoperative home care for esophageal atresia—a survey. *J Pediatr Surg* 2000;35:279–281.

Lai JY, Sheu JC, Chang PY, et al. Experience with distal circular myotomy for long-gap esophageal atresia. *J Pediatr Surg* 1996;31: 1503–1508.

Livaditis A, Radberg L, Odensjo G. Esophageal end-to-end anastomosis. Reductions of anastomotic tension by circular myotomy. *Scand J Thorac Cardiovasc Surg* 1972;6:206–214.

35

CAUSTIC ESOPHAGEAL INJURIES

ANNE C. FISCHER

Approximately 34,000 caustic injuries occur annually and represent a significant public health issue. Caustic ingestions are the leading toxic exposure in children and are surpassed only by analgesic drugs in adults. Children account for the majority of poison exposures, 74% of which are ingestions. The age distribution is bimodal, occurring as accidental ingestions in children under 5 and as suicide attempts in adults over 20. The ingestion of corrosive agents can cause a devastating injury to the esophagus and stomach. The resultant injury pattern is a challenging management and reconstruction problem. Prior to 1960, lye was crystalline and caused significant burns primarily localized to the oropharynx due to the adherence of the crystals to the mucosa. The immediate pain elicited from the oropharyngeal burns induced a protective rapid expulsion of the crystals, limiting the extent of the injury. The introduction of commercially available concentrated liquid lye markedly increased the severity and incidence of esophageal injury, which previously constituted only 10% to 25% of crystalline ingestions. The similarity of liquid lye to milk and the storage of liquid lye, as well as other caustic cleaners, in food or drink containers further contributed to the escalating incidence of corrosive exposures. Despite legislation to reduce the concentration of liquid lye, from 35% down to 5% NaOH, and to ensure childproof safety measures, the variety of commercially available corrosives are of sufficient strength to continue to create a public health hazard.

The extent of injury depends on the type of corrosive, its concentration, quantity, and duration of exposure. Household bleach, liquid laundry detergents, and ammonia usually result in mild esophageal burns since they are weak bases at low concentrations. Ingestions of strong alkalis such as liquid lye, Clinitest tablets (Bayer, Elkhart, Indiana), or button batteries are associated with the most deaths since they represent the highest concentration of a strong base. Lye is odorless and tasteless; thus, accidental large ingestions of concentrated liquid lye do not always evoke the protective emetic reflexes caused by crystalline ingestion. The high viscosity of the liquid results in a slow transit time with prolonged exposure and deeper tissue penetration.

Alkalis produce a solvent effect, a *liquefactive necrosis* with rapid tissue penetration. The most significant injuries occur at a pH exceeding 11. An alkaline ingestion causes a violent regurgitation against a closed cricopharyngeus, typically reexposing the esophageal mucosa to further injury after the initial insult. In contrast, the odor and bitter taste of strong acids induce a rapid expectoration that is somewhat protective. The lack of viscosity of acids is associated with a rapid transit time for the nonexpulsed portion of the ingestion. The rapid transit of acids is associated with relative esophageal sparing. Thus, acids usually spare the oropharynx and esophagus, causing skip lesions and a higher incidence of distal perforations.

Acids cause a *coagulation necrosis* that results in a superficial eschar, and this coagulum limits the extension of further mucosal penetration beyond the surface burn. Strong acids are found in battery fluids, antirust compounds, and swimming pool cleaners (Table 35.1). A caveat is that the ingestion of highly concentrated sulfuric or hydrochloric acid does cause esophageal injury in about half of cases. Hydrofluoric acid is another notable exception because it produces liquefactive necrosis and immediate life-threatening disturbances of calcium metabolism.

CLINICAL SYMPTOMS

The most common features of ingestions are oropharyngeal burning, odynophagia, dysphagia, and chest pain. Clinical symptoms are poor predictors of the degree of injury. Stridor is indicative of laryngeal and epiglottal edema. Drooling in the setting of stridor is highly suggestive of esophageal injury. Dysphagia and hematemesis are further suggestive of esophageal injury. Retrosternal pain radiating to the back and acute epigastric pain herald a full-thickness injury to the esophagus or stomach, respectively. Sloughing of the esophageal mucosa elicits hematemesis. Hemodynamic instability with systemic signs such as a change in

A. C. Fischer: Department of Surgery, Division of Pediatric Surgery, Johns Hopkins Hospital, Baltimore, Maryland.

TABLE 35.1. COMMON CAUSTIC EXPOSURES

Chemical Agent	Source
Alkaline	
Ammonia	Toilet bowel cleaners, hair dyes, floor strippers, glass cleaners
Sodium hydroxide	Clinitest tablets, detergents, laundry powders, paint removers, drain cleaners, button batteries
Sodium borates, carbonates, phosphates	Detergents, electric dishwashers, water softeners
Sodium hypochlorite	Bleaches, cleaners
Acid	
Hydrochloric acid	Swimming pool cleaners, metal and toilet bowel cleaners
Hydrofluoric acid	Antirust products
Sulfuric acid	Automobile batteries, drain cleaners

mental status, fever, and tachycardia typically follow massive ingestions. Severe injuries with peritoneal signs, cervical crepitance, and retrosternal pain radiating to the back are ominous findings consistent with esophageal perforation and impending mediastinitis. A pleural effusion or the combination of acidotic serum (pH <7.2) and an elevated gastric pH (>7.3), further substantiates the severity of injury.

In corrosive injuries, intense pylorospasm and gastric atony limit passage into the duodenum, which results in pooling of the material in the antrum and fundic sparing. Large volume ingestions can overcome the reflex pylorospasm and extend into contiguous structures beyond the duodenum. All areas of esophageal anatomic narrowing are potential areas of prolonged contact resulting in circumferential injuries and severe strictures. This occurs at the cricopharyngeus, the aortic arch, tracheal bifurcation, and distal esophagus. Ninety-five percent of severe strictures occur in the distal esophagus, sparing the constricted lower esophageal sphincter.

IMMEDIATE INTERVENTION

The primary goals of management are to identify the severity of injury and minimize the extension of injury. The type and amount of corrosive ingested should be identified in the history. The initial priority is airway assessment and stabilization with fluid resuscitation. Direct visualization of the oropharynx and a laryngoscopic examination are the initial steps in evaluating the extent of injury. The airway should be visualized with a fiberoptic nasopharyngoscope. Stridor strongly suggests laryngeal insult and mandates orotracheal intubation. If there are signs of laryngeal edema or changes in mental status, an airway should be rapidly established by oral endotracheal intubation or, less commonly, by tracheostomy. The presence or absence of oropharyngeal burns is not an indicator of distal esophagogastric injury. A third or more of severe esophageal lesions occur in the absence of any stigmata of oropharyngeal burns. Blind passage of a nasogastric tube or blind nasopharyngeal intubation are contraindicated.

Measures to dilute or neutralize the corrosive agent are contraindicated. Ingestion of water or milk can stimulate vomiting which causes reexposure to the corrosive agent. Alkalis cause such rapid tissue penetration that immediate attempts at dilution are unsuccessful. With concentrated acid injuries, large volumes of water may dilute and successfully neutralize the acid only if given immediately after the ingestion; however, attempts to neutralize acids or alkalis cause an exothermic reaction, enhancing the destruction of surrounding tissue. Therefore, all oral intake should be prohibited. Activated charcoal interferes with subsequent endoscopy and further complicates management. Syrup of ipecac, a proemetic agent, is also contraindicated because the resulting emesis reexposes the esophagus to the caustic agent. Plain films of the chest and abdomen readily identify specific operative indications such as pneumoperitoneum, pneumomediastinum, and pleural effusions, all associated with full-thickness injury and necessitating immediate operative intervention.

Unusual ingestions bear comment. The ingestion of concentrated hydrofluoric acid can cause significant gastritis and life-threatening calcium disturbances. The risk of perforation by passage of a nasogastric tube is markedly lower than the risk of death by systemic absorption of hydrofluoric acid. Uniquely in this exposure, blind nasogastric decompression to evacuate the stomach is acceptable because these exposures are otherwise universally fatal. Button batteries, such as those in hearing aids, watches, and computer games, are likewise solid caustic ingestions common to children. Each contains concentrated caustic alkalis similar to crystalline lye with a potential for leakage, significant burns, and pressure necrosis. The majority pass through to the colon within 4 days. Thorough evaluation is mandatory because a delay in diagnosis can result in an aortoesophageal perforation. Patients are abruptly symptomatic and require emergent bronchoscopy for batteries in the airway. Intact batteries that pass through the pylorus in asymptomatic patients can be followed with serial stool examinations for up to 7 days. In children under 6 years of age, batteries larger than 15 mm are not likely to pass the pylorus spontaneously. Failure to pass the pylorus within 48 hours or to be recovered in the stool within 7 days requires evaluation serially by radiography and retrieval by endoscopy.

The rapidity of the caustic process is such that mucosal injury is easily demonstrable by the time of hospital evaluation. Early endoscopy is the gold standard for the evaluation of caustic injuries and should occur within the first 12 to 24 hours. The reason for early endoscopy is that most perforations occur in a delayed fashion around the second to third day after injury, when the wound weakens with friable granulation tissue. Endoscopy is indicated in all patients with stridor, all intended suicidal ingestions, and any symptomatic children (vomiting, drooling). Endoscopy is not essential in patients already meeting operative criteria with evidence of esophageal or gastric perforation or mediastinitis. The most frequent exposures in children are mild alkalis, such as household bleach. Endoscopy is not necessary in such a mild injury if the child is asymptomatic. Accidental bleach ingestion necessitates clinical evaluation for 24 hours to ensure normal esophageal function and endoscopy for symptoms such as dysphagia or drooling (Fig. 35.1). Available data support the management of unintentional injuries in children based on clinical symptoms or injury pattern alone.

Caustic injuries are classified endoscopically in the same manner as surface thermal injuries (Table 35.2). First-degree injuries are superficial, and the mucosa sloughs without scar or stricture. Second-degree injuries penetrate through the mucosa to the muscular layer, and within days the sloughing results in deep ulcerations. Second-degree injuries can be subclassified by the presence of circumferential injury (IIB) as opposed to linear or patchy areas (IIA). Third-degree injuries involve full-thickness penetration, with mediastinitis or peritonitis usually occurring within 48 hours. Grade I and IIA injuries do not evoke strictures. All grade III injuries and more than 70% of grade IIB injuries have some degree of progression to strictures.

The limitations of endoscopy are (a) the presence of circumferential burns that preclude full visualization, (b) the unrecognized progression of caustic injuries resulting in delayed perforation at 7 to 14 days, and (c) the difficulty in reliably distinguishing grade IIB from grade III injuries. Differentiation between second- and third-degree injuries may be difficult, but third-degree injuries are often distinguished by the presence of gray friable tissue, thrombosed submucosal vessels, and extensive black eschar. Estrera and associates showed that three out of eight grade IIB patients

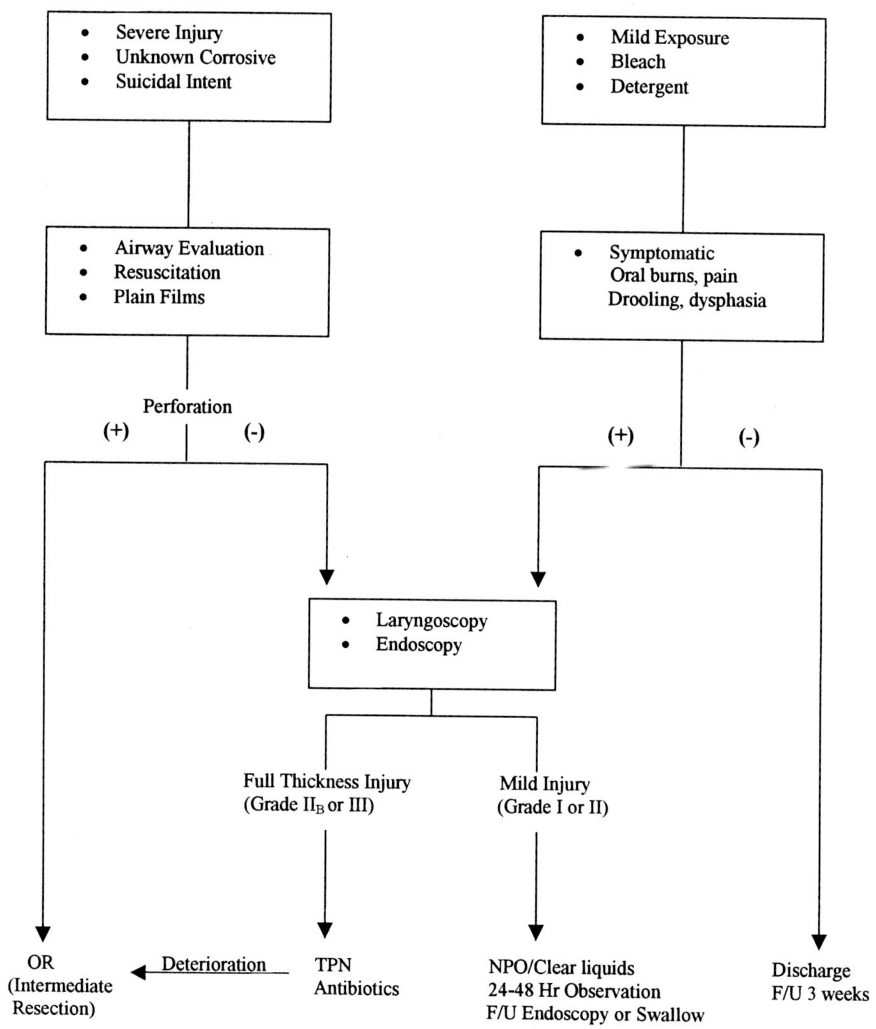

FIGURE 35.1. Acute caustic ingestion. Treatment algorithm.

TABLE 35.2. CLASSIFICATION OF CAUSTIC INJURY

Grade	Degree of Injury	Endoscopic Characteristics
I	Superficial mucosal burn	Mucosal edema and hypermia
IIA	Transmucosal injury	Patchy ulcerations, exudates, mucosal slough
IIB	Transmucosal injury	Circumferential injury
III	Transmural injury, periesophageal or perigastric extension	Deep ulcerations, black or gray discoloration, full-thickness necrosis

Modified from Estrera A, et al. Corrosive burns of the esophagus and stomach: a recommendation for an aggressive surgical approach. *Ann Thorac Surg* 1986;41:276; with permission.

actually have full-thickness injuries (grade III) requiring immediate surgery. Endoscopy up to the site of maximal esophageal injury provides the ideal evaluation to direct therapy (Fig. 35.1) and minimizes the risks of iatrogenic perforation. Contrast radiography is a method of identifying grade III injuries and is performed first with water-soluble contrast followed by thin barium contrast. Dye extravasation is diagnostic for perforation. Because endoscopy is limited to superficial mucosal evaluation only, laparoscopy can assist in documenting full-thickness injury. Laparoscopy, in contrast to laparotomy, cannot evaluate specifically the posterior serosal aspect of the stomach, which is confined to the lesser sac. In summary, the evaluation following a corrosive ingestion should include examination of the entire upper gastrointestinal tract by endoscopy or other noninvasive radiographic methods. Early surgical exploration is essential for visceral perforation or necrosis of surrounding structures.

SURGICAL MANAGEMENT AND INTERVENTION

The extent of tissue injury dictates management. The severity of the endoscopic grade of injury correlates with the expected incidence of subsequent strictures. Endoscopic grades of injury exceeding grade IIA are associated with the complications of esophageal perforation, infection, and stricture. Limiting the severity of injury is important because esophageal replacement can be problematic and is less satisfactory than retention of a damaged but functional esophagus.

Most investigators recommend the judicious use of antibiotics such as penicillin, ampicillin, or clindamycin to cover the oropharyngeal flora, because tissue disruption provides a source of bacteremia. Tissue turnover and remodeling from caustic burns is significant, and delayed perforation of the esophagus may occur at the height of remodeling, between 7 and 14 days postingestion. Fever and impending perforation may be partially masked by prophylactic antibiotics. However, the use of antibiotics is advocated for all patients also receiving corticosteroids to decrease the higher incidence of associated infection.

The role of corticosteroids was purported to arrest inflammation and prevent strictures. In the 1960s, the introduction of steroids to reduce the inflammatory response combined with antibiotics to reduce infection resulted in reduced mortality. More recent controlled trials have shown no benefit; therefore, the use of steroids remains controversial. A controlled trial by Anderson, et al. indicated that corticosteroids do not prevent strictures because a similar number of strictures developed in children receiving steroids (10 of 31) as in the control population (11 of 29). In grade I and IIA injuries there are no associated strictures, and steroids provide no benefit. Grade III injuries evolve into strictures regardless of therapy; thus, steroids do not provide a definitive long-term benefit. One might consider the use of steroids in grade IIB injuries; however, they are of unproven efficacy and may have a detrimental effect by masking an evolving perforation or delaying the diagnosis of infection. Future randomized studies that focus on grade II injuries may help clarify the value of steroids.

Empiric gastric acid suppression with histamine (H_2) blockers is recommended to decrease acid reflux, and possibly decrease stricture rates. No clinical studies have evaluated collagen synthesis inhibitors such as N-acetylcysteine. These experimental lathyrogenic compounds are designed to inhibit stricture formation. Intravenous alimentation is essential in those with perforations and delayed enteric feedings. Gastrostomy or jejunostomy provides a nutritional conduit. Gastrostomies are placed in children with severe injuries to provide enteral feeds and a route for retrograde dilatations. If a grade I or IIA injury is found, the patient may be started on liquids in 48 hours, progressing to regular diet. Grade IIB and III injuries should be observed for at least 48 hours and started on hyperalimentation. Vigilant observation is essential to detect delayed perforations and acute aortoesophageal fistulas.

Early identification of patients with full-thickness injuries to the upper digestive tract is critical for immediate resection of devitalized organs and limiting further extension of the corrosive injury. The decision to perform emergent surgery is dictated by radiographic signs of perforation, the presence of peritoneal signs, or endoscopic stigmata of a full-thickness injury. Delaying surgical repair has been associated with increased morbidity and mortality. Identifying the subtle evolution of corrosive injuries in patients who have not manifested evidence of significant tissue damage initially is challenging. The overall mortality rate is high but has been reduced from 20% to 3% over the past 20 years due to improved and timely surgery and the early introduction of parenteral nutrition and antibiotics. The morbidity of full-thickness esophageal necrosis remains high, with a 20% mortality rate. In the absence of perforation, no single criterion can identify patients who require surgery. A depressed or agitated mental status, shock, persistent acidemia, or coagulation disorders are usually associated with severe findings intraoperatively. Some surgeons advocate routine laparoscopy or laparotomy for patients with grade IIB and III burns of the esophagus for evaluation of serosal surfaces to determine a full-thickness injury.

The operative field should span from the mandible to the pelvis to accommodate cervical, thoracic, and abdominal approaches. Emergent operative intervention is best approached through the abdomen with complete visualization of the stomach and contiguous structures. Black eschar and thrombosis of the submucosal vessels indicate full-thickness gastric injury and warrant consideration of a total gastrectomy. Severe gastric injury is often associated with an equally severe esophageal injury. An emergent esophageal resection can be performed via a transhiatal approach, thus avoiding a thoracotomy. A transhiatal dissection for a total esophagogastrectomy is facilitated by the extensive acute periesophageal edema. A cervical esophagostomy is created, and a feeding jejunostomy is placed for enteral feeds. Delaying resection in the setting of third degree burns and perforation is associated with 100% mortality. Tracheoesophageal fistulas can occur within the first week of injury and necessitate a tracheostomy, a cervical esophagostomy, and a gastrostomy. After immediate and urgent resection, reconstruction is delayed for several months.

The reconstruction of a destroyed esophagus is challenging and requires the use of a substernal isoperistaltic colon interposition with the right or transverse colon or a reversed gastric tube. Gastric tubes may be of inadequate length, usually due to the original injury and associated stricture; furthermore, a gastrostomy may limit a gastric tube reconstruction. Other disadvantages are dumping symptoms following the usual pyloroplasty and reflux esophagitis occurring above the esophagogastric anastomosis. A colon interposition is the most widely used anatomic reconstruction. It provides a similar anatomic reservoir and dependable blood supply. Redundancy and stasis may present as late complications. Microvascularized free tissue jejunal grafts are excellent reconstructive bridges for minimal defects, particularly those in the hypopharynx, and are used in conjunction with the above surgical techniques.

LATE SEQUELAE

Long-term complications from a caustic ingestion include esophageal stricture and the potential for malignant transformation. Progressive dysphagia usually indicates a stricture, which can be documented radiographically or endoscopically. Bougienage is useful in the setting of a documented stricture more than 4 weeks after ingestion. Earlier dilations carry a high risk for iatrogenic perforations. Dilatation should be performed every other week, aiming for passage of a 46 to 50 French dilator in adults and a 32 to 36 French dilator in toddlers. High rates of perforation after bougienage and balloon dilatation underscore the difficulty in dilating corrosive strictures. Other risks include pulmonary aspiration and recurrent dysphagia. Intractable strictures require a bypass operation, resection, or esophagoplasty.

Persistent strictures or iatrogenic perforation may require an esophagectomy with an esophagogastric anastomosis or colon interposition. An esophageal bypass leaves the native esophagus *in situ* with the reconstruction of a new esophageal conduit and risks the formation of a mucocele in the isolated remnant.

In general, caustic esophageal burns are regarded as premalignant. The risk for carcinomatous degeneration in the strictured residual esophagus is said to be up to 1,000-fold higher than the expected frequency in the general population. Marchand in 1955 was unable to document any cases of carcinoma in the follow-up of 133 patients; however, the interval between injury and the development of cancer averages more than 40 years. Tumors are usually squamous cell cancers and typically develop in the midesophagus. Long-term annual follow-up of patients with grade IIB and III injuries is warranted. Persistent or recurrent dysphagia after a caustic ingestion should be evaluated annually, with both endoscopy and barium swallow. Periodic endoscopic brushings and biopsies are essential in evaluating the retained segment or documented stricture.

In summary, the ingestion of corrosives continues to require emergent medical and surgical intervention despite preventive strategies. The initiation of broad-based prevention strategies can increase public awareness and reduce the incidence of severe injuries. In Finland, a ban on lye effectively reduced the incidence of severe esophageal burns. Children tend to ingest caustic agents primarily by accident; thus, massive or life-threatening cases are fortunately rare. The lowest morbidity and mortality results from the early recognition of the extent and spectrum of caustic injuries and aggressive early surgical intervention.

SUGGESTED READINGS

Anderson KD, Rouse TM, Randolph JG. A controlled trial of corticosteroids in children with corrosive injury of the esophagus. *N Engl J Med* 1990;323:637–640.

Cattan P, Munoz-Bangrand N, Berney T, et al. Extensive abdominal surgery after caustic ingestion. *Ann Surg* 2000;231: 519–523.

Choi RS, Lillemoe CW, Lund DP, et al. Esophageal replacement in children who have caustic pharyngoesophageal strictures. *J Pediatr Surg* 1997;32:1083–1088.

Ein SH. Gastric tubes in children with caustic esophageal injury. *J Pediatr Surg* 1998;33:1363–1365.

Estrera A, Taylor W, Mills LJ, et al. Corrosive burns of the esophagus and stomach: a recommendation for an aggressive surgical approach. *Ann Thorac Surg* 1986;41:276–283.

Haller JA, Andrews HG, White JJ. Pathophysiology and management of acute corrosive burns of the esophagus: results and treatment in 285 children. *J Pediatr Surg* 1971;6:578–584.

Hugh TB, Kelly MD. Corrosive ingestion and the surgeon. *J Am Coll Surg* 1999;189:508–522.

Rao RB, Hoffman RS. Caustics and batteries. In: Goldfrank LR, et al., eds. *Toxicologic emergencies, 6th ed.* New York: Appleton & Lange, 1998:1399–1420.

Sugawa C, Lucas CF. Caustic injury of the upper gastrointestinal tract in adults: a clinical and endoscopic study. *Surgery* 1989;106: 802–807.

36

ESOPHAGEAL FOREIGN BODIES

ELLEN S. DEUTSCH

Young children explore the world with their hands and their mouths. Lack of complete dentition, limited oromotor control and immature judgment each may contribute to the ingestion of a foreign body. Many foreign bodies pass uneventfully through the digestive system, but some become lodged in the esophagus and require surgical removal.

DIAGNOSTIC APPROACH

Most children who ingest foreign bodies are under 3 years of age, and most esophageal foreign bodies in children are coins. Patients may be asymptomatic, or they may have dysphagia, emesis, or, in some cases, stridor, fever, or a cough aggravated by eating. Lodgment most commonly occurs just below the cricopharyngeus muscle, at the level of esophageal compression by the aortic arch and left main bronchus, or at a stricture.

Two-view radiographs of the neck and chest are often useful in identifying both the location and shape of a foreign body, as well as sequelae, such as an esophageal air-fluid level, prior to endoscopy (Fig. 36.1). A barium esophagram usually demonstrates the presence of a nonradiopaque foreign body, and also helps identify any underlying atresia or stenosis, which can contribute to foreign body lodgment. Water-soluble contrast may be indicated if a fistula, perforation, or aspiration is suspected (Fig. 36.2). Radiologic signs suggestive of perforation include extraluminal foreign bodies, retropharyngeal air, widening of the retropharyngeal soft tissue, or leakage of contrast.

In asymptomatic patients, a 24-hour period of observation is usually safe. Radiographic evaluation may then need to be repeated. Coins that reach the stomach are likely to pass through without complication and may be followed radiographically. Button batteries, sharp objects, and objects causing bleeding, acute or severe airway compromise, or significant pain or dysphagia must be removed emergently.

E. S. Deutsch: Departments of Otolaryngology–Head and Neck Surgery and Pediatrics, Thomas Jefferson University, Philadelphia, Pennsylvania; and Department of Surgery, Alfred I. duPont Hospital for Children, Wilmington, Delaware.

TECHNICAL APPROACH

Rigid pediatric esophagoscopes contain a side-channel oriented such that stiff plastic suction catheters or narrow, flexible alligator or biopsy forceps can be inserted into the lumen alongside a Hopkins rod telescope, allowing simultaneous magnification, visualization, and distal illumination. Alternatively, telescopes, light carriers, metal suction catheters, optical forceps, or other grasping instruments can be placed within the lumen of an open tube esophagoscope.

An experienced endoscopist might be able to retrieve a proximal esophageal foreign body during episodes of apnea, but in general, patients undergoing rigid esophagoscopy should be intubated, allowing control of the airway and minimizing time constraints. Taping the endotracheal tube to the left oral commissure facilitates passage of endoscopic instruments and helps to avoid inadvertent extubation.

The esophagus begins at the cricopharyngeus muscle and extends to the gastroesophageal junction at the diaphragmatic hiatus. The wall of the esophagus is thin and lined by a shiny, pale pink mucosa laced with fine blood vessels. Normally the lumen of the esophagus is collapsed in a flattened or stellate pattern. According to Jackson, a straight rigid tube with a diameter of 7 mm should pass freely within a normal infant's esophagus, and one that is 10 mm within a normal adult's esophagus.

The diameter of the esophagus is normally reduced at four points: the cricopharyngeus, the crossing of the aorta, the crossing of the left mainstem bronchus, and the hiatus esophagus at the diaphragm. The average distance to these points from the upper teeth, according to age, are shown in Fig. 36.3. A fifth narrowing of the esophageal lumen occurs just below the cricopharyngeus, at the superior aperture of the thorax, and is probably produced by the crowding of the numerous organs that enter or leave the thorax through this aperture.

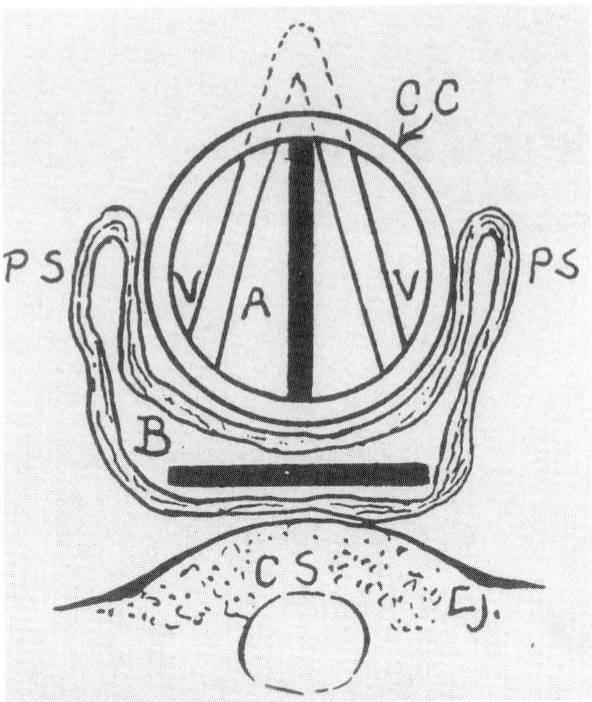

FIGURE 36.1. Diagram illustrating that a coin lodged in the proximal esophagus will lie in a coronal plane, whereas a coin lodged in the proximal airway will lie in a sagittal plane. (Reprinted from Jackson C, Jackson CL. *Diseases of the air and food passages of foreign-body origin.* Philadelphia: WB Saunders, 1936; with permission.)

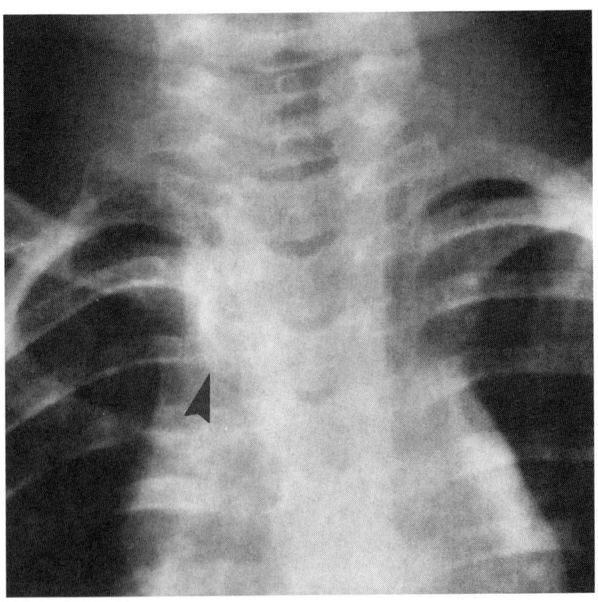

FIGURE 36.2. Radiograph demonstrating residual barium contrast coating a foreign body lodged in the proximal esophagus in a child with an esophageal stricture. (Courtesy of Gerald Mandel, M.D.)

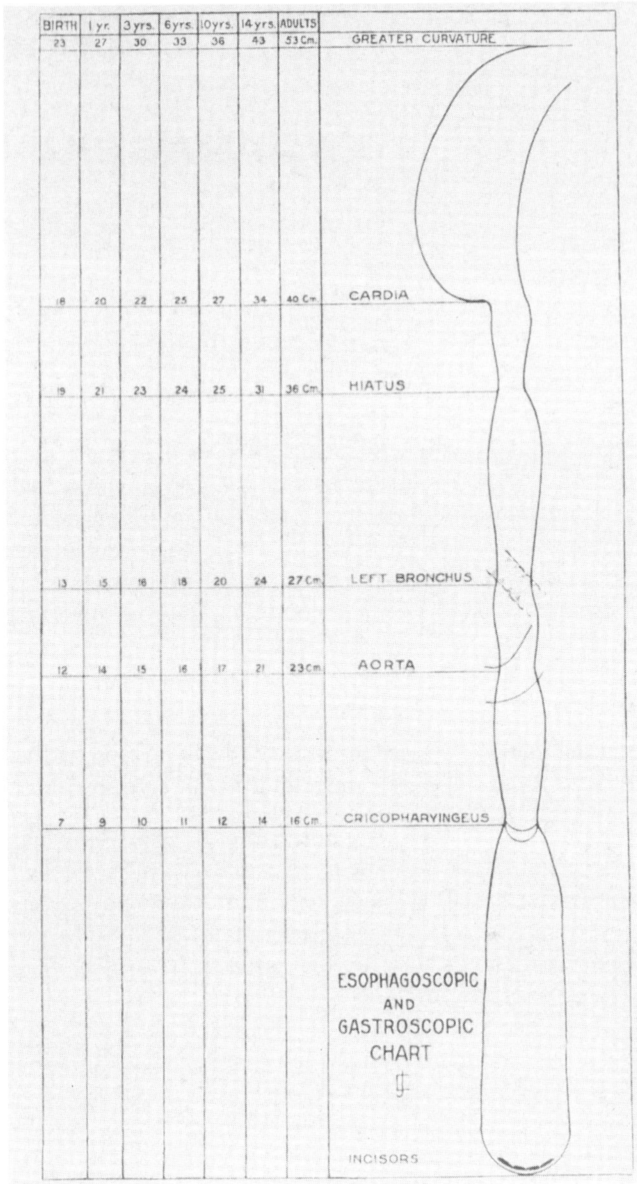

FIGURE 36.3. Jackson's chart of approximate distances of esophageal narrowings from the upper incisors at various ages. (Reprinted from Jackson C. Bronchoscopy and esophagoscopy. In: *A manual of peroral endoscopy and laryngeal surgery.* Philadelphia: WB Saunders, 1922: with permission.)

Advances in illumination and optics have facilitated the development of rigid esophagoscopy; however, an understanding of optimal patient positioning derives from the insight of physicians working in collaboration with sword swallowers. The two "crucial moments" during sword swallowing occur during passage of the sword at the upper and lower esophageal sphincters. The sword swallower must optimize the position of the proximal esophagus by voluntary anterior displacement of the lower jaw, hyoid bone, and tongue base, and simultaneously accommodating the forward direction of the distal esophagus. During modern rigid esophagoscopy, these alignments are achieved by changing the position of the patient's head and neck as insertion of the esophagoscope progresses.

In the "high-low" technique described by Jackson, the position of both the endoscopist and the patient's head and neck relative to his body change as the endoscopy proceeds. Initially, the patient's head is elevated into the "high" position, and the endoscopist stands cephalad to the patient. When available, a trained assistant sequentially adjusts the position of the patient's head. An alternative is to maintain head position by placing a firm support under the patient's head, and flexing and eventually extending the joint of the operating room table beneath the patient's neck.

Initially the esophagoscope is nearly vertical, with the long end of the bevel positioned anteriorly. As the esophagoscope is advanced along the right side of the tongue and down the posterior pharyngeal wall, the long bevel is used to lift the tongue base, endotracheal tube, and arytenoids in advance of the esophagoscope, and the position of the esophagoscope will approach horizontal. The esophagoscope follows the natural food passage: just as the epiglottis splits a bolus of food and the two portions drift laterally into the pyriform sinuses, the esophagoscope is introduced via the right pyriform sinus. A lifting motion imparted to the tip of the esophagoscope by the left thumb will expose the rounded right arytenoid eminence. The tip of the esophagoscope should now be directed somewhat toward the midline, following the funnel shape of the hypopharynx. The endoscopist's right hand remains at the proximal end of the esophagoscope to control the angle of insertion and progression of the esophagoscope, as well as the position of the telescope within the esophagoscope, and to manipulate side channel suctions or other equipment. The endoscopist's left hand is positioned at the alveolar ridge or maxillary teeth. The fingers of the left hand advance the esophagoscope and maintain an awareness of a space between the esophagoscope and the patient's teeth, and the left thumb lifts the tip of the esophagoscope. The cricopharyngeus is entered without force. Once the esophagoscope is introduced through the esophageal introitus and cricopharyngeus, the endoscopist sits and the head of the operating table is lowered below horizontal. At this point, the esophagoscope can be rotated so that the side-channel port is on the right, facilitating passage of suction catheters or instruments with the endoscopist's right hand. While instruments are manipulated with the right hand, the left hand maintains the appropriate position of the scope. The esophagoscope is gently advanced with the left hand, following the lumen.

The esophagoscope should glide easily through the thoracic esophagus. After the impressions or pulsations from the aorta and the left bronchus are passed, the lumen of the esophagus seems to disappear anteriorly. The patient's head is lowered and moved horizontally to the right so that the axis of the tube corresponds to the axis of the lower third of the esophagus. As the esophagus deviates to the left and turns anteriorly, the hiatus is usually apparent as an anteriorly placed narrowing. The patient's head and shoulders are supported by the head of the table, which at this point will be below the plane of the rest of the table. In addition to its anterior curvature, the lower third of the esophagus turns strongly to the left, so an esophagoscope inserted from the right angle of the mouth, when introduced into the stomach, points in the direction of the left anterior superior iliac spine. As the hiatus is passed, the stellate pattern of the esophagus is replaced by the deeper red velvety gastric mucosa and prominent rugal folds.

To grasp a foreign body during rigid esophagoscopy, the jaws of the forceps are inserted beyond the tip of the esophagoscope before they are opened and they may be used to push surrounding mucosa away from the foreign body. If the foreign body is too large to be withdrawn through the lumen of the esophagoscope, the esophagoscope is advanced to shield the foreign body. Sharp objects should be sheathed, or rotated so that the point trails (Fig. 36.4). A blunt foreign body may be held tightly against the opening of the esophagoscope, and the esophagoscope and foreign body withdrawn simultaneously, cephalad, in the

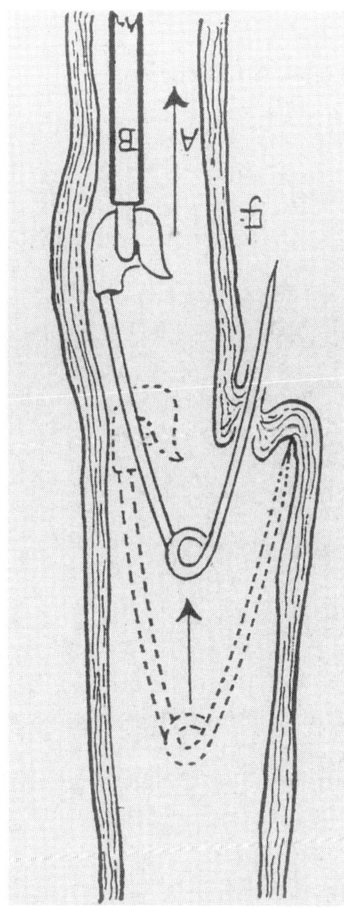

FIGURE 36.4. Schematic drawing of what will happen from ignoring the dictum "Advancing points perforate; trailing points do not." (Reprinted from Jackson C. Bronchoscopy and esophagoscopy. In: *A manual of peroral endoscopy and laryngeal surgery, 2nd ed.* Philadelphia: WB Saunders, 1927; with permission.)

plane of least resistance. Once proximal to the cricopharyngeus, the esophagoscope is tilted approximately 90 degrees to continue in an anterior direction through the pharynx and oral cavity. During the last phase of the maneuver, it may be more comfortable for the endoscopist to resume standing.

Specular esophagoscopy is the inspection of the hypopharynx and upper esophagus with an esophageal speculum or a long laryngoscope. The larynx is exposed as in direct laryngoscopy, the right pyriform sinus is identified, and the tip of the speculum is gently insinuated to the cricopharyngeal constriction. Slight flexion at the occipitoatloid joint may be helpful. Moderate anterior or upward traction pulls the cricoid away from the posterior pharyngeal wall and opens the lumen of the esophagus. The speculum has the disadvantage of limited length, so that should the foreign body move downward it cannot be followed with this instrument.

When feasible, the use of a "rat-toothed" forceps will allow the foreign body to swivel into the plane of least resistance. All U.S. coins have a rim, facilitating the surgeon's ability to grasp them.

POSTOPERATIVE CARE

Following uncomplicated removal of an asymptomatic coin, most patients can be fed once they have recovered from anesthesia. In the case of an atypical foreign body, difficult extraction, or significant underlying disease, patients may be observed and not fed for varying lengths of time. A chest radiograph should be obtained to evaluate the possibility of free mediastinal air or pleural effusion, infiltrate or pneumothorax. Either or both hemithoraces may be affected. If perforation is suspected, contrast esophagraphy should be performed, first with water-soluble contrast and then with thinned barium solution.

ALTERNATIVE METHODS

The use of rigid esophagoscopes with Hopkins rod telescopes remains the gold standard for evaluating and removing esophageal foreign bodies, but other methods have been advocated and may be useful in selected circumstances. Pharmacologic agents such as nifedipine have been used with varying degrees of success to facilitate the passage of an impacted foreign body by manipulating esophageal muscular tone. Glucagon does not appear to be effective in the dislodgment of esophageal coins in children. Enzymatic digestion of a meat bolus with papain (Adolph's Meat Tenderizer; Lipton, Englewood Cliffs, New Jersey) has largely been abandoned because of an unacceptable complication rate. Emetic agents are ineffective and unsafe. Blind bougienage with Maloney dilators and insertion of nasogastric tubes to push the object into the stomach are occasionally used, but current opinion favors abandoning these methods as lacking safety and efficacy. Nonendoscopic removal of foreign bodies does not allow evaluation of esophageal injury or visualization of multiple or radiolucent foreign bodies.

Fiberoptic esophagascopes are sometimes used to remove selected foreign bodies. Special adaptations include using suction or a protector hood secured to the tip of a fiberoptic esophagoscope, or performing retrograde esophagoscopy from a gastrostomy. Fiberoptic esophagoscopes are limited in their ability to visualize the region of the introitus and cricopharyngeus, where foreign bodies frequently become impacted.

In comparing the results of various techniques, one must consider comparable foreign bodies, as well as whether complications may result from the foreign body itself, from anesthesia or sedation, or from instrumentation. Berggreen et al. reported that rigid esophagoscopy with the use of general anesthesia was more likely to be successful than all other techniques combined in both adults and children, and that differences in complication rates were not statistically significant. Rarely, foreign bodies are so large or sharp that lateral pharyngotomy is necessary; and foreign bodies that have migrated into the soft tissues of the neck may require open neck exploration.

PITFALLS

Assembling the telescope within a pediatric esophagoscope with a locking bridge results in the tip of the telescope protruding beyond the opening of the esophagoscope, limiting visualization. Alternatively, the telescope can be secured within the esophagoscope by inserting it through a perforated rubber cap. This is less stable than a locking bridge, but allows the tip of the esophagoscope to distend the esophageal lumen in advance of the telescope, improving visualization (Fig. 36.5). Using this technique, the grip in the right hand must remain relaxed; clenching the fingers will cause the tip of the telescope to protrude beyond the tip of the esophagoscope.

The operating room table should have a movable joint under the patient's neck, so the patient's neck and head position can be adjusted as the procedure progresses. The end of the table should protrude so the endoscopist can sit comfortably with his or her legs beneath the head of the table as needed during the procedure.

To avoid perforation, the esophagoscope and any esophageal instruments should be advanced only when the lumen of the esophagus is visible, and the distal end of the instrument is visible within the esophageal lumen.

A side-channel suction can be used to aspirate secretions that interfere with visualization, and can be withdrawn slightly but left within the esophagoscope when not

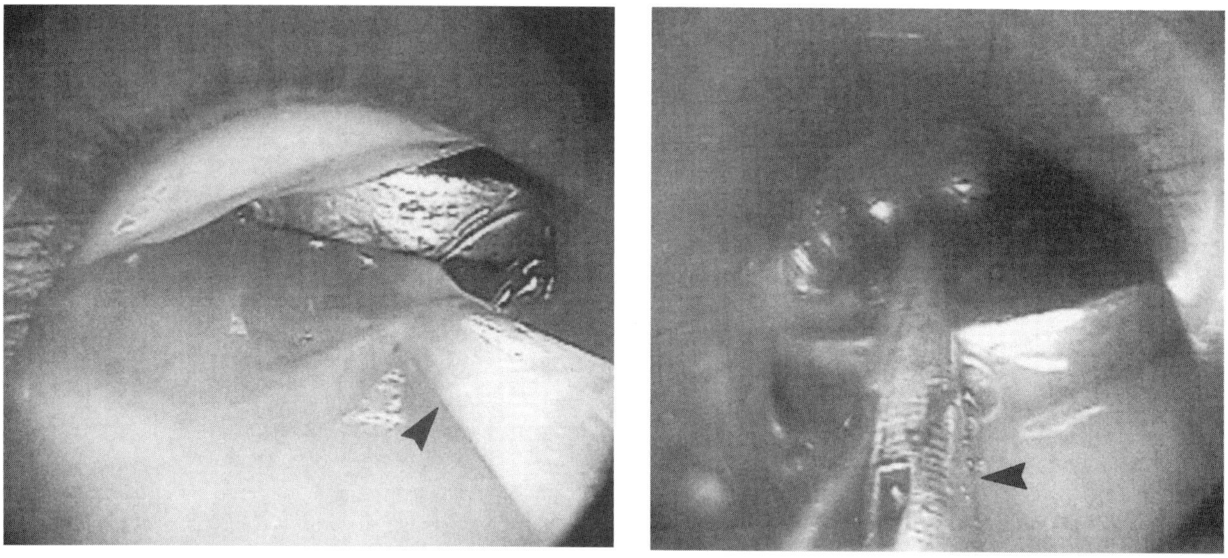

A C

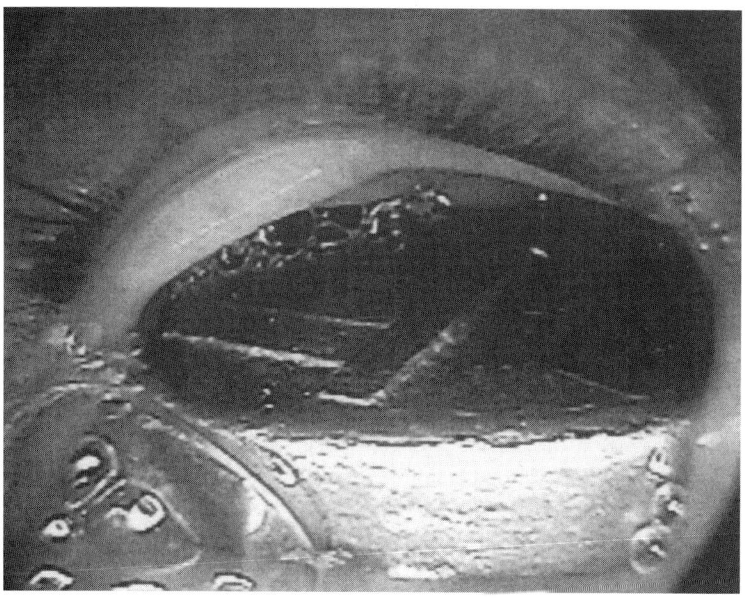

B

FIGURE 36.5. Visualization of a coin lodged in the esophagus. **A:** Note the suction catheter used to aspirate secretions interfering with visualization. **B:** View of coin. **C:** Coin grasped with a side-channel alligator forceps immediately prior to removal.

in active use. If the telescope is held in position by a rubber cap, the length to which the telescope is inserted into the esophagoscope can be varied by the endoscopist. If the esophagoscope becomes flooded with secretions, then the telescope can be partially withdrawn proximally, and the suction catheter can be positioned with good visualization. Withdrawing the telescope a few centimeters also allows visualization of side-channel instruments as they are advanced, before they project into the lumen of the esophagus.

Foreign bodies may be surrounded and obscured by granulation tissue, and some that escape detection during prograde endoscopy can sometimes be found while slowly withdrawing the esophagoscope. After foreign body removal, it is reasonable to repeat the endoscopy to evaluate the possibility of mucosal erosions or additional foreign bodies, as well as underlying strictures or other lesions, especially if the foreign body was atypical.

Button batteries, commonly used in hearing aids, watches, electronic devices, greeting cards, toys, and even novelty clothing items designed for children, can cause significant injury when lodged in the esophagus. Battery discharge state is not related to patient outcome. The patient who has ingested a button cell battery should undergo two-view radiographs of the neck and chest to determine its location. Batteries lodged in the esophagus should be removed emergently, because burns may occur as early as 4 hours after ingestion, and perforation as soon as 6 hours after ingestion. Fatalities have been reported. Removal should be performed endoscopically to allow direct visualization. The battery should be identified by size and imprint code, or by evaluation of a duplicate, measurement of the battery compartment, or examination of the product, packaging, and instructions. If the chemical system cannot be identified from packaging or product instructions, it can be determined from the imprint code by calling the National Button Battery Ingestion Hotline at 202-625-3333. When mercuric oxide cells are ingested, blood and urine mercury levels are necessary only if the cell is observed to split in the gastrointestinal tract or radiopaque droplets are evident in the gut.

COMPLICATIONS

Sharp objects have a perforation rate of 15% to 35%, but even coins can cause stridor, esophageal erosion, aortoesophageal or tracheoesophageal fistulas, mediastinitis, or paraesophageal abscess. Other complications of esophageal foreign bodies include esophageal edema, laceration or erosion, hematoma, granulation tissue, retropharyngeal abscess, mediastinitis, migration of the foreign body into the fascial spaces of the neck, arterial-esophageal fistulas with massive hemorrhage, respiratory problems, strictures, and proximal esophageal dilation.

Esophageal perforation may occur as a result of instrumentation or as a consequence of ulceration or erosion of the esophageal wall from the foreign body. Perforations most commonly occur at the weakest points of the esophageal wall, such as the area just below the cricopharyngeus, the distal one fifth, or the site of any local lesion that weakens the wall. Symptoms include retrosternal pain, back pain, and fever. Subcutaneous emphysema may be evident on physical examination. Because the retrovisceral space and the superior mediastinum have few tissue barriers, infection following rupture spreads rapidly and extensively and may result in septic mediastinitis.

Perforation caused by esophagoscopy can often be managed by prohibiting oral intake, and administering antibiotics and intravenous fluids. A feeding jejunostomy is occasionally indicated. If the tear is large or there is evidence of infection in the pleural space or mediastinum, surgical repair and drainage should be performed urgently. A pleural effusion necessitates drainage. The associated mortality rate is high and is greater in patients under 10 years of age or if recognition is delayed 24 hours or longer.

Other potential complications of esophagoscopy include cricoarytenoid joint dislocation and bleeding. Insufflation used during fiberoptic esophagoscopy can cause abdominal distension, contributing to respiratory compromise. Judicious choice of instrument diameter and length, maintaining visualization of the esophageal lumen, and gentleness of touch will help prevent complications.

FOLLOW-UP

Most patients who have undergone atraumatic removal of asymptomatic esophageal coins do not require additional follow-up; however, children with atypical impactions may have predisposing conditions such as esophageal strictures or neuromuscular disturbances. Patients are instructed to return for follow-up if they have risk factors for esophageal stricture or have dysphagia or signs or symptoms of esophageal perforation, in which case a barium swallow or additional swallowing evaluations may be useful.

SUGGESTED READINGS

Berggreen PJ, Harrison E, Sanowski RA, et al. Techniques and complications of esophageal foreign body extraction in children and adults. *Gastrointest Endosc* 1993;39:626–630.

Hawkins DB. Removal of blunt foreign bodies from the esophagus. *Ann Otol Rhinol Laryngol* 1990;99:935–940.

Huizinga E. On esophagoscopy and sword-swallowing. *Ann Otol Rhinol Laryngol* 1969;78:32–39.

Jackson C. Bronchoscopy and esophagoscopy. *A manual of peroral endoscopy and laryngeal surgery.* Philadelphia: WB Saunders, 1922. (Chevalier Jackson's writings are especially valuable for understanding patient positioning and anatomy.)

Litovitz T, Schmitz BF. Ingestion of cylindrical and button batteries: an analysis of 2382 cases. *Pediatrics* 1992;89(Part 2):747–757.

Loh KS, Tan LK, Smith JD, et al. Complications of foreign bodies in the esophagus. *Otolarnygol Head Neck Surg* 2000;123:613–616.

Lore JM Jr. *An atlas of head and neck surgery, 3rd ed.* Philadelphia: WB Saunders, 1988.

Mehta DI, Attia MW, Quintana EC, et al. Glucagon use for esophageal coin dislodgment in children: a prospective, double-blind, placebo-controlled trial. *Acad Emerg Med* 2001;8:200–203.

Myer CM III. Potential hazards of esophageal foreign body extraction. *Pediatr Radiol* 1991;21:97–98.

Steiner W. Techniques of diagnostic and operative endoscopy of the head and neck. Tracheoscopy, bronchoscopy, esophagoscopy, medistinoscopy, interdisciplinary panendoscopy. *Endoscopy* 1979; 11:151–157.

Winkler AR, McClenathan DT, Borger JA, et al. Retrograde esophagoscopy for foreign body removal. *J Pediatr Gastroenterol Nutr* 1989;8:536–540.

37

ACHALASIA

ALAN P. LADD
L.R. SCHERER III

Achalasia may be defined as irregular or absent peristalsis of the esophagus with associated hypertonicity and failure of relaxation of the lower esophageal sphincter (LES). Esophageal achalasia is a relatively rare problem in children, with those under 15 years of age making up only 4% to 5% of the symptomatic cases. This condition accounts for only 0.7% of cases among children with esophageal symptoms and is extremely rare among those less than 1 year of age. Expertise in the treatment of achalasia relies on the infrequent exposure to children with such an affliction and in compilation of approaches and outcomes from multicenter data.

DIAGNOSTIC IMAGING

Children with the diagnosis of achalasia maintain a duration of symptoms that often approaches 3 years. Presenting symptoms include regurgitation of food, dysphagia, and failure to thrive, and depend on the patient's age and cognitive function. Respiratory difficulties also may be present and are often the result of chronic aspiration.

Screening roentgenograms in children with this disorder are routinely normal. Occasional diagnoses of a mediastinal mass (24%) or abnormal thoracic air-fluid levels (21%) may be found. Evaluation of the esophagus with achalasia by way of a barium esophagram will demonstrate a smooth narrowing of the distal esophagus with dilatation of the proximal esophagus. Stricture from gastric reflux disease must be ruled out in such cases with upper endoscopy and will reveal normal mucosa of the esophagus, an easily passable esophageal narrowing, and no evidence of reflux disease in those with achalasia.

Esophageal manometry is used to discern the relative impairment of esophageal motility and to definitively demonstrate achalasia through the lack of relaxation of the LES to physiologic stimuli. LES pressures above 25 mm Hg are often recorded. Manometry also reveals lower amplitudes to the primary and secondary esophageal contractions, as well as segmental nonpropulsive or absent contractions of the esophagus in the majority of patients.

A. P. Ladd and **L. R. Scherer III:** Department of Surgery, Indiana University School of Medicine; and Department of Surgery, J.W. Riley Hospital for Children, Indianapolis, Indiana.

PREOPERATIVE CONSIDERATIONS

Historical reports have alluded to the use of pharmacotherapy in the treatment of achalasia. Studies, mostly from the adult population, show discouraging results from the use of agents such as nifedipine, verapamil, and isosorbide dinitrate with regard to their efficacy and side effects. Administration of botulinum toxin into the gastroesophageal region of the esophagus has shown short-lived usefulness on the order of months to years. This intervention requires general anesthesia with concurrent endoscopy for administration, often necessitating numerous injections for treatment failure or eventual loss of effect. At this time, the utility of botulinum toxin injections for achalasia should be reserved for patients who would not tolerate more invasive techniques.

Dilatation of the LES offers another avenue of treatment with the possibility of avoiding operative intervention. Through the application of intraesophageal pressures on the magnitude of 15 to 25 psi by either pneumatic or hydrostatic dilatation, disruption of the circular muscular complex of the LES occurs. Success rates of 25% to 73% have been reported, often using numerous treatments. Long-term results from this technique are inferior to those of surgical intervention, but the technique has been used by some clinicians as a means of screening those patients who will require definitive surgical intervention. Sequential bougienage has no place in the preoperative treatment of children with achalasia.

Upon the diagnosis of achalasia in an infant or child, only surgical intervention should be considered for definitive, long-term care.

SURGICAL TECHNIQUE

Our operative technique of thoracoscopic esophagomyotomy follows a modified technique described by Pellegrini. The patient is ventilated with a double-lumen endotracheal tube or with right mainstem bronchus intubation and placed in a right lateral decubitus position with appropriate padding of the head and pelvis. The left lung is allowed to collapse, and entrance into the chest is begun through a small incision in the third intercostal space just anterior to the posterior axillary line. A hemostat is used to bluntly dissect through the chest wall and into the thoracic cavity. A 5-mm trocar is then inserted into the chest through this tract. A 5-mm telescope may then be used to verify lung collapse and document any adhesions present. Additional trocars are then placed in a diamond configuration (Fig. 37.1). A 10-mm trocar is placed in the fifth intercostal space at the posterior axillary line for a working telescopic port. This is followed by placement of a 5-mm trocar in the sixth intercostal space along the anterior axillary line to be used for retraction and separation. A second 10-mm trocar is placed in the midaxillary line in the seventh intercostal space to be used as an operating port.

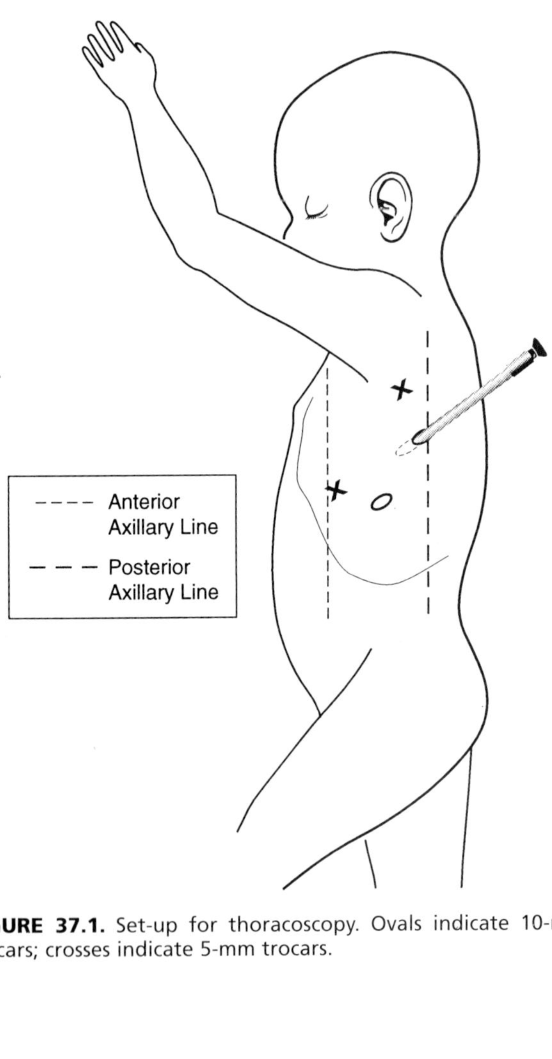

FIGURE 37.1. Set-up for thoracoscopy. Ovals indicate 10-mm trocars; crosses indicate 5-mm trocars.

The inferior pulmonary ligament is divided, allowing for retraction of the lung anteriorly with a fan retractor. The exposed mediastinal pleura is identified overlying the posterior pericardium and the aorta. Thoracoscopic shears or electrocautery are used to divide the pleura in this area. With the passage of an esophagoscope through the mouth, the esophageal location may be identified between the pericardium and aorta, with insufflation and mechanical pressure on the left lateral esophageal wall. Hook electrocautery is used to divide the esophageal muscularis, continuing the dissection through to the division of the circular muscular layer. Once this level has been reached, bipolar endoshears may be used to carry the dissection cephalad to the level of the inferior pulmonary vein and distally to the diaphragmatic hiatus. A two-handed technique, in which the surgeon uses his left hand to grasp the muscularis and the right hand to perform the dissection with electrocautery and shears, expedites the operation. Orientation of the dissection along the anterolateral aspect of the esophagus preserves the nearby anterior vagus nerve. The endoscope is invaluable during this dissection in both exposing the esophagus and directing the depth and length of dissection. During the distalmost portion of the dissection, the diaphragm should be retracted downward and the esophagus pulled cephalad. One must appreciate the change in orientation of the esophageal muscularis fibers and thinner mucosa in this region during dissection. The myotomy is carried approximately 0.5 cm onto the stomach, reaching the point of complete LES relaxation verified by endoscopy. Blunt dissection is used to elevate the muscularis from the underlying mucosa in order to allow its complete separation and avoid reannealing. A thoracostomy tube is placed through the dependent trocar site at the conclusion of the procedure. It may be removed on the first postoperative day.

COMPLICATIONS

Operative success in this palliative intervention lies in the LES dissection. One must confirm division of the distal circular muscle fibers of the LES. This is easily accomplished with the use of upper endoscopy. Dissection is carried onto the gastric wall until complete relaxation of the LES is verified to achieve this goal. Extension onto the cardia of the stomach must remain limited to less than 1.0 cm in order to minimize postoperative gastroesophageal reflux. We favor the above technique because the thoracoscopic approach minimizes injury to the antireflux mechanism of the diaphragmatic crura, and thus reduces problems with postoperative gastroesophageal reflux.

Violation of the mucosal layer during dissection should be immediately addressed. A thoracic esophageal mucosa injury necessitates a primary repair through either thorascopic maneuvers or open thoracotomy. Drainage of the thoracic repair is essential. The integrity of the repair should be confirmed through barium esophagraphy on postoperative day 5, prior to initiation of enteral feeds.

Operative intervention following trials of hydrostatic or pneumatic dilatation efforts must be performed with caution. Full-thickness scarring of the submucosa to the muscularis layers may result from the dilatory trauma. Dissection planes are thus obscure and increase the rate of operative perforation. Extreme diligence in dissection must be carried out in these difficult cases.

POSTOPERATIVE CARE

Narcotic or neuraxial opioid analgesia is recommended postoperatively in addition to nonsteroidal (i.e., ketorolac) injections during hospitalization. In uncomplicated cases, oral liquids may be initiated the first postoperative day. Diet may be advanced as tolerated with discharge by the third or fourth postoperative day. Early pulmonary physiotherapy by way of incentive spirometry and indirectly with early ambulation will minimize pulmonary complications.

FOLLOW-UP

Persistent dysphagia may afflict up to 10% of patients from incomplete myotomy. Similarly, gastroesophageal reflux occurs at a rate of nearly 15% to 20% in those patients undergoing esophagomyotomy without simultaneous fundoplication. These children should be followed regularly within the first year to verify successful intervention. Continued dysphagia should be reevaluated with barium esophagram and esophageal manometry to discern anatomic from functional etiologies. Treatment is then directed accordingly.

Partial gastroesophageal fundoplication may be required in those with proven postoperative reflux disease. Care should be taken to avoid violation of the exposed submucosal layer of the esophagus during repair as well as to prevent reapproximation of the muscularis layers. Laparoscopic Toupet or Dor partial gastric fundoplications are adequate in this situation.

Long-term follow-up also must be continued in light of the patient's underlying esophageal dismotility and possible reflux. A well-documented risk of esophageal adenocarcinoma has been estimated to occur in 5% to 10% of patients with achalasia. Routine esophagoscopy should be considered in patients with or without symptoms of gastroesophageal reflux disease.

SUGGESTED READINGS

Holcomb GW, Richards WO, Riedel BD. Laparoscopic esophagomyotomy for achalasia in children. *J Pediatr Surg* 1996;31:716–718.

Myers NA, Jolley SG, Taylor R. Achalasia of the cardia in children: a worldwide survey. *J Pediatr Surg* 1994;29:1375–1379.

Nakayama DK, Shorter NA, Boyle JT, et al. Pneumatic dilatation and operative treatment of achalasia in children. *J Pediatr Surg* 1987; 22:619–622.

Pellegrini C, Wetter LA, Patti M, et al. Thoracoscopic esophagomyotomy: initial experience with a new approach for the treatment of achalasia. *Ann Surg* 1992;216:291–299.

Vane DW, Cosby K, West K, et al. Late results following esophagomyotomy in children with achalasia. *J Pediatr Surg* 1988;23: 515–519.

38

ESOPHAGEAL PERFORATION

SIGMUND H. EIN

Esophageal perforation can occur in the newborn period, in older children, usually from foreign bodies, and during esophageal dilatation.

In the *newborn*, the rare esophageal perforation is almost always iatrogenic and typically occurs during attempted tracheal intubation or during attempted passage of a nasogastric tube. Both of these events are known to be difficult and are often unsuccessful. Bloody mucus noted immediately upon oral suctioning is usually the key sign that a perforation has occurred. The perforation is usually in the hypopharynx or upper esophagus, and extravasation of the oral secretions or initial feeds into the neck may cause respiratory distress, coughing, choking, sputtering, or turning blue. This extravasation into the soft tissues of the neck may produce crepitation on examination. There also may be extravasation if the mediastinum is torn, which causes the usual symptoms and signs of mediastinitis: fever, respiratory distress, esophageal obstruction and sepsis, and even the false impression of an obstruction leading to the equally false diagnosis of an esophageal atresia. In the latter case, the nasogastric tube may lie in the false passage with the tip stopping at the "obstruction."

Apart from the usual resuscitation of any baby with an upper airway problem or sepsis, chest radiography (including the neck) will show most of the above, if one is looking for it. If one is suspicious of a false passage mimicking an esophageal atresia, esophagram with water-soluble material or instillation of the contrast material down the nasogastric tube is indicated. When such a diagnosis is proven either by radiologic study or inadvertent thoracotomy (for a mistaken esophageal atresia), the nasogastric tube (if it is still in place) must be removed, and 1 week of broad-spectrum antibiotics (we prefer triple antibiotics) started, as well as total parenteral nutrition. Of course, if there is a perforation into the pleural cavity (almost always the right side), a chest tube to treat the pyopneumothorax is necessary; it should be left in as for a leaking esophageal atresia anastomosis. Another option for nutrition is to carefully pass a feeding tube into the stomach in the Radiology Department. Breast milk or formula can then be dripped through this tube.

The follow-up investigations are much like those for a leaking esophageal atresia anastomosis: a weekly water-soluble esophagram until the leak has healed (usually in 1–2 weeks) as well as antibiotic coverage until the leak has healed. Then all tubes can be removed and the baby fed in a normal fashion. It is unusual for the neck or mediastinum to require drainage, and I have never seen any long-term consequences from such perforations.

Foreign body perforations of the esophagus are uncommon in my experience, and usually occur in infants and toddlers. There is often an acute episode (in retrospect, a choking episode) and then the sudden or more chronic dysphagia for solids. The history of any of the above warrants chest radiography in case the foreign object is radiopaque, and even if the chest radiograph is normal, probably a water-soluble esophagram. If anything suspicious is seen, computed tomography and esophagoscopy are warranted.

If a foreign body is diagnosed, it can then be removed by esophagoscopy or, failing that, thoracotomy. If, however, the foreign body remains unnoticed and undiagnosed, it may cause an esophageal obstruction, or erode through the esophageal wall into the mediastinum, creating a tracheoesophageal/bronchial fistula or mediastinal abscess. The fistula can create a formidable problem, but fortunately its occurrence is rare. Obviously the foreign body must be removed and the fistula given a chance to close; this will require endoscopy and a nasogastric feeding tube or a gastrostomy. These tracheoesophageal fistulas are often mucosally lined (by the time they are discovered and the foreign body removed) and therefore will probably not close spontaneously. The other options are then operative closure (usually quite an undertaking, often fraught with complications and a unique lack of success), or the use of glue (with or without the passage of a stent) either via the esophagus or airway. The latter method requires the skill and patience of a very good Interventional Radiologist or endoscopist (Pediatric General Surgeon, Pediatric Otorhinolaryngolo-

S. H. Ein: Department of Surgery, Division of General Surgery, Faculty of Medicine, University of Toronto; and Division of General Surgery, The Hospital for Sick Children, Toronto, Ontario, Canada.

gist). Only as a last resort, when all else fails (I have only seen this on one or two occasions) is the sacrifice of the esophagus to permanently close the fistula. This will, of course, later require the creation of an esophageal substitute of the surgeon's choice (presently colon, gastric pull-up, or gastric tube). I prefer a gastric tube.

Probably the most common cause of an esophageal perforation is iatrogenic and occurs at *esophageal dilatation* for a stricture. Most, but not all, of the esophageal dilatations at our hospital are performed by Otorhinolaryngologists. The stricture usually results from repair of an esophageal atresia, gastroesophageal reflux, or caustic ingestion. The surgeon almost always knows (no matter who does it or how it is done) that he or she has perforated the esophagus. In such cases, the procedure must be stopped (even if there is only a suspicion of a perforation) and chest radiography performed to rule out a pneumothorax. This is followed by a water-soluble esophagram. Once the perforation is confirmed, the treatment is the same as outlined earlier in this chapter.

Over the past four decades at the Hospital for Sick Children in Toronto, almost all of these esophageal perforations have been treated nonoperatively, and quite successfully. The few esophageal perforations that have been treated operatively have uniformly releaked, and then the infant or child was faced with a thoracotomy incision (sometimes infected), as well as the leaking esophagus. My observation is that the esophageal perforations treated nonoperatively have always healed. One of the theories behind this successful, nonoperative treatment of esophageal perforations is the so-called resistance to a diffuse mediastinitis in many children whose mediastinum is "burned out" from previous surgery or inflammation. The planes are all sealed, so the perforation does not have far to go, and of necessity tends to be fairly well localized. Although we have talked about this at our hospital, it has never been put in print until now. It has been our (i.e., Departments of General Surgery and Ear, Nose, and Throat) clinical impression that once a dilated esophageal stricture has been perforated, it seldom needs to be dilated again after it heals. Of course, it must never be the intention of the dilator to be that aggressive or cavalier.

Although esophageal perforations due to *trauma* and *forceful vomiting* are exceedingly rare in the pediatric population, their investigation and treatment should be the same as stated above, with the even rarer exception of an operative repair, if the trauma causes additional damage to other mediastinal structures. In that case, esophageal repair with interrupted sutures is certainly warranted. However, the chances of this happening will be rare. Dr. Naclerio stated it very well almost 30 years ago: "Esophageal wounds secondary to penetrating or crushing trauma to the chest or abdomen occur infrequently principally because the esophagus is in a relatively protected paravertebral position. Also, if the injury is such as to damage the esophagus, major damage to the heart, aorta, or some other great vessel is usually also present and these wounds will in themselves frequently lead to immediate or early fatality." I cannot remember the last traumatic (puncture or blunt trauma) esophageal perforation at the Hospital for Sick Children, Toronto (a major pediatric trauma referral center), over the past 34 years, and in reviewing pediatric surgical publications in a similar time span (1967–2001), fewer than 10% had injuries to two of three major systems in the chest, with the airway being the most common and the esophagus being the most rare.

SUGGESTED READINGS

Blair GK, Filler RM, Theodorescu D. Neonatal pharyngoesophageal perforation mimicking esophageal atresia: clues to diagnosis. *J Pediatr Surg* 1982;22:770–774.

Ein SH. Gastric tube. In: Spitz L, Coran AG, eds. *Rob and Smith's operative surgery—pediatric surgery.* London: Chapman, 1995: 143–151.

Ein SH. Gastric tubes in children with caustic esophageal injury: a 32-year review. *J Pediatr Surg* 1998;33:1363–1365.

Ein SH, Friedberg J. Esophageal atresia and tracheoesophageal fistula: review and update. *Otolaryn Clin North Am* 1981;14:249–291.

Ein SH, Friedberg J, Chait P, et al. Traumatic tear of aorta, trachea and esophagus in a seven year old with survival. *J Pediatr Surg* 2002;37(1):E1.

Naclerio EA. *Chest injuries: physiologic principles & emergency management.* New York: Grune & Stratton, 1971:297.

Pieretti R, Shandling B, Stephens CA. Resistant esophageal stenosis associated with reflux after repair of esophageal atresia: a therapeutic approach. *J Pediatr Surg* 1974;9:355–357.

Simpson JS, Ruff T, Fearon B. Esophageal perforation during endoscopy in children. *Ann Otol Rhinolaryngol* 1974;83:1–4.

39

ESOPHAGEAL REPLACEMENT

ERIC R. SCAIFE
DALE G. JOHNSON

Esophageal replacement, either for congenital deficiencies in esophageal length or to repair esophageal injury or destruction, remains a surgical challenge and the subject of continuing controversy. The first successful esophageal replacement in a child was accomplished by W.A. Ladd, the father of pediatric surgery in the United States, who in 1939 treated an infant with esophageal atresia and tracheoesophageal fistula (EA-TEF). A gastrostomy was performed at 24 hours, extrapleural division of the TEF at 4 months, and esophageal replacement with presternal skin tube at 4 years. In the same year, N.L. Levin also treated an EA-TEF patient with gastrostomy at 72 hours and extrapleural division of the TEF at 5 weeks of age. Esophageal replacement in this patient was later accomplished by jejunal interposition at 12 years of age. In 1946, G.H. Humphreys II performed a mediastinal jejunal interposition in an 11-year-old child with EA-TEF who had undergone tube gastrostomy for esophageal replacement as an infant. Partial necrosis of the graft delayed the planned upper anastomosis for 5 years when continuity was finally established between the upper esophagus and the interposition, and oral feedings were first taken at 16 years of age.

Surgeons working with adult patients approached the technical challenges of esophageal replacement beginning early in the 20th century. Gastric tube replacement was described as early as 1905, whereas reports of skin-lined tubes, jejunal interposition, and colon transplants appeared before 1922. The techniques for colon esophageal replacement in the retrosternal, intrapleural, or posterior mediastinal positions all were developed after 1948. Gastric transposition in the posterior mediastinum, initially advocated by Adams and Phemister in 1938 and Sweet in 1945, has become the current favorite for esophageal replacement in adults, and has strong advocates as the procedure of choice in children.

E. R. Scaife and **D. G. Johnson:** Department of Surgery, Division of Pediatric Surgery, University of Utah School of Medicine; and Division of Pediatric Surgery, Primary Children's Medical Center, Salt Lake City, Utah.

The optimal approach to esophageal replacement remains highly dependent on the anatomy of the patient and the preferences of the surgeon. In the pediatric patient, gastric transposition, gastric tube, and colon interposition are the most popular techniques. Colon interpositions can vary in their route (substernal or mediastinal) and their blood supply (right colic or left colic). The most recent option in current debate involves techniques designed to achieve primary esophageal salvage. Data are insufficient at this time to rate one approach as clearly superior to all others. Therefore, this discussion will focus on our experience and preferences.

INDICATIONS

The congenital anomaly most commonly associated with esophageal replacement is primary EA with a long gap. Except for the occasional tracheal trifurcation or bronchoesophageal fistula, EA-TEF can usually be managed with primary repair. Although occasionally needing to be repaired in stages, this condition seldom requires esophageal replacement. The rare congenital esophageal stenosis involving a long segment and multiple cartilage rings may require resection and distal replacement, but the majority can be managed with direct anastomosis.

Injury of the esophagus from caustic ingestion can cause reversible mucosal injury, submucosal and muscular scarring leading to variable degrees of stricture, or total destruction of the esophagus with acute perforation. The extent of the injury depends on the strength and volume of the agent ingested and the duration of contact. Although caustic injury is the most common indication for esophageal replacement in children in developing countries, child safety regulations have made these injuries a rarity in the United States.

Untreated reflux esophagitis also can cause esophageal strictures that are not responsive to dilatation and antireflux surgery. Such severe strictures represent full-thickness injury with scar contracture and are often best treated by esophageal replacement.

DIAGNOSIS

The clinical presentation of EA is well known, and delivery room examination and diagnosis should be the standard of care. Inability to pass a nasogastric tube should lead to radiographic confirmation of a blind air-filled upper esophageal pouch. Classic symptoms of excessive salivation, coughing, respiratory distress, and regurgitation of feedings never develop if appropriate diagnostic tube insertion has been performed at birth. This maneuver is indicated for all infants and will identify both EA and EA-TEF. The presence of a blind upper pouch and the absence of bowel gas on a plain abdominal radiograph are essentially diagnostic of pure EA. The esophageal gap is confirmed by distal contrast study via gastrostomy.

If the upper esophageal pouch appears short and does not reach T2 in the chest, the possibility of an upper pouch TEF must be considered. Esophageal contrast studies risk aspiration and may yield falsely negative results. Endoscopic probing of the esophageal pouch most accurately confirms the diagnosis. Tracheoscopy is less accurate because the upper pouch fistula passes obliquely downward from esophagus to trachea, making visualization difficult without a retrograde view. Esophagoscopy can be performed either at the time of gastrostomy for the patient with isolated EA or at the time of fistula repair if a distal TEF is present.

Congenital strictures of the esophagus usually require both radiographic contrast studies and esophagoscopy for accurate preoperative diagnosis.

Caustic burns of the esophagus should be evaluated by flexible esophagoscopy within the first few hours of injury. The risk for perforation is minimal in the early stage if the endoscopist is experienced and if the scope is not advanced past areas of severe injury. Information regarding extent of injury is critical for determining subsequent duration and type of management.

Reflux strictures are evaluated by contrast esophagraphy, esophagoscopy, esophageal biopsy, 24-hour pH monitoring, therapeutic trial by proton pump inhibiting agents, and trial dilatations. Differentiation from achalasia is occasionally difficult but can usually be established based on a combination of diagnostic studies. Esophageal manometry also may sometimes be helpful.

PREOPERATIVE PREPARATION

The most immediate surgical concern in a baby with pure EA is the placement of a gastrostomy tube within the first few days of life. Technical aspects of the gastrostomy construction can be challenging, because the stomach in some infants may be so small the gastric fistula site barely reaches the abdominal wall. The gastrostomy is necessary as a route for nutrition, and the graduated bolus feedings serve the additional function of stretching the unused stomach and the distal esophageal segment. The upper pouch is managed with sump tube suction to prevent overflow aspiration of oral secretions. We try to avoid cervical esophagostomy because of our preference for eventual placement of the upper coloesophageal anastomosis in an intrathoracic, posterior mediastinal position.

During the sabbatical between gastrostomy and the definitive repair, some surgeons have advocated daily bougienage. In our experience, this is no more effective than waiting 6 to 12 weeks for spontaneous growth. We also suspect that the bougie can cause inflammation and edema, which may present a technical disadvantage at the time of anastomosis. Attempts to stretch the lower esophageal segment via gastrostomy likewise are seldom successful, even under fluoroscopy, and the procedure offers significant risk for perforation.

Preoperative contrast study of the stomach is useful to evaluate the adequacy of gastric stretching and to demonstrate the length of the lower esophageal segment. The lateral chest film with a bougie in the upper pouch and contrast in the lower pouch allows an estimate of the gap length and is useful on serial films to evaluate for a progressive decrease in gap length and the possibility of direct anastomosis or esophageal replacement. The final decision about the most appropriate type of reconstruction is not made until tension between the two esophageal segments is tested by traction after extrapleural exposure.

The ideal time to perform the definitive repair varies according to surgeon's preference. Although it is possible to reconstruct some large infants as early as 3 weeks of age, we prefer to delay esophageal reconstruction for 6 to 12 weeks after birth. The delay permits growth of the upper pouch and distention of the stomach and distal segment. The vascular arcade of our preferred colon replacement segment is also better developed at that age.

The date of the operation prompts an additional set of considerations to prepare the child for major surgery. Mechanical bowel preparation is performed for 24 hours preoperatively, whenever esophageal replacement is a possibility. Systemic antibiotics with aerobic and anaerobic organism coverage are started within 30 minutes of making the incision. Blood should be available on standby, but transfusion is not always needed.

TECHNICAL APPROACH

Patients with long-gap EA are positioned in a right-side-up thoracotomy position. The right neck, arm, chest, and abdomen are painted with povidone-iodine solution. Sterile draping then extends from the chin and occiput to the pelvis, and from midline to midline on the chest, plus the entire anterior surface of the abdomen. The right arm and hand are prepared into the field and covered with stockinet. Patient positioning must allow shifting from the right lateral position for the intrathoracic work, to the oblique abdominal position, and back several times during the procedure.

The initial skin incision is a right posterolateral thoracotomy skin incision overlying the fifth intercostal space. The latissimus dorsi muscle is incised, but the serratus anterior is mobilized and preserved. The chest is entered extrapleurally through the fourth intercostal space to mobilize the upper pouch and through the seventh or eighth intercostal space to expose the distal segment. An abdominal incision is not made until the feasibility of a direct esophageal end-to-end anastomosis has been determined.

Upper pouch dissection and traction are facilitated by placement of a 14 French rubber catheter in the pouch. Two silk sutures are then passed through the base of the pouch and through the indwelling catheter. This allows traction on the pouch without tearing of esophageal tissue. The upper pouch always shares a short segment of common wall with the trachea, and this must be incised sharply without injuring the trachea or the esophagus. In the rare circumstance of an upper pouch fistula, which should have been identified by intraoperative esophagoscopy and catheter stenting of the fistula, any existing TEF can be closed at this time. Upper pouch fistulas are virtually always associated with a short upper esophagus, and the surgical approach in such cases may be facilitated by an additional supraclavicular incision.

The distal esophagus is exposed extrapleurally through the seventh intercostal space, but the residual segment may be small and difficult to identify in the posterior mediastinum. It is therefore helpful to pass a Bakes common duct dilator through the gastrostomy from below and then guide the dilator into the distal esophagus with a hand in the mediastinum. Once identified, the distal esophagus also can be tagged with traction sutures to assist mobilization. Care must be taken to avoid injury to the vagus nerves during this distal dissection.

Traction on both segments of the mobilized esophagus will allow the experienced surgeon to decide whether a primary anastomosis is feasible and appropriate. The majority of series describing primary anastomosis report a high complication rate, including anastomotic leak, stricture, poor esophageal motility, and intractable reflux associated with displacement of the gastroesophageal junction into the chest. Mortality also has been reported at 25% to 40%.

An exceptional experience with direct anastomosis for long-gap esophageal defects is that of Foker and Linden, who assert that all cases of congenital EA can be managed by direct anastomosis. They have developed a technique whereby traction sutures on both the upper and lower esophageal ends are brought out through the chest wall and tied over buttons. The sutures are progressively tightened over the course of 1 to 3 weeks. Not all of their patients had isolated EA without a distal fistula, however, and the more commonly used staged approach would have perhaps yielded comparable results. Their reported success with the small number of patients with isolated EA with a long gap is nevertheless intriguing. The investigators reported only one early anastomotic leak among 93 patients meeting their definition of a long-gap defect. Five of 17 anastomotic strictures were subsequently resected, and 15 of 17 long-gap patients eventually required fundoplication for intractable reflux. This report is certainly provocative, but at this writing there are no comparable reports from other centers using this technique.

Our preference is to perform primary anastomosis only when the ends can be brought together with tension that is not extreme and which should allow a secure anastomosis using our standard anastomotic technique. We feel that a well-executed replacement is superior to a misguided attempt at direct anastomosis when the conditions are not favorable.

A right upper quadrant transverse incision is made and extended across the midline below the gastrostomy. The gastrostomy fistula is not taken down, and the stomach is left attached to the anterior abdominal wall. The colon and mesocolon are inspected to make sure that the vascular arcade appears intact and there has been no mesenteric vascular injury from any previous surgery. Trial clamping of the right colic and middle colic vascular pedicles may be considered if there is doubt about adequacy of the marginal vessels connecting the left and middle colic blood supply. The goal is to construct a graft using an isoperistaltic segment of transverse and left colon based on a left colic artery vascular pedicle.

If the blood supply is judged to be adequate, the middle colic vessels are doubly ligated and divided near their origin to preserve marginal flow, and the omentum is removed close to the serosa of the colon and discarded. The course of the planned interposition is then prepared by bluntly dissecting a tunnel beneath the splenic vessels and the tail of the pancreas, behind the stomach, and through the esophageal hiatus into the posterior mediastinum. Three Penrose drains are then passed through the hiatal tunnel, behind the stomach, and behind the pancreatic tail. Gentle traction on this harness of drains lifts the pancreas and stomach forward and opens the hiatal tunnel. This maneuver facilitates the eventual transfer of the colon segment and its vascular pedicle into the posterior mediastinum.

To isolate an adequate length of colon, the first of two measuring procedures is performed. A long silk suture is used to measure the distance from the upper esophageal pouch, through the mediastinum, to the left colic blood supply. This length of suture is then laid upon the colon, starting at the left blood supply. The end of the suture defines the transection point, which will become the proximal anastomosis. Almost invariably, the proximal division of the colon will be near the hepatic flexure (Fig. 39.1). It is always possible to trim excess length if the measurement is not exact, but a segment cut too short cannot be recovered.

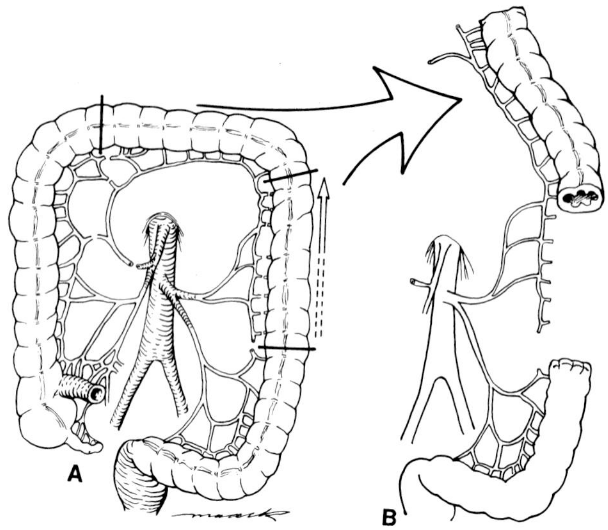

FIGURE 39.1. A: The colon interposition segment. After the first measurement, the colon is divided near the hepatic flexure and the descending colon. The distal portion of the conduit is eventually trimmed (*broken arrow*), so that the graft will perfectly bridge the gap between the proximal and distal esophageal pouches. The graft is fed off of the left colic artery. The middle colic artery is divided near its origin, and the transverse colon is perfused via marginal artery. **B:** When the distal portion of the graft is trimmed, it is critical to accurately divide the small end vessels close to the wall of the colon to be discarded. Accurate division protects the adjacent main vascular pedicle.

The colon is divided at the measured proximal site by application of a gastrointestinal stapling device. The distal division is also executed by stapling and is designed to preserve with the pedicle as many of the left colic vascular elements as possible. Usually there are two or three significant branches that can be incorporated as blood supply for the transposed colon graft.

Traction sutures are then placed at the proximal end of the colon segment, two sutures on the mesenteric side and one antimesenteric for orientation. It is helpful to also run a longitudinal tacking suture loosely through the taenia to maintain orientation and to prevent spiral rotation as the segment is pulled through the tunnels into the posterior mediastinum. Spiral twisting is easily overlooked and can result in luminal obstruction or vascular compromise. With the traction and orientation sutures in place, the colon segment is then drawn into the chest and more precise measurements are then made for the proximal and distal sites of transection that will allow colon interposition between the proximal and distal esophagus without anastomotic tension but also without redundancy. The transection levels are marked with sutures. The proximal end may not require trimming if the first measurement was accurate.

Following the second measurement, the colon segment is drawn back into the abdomen for preparation of the vascular pedicle. A short segment of the distal colon transplant is then discarded from the level of distal transection to the suture marking the distal anastomosis for the interposition. Technically, this is one of the most critical aspects of the operation because of the risk for compromise of the vascular pedicle. The end vessels leading from the marginal arcade to the colon must be divided very close to the colon wall, and we prefer to use fine, bipolar electrocoagulation forceps to minimize heat transfer or possible injury to the remaining pedicle.

The right and left colon segments are reanastomosed in two layers before the graft is transferred to the chest. The mesenteric defect is closed over the vascular pedicle before the abdomen is closed at completion of the operation.

Once the distal colon segment has been removed, the graft is transferred again through the hiatus and into the posterior mediastinum. The hiatus needs to be enlarged only minimally to allow this transfer, and once the interposition segment is in the chest, the vascular pedicle lies to the left and posterior to the esophagus (Fig. 39.2). The retroperitoneal course of the pedicle behind the stomach and pancreas protects the pedicle from injury during any future abdominal procedure and also forms the shortest and most direct route to the mediastinum.

The upper anastomosis is performed in the upper mediastinum using the fourth intercostal incision. The graft will lie in the normal anatomic position for the esophagus. Avoidance of initial cervical esophagostomy minimizes the potential for recurrent nerve injury and also prevents graft pinching at the thoracic outlet, which is sometimes encountered with intrathoracic rather than mediastinal interpositions. For this operation we prefer a two-layer interrupted anastomosis using 5-0 and 6-0 suture.

The distal anastomosis is technically more difficult because of location and size disparity between the small esophagus and the colon segment. This anastomosis is also performed in two layers with fine interrupted suture. The esophageal segment is cut obliquely to lessen size disproportion, and an additional anterior incision may be necessary to eliminate anastomotic puckering. When the lower esophageal segment is very short, we have found it useful to slide the anastomosis through the hiatus to perform the anastomosis from the abdominal side. Whenever possible, this lower anastomosis is wrapped with an anterior fundoplication of stomach to reinforce the suture line and to minimize postoperative gastroesophagocolic reflux. We make a point to avoid vagal nerve injury at the time of distal anastomosis. We generally place two chest tubes in the extrapleural space, one at the level of each anastomosis, and the wounds are closed in the standard fashion.

Some clinicians have advocated resection of the distal esophageal remnant with direct anastomosis between the colon and the fundus of the stomach. Unless there is virtually no distal esophagus remaining, as is often the case with caustic burns, we think both control of reflux and swallowing function are better when the graft is interposed between the upper and lower esophageal segments. Some

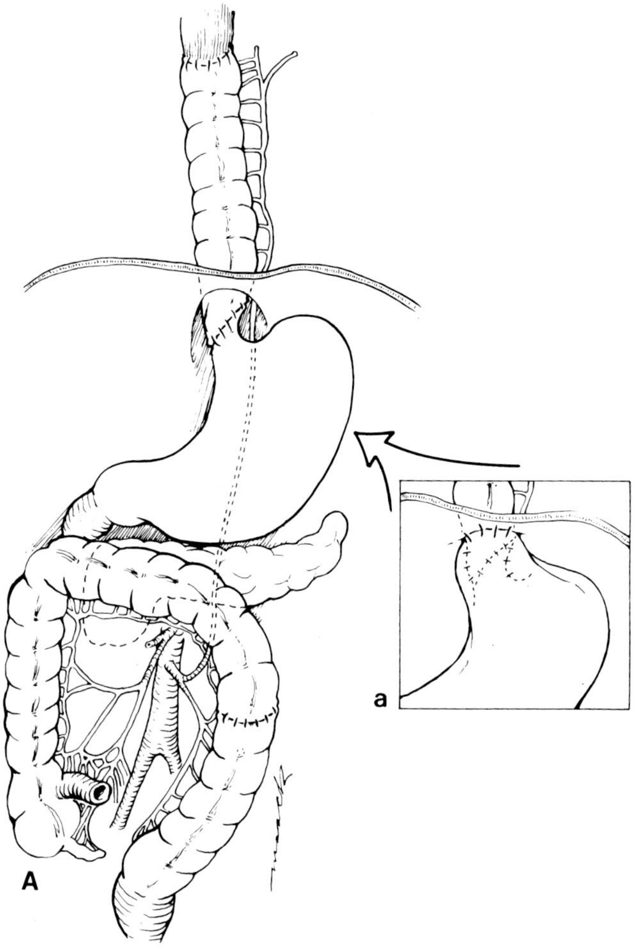

FIGURE 39.2. A: The completed colon interposition. The vascular pedicle is based off of the left colic artery and passes behind the pancreas and stomach in the retroperitoneum and exits the abdomen through the esophageal hiatus. The small distal esophageal stump is cut obliquely in order to transition the size discrepancy between it and the colon. **a:** An anterior fundoplication is fashioned to minimize gastrocolic reflux. The dotted lines represent the suture lines covered by the fundoplication. The wrap is sewn to the left side of the esophagus, then across the anterior surface of the esophagus, next to the right side, and finally the anterior surface of the wrap is sewn to the diaphragm. The vascular pedicle prevents a 360 degree fundoplication; in addition, a 360 degree wrap is obstructive underneath an aperistaltic conduit.

clinicians also advocate pyloroplasty to prevent delayed gastric emptying, but it is not part of our operation. In our opinion, the safety and effectiveness of pyloroplasty has not been proven by the current evidence. We have occasionally performed pyloromyotomy, because there is little evidence that it is harmful, but we have little evidence that it makes a difference.

Esophageal replacement for severe reflux stricture or caustic burn seldom allows preservation of a distal esophageal segment; therefore, the lower anastomosis is cologastric rather than coloesophageal. The damaged esophagus is resected from a right retropleural approach whenever possible. Inflammatory reaction from the primary injury, however, may make an intrapleural approach a necessity. The majority of patients will have a usable segment of upper esophagus within the chest, and in such cases we prefer to perform an intrathoracic proximal anastomosis. Chemical or inflammatory destruction of the upper and midesophagus can result in adherence to the adjacent trachea, requiring a careful dissection for esophagectomy without tracheal injury. We therefore do not consider the technique of blunt esophagectomy from the cervical and subhiatal approach appropriate, even if the injury is high enough to require anastomosis to the cervical esophagus or the pharynx. The transthoracic exposure also allows visualization and positioning of the graft with its vascular pedicle throughout the entire mediastinum, thus reducing the chance of an unrecognized twist.

The distal cologastric anastomosis is constructed well within the abdomen and to the anterior portion of the high gastric fundus. It is our clinical, albeit unproven, bias that reflux is more likely to occur when the anastomosis is situated in a posterior dependent position on the fundus. We postulate that the tendency to reflux may be lessened by a smaller fluid residual in the anterior fundus and that the anterior anastomosis, with several centimeters of subhiatal colon, may be dynamically compressed between the stomach and liver. Technically, it is more difficult to construct the anastomosis in the anterior position because the vascular pedicle courses behind the pancreas and gastric body. It is therefore essential that the trimming of the distal graft segment be sufficient to allow anterior relocation of the isolated vessels that are inferior to the colon segment at the same time the graft's distal end is sufficient to maintain 6 to 9 cm of length below the hiatus. Attempts at partial fundoplication at the cologastric anastomosis have been reported but have not been effective in our hands.

It is our preference to perform esophageal replacement at the time of esophagectomy, thus avoiding in most cases the necessity for temporary cervical esophagostomy. In the rare case of severe caustic injury involving acute destruction and perforation of the esophagus, the patient's condition may require emergency esophagectomy, diverting cervical esophagostomy, and staged reconstruction. The diverting cervical esophagostomy should be performed on the right side to avoid the thoracic duct on the left. Ipsilateral or bilateral traction injury to the recurrent nerves presents a real hazard during exteriorization of the upper esophagus. Rarely, the viable segment of cervical esophagus will be too short to reach the skin surface, and sump-tube drainage will be necessary to promote fistula formation. Concentrated acids as well as alkaline agents are likely to cause partial gastric necrosis, and the portion of damaged stomach should be resected at the time of emergent esophagectomy, esophagostomy, and gastrostomy. Delayed esophageal reconstruction in such cases may require an extramediastinal position of the colon graft because of mediastinal scarring following emergency resection.

POSTOPERATIVE CARE

Colon graft decompression is maintained for 5 to 7 days by means of a soft plastic sump tube placed on gravity drainage and irrigated each shift to maintain patency. This prevents gaseous distention of the transplanted segment in the setting of negative intrathoracic pressure. The gastrostomy is maintained on gravity drainage until a water-soluble contrast study is performed on postoperative day 5 to exclude an anastomotic leak. The chest tubes are maintained for the same interval. Nutrition is supported by intravenous infusion at least until the anastomoses are proven intact, and then gastrostomy feeds are initiated. Oral feeds are advanced from liquids to diet as tolerated. Intravenous antibiotic prophylaxis is continued for 48 hours or until the patient is afebrile and without clinical suspicion of infection.

COMPLICATIONS

The most devastating complication is graft ischemia. A necrotic graft must be resected and a diverting esophagostomy performed. It will prove to be a rare complication, if the operation is performed carefully and the vascular pedicle is not kinked or torsed. Failure to recognize it in a timely fashion, however, can result in death.

Perhaps the most frequent early complication is anastomotic leak. Anastomotic leaks are reported to occur in up to 40% of cases. The vast majority of leaks are small and heal with conservative management. Leaks can lead to significant anastomotic stricture, however, and children should have follow-up examinations that focus on this possibility. Pneumonia and intravenous catheter infections are not rare but are easily managed. Unusual complications of mediastinitis, empyema, peritonitis, and intestinal obstruction are all possible but are nearly always avoided by careful operative technique and management.

RESULTS

Colonic interposition is a complex operation that requires a commitment to long-term follow-up. Reflux of gastric contents into the graft probably occurs in most patients, although our recent addition of anterior fundoplication over the lower anastomosis has eliminated radiographic reflux in the small number of patients we have studied. More interestingly, endoscopic evidence of mucosal inflammation in the distal colon-esophagus is rare in our experience. We have not experienced postinterposition reflux strictures, and we do not keep our patients on acid-suppressing medication. Progressive redundancy of an intrathoracic colon graft requiring subsequent segmental resection has been reported by others but has not occurred in our 30-year experience. Proper measurement and careful adjustment of graft length at the initial operation seem to minimize the problems of postoperative redundancy, poor emptying, dysphagia, and halitosis. In our opinion, placement of the graft in the posterior mediastinum rather than the left chest also allows a straighter course, a shorter graft, and better emptying.

Long-term growth retardation and oral aversion have been associated with esophageal replacement, but again, this has not been our experience. Operation at an early age and without the necessity of cervical esophagostomy seems to eliminate the development of oral aversion and the need for supplemental gastrostomy feedings. It is not our experience that these children fall out of normal range on the standard growth charts. It is possible that our efforts to preserve vagal innervation are helpful, but this is only speculation. We have used occasional antegrade dilatation of the upper anastomosis and retrograde bougie or antegrade balloon dilation of the lower anastomosis on a few patients early postoperatively, but we have not been troubled with chronic strictures. There have been no stricture resections or reanastomoses.

In summary, esophageal replacement techniques continue to evolve as clinical experience accumulates. The indications for esophageal replacement remain relatively rare, however, and case numbers and surgical experience are limited even for major referral centers. Our own choice of procedure has changed with increasing personal and reported experience, and with continuing technical advances, our options for the future must remain open. Restoration of esophageal continuity with native esophagus has been an attractive concept, but few surgeons have thus far been able to achieve this goal without a high complication rate. A variety of techniques for esophageal replacement have therefore been described. This chapter describes a technique of colon interposition that has minimized, in our experience, problems associated with anastomotic leak and stricture, graft redundancy, eating and swallowing abnormalities, and inflammatory complications of acid reflux.

SUGGESTED READINGS

Bassiony IE, Bahnassy AF. Transhiatal esophagectomy and colonic interposition for caustic esophageal stricture. *J Pediatr Surg* 1992; 27:1091–1095.

Campbell JR, Webber BR, Harrison MW, et al. Esophageal replacement in infants and children by colon interposition. *Am J Surg* 1982;144:29–33.

Foker JE, Linden BC, Boyle EM Jr, et al. Development of a true primary repair for the full spectrum of esophageal atresia. *Ann Surg* 1997;226:533–543.

Freeman NV, Cass DT. Colon interposition: a modification of the Waterston technique using the normal esophageal route. *J Pediatr Surg* 1982;17:17–21.

Howard R, Myers NA. Esophageal atresia: a technique for elongating the upper pouch. *Surgery* 1965;58:725.

Ladd WE. The surgical treatment of esophageal atresia and tracheoesophageal fistulas. *N Engl J Med* 1944;230:625.

Orringer M, Marshall B, Iannettoni M. Transhiatal esophagectomy for treatment of benign and malignant esophageal disease. *World J Surg* 2001;25:196–203.

Spitz L, Kiely E, Sparnon T. Gastric transposition for esophageal replacement in children. *Ann Surg* 1987;206:69–73.

Stone MM, Fonkalsrud EW, Mahour GH, et al. Esophageal replacement with colon interposition in children. *Ann Surg* 1985;203: 346–351.

Sweet R. Subtotal esophagectomy with high intrathoracic esophagogastric anastomosis in the treatment of the extensive cicatricial obliteration of the esophagus. *Surg Gynecol Obstet* 1946;83:417–427.

Yudin SS. The surgical construction of 80 cases of artificial esophagus. *Surg Gynecol Obstet* 1944;78:561–583.

40

ESOPHAGEAL DUPLICATION

MICHAEL J. GORETSKY
MICHAEL D. KLEIN

The most common enteric duplication in the mediastinum is an esophageal duplication. Most esophageal duplications are cystic, enclosed within the muscular wall, and do not communicate with the lumen. Sixty percent occur in the lower third of the esophagus, and the remainder are equally divided among the upper and middle third. They seldom attain large size and are usually not obstructive. When esophageal duplications occur in the upper esophagus they are usually associated with cervical vertebral anomalies, which may even be unstable. Rarely, a duplication of the esophagus may communicate with the airway and be associated with cough or recurrent pneumonia. They also have been reported to communicate below the diaphragm with the jejunum or even the biliary tree. In these cases they may be associated with bilious emesis or abdominal pain.

The esophagus is derived from multipotential foregut tissue. The duplication cyst is an anomaly that occurs during differentiation of the larynx, trachea, and bronchi from the primitive foregut. This usually occurs around the 4th to 8th week of gestation. Gastric mucosa, respiratory epithelium, and squamous epithelium may all be found in the duplication cyst, although gastric mucosa is more common.

It is believed that during embryogenesis, vacuoles form in the foregut during the solid-tube stage of development. These should normally coalesce longitudinally to form a lumen. If there is a failure of coalescence, a cyst is left adjacent to the esophagus, sharing with it a common wall.

The incidence of esophageal duplication is approximately one in 25,000 live births. Such duplications constitute about 10% of all mediastinal tumors, and usually are located on the right side. Esophageal duplications are rarely symptomatic; however, they may occasionally cause dysphagia, chest pain, regurgitation, failure to thrive, recurrent pneumonias, or airway obstruction. Only 10% communicate with the esophageal lumen, and these may increase significantly due to secretions. If there is gastric mucosa, acid secretions may lead to bleeding, ulceration, or perforation. Vertebral anomalies have been associated with esophageal duplications, and when present may be associated with neurologic deficits, scoliosis, root compression, or pain. Infection may occur, especially if there is a communication, and rarely a malignancy may be present.

Esophageal duplications are usually found serendipitously on a chest radiograph or a computed tomography (CT) scan obtained for another purpose. On a chest radiograph the duplication will present as a radiolucent cyst (Fig. 40.1), usually just above the diaphragm to the left of midline. An esophogram (Fig. 40.2) demonstrates a smooth extrinsic mass indenting the column of contrast but not obstructing it. The differential diagnosis usually includes a pericardial cyst, bronchogenic cyst, and lymphangioma. The diagnosis can usually be made definitively via CT (Fig. 40.3).

Although most patients are asymptomatic, we recommend elective surgery in all cases where there are no contraindications. There is always the possibility of developing symptoms and complications during the natural course of the disease, and the definitive diagnosis cannot be made without a surgical specimen. Complete excision of the cyst is the treatment, and recurrences can occur if the cyst is incompletely removed.

Cyst excision can be performed using either an open approach or a minimally invasive approach. With an open approach, a posterolateral thoracotomy should be performed. Most lesions can be approached from the right side. If the cyst is in the distal esophagus, the left side may be more advantageous. The esophagus is isolated above and below the cyst, taking care to identify and preserve the vagus nerve. The muscular coat is opened and the cyst is "shelled" out without disturbing the esophageal mucosa. The muscle may be reapproximated. There has been a case report of a pseudodiverticulum developing in an area where the muscle had not been reapproximated.

M. J. Goretsky: Department of Surgery, Eastern Virginia Medical School; and Department of Surgery, Children's Hospital of the King's Daughters, Norfolk, Virginia.

M. D. Klein: Department of Surgery, Wayne State University; and Department of Surgery, Children's Hospital of Michigan, Detroit, Michigan.

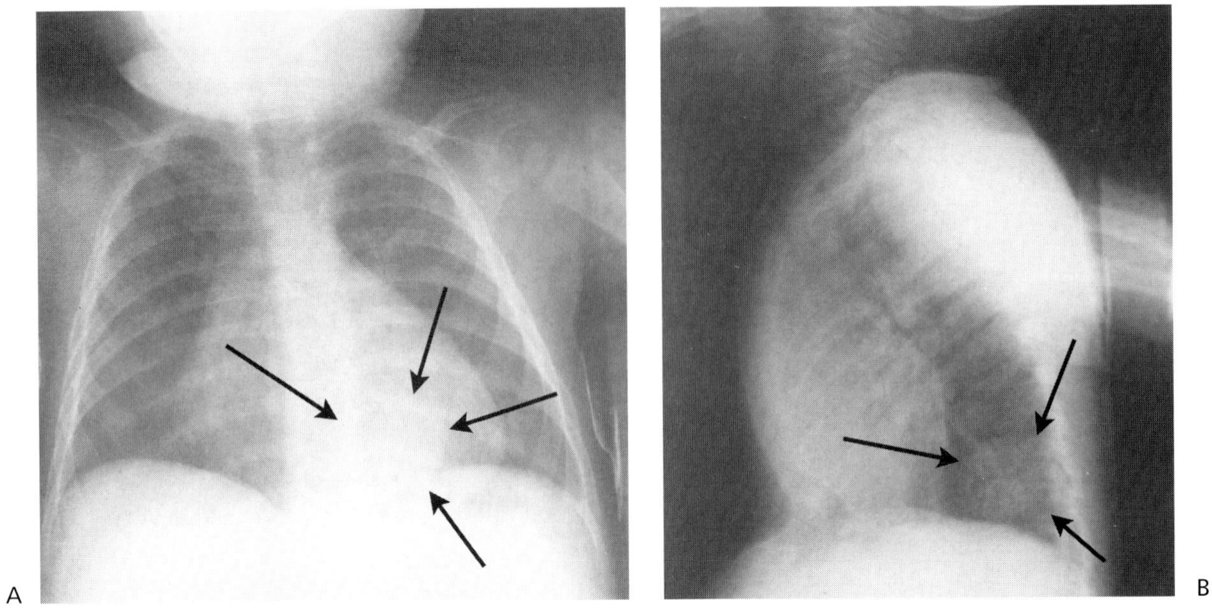

FIGURE 40.1. **A:** Radiolucent mass in the left base on a posteroanterior radiograph. **B:** On a lateral radiograph the mass is in the posterior mediastinum.

Minimally invasive surgery is feasible in most cases. Contraindications to thoracoscopy include mediastinal shift and compressive cysts leading to lung distention. The main advantages of thoracoscopy are reduced postoperative pain, earlier recovery and hospital discharge of the patient, and a superior cosmetic result. Thoracoscopic resection is reasonable for these cysts because they tend to be hypovascular. Care must still be taken to identify the vagus and phrenic nerves. Muscular fiber separation and submucosal dissection may be more difficult by thoracoscopy than thoracotomy due to the lack of tactile feedback, theoretically making injury to the esophagus more likely. Transillumination with a flexible esophagoscope may facilitate the dissection and aid in preserving mucosal integrity. A chest tube may be left to assure lung reexpansion, or the air may be evacuated through a catheter that is removed prior to skin closure. Complications and sequelae are rare.

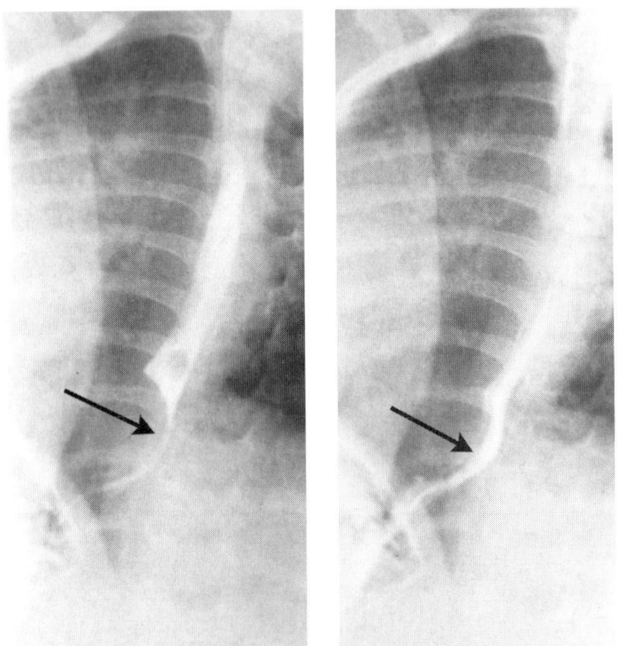

FIGURE 40.2. An esophagram shows a smooth extrinsic mass indenting the esophagus but not obstructing it.

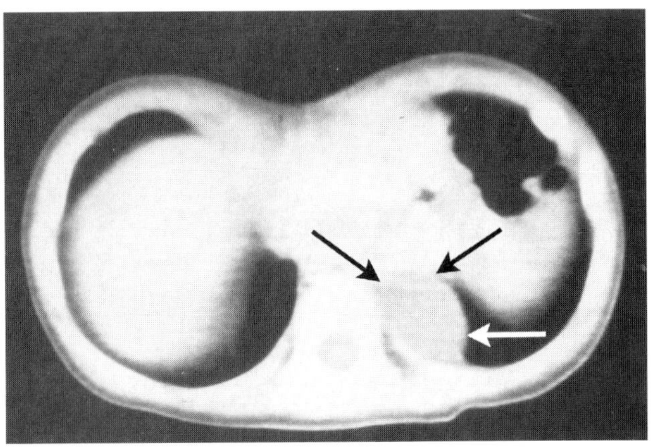

FIGURE 40.3. A computed tomography scan confirming the diagnosis of an esophageal duplication cyst.

SUGGESTED READINGS

Dresler CM, Paterson GA, Taylor BR, et al. Complete foregut duplication. *Ann Thorac Surg* 1990;50:306–308.

Michel JL, Revillon Y, Montupet P, et al. Thoracoscopic treatment of mediastinal cysts in children. *J Pediatr Surg* 1998;33:1745–1748.

Snyder CL, Bickler SW, Cittes CK, et al. Esophageal duplication cyst with esophageal web and tracheoesophageal fistula. *J Pediatr Surg* 1996;31:968–969.

Stewart RJ, Bruce J, Beasley SW. Oesophageal duplication cyst: another cause of neonatal respiratory failure. *J Paediatr Child Health* 1993;29:391–392.

SECTION VI

STOMACH AND SMALL INTESTINE

41

GASTROESOPHAGEAL REFLUX DISEASE

CATHERINE RICHARDS
LEWIS SPITZ

Gastroesophageal reflux (GER) is a common problem in children, and antireflux surgery provides effective control when medical treatment fails. However, postoperative complications are common; an understanding of the underlying physiology is invaluable in selecting patients for surgery and the management of postoperative symptoms.

PHYSIOLOGY OF THE ESOPHAGOGASTRIC JUNCTION

The lower esophageal sphincter (LES) and the sling of the right crus act in an integrated manner to control competence at the gastroesophageal junction. The LES maintains a resting tone 10 to 30 mm Hg above gastric pressure, and lower esophageal sphincter pressure (LESP) increases in response to situations where gastric pressure increases. The LES relaxes in association with specific reflexes such as swallowing, belching, and vomiting. The right crus of the diaphragm encircles the distal esophagus and acts as a pinchcock around the LES. Contraction of the crus is responsible for the cyclical increase in resting pressure in phase with inspiration, and also occurs during other activities that increase abdominal pressure, such as coughing. Reflex relaxation of the crus accompanies relaxation of the LES.

MECHANISMS OF GASTROESOPHAGEAL REFLUX

Gastroesophageal reflux is the *effortless* passage of gastric contents up the esophagus. It occurs when the mechanisms of esophagogastric competence malfunction or are overcome. Episodes of GER occur in normal individuals without significant consequences. Gastroesophageal reflux disease (GERD) occurs when the degree of reflux results in significant symptoms or harm to the patient. Its development depends on the balance between factors promoting reflux and the ability of the esophagus to clear/resist acid-pepsin exposure. The main factor involved in the causation of reflux disease is dysfunction of the LES complex.

The most common mechanism of a reflux event is "transient relaxation": basal LESP is normal, but reflux occurs during an episode of a sudden, brief decrease in pressure to near zero, which is not triggered by swallowing. Transient relaxations occur in asymptomatic individuals, but they are more frequent in patients with GERD, and account for the majority of reflux episodes. Transient relaxation is a vagal reflex; gastric distension stimulates mechanoreceptors in the fundus, especially around the cardia. The physiologic role of transient relaxation is in belching, and it is accompanied by complete inhibition of the crural diaphragm. Less frequently, reflux episodes are associated with a reduced basal LESP.

Other factors contributing to GERD include anatomic abnormalities such as sliding hiatus hernia, which spatially dissociates the crus from the LES. In addition, esophageal dysmotility, delayed gastric emptying, elevated intraabdominal pressure, central nervous system impairment, and the insertion of a feeding gastrostomy tube also may promote GERD.

MEDICAL THERAPY FOR GASTROESOPHAGEAL REFLUX DISEASE

The majority of children with GERD respond to medical therapy:

1. Small volume feedings or continuous tube feedings, to reduce the volume available to reflux and to reduce the stimulus to transient relaxations
2. Feed thickeners to reduce the ease with which liquids reflux

C. Richards: Department of Pediatrics, University Hospital, Lewisham, London, United Kingdom.

L. Spitz: Department of Pediatric Surgery, Institute of Child Health, University College London, Great Ormond Street Hospital, London, United Kingdom.

3. Upright posture, using gravity to reduce reflux and promote esophageal emptying
4. Reduction of the acidity of refluxed material using antacids, histamine receptor antagonists, or proton pump inhibitors
5. Motility agents, to improve gastric emptying, esophageal peristalsis, and LES function

SURGICAL THERAPY FOR GASTROESOPHAGEAL REFLUX DISEASE

Surgical treatment of GERD is indicated if an adequate trial of medical treatment fails to control symptoms, and in the presence of complications such as severe esophageal ulceration, Barrett's esophagus or stricture, chronic pulmonary disease or recurrent aspiration pneumonia, acute life-threatening events, or persistent failure to thrive despite maximal medical therapy. Neurologically normal children often improve with increasing age, and if symptoms can be controlled medically, we adopt a conservative approach. Surgical treatment is more frequently required in the neurologically impaired. Our preferred surgical management of GERD is the Nissen fundoplication, with or without gastrostomy.

DIAGNOSTIC APPROACH

The most common symptom of GERD in children is regurgitation or "vomiting" of feeds. Esophagitis may cause pain or acute or chronic bleeding, and may lead to stricture formation and dysphagia. Respiratory symptoms include reflex apnea and acute life-threatening events, and recurrent episodes of aspiration with pneumonia and chronic lung disease.

Many of the symptoms of GERD also may be due to other causes; if a child responds to simple medical treatment, it may be appropriate to avoid invasive investigations. However, children who are being considered for surgery require thorough investigation to identify as far as possible those whose symptoms are due to GERD. A major pitfall is to perform fundoplication on a vomiting child whose main problem is activation of the emetic reflex. We take a detailed clinical history of the nature, frequency, and amount of any "vomit," together with any accompanying symptoms such as pallor, salivation, sweating, or retching, which indicate activation of the emetic reflex rather than GERD. We plan our investigations to detect the presence and severity of GER, any underlying cause, and the presence of complications. Essential investigations include the following:

1. *Contrast swallow and meal,* to identify any anatomic abnormalities or causes of obstruction (e.g., esophageal stricture, midgut malrotation, or duodenal web). GER may be observed on contrast radiography, but may be missed because the study covers a limited time period. Conversely, if the emetic reflex is activated, then reentry of contrast into the esophagus during retching and vomiting may be misinterpreted as GER, and associated elevation of the gastroesophageal junction may be misinterpreted as a hiatal hernia. Surgical treatment should not be performed for "GER" diagnosed solely by radiography.
2. *24-hour intraesophageal pH monitoring.* This is a more sensitive method of diagnosing reflux and allows a *quantitative* assessment; even normal individuals experience reflux episodes daily. Patients with vomiting symptoms and mild reflux on pH study (i.e., <10% of the time) do not do well with antireflux surgery. The clinician should be wary of patients with severe vomiting symptoms and mild reflux on pH study. The presence of GER per se, does not imply that it is the cause of their symptoms, and does not guarantee that a fundoplication will offer symptomatic relief. It is sometimes useful to combine the pH study with a sleep study when there is concern that reflux is causing recurrent apnea.
3. *Esophagogastroduodenoscopy and biopsy* to reveal any gastritis, active infection with *Helicobacter pylori,* or food intolerance such as gluten enteropathy that may be contributing to symptoms. These should be treated first, and the patient reassessed, before considering surgical intervention for reflux.

Other investigations that may be useful include the following:

1. *Measurement of gastric emptying rate.* A marked delay may foretell a more generalized dysmotility or activation of the emetic reflex. It may indicate the need for prokinetics and will serve as a baseline if there are postoperative problems. Patients with a marked delay in gastric emptying may be better fed directly into the jejunum (i.e., feeding jejunostomy).
2. *Technetium-labeled milk scan with delayed imaging.* In selected cases, this may distinguish whether aspiration is due to GER or a swallowing disorder.
3. *Surface electrogastrography.* This noninvasive method of recording gastric electrical activity is not widely available, but may prove useful in identifying children with specific motility disturbances or a sensitive vomiting reflex.

Patients with GERD resistant to medical therapy or with life-threatening events are candidates for surgery.

ANTIREFLUX PROCEDURE

We perform an open floppy Nissen fundoplication. Preoperative preparation comprises a standard period of fasting and crossmatch of 1 unit of blood. We give a single dose of antibiotics (e.g., benzylpenicillin and an aminoglycoside) with induction of anesthesia and pass a standard-sized nasogastric tube.

We use a midline vertical incision; it is usually possible to gain good access by simple retraction of the left lobe of the liver, without formal mobilization. The upper short gastric vessels are divided to mobilize the fundus sufficiently for a loose wrap. We dissect the esophageal hiatus, identifying and preserving both vagal trunks and exposing both limbs of the crus. We repair the crura with nonabsorbable sutures, until the hiatus accepts only the esophagus plus a fingertip. Crural repair is important even when there is no hiatal hernia, because the dissection will allow the crura to separate and omission of the hiatal hernia repair is associated with a high failure rate. We then pass the gastric fundus behind and around the abdominal esophagus; to achieve a "floppy" wrap, the fundus must sit comfortably in the wrapped-around position without the need for traction. We stitch the wrap (2–4 cm according to the size of the child) in two layers with a nonabsorbable suture—the first layer fundus-esophagus-fundus, the second fundus-fundus—avoiding the anterior vagal trunk. Suturing the wrap to the esophagus should prevent slippage. We do not stitch the wrap to the diaphragm. An adequate wrap and hiatal hernia repair should maintain the wrap position, unless diaphragmatic forces are excessive. In this situation, a "diaphragmatic hitch" has the potential to cause disruption.

We also perform a gastrostomy (Stamm type) in children with dysphagia, those with increased caloric requirements, and in neurologically impaired children who cannot swallow safely. In addition to feeding, the gastrostomy tube is useful for release of gas and relief from emesis, and is readily converted to a transpyloric jejunostomy tube if required. If not used, it is easily removed, with the expectation that the stoma site will close spontaneously in a short period of time.

Postoperatively, the child returns to the ward with the nasogastric or gastrostomy tube on free drainage; most are ready to recommence enteral fluids on the second postoperative day (tube or oral, as appropriate). We order routine chest physiotherapy for children with lung disease.

Complications

Complications are common after antireflux surgery, especially in the neurologically impaired child. Nonprocedure-related complications include postoperative pneumonia, wound infection, and small bowel obstruction. We warn the parents specifically about the possibility of small bowel obstruction, because many children are unable to vomit following fundoplication, although they can still retch. These children are at risk of delayed diagnosis and mortality from intestinal obstruction, and other features such as repeated retching, abdominal distension, and bile aspirates from the gastrostomy must be emphasized.

Complications specific to antireflux surgery and commonly associated with recurrent reflux include wrap disruption, hiatal hernia (often associated with wrap disruption), and wrap slippage (the wrap slides down off the esophagus onto the stomach).

Dysphagia may be a problem in the immediate postoperative period. A number of factors may be responsible: a wrap that is too tight or too long, postoperative edema, impaired migration of the cardia during swallowing, primary esophageal dysmotility (especially children with esophageal atresia), esophageal dysmotility secondary to dissection and mobilization at the hiatus, inhibition of swallow-induced relaxation of the LES, or preexisting peptic stricture. It usually improves spontaneously. Persistent cases (>6–8 weeks after operation) may respond to one or more dilatations (the risk is that a dilatation may cause wrap disruption); resistant cases may need redo fundoplication.

Many patients are unable to belch following antireflux surgery, which may lead to gas trapping in the stomach and gas bloat syndrome. This generally improves with time, and can be relieved by venting the gastrostomy tube. Difficulty in belching is not surprising, considering that the most common mechanism of GER, the transient relaxation, is related to the belch reflex. Failure to belch may be a result of a valvelike effect of the wrap, impaired stimulus to transient relaxations due to denervation, scarring or deformity of the fundus, or the presence of the muscular cuff around the abdominal esophagus. It is noteworthy that following fundoplication, percentage acid reflux time is *significantly less* than normal controls. Similarly, many children are unable to vomit after fundoplication, although the emetic reflex may still be activated, with the associated prodromal symptoms and retching. Only the end stage of the reflex is blocked.

Other potential effects of fundoplication include vagal injury, ranging from division of a major trunk, to injury to minor branches or individual fibers. Some investigators have reported an increased gastric emptying rate in some patients following fundoplication; others have reported no change for liquids or solids. A few children have been shown to have dumping after fundoplication. "Early" dumping is attributed to rapid gastric emptying, leading to a hyperosmotic load to the jejunum, with fluid shifts and a sympathetic response; "late" dumping is attributed to early hyperglycemia due to rapid gastric emptying followed by late reactive hypoglycemia. You cannot reliably diagnose dumping clinically (but by gastric emptying studies and a prolonged glucose tolerance test), because the symptoms are not specific and overlap with those of activation of the emetic reflex from any cause.

Chronic retching/recurrent vomiting in the absence of GER is a common postoperative problem, and its significance is frequently unappreciated. It is due to activation of the emetic reflex. Many children undergoing fundoplication appear to have increased sensitivity to activation of the emetic reflex. This is often already present preoperatively but appears worse after surgery. The emetic reflex is a very different physiologic process from GER. The prodromal phase is characterized by nausea, sweating, salivation, tachycardia, and peripheral vasoconstriction. During the motor phase, retching is followed by vomiting, associated with powerful contraction of the diaphragm and abdominal wall muscles. Gastrointestinal events include retrograde intestinal peristalsis, LES and gastric relaxation and elevation of the gastroesophageal junction through the diaphragmatic hiatus into the thorax. The emetic reflex will be discussed further below, in relation to diagnostic pitfalls and causes of wrap failure.

Diagnostic Pitfalls

It is not sufficient simply to show that a child has GER before proceeding to antireflux surgery. It is essential to show as far as possible that the reflux is the cause of the child's symptoms, as indicated by the investigations above. Central apnea, pharyngeal incoordination, tracheoesophageal fistula, *Helicobacter* infection, food intolerance, or intestinal dysmotility will not respond to antireflux surgery.

A number of children (both neurologically normal and impaired), have an intrinsically sensitive emetic reflex that is responsible for their vomiting symptoms but is frequently confused with GERD. These children often have relatively mild reflux on pH study, but this is incidental or only one small part of the overall problem, and should alert you that there may be other, more significant pathology. Contrast radiography may be misleading in these children. During activation of the emetic reflex, retching and vomiting are accompanied by relaxation of the LES and elevation of the gastroesophageal junction into the thorax. This can give a radiograph the appearance of a wide-open gastroesophageal junction, hiatal hernia, and free reflux. Contrast radiography is useful in showing the anatomy but unreliable in the diagnosis of reflux. False negative results are well recognized, and we believe there are false positive results also. A 24-hour pH study gives a much better indication of the severity of GER.

We have found that many of these children with a sensitive reflex can be identified by a careful clinical history. Activation of the vomiting reflex is accompanied by a number of symptoms and signs that are absent in GER, which is *effortless*. The most obvious is the presence of retching. Other more subtle features, as described above, include nausea, pallor (due to peripheral vasoconstriction), sweating, and drooling or increased swallowing (due to increased salivation). In the presence of these symptoms we are reluctant to perform anti-reflux surgery, since it does not address the underlying problem and may make symptoms worse, since these children will continue to retch but will be unable to vomit. We believe that it is this group of children who are at high risk for retching following antireflux surgery, and they are best managed by the alternative strategies that we have found effective in the management of postfundoplication retching.

Our strategy for managing post-Nissen emetic symptoms (e.g., retching) starts with the use of conventional antiemetics such as domperidone (dopamine D_2 receptor antagonist). If domperidone alone is insufficient, we add a 5-HT_3 receptor antagonist (e.g., ondansetron, granisetron). These are established for use in the control of short-term vomiting in children (e.g., that related to surgery, chemotherapy, and cyclical vomiting syndrome). Although not recognized for long-term use, this might be justified for children with a limited life expectancy and distressing symptoms resistant to other forms of management. We also use continuous gastric feeding to reduce stimulation of gastric vagal afferents compared with bolus feeds. Many parents notice that their child retches with boluses, but not on continuous feeds. In children who are symptomatic despite antiemetics and continuous gastric feeds, the next step is to avoid all gastric afferent stimulation by feeding directly into the jejunum, either via a transpyloric gastrojejunostomy tube (easy to place if the patient already has a gastrostomy tube) or a direct jejunostomy tube. This generally results in a marked improvement of symptoms.

Causes of Wrap Herniation or Disruption

Crural repair is an important component of antireflux surgery, with a high rate of failure and wrap migration if it is omitted. In addition, several investigators have reported disruption or herniation of the fundoplication wrap in association with diaphragmatic stressor forces (e.g., activation of the emetic reflex secondary to gastrointestinal obstruction, uncontrolled seizures, persistent coughing, or weight lifting). During emesis the gastroesophageal junction is elevated through the diaphragmatic hiatus, and contraction of the diaphragm and abdominal wall generates a transdiaphragmatic pressure gradient of 200 mm Hg or more. Repeated episodes of retching will generate large forces that will drive the gastroesophageal junction and gastric fundus through the diaphragmatic hiatus into the thorax and pull the wrap apart. Clinically, the child retches repeatedly postoperatively. As the wrap fails, the child may subsequently develop recurrent vomiting. In this situation, stitching the fundus to the dome of the diaphragm may compound the disruptive forces on the wrap, because the diaphragm itself contracts strongly during retching and vomiting.

We believe that the relatively high failure rate of fundoplication in neurologically impaired children is a direct consequence of repeated activation of the emetic reflex and retching, which is common in this group. Those children whose primary problem is a hypersensitive emetic reflex often have postoperative retching, leading to wrap disruption. If these children can be identified preoperatively, inappropriate surgery may be avoided, and complication rates reduced.

ROLE OF THE GASTRIC EMPTYING PROCEDURE IN GASTROESOPHAGEAL REFLUX DISEASE

Delayed gastric emptying is sometimes associated with GER. This may reflect a generalized foregut dysmotility and may contribute to the severity of reflux. The effect of fundoplication upon gastric emptying rate also varies. Some investigators perform a gastric emptying procedure with fundoplication on the grounds that (a) delayed gastric emptying is associated with postfundoplication symptoms and that (b) delayed gastric emptying may promote wrap breakdown and hence recurrent reflux. However, the physiologic basis of delayed gastric emptying must be considered. It may be due to primary dysmotility, in which case a drainage procedure such as pyloroplasty *might* be beneficial, but must be balanced against the disturbances that it may induce: excessively rapid gastric emptying and dumping syndromes, or duodenogastric bile reflux. Other methods of circumventing the problem are more appropriate (e.g., continuous feeds, jejunal feeds, prokinetics). The effect of Nissen fundoplication on gastric emptying appears variable, and we avoid a drainage procedure as part of an initial operation, but assess the child after the antireflux procedure.

Moreover, delayed gastric emptying may be a result of activation of the emetic reflex, and accounts for the reported association between delayed gastric emptying postoperatively with symptoms such as retching or dyspepsia. In this situation, a gastric drainage procedure is inappropriate—there is no obstruction to gastric emptying, and a pyloroplasty cannot relieve symptoms of emesis. Antiemetic therapy is more logical.

There is concern in the literature that reduced gastric capacity and delayed gastric emptying may lead to increased intragastric pressures and risk of wrap disruption. However, even in situations where gastric pressures are higher than normal, truly excessive pressures are unlikely to occur. Orally fed children will stop when they feel full; bolus gastrostomy feedings are not subject to excessive pressures if administered by gravity and the tube is vented to the atmosphere after feeding. The vented gastrostomy tube serves as a manometer; feed does not flow back under pressure except during events such as crying or coughing, when intraabdominal or intragastric pressure is increased by contraction of the abdominal wall muscles and diaphragm. Continuous feedings through a pump should be administered at realistic pressure settings. If gastric capacity is reduced, it should be possible to compensate with smaller boluses or continuous feeds.

In contrast to distension by feeds, a source of much more significant excessive pressures is the much greater pressures that are generated when the emetic reflex is activated, and other events such as generalized convulsions or bouts of coughing. These will not be helped by a gastric drainage procedure.

CONCLUSIONS

Gastroesophageal reflux disease is primarily due to dysfunction of the LES–crus complex. Patients resistant to maximal medical therapy or with severe, life-threatening complications are candidates for antireflux surgery. Postoperative complications are common, but there is potential to reduce the incidence by careful preoperative selection, avoiding surgery in patients whose primary problem is activation of a sensitive emetic reflex, rather than GERD.

SUGGESTED READINGS

Andrews PLR. Vomiting: a gastro-intestinal tract defensive reflex. In: Andrews PLR, Widdicombe JG, eds. *Pathophysiology of the gut and airways.* London: Physiological Society, Portland Press, 1993: 97–113.

Butterfield WC. Current hiatal hernia repairs: similarities, mechanisms, and extended indications—an autopsy study. *Surgery* 1971; 69:910–916.

Mittal RK, Balaban DH. The esophagogastric junction. *N Engl J Med* 1997;336:924–932.

Mittal RK, Holloway RH, Penagini R, et al. Transient lower esophageal sphincter relaxations. *Gastroenterology* 1995;109: 601–610.

Richards CA, Andrews PLR, Spitz L, et al. Nissen fundoplication may induce gastric myoelectrical disturbance in children. *J Pediatr Surg* 1998;33:1801–1805.

Richards CA, Carr D, Spitz L, et al. Nissen-type fundoplication and its effects on the emetic reflex and gastric motility in the ferret. *Neurogastroenterol Motil* 2000;12:65–74.

Richards CA, Milla PJ, Andrews PL, et al. Retching and vomiting in neurologically impaired children following fundoplication: predictive pre-operative factors. *J Pediatr Surg* 2001 Sep;36(9): 1401–1404.

Spitz L. Gastroesophageal reflux: Nissen fundoplication. In: Spitz L, Coran AG, eds. *Rob and Smith's operative surgery, paediatric surgery, 5th ed.* London: Chapman & Hall Medical, 1995:265–273.

42

LAPAROSCOPIC FUNDOPLICATION

J. DUNCAN PHILLIPS

DIAGNOSTIC APPROACH

Children without neurologic impairment usually require an extensive workup for gastroesophageal reflux disease (GERD) in order to exclude other gastrointestinal disorders (such as malrotation and esophageal achalasia), to objectively quantitate the severity of GERD, and to assess response to medical therapy. The workup typically includes a contrast upper gastrointestinal radiographic series and a 24 hour ambulatory pH probe study. Other tests might include a nuclear medicine gastric scintiscan, flexible esophagogastroduodenoscopy with esophageal biopsies, or esophageal manometry. GERD refractory to a 6-week trial of maximal medical therapy or GERD causing life-threatening symptoms (such as episodes of apnea/bradycardia or recurrent pneumonias) warrant consideration of fundoplication.

Neurologically impaired children, such as those with mental retardation, cerebral palsy, or other degenerative neurologic disorders, are often referred for gastrostomy tube (GT) placement for feeding. In these patients, a clinical history of recurrent episodes of regurgitation, combined with an upper gastrointestinal radiographic series demonstrating GERD, is often sufficient workup.

Laparoscopic fundoplication is a technically challenging advanced procedure. In general, the technical difficulty increases as the size of the patient decreases. Children weighing less than 10 kg are moderately difficult, and those weighing less than 5 kg are usually very difficult. The operation has been reported in children as small as 1.2 kg. I have successfully performed the procedure on children down to 3 kg body weight but prefer the traditional open fundoplication on smaller children.

PREOPERATIVE PREPARATION

Most children can be admitted from home on the day of surgery. Rarely, children with chronic lung disease such as cystic fibrosis or recurrent aspiration pneumonias require preoperative hospitalization for pulmonary toilet and intravenous antibiotics. Perioperative blood transfusions are typically not required, but preparing a "type and screen" is not unreasonable. Because the surgeon's initial laparoscopic view of the stomach is from the umbilicus, up and over the transverse colon, neurologically impaired children with chronic constipation and a dilated large intestine may present an added challenge. Several enemas, given the night before surgery by the parents or other caregivers, can help decompress the transverse colon.

J. Duncan Phillips: Department of Surgery, University of North Carolina at Chapel Hill; and Department of Surgery, North Carolina Children's Hospital, Chapel Hill, North Carolina.

TECHNICAL APPROACH

Without proper preparation, laparoscopic fundoplication in small children can be a grueling 5-hour procedure, straining the patience of even the most mature pediatric surgeon and operating room (OR) staff. To perform a laparoscopic fundoplication, the pediatric surgeon should be an experienced laparoscopist and should have done advanced training, either in an advanced laparoscopy course or in his or her residency or fellowship. It cannot be overemphasized that this is a challenging, advanced procedure.

Laparoscopic instruments appropriate to the size of the individual patient are crucial. For most children weighing over 10 kg, one can usually use standard 5-mm diameter laparoscopic instruments available in most ORs and used by general surgeons to perform laparoscopic procedures in adults. Shafts are typically about 30 cm long. Instruments should be sturdy, insulated, and roticulating and should include several curved dissectors (Maryland or Kelly-type), several atraumatic graspers (Hunter bowel graspers work well), several fine Babcock clamps, a curved Metzenbaum scissors, a hook cautery (disposable or reusable), a knot pusher, a needle driver, and a liver retractor. I prefer the 60-mm triangular liver retractor made by Snowden Pencer (Genzyme Surgical Products, Fall River, Massachusetts). Most disposable balloon-type liver retractors require the use of a 10-mm trocar and are therefore less than ideal in children. Laparoscopes should be either 30 or 45 degrees (a 0 degree scope is unacceptable), and either 3.5 or 5 mm diameter.

For children weighing less than 10 kg (and especially those under 5 kg), 5-mm instruments are insufficient. A set of pediatric laparoscopy instruments, with 2- to 3-mm diameter shafts, must be purchased by the hospital for use. Although several companies currently market such instruments, I prefer the Storz ClickLine (Karl Storz Endoscopy America, Culver City, California) set of 3-mm diameter, 20-cm lengths. The instruments' shafts are fully insulated, and each instrument has a cautery plug, so that monopolar current can be delivered to tissue that is grasped or touched. Laparoscopes should be either 30 or 45 degrees and short. Storz markets a 4-mm diameter, 18-cm long scope.

Cameras should be three chip or better. Light sources should be xenon. The Achilles heel of pediatric laparoscopy remains the fiberoptic light cord with multiple broken fibers. If illumination is inadequate during a procedure, this should be the first suspect.

Large trocars, with diameters of 10 to 12 mm, are to be avoided in children. For children weighing over 10 kg, disposable (plastic) 5-mm trocars are preferred because reusable stainless-steel trocars are quite heavy and tend to flop over awkwardly when used in children with their thin abdominal walls. Most commercially available disposable trocars are 100 mm in length and therefore also tend to be awkward to use. However, the Innerdyne Company (Auto Suture Company, a division of United States Surgical Corporation, Norwalk, Connecticut) now markets a short, 70-mm long, radially expanding access device (STEP), which is inserted over a Veress needle and dilates, rather than cuts, the muscle layers of the abdominal wall during insertion.

For children weighing less than 10 kg (and especially those <5 kg), a combination of 5-mm Innerdyne devices and reusable stainless-steel 3 mm trocars is typically used. The pediatric laparoscopy set should include at least five small reusable trocars.

SURGICAL TECHNIQUE

Anesthesiologists familiar with the care of small children are absolutely essential. Prolonged mask ventilation during induction should be avoided due to its tendency to cause gastric and small intestinal dilatation. Nitrous oxide should be avoided due to its tendency to cause dilatation of the transverse colon. Endotracheal intubation and muscle paralysis during the procedure are essential.

SETUP

Two monitors should be positioned at the head of the table. After intubation, an orogastric tube should be inserted by the anesthesiologist and the child should be moved down toward the foot of the table. Larger children (>50 kg) can be positioned like adults, with the legs spread apart and the surgeon standing between the legs. Infants (<5 kg) can be positioned with their legs draped over the end of the OR table, with the surgeon standing next to the child's bent knees. For all other children, the surgeon stands to the patient's right side, with the assistant standing opposite. For smaller children, several folded towels placed beneath the patient will help elevate the child up and off the OR table and prevent impingement of the full range of motion of the laparoscopic instruments.

If a GT is to be placed, I indicate the proposed skin site with a marking pen prior to insufflation of the abdomen because insufflation tends to distort the abdominal wall and shift the site. The site is typically in the left upper quadrant (LUQ), several centimeters below the costal margin and lateral to the midline.

Local anesthesia is injected intradermally at each trocar site. I prefer 0.25% bupivicaine with epinephrine. A 5-mm umbilical incision is made first. In children weighing less than 5 kg, one can often dissect with electrocautery through the umbilical fascia and enter the peritoneal cavity under direct vision. A 5-mm umbilical trocar is inserted, and carbon dioxide is insufflated. For patients weighing less than 5 kg, I use an insufflation pressure of 10 mm Hg. For patients weighing 5 to 20 kg, I use approximately 12 mm Hg. Patients over 20 kg can usually tolerate a pressure of 14 or 15 mm Hg. The 5-mm disposable trocar must have a reducer cap available, so that 2- and 3-mm instruments can be inserted, if necessary. Both Innerdyne (STEP access devices) and Ethicon Endosurgery (Cincinnati, Ohio) make such reducer caps.

The 30 or 45 degree laparoscope is inserted, and a brief inspection of the peritoneal cavity should be performed, with particular attention to the underlying intestine to verify that there is no evidence of intestinal or vascular injury from the initial blind trocar insertion. Local anesthesia is then injected at each trocar site, with laparoscopic visualization so that a bleb of peritoneum can be raised by the local anesthetic agent at each site.

Under laparoscopic visualization, four additional trocars are inserted: LUQ (at the proposed gastrostomy site, in those patients), right upper quadrant (RUQ), right anterior axillary line (RAAL), and left anterior axillary line (LAAL). The liver retractor is then inserted through the RAAL trocar and opened. It is inserted beneath the left lateral segment, which is then retracted anteriorly and superiorly. I clamp a scope holder onto the right rail of the OR table, at approximately the level of the patient's right shoulder, to hold the liver retractor in position. The laparoscope is then moved to the LUQ trocar, and the table is tilted into a fairly steep reverse Trendelenburg position and tilted slightly to the right. The surgeon, standing to the patient's right side (or between the legs), operates with his or her left hand controlling an atraumatic grasper in the RUQ trocar and his or her right hand controlling the instrument inserted through the umbilical trocar. The assistant, standing on the patient's left, operates with his or her left hand on the laparoscope (inserted in the LUQ trocar) and his or her right hand controlling the instrument in the LAAL trocar. In this way, the surgeon and assistant avoid crossing hands during the procedure.

Using the atraumatic grasper, the surgeon grasps the gastrohepatic ligament and pulls it anteriorly, tenting it up. The hook cautery is then used to open a window in the ligament. The window is then enlarged superiorly, with cautery, to the right crus of the diaphragm. Care is taken to not injure the left gastric artery and vein, which can lead to bothersome bleeding. The assistant grasps the anterior gastric wall and gently retracts it inferiorly and to the left, to provide slight tissue traction. Peritoneum along the anterior surface of the right crus is then incised with cautery. If one stays right on the surface of the crus, the chance of esophageal injury is minimized. The cautery is then used to incise the peritoneum on the anterior surface of the gastroesophageal junction (GEJ). This is facilitated by having the assistant grasp the phrenoesophageal fat pad and pull it anteriorly and inferiorly.

Because dissection of the GEJ is much easier from the left side of the esophagus, one should not spend too much time on the right. Attention is then turned to the short gastric vessels. It is easiest to begin their division at the most inferior short gastric vessel. The surgeon gently grasps the anterior gastric wall at the level of the most inferior short gastric vessel and retracts it to the right. The assistant grasps the omentum or adjacent fatty tissue and retracts it to the left. The hook cautery is then used to "hook and cook" the first short gastric. As long as the vessel is held by the surgeon and assistant under slight tension while it is cauterized, it will usually divide easily, and the two cauterized ends will fall away and not bleed. In larger patients, some surgeons choose to use the 5-mm harmonic scalpel to divide the short gastric vessels. Retraction on the stomach by the surgeon's left hand should be inferiorly and to the right. Once the first one or two short gastric vessels are divided, one can usually see easily into the lesser sac, visualizing the pancreatic tail. This "opens up" the dissection, allowing the assistant to move sequentially along to each short gastric vessel, providing lateral traction for the surgeon. The dissection continues all the way to the GEJ. The surgeon then uses the hook cautery (or harmonic scalpel, if preferred) to incise peritoneum along the anterior edge of the left crus. There are almost always "adhesion-like" tissues between the posterior wall of the fundus and the retroperitoneum, superior to the highest short gastric and inferior to the left crus. These tissues should be divided.

Once the fundus is fully mobilized, the surgeon returns to the right crus to create a retroesophageal window. Using both the right and left instruments, the surgeon bluntly dissects straight to the left. To avoid esophageal injury, it is best to begin the window on the anterior edge of the right crus, staying as far posterior to esophagus as possible. When the dissection is nearly through the retroesophageal tissue, a bluish purple object (the spleen) often appears through the thinned-out tissue, confirming successful window creation. The assistant can aid in this step by grasping the phrenoesophageal fat pad and gently pulling anteriorly and inferiorly.

There is a tendency to follow the direction of the shafts of the surgeon's instruments and thus dissect upward and to the left, inadvertently entering the left pleural cavity, creating a pneumothorax. An anesthesiologist unfamiliar with pediatric laparoscopic fundoplications should be warned preoperatively of this possibility, and should notify the surgeon immediately of any sudden decrease in oxygen saturation, as measured by continuous pulse oximetry. If recognized quickly, a small chest tube (10 or 12 French) can be inserted anteriorly by the surgeon to treat such a complication, thus avoiding conversion to the open technique.

Once both instruments have successfully poked through the retroesophageal tissue, one can gently spread the instrument tips superiorly and inferiorly (the so-called "chop stix" maneuver) to widen the window. This usually allows visualization of both the anterior and posterior vagus nerves, adherent to the esophagus. The assistant will usually notice a gradual, progressive "give" as the window is widened, allowing the intraabdominal esophagus to be "lengthened" several centimeters.

Although adult laparoscopic fundoplication procedures typically require the insertion of a small Penrose drain or Silastic vessel loop to encircle the esophagus for downward traction, this is usually not necessary in children. The assistant can grasp the phrenoesophageal fat pad and pull laterally, allowing good visualization of the crura for suturing.

For crural approximation, I usually prefer to use 18-inch long, 2-0 Ethibond suture on RB-1 needles (with one of the double-arm needles cut off and the suture material left full length). These needles can be dragged into the peritoneal cavity with a 2- to 3-mm needle driver, inserted through the 5-mm umbilical trocar. The needle driver should grasp the suture material 1 to 2 cm distal to the needle. For infants, 3-0 Ethibond can be used. I tend to use the antrum of the stomach as my table to load the needle into my needle driver. Frequently bumping the tips of the instruments against the antrum gives the surgeon tactile feedback and a sense of depth perception. To allow better visualization of the right crus while suturing, the surgeon should use his or her atraumatic grasper to gently push the caudate lobe of the liver to the right. Once the stitch is placed through the crura, the surgeon grasps the suture material with the needle driver and gently pulls the needle out through the umbilical trocar.

The anesthesiologist should remove the orogastric tube and insert a large esophageal bougie before beginning crural approximation. The extracorporeal knot-tying technique is used. Because Ethibond is coated, I usually tie five knots before cutting. The tip of the knot pusher can easily become stuck on the serosa or pericolonic fat of the transverse colon during this step. The surgeon should introduce the knot pusher through the umbilical trocar and then intentionally angle it up and over the transverse colon before touching the tip down to the crural knots. Additional sutures should be placed and tied until snug against the posterior wall of the esophagus, with the bougie in place.

The bougie should then be pulled back into the thoracic esophagus. With the assistant pulling the phrenoesophageal fat pad anteriorly, the surgeon slides an atraumatic grasper through the retroesophageal window and grasps the fundus, gently pulling it from left to right, through the window. If the fundus has been adequately mobilized, it will tend not to snap back to the left, but rather, stay to the right of the esophagus, even when released. To assure that the fundus has not been twisted during this maneuver, the surgeon can grasp the fundus of the stomach both to the left and right of the esophagus and slide it back and forth gently (the so-called "shoe shine" maneuver).

Ethibond sutures can then be inserted to perform the wrap itself, taking a seromuscular bite of fundus to the left of the esophagus, anterior esophageal wall, and then seromuscular fundus to the right of the esophagus. Before each suture is tied, the bougie should be advanced by the anesthesiologist into the stomach. The wrap is typically made to be 1.5 to 2 cm in length. The suture line usually ends up at approximately the 10 o'clock position on the esophagus (with the anterior surface of the esophagus being the 12 o'clock position). The surgeon can check the length of the wrap by placing an instrument adjacent to the fundoplication valve and making a visual estimate (on the tip of the instrument) of its length. The surgeon then temporarily removes the instrument and can use a ruler to measure the visual estimate on the instrument.

Once the wrap is of sufficient length, the bougie is removed by the anesthesiologist and several additional sutures are placed to the right of the esophagus, securing the fundus to the crura at the crural approximation site. A nasogastric (NG) tube is inserted by the anesthesiologist.

If a GT is to be inserted, the laparoscope is relocated to the umbilical trocar, the liver retractor is removed, and the GT is placed through the LUQ trocar site. I prefer the technique described by Georgeson to introduce a gastrostomy "button." The stomach is insufflated by the anesthesiologist via the NG tube, the anterior gastric wall is grasped via the LUQ trocar site and pulled up to the anterior abdominal wall, 0 or 2-0 Prolene sutures are placed superior and inferior to the proposed gastrostomy site to secure the anterior gastric wall to the anterior abdominal wall, and then the grasper and trocar are removed. A finder needle is inserted through the LUQ trocar site and into the gastric lumen. Through the finder needle, a guide wire is advanced and a series of gastrostomy dilators are sequentially advanced over it to dilate the tract from the skin into the stomach. The smallest dilator can then be inserted into the button and then slid over the guide wire into the stomach before its balloon is inflated. The Prolene sutures are then tied over the wings of the button to secure it in place.

Trocars are removed under laparoscopic guidance so that no inadvertent abdominal wall bleeding is missed. Fascial closure at each trocar site is typically achieved by inserting the grooved director into the abdominal cavity.

POSTOPERATIVE CARE

If a GT is inserted, the NG tube can be removed intraoperatively. In patients without GTs, an NG tube is typically left to suction for 24 hours postoperatively before beginning oral feeding.

Neurologically normal children can usually begin taking a liquid diet on the first postoperative day and are discharged home on the first or second postoperative day. They are instructed to follow a "no chunk diet" (soft, mushy foods) for approximately 1 month to avoid food sticking at the Nissen valve. Edema of the Nissen valve typically subsides over a period of 3 to 4 weeks. Occasionally, children with preexisting esophagitis require continuation of acid-suppressive medications for 6 to 8 weeks postoperatively to allow full esophageal healing.

Neurologically normal children can usually return to normal activity, including school and physical education within 7 to 10 days.

Neurologically impaired children and those with other complex medical illnesses often experience dysmotility of multiple sections of the gastrointestinal tract and therefore are prone to postoperative digestive disturbances, including gas bloat syndrome, retching, high gastric residuals, and constipation. This can be frustrating to caregivers and physicians. Promotility agents, such as metoclopramide, can aid gastric emptying in some patients. Other patients, refractory to medications, may require a period of continuous drip feedings via the GT, in order to decrease stretch of the stomach. Caregivers should be instructed to vent the GT frequently to allow gas to expel from the stomach.

RESULTS

When originally described, laparoscopic fundoplication was felt to be less prone to failure than the tradition open procedure due to better intraoperative visualization of the crural approximation and fundoplication sutures. However, it is becoming increasingly apparent that the long-term failure rate of the laparoscopic approach appears similar to that of the traditional open approach, with an overall failure rate of about 10% in neurologically normal children and somewhat higher (perhaps 15%–20%) in the neurologically impaired.

SUGGESTED READINGS

Allal H, Captier G, Lopez M, et al. Evaluation of 142 consecutive laparoscopic fundoplications in children: effects of the learning curve and technical choice. *J Pediatr Surg* 2001;36:921–926.

Esposito C, Montupet P, Amici G, et al. Complications of laparoscopic antireflux surgery in childhood. *Surg Endosc* 2000;14:622–624.

Esposito C, Montupet P, Reinberg O. Laparoscopic surgery for gastroesophageal reflux disease during the first year of life. *J Pediatr Surg* 2001;36:715–717.

Georgeson KE. Laparoscopic fundoplication and gastrostomy. *Semin Laparosc Surg* 1998;5:25–30.

Lobe TE. Laparoscopic fundoplication. *Semin Pediatr Surg* 1993;2:178–181.

Meehan JJ, Georgeson KE. The learning curve associated with antireflux surgery in infants and children. *J Pediatr Surg* 1997;32:426–429.

Rothenberg SS. Experience with 220 consecutive laparoscopic Nissen fundoplications in infants and children. *J Pediatr Surg* 1998;33:274–278.

Van der Zee DC, Bax NM, Ure BM. Laparoscopic fundoplication in children. *Surg Endosc* 2000;14:1103–1104.

43

THE THAL FUNDOPLICATION

KEITH W. ASHCRAFT

RATIONALE

The normal or physiologic function of the lower esophageal sphincter (LES) is to allow the unrestricted passage of food or drink from the esophagus into the stomach. The normal LES also relaxes to allow eructation of swallowed air or to allow vomiting when appropriate. Gastroesophageal reflux (GER) may be defined simply as the *inappropriate* return of gastric contents into the esophagus. GER is an exceedingly common condition both in adults and children. It is primarily an anatomic disorder that becomes much more difficult to manage as the complications of inflammation and scarring progress. Because the pressure gradient between the mediastinum and abdominal cavities is increased by both the patient's weight and activity, obesity and those activities that increase intraabdominal pressure are factors that aggravate GER and reduce the chances for successful treatment.

Once hardly considered to be a disease or disorder affecting pediatric patients, GER is now one of the major causes of morbidity in children not due to infections. It has been recognized as a factor in malnutrition, respiratory disorders, otitis, and all the manifestations of esophageal mucosal erosion or esophagitis. It may be one of the major causes of "colic" in babies. Both medical and surgical therapy for GER is directed toward symptomatic relief.

The medical therapy for GER is directed toward reducing the production of gastric acid or enhancing prograde emptying of the stomach. However, the medications are expensive and carry some risk for side effects. The risk for serious side effects may be small, but the fact that the medications must be continued *ad infinitum* are of concern. Unrecognized or improperly treated GER may result in esophageal stricture or even sudden death due to laryngospasm. Many parents are unwilling to accept the risk of medical therapy, so surgical treatment of GER in children has become one of the most commonly performed procedures in pediatric surgery.

K.W. Ashcraft: Department of Surgery, Children's Mercy Hospital, Kansas City, Missouri.

A surgical procedure should produce a result that mimics the natural anatomy and function as nearly as possible. In very few areas does the surgeon have a choice of such different procedures as in the surgical treatment of GER. The fact that everybody has some postprandial LES relaxation has been taken into account in the most definitive of tests for GER: extended esophageal pH monitoring. The episodes of reflux that occur within 2 hours of ingestion of food are not counted in the scoring of reflux episodes or severity. Given that some reflux is not only normal but necessary, it is the partial wrap surgical procedures for GER that best provide "normalcy."

I suspect that many of the proponents of the complete wrap simply learned that one procedure and have not considered changing. I have heard from many of my colleagues in pediatric surgery that they cannot make the Thal partial-wrap "work" or that the failure rate is excessive. This may be based on the misconception that any demonstrable reflux by contrast study in the postoperative Thal patient is interpreted as a sign of failure. This finding would certainly be indicative of failure in the postoperative Nissen fundoplication.

Contrast radiographic studies either for preoperative evaluation or for follow-up are acute studies that generally take place within the postprandial period discounted by the extended pH study. Although contrast radiography absolutely should precede any operative approach to correction of GER, it is more useful to determine the angle of His and the ability or inability of the GE junction to open or relax than it is for diagnosis of GER. The observation of an obtuse angle of His is the best diagnostic sign of GER on a contrast study.

The best test of success for any fundoplication procedure is the assessment of symptomatic relief. If the patient no longer has the GER symptoms he or she had preoperatively, no longer requires medication to counteract acid, and does not have obstruction to the passage of food or to eructation and vomiting, the procedure may be termed successful.

There has been a recent swing toward minimally invasive surgery performed using multiple incisions and long (and often low-quality) instruments, while observing the whole process on a video monitor. Although shortened hospital stay and more rapid return to work have been arguments for the economic feasibility of such techniques, the intraoperative time and costs often waste the economies gained. Minimally invasive surgery is a relative term. I maintain that my approach to the Thal fundoplication is a minimally invasive approach that carries with it the distinct advantages of a close personal relationship with the tissues to be rearranged. Using a transverse, upper abdominal incision, only the viscera above the transverse colon are exposed or handled. The rectus muscles are cut rather than stretched as in the usual midline approach, and postoperative pain is much reduced as a result. Intestinal motility is not interrupted, and the patient does not require nasogastric drainage. The patient may almost always be discharged within 48 hours. Knots are tied the way they should be tied: by hand. Continuous suture techniques distribute tension better than do multiple interrupted sutures. The one disadvantage is that adhesions between stomach and liver are more intense than with endoscopic techniques.

The *Thal fundoplication* is created by applying the free wall of the gastric fundus to the anterior aspect of the intraabdominal esophagus and is also known as the Dor-Nissen procedure or the Boix-Ochoa procedure. The same physiologic result theoretically may be anticipated using the posterior, partial wrap fundoplication (Toupet), but much more dissection is required. Additionally, overdistension of the stomach following the Toupet procedure may angulate the intraabdominal esophagus to the point of obstruction. Proponents of a partial wrap believe that a successful wrap cures the problem of GER and yet leaves the patient with the ability to vomit and to burp if the need arises. Some pediatric patients, particularly those who have severe neurologic impairment, are perhaps better served by a complete wrap (Nissen) because there is little hope of any conscious control of the GE junction or of significant oral intake. Commonly, any fundoplication is accompanied by a gastrostomy used for feeding or gastric decompression in these patients.

Our experience with the Thal fundoplication has been entirely with open procedures. In my personal experience with over 1,000 Thal fundoplications, we have not used postoperative nasogastric drainage, oral liquids are started within 12 hours of operation, and the patient is discharged within 48 hours in the vast majority of cases. Several endoscopic surgeons in the United States have accumulated significant endoscopic experience with the Thal fundoplication, but their time to feeding and discharge is not significantly shorter than ours. The benefit, therefore, is probably related to the issue of one transverse abdominal scar versus several smaller ones. There is no question that the endoscopic procedure requires increased costs of equipment and supplies.

We require a barium study in all patients prior to operation to exclude the possibility of achalasia. One percent of our total institutional experience of 2,000 GER patients have had concomitant achalasia and have required a distal esophageal myotomy in conjunction with the Thal fundoplication.

SURGICAL TECHNIQUE

The patient is best anesthetized expeditiously and without distending the stomach or the gut with nitrous oxide. A nasogastric tube of appropriate size is passed by the anesthesiologist for purposes of intraoperative gastric decompression and to aid in the tactile identification of the GE junction. The tube also provides some rigidity for the esophagus during the creation of the fundoplication, preventing distortion of the GE junction during the suturing process.

1. An upper abdominal transverse incision is made from the left costal margin at the nipple line to the opposite costal margin, dividing both left and right rectus muscles. The abdomen is entered cephalad of the transverse colon and the small intestine is protected from exposure by the mesocolon. Sufficient relaxation is required to prevent the patient from "bucking" and eviscerating himself.
2. The anterior free wall of the stomach is grasped with a gauze pad and retracted downward. The left lobe of the liver is also grasped and dissected free from the underside of the left hemidiaphragm. The liver is folded downward and retracted to the right by the second assistant.
3. Incision of the peritoneum at the hiatus is executed in a transverse direction, and a blunt dissector is used to spread the areolar tissue on either side of the easily seen and palpated esophagus. The dissector is passed behind the esophagus from the right to the left, grasping and pulling through a Dacron tape that will be used for traction purposes. Using this tape retractor, the esophagus is lifted and the posterior (right) branch of the vagus nerve identified. If the posterior vagus nerve has not been included within the tape, the tape is repositioned.
4. Using the tape, the GE junction is retracted downward while the hiatus on either side of the esophagus is pushed in a cephalad direction. The hiatus is not intentionally enlarged during the mobilization of the lower 2 to 4 cm of esophagus.
5. Using an "S" or small Richardson retractor, the distal esophagus is retracted to the patient's left by the first assistant, exposing both limbs of the crura behind. The crura are approximated using a figure-of-eight suture of permanent material. It is important to leave a space behind the esophagus so that the hiatus is not narrowed excessively. It is important not to tie this hiatus closing suture too tightly or muscle necrosis will result in a

larger hiatus than was originally present. The hiatus suture is tied with its needle still attached so that it may now be used to anchor the posterior wall of the esophagus to the hiatus. This additional posterior fixation of the distal esophagus within the abdominal cavity adds to the effectiveness of the procedure.

6. The retractor is removed from behind the esophagus, and the Dacron tape ends are separated. A permanent suture [we prefer 2-0 or 3-0 polytetrafluroethylene (PTFE)] is placed and tied at the GE junction on the left. The fundoplication is created using a continuous suture technique going up the left side of the esophagus, suturing stomach to esophagus. As the suture line crosses over the front of the esophagus to reach the right side, the suture line incorporates stomach, esophagus, and hiatus. As the right side of the esophagus is reached, the suture line is turned caudally to reach the lesser curvature GE junction, where it is tied. Thus, an inverted "U" suture line is created holding the anterior free wall of the stomach to the anterior free wall of the intraabdominal esophagus. When complete, the esophagus has been sutured to the anterior half of the esophageal hiatus by the fundoplication suture and to the repaired hiatus posteriorly by the hiatus suture. It is not necessary to divide any of the short gastric vessels to perform this fundoplication.
7. The length of the fundoplication is assessed by palpating the nasogastric tube through the layers of stomach applied to the esophagus. The nasogastric tube is removed, the liver replaced in its bed, and the wound closed. Boix-Ochoa attaches the gastric fundus to the underside of the left hemidiaphragm to exaggerate the angle of His prior to replacing the liver and closure, a part of the procedure we have not found necessary. We do not establish a gastrostomy except for the patient who needs to be fed by gastrostomy postoperatively. Many younger patients who have a complete-wrap fundoplication require a gastrostomy to prevent gastric bloating, a sometimes serious result of this type of GER procedure.

POSTOPERATIVE CARE

The patient is offered clear liquids 6 to 8 hours after leaving the recovery room and is offered a diet for age the following morning. Once the patient is taking sufficient fluid, he is discharged, sometimes as early as 24 hours postoperatively. Virtually all patients who are not complicated by other disorders are out of the hospital within 48 hours.

RESULTS

As a group, we performed 2,078 Thal fundoplications in 1,915 patients between the years of 1974 and 1999. Seventy-eight percent of the patients were neurologically intact, and 60% were under 1 year of age at the time of the initial procedure. Four percent of the patients had esophageal atresia, and 1% had achalasia.

- Approximately 90% of patients are able to burp and to vomit within 2 weeks following the procedure.
- Those patients with severe esophagitis are more likely to suffer transient distal esophageal edema and obstruction requiring a liquid diet for more than a few days.
- Only three patients have required reinsertion of the nasogastric tube for the gas-bloat complication that resolved within 24 hours.
- Two deaths occurred early in our experience as a result of the surgical procedure, both due to unrecognized small bowel obstruction in severely impaired children.
- Seventy-five patients required a repeat fundoplication because of recurrent hiatal hernia with herniation of an intact wrap or disruption of the wrap.
- Three of these patients required a third fundoplication
- One patient had four Thal fundoplications in an attempt to reduce the multiple complications of a failed esophageal atresia repair.

FOLLOW-UP

Initially we performed a repeat barium study 4 months postoperatively to demonstrate that the wrap was intact. Recently we perform follow-up studies only if symptoms recur.

REOPERATION FOR RECURRENT GER

Recurrence of GER has been due almost equally to disruption of the fundoplication suture line and to recurrence of the hiatal hernia. The first 400 patients did not have a mandatory hiatus closure, which we call the "limiting stitch" and which we now place in all patients. The recurrence rate was 7% in those initial 400 patients. Of late, the recurrence rate is 2% to 3%, mostly because of fundoplication disruption. For some inexplicable reason we often found the PTFE suture to be broken and the stomach separated from the distal esophagus. We have not found in any patient adhesions between the stomach and esophagus sufficient to prevent recurrent GER in the event of a suture failure.

Reoperation is often complicated by extensive adhesions between the stomach and the underside of the liver. It is imperative to dissect all the adhesions both for visibility and for the necessary mobility to redo the fundoplication. All steps of the original procedure must be followed if one is to anticipate success. Clearly a thoracic approach for repeat fundoplication would not be feasible because of the gastrohepatic adhesions. Only in cases of extreme neurologic dysfunction have we converted a Thal procedure to a Nissen.

SPECIAL SITUATIONS

When faced with the request for a feeding gastrostomy in a *neurologically impaired* patient, we nearly always perform a concomitant fundoplication. This is done because most patients when fed by gastrostomy will begin to reflux even without prior evidence of GER. To perform a fundoplication in the presence of an established gastrostomy increases the likelihood of a wound infection and dehiscence. Reflux is a significant problem in approximately 50% of patients having repair of *esophageal atresia*. In most of these patients a fundoplication is necessary. It is important that the fundoplication not obstruct the passage of food or drink because the motility of the distal esophagus is abnormal in these patients. We think that the partial wrap fundoplication is certainly best for these patients.

LONG-TERM RESULTS

Several years ago we studied 23 patients more than 10 years after they had undergone Thal fundoplication. Many of the patients originally underwent surgery as babies and had grown into their teens. The patients were selected on the basis of availability and willingness to undergo both a contrast radiographic study and a 24-hour pH study. The selection resulted in data that were not generally reliable for the entire population, but we found that approximately one third had a small, presumably "traction" diverticulum at the level of the esophageal hiatus, but all had normal pH study result. All were asymptomatic.

SUMMARY

The Thal fundoplication and its related partial wrap fundoplications have resulted in short- and long-term results equal to or better than the published results of the complete wrap. The complications relating to gastric overdistension are not seen with the partial wrap procedures, and patient and parent satisfaction is quite high.

SUGGESTED READINGS

Boix-Ochoa J, Marhuenda C. Gastroesophageal reflux. In: Ashcraft KW, Murphy JP, Sharp RJ, et al., eds. *Pediatric surgery, 3rd ed.* Philadelphia: WB Saunders, 2000.

Caniano DA, Ginn-Pease ME, King DR. The failed antireflux procedure: analysis of risk factors and morbidity. *J Pediatr Surg* 1990; 25:1022–1026.

Fonkalsrud EW, Ashcraft KW, Coran AG, et al. Surgical treatment of gastroesophageal reflux in children: a combined hospital study of 7,467 patients. *Pediatrics* 1998;101:419–422.

Jolley SG, Herbst JJ, Johnson DG, et al. Patterns of postcibal gastroesophageal reflux in symptomatic infants. *Am J Surg* 1979;138: 946–950.

Ramachandran V, Ashcraft KW, Sharp RJ, et al. Thal fundoplication in neurologically impaired children. *J Pediatr Surg* 1996;31:819–822.

Snyder CL, Ramachandran V, Kennedy AP, et al. Efficacy of partial wrap fundoplication for gastroesophageal reflux after repair of esophageal atresia. *J Pediatr Surg* 1997;32:1089–1092.

Turnage RH, Oldham KT, Coran AG, et al. Late results of fundoplication for gastroesophageal reflux in infants and children. *Surgery* 1989;105:457–464.

Vane DW, Harmel RP Jr, King DR, et al. The effectiveness of Nissen fundoplication in neurologically impaired children with gastroesophageal reflux. *Surgery* 1985;98:662–666.

44

PERCUTANEOUS ENDOSCOPIC GASTROSTOMY

WILLIAM S. COBB
MICHAEL W.L. GAUDERER

Gastrostomy, from the Greek *gaster* (stomach) and *stomoun* (mouth), is defined as the surgical creation of an artificial opening into the stomach. The procedure dates back over 100 years, and some of the first patients were children who swallowed corrosive materials. Percutaneous endoscopic gastrostomy (PEG) was developed over 20 years ago to provide gastric access by using a sutureless technique that approximates the stomach to the anterior abdominal wall without the need for a celiotomy. Although extensively performed, PEG does not fully replace the gastrostomy with celiotomy, a procedure that is still required in certain patients, such as those with esophageal atresia without fistula or corrosive esophageal stricture. Over the years, gastrostomy has been considered a technically "basic" procedure; however, the complications of an improperly placed gastrostomy, including one placed using the percutaneous technique, can result in serious acute complications or chronic sequelae that defeat the purpose of facilitation of care.

INDICATIONS

The most common indication for percutaneous endoscopic gastrostomy in infants and children is long-term enteral feeding. Other well-established indications include gastric decompression and the administration of medications.

Gastrostomy for enteral feeding has two prerequisites. The upper gastrointestinal tract must be functional, and the need for feeding must be long-term, preferably years rather than months. If the length of time is short, the risk versus benefit of PEG compared with nasogastric feeds must be proven. Patients benefiting from gastrostomy for long-term feeding consist of those with the inability to swallow and those with the inability to consume adequate oral nutrition. The first group comprises the greatest number of patients and includes the neurologically impaired, those with head and neck tumors, and victims of major trauma. The latter group, or those who can swallow but are unable to consume adequate amounts, includes patients with anorexia secondary to malignancy, the severely debilitated (cystic fibrosis, Crohn's disease), and those requiring unpalatable diets (patients with short-gut syndrome or metabolic disorders).

Malnutrition resulting from dysphagia is common among children with developmental deficiencies that impair their ability to consume adequate oral nutrition. The best approach to these children is a multidisciplinary one. In addition to the primary care physician, involvement may require a dietitian, child psychologist, occupational therapist, speech therapist, pediatric gastroenterologist, and pediatric surgeon. A gastrostomy should be considered in those patients in whom return to complete oral feeding will exceed 3 to 4 months, in children who consistently take longer than 30 to 40 minutes to consume a meal because of dysphagia, and in those in whom aspiration during feeding is a frequent occurrence.

The manifestation of gastroesophageal reflux (GER) secondary to foregut dysmotility is commonly found among neurologically impaired children both before and after gastrostomy. There is considerable debate in the literature about whether these children should routinely have a gastrostomy with fundoplication or a gastrostomy alone. Preoperative evaluation including pH monitoring, barium swallow, and manometry is indicated. However, the findings may or may not be predictive of a favorable outcome after gastrostomy. We employ an antireflux procedure with a gastrostomy for patients with severe reflux, defined as those with inability to tolerate nasogastric feeds over a 4-week period. In all other patients, we place a PEG initially and reevaluate them carefully with frequent follow-up vis-

W. S. Cobb: Department of General Surgery, Greenville Hospital System, Greenville, South Carolina.

M. W. L. Gauderer: Department of Pediatric Surgery, University of South Carolina, School of Medicine, Columbia, South Carolina; and Department of Pediatric Surgery, Children's Hospital, Greenville Hospital System, Greenville, South Carolina.

its. If reflux is a major problem, an antireflux procedure is added later, usually without taking down the original gastrostomy. There are several reasons for starting the management with a gastrostomy only. Not all patients will have or develop symptomatic reflux, and those with mild GER can be managed medically. In cases of traumatic brain injury, the healing of the neurologic abnormality may parallel improvement in reflux symptoms. In some instances, removal of the nasogastric tube improves the symptoms of reflux. The placement of a PEG may improve nutritional status in the child who later may require an additional surgical procedure. The improved nutritional status after PEG may improve gastric emptying and ameliorate the symptoms of reflux.

Among patients with a malignancy, malnutrition frequently occurs as a result of anorexia, nausea, vomiting, and mucositis of chemotherapy and radiation treatment. Malnourished children have an increased risk for infection and less tolerance for intensive chemotherapy. Gastrostomy provides an alternative route for enteral nutrition, with improved comfort and cosmesis over the nasogastric route, and, when compared with parenteral routes, improved cost with fewer side effects.

Percutaneous endoscopic gastrostomy tube feeding has been used successfully in improving malnutrition associated with cystic fibrosis, chronic cholestasis, and Crohn's disease. The safety of gastrostomy placement in patients with Crohn's disease has been demonstrated with no increased incidence of peristomal disease or formation of gastrocutaneous fistula after removal of the gastrostomy tube.

Recently, gastrostomy tube placement has been shown to facilitate the administration of highly active antiretroviral therapy in pediatric patients infected with the human immunodeficiency virus. In this population, gastrostomy was well tolerated and improved adherence to complicated medication regimens.

Gastrostomy for decompression is less commonly performed; however, when it is used selectively, the outcome is favorable. Because prolonged nasogastric suctioning is poorly tolerated by patients with underlying pulmonary disease and by those among whom prolonged decompression is anticipated, placement of a PEG may be preferable. With a gastrostomy, the fluid output may be considerably less than with a nasogastric tube. This phenomenon is related to the irritation of the nasogastric tube, which causes excessive swallowing.

PREOPERATIVE PREPARATION

Preoperative assessment at our institution includes the assistance of the gastroenterology service. The children are evaluated for foregut motility, specifically GER. Studies include 24-hour pH monitoring, barium swallow, manometry, and, in select cases, gastric emptying studies. A trial period of nasogastric tube feeding is instituted for 2 to 4 weeks. Patients who tolerate these feedings are candidates for PEG. If the nasogastric tube feeding trial is not tolerated, a gastrostomy with an antireflux procedure is recommended. The physical examination includes careful inspection of the oropharynx and abdomen. Prior gastric surgery, previous correction of malrotation that places the cecum in the left upper quadrant, and scoliosis distort the anatomy and warrant special consideration. The level of the liver edge is also appreciated.

Absolute contraindications to PEG are the inability to perform upper tract endoscopy safely and the inability to identify transabdominal illumination and a clear anterior gastric wall indentation. Coagulopathy, ascites, and intraabdominal infection, if severe, may make the procedure inadvisable.

TECHNICAL APPROACH

In our institution, the procedure is performed in the operating suite. For children, general endotracheal anesthesia is used because the gastroscope tends to compress the trachea. Older children, who are capable of maintaining their airway during endoscopy, may receive intravenous sedation. A single intravenous dose of a broad-spectrum antibiotic is given shortly before the start of the procedure. We use the smallest upper endoscope available. For infants and small children, a 15 or 16 French PEG catheter is recommended. For all others we employ a 20 French PEG tube. The internal retaining portion of the PEG tube should collapse enough to pass atraumatically through the esophagus of the child.

Two operators are required: an endoscopist and a surgeon. The child is placed in the supine position. The abdomen is prepared and draped in standard surgical fashion. A suitable place for the gastrostomy is carefully chosen. A site over the left upper rectus muscle, one-third the distance of a line between the midportion of the inferior costal margin and the umbilicus, is marked as an initial guideline. The site is then modified, depending on where the greatest transillumination is seen. Endoscopy is then performed with brief inspection of the esophagus and stomach, minimizing air insufflation of the upper gastrointestinal tract. Excessive air in the small bowel can raise the colon and place it between the stomach and abdominal wall. Insufflation of the stomach brings the anterior gastric wall in contact with the abdominal wall and, more importantly, mobilizes the colon, spleen, and liver away from the gastrostomy site. The tip of the endoscope is directed at the proposed site. With the overhead lights dimmed, digital pressure is applied to the gastrostomy site. Transillumination and a distinct anterior gastric wall indentation are key elements before proceeding. The intragastric "mound" must be clearly visualized. If not, the finger is repositioned until the clearest indentation is seen.

When the gastrostomy site has been chosen, local anesthetic is used to create a skin wheal. A 25-gauge needle can be directed into the stomach to create a wheal on the gastric mucosa and display the correct angle and point of entry for the larger angiocatheter. A small incision, approximately 1 cm, is made in the skin in a transverse fashion. During this time, the endoscopist advances the polypectomy snare through the endoscope into the stomach. A curved hemostat with the prongs slightly open is used to apply pressure at the incision to recreate the intragastric mound (Fig. 44.1). The endoscopist opens the snare to encircle the mound. Under endoscopic visualization, the surgeon inserts the 18-gauge cannula between the prongs of the hemostat in the center of the incision to pierce the fascia, muscle, peritoneum, and anterior gastric wall (Fig. 44.1, insert). Rapid insertion of the cannula needle and the maintenance of gastric insufflation during insertion are important elements to prevent separation of the stomach from the abdominal wall.

The snare is loosely closed around the cannula and the needle removed. The surgeon inserts the plastic-covered, looped wire through the sheath. The endoscopist then closes the snare tightly around the looped wire, and, to prevent kinking, which would make passage of the guide wire difficult, takes care not to grasp the plastic sheath. Once the wire is seen advancing through the sheath into the stomach, the sheath may be removed to facilitate grasping the wire. As an alternative to the snare, biopsy forceps may be used to grasp the looped, plastic-covered wire. When the wire loop has been secured, the endoscopist removes the scope, pulling it through the mouth (Fig. 44.2). The guiding tract for passage of the PEG catheter is thus established.

The wire loop of the PEG catheter and the plastic-covered, looped guide wire are interlooped. Water-soluble lubricant is placed on the catheter. The surgeon applies steady traction to the transabdominal portion of the plastic-covered wire and brings the catheter through the patient's mouth, esophagus, and stomach (Fig. 44.3). The commercially available catheters are long; therefore, the tapered tip of the catheter will emerge through the abdominal skin before the "mushroom" end of the gastric retainer enters the mouth. Lubricant may be applied to the mushroom tip to ease passage. The markings on the catheter allow the surgeon to estimate the location of the gastric retainer.

The endoscope is reinserted to assess the position of the retaining mushroom. Tension on the outside catheter is applied to judge the loose approximation of the gastric and abdominal walls. The catheter is spun to ensure that the retainer is not embedded in the gastric mucosa. The external retaining crossbar and immobilization ring are applied to the catheter with the help of the hemostat. Pressure of the outer, retaining crossbar should not cause indentation

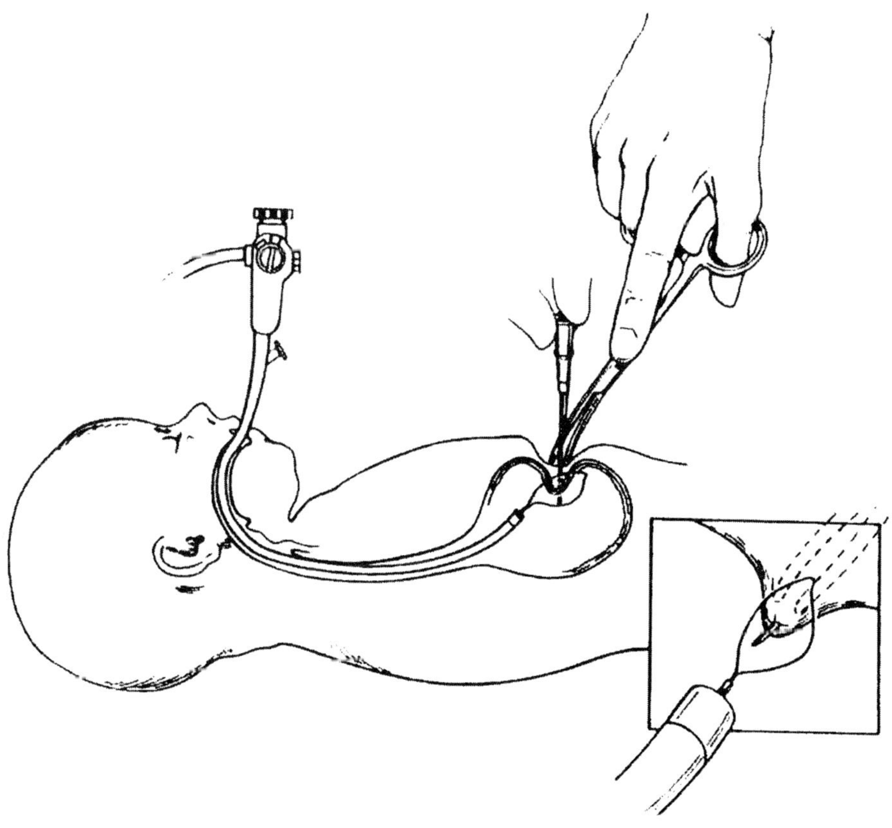

FIGURE 44.1. After determining the appropriate site and making the skin incision, the surgeon applies a hemostat to maintain the intragastric indentation. The cannula is placed in the incision between the slightly spread prongs of the hemostat and then firmly thrust through the abdominal and gastric walls, exiting through the tip of the mound into the loop of the polypectomy snare (insert). From Gauderer MWL, Stellato TA. Percutaneous endoscopic gastrostomy in children: the technique in detail. *Pediatr Surg Int* 1991; 6:82–87, with permission.

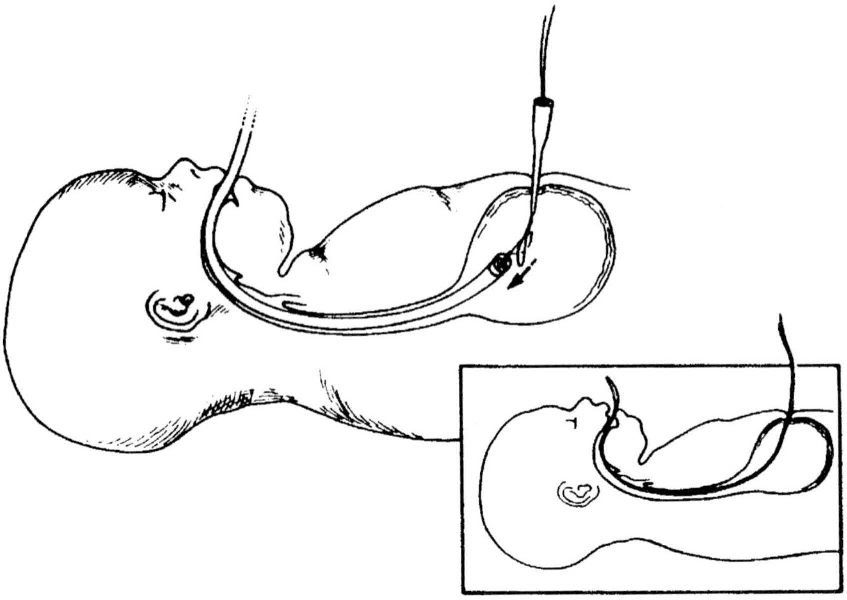

FIGURE 44.2. The needle is removed and the looped, plastic-covered wire inserted through the cannula. The snare is tightened around the wire. The scope is then pulled back through the stomach and esophagus, establishing the guiding tract (insert). From Gauderer MWL, Stellato TA. Percutaneous endoscopic gastrostomy in children: the technique in detail. *Pediatr Surg Int* 1991;6:82–87, with permission.

of the skin (Fig. 44.3, insert). The endoscope is removed. The catheter is cut to size and the feeding adapter attached. Sutures are not required, but 2 × 2 inch gauze and tape can be used to cover and secure the catheter.

The most widely performed PEG procedure is the original "pull" technique described here. Alternative placements include the "push" technique, in which a catheter is advanced over a guide wire, and the "poke" technique, in which the catheter is placed through the abdominal wall rather than through the esophagus. Because the stomach is pushed away from the abdominal wall during the placement, T-fasteners may be necessary with this approach. In the nonendoscopic or radiographic procedures, early dislodgment of relatively thin catheters can occur.

Laparoscopy can be combined with the PEG technique to add an element of safety if the anatomic relationships are unclear. If there are any questions concerning safety, an open gastrostomy should be performed.

POSTOPERATIVE CARE

A small sponge and tape are sufficient to cover the incision site. On postoperative day 1, the external retainer bar is loosened to accommodate the anterior abdominal wall edema, but, at the same time, ensure a "snug" fit against the skin without causing indentation. The wound dressing is removed; no ointments or salves are needed. Feedings are

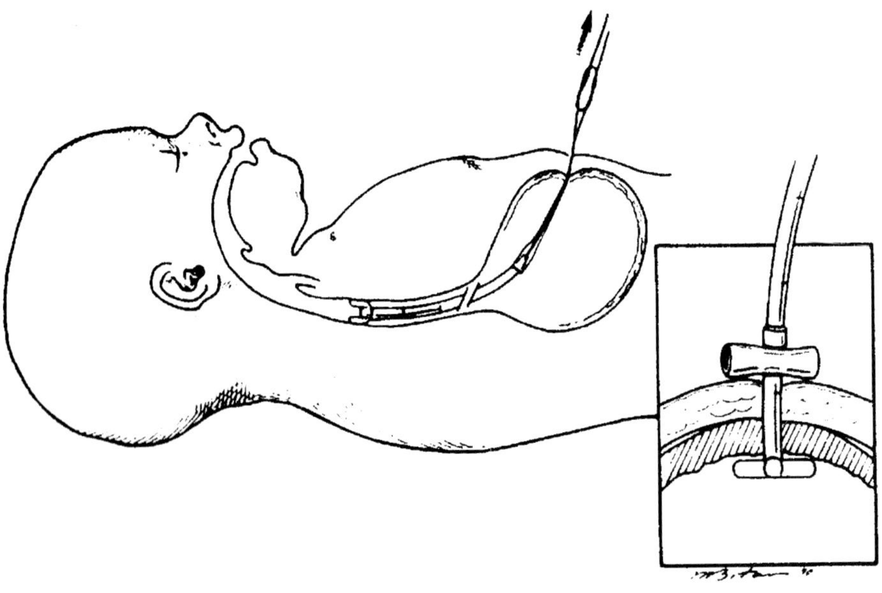

FIGURE 44.3. The percutaneous endoscopic gastrostomy catheter is attached to the guiding wire by interlocking the two loops. Traction is applied to the abdominal end of the wire, guiding the catheter through the esophagus, stomach, and across gastric and abdominal walls. Once the gastric and abdominal walls are in loose contact, the external crossbar and immobilizing ring are slipped over the catheter and guided to the skin level (insert). From Gauderer MWL, Stellato TA. Percutaneous endoscopic gastrostomy in children: the technique in detail. *Pediatr Surg Int* 1991;6:82–87, with permission.

begun after 12 to 24 hours, although, theoretically, feedings could be started immediately because there is no ileus. Delay in feeding allows for careful abdominal examination of an empty gastrointestinal tract to rule out peritonitis; delay also reduces postprocedure emesis from anesthetic agents or pain and permits sealing of the tract around the PEG tube. Initially, small amounts of dilute formula or breast milk are used. Advancement to full concentration and volume ensues over 1 to 2 days.

To facilitate management and reduce the complications associated with conventional long gastrostomy tubes, conversion to a skin-level device is recommended. Skin-level devices such as the initial "button" developed in 1982 continue to be used with success. However, these devices require removal of the initially placed PEG tube after a suggested waiting period of 3 months. The conversion from long tube to skin-level device can result in pain, tract damage, and, possibly, separation of the stomach from the abdominal wall. The Genie PEG system (Bard Interventional Products, Billerica, MA) was developed to circumvent tube replacement problems. The initially placed long tube is left *in situ,* and an external port valve is applied. The Genie kit contains the equipment necessary for the change to a skin-level device. After removing the external retainer bar, a nontraumatic plastic hemostat clamps the catheter shaft just above the skin level. The tubing is divided above the hemostat, allowing for enough room to fit the nozzle of the valve. The nozzle slides into the end of the cut tubing, and the plastic clip secures the valve to the catheter. If valve failure should occur, only the port-valve, not the entire tube, is changed.

COMPLICATIONS

Complications of gastrostomy consist of those related to the operative technique, care of the stoma, and the catheter itself.

Operative Technique

Separation of the stomach from the abdominal wall is the most serious complication; it can result in death if recognition is delayed. It most commonly occurs after early reinsertion of the gastrostomy tube before adhesion of the gastric and abdominal walls has occurred. While attempting to reinsert a tube, the surgeon pushes the stomach away from the abdominal wall. In the event of premature removal, gentle probing of the tract with placement of a small (12–14 French) Foley catheter is acceptable. A contrast study through the Foley catheter under fluoroscopy must be performed to ensure the intragastric position of the tube and the absence of intraperitoneal leakage. Any question concerning position of the tube requires laparotomy.

Hemorrhage following PEG placement is rare. It can result from injury to the gastroepiploic vessels, gastric varices, or superficial epigastric vessels during needle puncture. It is usually self-limiting because of the compressive action of the gastrostomy tube. Initially, bleeding can be managed with traction on the tube. If this maneuver fails, repeat endoscopy should be performed to evaluate gastric sources of bleeding separate from the gastrostomy site.

Infection remains a complication of gastrostomy. Theoretically, the risk arises from carrying the oropharyngeal secretions through the gastric and abdominal wall. It is usually limited to the skin and subcutaneous tissue; however, deep infections involving the entire thickness of the abdominal wall can occur. Higher infection rates are seen among obese patients, those receiving steroids, and immunosuppressed children. Preventive measures include making the skin incision slightly larger than the diameter of the tube to allow drainage and to administer preoperative antibiotics.

Injury to other organs, most notably the colon, is another major complication of the PEG procedure. The incidence is reported as 2% to 3%, but should be lower if careful preventive steps are taken. The transverse colon may lie across the stomach with under- or overinflation of the stomach. If the transverse colon is in front of the stomach, transillumination is impaired. Passage of the PEG catheter through the liver has been reported, but usually without any adverse effects.

Pneumoperitoneum is commonly seen on post-PEG abdominal films. This finding is usually innocuous and does not require special attention.

Proper placement of the catheter is important. Catheters placed in the gastric antrum have an increased chance of causing pyloric occlusion, especially with balloon catheters. Because of the dependent position, there is also an increased potential for leakage. Catheters placed too high may interfere with later fundoplication procedures. Catheters placed too close to the rib cage also interfere with later fundoplication and cause pain. We recommend placing catheters in the midportion of the stomach, halfway between the greater and lesser curvatures.

Care of the Stoma

Formation of granulation tissue is by far the most common problem encountered. If treated early when the condition is mild, a few applications of silver nitrate are usually curative. It is therefore important to inform the patient and family of the possibility and encourage early treatment. Unfortunately, it is common to see the patient only after a heaping mound of "proud flesh" has grown around the catheter. Skin irritation and leakage of gastric contents follow. Many times physicians culture the area and prescribe antibiotics, often antipseudomonal agents. This is unnecessary. In severe conditions, silver nitrate applications alone are not adequate. This situation requires local excision and cauterization with the aid of local anesthetic. Once epithelization of the tract occurs, granulation tissue will not form. We have had good results with the prophylactic application of a combination of nystatin and triamcinolone acetonide cream to prevent the formation of and reduce the amount of already formed granulation tissue.

Skin irritation and moniliasis also can be a problem. This is particularly true if occlusive dressings are used. Therefore, the gastrostomy site should be kept open and dry. The skin around the site should be washed with soap and water, and, if irritated, dried with a hair dryer. Ointments and other creams, except for the treatment of moniliasis, should be avoided. Early conversion to a skin-level port-valve helps prevent these problems.

Accidental removal of the PEG catheter is uncommon. However, delay in the reintroduction of the gastrostomy catheter can result in closure of the tract in a relatively short time. Therefore, parents should be instructed in how to avoid accidental removal as well as in inserting a replacement catheter. We instruct them in how to reinsert a Foley catheter at home, and we subsequently replace the catheter in the office with a skin-level device if the tract is already mature.

Trauma during reinsertion of a gastrostomy catheter can result from improper technique. Damage to the spleen, liver, or pancreas can occur, especially in small children, given the short distance between the abdominal wall and these organs. Gentle insertion with the introducer directed at the gastric cardia reduces the chance of injury. Occasionally, gradual widening of the tract with Hegar dilators is necessary.

Catheter-Related Problems

Tube plugging is usually preventable. After each use, the tube must be flushed with water. If plugging should occur, forceful irrigation is successful in most cases. Soda water or meat tenderizer and saline may be instilled in attempts to unclog the tubing. If these maneuvers fail in a well-healed gastrostomy tract, the tube is changed.

Gastrostomy leakage is more commonly seen in children than in adults because of the thinner abdominal wall musculature; however, leakage following PEG is uncommon. The main cause of leakage is the enlargement of the stoma by the pivoting action of a gastrostomy tube that is too large or too stiff. Excessive granulation tissue also contributes to this problem. Placement of the gastrostomy in the midline contributes to the chance of leakage because the abdominal wall is thinner at this site without the underlying rectus musculature. Immobilization of the catheter with the retainer bar helps to reduce widening of the stoma. Contrary to popular approach, a larger tube does not help the problem; it actually compounds it for the reason described above. A helpful, initial step in controlling leakage is to replace the tube with a smaller one to allow the stoma to shrink, and then replace the initial tube. If all simple measures fail, a new PEG is placed close to the original, leaking stoma, which is then closed extraperitoneally. Before closure, a large, curved needle can be inserted into the leaking stoma, traversing the gastric and abdominal walls. Once the tract is established, a PEG catheter is attached to the suture and pulled into place.

All catheters eventually deteriorate. This is particularly evident with latex products. Foley latex catheters may degrade in as little as a few weeks. The newer, silicone rubber catheters have helped to ameliorate this problem. Internal migration of the catheter is particularly common with Foley-type catheters if an external retainer is not used. The usual presentation is that of gastric outlet obstruction, with epigastric pain and vomiting, or increased leakage around the tube and shortening of the visible catheter length. The problem is easily corrected by deflating the balloon and pulling the catheter back. Therefore, external retainer bumpers should be used with all long gastrostomy tubes. For these reasons, we do not recommend the use of Foley catheters in children.

A persistent gastrocutaneous fistula after removal of the gastrostomy tube is a common problem if the catheter has been in place longer than 9 to 12 months. If the catheter has been in place for shorter periods, the stoma will typically close spontaneously hours to days after removal of the tube. If drainage persists beyond several weeks, simple techniques such as silver nitrate application and electrocautery under local anesthesia may be tried. Failing these maneuvers, surgical closure is required. Excision of the tract without entering the abdominal cavity, followed by a layered closure, is simple and very effective.

CONCLUSION

Percutaneous endoscopic gastrostomy was developed to simplify catheter placement and to reduce the number of complications associated with open gastrostomies. This goal has been largely achieved, and the approach has benefited countless patients, especially those who require long-term feeding. It is important, however, to stress that any child in whom a gastrostomy is placed must be carefully followed, preferably by the team who was initially involved in the indication of the procedure. Stoma care, nutritional adjustments, and periodic monitoring for the development of gastroesophageal reflux are key in the follow-up of these children. With a properly indicated, correctly placed, and carefully followed PEG, results are generally very satisfying.

SUGGESTED READINGS

Boyle JT. Nutritional management of the developmentally disabled child. *Pediatr Surg Int* 1991;6:76–81.

Gauderer MWL, Abrams RS, Hammond JH. Initial experience with the changeable skin-level port-valve: a new concept for the long-term gastrointestinal access. *J Pediatr Surg* 1998;33:73–75.

Gauderer MWL, Ponsky JL, Izant, RI Jr. Gastrostomy without laparotomy—a percutaneous endoscopic technique. *J Pediatr Surg* 1980;15:872–875.

Gauderer MWL, Stellato TA. Gastrostomies: evolution, techniques, indications, and complications. *Curr Prob Surg* 1986;23:661–719.

Gauderer MWL, Stellato TA. Percutaneous endoscopic gastrostomy in children: the technique in detail. *Pediatr Surg Int* 1991;6: 82–87.

Gauderer MWL. Feeding gastrostomy or feeding gastrostomy plus antireflux procedure? [Editorial] *J Pediatr Gastroenterol Nutr* 1988;7:795–796.

Gauderer MWL. Twenty years of percutaneous endoscopic gastrostomy: origin and evolution of a concept and its expanded applications. *Gastrointest Endosc* 1999;50:879–883.

Gordon JM, Langer JC. Gastrocutaneous fistula in children after removal of gastrostomy tube: incidence and predictive factors. *J Pediatr Surg* 1999;34:1345–1346.

Sulaeman E, Udall JN Jr, Brown RF, et al. Gastroesophageal reflux and Nissen fundoplication following percutaneous endoscopic gastrostomy in children. *J Pediatr Gastroenterol Nutr* 1998;26: 269–273.

Williams SGJ, Ashworth F, McAlweenie A, et al. Percutaneous endoscopic gastrostomy feeding in patients with cystic fibrosis. *Gut* 1999;44:87–90.

45

HYPERTROPHIC PYLORIC STENOSIS

STEPHEN G. MURPHY

HISTORY

In a 1717 presentation to the Royal Society of London of an autopsy report of a 5-month-old, Dr. Patrick Blair succinctly summarized the fundamental characteristics of pyloric stenosis: "... his Mother told me he seemed to be healthy till he was about one month old when he was seized with a violent vomiting... he seemed to have a great appetite taking whatever food was offered him... but he immediately threw it all up again... the pylorus and duodenum were so cartilaginous that no nourishment could have passed into the intestines."

In the first U.S. account of this malady in 1788, Dr. Hezekiah Beardsley reported to the Medical Society of New Haven: "A child... in the first week of its infancy was attacked with a puking... the child ejected whatever was received into the stomach... at autopsy, the pylorus was invested with a hard substance or schirrosity which completely obstructed passage into the duodenum." In Germany in 1887, Dr. Harold Hirschsprung presented two cases of pyloric stenosis. In 1898, the first successful gastroenterostomy for pyloric stenosis was performed. Extramucosal pyloroplasty was performed in the early 1900s by Nicoll, Fredet, Weber, and Ramstedt. All reapproximated the muscle transversely. In 1911, after operating on a baby with pyloric stenosis, Ramstedt wrote "... the wound edges parted vigorously and I had the impression that by this the narrowing was relieved... I decided that in the next case I would employ no suturing of split muscles, but would leave the incision gaping and unsutured." Ramstedt performed this procedure on June 18, 1912. In 1910, published mortality for Weber's series of gastroenterostomy for treatment of pyloric stenosis was 61%. In 1946, Ladd reported on 225 patients treated by pyloromyotomy with no deaths.

S.G. Murphy: Department of Surgery, Thomas Jefferson University, Philadelphia, Pennsylvania; and Department of Surgery, Alfred I. duPont Hospital for Children, Wilmington, Delaware.

EPIDEMIOLOGY

The incidence of hypertrophic pyloric stenosis (HPS) ranges from 2 to 4 per 1,000 live births. There is a male predominance at a ratio of 4 to 1. Whites are more often affected than blacks or Asians. Over 90% of cases are sporadic, but approximately 7% are familial. A mother who had HPS as an infant transmits the risk of developing HPS to her offspring: 19% for boys, 7% for girls. A father with HPS also transmits an increased risk to his progeny: 5% for boys and 2.5% for girls. An increased risk for development of HPS has been reported with blood types B and O. Associated anomalies are extremely rare and are predominantly limited to case reports.

ETIOLOGY

The cause of pyloric stenosis has yet to be determined. The classic teaching purported that milk curds propelled against the pylorus lead to mucosal swelling. This is followed by hypertrophy of the circular muscle, which creates a vicious cycle of more muscle hypertrophy and a progressive gastric outlet narrowing. The lesion is not generally seen at birth, but takes a few weeks to develop. Numerous investigators have sought to shed light on the cause of pyloric stenosis. Inquiries have focused on characteristics of the pyloric region, ganglion cells, levels of various neuropeptides, including vasoactive intestinal polypeptide, gastrin, substance P, and serotonin, as well as reduced levels of nitric oxide synthetase in the circular smooth muscle. Histologic evaluation reveals thickening of the inner layer of smooth muscle. This is due to hypertrophy, not to hyperplasia. The mucosa is normal.

PRESENTATION

Pyloric stenosis typically develops in an otherwise healthy child who feeds normally at birth. At 2 to 6 weeks of age, the child develops progressively forceful vomiting. This begins as intermittent feeding intolerance and is often treated by the pediatrician by changing formula. With time, as the gastric outlet obstruction becomes more significant, the course progresses to forceful vomiting with, or shortly following, feeding. The emesis is essentially always nonbilious because the obstruction is proximal to the ampulla of Vater. Blood-tinged emesis indicates gastric irritation and is seen in up to 10% of cases. After vomiting, the baby is hungry again. Most babies do not appear ill unless dehydration becomes severe.

An increasing awareness of this entity by primary care physicians has led to timelier surgical referral. Most babies can be kept hydrated by oral intake early in the course when gastric outlet narrowing is not critical. Profound dehydration and malnutrition were more prevalent years ago.

A history of progressive, projectile, nonbilious emesis in an infant 2 to 8 weeks of age is almost pathognomonic of HPS.

DIAGNOSIS

Obtaining a characteristic history is helpful in diagnosing pyloric stenosis. However, HPS should be differentiated from gastroesophageal reflux. Projectile vomiting also can be a manifestation of increased intracranial pressure.

The physical examination may be diagnostic. The abdomen should be observed for waves of gastric peristalsis. Success in palpation depends on the expertise, patience and persistence of the examiner. Nasogastric decompression can help when the stomach is dilated. The olive is virtually impossible to feel in a crying baby. Allowing the infant to take a pacifier or some glucose water may relax the abdominal wall sufficiently. If an olive is palpable, the diagnosis is confirmed and imaging becomes superfluous.

The examination is best performed in a quiet, comfortable setting. The infant must be kept warm, and the examiner may place a hand under the baby's buttocks to gently flex the spine and soften the abdomen. The pylorus is a midline structure. With gentle sweeping motions deep in the abdomen, the olive can be coaxed out of its hiding place under the liver.

IMAGING

Ultrasonographic evaluation has supplanted swallowed contrast as the preferred imaging study. Ultrasonography avoids radiation exposure and the risk of aspiration of contrast. It is reproducible and reliable. Examination is best performed in the right decubitus position to displace fluid to the antrum. Pyloric muscle thickness of 4 mm or greater, an immobile pyloric channel length greater than 1.6 cm, or a pyloric diameter of 1.4 cm are compatible with pyloric stenosis. Sensitivity is greater than 95%, with 100% specificity. An upper gastrointestinal contrast study is also accurate but subjects the patient to radiation. It also requires administration of contrast to a patient with a gastric outlet obstruction with some inherent risk of aspiration. Typical contrast findings are an elongated stringlike pyloric channel and the impression of the enlarged pyloric muscle upon the antrum and duodenum. Many babies are referred from the pediatrician, with ultrasonography already completed.

The preferred diagnostic study is physical examination; however, most patients will have been referred for an imaging study. When the history is suggestive of pyloric stenosis, ultrasonography is the preferred study. If other diagnoses (reflux, malrotation, obstruction) are being considered, an upper gastrointestinal contrast study can provide more information.

LABORATORY EVALUATION

The characteristic presentation of prolonged gastric outlet obstruction is that of hypokalemic, hypochloremic metabolic alkalosis. Loss of gastric acid secondary to emesis contributes to the alkalosis, but the primary driving force for the electrolyte derangement is dehydration. With dehydration, aldosterone production is stimulated. Physiologically, the patient is in a sodium-avid state: conserving sodium is conserving volume. The effect of aldosterone on the distal tubules favors reabsorption of sodium. Hydrogen and potassium are excreted to maintain electroneutrality. This accounts for the classic paradoxic aciduria, an indicator of severe dehydration. A few babies with pyloric stenosis (<5%) have an indirect hyperbilirubinemia on presentation. This is due to a transient deficit in glucuronyl transferase activity that promptly returns to normal with hydration, treatment, and resumption of feedings.

MANAGEMENT

There is no urgency to operate on a child who is known to have pyloric stenosis. It is far more important to correct the dehydration and electrolyte derangement. The compensation for severe metabolic alkalosis is respiratory acidosis, which is produced by hypoventilation. Therefore, the baby with severe metabolic alkalosis will not breathe well postoperatively. The severity of the serum electrolyte anomalies dictates the vigor of the resuscitation. For severe dehydration, the baby should receive crystalloid fluid boluses of 20 mL/kg. Half normal saline solution with potassium is administered at a rate of up to twice the maintenance dose, with additional boluses of normal saline to maintain a good urine output. A low potassium level indicates a critical depletion of body stores—potassium must be added to the intravenous solution. Surgery should be deferred until the serum bicarbonate approaches a normal level. Most surgeons and anesthesiologists would agree to proceed with operation when the HCO_3 level is 28 mEq/L or less, and the chloride is greater than 98 mEq/L. A high measured potassium level is nearly always due to hemolysis. The measurement should be repeated to avoid the unnecessary and potentially dangerous omission of intravenous potassium administration. For a severely dehydrated baby, correction of electrolyte imbalance may take days, although the more typical patient can be corrected overnight.

Medical management of HPS is possible but is reserved for patients who are poor operative risks. This method requires prolonged (6 months to a year) postpyloric feeding via a feeding tube. Correction by Ramstedt pyloromyotomy is simple, safe, and effective, and rapidly returns the patient and family to a normal life.

OPERATIVE CORRECTION

Ramstedt pyloromyotomy has been performed since 1912 with superlative results. Choices of incisions include the standard right upper quadrant transverse incision (1 cm superior to the umbilicus and 1 cm to the right of midline), the Robertson subcostal incision, or a periumbilical approach. The rectus muscle may be retracted or divided. The thickened pylorus is easily delivered into the wound by using a wet sponge to grasp the stomach and torquing the pyloric olive into the wound (Fig. 45.1). Pertinent anatomy includes the pyloric vein of Mayo, which is adjacent to the boundary demarcating thick white pyloric muscle from pink duodenum, and the avascular plane on the anterior surface of the pylorus. The incision should be placed in the anterior avascular plane and extended onto the stomach to avoid risk of recurrence. The incision should start just proximal to the vein of Mayo, not at it. Perforations of the mucosa should be rare but usually occur at the duodenal border of the pylorus. At this point the duodenal mucosa protrudes back toward the stomach and is easily injured. By performing the initial myotomy in the center of the olive and approaching the duodenal aspect last, this risk is minimized. The myotomy may be performed with a Benson pyloric spreader, the back-handle of a scalpel, or with an upturned, curved hemostat. The procedure is complete when the donut-shaped outlet of the pylorus is converted to a "C" shape. The cut edges of pyloric muscle should move independently of one another. The mucosa should bulge nicely into the incision, with no transverse bands of muscle remaining. It is not a tragedy to make a small hole in the mucosa, but it is potentially fatal not to recognize this injury. Milking gastric contents through the duodenum and pouring saline over the mucosa detects bubbling if there is a leak. Bleeding from the cut muscle edges will stop once the pylorus is placed back inside the abdominal cavity. A laparoscopic approach is used in many centers, but it is difficult to improve upon the excellent long-term track record of the Ramstedt pyloromyotomy.

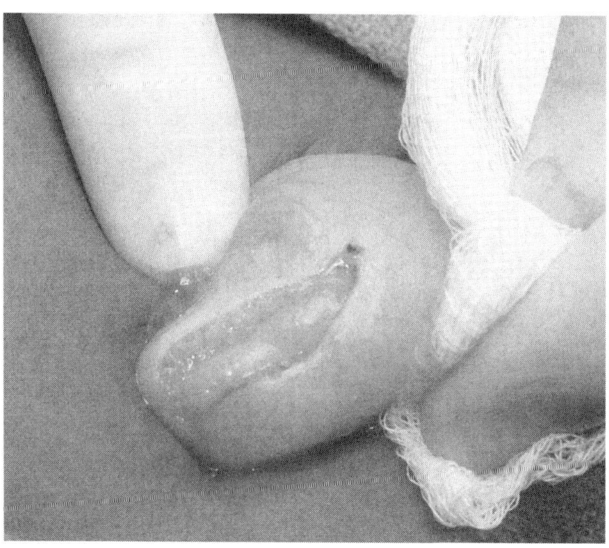

FIGURE 45.1. Operative photograph of pyloromyotomy depicting mucosa protruding through divided thickened pyloric muscle.

FEEDING

Feeding is safely initiated within 6 hours postoperatively. The initial feeding at our institution is Pedialyte (Abbott Laboratories, Abbott Park, Illinois). Feedings are administered every 2 hours and increased gradually in volume and formula strength. With this regimen, the majority of infants are advanced to full feedings within 24 hours after pyloromyotomy.

QUANDRIES

Rarely, ultrasonography demonstrates pyloric stenosis but a mass is not palpable with the baby under general anesthesia. Options include proceeding with operation, reassessing with ultrasonography in the operating room, or waking the baby up. Our experience has suggested that ultrasonography may be more accurate than palpation. Confirming the result with ultrasonography in the operating room before incision seems reasonable.

What if a hole is made in the duodenal mucosa during the procedure? The traditional recommendation for this injury included closure of mucosa, followed by closure of pyloric muscle over mucosa. The pylorus was then turned 90 degrees, and the myotomy repeated. A safe alternative approach is to close the mucosa with simple stitches and lay an omental patch over it. This is effective, and the baby may be fed the next day.

What if the baby vomits frequently postoperatively? The vast majority of babies will tolerate feeding within 48 hours postprocedure. Some babies vomit for longer periods, such as those with gastritis or prolonged preoperative emesis. As long as the baby is gaining weight, we reassure parents. Babies with gastritis often improve with histamine–2 blocker therapy. What if the vomiting is forceful and prolonged postoperatively? Recurrent (or persistent) pyloric stenosis should be a rare occurrence, preventable by carrying the myotomy onto the stomach. If one is considering residual obstruction, ultrasonography is not a good test—even babies who are well will have bulky pyloric muscle postoperatively. The pyloric muscle remains thickened for up to 6 months after pyloromyotomy, gradually returning to normal thickness. The upper gastrointestinal series may be helpful in this setting, but is also often abnormal.

OUTCOME

The most common complication is wound infection, occurring in 1% to 2% (some series report rates as high as 16%). After pyloromyotomy, most babies feed well and resume normal weight gain. No study has demonstrated a consistent negative effect on gastric emptying. Wound dehiscence secondary to malnutrition is of historic interest. This complication would now be ascribed to technical error. Perforation and recurrence should be rare events. Perforation occurs in less than 1% of cases. Recurrence is attributed to inadequate initial myotomy, that is, not carrying the myotomy a sufficient distance onto the stomach. Over 90% of our babies are discharged to home and are feeding well within 48 hours after pyloromyotomy. Mortality from pyloromyotomy should be nil and is zero in most pediatric specialty centers. In a recent collective review, the incidence of wound infection and mucosal perforation was higher when the procedure was performed by general surgeons compared with pediatric surgeons.

SUGGESTED READINGS

Brain A, Roberts D. Who should treat pyloric stenosis: the general or specialist pediatric surgeon? *J Pediatr Surg* 1996;31:1535–1537.

Crabbe D. Infantile hypertrophic pyloric stenosis. In: Stringer MD, Oldham KT, Mouriquand PDE, et al., eds. *Pediatric surgery and urology: long term outcomes.* Philadelphia: WB Saunders, 1998: 264–271.

Hight DW, Benson CD, Philippart AI, et al. Management of mucosal perforation during pyloromyotomy for infantile pyloric stenosis. *Surgery* 1981;90:85–86.

Keller H, Waldmann D, Greiner P. Comparison of preoperative sonography with intraoperative findings in congenital hypertrophic pyloric stenosis. *J Pediatr Surg* 1987;22:950–952.

Najmaldin A. Early experience with laparoscopic pyloromyotomy for infantile hypertrophic pyloric stenosis. *J Pediatr Surg* 1995;30: 37–38.

Ramstedt C. Zur Operation der angeborenene Pylorus Stenose. *Med Klin* 1912;8:1702–1705.

Ravitch MM. The story of pyloric stenosis. *Surgery* 1960;48:1117–1143.

Yoshizawa J, Eto T, Higashimoto Y, et al. Ultrasound features of normalization of the pylorus after pyloromyotomy for hypertrophic pyloric stenosis. *J Pediatr Surg* 2001;36:582–586.

46

DUODENAL ATRESIA

DANIEL von ALLMEN

DIAGNOSTIC APPROACH

The diagnosis of duodenal atresia is most commonly made prenatally. Although the use of prenatal ultrasonographic examination is not universal, it is so ubiquitous that many cases are identified before birth. The ultrasonographic diagnosis can be made as early as 20 weeks' gestation and is more frequently made in fetuses with multiple anomalies. Polyhydramnios is present in as many as 60% of mothers of fetuses with high intestinal obstruction, increasing the likelihood that more focused prenatal evaluation will identify the abnormality. The ultrasonographic characteristics of duodenal atresia include the presence of polyhydramnios, a dilated stomach and duodenal bulb ("double bubble"), and decreased meconium in the distal bowel. The ability to identify a proximal bowel obstruction on prenatal ultrasonography is high in experienced hands, although the exact cause may not be obvious and the differential diagnosis includes duodenal atresia, duodenal duplication, choledochal cyst, and proximal jejunal atresia. An annular pancreas also may be present. Conversely, the absence of typical findings does not rule out the presence of duodenal atresia or duodenal stenosis with or without a "windsock"-type abnormality.

Infants who are not diagnosed prenatally present with vomiting within the first few hours of life or with the initiation of feedings. In the majority of cases the vomiting is bilious, because the duodenal obstruction is distal to the ampulla of Vater in 85% of cases. Typically the infant's abdomen is not particularly distended on physical examination because of the proximal nature of the obstruction. A plain radiograph of the abdomen shows dilation of the stomach and first portion of the duodenum with no gas in the distal intestine (double bubble sign). The accuracy of this simple examination can be increased by aspirating the gastric contents and injecting 40 to 60 mL of air into the stomach via a nasogastric tube prior to taking the film (Fig. 46.1).

D. von Allmen: Department of Surgery, Division of Pediatric Surgery, University of Pennsylvania School of Medicine; and Department of General and Thoracic Surgery, Children's Hospital of Philadelphia, Philadelphia, Pennsylvania.

The differential diagnosis for patients with bilious vomiting or bilious nasogastric aspirates includes malrotation with volvulus, more distal atresias, and Hirschsprung's disease. The diagnosis of malrotation with volvulus must be made immediately to avoid loss of the midgut, but volvulus is unlikely in stable infants with a dilated first portion of the duodenum noted on prenatal ultrasonography, a classic double bubble sign, and no distal bowel gas on postnatal radiographic studies. In contrast to infants with an acute volvulus, infants with duodenal atresia do not appear ill. Radiologic contrast studies are not usually required to confirm the diagnosis of duodenal atresia but should be obtained if the question of malrotation and volvulus exists.

Patients with nonbilious vomiting may present some confusion because the majority of duodenal atresias occur beyond the ampulla of Vater. However, in 15% of cases the atresia is more proximal and the emesis is nonbilious. In

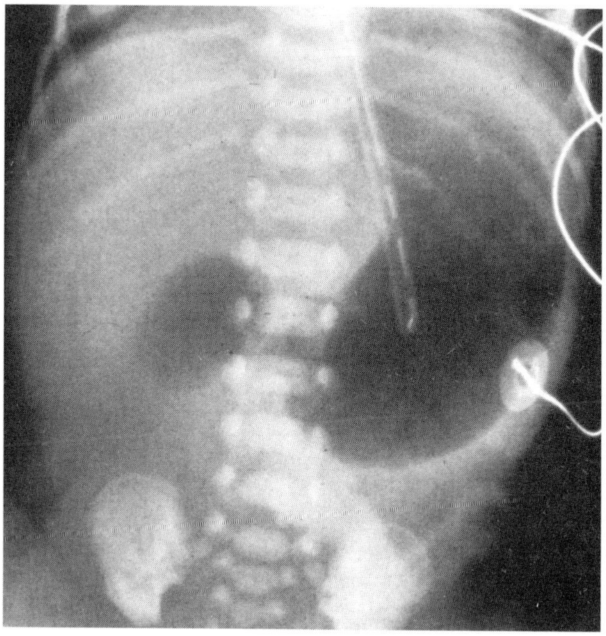

FIGURE 46.1. Abdominal radiograph of a newborn with duodenal atresia demonstrating a "double bubble" after injection of air into the stomach via the nasogastric tube.

these patients, pyloric atresia, antral webs, and duodenal stenosis are all in the differential diagnosis. A high index of suspicion based on prenatal ultrasonography and the appearance of postnatal plain films usually leads to the correct diagnosis without an extensive workup.

PREOPERATIVE PREPARATION

Infants diagnosed prenatally are transported to the neonatal intensive care unit immediately following delivery. Intravenous fluids and nasogastric decompression are initiated, and plain films of the abdomen are obtained after injecting a small amount of air into the nasogastric tube. Bilious or nonbilious vomiting in an undiagnosed postnatal patient should immediately prompt similar management, and arrangements should be made to transfer the child to a facility with pediatric surgical support if it is not available at the institution at which the child was delivered. Patients with characteristic prenatal ultrasonographic findings and postnatal plain film findings of duodenal atresia do not require immediate surgery and should undergo evaluation for associated anomalies. Approximately 30% of patients with duodenal atresia have trisomy 21 and 20% have significant cardiac anomalies. Knowledge of these anomalies prior to surgery can affect both the anesthetic and surgical management of the child. Cardiology and genetic consultation are appropriate, and an echocardiogram should be obtained if there is any question of an associated cardiac defect. Regardless of the cardiac status of the infant, prophylactic antibiotics should be given prior to operation. I prefer ampicillin and gentamicin, although a cephalosporin is probably adequate.

SURGICAL MANAGEMENT

The abdomen is entered through a supraumbilical right-sided transverse incision. A thorough exploration of the peritoneal cavity is important to confirm the diagnosis and identify any associated anomalies. Malrotation may accompany the duodenal atresia in as many as 40% of patients, and a formal Ladd procedure should be performed prior to repairing the atresia. The lesser sac should be opened and the duodenum mobilized laterally with a Kocher maneuver to allow inspection of the pancreas and the entire course of the duodenum. An annular pancreas may be present in as many as 40% of patients. The annular pancreas usually obscures the actual site of the bowel obstruction, but the pancreatic tissue should not be divided because it contains a significant pancreatic duct. Embryologically, rotation of the ventral anlage of the pancreas occurs at the time of duodenal recannalization, which may explain the association between the two abnormalities. A preduodenal vein may be present and is also associated with anomalies of the vena cava and biliary tree.

Three types of atresias of the duodenum are found. In type I atresias an intrinsic web is present at the level of the ampulla of Vater. In some cases this web may balloon into the lumen to form a windsock-type deformity. In type II atresias a solid cord of tissue is present between the proximal and distal bowel, and in type III atresias, the bowel segments are completely separated. Usually an abrupt change in the caliber of the duodenum identifies the site of the obstruction. The first portion of the duodenum is thickened and dilated, and the second portion is decompressed and narrow. In rare cases, the obstruction may be more distal, requiring exposure of the third and fourth portions of the duodenum and mobilization of the ligament of Trietz.

For the actual repair, I prefer a diamond-shaped duodenoduodenostomy as described by Kimura. A transverse incision is made in the dilated proximal duodenum. The lumen should be explored to identify the site of obstruction because a windsock-type deformity of the web may cause confusion as to the actual level of obstruction. A longitudinal incision is made in the collapsed duodenum distal to the site of obstruction. Bile is usually seen on only one side of the web, but the presence of pancreatic divisum or a small fenestration in the web may result in bile being present on both sides of the obstruction. Milking the gallbladder usually demonstrates the presence of bile in at least one segment of the duodenum and rules out associated biliary atresia. I do not manipulate the web because the ampulla is frequently located on the medial margin. Others resect the lateral margin of the web, but I prefer to bypass the lesion and avoid risking injury to the ampulla or bile duct. Prior to completing the anastomosis, a small red rubber catheter is advanced into the distal duodenum and saline injected slowly to confirm patency of the small bowel to the ileocecal valve. The diamond-shaped anastomosis is then performed in a single layer with 5-0 PDS suture. A broad, widely patent anastomosis is achieved.

The duodenum proximal to the obstruction may be grossly dilated. These patients often have significant feeding problems postoperatively because of poor emptying through the anastomosis. In these cases, I taper the duodenum using a gastrointestinal stapling device. A large-bore tube is inserted retrograde into the proximal duodenum, and the stapler is used to resect the antimesenteric border. Others prefer to imbricate the redundant duodenum rather than resect any portion of the bowel. Placement of a drain is seldom indicated.

Although transanastomotic feeding tubes have fallen out of favor with some surgeons, I frequently pass a soft silastic tube distal to the duodenal anastomosis in patients with significant proximal duodenal dilation. For patients with associated anomalies, especially cardiac anomalies, consideration is also given to placing a gastrostomy tube to facilitate postoperative feedings. This is particularly true for patients with trisomy 21 because of the high risk of delayed oral feeding. When a gastrostomy tube is placed, the silastic jejunostomy tube can be brought out through the abdominal wall adjacent to the small gastrostomy tube as an alternative to the larger stiffer commercially available gastrojejunostomy tubes.

Duodenal atresia can occur in conjunction with esophageal atresia. In these cases, I prefer to place a gastrostomy tube and repair the duodenal atresia first, if technically possible. The esophageal atresia can then be addressed at a subsequent thoracotomy without concern for a distal bowel obstruction. This approach may be impossible for premature patients with a large tracheoesophageal fistula that complicates positive pressure ventilation. In these cases the fistula must be ligated first with repair of the esophageal atresia if possible. The duodenal atresia repair is performed when the child is more stable.

A diamond-shaped or side-to-side duodenoduodenostomy is sufficient to relieve congenital duodenal obstruction in nearly all cases regardless of the cause. In rare cases, for example, in some patients with a preduodenal portal vein, a traditional side-to-side retrocolic duodenojejunostomy may be indicated. Although drainage is typically adequate after this procedure, the incidence of long-term complications such as blind-loop syndrome and obstruction are higher.

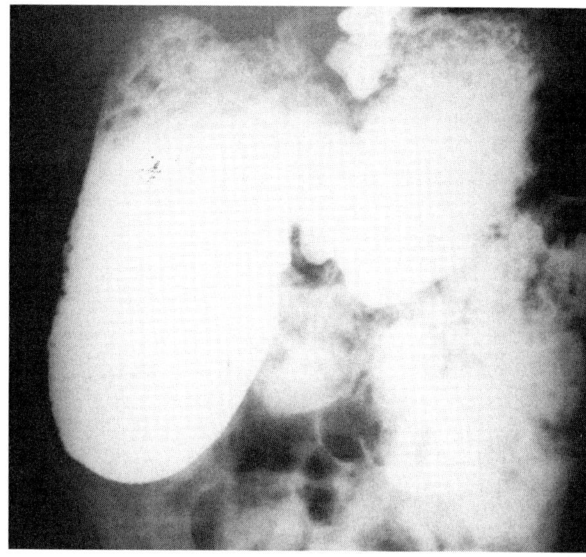

FIGURE 46.2. Upper gastrointestinal tract study of a teenager with massive dilation of the first portion of the duodenum following duodenal atresia repair as an infant. A colon interposition is also present from an associated esophageal atresia.

POSTOPERATIVE MANAGEMENT

Prophylactic antibiotics are discontinued shortly after surgery unless there is another indication for antibiotic therapy. Nasogastric decompression is continued until evidence of bowel function returns. Typically the nasogastric drainage remains bilious despite a patent anastomosis and return of peristalsis because of an incompetent pylorus. Once evidence of bowel function returns, feedings are initiated as continuous drip feeding through an indwelling feeding tube. In my experience, the transanastomotic feeding tube allows the child to reach goal feedings more quickly. Delayed gastric emptying is common and may slow advancement of gastric feedings. Conversion to oral feedings can be accomplished in a stepwise manner based on the individual child's clinical course.

COMPLICATIONS AND LONG-TERM OUTCOME

Major complications such as a leak from the duodenoduodenostomy are uncommon, and long-term mortality is usually related to associated anomalies. Most patients achieve full oral feedings, and late complications are rare. Several cases of late intestinal obstruction at the duodenoduodenostomy site years after the primary surgery have been reported. In these cases the proximal duodenum is massively dilated (Fig. 46.2), and treatment consists of plication of the dilated bowel rather than some type of bypass. Results following plication are excellent. Other late complications include bile reflux gastritis, gastroesophageal reflux, and blind loop syndrome.

SUGGESTED READINGS

Adzick NS, Harrison MR, deLorimier AA. Tapering duodenoplasty for megaduodenum associated with duodenal atresia. *J Pediatr Surg* 1986;21:311–312.

Dalla VL, Grosfeld JL, West KW, et al. Intestinal atresia and stenosis: a 25-year experience with 277 cases [Review]. *Arch Surg* 1998; 133:490–496.

Ein SH, Kim PC, Miller HA. The late nonfunctioning duodenal atresia repair—a second look. *J Pediatr Surg* 2000;35:690–691.

Grosfeld JL, Rescorla FJ. Duodenal atresia and stenosis: reassessment of treatment and outcome based on antenatal diagnosis, pathologic variance, and long-term follow-up. *World J Surg* 1993;17:301–309.

Hayden CKJ, Schwartz MZ, Davis M, et al. Combined esophageal and duodenal atresia: sonographic findings. *AJR* 1983;140:225–226.

Kimura K, Mukohara N, Nishijima E, et al. Diamond-shaped anastomosis for duodenal atresia: an experience with 44 patients over 15 years. *J Pediatr Surg* 1990;25:977–979.

Lawrence MJ, Ford WD, Furness ME, et al. Congenital duodenal obstruction: early antenatal ultrasound diagnosis. *Pediatr Surg Int* 2000;16:342–345.

Pameijer CR, Hubbard AM, Coleman B, et al. Combined pure esophageal atresia, duodenal atresia, biliary atresia, and pancreatic ductal atresia: prenatal diagnostic features and review of the literature [Review]. *J Pediatr Surg* 2000;35:745–747.

Spigland N, Yazbeck S. Complications associated with surgical treatment of congenital intrinsic duodenal obstruction. *J Pediatr Surg* 1990;25:1127–1130.

47

INTESTINAL ATRESIA

TODD A. PONSKY
KURT D. NEWMAN

Congenital atresia of the jejunum or ileum is a rare entity but is one of the most common causes of small bowel obstruction in the newborn. Goeller first described ileal atresia in 1684. During the past several decades, the pathophysiology and natural history of the disease have become more clearly understood. Intestinal atresia occurs with a reported incidence that varies from 1 in 330 to 1 in 1,500 live births, and affects equal numbers of boys and girls. It occurs with equal distribution throughout the small intestine. Colonic atresia also can occur but is much less frequently described.

The first evidence of embryonic intestine can be seen around the third week of gestation. The primitive gut undergoes several transformations during development. The midgut elongates enormously and disproportionately, causing it to herniate from the coelom early in gestation. As it returns to the abdomen starting in the 10th week, rotation and fixation to the posterior body wall occurs. During this time, there is a rapid proliferation of intestinal epithelium. In rare instances, this can lead to occlusion of the intestinal lumen, which usually resolves by recanalization. Failure of recanalization is one theory proposed as to the etiology of type I atresias, in which there is continuity of the bowel and the lumen is occluded by a web or diaphragm.

Small bowel atresia is a congenital occlusion of the intestinal lumen that causes a complete obstruction. Although duodenal atresia is technically a "small bowel atresia," it is now understood to be a distinct entity with a completely different pathophysiology, presentation, and treatment than jejunoileal atresias. Children with jejunoileal atresia typically have no other associated extraintestinal anomalies. Children with duodenal atresia, on the other hand, have a significantly higher incidence of associated congenital anomalies, such as trisomy 21 and cardiac anomalies. This suggests that duodenal atresia results from an earlier and perhaps more global insult than jejunoileal atresias.

Although generally considered together, recent data suggest that jejunal atresia and ileal atresia may be distinct entities as well. Although rare, extraintestinal anomalies appear to be more common in patients with jejunal atresia. Jejunal atresias are also more likely to be multiple (67%) than ileal atresias (25%). Nevertheless, the presentation, treatment, and natural history of the two are sufficiently similar that they will be considered together here.

PATHOPHYSIOLOGY

In 1900, Tandler proposed that intestinal atresia resulted from failure of recanalization of the solid cord stage of intestinal development. This was supported by the work of others who suggested that epithelial plugging and failure of recanalization was the cause. However, the theory could not account for the observation that there was often a physical separation of the ends of the atretic bowel or a fibrous cord connecting the two. Furthermore, Louw and Barnard realized in 1955 that bile pigments were often found distal to the atretic segment. Fetal bile secretion begins around the 11th week of gestation, which is significantly later than the recanalization of the solid cord stage. In 1912, Spriggs first suggested that jejunoileal atresia resulted from mesenteric vascular accidents that occur relatively late in development. Louw and Barnard, again in 1955, substantiated this theory by demonstrating that 2 weeks after ligating mesenteric vessels in fetal dogs, intestinal atresia developed in the same pattern seen in humans; specifically, a V-shaped mesenteric gap defect was seen.

The prevailing theory is that the majority of cases of jejunoileal atresias are the result of late mesenteric vascular accidents. The segment of bowel becomes ischemic and is subsequently resorbed by the fetus. Because the bowel contents are sterile and enzymatically inert, peritonitis is rare and sepsis does not occur. These vascular accidents are proposed to be secondary to *in utero* volvulus, malrotation, gas-

T. A. Ponsky: Department of Surgery, The George Washington University School of Medicine, and The George Washington University Hospital, Washington, D.C.

K. D. Newman: Departments of Surgery and Pediatrics, The George Washington University School of Medicine; and Department of Surgery, Children's Hospital, Washington, D.C.

troschisis, intussusception, or internal hernia. All of these have been reported. It is reported that up to 23% of infants with gastroschisis have an associated bowel atresia. In addition, approximately 12% of patients with intestinal atresia also have cystic fibrosis, suggesting that in some cases meconium ileus may be the cause. Another theory, proposed by Walker et al. in 1993, suggests that a primary immunodeficiency disorder may be the cause in some cases.

Intestinal atresias were originally classified by Louw into three types. The current classification scheme is a modification of Louw's system, and describes five types (Fig. 47.1). Type I is a membranous obstruction with intact bowel and mesentery. There is no decrease in bowel length and no mesenteric gap. These may result from incomplete recanalization of the embryonic gut. Type II describes two blind ends separated by an atretic fibrous cord with an intact mesentery. Type IIIa is complete separation of the blind ends by a V-shaped mesenteric defect. Type IIIb is characterized by a more extensive mesenteric defect, in which there is an "apple-peel" or "Christmas-tree" deformity of the small bowel and the bowel receives its blood supply in a retrograde manner from the ileocolic or right colic artery. Type IV is used to describe multiple atresias and occurs in about one fourth of cases. Although the degree of separation of the bowel segments and the size of the mesenteric gaps vary, the pattern of the isolated small bowel segments may have a "string-of-sausage" appearance. Types II and IIIa account for most cases of intestinal atresia and generally have the best results after treatment. Type IIIb and type IV patients are treated successfully in most cases, but these patients are at significant risk for complications, including leak, stricture, sepsis, and short bowel physiology. Together, they account for approximately one third of intestinal atresias.

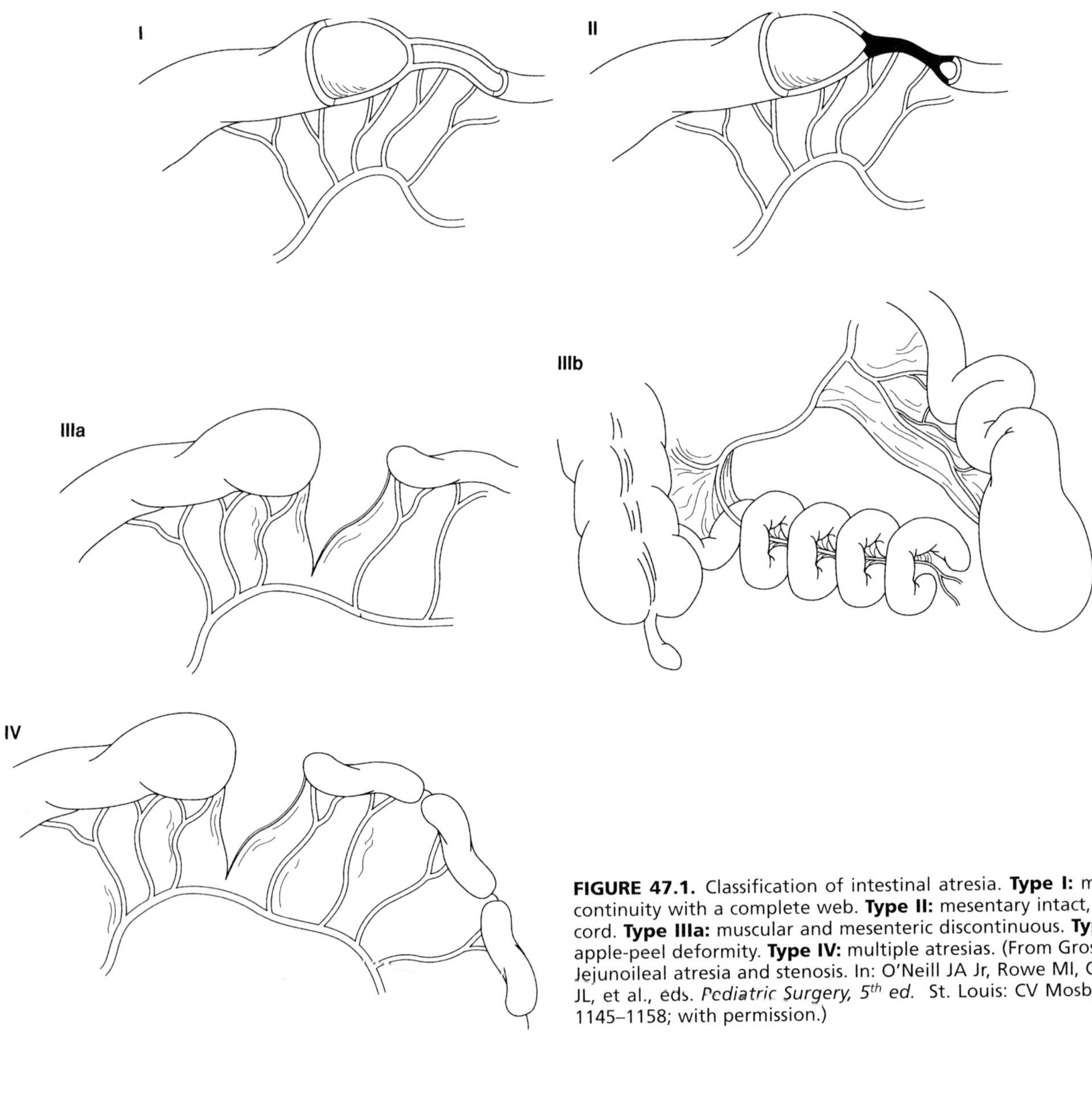

FIGURE 47.1. Classification of intestinal atresia. **Type I:** muscular continuity with a complete web. **Type II:** mesentary intact, fibrous cord. **Type IIIa:** muscular and mesenteric discontinuous. **Type IIIb:** apple-peel deformity. **Type IV:** multiple atresias. (From Grosfeld JL. Jejunoileal atresia and stenosis. In: O'Neill JA Jr, Rowe MI, Grosfeld JL, et al., eds. *Pediatric Surgery, 5th ed.* St. Louis: CV Mosby, 1998: 1145–1158; with permission.)

DIAGNOSIS

The diagnosis of intestinal atresia is occasionally suspected on the basis of antenatal ultrasonography. Findings suggestive of an atresia are identified in only approximately 30% of cases. Polyhydramnios is seen in approximately 16% of cases, usually in the presence of a proximal atresia. Occasionally, dilated loops of bowel are visualized, suggesting the presence of obstruction. Overall, the diagnostic accuracy of prenatal ultrasonography for bowel atresia is relatively low, averaging 42% in reported series.

The diagnosis of intestinal atresia is usually made within hours of birth. It should be considered in the differential diagnosis of any newborn who presents with a clinical picture of bowel obstruction. Typically, infants with jejunoileal atresia develop abdominal distension and bilious emesis. The vomiting is usually immediately postprandial. Most of these infants fail to pass meconium; however, passage of meconium does not exclude the diagnosis. On examination, there is typically upper abdominal distension and tympany. As would be expected with any small bowel obstruction, abdominal distension is more frequently seen with the more distal ileal atresias (98% of cases) than with the more proximal jejunal atresias (78%). A digital rectal examination should be performed when feasible. In addition to ruling out rectal causes of the obstruction such as imperforate anus, the presence of white mucoid material per rectum suggests the presence of an obstruction distal to the ampulla of Vater. Jaundice occurs in 33% of patients with jejunal atresia and 20% of patients with ileal atresia. The etiology of this indirect hyperbilirubinemia in these patients is unclear. In some cases of type I atresia, microperforations in the web allow for passage of air and some stool, resulting in a delay in the diagnosis for months or years.

Plain radiographs may show dilated air-filled loops of proximal bowel with no air in the rectum. If an extremely dilated loop of bowel is seen, the diagnosis of intestinal atresia can reliably be made and no further imaging studies are necessary. If, on the other hand, multiple equally dilated loops are seen, a contrast enema may be necessary to exclude diagnoses that can be treated nonsurgically (meconium plug syndrome, meconium ileus) or with a diverting colostomy (Hirschsprung's disease). If the enema reveals a small-caliber, unused, or "microcolon," the likelihood of a long-standing proximal obstruction such as an atresia is increased. However, a proximal obstruction can result in a normal-caliber colon due to the secretion of mucus and succus entericus by the distal bowel.

At this point, the decision to proceed with operation for a bowel obstruction regardless of cause can usually be made with confidence. There are rare circumstances, for example, in the presence of a partial small bowel obstruction or in the rare case of an ileus simulating an obstruction, in which an upper gastrointestinal series or enteroclysis study may be useful. When in doubt, it is usually best to recommend laparotomy, because the accuracy of these studies in newborns is questionable and the risks are proportionately greater.

TREATMENT

The initial management of jejunoileal atresia consists of optimizing the physiologic status of the baby before surgery. First we insert an orogastric tube to prevent aspiration and progression of bowel dilatation. Fluid resuscitation is begun intravenously. Maintenance fluids should be supplemented with replacement of gastric losses. The child is kept warm in an isolette or radiant warmer bed. Broad-spectrum intravenous antibiotics should be started, typically ampicillin and gentamicin. Any additional laboratory abnormalities are corrected. Following physiologic optimization, the child is taken to the operating room for laparotomy. We prefer a right upper quadrant transverse incision and begin the operation by inspecting the bowel carefully, looking for multiple atretic lesions. If there is any doubt, we pass a soft rubber catheter or instill saline into the lumen of the bowel to exclude additional obstructions. After confirmation of distal patency, the ends of the atretic bowel are resected, along with a portion of the dilated proximal segment. A primary hand-sewn anastomosis is usually technically feasible, performed in the usual fashion according to surgeon's preference. There is usually a significant size discrepancy between the two ends to be joined. Spatulation of the distal bowel, creation of an end-to-back anastomosis, or tapering of the proximal segment may be necessary to create a safe anastomosis. Temporary decompressive enterostomy is almost never necessary, except in the rare case of an exceedingly ill infant who cannot withstand a longer operation or when the bowel ends are of questionable viability and a second-look procedure is planned in an attempt to retain bowel length. The mesenteric defect should be closed carefully to prevent an internal hernia.

The main principle of the surgical therapy of jejunoileal atresia is removal of compromised small bowel while preserving bowel length and function. The atretic lesions are sometimes associated with a primary lesion such as volvulus, gastroschisis, or intussusception. It may thus be necessary to remove not only the atretic lesion but also to correct the primary lesion. Occasionally, this will make a short bowel syndrome a concern. The function of the remaining bowel must also be a consideration. There is often a dilated, hypertrophied, and aperistaltic proximal bowel segment. A frequent postoperative complication is small bowel enteropathy due to the presence of this enlarged segment. We prefer to resect most of this dilated dysmotile segment prior to creating an anastomosis. If resection will likely result in short bowel syndrome or if the atresia is close to the ligament of Treitz, the proximal segment should be preserved. This can be accomplished by tapering the dilated segment using a gastrointestinal stapling device, partial excision, and a long suture line, or by simple plication.

In cases of an apple-peel deformity (type IIIb), an anastomosis is usually still feasible. Careful attention must be directed to preserving the long and often tenuous distal blood supply to the bowel, which depends entirely on a long marginal mesenteric branch from the ileocolic artery. These anastomoses are more prone to ischemia, leak, and stricture and demand technical diligence and gentle handling of tissues. The same can be said for cases of multiple atresias (type IV) in which multiple anastomoses are required, with a relatively high incidence of technical complications.

Children with gastroschisis and associated bowel atresia are usually best treated with primary reduction and repair of the abdominal wall defect. We prefer to delay definitive treatment of the atresia for at least 6 weeks, which allows for bowel wall thickening and inflammation to subside. Likewise, patients who have failed to demonstrate bowel function 6 to 8 weeks after repair of a gastroschisis should undergo contrast studies to exclude intestinal atresia.

Postoperative care is generally standard as for any laparotomy in a newborn. Attention should be directed to fluid balance and temperature homeostasis. A nasogastric tube is used for decompression until bowel function is demonstrated. Antibiotics are continued for 24 to 48 hours. Infants with short bowel, apple-peel deformities or multiple atretic segments will likely require a prolonged course of parenteral nutrition; therefore, most will require long-term central venous access.

Patients should be followed on an outpatient basis by the surgical service until full enteral nutrition is tolerated and adequate weight gain is demonstrated. Thereafter, periodic visits to ensure adequate growth and development as well the absence of symptoms or signs suggestive of enteropathy or obstruction are recommended.

RESULTS AND COMPLICATIONS

Overall, infants with intestinal atresia do well after surgical treatment. Most have normal gut function and receive all of their nutrition enterally, with normal somatic growth and cognitive development. With current therapy, children with jejunoileal atresia have a very low mortality rate. Grosfeld et al. reported a large series of infants with intestinal atresia in 1998. They observed an operative mortality rate of 0.8%, and the long-term survival rate was 84%. Postoperative complications included short bowel syndrome (defined as <40 cm of bowel), adhesive small bowel obstruction, ileus, enterostomy prolapse, pneumonia, and wound infection. Of the 16% of children who suffered late deaths, all were dependent on parenteral nutrition and 80% died from sepsis. Although 70% of patients who had late deaths had short bowel syndrome, 81% had type IIIa, IIIb, or IV lesions.

Most of the complications that occur after surgical therapy of intestinal atresia are diagnosed and treated in a straightforward manner. Anastomotic leak, recurrent stricture, adhesive small bowel obstruction, and intraabdominal abscess are treated according to standard principles. Recurrent enteropathy or stasis due to a residual dilated segment of proximal bowel can sometimes be treated with bowel rest and antibiotics to treat bacterial overgrowth until the bowel returns to normal caliber. This may not occur in all cases, and primary resection and reanastomosis or tapering enteroplasty is often necessary.

SUGGESTED READINGS

Dalla Vecchia LK, Grosfeld JL, West KW. Intestinal atresia and stenosis: a 25 year experience with 277 cases. *Arch Surg* 1998;133:490–496.

Heij HA, Moorman-Voestermans CG, Vos A. Atresia of jejunum and ileum: is it the same disease? *J Pediatr Surg* 1990;25:635–637.

Louw JH, Barnard CN. Congenital intestinal atresia: observation on its origin. *Lancet* 1955;2:1065.

Masumoto K, Suita S, Nada O, et al. Abnormalities of enteric neurons, intestinal pacemaker cells, and smooth muscle in human intestinal atresia. *J Pediatr Surg* 1999;34:1463–1468.

Sweeney B, Surana R, Puri P. Jejunoileal atresia and associated malformations: correlation with the timing of in utero insult. *J Pediatr Surg* 2001;36:774–776.

Tam PK, Nicholls G. Implications of antenatal diagnosis of small intestinal atresia in the 1990s. *Pediatr Surg Int* 1999;15:486–487.

Tandler J. Zur Entwicklungsgeschichte des menschlichen duodenum in fruhen embryonalstadien. *Morphol Jahrb* 1900;29:187.

Walker MW, Lovell MA, Kelly TE, et al. Multiple areas of intestinal atresias associated with immunodeficiency and post-transfusion graft vs. host disease. *J Pediatr* 1993;123:93.

Ward HC, Leake J, Milla PJ, et al. Brown bowel syndrome: a late complication of intestinal atresia. *J Pediatr Surg* 1992;27:1593–1595.

Weber TR, Vane DW, Grosfeld JL. Tapering enteroplasty in infants with bowel atresia and short gut. *Arch Surg* 1982;117:684–688.

48

ALIMENTARY TRACT DUPLICATIONS

ANDRÉ HEBRA

Alimentary tract duplications are uncommon anomalies that can affect any portion of the gastrointestinal tract. The condition also has been called *enterogenous cyst, accessory enteric formation, ileum duplex, foregut cyst, and intestinal diverticula*. The term *duplication of the alimentary tract* was used by Gross in 1952 to include all the various descriptions of this unique embryologic anomaly. This anomaly is characterized by the presence of a cystic or tubular structure lined by normal gastrointestinal mucosa and having smooth muscle walls like those of the intestines.

The embryologic event that gives rise to duplications has yet to be fully understood. Several theories have been proposed, the so-called "diverticular theory," the theory of "aberrant luminal recanalization," and the theory by Saunders in which the incomplete separation of the foregut and notochord resulted in foregut duplications with associated vertebral anomalies. Bentley described the "split notochord syndrome" to clarify the coexistence of vertebral anomalies and neuroenteric cysts in the dorsal, lumbar, and sacral spine. Possible abnormalities related to failure of regression of the neuroenteric canal are complete dorsal enteric fistula, diastematomyelia (fibrous cord), intraspinal enteric cyst, and enteric duplications. Mellish, Koop, and others independently observed the coexistence of intestinal atresias and duplications and proposed the theory of vascular insult as the cause for the atresia and duplication. Most recently, Alrabeeah took Saunders' theories and expanded them to explain neuroenteric cysts at all spinal levels. Another interesting observation is that certain duplications appear to represent partial twinning, particularly tubular duplications of the terminal ileum and colon. No single theory can explain all the variations seen in the various types of gastrointestinal duplications. As a rule, duplications typically lie in close proximity to the alimentary tube and frequently share a common muscular wall and common blood supply. The usual location is on the mesenteric side of the viscera, in contrast to vitelline duct remnants, such as Meckel's diverticula, which lie on the antimesenteric aspect of the bowel.

Classically, duplications have been defined by three characteristics: (a) contiguity with and strong adherence to some part of the alimentary tract (from tongue to anus), (b) smooth muscle coat, and (c) mucosal lining consisting of one or more types of cells usually found in the alimentary tract (or the upper respiratory tract in the case of some foregut duplications).

Interestingly, the epithelium present is frequently not native to the part of the tract at which the duplication occurs. The most common ectopic epithelium lining duplications are gastric and pancreatic epithelium. Ectopic mucosa is identified in 25% to 50% of all cases, more commonly when the duplication is in the small intestine.

Intestinal duplications have been described in the following locations: pharynx, esophagus, stomach, duodenum, jejunum, ileum, colon, appendix, rectum, and anal canal. The most common types are ileal, followed by esophageal and colonic duplications. Pharyngeal and anal duplications are extremely rare. Pharyngeal duplications typically possess both a striated and smooth muscle coat, and are adherent to the most rostral part of the alimentary tract, the tongue. Gastrointestinal duplication cysts may contain esophageal, gastric, intestinal, colonic, and respiratory epithelium. The most commonly found ectopic mucosa is of the gastric type. Duplications also may be classified into *tubular* (20%) or *cystic* (80%), depending on their appearance. The tubular type is longer and usually communicates with the segment of intestine with which it is associated. The cystic type is usually filled with clear serum-like fluid that does not necessarily communicate with any segment of the gastrointestinal tract.

A. Hebra: Department of Surgery, University of South Florida, and Minimally Invasive Pediatric Surgery Program, All Children's Hospital, St. Petersburg, Florida.

DIAGNOSTIC APPROACH

The clinical presentation of gastrointestinal duplications is variable, depending primarily on the type and location of the lesion. Patients may be completely asymptomatic or may present with signs and symptoms of intestinal obstruction. A mass discovered on physical examination or radiologic examination of the chest or abdomen is a common feature. The presence of pain usually indicates a complication, such as intestinal obstruction due to volvulus or intussusception, peptic ulceration, or perforation. Figure 48.1 is a plain abdominal radiograph of an infant with abdominal distension and vomiting. The radiograph shows a pattern of small bowel obstruction characterized by the presence of multiple dilated loops of intestines. Figure 48.2 is a view of the barium enema performed on the same patient demonstrating the presence of a round filling defect at the cecum, which was found to be an ileal duplication cyst. Vomiting in patients with gastrointestinal duplication may result from compression of the adjacent bowel lumen, especially in duplications of the pylorus, duodenum, or small bowel. Occasionally an intussusception may result from a duplication cyst. Such lesions also may lead to gastrointestinal hemorrhage. Bleeding may be sudden, severe, and painless, as noted with the more common Meckel's diverticulum. Rectal bleeding associated with severe abdominal pain would more likely indicate intussusception or volvulus. Anemia may result from chronic blood loss into the intestine. Intrathoracic duplications can cause respiratory distress owing to compression of the tracheobronchial tree or lung, or dysphagia, if the esophagus is narrowed. Presacral enteric cysts can cause constipation or can prolapse through the anus. Neurologic signs of spinal cord compression may result from intraspinal cysts. Myelomeningocele is present with some duplications, especially the thoracic variety.

Table 48.1 summarizes the experience at the Children's Hospital of Philadelphia (126 cases between 1950 and 1995) which demonstrated the relative incidence based on location in the gastrointestinal tract as follows: esophagus (20%), stomach (9%), duodenum (6%), jejunum (10%), ileum (33%), colon (15%), rectum (3%), combined (3%), and anal/pharyngeal (1%). In addition, the age range at the time of diagnosis for patients evaluated after 1987 was between prenatal and 8 years of age, with more than 50% diagnosed before 1 month of age. The availability of prenatal ultrasonography has improved our ability to establish an accurate prenatal diagnosis. Almost one third of all cases of intestinal duplication are now diagnosed prenatally.

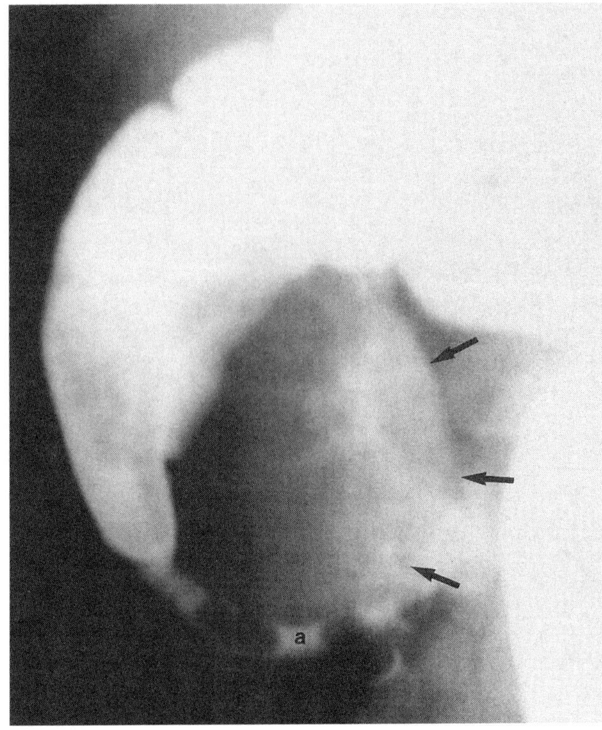

FIGURE 48.2. Barium enema of the same patient described in Fig. 48.1 (magnified view of the right lower quadrant). The study shows a soft tissue mass (*arrows*) abutting the cecum and appendix (*a*). This proved to be a cystic cecal duplication.

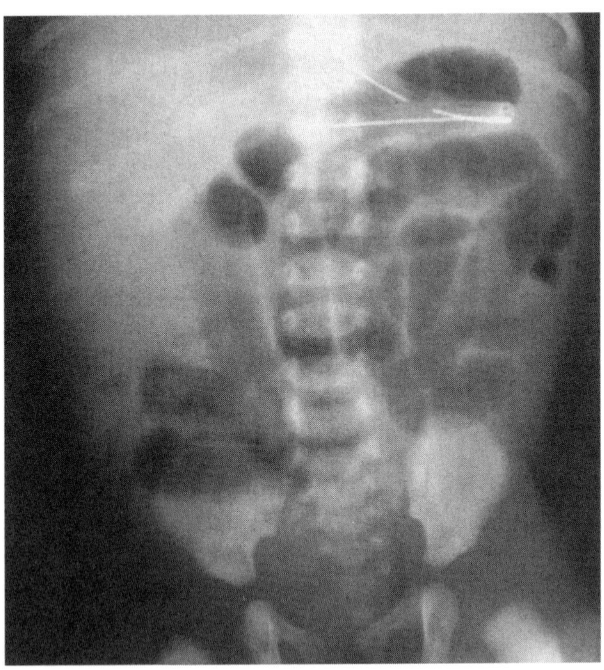

FIGURE 48.1. Plain abdominal radiograph of an infant with acute onset of abdominal distension and bilious vomiting. The radiograph shows moderately dilated loops of small bowel, suggestive of a small bowel obstruction.

TABLE 48.1. SUMMARY OF THE EXPERIENCE WITH 126 CASES OF GASTROINTESTINAL DUPLICATIONS TREATED AT THE CHILDREN'S HOSPITAL OF PHILADELPHIA

Location	% of Cases	Structure	Clinical Presentation	Surgical Treatment
Thoracic	20%	Cystic	Asymptomatic; respiratory distress; associated with TEF; abdominal pain; incidental finding	Complete excision (95%); marsupialization (5%)
Gastric	9%	Cystic	Vomiting; hematemesis	Complete excision (85%); partial excision with mucosal stripping (10%); internal gastric drainage (5%)
Duodenal	6%	Cystic	Vomiting; abdominal pain	Partial excision with mucosal stripping (100%)
Jejunoileal	43%	Cystic (80%) Tubular (20%)	Vomiting; abdominal pain; intussusception; volvulus; rectal bleeding; abdominal distension; acute abdomen	Excision with partial resection of normal bowel (80%); partial excision with mucosal stripping (20%)
Colonic	15%	Cystic (25%) Tubular (75%)	Vomiting; volvulus; urinary retention; incidental finding; megacolon; asymptomatic	Complete excision (25%); excision with partial resection of normal bowel (30%); excision and temporary colostomy (25%); left intact (10%); internal drainage (10%)
Rectal	3%	Cystic	Colonic distension; asymptomatic	Complete excision (90%); colostomy and delayed resection (10%)
Thoracoabdominal	3%	Tubular	Vomiting; abdominal mass; thoracic mass	Thoracoabdominal approach, excision
Pharynx or anal	1%	Cystic	Mass	Complete excision

Although contrast studies of the esophagus, stomach, duodenum, small bowel, and colon, as well as computed tomography (CT) and magnetic resonance imaging, have been used in the workup of patients with suspected gastrointestinal duplication cysts, the diagnostic test of choice is ultrasonography. The finding of an echogenic inner mucosal layer and hypoechoic outer muscular layer on real-time ultrasonography are highly suggestive of a duplication cyst. When the ultrasonographic findings are typical for duplication, no further imaging study is indicated. Figure 48.3 demonstrates the classic appearance of a duplication cyst on ultrasonography. The CT scan appearance of the same cyst is shown in Fig. 48.4. In the past 20 years, prenatal ultrasonography has become an important diagnostic tool in demonstrating the presence of gastrointestinal duplications as early as 20 weeks of gestational age (Fig. 48.5). In the case of esophageal/thoracic duplication cysts, the CT scan may be more useful in establishing the diagnosis because the ribs limit the visual resolution of ultrasonography. The CT scan can demonstrate the cystic nature of the mass and its relationship to adjacent structures. It also allows for imaging and evaluation of the spine, pulmonary parenchyma, airway, and adjacent structures. Enhancement of the outer rim of the cyst with intravenous contrast and no enhancement of the central core is typical. This peripheral enhancement distinguishes this cyst from a neurogenic tumor. Myelography should be performed for those lesions with suspected communication to the vertebral

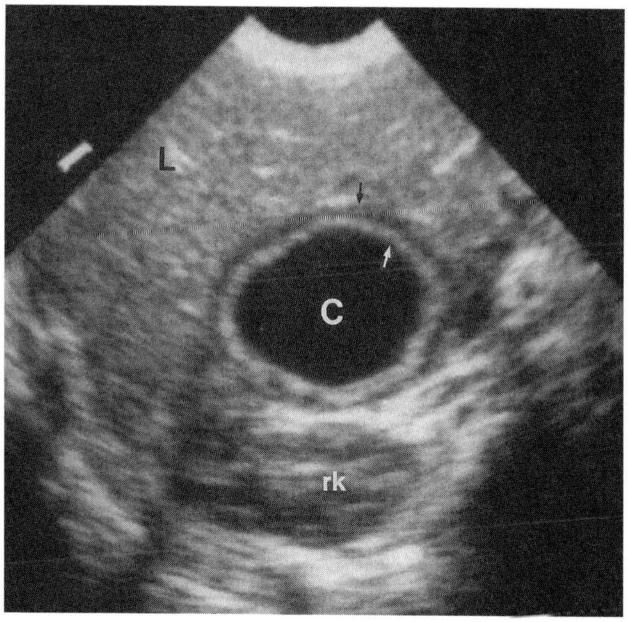

FIGURE 48.3. Ultrasonographic appearance (transverse view) of the right abdomen in a child with hematemesis caused by a gastric duplication. A large duplication cyst (*C*) with a hyperechoic inner mucosa (*white arrow*) and a hypoechoic muscular outer layer (*black arrow*) is seen in the region of the second portion of the duodenum, adjacent to the liver (*L*) and anterior to the right kidney (*rk*).

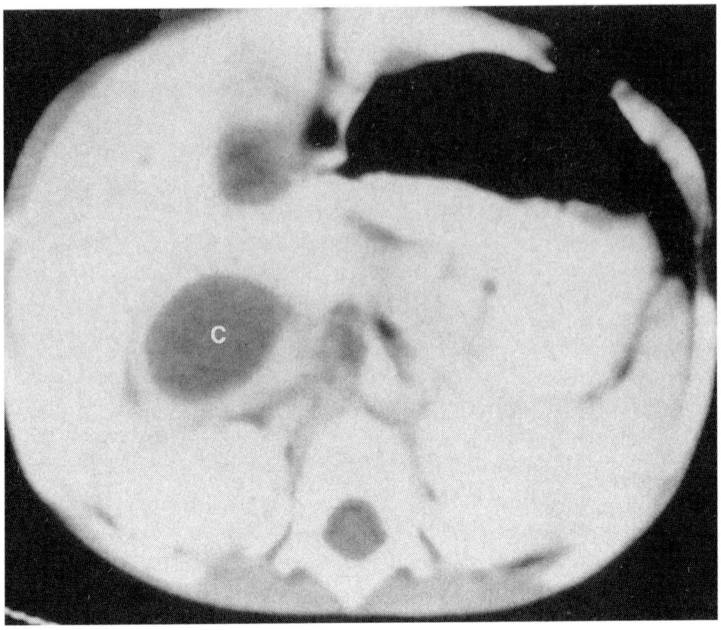

FIGURE 48.4. Computed tomographic (CT) image of the abdomen of the same child discussed in Fig. 48.3. The CT scan (with contrast) shows a thick-walled duplication cyst (*C*) in the anterior pararenal space. Operative exploration demonstrated the presence of an antral duplication cyst.

column. A Y-shaped splitting of the lower vertebrae and sacrum is seen with some hindgut duplications. Radioisotope scans using technetium isotopes are useful if the clinician is interested in determining the presence of ectopic gastric muscosa.

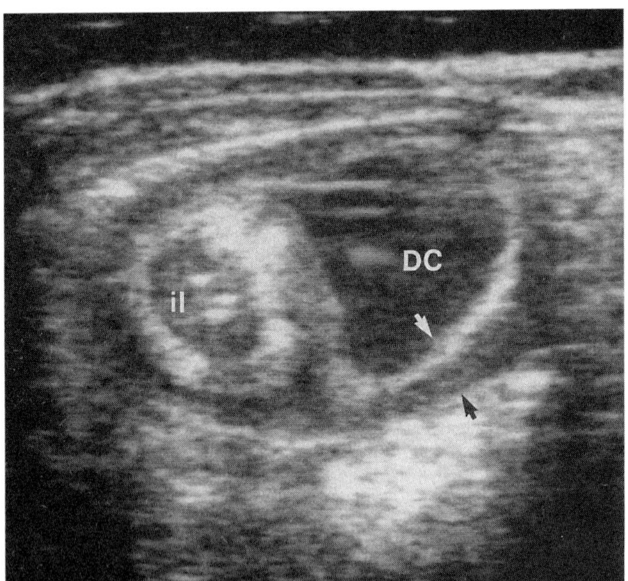

FIGURE 48.5. High-resolution sonogram (transverse view) of the right lower quadrant in a fetus with a cystic mass diagnosed at the time of prenatal fetal ultrasonography. A duplication cyst (*DC*) was found to be contiguous with the normal ileum (*il*). Note the sonographic appearance of bowel wall. Both the ileum and the duplication cyst display a hyperechoic, inner mucosal layer (*white arrow*) and a hypoechoic, outer muscular layer (*black arrow*).

PREOPERATIVE PREPARATION

When the appropriate diagnosis is established prior to operative treatment, minimal preparation is necessary. Patients should be given preoperative antibiotics, such as a first- or second-generation cephalosporin or ampicillin and gentamicin. For duplications involving the colon and rectum, a standard preoperative bowel preparation is appropriate in order to minimize the occurrence of complications related to bowel resection. As previously mentioned, when dealing with thoracic duplications, the patient should undergo abdominal ultrasonography to rule out the possibility of an associated abdominal lesion or communication. A staged approach may be necessary in selected cases of combined thoracoabdominal duplications. If vertebral anomalies are identified, consultation with neurosurgery prior to operative exploration is indicated in order to determine if any further imaging of the spinal canal is necessary.

TECHNICAL APPROACH

Because gastrointestinal duplications have such wide anatomic variation depending on their location and type, several different surgical techniques may be required for their management. The goal of surgery is to achieve complete surgical excision, without causing any harm to the surrounding structures. Typically, cystic duplications can be completely removed. However, when the enterogenous cyst is within the mesentery, its removal may cause significant disruption to the visceral blood supply of the adjacent bowel. This may necessitate the resection of normal intestine together with the resected duplication. Complete removal of duodenal duplications may endanger the bile ducts or pancreas. They are thus managed more safely by marsupialization of the cyst into the duodenum through an anastomosis of the common walls or by partial cystectomy and stripping the mucosa from the residual cyst wall. Tubular duplications of the hindgut may not need to be removed if they are capable of normal function. However, if the tubular malformation contains a point of obstruction or aberrant termination of one or both lumens, it may require surgical removal. Tubular duplications of the upper gastrointestinal tract and small bowel so often contain gastric mucosa that they should be removed completely to prevent bleeding from peptic ulceration. A rare form of duplication is the so-called *combined type* that is frequently located between the chest and abdomen. In such cases, a thoracoabdominal surgical approach is usually necessary. One must remember that a dorsal enteric fistula may be present between the duplication (alimentary tract) and the skin of the back, passing through a bifid spinal cord and vertebral column. Such fistulas occur more often in the thoracic area than in the lumbosacral area.

When complete resection of a duplication is not possible without sacrificing a large amount of normal intestine, one should remove the mucosa by stripping it from the muscle layers of the duplication without disturbing the essential blood supply to the adjacent intestine. The seromuscular tube that is left behind usually collapses and should not cause any problems.

Thoracic duplications are usually located in the right posterior mediastinal space, in close relationship to the esophagus, but they rarely communicate with its lumen. Simple surgical excision can be easily accomplished in the majority of such patients. However, one must note that several cases of thoracic duplication cysts have been reported to communicate with the proximal small bowel via the esophageal hiatus and can present with severe gastrointestinal hemorrhage due to bleeding from peptic ulceration. For this reason, it is recommended that patients with thoracic duplications undergo abdominal ultrasonography to evaluate for the possible presence of an associated intestinal duplication. In cases of combined duplications, a staged surgical approach may be necessary to achieve complete and safe removal of the lesions. In the past 5 years, several reports have described the use of thoracoscopy for diagnosis and excision of thoracic duplications, with excellent results. When using thoracoscopy, the patient should be placed in a lateral decubitus position, and selective lung ventilation is preferred to facilitate the visualization of the lesion in the posterior mediastinal space. Needle aspiration under thoracoscopic guidance will aid in decreasing the size of larger lesions, which can then be easily separated from the esophageal wall by means of careful sharp and blunt dissection using endo-scissors and laparoscopic graspers. Because such lesions typically shell out quite easily, one should consider using thoracoscopy instead of thoracotomy in the management of simple thoracic duplication cysts.

Jejunal and ileal lesions are the most common type of gastrointestinal duplications in children. They usually share a common muscular wall with the adjacent bowel and are located on the mesenteric side. Mesenteric vessels pass on both surfaces of the duplication to supply both it and the overlying intestine. They may look like mesenteric and omental cysts, and differentiation may not be possible until complete histologic assessment of the removed lesion has demonstrated the presence of muscular and mucosal layers. The traditional approach is to perform a laparotomy and excise the lesion. Because of the close relationship to the native intestine and possible compromise to its blood supply, removal of the adjacent normal bowel is often necessary. If complete excision cannot be accomplished, mucosal stripping must be performed because acid peptic ulceration from ectopic gastric muscosa can lead to severe intestinal bleeding. This is in contrast to colonic tubular duplications, which rarely contain ectopic mucosa and can be treated by internal drainage only. Small bowel duplications also may be associated with intestinal atresia in infants. In selected cases, laparoscopy may be helpful in establishing the diagnosis of a small bowel duplication cyst. Laparoscopic surgical excision may be attempted but is technically much more demanding than thoracic duplications. A combined open and laparoscopic approach may be used. In such cases, the segment of intestine containing the duplication can be precisely identified during laparoscopy, and the bowel with the duplication cyst can be resected and reanastomosed using a small abdominal incision (minilaparotomy). The entire small bowel and colon can be inspected laparoscopically for the presence of any additional lesions.

In some cases of tubular duplications, the length may vary greatly from just a few centimeters to as long as the entire small bowel. The communication may be at the proximal or the distal end or at several points in between. If the only communication is at the cephalic end, the lumen may become distended and cause compression of the adjacent intestine. Complications can include obstruction, intussusception, perforation, and even peptic ulceration, as seen with a Meckel's diverticulum. Tubular duplications of the colon (hindgut) are more likely to have unobstructed lumens and function normally. The entire colon may be "double" and drain through a single anal opening. Occasionally double external genitalia may accompany this malformation. Several cases have been reported in association with imperforate anus. Figure 48.6A illustrates the occurrence of a cecal duplication in a 1-year-old child who presented with an abdominal mass. In this particular case, it was possible to perform laparoscopic exploration with aspiration of the fluid contained in the cyst. This allowed for significant reduction in the size of the mass with subsequent exteriorization of the cecum and associated duplication cyst through a small abdominal incision (Fig. 48.6B). This cystic mass was than resected from the mesenteric side of the cecum (Fig. 48.6C). It was not necessary to perform cecal

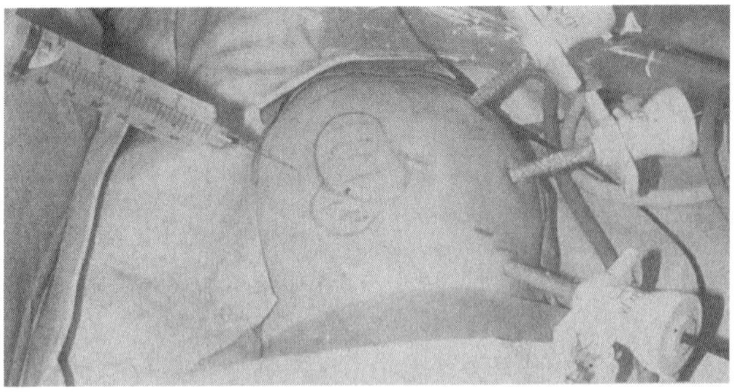

A

FIGURE 48.6. **A:** One-year-old child with a palpable right lower quadrant abdominal mass diagnosed as a cecal duplication by ultrasonography. The mass outline was drawn on the abdominal wall. Laparoscopic exploration was performed with percutaneous cyst aspiration to allow for reduction in the size of the mass (note syringe with clear fluid being aspirated). **B:** The cecum was exteriorized under laparoscopic guidance, and the decompressed cecal duplication is seen on the mesenteric side of the cecum, separate from the appendix (seen in the lower right). **C:** The opened cecal duplication is being resected from the cecum. Note the normal-appearing mucosa within the cecal duplication cyst.

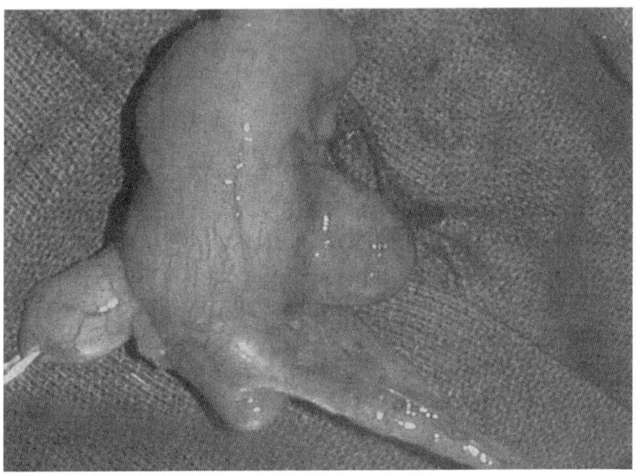

B

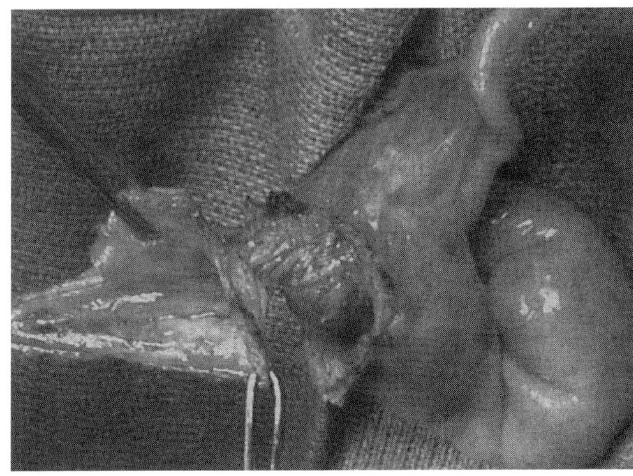

C

resection with colocolostomy, although it is not unusual that resection of the adjacent bowel is necessary when removing a duplication cyst. In cases of long tubular colonic duplication, internal drainage can be an effective alternative when complete resection is not possible. The typical rectal duplication is cystic and presents as a gradually enlarging mass adjacent to but not involving the anal canal. They usually present with signs of intestinal obstruction and may resemble a sacrococcygeal teratoma.

Duplications of the stomach may be completely asymptomatic, unless the gastric outlet is obstructed or rupture occurs. Figure 48.3 is a sonogram of an antral duplication cyst. Large gastric cysts can present as an asymptomatic palpable abdominal mass. Small cysts near the pylorus may mimic pyloric stenosis. Mucosal ulceration may develop due to the presence of ectopic gastric mucosa. The treatment involves simple resection of the duplication. The normal stomach should be easily spared during resection, primarily due to its rich blood supply. Occasionally a partial gastrectomy is necessary to remove this congenital anomaly.

Duplication cysts attached to the duodenal wall are more challenging because they are usually located in the posteromedial wall and are fused by a common muscularis to the duodenum. They are frequently embedded in the pancreas. Obstruction of the duodenum is the usual clinical picture. During surgery, extreme caution must be used to avoid injury to the adjacent structures, including common bile duct, ampulla, pancreatic duct, and the duodenum itself. Selected cases also can be treated by internal drainage using a Roux-en-Y loop of jejunum. Another treatment option when complete resection is not possible is to perform a mucosectomy of the cyst, leaving its seromuscular coat behind. Recent advances in therapeutic endoscopy have allowed the use of endoscopic retrograde cholangiopancreatography techniques for providing internal drainage of duodenal duplication cysts that are not amenable to safe surgical resection. Using the knife papillotome, the gastroduodenal wall can be incised and internal drainage can be effectively achieved. However, bleeding is a common complication.

Table 48.1 summarizes the clinical experience at the Children's Hospital of Philadelphia with 126 cases of gastrointestinal duplications. The relative incidence of the different types of duplications, the clinical presentation, and surgical treatment performed for each type are also tabulated.

POSTOPERATIVE CARE

The pitfalls may be summarized as follows:

1. One must remember that malignant tumors in duplications may develop later in life (typically after 30 years of age). Reports of such occurrences have included cases of

adenocarcinoma (the most commonly found malignancy), squamous cell carcinoma, and even carcinoid tumors. For this reason, removal of even asymptomatic duplication cysts is indicated. If this cannot be accomplished safely, mucosectomy should be considered.
2. Patients with thoracic duplications should undergo abdominal ultrasonography to identify possible associated intestinal duplications.
3. When dealing with duodenal duplications, cholangiography may be necessary to determine the relationship of the cyst to the pancreaticobiliary tree. Due to complex anatomic relationships, surgical excision may not be possible.
4. The mucosa of duplications of the small bowel is more likely to contain ectopic gastric mucosa than duplications of the colon. Acid peptic ulceration may result if complete mucosectomy is not performed. Tubular colonic duplications may be treated with simple internal drainage because they are less likely to contain ectopic gastric mucosa.
5. Associated anomalies, such as cloacal extrophy, genitourinary abnormalities, spina bifida, imperforate anus, and even the VACTERL association (abnormalities of vertebrae, anus, cardiovascular tree, trachea, esophagus, renal system, and limb buds) can be found in patients with gastrointestinal duplications, particularly when involving the colon and rectum.
6. Jejunoileal duplications may be associated with intestinal atresias.
7. Multiple gastroenteric duplications may occur in a single individual.
8. Neuroenteric cysts can cause neurologic signs of spinal cord compression, and myelomeningocele may be present with some duplications, especially the thoracic variety. Vertebral anomalies, such as spina bifida and missing or hemivertebrae, accompany many thoracic and abdominal duplications.

COMPLICATIONS

Due to the many surgical approaches available to treat duplications (depending on location, type, size, relationship to adjacent structures, and associated anomalies), complications can vary greatly. As a rule, duplications in children are considered benign lesions, and the surgical procedure should not be more radical than necessary to eliminate the patient's complaints and prevent further recurrence.

FOLLOW-UP

Patients should be followed until complete resolution of symptoms and full recovery from surgery has been documented. Complete excision of the duplication should be possible in approximately 80% of all cases. If complete removal of the duplication is not possible, long-term follow-up may be necessary to ensure that the patient will not develop a recurrent cyst from the residual lesion. If ectopic gastric mucosa was left with the duplication, the patient may benefit from histamine blockers to prevent the development of peptic ulceration. Such patients also should be monitored for the possible development of malignant changes during adulthood. The overall prognosis of patients with intestinal duplications is considered excellent.

ACKNOWLEDGMENT

I am thankful for the contributions of radiographic and ultrasound images provided by Dr. Richard D. Bellah, Director, Division of Ultrasound, Children's Hospital of Philadelphia, Philadelphia, Pennsylvania.

SUGGESTED READINGS

Bentley JFR, Smith JR. Developmental posterior enteric remnants and spinal malformations, the "split notochord syndrome." *Arch Dis Child* 1960;35:76–86.
Bishop HC, Koop CE. Surgical management of duplications of the alimentary tract. *Am J Surg* 1964;35:76–86.
Chuang MT, Barba FA. Adenocarcinoma arising in an intrathoracic duplications cyst of foregut origin. *Cancer* 1981;47:1887–1890.
Dillon PW, Cilley RE. Video-assisted thoracoscopic excision of intrathoracic masses in children: report of two cases. *Surg Laparosc Endosc* 1993;3:433–436.
Favara BE, Franciosi RA. Enteric duplications. Thirty-seven cases: a vascular theory of pathogenesis. *Am J Dis Child* 1971;122: 501–506.
Gross RE, Holcomb GW Jr, Farber S. Duplications of the alimentary tract. *Pediatrics* 1952;9:449–468.
Holcomb GW, Gheissari A. Surgical management of alimentary tract duplications. *Ann Surg* 1989;209:167–174.
Ladd WE, Gross RE. Surgical treatment of duplications of the alimentary tract: enterogenous cysts, enteric cysts, or ileum duplex. *Surg Gynecol Obstet* 1940;70:295.
Lamont AC, Starinsky R. Ultrasonic diagnosis of duplication cysts in children. *Br J Radiol* 1984;57:463–467.
Traif IA, Khan MH. Endoscopic drainage of a duodenal duplication cyst. *Gastrointest Endosc* 1992;38:64–65.

49

ANOMALIES OF INTESTINAL ROTATION AND FIXATION

BRAD W. WARNER

An understanding of abnormalities of intestinal rotation and fixation is vital to pediatric surgeons, because the majority of these problems become clinically evident during infancy and childhood. Normal rotation of the midgut consists of the duodenojejunal junction (ligament of Treitz) rotating 270 degrees in a counterclockwise direction around the superior mesenteric artery to fix into a final position that is to the left of the spine and at or above the level of the pylorus. Similarly, the ileocolic junction rotates 270 degrees in a counterclockwise direction around the superior mesenteric artery to lie in its normal location within the right lower quadrant. Interruption of any stage of intrauterine intestinal development may result in anatomic defects that set the stage for later obstruction or volvulus. Complete nonrotation of the midgut is the most frequently encountered anomaly and occurs when neither the duodenojejunal limb nor the cecocolic limb undergo rotation. This is the major cause of midgut volvulus.

Malrotation may clinically present in several different ways; however, the main symptom complexes may be grouped together as those related to acute volvulus, duodenal obstruction, intermittent or chronic abdominal pain, or as an incidental finding in an otherwise asymptomatic patient. Although the majority of patients present during the first month of life or prior to 1 year of age, malrotation may be clinically silent until adulthood. In a child under 1 year of age, bilious emesis should be assumed to be due to malrotation until proven otherwise.

DIAGNOSTIC APPROACH

The preoperative evaluation of malrotation/midgut volvulus is the radiologic determination of the position of the ligament of Treitz and its distance to the ileocecal junction. Several imaging studies are indicated in sequential order.

B. W. Warner: Department of Surgery, University of Cincinnati College of Medicine; and Division of Pediatric Surgery, Cincinnati Children's Hospital Medical Center, Cincinnati, Ohio.

Plain Abdominal Radiographs

Although plain abdominal radiographs cannot make the diagnosis of malrotation/midgut volvulus, they are usually the first step in the diagnosis of an infant with bilious emesis. If an obvious obstruction of the stomach, duodenum, or small bowel is seen, further radiographic studies are generally not needed and the patient should undergo expeditious exploration. On the other hand, in patients with malrotation/midgut volvulus, the plain abdominal radiographs are most often nonspecific. This study can neither rule in nor rule out a rotational abnormality. For this reason, further emergent evaluation is warranted.

Upper Gastrointestinal Series

The upper gastrointestinal (UGI) series is the gold standard test to make the diagnosis of malrotation. It is not necessary in patients with radiographic evidence of obstruction and is contraindicated if there is clinical evidence of peritonitis. Barium is considered the contrast agent of choice, although water-soluble agents may be used. Little useful information is gained by instilling contrast into a nasogastric tube on the ward and following its progress by serial plain radiographs of the abdomen. It is important that the study be conducted in the radiology department by a trained radiologist using fluoroscopy. In cases of volvulus, the site of obstruction is in the second or third portion of the duodenum and has the appearance of a bird's beak. If the duodenum is partially obstructed, a spiral or corkscrew configuration may be present.

In patients with malrotation but without volvulus, the UGI series is important to document the position of the duodenojejunal junction. The normal position ought to be to the left of the spine and at the level of the gastric antrum. In patients with nonrotation of the duodenum, the duodenojejunal junction is found on the right side of the spine and inferior to the duodenal bulb. Another finding suggestive of malrotation is that of all loops of the proximal jejunum being present on the right side of the abdomen.

Barium Enema

Although the barium enema has historically been considered the procedure of choice for the diagnosis of malrotation, it has several limitations, which make the UGI series a better test. A high and mobile cecum (which can suggest malrotation) is found normally in approximately 15% of infants without malrotation. The spot-film identification of the cecum may be difficult in infants because of the redundancy of the colon. Finally, and more important, duodenal obstruction due to malrotation may occur in the presence of a normally positioned cecum. Probably the most useful role for a contrast enema in a patient with suspected malrotation is to confirm the position of the cecum, thereby allowing for an estimate of the width of the mesenteric base (from the duodenojejunal junction to the cecum). A patient with a slightly low duodenojejunal junction and a normally positioned cecum would have a relatively broad-based mesentery and would be at low risk for volvulus. Alternatively, a high cecal position in a patient with a low duodenojejunal junction should be considered as a higher risk for volvulus.

Ultrasonography

Information regarding the orientation of the superior mesenteric vessels can also be obtained by ultrasonography and may be useful in suggesting the diagnosis of malrotation. Normally, the superior mesenteric vein (SMV) lies to the right of the superior mesenteric artery (SMA). If the SMV lies either anterior or to the left of the SMA, malrotation may be present. Unfortunately, this is inconsistent. Because malrotation may be present in patients with normal mesenteric vessel orientation and abnormal vessel orientation may not be associated with malrotation, ultrasonography must be considered to be suboptimal as a screening tool or definitive test for the diagnosis of malrotation. Its role may be confined to suggesting the need for a UGI series in a vomiting child referred for ultrasonography in which pyloric stenosis has been ruled out.

PREOPERATIVE PREPARATION

In the acutely ill child with a midgut volvulus/obstruction, urgent operative correction is indicated and little time should be needed for intravenous fluid resuscitation, placement of a nasogastric tube and Foley catheter, type and crossmatch for blood, and administration of broad-spectrum antibiotics. Time is critical in terms of small intestinal salvage.

In patients with malrotation but without volvulus or mechanical obstruction, the urgency for operative correction is somewhat lessened. Because it is unpredictable as to when and if a patient with malrotation will develop midgut volvulus, the operation need not be performed emergently. Early operation in neonates (within a day or two after diagnosis) would appear to be justified. Older children with intermittent symptoms over a prolonged period would be at lower risk for the development of volvulus within a few days after diagnosis. An operation could be done more electively in this situation.

TECHNICAL APPROACH

The operative technique for the management of midgut volvulus and malrotation generally involves six steps. The incision is usually made transversely in the right upper quadrant to directly address the duodenum.

Evisceration

Upon entering the peritoneal cavity, the entire bowel should be immediately delivered from the abdomen to identify the presence or absence of volvulus, obstruction from other causes, and the position of the cecum, and to enable safe performance of the subsequent steps of the procedure. Cloudy or turbid peritoneal fluid may be encountered and is usually the result of lymphatic obstruction induced by the volvulus. Alternatively, it may reflect bacterial contamination or purulent ascites from ischemic or necrotic bowel. Peritoneal fluid should be sent for Gram stain and cultures if this is a concern.

Detorsion of the Volvulus

If no volvulus is encountered, the subsequent steps for correction of the malrotation are undertaken (see the next four sections). In the vast majority of cases, the volvulus twists in a clockwise direction (as viewed from the surgeon's perspective looking down onto the abdomen). The direction of detorsion is therefore counterclockwise. It is helpful to remember the phrase "turning back the hands of time" when looking down upon the twisted bowel. After detorsion, the intestine may be congested, edematous, and some areas may appear necrotic. Placement of warm sponges and observation for a period may improve the appearance of the intestine where the vascular integrity has been compromised. If areas of the bowel are obviously necrotic, resection with creation of a stoma is performed. Because it is imperative to preserve as much intestine as possible, marginal or questionable segments of bowel should be left in place and a second-look procedure performed within 24 to 36 hours.

Division of the Ladd's Bands

Ladd's bands extend from the ascending colon (on the medial aspect of the duodenum in patients with malrotation) across the duodenum and attach to the posterior aspect of the right upper quadrant. In order to prevent extramural compression of the duodenum and recurrent obstruction, the bands must be lysed completely and on both lateral and medial aspects of the duodenum. To lyse the lateral bands, a generous Kocher maneuver is performed, and all bands should be divided to the level of the portal triad superiorly and to the duodenojejunal junction inferiorly. The medial bands are then lysed between the duodenum and the ascending colon.

Widening Mesenteric Base

The base of the mesentery in patients with malrotation is formed by the superior mesenteric artery running through the space between the duodenum and ascending colon. This mesenteric base is narrow and forms a pedicle on which the midgut can twist. In dividing the bands on the medial aspect of the duodenum, the distance between the duodenum and ascending colon is increased. With further sharp and blunt dissection to separate these structures, the base can be maximally broadened such that the tendency to twist is lessened. Adhesions are generally present between the leaves of the mesentery, and these should be divided.

Relieving Duodenal Obstruction

The duodenum may have a corkscrew configuration and is often twisted back upon itself. This should be fully freed for the entire length of the duodenum. One should be able to visualize the entire duodenum from the pylorus to the proximal jejunum and see no areas of obstruction. If there is significant concern, a balloon-tipped catheter may be passed through the pylorus into the distal duodenum. In a child with failure to thrive or known feeding problems, or if a significant amount of intestine must be resected, consideration should be given to placement of a gastrostomy tube. This is not necessary in the majority of cases.

Incidental Appendectomy

The cecum will ultimately lie on the left side of the abdomen after this procedure. The potential for diagnostic confusion is great if appendicitis develops later. Incidental appendectomy should therefore be performed. Inversion appendectomy is the preferred technique in infants because there is no entry into the gastrointestinal tract. The intestine should be replaced into the abdominal cavity with the small bowel lying entirely on the right side while the colon is positioned on the left. Due to the manipulation of the intestine, a paralytic ileus is expected and a nasogastric tube will generally be required for 1 to 2 days postoperatively.

POSTOPERATIVE CARE

The mortality rate for the operative correction of malrotation ranges from 3% to 9% and is increased in patients with volvulus, intestinal necrosis, prematurity, and the presence of other abnormalities. Survival has improved due to the advent of refined pediatric surgical intensive care and parenteral and enteral nutritional support. Furthermore, early diagnosis, heightened awareness of the significance of the presence of a volvulus or rotational anomaly, and urgency in management are the most important factors contributing to favorable outcome.

Recurrent volvulus is relatively infrequent, but should be of prime concern in patients who present with obstructive symptoms at any time postoperatively. Factors contributing to recurrent volvulus could possibly be due to inadequate adhesion formation within the peritoneal cavity to maintain fixation of the small intestine to the right side of the abdomen and the colon on the left. Recurrent volvulus also may occur if the mesenteric base has not been widened sufficiently. The incidence of recurrent volvulus has been reported to be less than 10%.

Gastrointestinal motility disturbances are common after operative correction of malrotation. Other postoperative complications include adhesive bowel obstruction (not due to volvulus), prolonged ileus, or bleeding from mesenteric vessels that were damaged during the operative dissection. The intestine may undergo reperfusion injury after detorsion of a significant volvulus with massive infusion of cytokines, bacteria, and other toxins into the systemic circulation. This may contribute to hemodynamic instability during the intraoperative or late postoperative period. Finally, midgut volvulus accounts for roughly 18% of cases of short gut syndrome in the pediatric population. Urgent recognition and management is the most important factor in preventing this complication.

SUGGESTED READINGS

Coombs RC, Buick RG, Gornall PG, et al. Intestinal malrotation: the role of small intestinal dysmotility in the cause of persistent symptoms. *J Pediatr Surg* 1991;26:553.

Devane SP, Smith VV, Bisset WM, et al. Persistent gastrointestinal symptoms after correction of malrotation. *Arch Dis Child* 1992; 67:218.

Filston HC, Kirks DR. Malrotation—the ubiquitous anomaly. *J Pediatr Surg* 1981;16:614.

Ford EG, Senac MO Jr, Srikanth MS, et al. Malrotation of the intestine in children. *Ann Surg* 1992;215:172.

Messineo A, MacMillan JH, Palder SB, et al. Clinical factors affecting mortality in children with malrotation of the intestine. *J Pediatr Surg* 1992;27:1343.

Powell DM, Othersen HB, Smith CD. Malrotation of the intestines in children: the effect of age on presentation and therapy. *J Pediatr Surg* 1989;24.777.

Spigland N, Brandt ML, Yazbeck S. Malrotation presenting beyond the neonatal period. *J Pediatr Surg* 1990;25:1139.

Stewart DR, Colodny AL, Daggett WC. Malrotation of the bowel in infants and children: a 15 year review. *Surgery* 1976;79:716.

50

NECROTIZING ENTEROCOLITIS

JOHN C. CHANDLER
SAMUEL D. SMITH

Necrotizing enterocolitis (NEC) is a neonatal disease process in which some portion of the bowel becomes gangrenous. This leads to sepsis and sometimes death, even in the face of early and aggressive treatment. The incidence of NEC has been reported to be up to 7.7% of all neonatal intensive care unit (NICU) admissions, or 1 to 3 per 1,000 live births. It is now the most common newborn surgical emergency, with a mortality that far exceeds that of any other operative gastrointestinal (GI) condition. A recent study of the mortality of necrotizing enterocolitis found that as overall infant mortality diminished due to improved neonatal intensive care and surfactant therapy, the mortality rate of NEC has increased from 11.5 to 12.3 per 100,000.

The cause is not known, and the pathophysiology is poorly understood. Molecular-level understanding of the disease might eventually provide some insight. In the ischemia/reperfusion injury model, hypoxic changes in the cells are compounded by the subsequent formation of oxygen free radicals and the release of inflammatory cytokines. A few inflammatory mediators—nitric oxide (NO) and platelet-activating factor (PAF)—bear mentioning, if only because they may play a prominent role in future therapy. Inducible nitric oxide synthase (iNOS) is significantly upregulated in enterocytes involved in the disease. In a study by Ford, iNOS was markedly diminished in five of seven patients at the time of stoma closure, but persistently elevated in two who died of the disease. Inhibitors of NO have been shown to blunt the intestinal injury in animal models of NEC. However, intravenous nitroglycerin, a nitric oxide donor, blunted the injury in a rabbit model of NEC. Rather than its presence or absence contributing to disease, the location and timing of its appearance probably determine its effects. PAF causes a NEC-like injury in rats. Furthermore, a PAF receptor agonist (WEB 2170) and a recombinant degrading enzyme (PAF-acetylhydrolase), have been shown to blunt that injury. Notably, breast milk contains PAF-acetylhydrolase.

J. C. Chandler: Departments of Surgery and Pediatrics, Greenville Hospital System, Greenville, South Carolina.

S. D. Smith: Department of Surgery, University of Arkansas for Medical Sciences; and Department of Pediatric Surgery, Arkansas Children's Hospital, Little Rock, Arkansas.

DIAGNOSTIC APPROACH

The "typical" infant with NEC is a preterm baby in the NICU, often with significant medical problems, and usually experiencing feeding intolerance or bloody stools. However, there is great variability: the infant can be full term, there may be no blood in the stool, and he or she may not yet have been fed. The early manifestations of NEC are signs of physiologic stress: episodes of apnea and bradycardia, temperature instability, and lethargy. A subtle period of respiratory decompensation can often be identified in the previous 12 hours. The presence of umbilical artery catheters or a history of a recent cardiac catheterization are known risk factors. Abdominal distension is usually progressive. This distension can compromise blood flow and compound the problem. Abdominal wall edema, erythema, and even crepitus are late findings that herald the presence of peritonitis.

It is important to remember that physical findings of NEC, especially in the smallest infants, can be difficult to identify due to the patient's small size, mechanical ventilation, sedation, or lethargy, and the presence of numerous monitoring lines, intravenous lines, and electrodes within the limited confines of an isolette. It is important not to let these factors hinder the clinician from getting an adequate physical examination.

The white count may be elevated, but is more often depressed because the available neutrophils are sequestered in the peritoneal fluid and there is a decreased ability to mobilize more. Infants with the lowest neutrophil counts typically have the worst prognosis. Thrombocytopenia is also a hallmark of severe disease. Radiographic findings include pneumatosis, ileus, persistent loops of small bowel, portal venous gas (PVG) or pneumoperitoneum. Alternatively, a gasless abdomen may indicate late disease.

Portal venous gas represents gas visible within the liver, branching as it follows the portal venous system. PVG may be fleeting, and there is disagreement about the associated prognosis. Anecdotally, it can be seen with greater frequency during ultrasonography, although the clinical importance of that finding has not been determined. Rowe found that pan-intestinal involvement was significantly more common in the presence of PVG in the very-low-birth-weight infant (VLBW, defined as <1,000 g or <28 weeks) than in the "standard" premature infant.

Ultrasonography is being used increasingly for assessing the presence and character of ascites, as well as to mark a location for paracentesis. This imaging modality may play a role in the future in determining the presence of intestinal ischemia by examination of the bowel wall, mucosa, and mesenteric vessels.

PREOPERATIVE PREPARATION

The treatment for uncomplicated NEC (i.e., no perforation or stricture) is medical. Feedings are held and an orogastric (Replogle) tube is placed to low intermittent suction for decompression of the bowel.

Broad-spectrum antibiotics are begun. The choice of antibiotics varies among practitioners, but gram-positive, gram-negative, and anaerobic coverage is required. We use ampicillin, gentamicin, and clindamycin. Culture results have been found to differ based on the size of the infant. VLBW infants are more likely to grow a variety of organisms. Anaerobes play a larger part in the VLBW infant than in other infants, but the reverse is true for *Escherichia coli.* Toxins from *Clostridium* species, *E. coli,* and coagulase-negative *Staphylococcus* have been isolated from stool samples during epidemics. Thankfully, vancomycin-resistant *Enterococcus* has so far been a rare event in these neonates. Neither the administration of intravenous immune globulin nor of enteral antibiotics has been shown to have benefit. Unfortunately, most premature infants have not received the benefit of immunoglobulin A from breast milk.

Fungal sepsis is a significant and potentially lethal factor in the morbidity of NEC, but is generally a late finding. A high index of suspicion for fungal infection should be maintained because these patients are immunosuppressed and are receiving broad-spectrum antibiotics.

Close observation is required, because changes may be dramatic. NEC can become fulminant and lead to death within hours of the first presenting sign. Clinical deterioration may be seen in the form of hemodynamic instability, respiratory failure, worsening acidosis, or thrombocytopenia. Serial physical examinations, laboratory studies (complete blood count, chemistries, and blood gases), and radiographs should be performed. Careful attention must be focused on fluid balances; blood products are transfused as necessary.

The infant should remain on bowel rest for at least 7 to 14 days, and total parenteral nutrition is used. Feedings are begun with an electrolyte solution and advanced slowly from dilute to full-strength formula with gradual increases in amount. Some surgeons prefer to conduct a contrast study prior to initiating feedings to look for strictures, a common occurrence following the development of circumferential ischemia in a segment of bowel. We believe it is reasonable to attempt feedings without a study, and then obtain a small bowel follow-through if not tolerated. A low threshold for withholding feedings should be maintained in the face of intolerance, because feedings can induce a recurrence.

Approximately 10% to 25% of infants will further deteriorate or fail to improve. Operative indications certainly include pneumoperitoneum and debris-filled ascites, indicative of intestinal perforation. Perforation strongly correlates with the presence of gangrenous bowel; abdominal wall erythema, a fixed abdominal mass, or a dilated loop of bowel persistent on radiography are weakly associated; clinical deterioration, persistent abdominal tenderness, profuse lower GI hemorrhage, gasless abdomen, and severe thrombocytopenia do not correlate with gangrenous bowel. PVG has been correlated with gangrenous bowel, and we use it as an indication for operative intervention.

Note that not all cases of pneumoperitoneum are the result of perforation from NEC—the perforated viscus may have another cause and may even represent a benign process. Occasionally, a benign pneumatosis coli leads to pneumoperitoneum and operation, although resection is not warranted in these cases.

TECHNICAL APPROACH

Exploratory laparotomy for NEC is performed for the following reasons: in response to failure to improve after peritoneal drainage (PD), as planned intervention shortly following PD, or as the primary intervention of choice.

Strong consideration should be given to operating at the bedside in the NICU. Recently, hypothermia has been described as inducing regional and systemic blood flow changes in piglets. These changes are prolonged beyond the time of returning to euthermia and may predispose to worsening NEC. Frawley et al. found that although mortality was clearly defined by the severity of illness, specific adverse events associated with transfer to the operating room included hypothermia, decreases in platelet counts, and deterioration of oxygenation and ventilation parameters, which could contribute to morbidity. Operating at the bedside avoids the stress associated with movement and hypothermia, and possible dislodgment of catheters and the endotracheal tube.

An upper transverse incision is chosen to allow maximal access to most of the intestinal tract. The extent of disease is determined: approximately half will have focal disease, one quarter each diffuse disease and pan-involvement.

In the case of focal disease, resection is undertaken and an end ostomy is brought out. Restoration of intestinal continuity following resection for NEC was previously discouraged, particularly in the VLBW infant. However, in clearly focal disease, if the viability of the bowel ends can be assured with a good degree of certainty, primary anastomosis has been undertaken. Especially in the case of an isolated ileal perforation, this picture likely represents a more benign spectrum of the disease in which the vascularity of the bowel is only temporarily and marginally compromised.

For NEC totalis, in which most of the bowel from the ligament of Treitz to the midtransverse colon is necrotic, the choice, although grim, is to avoid a massive resection and plan a "second-look" exploration 24 to 48 hours later if the neonate survives such a catastrophic event. Often, when confronted with this occurrence, neonatologists and parents understand the prognosis and opt to withdraw support. One must remember that in this Internet age, parents may pose the question of intestinal transplantation, and you should know your position on this. We currently do not feel that it is an acceptable alternative.

Difficult choices must be made when faced with disease of multiple segments, because the goal of saving as much viable bowel as possible conflicts with the desire to remove one long segment with all the necrotic bowel. Options include (a) proximal enterostomy without resection (clearly setting the stage for multiple surgeries), (b) the "clip and drop back" technique (multiple necrotic segments are resected, leaving the ends of viable bowel intraperitoneal and clipped or stapled, with planned laparotomy for reanastomosis in 48 to 72 hours), and (c) placing short segments of bowel in continuity over a small feeding tube without suturing (continuity usually ensues). No single technique is applicable to all infants, and the pediatric surgeon must be able to accommodate the technique to the situation.

Peritoneal drainage has gained increasing importance in the management of the VLBW infant with NEC as either a stabilizing procedure or as a potentially definitive treatment. As a rule, we consider PD primary treatment for infants weighing less than 1,000 g or those weighing more than 1,000 g who are too unstable to undergo laparotomy. We have found this to be a bridging technique, part of the resuscitation, expecting formal laparotomy within 72 hours. The only exception would be those infants weighing less than 1,000 g who have never been fed; these are the patients who may get away with PD only if their general condition stabilizes rapidly.

Peritoneal drainage is performed in the NICU, administering local anesthesia and muscle relaxation as needed. A small (<1 cm) right lower quadrant incision is made. After evacuation of gas and fluid, a Penrose drain is carefully inserted into the peritoneal cavity and sutured to the skin. A marked improvement in the patient's condition usually can be noted within 24 hours, with less hemodynamic instability and reduced acidosis. Drains are gradually removed over 7 to 10 days unless meconium or significant purulent material is still draining. Occasionally, a second drain is placed on the contralateral side. The antibiotics should be continued until the time of drain removal, and coverage may be adjusted based on culture results. Nasogastric suction is continued until patency and integrity of the GI tract is confirmed by a nonionic upper GI series.

The occasionally successful outcome of PD alone requires us to reevaluate our established surgical principles regarding intestinal ischemia and intraabdominal sepsis. VLBW infants appear to have unusual characteristics. Fetal wound healing and underdeveloped host defense mechanisms may contribute to the ability to overcome an otherwise catastrophic event and the continued presence of gangrenous bowel. The milieu of the neonatal abdomen appears to be markedly different from that of adults, as the rate of postoperative intraabdominal sepsis and abscess formation is remarkably low, often less than 5%. It is becoming clear that the infants who survive with drainage as the only surgical therapy may have a different, more benign disease with limited involvement and an isolated perforation.

POSTOPERATIVE CARE

Although the mortality rate for all infants with NEC requiring surgery has improved, it remains substantial (25%–40%). Infants weighing less than 1,000 g have the highest mortality rates (35%–50%). Prognosis may best be predicted by Sonntag's modification of the classification system originally developed by Bell. In his study of 50 VLBW infants (580–1,475 g), all infants who died were in Bell category III (advanced NEC with or without perforation), although less than half the babies in that category died. It was determined that within that category, mortality correlated with the number of organs failed: all those who died had failure of four or more organ systems other than the GI tract (cardiovascular, respiratory, hepatic, microvascular, renal, or coagulation). In particular, those with capillary leak syndrome (tachycardia of >180 beats/min persisting over 12 hours or weight gain exceeding 150 g/kg body weight over 1 day or 300 g/kg over 3 days) had a mortality rate of 80%. A retrospective study of our own patients found that mortality was strongly correlated with having been fed previously.

Laparotomy is also often required after the acute stage, because strictures occur in 20% to 25% and fistulas and abscesses also occasionally occur.

Short bowel syndrome, with its attendant metabolic, endocrinologic, and immunologic implications, is a well-described complication. Intestinal transplantation has met with modest success, and its strongest advocates, those at Pittsburgh, state that it is quickly becoming the standard of care for the treatment of intestinal failure, with or without simultaneous liver transplantation. One must remember that such transplant procedures in infants under 1 year of age carry significant morbidity and mortality with very limited long-term survival. The loss of the ileocecal valve alone does not appear to affect outcome, but the loss of most of the colon and terminal ileum is associated with a higher risk for developing short bowel syndrome.

Considerable, and progressively more, attention is being given to the neurocognitive development of premature infants as they enter childhood and adolescence. Although it would be difficult to separate the effects of NEC and its sequelae in the premature infant from those of other medical complications (intraventricular hemorrhage, retinopathy of prematurity, chronic lung disease, and others), it is becoming clear that medical complications play a significant role in the impairment of cognitive abilities and that such effects may be more important than psychosocial determinants.

PREVENTION

Even if the questions of treating NEC were to be answered, it is likely that the best "cure" will remain prevention. Although isolation of a common offending organism is rarely accomplished, infection control practices seem to limit the size of clusters of the disease. Some believe that routine "prophylactic" acid suppression is to be avoided, because the acid environment of the stomach affords some degree of protection. Breast milk seems to provide protection against NEC (and also throughout life against Crohn's disease, ulcerative colitis, and diarrheal illnesses). Important components of breast milk include immunoglobulin A, PAF-acetylhydrolase, and various oligosaccharides and glycoconjugates that may prevent intestinal attachment by pathogens. Although it seems prudent to slowly advance feedings in the smaller infants, the evidence of the utility of various regimens in the prevention of NEC is contradictory.

There is strong evidence that maternal glucocorticoids administered antenatally to women in preterm (weeks 24–34) labor decreases the incidence of subsequent NEC, but there is obviously a limited temporal window for effectiveness. This may represent an acceleration of the maturation of the gut, or may simply be the result of a reduced incidence of hypoxic stress. The addition of antibiotics to steroids administered to mothers with preterm premature rupture of the membranes substantially reduces the subsequent episodes of NEC and other causes of morbidity.

CONCLUSION

Care of the infant with NEC can be one of the greatest challenges for the pediatric surgeon. Our ability to fully understand and control NEC is elusive. Although operative intervention is frequently necessary, the management of this disease requires the collaborative efforts of neonatologists and surgeons in order to improve outcomes.

SUGGESTED READINGS

Ahmed T, Ein S, Moore A. The role of peritoneal drains in the treatment of perforated necrotizing enterocolitis: recommendations from recent experience. *J Pediatr Surg* 1998;33:1468–1470.

Ford H, Watkins S, Reblock K, et al. The role of inflammatory cytokines and nitric oxide in the pathogenesis of necrotizing enterocolitis. *J Pediatr Surg* 1997;32:275–282.

Frawley G, Bayley G, Chondros P. Laparotomy for necrotizing enterocolitis: intensive care nurshrey compared with operating theatre. *J Paediatr Child Health* 1999;35(3):291–295.

Kosloske AM. Epidemiology of necrotizing enterocolitis. *Acta Paediatr Suppl* 1994;396:2–7.

Sonntag J, Wagner MH, Waldschmidt J, et al. Multisystem organ failure and capillary leak syndrome in severe necrotizing enterocolitis of very low birth weight infants. *J Pediatr Surg* 1998;33:481–489.

51

PERITONEAL DRAINAGE FOR NECROTIZING ENTEROCOLITIS

REED A. DIMMITT
R. LAWRENCE MOSS

A 10-day-old infant was born prematurely at 26 weeks' gestation with a birth weight of 860 g. He required ventilatory support in the delivery room. After admission to the neonatal intensive care unit (NICU), he received exogenous surfactant, positive pressure ventilation, and had umbilical lines placed. He received no enteral feeding, and total parenteral nutrition was started on the second day of life. Ampicillin and gentamicin were empirically given for the first week. Dopamine and hydrocortisone were required to treat severe hypotension at 5 days of age. He had documented closure of a patent ductus arteriosus with indomethacin. This morning he was noted to have abdominal distention with occult blood in his stool. Morning laboratory tests revealed leukopenia and thrombocytopenia. He requires pressor support and has both a respiratory and metabolic acidosis. Serial flat anteroposterior abdominal radiographs show pneumatosis, and a recent left lateral decubitus film demonstrated free air. You are called for a consultation to discuss the surgical options available.

Advances in perinatal and neonatal medicine have resulted in greater numbers of very-low-birth-weight (VLBW) infants surviving initial resuscitation. These are the patients who are at the greatest risk for necrotizing enterocolitis (NEC). Even with appropriate nonoperative management of NEC, almost half of the smallest and least stable babies require surgical intervention for their disease.

Necrotizing enterocolitis is the most common intestinal emergency in the premature infant. NEC occurs in 1% to 5% of patients admitted to the NICU. While the outcomes from other diseases of extreme prematurity have improved over the past two decades, the mortality rate of 35% to 50% for perforated NEC is largely unchanged. Most surgeons agree regarding the indications for operation, but there is much debate about the preferred procedure.

INDICATIONS FOR PERITONEAL DRAINAGE

Historically, the surgical management of neonates with perforated NEC has been laparotomy with resection of necrotic bowel and stoma creation. In the 1970s, pediatric surgeons were called on to operate on progressively smaller and more premature babies with perforated NEC. These critically ill VLBW infants had a mortality rate of over 50% following operation. Some surgeons suggested that application of classic surgical techniques in these very small babies might not be indicated. Surgeons began to ask if the operation was "doing more harm than good."

In 1977 Ein and colleagues at Toronto's Hospital for Sick Children first reported the use of primary peritoneal drainage (PPD) for perforation in VLBW infants. They treated five patients weighing between 760 and 1,600 g who were described as septic and too unstable to undergo laparotomy. To the surprise of Ein and his colleagues, three of these five "moribund" babies survived. One of the three developed an intestinal stricture that was repaired electively 6 weeks later. The two infants who did not survive died of causes unrelated to NEC, and their gastrointestinal tracts were intact at autopsy. Although this report was anecdotal, the success of peritoneal drainage was impressive compared with the 35% to 55% mortality rate associated with conventional surgical treatment. The technique was widely criticized in the pediatric surgical community. This led to a comment from Ein that peritoneal drainage should only be used as a temporizing procedure in the "sickest" premature infants, with the intention of

R. A. Dimmitt: Department of Pediatrics, University of Alabama at Birmingham; and Department of Pediatrics, NICK– Children's Hospital of Alabama, Birmingham, Alabama.

R. L. Moss: Department of Surgery, Yale University School of Medicine; and Department of Surgery, Yale–New Haven Children's Hospital, New Haven, Connecticut.

stabilizing the baby until formal laparotomy could be safely performed.

As experience with PPD increased, many babies treated with this "temporizing" procedure did not appear to need a subsequent laparotomy. The institution originating the procedure reported their updated experience in 1980. They described 15 patients who underwent peritoneal drainage with the intention of proceeding to laparotomy within 24 to 48 hours. Forty percent of these patients improved so markedly that laparotomy was not performed and they completely recovered without further intervention.

Primary peritoneal drainage has never been studied in a controlled fashion, nor has it been compared with laparotomy in a trial. In fact, every center using peritoneal drainage reports selection bias in patient assignment. A recent review of the published experience of the use of peritoneal drainage for perforated NEC revealed that patients undergoing this procedure were significantly smaller and more premature (Table 51.1). Using techniques of metanalysis, these data were pooled. Because of the marked selection bias and the lack of published information as to why patients were assigned to peritoneal drainage versus laparotomy, the effectiveness of the two techniques could not be determined. The principle investigators from each institution used peritoneal drainage in patients with a greater expected risk for death. The fact that this "sicker" group of patients did better than predicted raises the question of whether peritoneal drainage may be superior to laparotomy. To answer this question, a multicenter, randomized, controlled clinical trial is currently accruing patients. If this trial is successful, the best treatment for this severe disease of premature infants may be determined.

PREOPERATIVE PREPARATION

Most patients are hypovolemic and require vigorous fluid resuscitation and correction of acid-base imbalance. The acidemia in severe NEC is often mixed, with a respiratory component from hypoventilation as well as a metabolic contribution from hypoperfusion. Capillary refill time is a sensitive indicator of cardiac output in this population. Peripheral arterial access should be established for accurate measurement of systemic blood pressure and arterial blood gases. A rule of thumb is that the mean arterial blood pressure should be the corrected gestational age in weeks, and a diastolic blood pressure of 20 mm Hg or greater is needed for adequate cerebral blood flow.

Resuscitation with isotonic crystalloid fluid is recommended initially, but colloid use may become necessary secondary to capillary leak and subsequent hypoalbuminemia with third space fluid accumulation. Packed red blood cell transfusion (10–15 mL/kg) is also appropriate in the presence of anemia. If there is evidence of coagulopathy, administration of platelets, fresh-frozen plasma, or cryoprecipitate may be indicated. Sodium bicarbonate should be given in severe metabolic acidosis. Pressor support may be necessary when hypoperfusion persists despite adequate fluid administration.

After obtaining blood cultures, broad-spectrum antimicrobial therapy appropriate to cover bowel flora should be initiated. Although ampicillin and gentamicin would be appropriate choices, the common use of these antibiotics in the NICU typically results in the development of resistant organisms. NEC is usually acquired while in the NICU; therefore, antibiotic therapy may be guided by patterns of resistance seen in the individual unit. In addition, VLBW infants are at risk for bacteremia from coagulase-negative

TABLE 51.1. TYPE OF OPERATION, GESTATIONAL AGE (GA), BIRTH WEIGHT (BW), AND SURVIVAL WITH PERFORATED NECROTIZING ENTEROCOLITIS: PUBLISHED DATA

	Primary Peritoneal Drainage				Laparotomy			
Author	n	GA (wk)[a]	BW (g)[a]	Survival	n	GA (wk)[a]	BW (g)[a]	Survival
Cheu	51	29	1,158	18 (35%)	41	32	1,875	31 (76%)
Takamatsu	4	27	808	4 (100%)	0	0	0	0
Morgan	29	27	994	23 (79%)	20	32	1,854	18 (90%)
Azarow	44	28	1,100	27 (61%)	42	31	1,700	24 (57%)
Snyder	12	29	1,134	3 (25%)	91	31	1,628	52 (57%)
Lessin	9	25	615	6 (67%)	0	0	0	0
Ahmed	23	27	910	10 (43%)	22	35	2,271	19 (86%)
Rovin	18	28	1,118	16 (89%)	10	29	1,274	9 (90%)
Downard	24	26	794	19 (79%)	9	30	1,510	7 (78%)
Dimmitt	17	25	677	7 (41%)	9	26	807	5 (56%)
Total	231	27 (0.5)	931 (63.2)	133 (58%)	244	31 (0.9)	1,615 (155)	165 (68%)

[a]Values are means (standard error of the means).
Reprinted from Moss RL, Dimmitt RA, Henry MC, et al. A meta-analysis of peritoneal drainage and laparotomy in perforated necrotizing enterocolitis. *J Pediatr Surg* 2001;36(8):1210-1213.; with permission.

Staphylococcus. Thus, empiric treatment with vancomycin and a third-generation cephalosporin is an appropriate regimen. Acquisition of anaerobic flora occurs as early as 1 week of age; therefore, a third agent to cover these organisms may be warranted. Because of the severity of the disease and the need for long-term coverage with broad-spectrum antibiotics, patients undergoing peritoneal drainage are at risk for fungal sepsis. Amphotericin, either empirically or with proven culture, may be necessary later in the course of treatment.

Some patients with tense pneumoperitoneum may have difficulty in diaphragmatic excursion. It may be necessary to relieve the increased abdominal pressure to allow adequate ventilation. A 22-gauge intravenous catheter can be inserted into the midabdomen, allowing stabilization prior to operation.

TECHNIQUE

The VLBW infant with NEC should only undergo peritoneal drainage after appropriate medical stabilization. Some clinicians recommend taking infants with perforated NEC to the operating room for drainage. We prefer to perform peritoneal drainage in the NICU. This approach minimizes complications during transport to the operating room, including the serious complication of hypothermia.

Because the procedure is relatively short, satisfactory anesthesia can be accomplished by using a combination of systemic and local agents. The regimen of intravenous narcotics, benzodiazepines, and short-acting paralytics with local instillation of lidocaine at the incision site is an appropriate choice. This provides adequate analgesia and relaxation without compromising cardiovascular function.

We keep the baby under an open warmer to prevent hypothermia. We then place the baby supine and turned slightly to the left (Fig. 51.1). The abdomen is then washed with warmed iodine solution. We make our incision in the right lower quadrant just below the level of the umbilicus. Other clinicians suggest a left lower quadrant incision to avoid the liver. Whichever technique is used, it is critically important that the surgeon palpate the liver edge prior to making the incision so that injury to the delicate premature liver is avoided.

We then use the knife to make a 0.5- to 1-cm incision through the skin and muscle layers. Cautery is not necessary. We identify the peritoneum, grasping it with two forceps, and enter the peritoneal cavity bluntly with a hemostat (Fig. 51.2). Typically, a large quantity of bile, stool, and pus is immediately expressed. Because the objective of peritoneal drainage is to clear the peritoneal cavity of toxins, we believe irrigation with warm saline is important. A 22-gauge angiocatheter (without needle) is advanced into all four quadrants of the abdomen and flushed until the drainage is clear. Again, great care is taken to avoid liver injury. Next, we use a hemostat to advance a ¼-inch Penrose drain into all four quadrants of the abdomen (Fig. 51.3). The drain is sutured to the skin to prevent it from falling out, and a safety pin is attached to the drain to prevent it from falling in.

As mentioned previously, peritoneal drainage has almost universally been used in the smallest and most unstable

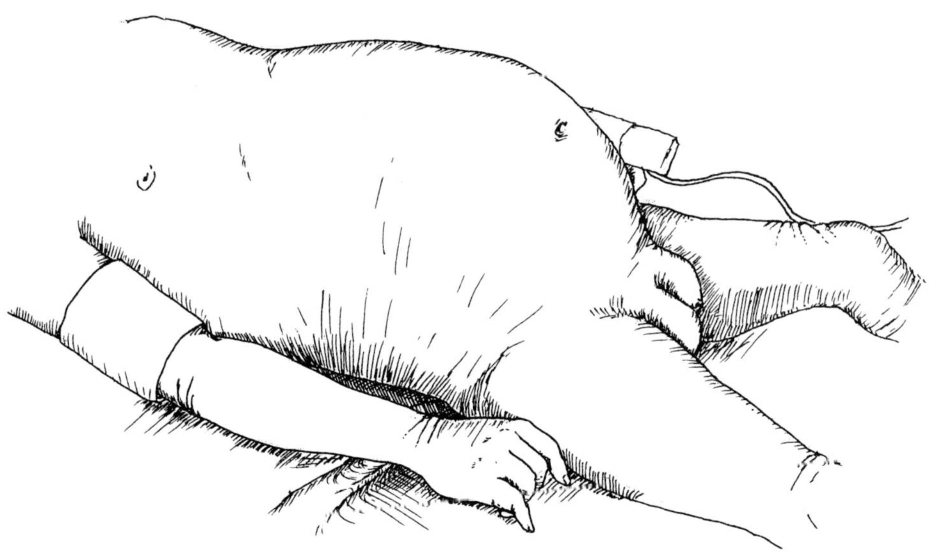

FIGURE 51.1. The patient is placed supine under a radiant warmer prior to the abdominal incision. In addition, the baby is turned slightly to the left to allow easier access to the right lower abdominal quadrant.

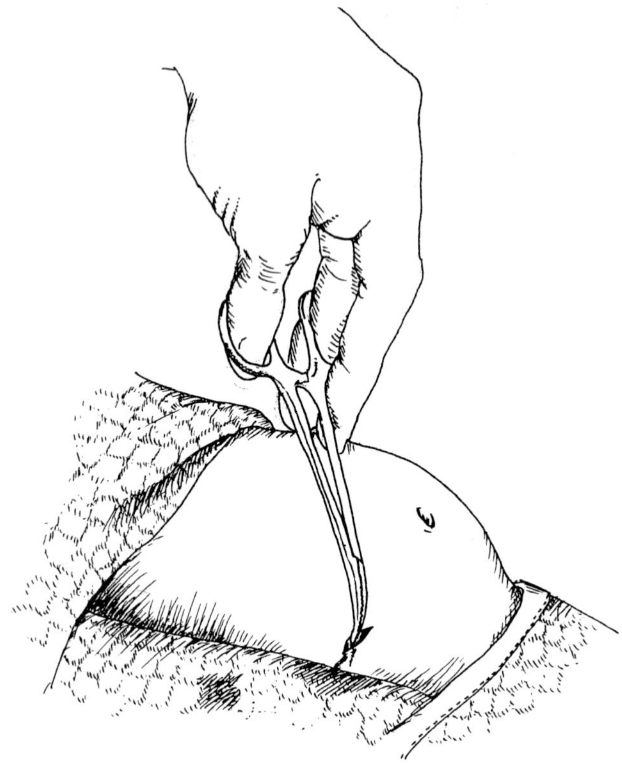

FIGURE 51.2. An incision (0.5–1 cm) is made through the skin and muscle layers. After grasping the peritoneum, the peritoneal cavity is bluntly entered with a hemostat.

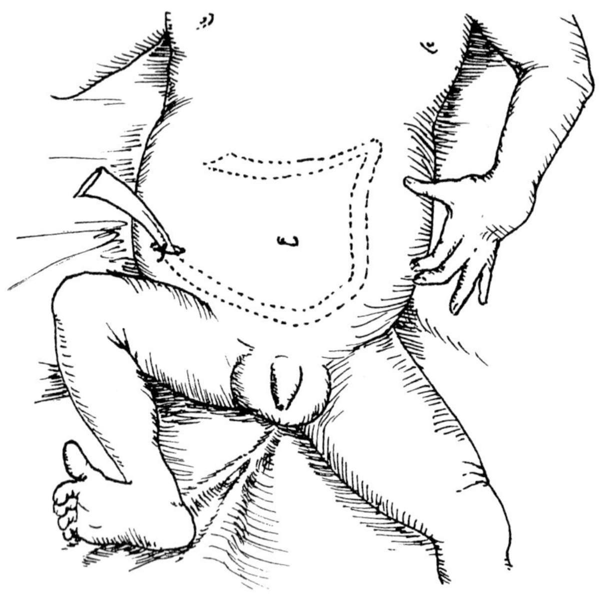

FIGURE 51.3. After warm saline lavage of the peritoneal cavity, a ¼-inch Penrose drain is placed. The drain should be directed inferiorly to avoid the liver. It is important that the drain communicates in all four quadrants. The drain is then sutured to the skin.

patients. Patients usually do not immediately improve and typically require continued intensive support. These infants show continued clinical and laboratory evidence of ongoing sepsis. A retrospective study of 17 patients treated with peritoneal drainage was unable to predict survival by the severity of the early postoperative period. In fact, most patients who ultimately recover get worse before they get better.

Some institutions uniformly perform a planned laparotomy after peritoneal drainage. This second operation is performed when the patient's clinical status improves. Other surgeons recommend additional surgical intervention if there is not rapid improvement after peritoneal drainage. We believe early laparotomy following drainage is not useful for several reasons. First, most patients experience clinical deterioration with ongoing signs of systemic sepsis early after peritoneal drainage. Thus, it is difficult to differentiate which infants to treat with a "salvage laparotomy." Second, if peritoneal drainage was chosen over laparotomy because of clinical instability, it seems counterintuitive to perform a salvage laparotomy when a patient is more unstable. A case series of a small number of patients undergoing salvage laparotomy reported a 100% mortality rate with a long protracted postoperative course. None of the patients tolerated enteral nutrition, and all died of NEC-related complications.

Based on the current data available, we recommend that when the choice of peritoneal drainage is made, salvage laparotomy should not be performed for perceived failure. It appears that patients treated with peritoneal drainage follow the rule of one thirds: one third will die of their disease, one third will survive with no additional surgical intervention, and one third will require late elective exploration for relief of mechanical obstruction.

LONG-TERM OUTCOME

Patients who undergo surgical intervention for NEC have a high probability of long-term adverse outcomes. The most common intestinal complication after laparotomy is short-bowel syndrome (25%). Short-bowel syndrome is rarely a complication following peritoneal drainage because no resection is performed.

Feeding intolerance during the advancement of enteral nutrition can be due to mechanical obstruction. If a bowel obstruction is suspected, contrast studies should be undertaken to look for a stricture. Strictures occur in areas of the intestine that are severely ischemic and heal by scarring and contraction. Strictures are best treated by elective resection and anastomosis once the baby is clinically stable and has reached a weight of at least 2 kg. The development of adhesive small bowel obstruction after peritoneal drainage is apparently rare. We have not observed it in our experience, and it is not reported as a cause in large series of children with bowel obstructions.

As many as 50% of patients who survive surgically treated NEC develop neurodevelopmental delay. NEC is not believed to be directly causative. Any condition that results in prolonged hospitalization has been shown to place neonates at risk. In a matched cohort study, no difference in the Bailey Scales of Infant Development was seen in patients surviving severe NEC compared with patients who had similar hospital stays without NEC.

CONCLUSION

Necrotizing enterocolitis remains a serious cause of morbidity and mortality in VLBW infants. Peritoneal drainage offers a viable and less invasive alternative to laparotomy in this critically ill group of patients. Peritoneal drainage has generally been used in the sickest and most unstable patients and produced survival rates better than expected. Available data comparing peritoneal drainage with laparotomy are anecdotal, retrospective, and not controlled. The true role of peritoneal drainage is not yet defined. A randomized trial currently underway may help determine the best treatment for infants with perforated NEC.

SUGGESTED READINGS

Albanese CT. Necrotizing enterocolitis. In: O'Neill JA, Rowe MI, Grosfeld JL, et al., eds. *Pediatric surgery, 5th ed.* St. Louis: Mosby-Year Book, 1998:1297–1320.

Bell MJ, Ternberg JL, Feigin RD, et al. Neonatal necrotizing enterocolitis: therapeutic decisions based upon clinical staging. *Ann Surg* 1978;187:1–7.

Dimmitt RA, Meier AH, Skarsgard ED, et al. Salvage laparotomy for failure of peritoneal drainage in necrotizing enterocolitis in extremely low birth weight infants. *J Pediatr Surg* 2000;35:856–859.

Ein SH, Marshall DG, Gervan D. Peritoneal drainage under local anesthesia for perforations from necrotizing enterocolitis. *J Pediatr Surg* 1977;12:963–967.

Holman RC, Stoll BJ, Clarke MJ, et al. The epidemiology of necrotizing enterocolitis infant mortality in the United States. *Am J Public Health* 1997;87:2026–2031.

Kosloske AM, Musemeche CA. Necrotizing enterocolitis of the neonate. *Clin Perinatol* 1989;16:97–111.

Morgan JL, Shochat SJ, Hartman GE. Peritoneal drainage as primary management of perforated NEC in the very low birth weight infant. *J Pediatr Surg* 1994;29:310–315.

Moss RL, Dimmitt RA, Henry MC, et al. A meta-analysis of peritoneal drainage and laparotomy in perforated necrotizing enterocolitis. *J Pediatr Surg* 2001;36(8):1210–1213.

Snyder CL, Gittes GK, Murphy JP, et al. Survival after necrotizing enterocolitis in infants weighing less than 1,000 g: 25 years' experience at a single institution. *J Pediatr Surg* 1997;32:434–437.

52

SHORT BOWEL SYNDROME: A MEDICAL AND SURGICAL PERSPECTIVE

MORITZ M. ZIEGLER

Short bowel syndrome has become a large part of the pediatric surgeon's daily practice for a variety of reasons. Our ability to nourish and sustain growth in the face of a short intestine with application of the artificial gut or total parenteral nutrition (TPN), as well as our ability to support the tiniest premature baby, has resulted in a cohort of patients who survive devastating gastrointestinal insults. The product of this survival is a series of patients who manifest both functional and anatomic short intestine and whose care provides the substance of this report.

HISTORIC PERSPECTIVE

The history of short bowel syndrome takes two parallel tracks. In the late 1800s and throughout the first half of the 1900s, the history of short bowel syndrome focused on a description of the pathophysiology of the intestinal track following massive enterectomy. Nicholas Senn in 1888 first reported diarrhea and malabsorption associated with extensive enterectomy. This observation was confirmed in the early 1950s when Clatworthy and colleagues described the growth of beagle puppies following more than a 50% enterectomy, with conventional nutritional therapy. Clinical papers outlined the survival of the selected few patients who also sustained various degrees of short bowel syndrome following a variety of insults.

In parallel with this physiologic history, the ability to nourish patients parenterally also developed. In 1944, Helfrick and Abelson reported on a 5-month-old child who was nourished exclusively intravenously for 5 days. The field then lay dormant until the classic description of Wilmore, Dudrick, Rhoads, Vars, and others working at the Hospital of the University of Pennsylvania and the Harrison Department of Surgical Research. In 1966, a child was admitted to the Children's Hospital of Philadelphia with intestinal atresia and secondary short bowel syndrome. Wilmore, et al. orchestrated her intravenous feeding with carbohydrate and protein hydrolysate, and this child became the first infant who was documented to grow and develop while fed exclusively by vein. This began the modern era of the management of short bowel syndrome facilitated by the application of parenteral nutrition.

ETIOLOGY OF SHORT BOWEL SYNDROME

Wilmore in 1971 wrote a literature review of short bowel syndrome and described a series of diagnoses associated with the entity. In this world literature review, the diagnoses included intestinal atresia, gastroschisis, vascular infarct, and midgut volvulus, the latter making up 60% of reported cases at that time. Over the subsequent 30 years, a series of reports have accrued from several children's centers in the United States and abroad. As these reports have sequentially occurred, there has been a transition from midgut volvulus as the most frequent etiology to a recognition of necrotizing enterocolitis as the most frequent cause of this entity today. In fact, a series of additional diagnoses have evolved that are summarized in Table 52.1. In essence, the three top diagnoses in this combined series include necrotizing enterocolitis (29.1%), midgut volvulus (27.1%), and intestinal atresia (22.9%). In addition, depending on the medical center reporting, a variety of diagnoses have surfaced as etiologies of short bowel syndrome. They include trauma, intestinal aganglionosis involving the small intestine, the rare case of congenital short bowel syndrome, meconium ileus, and the unusual case of an isolated vascular infarct. Necrotizing enterocolitis produces short bowel syndrome secondary to (a) massive intestinal loss at the initial resection and (b) absorption and motility dysfunction resulting from the ini-

M.M. Ziegler: Department of Surgery, Harvard Medical School; and Department of Surgery, Children's Hospital, Boston, Massachusetts.

TABLE 52.1. ETIOLOGY OF SHORT BOWEL SYNDROME: SUMMARY, 1972–2000, 13 SERIES

Aganglionosis	19 (4.4%)
Atresia	100 (22.9%)
Congenital	3 (0.7%)
Gastroschisis	43 (10.0%)
Meconium ileus	2 (0.5%)
Necrotizing enterocolitis	127 (29.1%)
Trauma	2 (0.5%)
Vascular infarct	6 (1.4%)
Volvulus	118 (27.1%)
Other	16 (3.7%)
Total	436

tial ischemic insult in the profoundly premature baby. Intestinal atresia is problematic in that not only is there the question of how much intestine is missing from the atretic area, but the proximal more dilated bowel at times demonstrates motility dysfunction. Successful management requires precise reconstruction to avoid delayed emptying of the distended loop with stasis, bacterial overgrowth, and secondary malabsorption. Volvulus remains a preventable form of short bowel syndrome; if properly diagnosed, the ravages of ischemic enteropathy can sometimes be averted. Again, not only is short bowel physiology secondary to loss of the infarcted bowel, but the ischemic insult may produce a functional absorptive and motility disorder of the remaining intestine.

EMBRYOLOGY: PATHOPHYSIOLOGY

The midgut is the embryologic origin of the small bowel. By the 14th week of gestation, the crypts and villi in the small bowel are complete in their development. By the 20th week of gestation, anatomic structure of the bowel is completed. Subsequently, during weeks 24 to 38 of gestation, the predominant alteration in the anatomy of the gastrointestinal tract is a substantial (1.7-fold) increase in intestinal length. Intestinal length increase continues throughout fetal, infant, and early childhood development. Table 52.2 summarizes an adaptation of data reported by Touloukian that compares small bowel and colon length with conceptual age. Throughout fetal development, the bowel continues to grow, a principle that has advantage when aggressively rehabilitating the child. Furthermore, this relationship of intestinal length to both conceptual age as well as body length of the infant (crown-heel length) is a useful measurement for predicting bowel length. A useful, albeit arbitrary, rule of thumb is that the predicted small bowel length in a newborn is approximately two and a half times the body length of the baby. For example, a 20-inch long neonate is expected to have approximately 50 inches or 125 cm of small bowel.

TABLE 52.2. ETIOLOGY OF SHORT BOWEL SYNDROME: CONCEPTUAL AGE AND BOWEL LENGTH

Category	Age (wk)	Small Bowel Length	Colon Length
Fetus	19–27	118 cm	23 cm
	27–35	177 cm	41 cm
Infant	>35	255 cm	49 cm
Adult		12–22 ft	4–5 ft

From Touloukian RJ, Smith GJ. Normal intestinal length in preterm infants. J Pediatr Surg 1983;18:720–723; with permission.

The pathophysiology of short bowel syndrome can be specifically linked to gastrointestinal physiology at each level of the gastrointestinal tract. In the presence of massive intestinal resection, the stomach secretes both an excessive volume and acid content of its fluid output. This hypergastrinemic state contributes to an alteration in small bowel luminal pH, inhibition of pancreatic digestive enzymes, and an irritation of perianal skin. This state, often seen early in short bowel syndrome, forms the basis for the application of either hydrogen ion antagonist or proton pump inhibitor medications in the early management of short bowel syndrome.

Jejunal loss has several ramifications. First, in the high jejunum are brush border hydrolytic enzymes, particularly the disaccharidases. Their loss impairs carbohydrate absorption, and intraluminal carbohydrate stasis forms a milieu for bacterial overgrowth, fermentation, osmotic diarrhea, and secondary malabsorption. Jejunal loss also may reduce the amount of cholecystokinin and secretin, a change that further impairs pancreatic and biliary secretion. There also may be a malabsorption of peptides and amino acids, which impairs the hepatic production of albumin and other acute phase proteins. This can have an adverse impact on liver structure and function. Another outcome of jejunal loss is calcium loss into the stool with excessive stool fat, a loss further exacerbated by vitamin D malabsorption. This is one of the causes of hypocalcemia and the metabolic bone disease that characterizes short bowel syndrome. The secondary hyperoxaluric state contributes to the development of oxalate urinary tract stones. There may be a secondary iron deficiency due to a deficient absorptive surface following jejunal loss, a deficiency exacerbated by chronic blood sampling and chronic gastrointestinal tract bleeding. There may also be a loss of trace metals such as zinc, chromium, manganese, and selenium, each producing a trace metal deficiency syndrome. Finally, with jejunal loss there can be a secondary loss of water-soluble vitamins of the B complex.

Ileal loss has the adverse impact of bile salt malabsorption, which in turn depletes the enterohepatic pool. Furthermore, such bile salt malabsorption can cause colonic irritation and secondary diarrhea. Finally, the increased lithogenicity of the bile related to this aberration may be the prime etiologic factor that increases the incidence of gallstones in the short bowel syndrome. Ileal loss also may contribute to vitamin B_{12} deficiency.

Colonic loss in the pediatric patient not only removes a source for water and mineral absorption, but there is some evidence that the colonic surface has a potential role in carbohydrate absorption.

In parallel to the adverse physiologic impacts of intestinal loss is the early and aggressive beneficial response of intestinal adaptation. Typically, within 12 to 24 hours of the enterectomy or gut insult, a process begins that includes small bowel cellular hyperplasia, villus hypertrophy, intestinal lengthening, altered intestinal motility, and hormonal change. It is known that hyperplasia is greater in the younger patient and greater in the ileum. It is also known that adaptation includes a change in bowel circumference, wall thickness, length, villus height, crypt depth, and cellular proliferation, as well as apoptosis, all of which substantially increase absorptive activity. Furthermore, there is an enhancement of absorptive enzyme action. Intestinal adaptation is facilitated by a variety of trophic influences, including intraluminal nutrients; various intrinsic gut hormones from the stomach, duodenum, biliary tract, pancreas, and intestine; bile acids; and even nongut hormones such as pituitary hormone, mineralocorticoids, testosterone, and thyroid hormone. Both intrinsic and extrinsic growth factors such as epidermal growth factor, gastrin, and enteroglucagon also stimulate adaptation.

MEDICAL MANAGEMENT OF SHORT BOWEL SYNDROME

In addition to delivering nutrients into the gut as well as intravenously, the medical management has focused on four specific areas: (a) the treatment of hypergastrinemia; (b) the management of bowel motility or transit time; (c) the treatment of the adverse impact of bile salts on the colon; and (d) the treatment of bacterial overgrowth in the intestinal lumen.

The treatment of hypergastrinemia has been typically managed with the administration of either a histamine blocker such as cimetidine or ranitidine or a proton pump inhibitor such as omeprazole. Typically, the state of excessive gastric acid and gastric volume output is transient, and the treatment directed at the problem need not be persistent.

The treatment of bowel motility has had variable success. Typically, diphenoxylate hydrochloride or loperamide hydrochloride has each been used in an effort to slow motility and prolong intestinal transit. They have met with variable results. Prokinetic agents also have been used to enhance gastric emptying as well as to enhance transit in the face of dilated intestinal loops that empty poorly. Metoclopramide is used most often today.

The application of cholestyramine resin occasionally has been useful to bind bile salts to diminish their irritation of the colon and minimize associated diarrhea. At times, other adjunctive agents also have been used in the medical management of short bowel syndrome, including such antisecretory agents as somatostatin given in an effort to diminish gut luminal output.

SURGICAL OPTIONS IN SHORT BOWEL SYNDROME

The surgical management of short bowel syndrome has typically been defined into four separate categories of approach. First, the establishment of continuity of the gastrointestinal tract should be a top priority and includes the closure of existing stomas. Second, surgical attention should be directed to eliminating gastrointestinal stasis by relieving intestinal obstruction, by considering tapering enteroplasty, or, where preservation of the mucosal surface is paramount, by considering an intestinal plication. A third principle is to prolong intestinal transit time. Operative interventions to achieve such goals include reverse intestinal pacing, the insertion of intestinal valves, the insertion of a reversed small bowel segment, or even a small bowel–colon interposition. Finally, enhanced mucosal surface area can be achieved by a variety of operative techniques. These techniques include intestinal lengthening using a Bianchi (autologous gastrointestinal reconstruction; AGIR) procedure, a Kimura (Iowa) procedure, a mechanical distraction, or a recirculating loop. Patch enteroplasty also has been used to enhance mucosal surface area. Intestinal transplantation, either using isolated small bowel or liver–bowel grafts, is a possible solution with great promise. Table 52.3 outlines a sequential historic description of various operative procedures for short bowel syndrome that have been developed in the pediatric patient.

Unfortunately, few prospective scientific studies have been conducted to validate these various operative approaches. However, principles of approach have been defined. In the patient with short intestinal length and associated liver dysfunction, whose risk for death is greatest, a prompt referral for intestinal transplantation would seem most prudent. In the child with short intestinal length but normal caliber bowel, a valve placement that produces distention and facilitates a subsequent lengthening procedure may be a consideration. The same patient with a dilated intestine may be amenable to a lengthening procedure. The child with moderate intestinal length and rapid transit may be best managed operatively by insertion of a valve or a reversed intestinal segment or even a colon–small bowel interposition. Finally, the patient with adequate intestinal length and dilated bowel may be best managed by relieving any existing obstruction or by considering a tapering enteroplasty or an intestinal plication.

TABLE 52.3. OPERATIVE ADJUNCTS IN HISTORIC PERSPECTIVE

1950															2000
	1959 Hammer reversed segment		1967 Budding recirculating loop		1970 Waddell nipple valve		1975 Camprodan recirculating loop		1981 Gladen, Kelly electrical pacing		1984 Vinograd tunneled valve	1989 Bianchi composite ileocolic loop		1994 Georgeson sequential intestinal lengthening	
		1965 Keller reversed segment		1968 Cywes S-shaped pouch		1971 Hutcher, Salzberg colon interposition		1980 Bianchi intestinal lengthening		1982 Weber tapering enteroplasty	1984 Glick, deLorimier colon interposition		1990 Kimura intestinal lengthening		1995 Georgeson wrapped valve

RESTORATION OF INTESTINAL CONTINUITY

The value of closing intestinal stomas may include an increased absorptive capacity, a prolonged transit time, an enhanced effect of short-chained fatty acids on the colon, and the avoidance of a stoma. In contrast, the adverse impact of premature closure of a stoma includes the facilitation of bile acid-induced secretory diarrhea, an enhanced opportunity for perianal excoriation, an increased incidence of nephrolithiasis, and the potential for inducing dietary restrictions. However, there is general consensus that in children with an intestinal stoma who are beginning enteral feedings, it is most often prudent to close that stoma before progressing with the feedings. This will take advantage not only of all of the small and large bowel length, but it will also interpose into the fecal stream the anal sphincter, a mechanism that has the salutary benefit of slowing intestinal transit and potentially improving intestinal absorption. Furthermore, the potential value of colonic absorption of selected nutrients, particularly carbohydrates, in the pediatric patient suggests a further nutrient value to closing intestinal stomas.

SLOWING INTESTINAL TRANSIT TIME

Slowing intestinal transit with small bowel reversed segments has been reported in the pediatric patient. In a series of children with measured small bowel length varying from 20 to 94 cm, four of five who had a reversed segment of 3 cm of length survived their short bowel syndrome. Using a 12-cm reversed segment in a series of adults, 50% of patients had substantial reductions in their TPN, and three of eight completely converted to oral nutrient support. The application of an intestinal valve is designed to increase small bowel transit time, and to decrease colon–to–small bowel reflux and potential bacterial colonization. It also has been designed to produce small bowel dilatation, making it amenable to a subsequent AGIR lengthening procedure. The most commonly used valves are intussuscepted valves, but because of their propensity to come undone, wrapping of the valve with a prosthetic material may be prudent. Other alternate mechanisms include the construction of a nipple valve or the construction of a subserosal small bowel insert into the large bowel, a tunnel valve technique originally developed for urinary vesicoureteral reflux. No specific trials of intestinal valves in the pediatric age group have been reported.

The application of the small bowel colon interposition is also designed to increase transit time; enhance carbohydrate, vitamin B_{12}, and fat absorption; and potentially enhance weight gain. The principles of this operation are to have an intact colon but a short small bowel. A piece of colon is implanted in the center of the small bowel, either in a properistaltic or antiperistaltic fashion. In a series of seven such colon interpositions performed at the University of California at San Francisco, four patients survived whose small bowel length varied from 15 to 63 cm.

ENHANCING MUCOSAL SURFACE AREA

The predominant operation to enhance mucosal surface area in the pediatric age group has been the Bianchi intestinal lengthening procedure (AGIR). This operation is designed to increase the intestinal mucosal surface area and to prolong intestinal transit. The down side of the operation may be an actual loss of intestinal mucosal surface because of the operative technique of division of the bowel in a longitudinal fashion using either an automated stapling device or a hand-sewn technique. As such, there can be impaired intestinal absorption and impaired intestinal adaptation. Selected studies also have demonstrated a prolonged hypergastrinemic state, an enhanced postprandial somatostatin output, and a diminished enteral glucagon secretion. Such bowel also has been found to impair propagation of a migrating motor complex. In a series of such patients reported by Bianchi himself, 9 of 20 patients whose small bowel length measured an average 62 cm survived, whereas 11 of 20 with an average small bowel length of 43 cm died. The lengthening procedure of the survivor group increased bowel length to an average 97 cm, whereas in the nonsurviving patients, the average length attained was 68 cm. Certainly in selected patients who require partial to continued TPN, an intestinal lengthening procedure may be that adjunctive operation which will free the patient from being TPN dependent. However, in the patient largely dependent on TPN, a lengthening procedure alone will not effectively remove them from their parenteral nutrient support.

Anecdotal reports of applying the Kimura (Iowa) procedure also exist. In addition to performing a Bianchi procedure with the blood flow to the longitudinally split intestine dependent on one leaf of the mesentery, a deserosalized antimesenteric segment of the split small bowel is connected to the undersurface of the rectus muscle or the liver, facilitating a parasitization of a secondary blood flow. This permits a subsequent horizontal division of the bowel. At least in one report, the sequential application of the AGIR followed by the Iowa procedure substantially reduced the need for parenteral nutrition. Other similar outcomes of patch enteroplasty using the colon onto small bowel mucosa have been reported for children with jejunal atresia.

MANAGEMENT PLAN OVERVIEW

When considering the severity of short bowel syndrome, outcomes typically are related to length and location of the remaining bowel, presence or absence of an ileocecal valve, mucosal integrity and function, motility of the remaining bowel, concomitant colonic disease, and, finally, time since the onset of the actual short bowel syndrome. With these factors in mind, each patient requires an individualized management plan, a plan that can be defined in a stepwise time interval. Table 52.4 summarizes my recommended plan.

After the initial operative or diagnostic procedure for short bowel syndrome, the initial parameters of any management plan are to define the anatomy of the residual bowel, including the approximate length of jejunum, ileum, and colon, as well as the presence or absence of the ileocecal valve. It is imperative to initially establish vascular access and to initiate TPN to facilitate nutritional rehabilitation and somatic growth. It is also important to establish an enteral access route early, whether by mouth, gastrostomy, or transnasal feeding tube. From the initiation of the management plan, it is important to consider oral stimulation to facilitate the oral and esophageal swallowing reflex.

Over the first month, TPN is imperative. However, it is also useful even after a couple of weeks into the syndrome to consider the initiation of enteral feeding. Whether this is nutritive to the gut or nutritive to the patient depends on the degree of gastrointestinal shortening. Between the first month and sixth month following the initiation of the syndrome, a comprehensive plan must be put in place. This would include continuation of TPN and potentially thereafter a gradual tapering of that route of support along with a concomitant gradual transition to enteral feedings with an incremental increase in feedings both by volume, number of hours, and caloric density. It is important during this period of time to initiate a plan to monitor as well as treat bacterial overgrowth and to plan for transitioning the patient and family to home care. There may be a role for selected nutrient replacement, especially of minerals, vitamins, and trace elements, and there is also an early role for pharmacologic therapies. These therapies include the treatment of the hypergastrinemic state, motility slowing agents, the administration of bile salt binding agents, and even the application of a cholagogue to enhance biliary secretion and minimize cholestatic TPN-induced liver disease. Then, during the rest of the first year of management, growth and nutritional outcomes must be closely monitored and managed. Particular complications of short bowel syndrome must be expected, including the recurrent problem of bacterial overgrowth and central line infections, nutrient deficiency states, liver dysfunction, gallstones, and even renal stones. Finally, I support the principle that only after 12 months of aggressive medical and nutritional management is the time appropriate to consider operative intervention. The operative procedures have been outlined above.

TABLE 52.4. PEDIATRIC SHORT BOWEL SYNDROME: MANAGEMENT PLAN

Initial
1. Define anatomy of residual bowel
   a. Length of jejunum, ileum, colon
   b. Presence/absence of ileocecal valve
2. Establish vascular access/initiate TPN
3. Establish enteral access
   a. Gastrostomy
   b. Oral stimulation

After 2–4 weeks
1. Continue TPN
2. Initiate enteral feedings

4 weeks to 6 months
1. Gradual transition to enteral feeds
2. Continue TPN-taper regimen
3. Monitor/treat bacterial overgrowth
4. Transition to home care
5. Selective nutrient replacement
6. Pharmacologic therapies: gastric acid inhibition, bile salt binding resin, motility slowing agents, cholagogue

6–12 months
1. Monitor growth and nutritional outcomes
2. Monitor complications of nutritional care and SBS: nutrient deficiency, gall stones, liver function, renal stones

After 12 months
Consider operative options:
- Short length/liver dysfunction → Refer for transplantation
- Short length/liver satisfactory → Lengthen
- Moderate length/rapid transit → Valve/reverse segment/colon interposition
- Adequate length/dilated → Relieve obstruction/tapering enteroplasty

OUTCOMES FROM SHORT BOWEL SYNDROME

The outcomes of short bowel syndrome have changed significantly since the initial report of Wilmore. At that time, the standard of 40 cm of remaining small bowel with an intact ileocecal valve would translate into approximately a 50% survival. Today, in both large series as well as anecdotal reports, the absolute small intestinal length associated with a predictable high-quality survival has diminished to 20 to 25 cm. What is less clear is whether or not the ileocecal valve plays a critical role in outcomes. There are data to suggest that short bowel syndrome management with an ileocecal valve will enhance the ability to wean from TPN, but there is little evidence to suggest that the presence or absence of an ileocecal valve will influence survival and eventual disease outcome.

The improved overall outcome from short bowel syndrome has occurred concurrent with a transition to survival of more critically ill patients, particularly the premature baby with necrotizing enterocolitis. However, these children also have the greatest morbidity from management of short bowel syndrome, including the development of cholestatic liver disease and progressive liver dysfunction requiring the eventual consideration of liver and/or liver–bowel transplantation.

None of the above data have taken into consideration the application of transplantation as an option for the short bowel syndrome. However, with small bowel transplantation, there is now a predictable survival rate that is quite favorable. Despite favorable survival rates and despite the high likelihood of weaning from TPN with a successful transplant, the complications of graft-versus-host-disease, lymphoproliferative disease, and allograft rejection have remained formidable morbidities whether for both an isolated small bowel or for a liver–bowel transplant.

SUMMARY

Short bowel syndrome in the pediatric patient accounts for a large portion of hospital inpatient days and a substantial portion of time expended by the pediatric surgeon. These children provide a unique opportunity for a surgeon to be a comprehensive, thorough, and complete physician, administering not only to the operative needs of the patient but to their physiologic, nutritional, and social needs as well. Substantial progress has been made in the management of this complex disease, and extremely innovative operative procedures have been applied to its management. It is less clear what impact these operations have on outcomes from short bowel syndrome. Furthermore, what is the eventual impact of intestinal transplantation on this disease? A considerable challenge awaits the pediatric surgical community to optimize the outcomes from this disease and its management.

SUGGESTED READINGS

Bianchi A. Intestinal loop lengthening—a technique for increasing small intestinal length. *J Pediatr Surg* 1980;15:145–151.

Chaet MS, Farrell MK, Ziegler MM, et al. Intensive nutritional support and remedial surgical intervention for extreme short bowel syndrome. *J Pediatr Gastroenterol Nutr* 1994;19:295–298.

Garcia VF, Templeton JM, Eichelberger MR, et al. Colon interposition for the short bowel syndrome. *J Pediatr Surg* 1981;16:994–995.

Gladen HE, Kelly KA. Electrical pacing for short bowel syndrome. *Surg Gynecol Obstet* 1981;153:697–700.

Glick PL, deLorimier AA, Adzick NS, et al. Colon interposition: an adjuvant operation for short gut syndrome. *J Pediatr Surg* 1984;19:719–725.

Grosfeld JL, Rescorla FJ, West KW. Short bowel syndrome in infancy and childhood. *Am J Surg* 1986;151:41–46.

Haymond HE. Massive resection of the small intestine: analysis of 257 collected cases. *Surg Gynecol Obstet* 1935;61:693.

Kurkchubasche AG, Rowe MI, Smith SD. Adaptation in short bowel syndrome: reassessing old limits. *J Pediatr Surg* 1993;28:1069–1071.

Thompson JS, Langnas AN, Pinch LW, et al. Surgical approach to short bowel syndrome. *Ann Surg* 1995;222:600–607.

Touloukian RJ, Smith GJ. Normal intestinal length in preterm infants. J Pediatr Surg 1983;18:720–723.

Venables CW, Ellis H, Smith ADM. Antiperistaltic segments after massive resections. *Lancet* 1966;2:1390–1394.

53

SUPERIOR MESENTERIC ARTERY SYNDROME

J. DAVID HOOVER
ROBERT M. ARENSMAN

Superior mesenteric artery syndrome, Wilkie's syndrome, and vascular compression of the duodenum all describe an entity in which the third portion of the duodenum is compressed by the overlying vessels, usually the superior mesenteric artery (SMA) or the middle colic artery.

DIAGNOSIS

Patients with SMA syndrome develop intermittent upper gastrointestinal obstruction with bilious emesis and malnutrition. The malnutrition is a key component of this entity. The SMA normally comes off the aorta at 44 degrees and crosses the duodenum 19 mm above the aorta. With loss of mesenteric fat, the angle may narrow to 8 degrees and the distance may decrease to 8 mm. Another factor that predisposes a given patient to obstruction is a prolonged recumbent position, for example, children in a spica cast or with severe neurologic impairment leading to prolonged bed rest.

The diagnosis is suspected when a child with known risk factors (weight loss, positional constraints) presents with bilious emesis. These children often present with profound malnutrition and severe electrolyte abnormalities (hypochloremia, hypokalemia, hyponatremia, alkalosis). Once electrolyte abnormalities have been addressed, the diagnosis is confirmed with radiologic studies. The classic study is a contrast upper gastrointestinal study with duodenography. This generally demonstrates an abrupt, nontapered cutoff of the duodenum in the midline with to-and-fro movement of contrast in the second portion of the duodenum suggestive of an obstruction. More importantly, there should be circumstantial evidence of a chronic duodenal obstruction, such as a dilated stomach and proximal duodenum with residual fluid despite an adequate interval for emptying. An indentation of the duodenum by the vessels is a normal variant and should not be considered sufficient evidence of an SMA syndrome without proper clinical and radiographic correlates. Recent literature supports the use of spiral computed tomography with intravenous and oral contrast and three-dimensional angiographic reconstruction. This obviates the need for angiography but allows spatial visualization of the artery and the site of the obstruction.

TREATMENT

Most patients with SMA syndrome are initially treated conservatively. Nonoperative management involves the placement of a nasojejunal feeding tube with the tip placed beyond the site of obstruction. Patients with a high-grade obstruction cannot tolerate their own secretions and also may require placement of a gastric tube for continuous gastric drainage. Because the gastric decompression volume may be large and contains most of the bile, it is important to refeed the gastric drainage into the jejunal feeding tube to prevent fluid losses and maintain normal enterohepatic biliary circulation. Enteral nutrition is the primary treatment, but parenteral nutrition can be used as a supplement if there is any question that the patient is tolerating or absorbing the enteral nutrition. As the patient gains weight, the obstruction gradually resolves. The gastric tube becomes unnecessary first, followed by removal of the feeding tube. This generally takes about 4 to 6 weeks, but may take longer, especially if the patient remains in a recumbent position.

Surgical therapy is rarely necessary. There are two procedures described for the treatment of SMA syndrome. The first is a release of the ligament of Treitz. The aim of this procedure is to alleviate the obstruction by moving the duo-

J.D. Hoover: Departments of Surgery and Pediatrics, Northwestern Memorial Hospital; and Department of Pediatric General Surgery, Children's Memorial Hospital, Chicago, Illinois.

R.M. Arensman: Departments of Surgery and Pediatrics, Northwestern University Medical School; and Department of Pediatric General Surgery, Children's Memorial Hospital, Chicago, Illinois denum from under the compressing artery. This is achieved by dividing the ligament of Treitz and mobilizing the duodenum so that it comes to lie to the right of the midline. The ascending colon is mobilized so the small bowel lies on the right side of the abdomen and the colon lies on the left side. This is similar to the Ladd procedure for malrotation. An appendectomy is performed because the appendix is generally displaced with this procedure. Patients often develop prolonged delayed gastric emptying and duodenal dysmotility after extensive mobilization of the duodenum. Nasojejunal and nasogastric tubes are often placed to provide postoperative decompression and allow early enteral feedings.

An alternative surgical approach is bypass of the obstructed segment. Enteric bypass is sometimes performed in conjunction with the release procedure and can be in the form of duodenojejunostomy or gastrojejunostomy. These are performed in standard fashion, using basic general surgical techniques. It should be emphasized that these are rarely performed procedures that are associated with significant complications and a significant rate of failure.

Medical management is attempted first, although placement of a nasojejunal feeding tube can sometimes be difficult. Positioning the child prone or even on all fours can allow passage of the feeding tube. Fluoroscopy is nearly always required. If the child cannot be maintained long-term with nasal tubes, then a gastrostomy with a jejunal tube through the gastrostomy tube may be used. Even if medical treatment lasts only a few days, it may provide enough nutrition to minimize the potential operative complications of enteric surgery in these malnourished patients.

If medical treatment fails, then operative intervention is used. Because these patients are malnourished, minimally invasive surgery is an attractive option. There is new literature that supports a laparoscopic approach for the ligament of Treitz release and even duodenojejunostomy.

Enteric bypass has the highest potential complication rate because an anastomosis is being performed on dilated, edematous, atonic bowel. Furthermore, when therapies are compared in a retrospective fashion, bypassed patients have a longer convalescence and longer time to return of bowel function than those patients treated with release alone.

SUMMARY

Superior mesenteric artery syndrome is a confounding problem of ongoing malnutrition and duodenal obstruction. It requires a high index of suspicion to make the diagnosis in a timely matter. Once the diagnosis is confirmed, every attempt is made to manage the obstruction without surgery. Should this fail, ligament of Treitz release or enteric bypass is undertaken.

SUGGESTED READINGS

Akin JT, Gary SW, Skandalakis JE. Vascular compression of the duodenum: presentation of ten cases and review of the literature. *Surgery* 1976;79:515–522.

Konen E, Amitai M, Itzchak Y. CT angiography of superior mesenteric artery syndrome. *AJR* 1998;171:1279–1281.

Ylinen P, Kinnumen J, Kockerstedt K. Superior mesenteric artery syndrome, a follow-up of 16 patients. *J Clin Gastroenterol* 1989;11: 386–391.

54

NEONATAL INTESTINAL OBSTRUCTION

MICHAEL L. NANCE

Bowel obstruction in the newborn is a surgical emergency. A successful outcome in this setting is often dependent on timely diagnosis and intervention. The differential diagnosis and ultimate decision to operate are based on a review of the available history, the findings on physical examination, and the results of diagnostic studies, if needed. After evaluation of the clinical information, however, not all neonates with a picture suggesting bowel obstruction will have an underlying cause requiring surgical attention (Table 54.1).

INITIAL ASSESSMENT

Evaluation begins with a review of maternal and familial history. A maternal history of diabetes mellitus, for example may be associated with small left colon syndrome in the newborn. Other factors, such as a familial history of cystic fibrosis or a known chromosomal abnormality, will impact the differential diagnostic possibilities. A family history of a prior congenital abnormality, such as Hirschsprung's disease, should raise the possibility of a similar occurrence in subsequent pregnancies. Increasingly, prenatal ultrasonography can be used to demonstrate abnormalities that may be associated with a bowel obstruction. Maternal polyhydramnios or a dilated gastric silhouette, for instance, may be seen with a proximal obstruction such as duodenal atresia or annular pancreas. This knowledge may help direct the perinatal course, perhaps including the decision to deliver at or near a center with capabilities to manage the newborn surgical issues.

Anatomically, intestinal obstruction can occur anywhere from the esophagus to the anus; thus, the presentation may vary significantly. Causes can be categorized broadly into a proximal or distal site of obstruction (Tables 54.2 and 54.3). The postnatal history and sequence of events leading to diagnosis are important. The hallmark of neonatal bowel obstruction is bilious emesis and abdominal distention, a presentation that should be considered malrotation with volvulus until proven otherwise. However, not all cases of obstruction present with bilious emesis (including malrotation) and not all newborns with bilious emesis have malrotation. In addition to malrotation with volvulus, bilious emesis also may be seen in the setting of a distal bowel obstruction such as Hirschsprung's disease or colonic atresia. A history of nonbilious emesis, in contrast, usually suggests a much more proximal site of obstruction (proximal to the ampulla of Vater), such as a duodenal atresia or pyloric web. Intestinal obstruction also may manifest initially not with emesis, but with delayed or no passage of meconium, as may be seen with conditions such as Hirschsprung's disease or imperforate anus. Although most causes of bowel obstruction in the newborn follow a characteristic course, variability does exist, and correlation of the newborn history with physical findings is essential.

Physical examination of the newborn with suspected bowel obstruction must be thorough to help characterize the problem and to identify other associated abnormalities. For instance, morphologic features suggesting Down syndrome may be noted in a newborn with suspected duodenal atresia. A cardiac murmur might suggest associated heart disease that can be seen in newborns with the VATER association and imperforate anus. The abdomen in a newborn with a bowel obstruction can be scaphoid if the obstruction is very proximal or distended if a blockage is more distal. The timing of abdominal distension is also important. Infants with conditions such as meconium ileus are usually born with significant abdominal distension.

TABLE 54.1. NONSURGICAL CONDITIONS MIMICKING INTESTINAL OBSTRUCTION

Sepsis (with ileus)
Hypothyroidism (with ileus)
Increased intracranial pressure (hydrocephalus, intracranial hemorrhage)
Uremia (polycystic disease, agenesis)
Meconium ileus
Meconium plug syndrome
Small left colon syndrome

M. L. Nance: Department of Surgery, University of Pennsylvania; and Department of Surgery, Children's Hospital of Philadelphia, Philadelphia, Pennsylvania.

TABLE 54.2. CAUSES OF NEWBORN INTESTINAL OBSTRUCTION (PROXIMAL)

Esophageal atresia
Duodenal atresia
Annular pancreas
Preduodenal portal vein
Jejunal/ileal atresia
Omphalomesenteric duct remnant
Incarcerated inguinal hernia
Malrotation with volvulus

TABLE 54.3. CAUSES OF NEWBORN INTESTINAL OBSTRUCTION (DISTAL)

Meconium ileus
Colonic atresia
Hirschsprung disease
Imperforate anus
Meconium plug syndrome
Small left colon syndrome

With other causes of bowel obstruction such as jejunal/ileal atresia, abdominal distension is a later finding, developing after initiation of feedings. Percussion of the abdomen may reveal dullness as might be associated with ascites or tympany with free intraabdominal air. Tenderness may be due to distension of the visceral peritoneum or irritation of the parietal peritoneum. The presence or absence of bowel sounds and the character of bowel sounds are not reliable indicators of a bowel obstruction in the newborn. As such, bowel sounds rarely add much information during the diagnostic evaluation. Abdominal wall erythema is a later finding and suggests perforation with focal inflammation. Confirmation of the presence and normal positioning of the anus is important in the newborn who fails to pass meconium. An imperforate anus is usually apparent on inspection but on occasion will be missed if a fistula is present and meconium on the perineum is interpreted as a normal perineum without visualizing the anal orifice. Although rarely a cause of bowel obstruction in the newborn, incarcerated hernia should be considered and ruled out by a thorough physical examination.

DIAGNOSTIC WORKUP

Radiologic studies are useful in evaluating the newborn with a suspected bowel obstruction. Radiologic assessment typically begins with an abdominal flat plate to determine the bowel gas pattern. In cases of suspected esophageal atresia, chest radiography is also performed and demonstrates a coiled nasogastric tube within the proximal pouch. In addition, radiographic evaluation helps determine if a tracheoesophageal fistula is present. The absence of abdominal gas suggests a pure esophageal atresia, whereas the presence of intestinal air confirms the presence of a fistulous communication. In other cases of suspected intestinal obstruction, a paucity of gas suggests a proximal obstruction such as a duodenal web or volvulus but may also be present in the setting of profound sepsis with an ileus. Typically, however, ileus is characterized by a uniform dilation of the bowel with air down to the rectum. In contrast, cases of intestinal obstruction often demonstrate bowel loops of varying size, a result of proximal distension and distal decompression. The finding of a "double bubble" suggests an obstruction just distal to the pylorus as with duodenal atresia or annular pancreas and represents the dilated stomach bubble and dilated proximal duodenum. Numerous dilated loops of bowel may be noted in the case of a distal bowel obstruction such as Hirschsprung's disease or colonic atresia. Absence of air in the rectum also may signify a distal obstruction. Additional views of the abdomen such as a cross-table lateral or decubitus film may reveal air-fluid levels or free intraperitoneal air. A cross-table lateral film obtained with the infant in the prone position may help detect the presence of air within the rectum. Areas of speckled calcification on a plain film may be observed with cases of complicated meconium ileus and perforation. In addition to routine plain films of the abdomen, a small volume of air can be instilled via the nasogastric tube to act as a contrast agent. This may further delineate the level of a proximal bowel obstruction. Finally, caution should be exercised in interpretation of the abdominal radiograph, because it is not possible to definitively distinguish dilated small bowel from dilated colon. Therefore, determining the level of obstruction based on plain film alone may be unwise.

Frequently, contrast-enhanced radiographic studies are needed to confirm the diagnosis during the workup of a newborn bowel obstruction. In the setting of bilious emesis for which a proximal obstructive source is suspected, an upper gastrointestinal series would be most diagnostic. If the source is thought to be distal, a contrast enema is the test of choice. In most cases, contrast can be refluxed through the ileocecal valve to provide information about the distal small bowel. On occasion, the clinical findings are insufficient to narrow the possible diagnoses, and both an upper gastrointestinal (UGI) series and a contrast enema are necessary. In this case, these concerns should be communicated to the radiologist, and a limited UGI series can be performed to determine the location of the ligament of Treitz; if results are normal, a contrast enema may follow. It must be remembered that a contrast enema, obtained in the first few days of life, may not demonstrate the characteristic transition zone associated with Hirschsprung's disease. In this case, clinical suspicion of Hirschsprung's disease merits suction rectal biopsy to exclude the diagnosis.

Additional diagnostic studies may be indicated during the evaluation. In a newborn with VATER features, for example, ultrasonography of the abdomen to evaluate the kidneys and the spine to exclude a tethered cord, as well as spine films to look for vertebral anomalies, will be necessary. In the newborn demonstrated to have a small left colon or meconium plug syndrome, or who is indeterminate for Hirschsprung's disease by contrast enema, a suction rectal biopsy is indicated.

Resuscitation should be ongoing during evaluation of the newborn with a bowel obstruction. If deterioration in a newborn's condition occurs during the evaluation for a possible bowel obstruction, urgent laparotomy must be considered. Nasal or orogastric decompression is mandated to minimize additional bowel distension and lessen the risk of aspiration at the time of anesthetic induction. In the child with esophageal atresia, a Replogle tube (with suction holes located only at the distalmost portion of the tube) is preferred for decompression of the pouch to prevent aspiration of secretions. Newborns with a possible bowel obstruction are maintained with nothing by mouth, and should be provided with maintenance intravenous fluids. Careful attention to the electrolytes is necessary because third spacing of fluids and nasogastric losses may be significant. In the newborn undergoing gastrograffin enema for possible meconium ileus, adequate hydration is necessary to prevent hemodynamic collapse that may develop following the intraluminal migration of fluids associated with the hydrophilic contrast agent. A specimen should be sent to the blood bank in preparation for operative intervention. Antibiotics are generally given to these patients to minimize the risk of bacterial translocation in the compromised or dilated bowel and because neonatal sepsis is often in the differential diagnosis. Specific bacterial endocarditis prophylaxis also may be indicated in this population. A newborn with an abnormal cardiac murmur may require an echocardiographic study prior to operative intervention to help guide fluid management during and after surgery.

Intraoperative management of an intestinal obstruction is guided by the pathology identified and is discussed in other chapters.

EDITOR'S NOTES

Bowel obstruction in the newborn can present in a variety of ways, ranging from subtle feeding intolerance to the rapid deterioration seen in some cases when bowel viability is compromised. Because there is no correlation between the severity of the presenting illness and the degree or nature of the obstruction, and specifically because even malrotation with midgut volvulus can present with seemingly minor symptoms, every newborn with suspected bowel obstruction should be evaluated thoroughly and emergently. A useful diagnostic approach is described nicely in this chapter.

Although the differential diagnosis of neonatal bowel obstruction is relatively finite and well understood by pediatric surgeons, generalizations and rigid application of a diagnostic algorithm should be avoided. Every child should be evaluated in a thoughtful and systematic way, considering the unique circumstances of their particular case. This is especially true of the patient with peritonitis or signs of impending clinical deterioration: these patients are better served by emergent resuscitation and laparotomy, rather than a trip to the medical imaging suite for a study. Likewise, unequivocal clinical or radiographic evidence of bowel obstruction is an indication for laparotomy, even when a specific diagnosis has eluded the radiologist.

Most of the time, a diagnosis can be made or suggested on the basis of physical examination and plain radiography, in which case contrast studies may be unnecessary. A thorough physical examination should be performed by the surgeon. Incarcerated inguinal hernia and imperforate anus should be specifically ruled out. Evidence of peritonitis or abdominal wall cellulitis are clear indications for laparotomy. Many patients, however, demonstrate few if any diagnostic clues as to the etiology of the obstruction, and will therefore need abdominal radiography. If the bowel gas pattern is nonspecific or normal, assuming the child is clinically stable, contrast studies may then be indicated.

The upper gastrointestinal study is useful only to document the normal location of the ligament of Treitz (to rule out malrotation) and is not used to define the cause or anatomic location of the obstruction. To attempt to do so results in a potentially dangerous delay in definitive management, places the child at risk for hypothermia and sepsis, fills the bowel with barium (which can cause problems at laparotomy), and is nearly always unnecessary. An exception might be the rare case of suspected ileus in which the likelihood of obstruction is felt to be extremely low but needs to be ruled out by a modified small bowel follow-through study.

In contrast, unless they require urgent laparotomy, many infants with what appears to be a distal bowel obstruction will benefit from a contrast enema. The goal is to rule out several specific conditions that may not require immediate operation, such as meconium plug syndrome or meconium ileus, and can help determine the more appropriate operation in some cases of Hirschsprung's disease. If the contrast enema reveals an unused colon (microcolon) the radiologist should convert to water-soluble contrast and reflux the contrast into the distal ileum to look for meconium ileus. In most other cases, the contrast enema is not intended to confirm the cause or location of the obstruction, but to diagnose or rule out the conditions described above. The diagnostic workup should be discussed with the radiologist ahead of time, especially if it is likely that both an upper contrast study and an enema will be required. Some clinicians may prefer to administer the contrast enema first, followed by a UGI series if the results of the enema are negative, whereas others would prefer to reverse the order of the studies.

The surgical management of specific causes of bowel obstruction are discussed elsewhere in this book. There are times when the cause of the obstruction is unknown prior to laparotomy. A standard approach is to explore the abdomen through a right upper quadrant transverse incision. This allows access to the anatomic sites most commonly involved with an obstruction: the duodenum, the mesentery, and the distal ileum. Perhaps Hirschsprung's disease is a condition not easily managed with this approach, but it is unusual not to have considered this diagnosis prior to exploration. If a sigmoid transition zone is found, the incision can be extended to the left side if necessary, or a second incision can be made in the left lower quadrant. The parents should be told what the most likely diagnoses are and that the treatment of the obstruction might involve bowel resection and primary anastomosis or creation of a stoma. Rarely does laparotomy reveal no evidence of a mechanical obstruction. A transition zone (most commonly in the distal ileum) should be sought and multiple seromuscular biopsy samples taken to rule out Hirschsprung's disease. Appendectomy has been traditionally recommended in these cases to provide tissue to confirm the presence of ganglion cells. However, unless the cecum is in an abnormal location, consideration should be given to preserving the appendix in the event that the patient develops severe chronic constipation, in which case the appendix may be a useful conduit for antegrade enema in the future.

–P.M.

SUGGESTED READINGS

Hernanz-Schulman M. Imaging of neonatal gastrointestinal obstruction. *Radiol Clin North Am* 1999;37:1163–1186.

Jona JZ. Advances in neonatal surgery. *Pediatr Clin North Am* 1998; 45:605–617.

Oldham KT. Introduction to neonatal intestinal obstruction. In: KT Oldham, PM Colombani, RP Foglia, eds. *Surgery of infants and children: scientific principles and practice, 1st ed.* Philadelphia: Lippincott-Raven, 1997:1181–1182.

Ross AJ. Intestinal obstruction in the newborn. *Pediatr Rev* 1994;15: 338–347.

Surgical Directives: Pediatric Surgery, edited by Peter Mattei. Lippincott Williams & Wilkins, Philadelphia © 2002

55

MECONIUM ILEUS

PETER MATTEI

Meconium ileus is a distal small bowel obstruction caused by inspissated meconium in the newborn. It is associated with cystic fibrosis in most cases, and up to 20% of newborns with cystic fibrosis present with meconium ileus. Although sometimes treatable by nonoperative means, many of these infants require laparotomy and can have ongoing difficulty with bowel function related to their cystic fibrosis. Presumably, enzymatic insufficiency leads to extremely viscous meconium that cannot pass through the ileum, although why some infants with cystic fibrosis develop meconium ileus and others do not remains unclear.

As with other causes of bowel obstruction, meconium ileus also can give rise to volvulus, ischemia, and perforation. This form of "complicated" meconium ileus can occur *in utero* and may result in intestinal atresia, short bowel syndrome, or meconium peritonitis, which itself can cause ascites, intraperitoneal calcifications, or meconium pseudocysts. Antenatal ultrasonography may detect dilated loops of bowel or ascites, but except for the occasional case of polyhydramnios related to a more proximal volvulus or atresia, most are not detected before birth.

DIAGNOSIS

Meconium ileus must be considered in the differential diagnosis of any newborn infant with a bowel obstruction or failure to pass meconium in the first few days of life. Most are otherwise well-appearing newborns who present with feeding intolerance or bilious emesis and progressive abdominal distension. The remainder of the physical examination is often unremarkable, and the family history is positive for cystic fibrosis in less than one third of cases. The differential diagnosis of newborn bowel obstruction includes intestinal atresia, volvulus, meconium plug syndrome, and Hirschsprung's disease.

P. Mattei: Department of Surgery, Thomas Jefferson University, Philadelphia, Pennsylvania; and Department of Pediatric Surgery, Alfred I. duPont Hospital for Children, Wilmington, Delaware.

The next step in the diagnostic workup is plain radiography of the abdomen. This usually demonstrates dilated air-filled loops of bowel consistent with a distal obstruction. A large amount of retained meconium with a ground-glass or soap bubble appearance (the Neuhauser's sign) is highly suggestive of meconium ileus (Fig. 55.1). On the other hand, the presence of air-fluid levels makes the diagnosis less likely, given that the highly viscous meconium does not layer out very easily. The presence of peritoneal calcifications suggests the diagnosis of complicated meconium ileus with *in utero* perforation and subsequent meconium peritonitis.

Patients who are clinically well with no evidence of perforation or ischemic bowel should be given a contrast enema. Prophylactic antibiotics (ampicillin and gentamicin) are given before the study is undertaken. A contrast study will confirm and treat meconium plug syndrome and might suggest the diagnosis of Hirschsprung's disease or small left colon syndrome. If the findings include a microcolon, then a diagnosis of intestinal atresia or meconium ileus is most likely. It is in this situation that the pediatric radiologist should attempt to reflux the contrast material into the ileum. If there are filling defects in the terminal ileum consistent with pellets of meconium, then the diagnosis of meconium ileus is confirmed. Further retrograde progress of the contrast column will reveal a much more dilated segment of ileum filled with meconium (Fig. 55.2). The contrast itself may help to evacuate the meconium and thus alleviate the obstruction.

The choice of contrast material probably matters very little, although the traditional recommendation is diatrizoate meglumine (Gastrografin, Schering Diagnostics, Berlin, Germany). Gastrografin formulations in the past included a wetting agent, polysorbate 80 (Tween-80, Unigema, New Castle, Delaware), which perhaps made it a superior solvent for evacuation of inspissated meconium. Current formulations do not contain Tween-80, and although its high osmolarity (1,900 mOsm/L) might give it a theoretic advantage, many clinicians feel that other agents may be just as effective (or ineffective). Others have added Tween-80 or acetylcysteine to the contrast material and feel

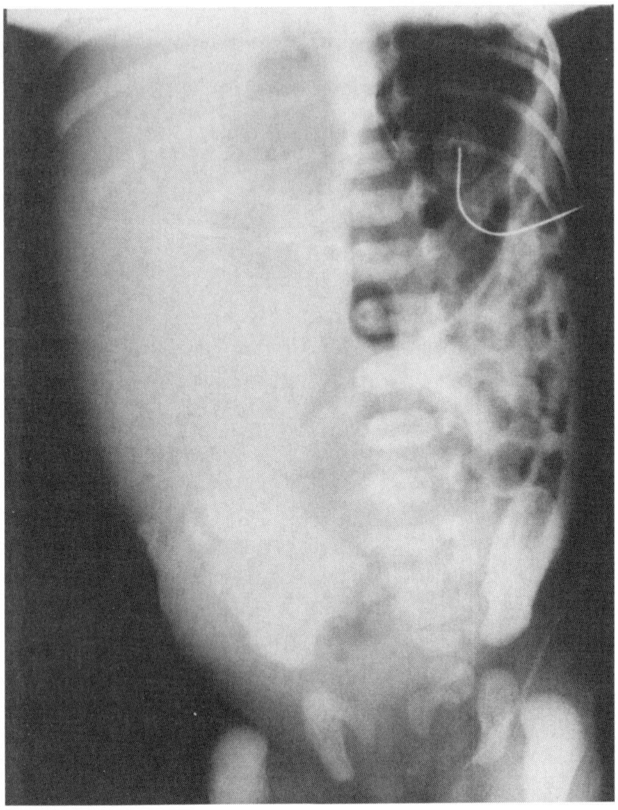

FIGURE 55.1. Plain radiograph of an infant with meconium ileus. Note the dilated loops suggestive of obstruction, the paucity of gas in the right lower quadrant, and the ground-glass appearance of meconium.

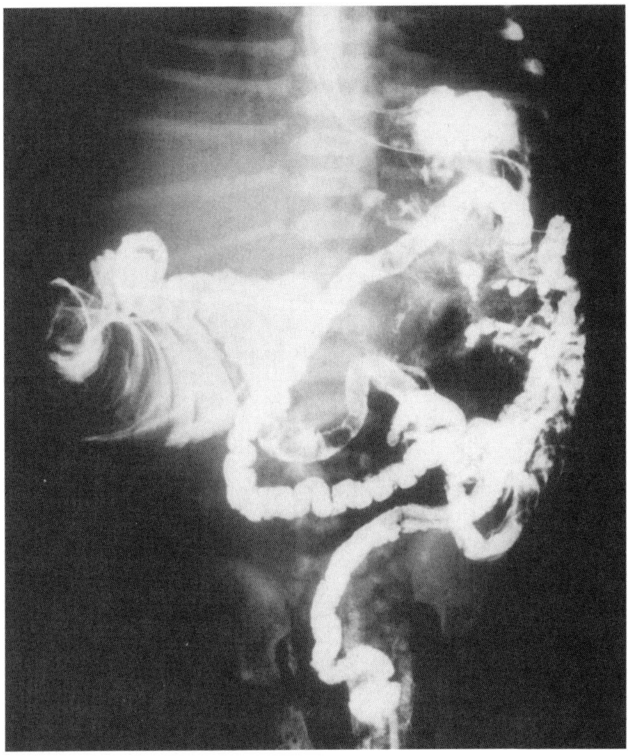

FIGURE 55.2. Contrast enema in a patient with meconium ileus. Note the small caliber of the unused microcolon, the filling defects in the ileum (meconium pellets) and the hugely dilated bowel proximal to the obstruction.

that this improves their results. Nevertheless, most of us are bound by the preferences and experience of the radiologists at our respective institutions, which I suspect is the most important factor of all. Some radiologists are comfortable with the technique and are therefore more aggressive, whereas others are less likely to keep trying due to a concern about the potential for a bowel perforation. Up to half or more of the babies with meconium ileus may have a successful clean-out with the contrast enema, although in most centers the actual success rate is probably lower.

Total colonic aganglionosis (long-segment Hirschsprung's disease) may present with a clinical and radiographic picture indistinguishable from meconium ileus. If the obstruction is alleviated by contrast enema, aganglionosis should be ruled out by suction rectal biopsy. If a laparotomy is performed, the appendix can be evaluated for the presence of ganglion cells, which will rule out colonic aganglionosis with rare exception. Not all babies with meconium ileus have cystic fibrosis, although the proportion who do not is unknown and likely varies considerably between populations. It is especially in these infants that aganglionosis coli needs to be ruled out with certainty.

The diagnosis of cystic fibrosis is best made by measurement of sweat chloride after the collection of sweat using pilocarpine iontophoresis. The test is not always useful, however, in the first few weeks of life. Genetic testing can be performed on a buccal smear or blood sample, but current genetic testing only detects approximately 95% of all mutations. Some state newborn screens include measurement of immunoreactive trypsinogen using standard blood collection blots, as used for other screening studies. However, the results often take weeks to process and need to be confirmed with more definitive tests because of a high false-positive rate. Nonetheless, all infants with meconium ileus are treated as though they have cystic fibrosis until the diagnosis can be ruled out with sweat chloride testing. General support and genetic counseling should be available for the families of these infants while the diagnosis is being confirmed.

TREATMENT

Nonoperative therapy is possible if the contrast enema is successful in clearing a significant amount of meconium, although sometimes the enema needs to be repeated. These patients are maintained on bowel rest initially. Adequate intravenous hydration is provided and is especially important if high-osmolarity enema solutions have been used.

Standard management includes 10% acetylcysteine (Mucomyst) administered by orogastric tube at a dose of 10 mL every 6 hours for up to a week. Acetylcysteine is a mucolytic that is particularly effective in loosening meconium in these babies. The enema should be repeated if signs of obstruction recur. These infants also need to be assessed frequently for evidence of bowel perforation related to the obstruction or the enemas. When all signs of obstruction have resolved, enteral feedings can be started and advanced cautiously. Pancreatic enzyme supplements are provided when feedings start.

Some babies with meconium ileus complicated by *in utero* perforation can be treated nonoperatively, although most require laparotomy. The exceptions are infants with peritoneal (or scrotal) calcifications on radiography who are presumed to have had meconium peritonitis but who show no signs of obstruction and are passing meconium spontaneously. These infants may warrant a cautious feeding trial in addition to a workup for cystic fibrosis. More often, the calcifications are identified in an infant being evaluated for obstruction, in which case laparotomy is indicated without further studies.

Patients who fail nonoperative therapy should undergo laparotomy. The parents are informed that the goal is to remove the inspissated meconium but that a bowel resection, stoma, or tube ileostomy may be necessary, depending on the operative findings. A transverse right upper abdominal incision is made, and the dilated ileum is delivered (Fig. 55.3). The cecum may need to be gently mobilized, and the peritoneum should be protected from contamination with moist packs. Simple meconium ileus, with no evidence of perforation, volvulus, or atresia, is best treated by irrigation. An enterotomy is made on the antimesenteric border of the dilated ileum for instillation of irrigation solution and evacuation of the meconium. Although saline solution is used by some surgeons with good results, the preferred irrigant is acetylcysteine. Acetylcysteine comes in 10% and 20% solutions and can be diluted with saline or water to a final concentration of 4%. A 10 or 12 French rubber catheter is used to instill the irrigation solution, which usually allows the tar-like meconium to be removed easily from the bowel lumen via the enterotomy (Fig. 55.4). The acetylcysteine also should be instilled distally to allow further evacuation of meconium from the colon. After removal of the meconium, the enterotomy is closed transversely in two layers and an appendectomy is performed. The pathologist should be made aware that the appendix needs to be evaluated specifically for the presence of ganglion cells. Histologic examination of the appendix also might reveal mucous plugging of the crypts and exuberant intraluminal mucinous material, which are suggestive of cystic fibrosis. At the conclusion of the procedure, especially if a large amount of meconium was seen to pass into the colon, a gentle anal dilatation and rectal irrigation should be performed.

Although enterotomy and bowel irrigation is a useful approach in most cases of simple meconium ileus, a modified technique is occasionally necessitated by the operative findings. In the past, it was common practice to treat all infants with meconium ileus with an ileostomy. This was felt to be necessary to facilitate postoperative irrigation and evacuation of meconium. Although no longer used rou-

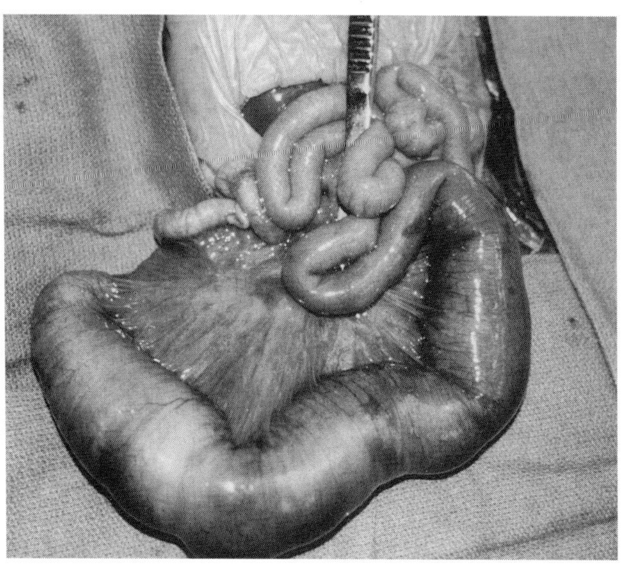

FIGURE 55.3. Operative findings in a patient with meconium ileus. There is a gradual tapering of the ileum, which is filled with inspissated meconium.

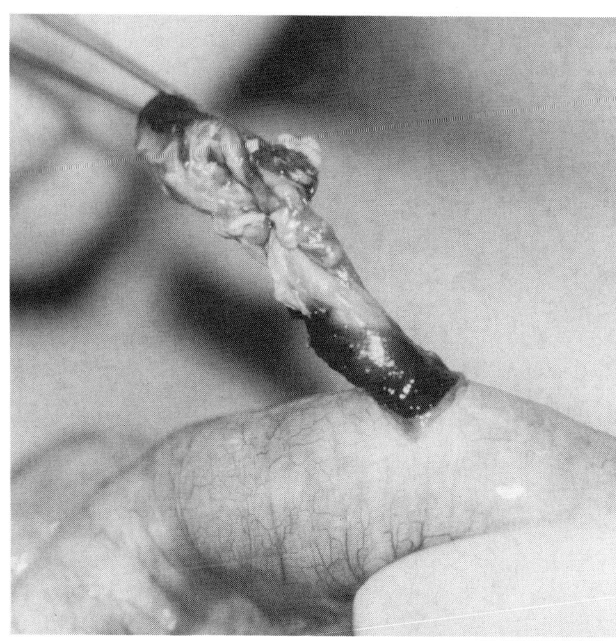

FIGURE 55.4. The meconium has the consistency of tar and can be pulled out from the lumen via the enterostomy in large pieces.

tinely, the various stoma operations described should be part of the armamentarium of the pediatric surgeon (Fig. 55.5). The Bishop-Koop ileostomy is a Roux-en-Y construct in which the distal limb is brought out as an end stoma and the proximal bowel is anastomosed end to side. This procedure produced excellent results, and was commonly used in the past. The Santulli-Blanc operation creates a proximal stoma and the distal bowel is sewn end to side to it. The Mikulicz operation was widely used at one time for many indications and consists of a double-barrel stoma in which the two ends are sutured together side to side for some length proximal to the end of the stoma. It was designed for bedside stoma closure in which the common wall was crushed and obliterated with a specially designed clamp (Mikulicz clamp) and the bowel ends were closed over the top. This operation is rarely used today. Another useful option is a tube ileostomy. A small-caliber rubber tube is placed through a small enterotomy and secured with a purse-string suture. The bowel is tacked to the fascia in standard fashion with the tube exiting through a small stab incision. This allows instillation of irrigant solution directly into the ileum without the creation of an ileostomy. Of course, a conventional end or loop ileostomy may be necessary if peritonitis or obstruction precludes a safe anastomosis after bowel resection or volvulus.

The approach to complicated meconium ileus is the same as for any complicated intestinal process, and includes an extensive lysis of adhesions, careful inspection of the bowel with possible bowel resection, and evacuation of inspissated meconium, if necessary. Perforations may be amenable to primary repair if a distal obstruction can be safely excluded. If a bowel resection is felt to be necessary, a judgment is made whether primary anastomosis is feasible or a stoma is necessary, based on the condition of the bowel, the likelihood of a distal obstruction, and the overall condition of the patient. The fibrous wall of the pseudocyst is debrided without sacrificing viable intestine. Meconium peritonitis can cause obstruction due to adhesions, requiring extensive adhesiolysis. The adhesions are typically dense and very vascular. It is not necessary to perform a radical debridement of all meconium or calcified plaque that is encountered, as long as the obstruction is relieved. Appendectomy should be performed to rule out long-segment Hirschsprung's disease and to avoid diagnostic confusion in the future. A gastrostomy should be considered in infants with complicated meconium ileus, especially if extensive

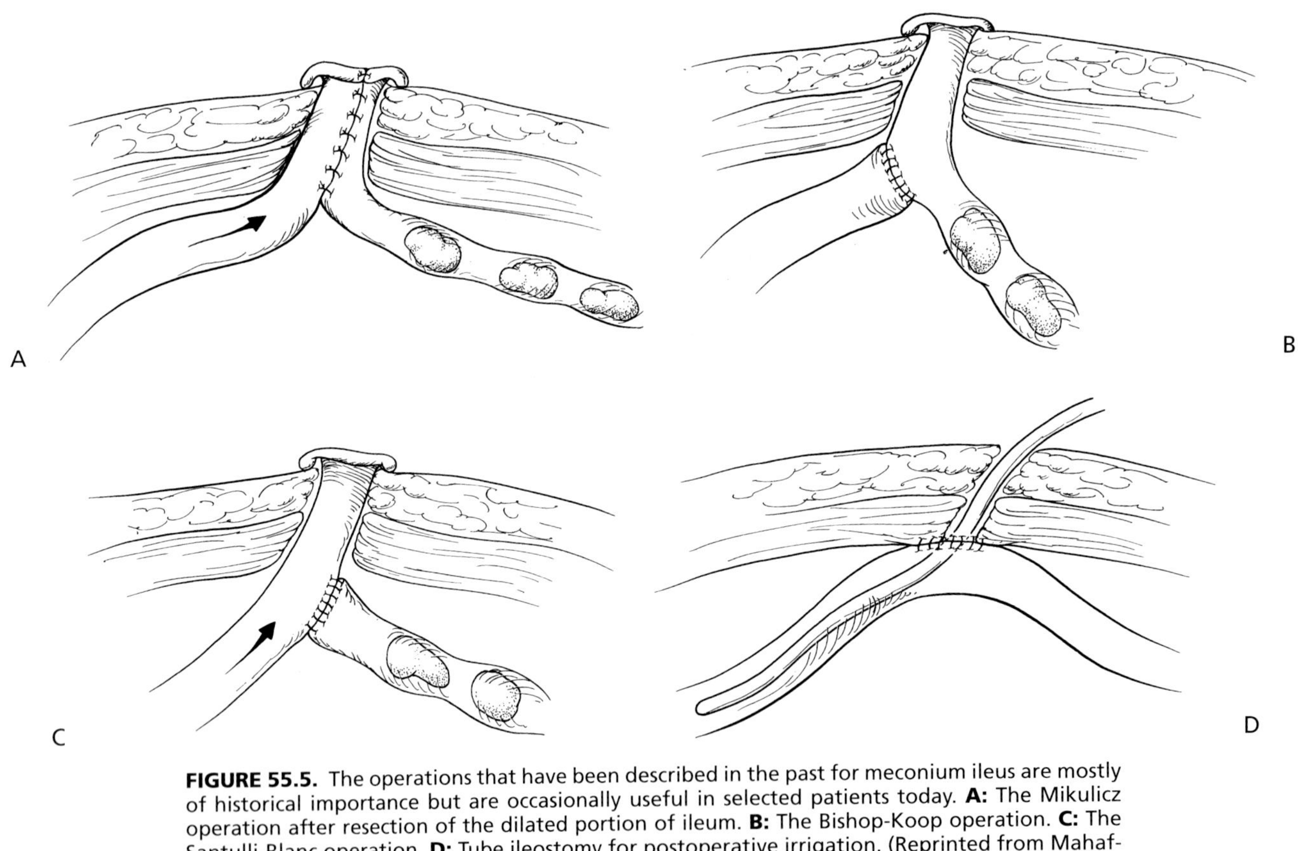

FIGURE 55.5. The operations that have been described in the past for meconium ileus are mostly of historical importance but are occasionally useful in selected patients today. **A:** The Mikulicz operation after resection of the dilated portion of ileum. **B:** The Bishop-Koop operation. **C:** The Santulli-Blanc operation. **D:** Tube ileostomy for postoperative irrigation. (Reprinted from Mahaffey SM. Meconium syndromes and cystic fibrosis. In: Oldham KT, Colombani PM, Foglia RP, eds. *Surgery of infants and children: scientific principles and practice.* Philadelphia: Lippincott-Raven, 1997; with permission.)

bowel resection is necessary. Most infants will also need central venous access for parenteral nutrition during the postoperative period.

POSTOPERATIVE CARE

Patients are initially on bowel rest and are given acetylcysteine by gastric tube as described above for nonoperative management. Rectal irrigations may be necessary as well. Most eventually establish a normal stooling pattern and can be advanced on feedings within 1 to 2 weeks. Patients should be maintained on parenteral nutrition in the meantime. Recurrence is uncommon and treatment can be attempted using contrast enema, if necessary. Reoperation may suggest the need for ileostomy and a more definitive workup for Hirschsprung's disease.

Infants with meconium ileus require an extensive workup involving multiple pediatric subspecialists, including gastroenterologists, geneticists, pulmonologists, and pediatric surgeons. Family support should include access to counseling services and social work assistance. Patients are initially followed in the surgery office as after any major abdominal procedure, and the surgeon may need to become involved again later for issues related to feeding access, central venous access and stoma care. Stomas can be taken down after the standard 4 to 6 weeks, according to the usual criteria of adequate weight gain and resolution of symptoms. A distal contrast study should be performed to rule out obstruction prior to reanastomosis.

Short-term complications are uncommon in infants with simple meconium ileus. Long-term complications are generally those common to patients with cystic fibrosis. Patients also may present years later with bowel obstruction. Those with a history of meconium peritonitis or laparotomy may have obstruction due to adhesions or segmental volvulus, but other diagnoses need to be considered. For example, patients with cystic fibrosis are more susceptible to intussusception. The intussusception can be of the conventional ileocolic variety seen in patients under the age of 3, but also may be ileoileal and can occur in older children. Appendicitis appears to be more common in patients with cystic fibrosis, and when associated with perforation and phlegmon can be a cause of bowel obstruction or severe ileus. Inguinal hernias are also more common in this population and, as in other patients, can be a cause of obstruction due to incarceration. High-dose pancreatic enzyme supplementation has been associated with the development of colonic strictures. These are diagnosed by contrast enema and are usually treated with resection and anastomosis. Finally, older patients may develop meconium ileus equivalent, an obstruction caused by inspissated stool in the ileum and colon. Many of these patients can be treated initially with decompression and enemas, although some eventually require laparotomy. The cause is unknown but is presumably related to the viscosity of intestinal mucus.

In summary, meconium ileus is a cause of bowel obstruction in the newborn and mainly affects infants with cystic fibrosis. The diagnosis is confirmed with contrast enema, which can sometimes also be therapeutic. Patients with complications related to the obstruction, including volvulus, perforation, or atresia, and those who fail nonoperative management require operative intervention. At laparotomy, the conventional approach for simple meconium ileus is to irrigate the bowel lumen with acetylcysteine through a small enterotomy, which facilitates evacuation of the highly viscous meconium. Patients with complicated disease may require bowel resection, tube enterostomy, or creation of a stoma, many varieties of which have been described over the years for management of the disease. Most patients respond well to therapy in the short-term but need to be followed closely for complications related to their underlying disease. This includes bowel obstruction, which has many potential causes in these patients.

SUGGESTED READINGS

DelPin CA, Czyrko C, Ziegler MM, et al. Management and survival of meconium ileus, a 30-year review. *Ann Surg* 1992;215:179–185.

Ein SH, Shandling B, Reilly BJ, et al. Bowel perforation with nonoperative treatment of meconium ileus. *J Pediatr Surg* 1987;22:146–147.

Kao SCS, Franken EA Jr. Nonoperative treatment of simple meconium ileus: a survey of the Society for Pediatric Radiology. *Pediatr Radiol* 1995;25:97–100.

Mak GZ, Harberg FJ, Hiatt P, et al. T-tube ileostomy for meconium ileus: four decades of experience. *J Pediatr Surg* 2000;35:349–352.

Noblett H. Treatment of uncomplicated meconium ileus by Gastrografin enema: a preliminary report. *J Pediatr Surg* 1969;4:190–197.

Rescorla FJ, Grosfeld JL. Contemporary management of meconium ileus. *World J Surg* 1993;17:318–325.

Ziegler MM. Meconium ileus. *Curr Prob Surg* 1994;31:731–777.

56

MECONIUM PLUG SYNDROME

ROBERT D. ACTON
ROBERT M. ARENSMAN

Meconium plug syndrome is a mechanical colonic obstruction that generally appears within the first 24 to 48 hours of life, and produces abdominal distension, feeding intolerance, and vomiting. Because the causes of neonatal colonic obstruction, both medical and surgical, are numerous and often have greater consequences than the diagnosis of meconium plug syndrome, it is imperative that the obstruction be expeditiously evaluated and the more serious causes of blockage eliminated (Table 56.1).

The modern description and naming of meconium plug syndrome is credited to Clatworthy. His description of nine patients with neonatal intestinal obstruction appeared in 1956. All but one presented by the third day of life; only two had passed small meconium smears; two underwent surgery for the diagnosis of Hirschsprung's disease (and were found to have normal ganglion cells), and all did well in follow-up. An additional 21 patients were reported in 1966. Again, the typical patient presented as an average-sized, full-term infant, with low intestinal obstruction and failure to pass meconium by the second day of life.

Meconium plug syndrome may have been first described in 1898 by Bertie, who reported on a case in which anal/rectal fibroepithelial plugs, once removed, resulted in normal childhood stools. Falls and Jaffe in 1931 described the incidence of rectal plugs at 1%, and reported that only 0.2% of infants had persistent difficulty. They also reported, however, that if the child had a perforation proximal to the plug, it was a lethal event, which Zachary confirmed in six additional reports in 1957.

It is hypothesized that meconium plug syndrome is part of a continuum of colonic obstructive disorders, and infants may present in different ways. Most infants with meconium plug syndrome present on their second or third day of life. They are most often full-term infants of normal weight, and they demonstrate vomiting, abdominal distension, and failure to pass meconium. Ninety-four percent of full-term infants pass meconium within the first 24 hours of life, and nearly 99% do so by 48 hours. However, in infants delivered at 33 to 38 weeks, only 80% pass meconium by the third day; at 29 to 32 weeks, 65%; and at less than 28 weeks, 57%. Meconium plug syndrome has been reported in preterm infants weighing 500 to 1,500 g and is often initially treated as necrotizing enterocolitis. In a retrospective review of the infants diagnosed with meconium plug syndrome at Children's Memorial Hospital between 1970 and 1980, 9 of 25 were preterm, 50% had jaundice, and 50% had maternal complications such as premature rupture of membranes, preeclampsia, third-trimester bleeding, elderly or teenage mother, and precipitous labor. Six infants ultimately proved to have cystic fibrosis, and one had Hirschsprung's disease. These facts demonstrate the spectrum of meconium disease in infants and emphasize the open mind required when pursuing the differential diagnosis of low intestinal obstruction in a newborn (Table 56.1).

The exact cause of meconium plug syndrome remains unknown, but many theories have been proposed. In Clatworthy's initial description, several of the meconium plugs had decreased tryptic activity leading to decreased liquefaction of normal meconium, permitting the formation of inspissated plugs. These infants later had normal tryptic activity in subsequent stools. However, his subsequent report noted that tryptic activity was present in many of the plugs in the obstructed group, yet was absent in normal infants not manifesting meconium plug syndrome, making decreased trypsin less likely as the cause. Magnesium use for maternal preeclampsia also has been implicated as a possible cause. This theory suggests that the use of magnesium to treat preterm labor and preeclampsia leads to hypermagnesemia in the fetus, colon smooth muscle relaxation, delayed transit, water absorption from meconium, and plugging. When tested in the laboratory, this chain of events did not reproduce plugs in rats or dogs, even with extremely high serum magnesium levels. It is likely that the

R. D. Acton: Department of Pediatric General Surgery, Children's Memorial Hospital, Chicago, Illinois.

R. M. Arensman: Departments of Surgery and Pediatrics, Northwestern University Medical School; and Department of Pediatric General Surgery, Children's Memorial Hospital, Chicago, Illinois.

TABLE 56.1. CAUSES OF NEONATAL COLONIC OBSTRUCTION

- Medical
  - Endocrine
    - Hypothyroid
    - Adrenal insufficiency
  - Functional intestinal obstruction in the premature infant
  - Hypoxic encephalopathy
  - Metabolic
    - Hypoglycemia
    - Hypercalcemia
    - Hypokalemia
    - Hypermagnesemia
    - Hypomagnesemia
  - Neonatal sepsis
  - Pharmacologic
    - Narcotics
    - Neuromuscular blocking agents
    - Tricyclic antidepressants
- Surgical
  - Anal/rectal stenosis or web
  - Colonic atresia
  - Hirschsprung disease
  - Imperforate anus with or without a fistula
  - Meconium plug syndrome
  - Meconium ileus
  - Necrotizing enterocolitis
  - Small left colon syndrome

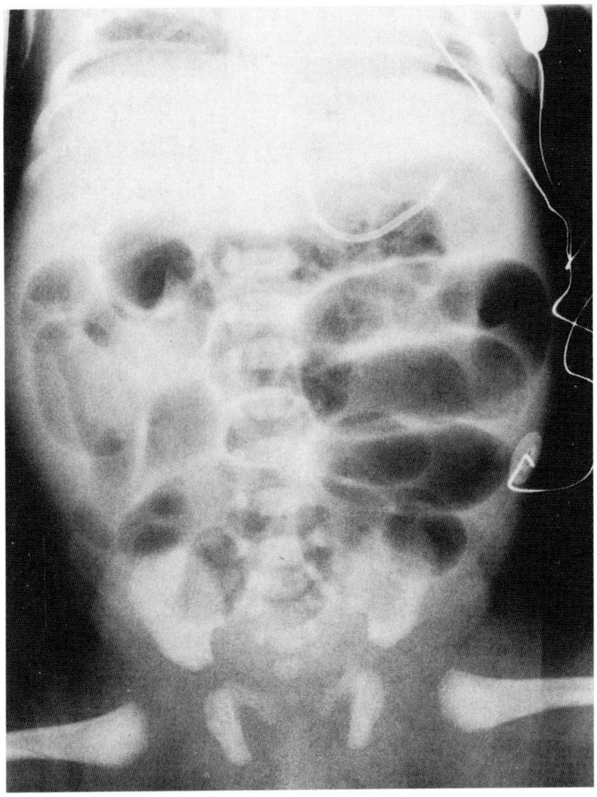

FIGURE 56.1. Anterior **(A)** and lateral abdominal radiographs **(B)** of a full-term female infant who presented on the second day of life with abdominal distension, vomiting, and failure to pass stool. Note the numerous dilated loops of bowel and lack of rectal gas. *Continued on next page*

association between magnesium and plugs is simply two common events occurring together with no inherent relationship. The true cause of meconium plug syndrome also may be a relative intestinal neurologic immaturity of the myenteric plexus that continues to mature even after birth. As with all biologic systems, there is a normal distribution pattern. Some infants have a relatively less mature colon and are unable to pass the initial meconium plug, but ultimately obtain normal colonic function.

DIAGNOSIS

The diagnosis of meconium plug syndrome begins with a medical history and a physical examination. When an infant presents with vomiting, abdominal distension, and lack of a meconium stool, it is imperative that life-threatening problems be excluded immediately. In practice, multiple diagnoses are pursued at the same time. The physical examination is performed to exclude an imperforate anus or any syndromic problems. Laboratory testing and a septic workup are instituted. At this point flat abdominal radiography is performed to exclude free gas within the abdominal cavity. If the diagnosis is meconium plug syndrome, this film usually shows a diffuse gas pattern and sometimes air-fluid levels (Fig. 56.1). If the initial radiograph suggests meconium plug problems, a contrast enema with an isoosmolar, water-soluble contrast medium (diluted Gastrograffin) is warranted. This is usually diagnostic and therapeutic at the same time. It demonstrates the meconium plug (Figs. 56.2 and 56.3) or suggests an alternative diagnosis (Table 56.1). Ultrasonography has been described as a method of detecting colonic obstruction *in utero,* but at present is not considered a technique with which to make the diagnosis of meconium plug syndrome in a newborn. Similarly, scoring systems have been developed to assist with making the diagnosis between meconium plug, meconium ileus, or Hirschsprung's disease based solely on the interpretation of plain radiographs. At present this system has not become widespread, so a contrast enema remains the preferred diagnostic method.

In the infant with confirmed and resolved meconium plug syndrome, a sweat chloride assay and rectal biopsy should be performed. A patient with either or both Hirschsprung's disease and cystic fibrosis can initially present with what appears to be simple meconium plug syndrome; the true diagnosis can be missed for an extended period of time.

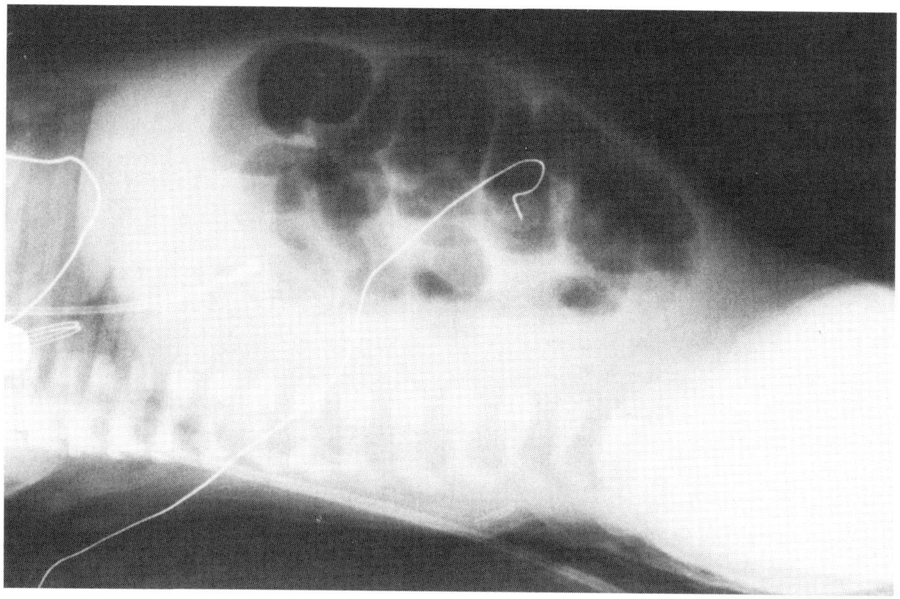

B

FIGURE 56.1. ***(Continued)***

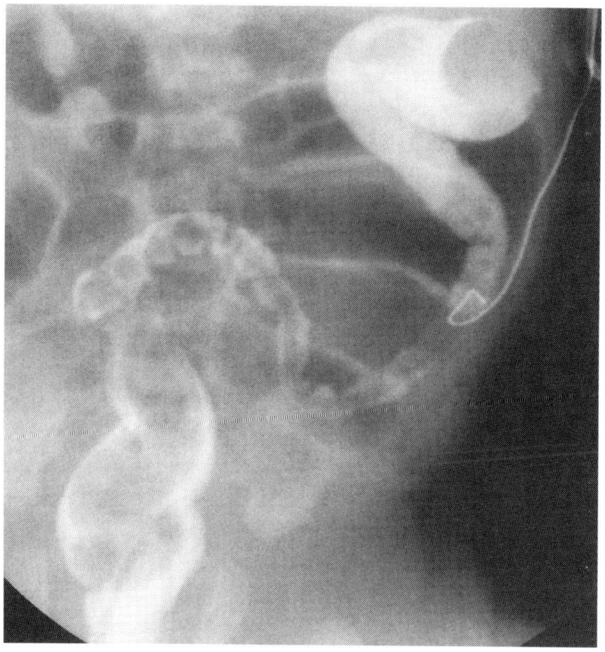

FIGURE 56.2. Gastrograffin enema of the same child; note the large meconium plug in the rectum and a second plug at the splenic flexure.

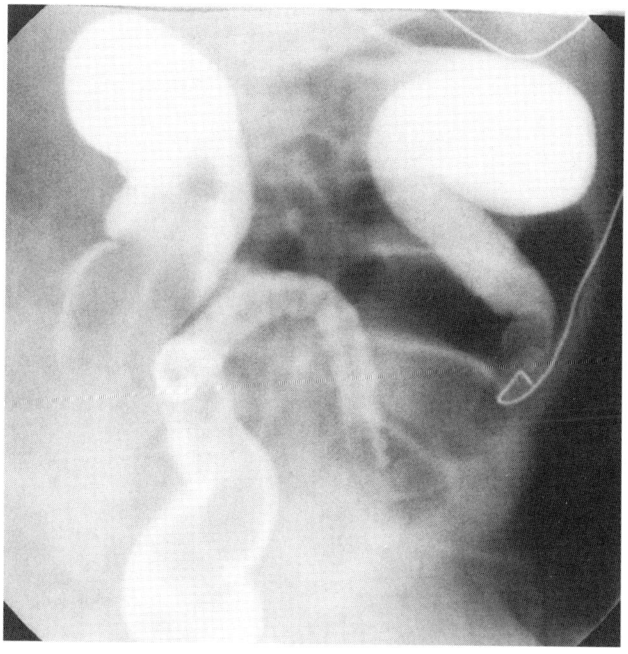

FIGURE 56.3. The plug previously at the splenic flexure now has been pushed back to the cecum. The rectal plug passed at the end of the procedure and the second later in the same day. The child continued to pass stool normally.

TREATMENT

The treatment of meconium plug syndrome begins at the time of the diagnostic enema. In Clatworthy's original description, dilute hydrogen peroxide was used for colonic irrigation to remove the obstructing meconium. This is no longer used in favor of water-soluble contrast under radiographic guidance. The plug almost always then passes upon completion of the initial contrast enema or within a few hours. For infants who have only meconium plug syndrome, no further therapy is required other than routine follow-up by their pediatrician.

Rarely, a newborn requires a second enema to fully clear all of the obstructing meconium. If perforation occurs, the child is treated with a standard exploration and diversion. Overall, infants with meconium plug syndrome live normal lives after treatment of this short-term problem.

SUGGESTED READINGS

Clatworthy HW, Howard WHR, Loyd J. The meconium plug syndrome. *Surgery* 1956;39:131–142.

Cooney DR, Rosevear W, Grosfeld JL. Maternal and postnatal hypermagnesemia and the meconium plug syndrome. *J Pediatr Surg* 1976;11:167–172.

Fuch JR, Langer JC. Long-term outcome after neonatal meconium obstruction. *Pediatrics* 1998;101:E7.

Hen J, Dolan TF, Touloukian RJ. Meconium plug syndrome associated with cystic fibrosis and Hirschsprung's disease. *Pediatrics* 1980;66:466–468.

Krasna IH, Rosenfield D, Salerno P. Is it necrotizing enterocolitis, microcolon of prematurity, or delayed meconium plug? A dilemma in the tiny premature infant. *J Pediatr Surg* 1996;31: 855–858.

Olsen M, Luck SR, Still JL, et al. The spectrum of meconium disease in infancy. *J Pediatr Surg* 1982;17:479–481.

Sherry NS, Kramer I. The time of passage of the first stool and first urine by the newborn infant. *J Pediatr* 1955;46:158–159.

57

MECKEL'S DIVERTICULUM

SHERIF G.S. EMIL
JEAN-MARTIN LABERGE

As Charles Mayo remarked in 1933, a Meckel's diverticulum is "frequently suspected, often looked for, and seldom found." When it is found, either incidentally during laparotomy or associated with abdominal pathology, it often produces a great deal of excitement. Procedures to treat complicated Meckel's diverticula are usually "fun" for the surgeon and result in an excellent prognosis for the patient. It is a lesion sometimes difficult to diagnose but often easy to treat.

All gastrointestinal surgical pathology can be classified into four categories: bleeding, obstruction, inflammation, and perforation. Complications related to a Meckel's diverticulum can produce any of these outcomes. In addition, it often presents incidentally during laparotomy. Finally, its embryologic origin, the omphalomesenteric duct, can present as an umbilical abnormality requiring elective treatment. We first discuss the approach to an incidentally discovered Meckel's diverticulum, followed by diagnosis and treatment of its complications, and ending with an approach to umbilical pathology.

INCIDENTAL MECKEL'S DIVERTICULUM

As a chief resident in general surgery, one of us (S.E.) operated on a young female prison inmate who presented with a clinical picture of early acute appendicitis. Exploration was performed through a small transverse right lower quadrant incision. A normal appendix was found and removed. Upon examination of the bowel, a normal appearing Meckel's diverticulum was found, which was removed as well. The next morning in attending rounds, half the staff supported these operative decisions, whereas the other half criticized them. The controversy of dealing with a noncomplicated Meckel's diverticula is unresolved.

Most surgeons use the suspicion of presence of ectopic mucosa as the main indication to resect an asymptomatic diverticulum. This suspicion arises when an area of pale grayish discoloration is seen in the diverticulum's wall, or the wall is simply thickened compared with adjacent healthy ileum. The rationale for this approach is the high incidence (60%–80%) of ectopic gastric or pancreatic tissue in symptomatic diverticula. Interestingly, diverticula resected based on palpation only demonstrate ectopic tissue in 30% to 50% of cases. There is also agreement that diverticula associated with fibrous vitelline artery remnants or omphalomesenteric bands should be resected, because both can result in small bowel obstruction. Symptoms are more common in males and in younger children. A narrow diverticular base may predispose a person to diverticular obstruction, inflammation, and perforation. Thus, some surgeons have used male gender, preadolescent age, or a narrow base as indications for resection. However, these indications are themselves controversial. Many surgeons would excise the diverticulum in any patient explored for abdominal pain when no other pathology is found, such as the one presented at the beginning of this section. Because the morbidity of future complications in all asymptomatic Meckel's diverticula probably equals the morbidity of removing all of them, the verdict is still open. It is therefore more useful for each surgeon to decide in advance when an incidental Meckel's diverticulum should *not* be removed. We would not remove an incidental diverticulum if it is broad based *and* feels exactly like the adjacent ileum. For those surgeons whose orientation is to remove all incidental diverticula, we would still caution them not to remove it in a patient undergoing surgery for acute life- or limb-threatening emergencies (e.g., major trauma, midgut volvulus, ovarian torsion), in a patient undergoing an elective operation in which the bowel is not opened (e.g., cholecystectomy, splenectomy), or in the presence of peritonitis (e.g., appendicitis, perforated Crohn's disease).

S.G.S. Emil: Division of Pediatric Surgery, University of California, Irvine College of Medicine, Irvine, California; and Department of Pediatric Surgery, Miller Children's Hospital, Long Beach, California.

J.M. Laberge: Department of Surgery, McGill University; and Division of Pediatric General Surgery, Montreal Children's Hospital, Montreal, Quebec, Canada.

BLEEDING

In large series of complicated Meckel's diverticula, bleeding and bowel obstruction are both common findings. Bleeding is secondary to mucosal ulceration, either in the diverticulum itself or in the ileum near the junction with the diverticulum. Bleeding associated with a Meckel's diverticulum is the most common cause of significant lower gastrointestinal hemorrhage in children. Although the bleeding is typically painless, intermittent, and massive, it can occasionally be chronic, presenting with iron deficiency anemia. We also have seen patients presenting with pain preceding or accompanying an acute bleeding episode. Rarely, a Meckel's diverticulum-induced ulcer can perforate and present with hemoperitoneum. Because mucosal ulceration is a gradual and time-consuming process, bleeding is an uncommon presentation in infants. The differential diagnosis of lower gastrointestinal bleeding in children includes inflammatory bowel disease, intestinal duplications, polyps, congenital vascular malformations, clotting disorders, infectious colitis, and upper gastrointestinal sources.

Many surgeons have had the unpleasant experience of operating on a patient with lower gastrointestinal bleeding and not finding the cause. This, in addition to the fact that the bleeding usually stops spontaneously, calls for adequate resuscitation and attempts at diagnosis. Intravascular volume should be replenished with crystalloids and packed red blood cells (RBCs) should be transfused if the patient is hemodynamically unstable or there is severe anemia with ongoing hemorrhage. Fresh frozen plasma should be transfused if an acquired coagulopathy has resulted. Intravenous ranitidine should be started in anticipation of the technetium 99m scan. A Foley catheter should be inserted to monitor urine production during resuscitation. It will also increase the yield of the scan by decompressing the bladder, where the isotope is accumulated, revealing a Meckel's diverticulum behind or adjacent to the bladder.

Unless another source of bleeding is suspected, the ^{99m}-Tc Meckel's diverticulum scan is the first diagnostic maneuver in a child with massive lower gastrointestinal hemorrhage. This scan detects ectopic gastric mucosa, and hence the presence of the Meckel's diverticulum, not the bleeding event itself. An intestinal duplication containing ectopic gastric mucosa also may yield a positive scan result. It is reasonable to perform the scan the first day after admission, when the patient has been stabilized and histamine blockers have been administered. Although results of this scan have traditionally been regarded as accurate in the presence of hemorrhage, recent literature has challenged this, citing a negative predictive value of only 74%. If results of the scan are negative but suspicion is still high, it can be repeated with pentagastrin stimulation or glucagon administration, both of which may enhance the scan's accuracy. If results of the second scan are also negative and the patient remains stable, a colonoscopy should be performed. It will identify inflammatory bowel disease, infectious colitis, colonic polyps, and vascular malformations of the colon, and may indirectly implicate the small bowel if blood is seen entering the colon through the ileocecal valve. Tagged RBC scans and angiograms are seldom needed in children. Contrast studies have no place in the workup.

Laparoscopy can serve as a diagnostic, as well as therapeutic, tool in the patient with ongoing bleeding, negative scan results, and noncontributory colonoscopy. Duplications can be diagnosed, and a Meckel's diverticulum that has escaped detection by scans will be evident. In the setting of hemorrhage, a Meckel's diverticulum is usually not inflamed and should be easy to dissect. In this circumstance, we would place the first trocar by open technique at the superior margin of the umbilicus to avoid injury to possible omphalomesenteric duct remnants. The blood supply to the diverticulum, which may be prominent if bleeding has occurred, is clipped and divided. Any adhesions should be freed. If the base of the diverticulum is narrow, an endo-GIA can be fired at the base at a 90 degree angle to the long axis of the ileum. The diverticulum can then be removed in an endo-bag. Some surgeons may criticize this approach, preferring to open the ileum, examine it for ulcers, and oversew them if found. We do not find this necessary for two reasons. First, the ulcers are often in the diverticulum itself and also often small enough to be discovered by the pathologist, not the surgeon. Second, most ulcers are no longer bleeding at the time of operation. In the absence of a continued peptic insult, the ulcer will promptly heal. If the diverticulum has a wide base or there appears to be fresh blood in the adjacent ileum, we would eviscerate the lesion and perform an extracorporeal resection, after slightly enlarging the supraumbilical incision.

If the diagnosis of a Meckel's diverticulum is made preoperatively, the patient is explored through a right lower quadrant, transverse, muscle-splitting incision. The distal ileum is followed to the diverticulum, which is delivered into the wound. If the base is narrow, a GIA stapler is used for resection. If the base is wide, stay sutures are placed transversely on each side. An elliptical longitudinal incision is made in the ileal wall, incorporating the base. If an actively bleeding ulcer is seen, it is oversewn. The ileum is then closed in one layer transversely with interrupted sutures. If the base is too wide to permit this, a short ileal resection is performed and an end-to-end anastomosis completed. The surgeon should insist on removing the entire diverticulum. Leaving any portion of its base risks leaving gastric mucosa behind, resulting in recurrent ulceration and bleeding.

One preoperative dose of gentamicin and clindamycin is given. Antibiotics are not continued postoperatively. The patient can be started on clear liquids the following day and advanced to a regular diet as tolerated, in the absence of an ileus. The patient should be discharged on iron if significant anemia has resulted. After resection of a Meckel's divertículum, we remind the parents of the 5% to 8% lifelong risk of small bowel obstruction from adhesions and describe the symptoms.

OBSTRUCTION

In our experience, obstruction has been a much more common complication of a Meckel's diverticulum. The obstruction can be caused by the diverticulum itself or by associated bands. The diverticulum usually causes obstruction by acting as a lead point for an intussusception, resulting in an ileoileal or ileoileocolic intussusception. Rarely, the diverticulum may obstruct the ileum by twisting on a narrow base, resulting in necrosis and an intense local inflammatory reaction or a long diverticulum looping around itself and "knotting" the ileum, setting the stage for an internal hernia. A fibrous band between the diverticulum and the umbilicus can extrinsically obstruct a loop of bowel or act as a focus for volvulus. A fibrous mesodiverticular band containing the blood supply to the Meckel's diverticulum can trap a loop of bowel between itself and the ileal mesentery, again producing an extrinsic obstruction.

Regardless of etiology, most obstructions precipitated by a Meckel's diverticulum present as a small bowel obstruction. The three "E's" of bowel obstruction—"IVee," "NGee," and "Folee" (intravenous line, nasogastric tube, and Foley catheter placement)—are promptly instituted. The latter is required to monitor urine output if the child presents with profound hypoperfusion, electrolyte abnormalities, or azotemia. In a child within the age range for idiopathic intussusception (3 months to 3 years), a barium enema is usually obtained to diagnose and treat this entity, as long as signs of peritonitis are absent. If a Meckel's diverticulum is acting as a lead point, the enema will either demonstrate the obstruction to be proximal to the ileocecal valve or will be unsuccessful in reducing an ileoileocolic intussusception. The patient should then be brought to the operating room. In children over 3 years of age, as in adults, a bowel obstruction in a virgin abdomen is an indication for laparotomy. Further diagnostic testing is unlikely to contribute much and will not change the course of action.

We explore such patients through a right transverse infraumbilical incision, after prophylactic clindamycin and gentamicin are administered. The small bowel is eviscerated, and the transition zone between distended and collapsed bowel promptly leads to the site and cause of the obstruction. If an intussusception is identified, an attempt at manual reduction is made. This is typically partially successful, but complete reduction is highly unlikely if a Meckel's diverticulum is serving as a lead point. En bloc resection of the intussusceptum and intussuscipiens is completed and bowel continuity is restored by end-to-end anastomosis. If bands to the umbilicus are causing obstruction either by extrinsic compression or volvulus, they should be resected along with the associated diverticulum. A mesodiverticular band-induced obstruction is also treated with resection of the diverticulum along with its blood supply. As in any operation for bowel obstruction, frankly necrotic bowel is resected. Bowel of borderline perfusion should be packed in warm sponges while the surgeon is performing the resection. It usually demonstrates marked improvement by the time the abdomen is ready for closure.

Aggressive hydration and adequate monitoring are continued postoperatively. Ampicillin, gentamicin, and clindamycin are continued for 48 hours if any intraoperative contamination has ensued. Nasogastric decompression is continued until the ileus has resolved. The patient is usually discharged on a regular diet 3 to 4 days after operation.

INFLAMMATION

Meckel's diverticulitis is the least likely complication to be suspected preoperatively. Most investigators state that the presentation is similar to acute appendicitis, with an inflamed Meckel's diverticulum discovered upon examination of the bowel after finding a normal appendix. In our experience, patients with this complication do not have the "typical" picture of appendicitis. They often have shifting, rather than localized, tenderness and tend to have more diffuse peritonitis after a relatively short history. Because of this, patients are often sent for sonography. Recently, sonographic stigmata of an inflamed Meckel's diverticulum have been described. The inflamed diverticulum often appears as a thick-walled teardrop-shaped structure or blind-ending sac filled with fluid.

The patient undergoes surgery after adequate hydration and administration of antibiotics. It is important to examine the patient under anesthesia. An inflamed or perforated diverticulum often results in an inflammatory mass or phlegmon that declares itself only after muscular relaxation is achieved. If such a mass is palpated, a right subumbilical transrectus incision centered over the mass is executed to expose it. If no mass is palpable, a Rocky-Davis incision is used. Omental and small bowel adhesions to the diverticulum and surrounding ileum can be substantial if perforation has occurred. Once the mass is delivered, one makes a decision whether a bowel resection is required or a simple diverticulectomy will suffice. If the surrounding ileum is inflamed or densely adherent or the diverticulum is very wide based, it is best to perform an en bloc resection of the bowel and perform an anastomosis between healthy ends. Otherwise, a diverticulectomy suffices. An incidental appendectomy completes the procedure.

Postoperatively, oral intake starts once the ileus resolves. Antibiotics are continued until the patient is afebrile for 24 hours and the white blood cell count and differential are normal.

UMBILICAL LESIONS

The most impressive of these lesions is the "ram's horn." This lesion exists when the ileum on each side of a wide, patent vitellointestinal tract prolapses through this tract. It is one of a spectrum of anomalies all caused by persistence of some portion of the vitellointestinal tract, also known as the omphalomesenteric duct. These anomalies may include ectopic intestinal mucosa at the umbilicus, an umbilical sinus, a subumbilical enteric cyst, an intraabdominal "trapped" cyst, or a tract or fibrous band attached to a Meckel's diverticulum or the ileum itself. Most of these lesions present shortly after birth. The trapped cyst usually presents as an inflammatory mass associated with peritonitis if it becomes infected. The remainder of the lesions either present as an asymptomatic umbilical mass or with umbilical drainage.

The surgeon's challenge is to differentiate these lesions from two other entities: umbilical granuloma and urachal remnant. If the sinus discharges fecal material or gas, or obvious intestinal mucosa is seen at the umbilicus, diagnosis is easy.

A urachal fistula may be identified by urinary drainage at the umbilicus. However, a blind urachal sinus draining mucus is more frequent. If there seems to be a sinus tract at the base of the umbilicus, an attempt should be made to cannulate it and perform a contrast study. We find a 24-gauge intravenous plastic cannula ideally suited for this test when the opening is small. This simple procedure often differentiates urachal from omphalomesenteric remnants.

An umbilical granuloma is a tuft of granulation tissue remaining at the umbilicus after cord separation. Topical application of silver nitrate is usually curative. Failure of resolution with such applications raises the suspicion of omphalomesenteric remnants. Large granulomas with a narrow base are best tied off at the base, resected, and submitted for pathology studies. Although the smooth mucosa of an omphalomesenteric duct remnant usually appears different from the redder, more irregular granulation tissue, the pathologist's findings can sometimes be surprising. If this is the case and the umbilicus has completely healed, we would perform an ultrasonographic examination. If this does not reveal any mass or bowel loop fixed under the umbilicus, we would not explore further.

The treatment of omphalomesenteric duct lesions is surgical excision. Unless they are polypoid as described above, we approach them through a transumbilical or an infraumbilical circular incision. We follow the mass or sinus to the fascia. If it extends deep to this plane, an inferior skin flap is raised and the linea alba is divided to enter the abdomen. The tract can then be followed to its connection with the ileum. It is divided flush with the bowel. If it ends in a Meckel's diverticulum, the diverticulum is excised along with the tract. The fascia is then closed with a running slow absorbable suture. The umbilical skin is either closed with simple 5-0 plain sutures or purse-string umbilicoplasty is performed, depending on the amount of umbilical skin remaining at the end of the procedure. An antibiotic-impregnated gauze pad is used as a wound dressing. Prophylactic antibiotics are used, but not continued postoperatively.

SUGGESTED READINGS

Amoury RA, Snyder CL. Meckel's diverticulum. In: O'Neill JA, Rowe MI, Grosfeld JL, et al., eds. *Pediatric surgery, 5th ed.* St. Louis: CV Mosby, 1998:1173–1184.

Beasley SW. Vitellointestinal (omphalomesenteric) duct anomalies. In: Spitz L, Coran AG, eds. *Rob & Smith's operative surgery: pediatric surgery, 5th ed.* London: Chapman & Hall, 1995:372–382.

Daneman A, Lobo E, Alton DJ, et al. The value of sonography, CT and air enema for detection of complicated Meckel's diverticulum in children with nonspecific clinical presentation. *Pediatric radiology* 1998;28:928–932.

St-Vil D, Brandt ML, Panic S, et al. Meckel's diverticulum in children: a 20-year review. *J Pediatr Surg* 1991;26:1289–1292.

Swaniker F, Soldes O, Hirschl RB. The utility of technetium 99m pertechnetate scintigraphy in the evaluation of patients with Meckel's diverticulum. *J Pediatr Surg* 1999;34:760–765.

58

INTUSSUSCEPTION

THOMAS V. WHALEN

Intussusception is most often a nonoperative disease. It is well known that this is a process that usually is seen in patients who are 5 to 18 months of age. That being said, one may see the disease in neonates and in older children. Certainly, intussusception also may be seen in patients of any age if there is a defined anatomic lead point. The process of intussusception in pediatric surgery in the defined age population is generally considered idiopathic. There are multiple theories as to what the actual pathogenesis of intussusception may be, but most describe hypertrophy of Peyer's patches in the mucosa of the small bowel.

DIAGNOSTIC APPROACH

The most important instrument in the diagnosis of intussusception is undoubtedly the telephone. This is because the classic history of intussusception is so important. In the defined age range, when the mother describes cyclic colicky abdominal pain with a periodicity of some 5 to 10 minutes in an otherwise healthy child, then clearly, on that history alone, the diagnosis of intussusception should be entertained. The presentation is occasionally more subtle, causing only the most experienced primary physician or emergency medicine physician to even consider the diagnosis. I believe, from at least a medicolegal standpoint, that if the word *intussusception* is found in any medical record in an emergency department or perhaps even mentioned in conversation between the primary physician and the surgeon, it then becomes mandatory to rule out that process. If one is referred a patient with a question of intussusception, that patient is generally otherwise healthy and early in the course of their pathologic process. There remain significant exceptions that will be discussed later. In the healthy, well-hydrated, nonseptic child, after placement of intravenous access one can proceed when necessary to radiologic confirmation of the diagnosis.

There is a small subset of patients with intussusception for whom one needs to rapidly prepare for operative intervention. This is the unusual late presentation of a patient who almost undoubtedly will have gangrenous bowel within the peritoneal cavity. These patients present as clearly critically ill. They are generally dehydrated and septic. Rapid intravenous access and appropriate broad-spectrum antibiotics should be initiated. After quick stabilization, the patient should be brought to the operating room without further delay. Obviously, this will be in the setting of a history that clearly reveals the nature of the process. Namely, the patient will have demonstrated a history of colicky abdominal pain that is then followed by a reduction in mental status as he or she becomes more dehydrated and septic. Frequently such patients also present with bilious emesis.

Currant jelly stool is perhaps the finding that is most clearly emblazoned in the minds of most medical students and general surgery residents. One should put the finding of currant jelly stool in its proper perspective; that is, it should only be seen in patients who present quite late in their course. Currant jelly stool is caused by the admixture of ischemic desquamated mucosal tissue with blood and stool. In our present health-care system, primary care providers and surgeons should be able to diagnose intussusception prior to this rather late pathophysiologic event.

Another ominous presentation of intussusception is seen when the intussuscepiens presents visibly at the anus. Anatomically this process has progressed from the ileocecal valve all the way past the dentate line and thus the presence of an ischemic segment of intestine is virtually assured. If the child does not manifest the more typical attendant signs and symptoms, the clinician risks making the grave diagnostic error of mistaking this very serious intussusception for an innocuous rectal prolapse. Generally, if one attempts to slide a cotton-tipped applicator or other small probe

T. V. Whalen: Departments of Surgery and Pediatrics, University of Medicine and Dentistry of New Jersey–Robert Wood Johnson Medical School, New Brunswick, New Jersey.

along the presenting mucosa, it will rapidly come to an impasse if the process is a rectal prolapse.

The role of radiologic evaluation in intussusception depends on the presentation of the particular patient in question. As mentioned above, certain critically ill patients should be rapidly prepared for the operating room with the intent of physiologic optimization and sepsis reduction but without any further diagnostic studies. This constitutes the relatively small proportion of patients with intussusception. Obviously the patient with a frank peritonitis, regardless of the history, should likewise be brought quickly to the operating theater rather than the radiology suite. Another class of patients who do not require the delay of radiographic diagnostic study are those with the appropriate history who have a palpable sausage-shaped mass. Just as the patient with the classic history for pyloric stenosis and a palpable "olive" does not require study (does any surgeon see such patients without ultrasonography having already been performed anymore?), the physical finding of such a mass in a patient suspected of having intussusception is an indication to proceed with operative therapy without further delay.

Is there a role for plain abdominal radiography? There undoubtedly is for at least two reasons. Most important is that when one clearly sees the right colon filled with air or stool, there cannot reasonably be an intussuscepiens in the same structure, and thus one has reasonably, quickly, and easily ruled out the process. The other finding on plain film is less clear-cut: evidence of a bowel obstruction. By definition, all infants and children with intussusception have a bowel obstruction, but most do not show evidence of the process on plain film. When I was a fellow in pediatric surgery, there was a clear directive from the chief of pediatric radiology that there would not be any attempt at reduction of patients who had clear evidence of a small bowel obstruction on the KUB or scout film. The basis of this opinion was that the risk for perforation would be increased in such patients where an attempt was made at hydrostatic reduction. I have long held that with appropriate criteria for safe nonoperative reduction, there is no higher risk for perforation of the intestine and that this particular contraindication need not apply.

If radiology is needed for diagnostic confirmation, the traditional method is barium enema. This does not preclude subsequent attempts at pneumatic reduction. The finding of a "coiled spring" at the lead of the process is diagnostic. Other modalities include ultrasonography and computerized tomography. Ultrasonography has clearly been demonstrated in the literature to be efficacious, but is highly dependent on the skill of the operator. If one needs to go to the extent of performing a computed tomography scan, then perhaps another diagnosis was the leading consideration prior to the study being performed.

PREOPERATIVE PREPARATION

Once the clinical diagnosis of intussusception is made, little preparation is required. Intravenous access is important, but antibiotic prophylaxis is only necessary when going to the operating room. Over the past two decades there has been a remarkable transition from hydrostatic reduction with a 1-meter column to pressure-regulated pneumatic reduction. This method gained popularity in North America after the seminal demonstration of its safety and efficacy at Shanghi Children's Hospital. However, use of this method would be indefensible were a perforation of the intestine to occur during attempted reduction of an intussusception, that was then followed by barium peritonitis. The success rate with nonoperative reduction should be approximately 70%. Occasional reports of success rates of 80% or more exist.

Whether the surgeon should be present at the time of reduction is a matter of opinion. Certainly most pediatric surgeons were trained to be present at the time of reduction, but in practice this is not always the case. A recent poll on a list server of international pediatric surgeons revealed that less than half are present for this procedure. It is a matter of conjecture as to whether this apparent trend in the care of the patient is based on the principle of quality of care or other factors, such as time constraints or the lack of reimbursement.

The definition of successful reduction is generally but not uniformly agreed upon. Most clinicians would insist that there be visualization of the terminal ileum, but a minority would suggest that edema at the ileocecal valve may preclude this provision. In either case, even in an era permeated by stringent length of stay guidelines, the child should be admitted after reduction for 24 hours of observation. It is frequent during such observation to see a temperature spike. No sequelae are seen, and a workup of the fever is unnecessary.

OPERATIVE CARE

Patients who fail operative reduction and those who satisfy the above-mentioned criteria for urgent operative intervention are prepared for laparotomy. After obtaining informed consent and administering prophylactic antibiotics, the patient is brought to the operating suite. I find that a transverse right lower quadrant incision is best. The intussusception can be manually "milked" back to the cecum, and then both intussusceptum and intussuscepiens are brought up through the wound. The key maneuver in reducing the intussusception is best illustrated by the time-honored teaching about the childhood toy, the Chinese finger cot. If one attempts to simply pull on each end of the intussusception it only tightens the constriction and can result in tearing of the bowel. The technique to assure rapid and simple reduction is to locate the area of the colon immediately distal to the intussusception and then to squeeze the lead point retrograde. The point of maximum difficulty, not surprisingly, is found at the cecum near the ileocecal valve. With persistent, sustained manual compression, one can almost hear the edema squeezing out of the bowel, and reduction is generally accomplished.

Two circumstances necessitate further operative intervention: the intussusception that cannot be reduced and the reduced intussusception that has bowel of either questionable viability or frankly apparent gangrene or perforation. These patients require bowel resection and should represent no more than 15% of patients presenting with this disease process. Although the decision to resect the ileocecal valve should not be made in a cavalier fashion, the morbidity of such a resection in an infant—namely, that of frequent loose stools and, to a lesser extent, mild nutritional implications—clearly should not be feared if there is reasonable suspicion that there may be a nonviable segment of the intestine that could subsequently be perforated. Although a second-look operation would not be out of the question in such an instance, in my opinion the morbidity attendant to that second-look operation is probably greater than that of ileocecal resection.

It is prudent after operative reduction of intussusception without resection to remove the appendix. Although general arguments may be made for or against incidental appendectomy, it is unacceptable to leave a patient, particularly an infant, with a right lower quadrant incisional scar with an appendix still in place. The life-long potential for a diagnostic dilemma or a dangerous delay in therapy is too great to justify leaving the appendix *in situ*.

Children older than those with classic intussusception present something of a challenge. Most will come to operation because of late presentation, failed nonoperative reduction, or concern about the possibility of a lead point. These patients may require resection but can at least be evaluated for a lead point by direct inspection of the bowel. If the intussusception is not reducible by contrast enema or if it is clearly more proximal than the ileocecal region, one must consider the possibility of a pathologic lead point such as a Meckel's diverticulum. Older children whose intussusception is reduced nonoperatively should be followed closely, but evaluation for a possible lead point can be difficult. Carefully performed contrast studies or imaging studies are occasionally useful but are no substitute for conscientious clinical follow-up.

POSTOPERATIVE CARE

General postlaparotomy management is followed in rather routine fashion after operative reduction of intussusception. Even in the age of managed care, demonstrated resolution of ileus in the hospital is clearly indicated when the acknowledged rate of recurrence of the process is 5%. This typically is seen within 24 hours of the operative procedure.

The patient having undergone bowel resection has no possible chance of recurrence of the primary ileocolic intussusception (except for the very small possibility of postoperative intussusception). Care of the patient, then, is no different than that of any patient after a limited bowel resection.

COMPLICATIONS

There is always the possibility of recurrence of the primary process. In the postoperative hours and days this occurrence may be rather insidious in that one is expecting some degree of ileus. Keys to recognition lie in heightened awareness and the anticipation that there should be resolution of ileus within 48 to 72 hours.

Other common postoperative complications include those of wound infection and hemorrhage. The former should follow the established wound classification standard statistics, and the latter should be rare indeed. The overall survival rate should approach 100%, except rarely among those with the most delayed diagnosis.

FOLLOW-UP

Long-term issues in the patient with a pneumatic or older hydrostatic reduction of an intussusception are nonexistent. If the child has undergone operative therapy, then the low likelihood of a subsequent adhesive bowel obstruction will clearly exist but there should be few other problems. In general, one postoperative visit 2 to 4 weeks after discharge is all that is needed.

SUGGESTED READINGS

Bratton SL, Haberkern CM, Waldhausen JH, et al. Intussusception: hospital size and risk of surgery. *Pediatrics* 2001;107:299–303.

Calder FR, Tan S, Kitteringham L, et al. Patterns of management of intussusception outside tertiary centres. *J Pediatr Surg* 2001;36: 312–315.

Laan M, Bax NM, Zee DC, et al. The role of laparoscopy in the management of childhood intussusception. *Surg Endosc* 2001;15: 373–376.

Lui KW, Wong HF, Cheung YC, et al. Air enema for diagnosis and reduction of intussusception in children: clinical experience and fluoroscopy time correlation. *J Pediatr Surg* 2001;36:479–481.

Tiao MM, Wan YL, Ng SH, et al. Sonographic features of small-bowel intussusception in pediatric patients. *Acad Emerg Med* 2001;8:368–373.

59

CROHN'S DISEASE

STEPHEN E. DOLGIN

Crohn's disease is an idiopathic inflammatory condition that can have protean manifestations but primarily affects the gastrointestinal tract. The disease most commonly presents in the second and third decades of life, but there is a second peak age of onset in the fifth and sixth decades. It can present at any age, including, although rarely, the first months of life.

Crohn's disease can affect every inch of the gastrointestinal tract from the mouth to the anus. The terminal ileum, often including the cecum, is the most frequent site of clinical involvement. The most common symptoms of Crohn's disease are abdominal pain, diarrhea, weight loss, anorexia, and growth retardation.

Growth retardation is a particularly important feature of this illness in the pediatric population. The causes are multifactorial and include inadequate enteral intake. Approximately 25% of children experience growth retardation before the direct gastrointestinal signs first appear. Growth retardation is important in considering resection for Crohn's disease in childhood, because a period of remission may allow a growth spurt, which is impossible after epiphyseal fusion.

PATHOPHYSIOLOGY

Intestinal inflammation due to Crohn's disease involves all layers of the intestinal wall. It begins with aphthous ulcers on the mesenteric side of the mucosal surface and progresses into the wall and finally through the serosa. Inflammation extends beyond the serosa with induration of the surrounding fat, including the mesentery. Long, deep, longitudinal ulcers are characteristic and often are accompanied by transverse ulcers, which together yield the cobblestone appearance evident on contrast studies and grossly on the luminal surface. Crohn's disease is segmental and can appear in multiple sites concomitantly.

S.E. Dolgin: Departments of Surgery, Pediatrics, Anatomy, and Functional Morphology, Mt. Sinai School of Medicine and Mt. Sinai Hospital, New York, New York.

The intestine "has the consistency of an eel in rigor mortis" (Dalziel, 1913). This descriptive phrase was written to describe an intestinal condition, undoubtedly Crohn's disease, several decades before the classic description by Crohn, Ginzburg, and Oppenhemier from the Mt. Sinai Hospital in New York in 1932.

The inflammatory process extending from the mucosa into the deeper layers of the wall accounts for obstruction, due to edema that narrows the lumen. The acute inflammatory process causes an initially reversible form of obstruction. After repeated episodes, fibrosis contributes to the obstructing process, which eventually becomes unresponsive to nonoperative interventions. The progressive advance of inflammation into and beyond the mesentery causes phlegmonous changes and abscesses. As inflammation encroaches on adjoining organs, fistulas develop.

The progressive nature of the inflammation extending beyond the serosal surface explains the characteristic findings in advanced Crohn's disease. The involved segment of intestine is indurated and hyperemic. The mesenteric fat seems to guard the inflamed intestine and "creeps" around toward the antimesenteric border of the intestine. The mesentery is thickened, making intestinal resection difficult, because the vessels are obscured by the excessive mesenteric fat. Adjoining viscera, including neighboring segments of intestine, vagina, or bladder, become adherent to the inflamed segment. An infected, edematous mass of intestine and surrounding fat without a fluid collection is designated as a phlegmon. True abscesses do arise not only between loops of intestine but in the retroperitoneum (such as psoas abscesses) and in the abdominal wall.

Recurrent disease, which is commonplace after resection, occurs most often at the neoterminal ileum, and frequently involves prior incisions or drainage sites, eventuating in enterocutaneous fistulas and abdominal wall abscesses.

The inflammation can distort the anatomy, making organs vulnerable to injury. The right ureter is particularly at risk during a secondary or tertiary ileocolic resection. For this reason, consideration should be given to retrograde catheterization of the ureters to help recognize and perhaps avoid ureteral injury. This consideration is highest before a reoperation or when there is known urinary tract involvement preoperatively. Computed tomography (CT) may yield important information about ureteral obstruction or distortion.

DIAGNOSIS

Crohn's disease typically presents with a subacute onset, and the diagnosis is usually not made until symptoms have persisted for some time. In addition to the common gastrointestinal symptoms (abdominal pain, diarrhea, anorexia, and weight loss), nonspecific signs include leukocytosis, elevated erythrocyte sedimentation rate, anemia, and hypoalbuminemia. The diagnosis is confirmed with gastrointestinal contrast studies. The upper gastrointestinal series with small bowel follow-through, particularly focusing on the terminal ileum, is the single most valuable diagnostic study. Colonic involvement should be assessed either with colonoscopy or a contrast enema. This is of particular relevance in planning a resection and assessing the prognosis preoperatively. Colonic Crohn's disease is not always as obvious grossly from the serosal surface as small bowel involvement, so preoperative assessment of the colon is mandatory.

If Crohn's disease is limited to the colon, it can be difficult to differentiate from ulcerative colitis. The distinction between these two forms of inflammatory bowel diseases is particularly relevant to the surgeon because ulcerative colitis is limited to the colon (and largely to the mucosa), cured by proctocolectomy, and most often treated by restorative proctocolectomy. Crohn's disease, to the contrary, affects all areas of the gastrointestinal tract (and all layers of the wall), often recurs after resection, and is not managed by restorative proctocolectomy.

HISTORY

When a surgeon sees a child for elective consideration of a resection for Crohn's disease (in distinction to the child with a complication dictating an operative approach) certain questions are useful in deciding about an operation. How much school has the child missed in the past year? What medicines have been taken and at what dose? Which of the multiple symptoms is the most bothersome? In other words, if the surgeon could cure one symptom, which would the patient pick. The nature of the pain should be clarified to help determine if partial obstruction is responsible.

Knowledge of the child's growth curve, weight changes, and present height and weight are pertinent. Lower abdominal pain, dysuria, or urinary tract infections raise the question of enterovesical fistula. The presence of pneumaturia by history is diagnostic.

PHYSICAL FINDINGS

The surgeon's examination focuses on the nutritional status, cutaneous findings, and effects of steroids. Many children with inflammatory bowel disease are moon faced, with acne, central obesity, and peripheral wasting. A careful examination of the perineum is obligatory. The abdominal examination may reveal tenderness, guarding, a mass, peritoneal signs, or evidence of intestinal obstruction.

INDICATIONS TO OPERATE

Although there are numerous specific complications that demand exploration, perhaps the most common indication is overall deterioration despite long-term (and at times toxic) medical management. The unfortunate expression often used for this nonspecific indication is "failure of medical management." This expression should be discarded.

The goal of the team caring for the child with Crohn's disease is to help maintain as normal a life as possible. This means attending school, playing sports, enjoying extracurricular activities and staying out of the hospital. The notion of a "failure of medical management" increases the disappointment and apprehension of the family facing an operation for the child with Crohn's disease. When a child has been failing to grow, missing school, and suffering deformity from the effects of medications, an operation can induce remission and allow a growth spurt. Even if Crohn's disease does recur, if the operation provides remission when there is still potential for growth, benefits may be life long. Recalcitrant avoidance of an operation results in chronic deterioration with progressive malnutrition. This eventuates in specific complications such as sepsis or obstruction, which will demand operative intervention. However, the patient may have become too sick to do as well as when the disease had been clearly refractory but not so advanced.

OBSTRUCTION

Initial episodes of small bowel obstruction secondary to Crohn's disease almost always resolve with gastrointestinal decompression. Antiinflammatory medications may help hasten resolution. Steroids mask peritonitis. However, in the child who has never been explored, there is no risk of intestinal ischemia from obstructing Crohn's disease. A trial of nonoperative management for obstructing Crohn's disease in a child never surgically explored is safe.

Once a child has been surgically explored, small bowel obstruction can reflect postoperative adhesions. Because adhesive small bowel obstruction can be complicated by ischemic necrosis, it is prudent for the surgeon to assume that the obstruction is secondary to adhesions in the child previously explored surgically for Crohn's disease. Peritoneal signs, failure to improve, and other signs of possible ischemia dictate surgical exploration in that setting. Complete small bowel obstruction rarely results from Crohn's disease and would suggest that the cause is adhesive. One of my patients was admitted to the hospital with intestinal obstruction months after a resection for Crohn's disease. Her obstruction was attributed to a recurrence and she was treated initially with decompression. Surgical exploration eventually revealed an ischemic adhesive obstruction that required a resection.

ABSCESS

The presence of an abscess in a child with Crohn's disease is usually established and defined by a CT scan. The operative approach should ordinarily be staged if resection is indicated. If, for instance, the abscess appears in the abdominal wall, simply establishing good drainage of the abscess is the proper first intervention. An enterocutaneous fistula is expected, because communication from the inflamed intestine is the underlying cause of the abscess in most cases.

Although percutaneous drainage of abscesses has gained widespread utilization, in a child with an abscess from Crohn's disease an argument can be made for open operative drainage in many cases. First, a child requires satisfactory sedation or general anesthesia even for percutaneous drainage. Second, the purulence may be thick, largely gastrointestinal contents and may drain much more effectively into the larger drain placed by the surgeon at an open procedure. One patient of mine with an abdominal wall abscess underwent percutaneous drainage that did not adequately relieve the abscess, delaying the effective step, which was a subsequent open drainage using a much larger catheter.

Once sepsis is controlled, the child can be discharged from the hospital. An enterocutaneous fistula is expected. Usually resection will be performed subsequently, but in a cleaner field on a patient in better overall condition. An attempt at a single operation to drain an abscess and perform primary resection with anastomosis in an infected field is fraught with danger.

FISTULAS

Although there are patients whose fistulas will heal when managed with medical therapy, fistulas usually eventuate in an operation. The best timing requires careful assessment of each patient.

When a child with one or more enterocutaneous fistulas is explored, I try to make an incision at a site separate from the fistulas. This allows easier entry into the abdominal cavity away from the fistula sites, which can be approached from proximal and distal orientations. After taking down the involved intestine, I debride the tract through the abdominal wall with umbilical tape as if it were dental floss and leave a loose packing in the site on the abdominal wall.

ACUTE PRESENTATION

Occasionally a child is explored for presumed appendicitis and terminal ileitis is found. The diagnosis of Crohn's disease should not be proffered with certainty in this setting because self-limited causes of inflammation, such as *Yersinia* or *Campylobacter* infection, may present in this manner.

If the cecum at the base of the appendix is not inflamed, appendectomy should be performed. A myth holds that appendectomy is inappropriate because it eventuates in a fistula from the appendical stump when Crohn's disease is present. Actually, postoperative fistulas in this setting almost always arise from the ileum itself and not the appendiceal stump. The possibility of a postoperative fistula when the ileum is not resected alerts the surgeon to handle the involved intestines delicately so as not to promote fistulization.

TECHNIQUE OF RESECTION

Resection for Crohn's disease with primary anastomosis should include only a few centimeters of grossly normal intestine. Histologic presence of Crohn's disease at the resection's margins does not impact on the risk of recurrence. Long margins of normal intestine should be avoided because they are not protective and waste potentially critical absorptive surface. When disease is limited to the terminal ileum, resection should be limited to an ileocecectomy.

The risk of anastomotic leaks in Crohn's disease emphasizes the need for a careful technique. When operating on a child with Crohn's disease, I have stopped using the single layer interrupted technique that many pediatric surgeons (including me) use in most other settings. A few patients of mine had intestinal leaks after resections for Crohn's disease. I decided that patients would be better served by a two-layer, hand-sewn anastomosis. The major advantage of the interrupted single-layer technique in children is to avoid stricturing, which is pertinent to neonates and infants. Because patients with Crohn's disease are usually older, their intestines are usually wide enough at the normal margins so that there is no disadvantage to the two-layer technique. I do, occasionally, use stapling devices. I do not routinely leave a drain.

PERIOPERATIVE MANAGEMENT

Most children undergoing surgery for Crohn's disease have received steroids in the recent past. I provide stress doses of methylprednisolone intravenously if the patient has received steroids during the 6 months prior to the operation. I taper the dose fairly rapidly postoperatively. Children are usually discharged home on a taper, receiving about 10 mg of prednisone daily.

Some surprising postoperative complications occasionally occur in children with Crohn's disease. These include phlebitis, kidney stones, and grand mal seizures. The causes of each of these may be multifactorial.

Phlebitis may result from an inherent coagulopathy in patients with inflammatory bowel disease. However, prolonged periods of bed rest secondary to chronic illness may be a contributing factor.

The formation of kidney stones in general is enhanced by periods of dehydration and bed rest. Steatorrhea promotes the formation of oxalate stones. Free fatty acids in the lumen scavenge calcium, which is then not available to chelate the luminal oxalate. Oxalate is then absorbed, rather than passed in the stool in its nonabsorbable calcified form. The high level of absorbed oxalate can eventuate in oxalate stones.

Although seizures can be initiated by electrolyte imbalance, most often no specific abnormality is present. Magnesium, calcium, and sodium concentrations are typically within normal ranges when a seizure occurs in a child with Crohn's disease. The reason for this association is obscure.

RISK OF RECURRENCE

There is no doubt that the likelihood of eventual recurrence after a resection for Crohn's disease is high, perhaps 50% in 3 to 5 years. At present, there is increasing hope that medications can confer prophylaxis. Some practitioners advocate pharmacologic intervention to reduce the risk of recurrence in all patients resected for Crohn's disease. Certainly, consideration should be given to pharmacologic intervention after a resection, weighing the toxicity of the medication against the evidence of efficacy. Our team has advocated some postoperative medication to reduce recurrence risk in all children undergoing resection for Crohn's disease in recent years.

PERINEAL DISEASE

Discussions of perineal involvement from Crohn's disease often warn about the dangers of operative interventions, stressing that wounds tend to heal poorly. Despite these provisos, undrained purulent fluid should not be tolerated, and abscesses must be drained. Some patients develop severe perirectal infections with or without rectal involvement of their Crohn's disease. In these patients, temporary diversion of the fecal stream may provide substantial benefit.

ROLE OF FECAL DIVERSION

In a severely malnourished or septic child who might do poorly with intestinal anastomosis, a staging procedure including ileostomy should be considered. Diversion of the fecal stream usually has a beneficial influence on distal Crohn's disease.

GASTRODUODENAL INVOLVEMENT

Upper abdominal symptoms are common in children with inflammatory bowel disease and often controlled with histamine blockers. When children with Crohn's disease undergo gastroduodenoscopy, histologic evidence of nonspecific inflammation is common. Granulomas are occasionally found. However, clinically significant symptoms from gastroduodenal Crohn's disease are rare, especially in children. Severe obstructing gastroduodenal Crohn's disease may require gastrojejunostomy, perhaps with vagotomy.

ROLE OF STRICTUREPLASTY

Because, ultimately, short gut syndrome can arise from long-standing Crohn's disease, especially after multiple resections, strictureplasty has gained popularity for obstructing disease. Strictureplasties seem most applicable to the chronic fibrotic form (a "burned out" type of Crohn's disease). They have been performed in segments of acute Crohn's disease, but concerns about a leak are increased. Strictureplasties are most applicable for the patient with multiple short obstructing fibrotic segments. Strictureplasty may have a somewhat limited role in pediatrics because pediatric patients are not often threatened by short gut from Crohn's disease, and the burned out type is less common. However, this intestinal sparing approach should be given some consideration, even in the youngest age groups, because children face the prospect of lifelong Crohn's disease.

CONCLUSION

The child with Crohn's disease needs a team of health-care personnel and physicians. Many of the symptoms are controlled with medications and dietary management. The disease is not primarily cured by operative intervention. However, the vast majority of patients will eventually undergo resection. These patients can be quite ill. A malnourished child on immunosuppressive medications heals poorly and is at risk of sepsis. Appropriately timed operations, occasionally staged, can be life saving and reduce the disease's morbidity.

SUGGESTED READINGS

Aufses AH Jr. Crohn's disease of the gastrointestinal tract. In: Scott HW Jr, Sawyers JL, ed. *Surgery of the stomach, duodenum, and small intestine, 2nd ed.* Blackwell Science, Oxford, UK 1991:795–811.

Crohn BB, Ginsberg L, Oppenheimer GD. Regional ileitis, a pathologic and clinical entity. *JAMA* 1932;99:1323–1328.

Dalziel TK. Chronic interstitial enteritis. *BMJ* 1913;2:1068–1070.

Griffiths AM, Wesson DE, Shandling B, et al. Factors influencing postoperative recurrence of Crohn's disease in childhood. *Gut* 1991;32:491–495.

Hellers G, Ewerth S, Bergstrand O. The incidence of fecal fistula following exploratory laparotomy and appendectomy in patients with ileocolic Crohn's disease. *Acta Chir Scand* 1980;500(suppl): 37–38.

Hyams JS. Crohn's disease in children. *Pediatr Clin North Am* 1996; 43:255–277.

60

ILEOSTOMY AND COLOSTOMY

MARY L. BRANDT
MICHAEL A. HELMRATH

Creation of an ostomy for decompression was first suggested by Littre in 1710, but not successfully performed until 1793, when Duret created a sigmoid colostomy in a child with imperforate anus. Although early diverting ostomies clearly decreased peritonitis and fistula formation after intestinal surgery, the ostomies themselves were associated with a high degree of morbidity and mortality. Underscoring this point, Amussat's lumbar colostomy procedure (1839) was considered successful because it had "only" a 40% associated mortality rate. Although mortality from ostomies is not an issue in modern times, morbidity from stoma formation remains a significant problem, occurring in a majority of patients. The long-term success of a stoma depends on the type of stoma created, the location selected for placement, careful attention to surgical technique, and the prevention and treatment of common complications.

TECHNICAL CONSIDERATIONS

Decompressive ostomies are used primarily in emergent situations of imminent bowel rupture or to protect a distal anastomosis. The most common decompressive ostomies in pediatric surgery are also completely diverting and include divided sigmoid loop colostomies, used for children with imperforate anus, and leveling colostomies, used for children with Hirschsprung's disease. Other purely decompressive ostomies include cecostomies, either matured or created with an indwelling tube, the transverse colon Turnbull "blow hole," occasionally used in the setting of toxic megacolon, and loop enterostomies placed proximal to distal disease or obstruction. Loop ostomies function to completely divert the fecal stream for about 4 to 6 weeks until spillover begins to occur as the posterior wall retracts, at which time they become decompressive only.

Diverting ostomies may be placed anywhere throughout the length of the bowel as end or divided loop ostomies. When the bowel is completely divided, as in the case of a bowel resection, the distal end can be oversewn and left in the peritoneal cavity, as in the Hartmann procedure, or brought out as a mucous fistula. The mucous fistula is decompressive if there is a known or potential distal obstruction, such as an imperforate anus, or a stricture from necrotizing enterocolitis. In babies with proximal jejunostomies with or without short gut syndrome, the mucous fistula also can be used to refeed the effluent from the proximal stoma.

Diverting stomas in the small bowel differ from colostomies in that the liquid consistency and high volume of stool can be corrosive to surrounding skin. To prevent skin breakdown, the stoma must be constructed so that it protrudes significantly from the abdomen. This technique, first described by Brooke for ileostomies, allows a more secure placement of the ostomy appliance and prevents skin breakdown. In the tiny premature infant with necrotizing enterocolitis, the formal maturation of a stoma is often difficult. In these cases, limited fixation of the exteriorized bowel to the skin may be sufficient. Ischemia of these fragile stomas is frequent in the immediate postoperative period. As long as the mucosa at the level of the fascia is viable, these stomas usually heal and function normally.

Ostomies also can be created to provide access to the colon for irrigation. In children with severe constipation due to malformations of the anus or spinal cord, a proximal colonic ostomy can be created for antegrade irrigation. Tube cecostomies, matured cecostomies, and continent appendicostomies have all been described for this purpose. The continent appendicostomy has become the most frequently used approach to the antegrade irrigation of the colon. In this procedure, the cecum is wrapped around the base of the appendix, much like a Nissen fundoplication, and the appendix is brought out through the base of the umbilicus. The redundant portion is removed and the appendix

M. L. Brandt and M. A. Helmrath: Department of Surgery, Division of Pediatric Surgery, Baylor College of Medicine; and Department of Pediatric Surgery, Texas Children's Hospital, Houston, Texas.

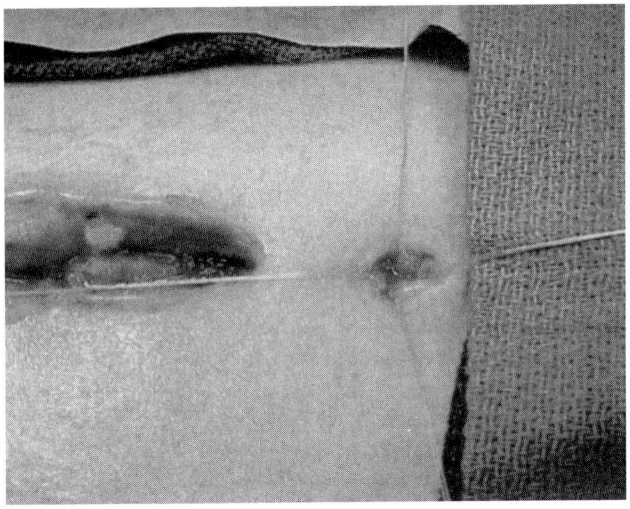

FIGURE 60.1. Maturation of the continent appendicostomy in the umbilicus.

matured as a stoma (Fig. 60.1). This allows catheterization of the umbilicus, and antegrade irrigation of the colon.

The location of the stoma on the abdominal wall is critical in preventing postoperative complications related to displacement or leakage of the ostomy appliance. For older children, the location of a stoma should be marked before surgery, with the patient or family helping. It is important to choose a site that is not in an abdominal crease in the sitting position and that is not too close to the costal margin or anterior iliac crest. The area selected should be flat to allow a good seal for the appliance. In obese patients, the stoma should exit on the most convex portion of the abdominal fat fold. Ideally, an ostomy should be brought through the lateral third of the rectus muscle, on a line roughly midway between the umbilicus and iliac crest or costal margin. The stoma should be exteriorized through its own separate incision through a carefully created, circular skin incision. The fascial incision should be linear, rather than cruciate, and large enough to easily allow the perpendicular passage of the bowel and its mesentery. There should be no tension on the bowel, which could lead to ischemia and retraction. The mucosa should be carefully approximated to the epithelium of the skin.

COMPLICATIONS

Dermatitis is the most common complication of ostomies. Most dermatitis can be prevented by proper placement of the stoma and creation of an adequate "nipple" in order to allow a good appliance fit. In addition, attention to skin care is essential, and careful instructions for the family are critical in preventing this complication. In instructing families to care for stoma sites, the analogy of diaper care is often helpful. As with the skin care of the perineum in a child in diapers, the site should be kept clean and dry at all times. The appliance may be left in place for 1 to 3 days, but should be changed whenever there is leakage. The appliance should be emptied when one-third full to prevent leakage. When changing the appliance, all the old adhesive must be removed and the site cleaned with soap and water. Excessive scrubbing will damage the skin and should be avoided. A hairdryer placed on the "cool" setting is often the least traumatic method of drying the site. If dermatitis develops, local wound care can be thought of as analagous to that of diaper rash. The area should be carefully and completely washed and dried. A protective ointment or cream (such as one that contains zinc oxide) or mechanical skin barriers around the stoma should be applied before the appliance is placed. Irritation from the corrosive enteric content also can be improved with stomahesive powder, which helps absorb fluid. Cellulitis should be treated with antibiotics (usually a first-generation cephalosporin) and monilial infections with mycostatin powder or ointment. Allergic dermatitis is unusual, but responds to treatment with topical steroid cream.

Other complications of stomas include peristomal hernias, prolapse, retraction, and stricture formation. Peristomal hernias are a common problem in older patients, occurring in 50% of patients within 5 years of creation of the stoma. The diagnosis of peristomal hernia is suggested by pain, bulging, and difficulty with defecation or irrigation. In obese patients a computed tomography scan may be needed to confirm the diagnosis. Treatment of these hernias is often difficult. Primary repair may be attempted but has a low success rate. The addition of a prosthetic mesh may be useful. However, definitive repair usually requires a takedown of the stoma and placement in a new location.

Prolapse and retraction of stomas are both common problems. Prolapse occurs due to a lack of fixation of the mesentery. This complication is most common in loop colostomies, particularly the distal end. Prolapse can usually be prevented by suturing a short segment of proximal and distal limbs together, or by plication of the distal end to create a smaller stoma. Once prolapse occurs, it is usually progressive and difficult to treat. Although various repair techniques have been proposed, including a buttressed suture and purse-string technique, surgical revision is often required for permanent stomas. Retraction of the stoma usually occurs due to excessive tension or from "skeletonizing" the intestine, both of which result in ischemia. Acute postoperative retraction is an emergency requiring immediate revision of the stoma. Chronic retraction may result in local wound care issues, but usually can be managed nonoperatively.

Strictures are another common complication of stomas. In newborns who require creation of a stoma to treat necrotizing enterocolitis, the incidence is as high as 50% to 60%. Patients with a stricture often present with diarrhea, because the obstructed bowel increases secretion, or with obstruction of the stoma by a piece of undigested food or a foreign body. Dilatation may be successful in treating some strictures, but revision of the ostomy is often required.

SUGGESTED READINGS

Al-Harbi K, Walton JM, Gardner V, et al. Mucous fistula refeeding in neonates with short bowel syndrome. *J Pediatr Surg* 1999;34: 1100–1103.

al-Salem AH, Grant C, Khawaja S. Colostomy complications in infants and children. *Int Surg* 1992;77:164–166.

Ball WS Jr, Kosloske AM, Jewell PF, et al. Balloon catheter dilatation of focal intestinal strictures following necrotizing enterocolitis. *J Pediatr Surg* 1985;20:637–639.

Borkowski S. Pediatric stomas, tubes, and appliances. *Pediatr Clin North Am* 1998;45:1419–1435.

Driver CP, Barrow C, Fishwick J, et al. The Malone antegrade colonic enema procedure: outcome and lessons of 6 years' experience. *Pediatr Surg Int* 1998;13:370–372.

Golladay ES, Bernay F, Wagner CW. Prevention of prolapse in pediatric enterostomas with purse string technique. *J Pediatr Surg* 1990;25:990–991.

Kosloske AM, Burstein J, Bartow SA. Intestinal obstruction due to colonic stricture following neonatal necrotizing enterocolitis. *Ann Surg* 1980;192:202–207.

Leong AP, Londono-Schimmer EE, Phillips RK. Life-table analysis of stomal complications following ileostomy. *Br J Surg* 1994;81: 727–729.

Makela JT, Turku PH, Laitinen ST. Analysis of late stomal complications following ostomy surgery. *Ann Chir Gynaecol* 1997;86: 305–310.

Mollitt DL, et al. Colostomy complications in children. An analysis of 146 cases. *Arch Surg* 1980;115:455–458.

Van Savage JG, Yohannes P. Laparoscopic antegrade continence enema in situ appendix procedure for refractory constipation and overflow fecal incontinence in children with spina bifida. *J Urol* 2000;164(part 2):1084–1087.

61

GASTROSTOMY

JOHN T. TOMICIC
FRANÇOIS I. LUKS

Creation of a gastrostomy is a common procedure performed by the pediatric surgeon. Despite the simplicity of the operation, considerable forethought must be applied regarding type, position, and technique to facilitate optimal nutrition and minimize the risk of complications. Indications for gastrostomy include swallowing disorders related to neuromotor dysfunction, congenital anomalies (e.g., pure, or type A esophageal atresia), chronic lung disease, and reflux esophagitis. Failure to thrive may be common to most of these indications, and often constitutes the main reason for a surgical consultation. This chapter reviews the techniques of open (Stamm) and laparoscopic gastrostomy.

Regardless of the indications, a functional gastrointestinal tract is required. Preoperative evaluation should ascertain presence or absence of gastroesophageal reflux (GER) and adequacy of gastric emptying. No single test is fool proof; we usually obtain an upper gastrointestinal contrast series (which might suggest GER or poor gastric emptying, and outlines gastroesophageal anatomy), a 24-hour pH study, and a nuclear gastric emptying scan. Esophageal manometry is seldom used in children, but flexible endoscopy may be used when esophagitis is suspected.

If moderate to severe GER is present preoperatively, a concomitant antireflux procedure may be necessary. In this case, an open or a laparoscopic approach (rather than percutaneous endoscopic gastrostomy, or PEG) is preferable. Although the very presence of a gastrostomy may cause or aggravate GER, we have not found this to be clinically important. In those cases in which GER becomes clinically significant after a gastrostomy, none of the techniques described below preclude the subsequent creation of an antireflux valve, either by an open or laparoscopic route. If severe GER and poor gastric emptying are present in neurologically impaired children, a jejunostomy (possibly with decompressing gastrostomy) may be preferred to allow adequate nutrition in a safe manner.

J. T. Tomicic: Department of Surgical Oncology, Boston University, Boston, Massachusetts; and Department of Surgical Oncology, Roger Williams Hospital, Providence, Rhode Island.

F. I. Luks: Departments of Surgery and Pediatrics, Brown Medical School; and Division of Pediatric Surgery, Hasbro Children's Hospital, Providence, Rhode Island.

OPEN GASTROSTOMY (STAMM)

The Stamm gastrostomy was described more than 100 years ago and, with few modifications, is still the most widely used technique in children. As with the other gastrostomy techniques, the site of the future stoma should be outlined beforehand, preferably two finger breadths below the costal margin (to avoid irritation by the tube or button). A small upper midline (our preference) or a left subcostal incision is made. Once the peritoneal cavity is entered, the stomach is gently mobilized and a site is chosen close to the incisura angularis (i.e., sufficiently proximal to the pylorus). Placing the gastrostomy toward the lesser curvature has been reported to decrease gastrostomy-associated GER. Two concentric purse-string sutures (2-0 or 3-0 silk) are loosely placed, such that they will be cinched and tied on opposite sides of the gastrotomy. This will allow the purse-string sutures to be used to anchor the stomach to the anterior abdominal wall (Fig. 61.1).

A 5- to 10-mm incision is made on the abdominal wall, at the chosen site, and the tract is created with a long clamp. The gastrostomy tube or "button" is passed through the abdominal wall. A small gastrotomy is made with electrocautery in the center of the purse-strings, and the tract is gently dilated. Making this tract too large may lead to leakage of gastric contents. The tube (14 French is appropriate for most infants and children) is introduced into the stomach, and the inner purse-string is tied. As the outer suture is tied, the gastric serosa is tightened around the catheter, creating a gastric tube. The needles should not be cut, because they will be used to anchor the stomach to the abdominal wall. Two additional seromuscular sutures are placed (in the remaining quadrants surrounding the gastrotomy), and the stomach is anchored to the anterior abdominal wall.

It is easier to introduce a gastrostomy tube (Foley balloon catheter, Pezzar, or Malecott) initially; if needed, it can

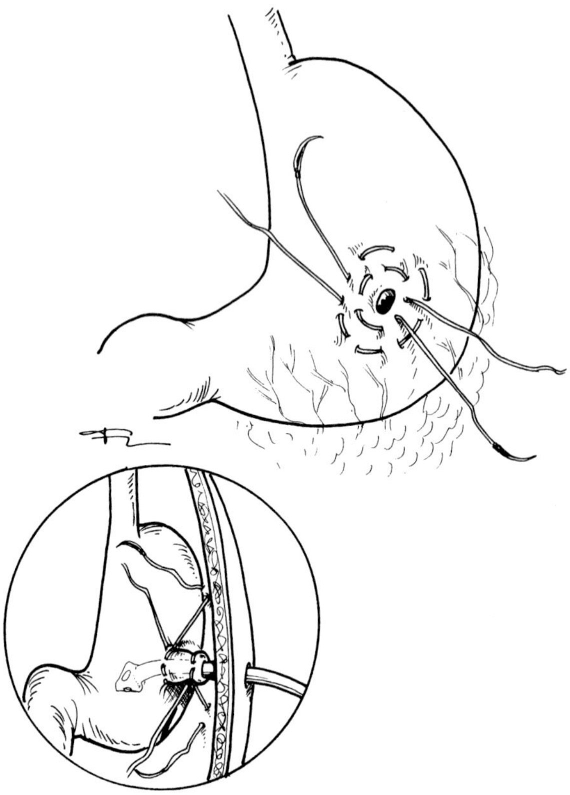

FIGURE 61.1. Open (Stamm) gastrostomy. Cinching the purse-string sutures creates a gastric cuff around the tube. Note **(insert)** that the purse-string sutures are used to tack the stomach to the anterior abdominal wall.

be replaced with a low-profile device after 4 to 6 weeks. However, parents often appreciate having a low-profile device placed primarily. This is technically more difficult, because the custom-fitted length of the tube does not allow a lot of manipulation. We have found that reinforcing the silicone rubber device with a blunt probe inside the lumen (taking care not to perforate the posterior gastric wall) facilitates the introduction of the device into the stomach. If a button is placed primarily, its length should be appropriate to the size of the child (exact measurement with a specialized device may be difficult intraoperatively). In general, a usable length of 1.0 to 1.2 cm is adequate for newborns and infants, 1.5 cm is best for toddlers, and older children may require a 2.0- to 3.0-cm tube. It is best to err on the longer side; the tube can be replaced with a more appropriate size at 4 to 6 weeks.

If a tube (cage- or mushroom-tipped Pezzar or Malecott, or balloon-tipped tube) is used, it should be pulled up snugly, without applying too much traction (which can cause necrosis and perforation of the stomach). Conversely, if the tube is not secured against the abdominal wall, the catheter may migrate distally with peristalsis, occluding the pylorus or the duodenum. The tube can be secured to the abdominal wall with a nylon suture, or preferably with a rubber nipple (to keep it perpendicular to the abdominal wall) or a fenestrated silicone rubber ring and fastener. When using a balloon (catheter or button), water should be used: the balloon is not airtight, and saline may crystallize and damage the balloon.

LAPAROSCOPIC GASTROSTOMY

Laparoscopic gastrostomy is a relatively noninvasive procedure that, unlike PEG, allows a concomitant antireflux procedure to be performed. Because it allows direct visualization of the gastric wall and the peritoneal cavity, it also may be preferred to a PEG if the operator is overly concerned about the possibility of colon or small bowel interposition between the stomach and the abdominal wall (which might be more difficult to notice in small children). Laparoscopic and open gastrostomies are comparable in technique, but laparoscopy may offer faster recovery. If a fundoplication is needed, this should be performed before the gastrostomy. If not, a two-port technique can be used. We use an umbilical port (5 or 10 mm diameter, depending on the patient's size) and a 30 degree telescope. A second (5-mm) port is placed at the gastrostomy site. The stomach is grasped at the future site of the gastrotomy, and two T-shaped anchor sutures are introduced on either side of the stoma. This is best accomplished while the stomach is distended with air, through a nasogastric tube, or occasionally with the help of a gastroscope (if concomitant endoscopy is performed). The anterior gastric wall is pulled up to the abdominal wall with the T-anchors, and the gastrostomy is created using a Seldinger technique (Fig. 61.2). A needle is

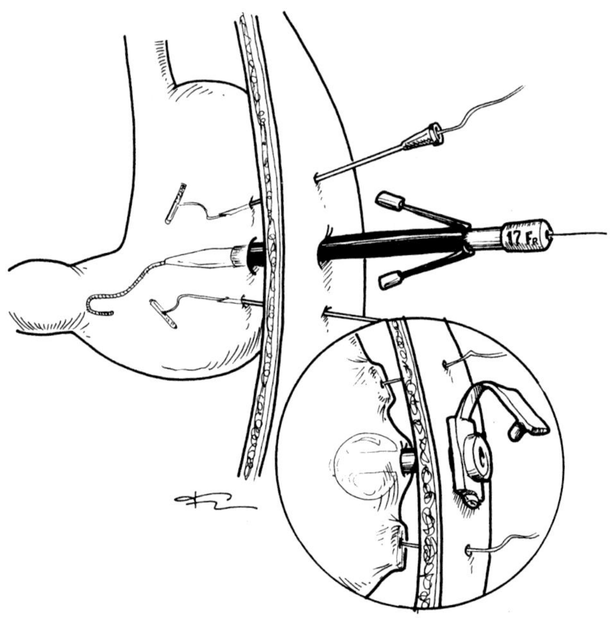

FIGURE 61.2. Laparoscopic gastrostomy. After hitching the stomach to the anterior abdominal wall with two T-anchors, a Seldinger technique is used to insert a 17 French peel-away sheath into the gastric lumen. **Insert:** A balloon gastrostomy button can be primarily introduced.

introduced into the stomach, followed by a guide wire and successive dilators (12, 14, and 17 French). The latter is fitted inside a peel-away sheath, through which the 14 French gastrostomy tube or button is introduced. We routinely introduce a 5-mm telescope through the peel-away sheath (17 French or 5.5 mm) to confirm its intragastric position. As with the open technique, placement of a gastrostomy tube is easier, but placement of a button primarily is often appreciated by parents and caretakers. In general, low-profile devices are easier to secure and cause fewer wound problems due to reduced torque at the insertion site.

POSTOPERATIVE CARE

Postoperative care is directed at educating the parents in wound cleansing and techniques to keep the gastrostomy tube patent. Most infections are limited to the skin, and most clear with meticulous wound care. A small amount of exudate around the tube is commonly caused by a reaction to the latex, and is managed effectively by cleansing the site with half-strength hydrogen peroxide and water once or twice a day. If a deeper or more widespread infection is suspected (erythema spreading along the abdominal wall, pain and tenderness beyond the immediate site, edema), prompt evaluation, antibiotic treatment, and possibly operative drainage may be indicated.

Frequent or constant leakage of gastric secretions or feeding solution causes irritation around the exit site. Constant moisture and exposure to acid may lead to peristomal swelling and further skin breakdown. If meticulous cleansing of the site is not sufficient, the addition of topical antibiotics (e.g., bacitracin) and the application of skin barriers may be necessary.

A common problem is the enlargement of the stomal site due to motion of the tube at the skin level. This is usually a result of improper stabilization of the tube, and is less common with low-profile devices. However, both tubes and buttons can cause irritation and formation of granulation tissue at the stoma site. This may be due to a combination of friction, foreign body reaction, and infection. The granulation tissue is pinkish red and friable, and produces a constant moisture, which may further contribute to skin irritation and local infection. Repeated application of silver nitrate most often allows the granulation tissue to slough and disappear. If this is unsuccessful, surgical cauterization or even excision may be required. With long-standing gastrostomies, the tract may be epithelialized with gastric mucosa, which can protrude through the site; it is important to differentiate it from granulation tissue, because simple cauterization is contraindicated.

Dislodgment of a gastrostomy tube is a common event, and it is important that the problem be addressed rapidly. The dislodged gastrostomy tube needs be replaced as soon as possible before the tract closes and reoperation becomes necessary. For tubes or devices that have accidentally become dislodged within the first 4 weeks of placement, immediate surgical consultation should be obtained, before any attempt is made to replace it. A solid tract may not yet have formed, and separation of the stomach from the abdominal wall and peritonitis are real problems. Even if the tube can be easily introduced, radiologic guidance may be helpful to assure proper placement within the stomach. Contrast should be injected through the catheter for confirmation of the tube's position before it can be used. Not uncommonly, early dislodgment (within the first postoperative days) requires surgical intervention.

In the mature tract, similar principles of caution apply, but false passage, leakage, and disruption are much less likely. Reinsertion is therefore safer, but radiologic confirmation is desirable, particularly if resistance was met during tube insertion. If reinsertion is delayed by even a few hours, the tract may have started to close down. Percutaneous dilation of the tract may then be necessary, or a smaller size tube may have to be inserted initially. This can be followed by replacement with the desired tube 24 to 48 hours later. If this cannot be accomplished, dilation under sedation or anesthesia, or even reoperation, may be required. The parents should remember to keep a record of the type and size of device, and should bring the dislodged tube (and ideally, a replacement device) with them at the time the child is being examined. Because balloon-tipped devices have a limited life expectancy, it is good practice to order an additional one (to be kept by the parents) at the time of replacement.

To prevent the stress and sense of urgency associated with the accidental dislodgment of a gastrostomy device, it is helpful to periodically monitor the status of the balloon. A button that is no longer taut, but shows some slack, may have a balloon that is slowly leaking. Similarly, the amount of water in the balloon should be checked once a week.

Finally, long-term gastrostomy devices may have to be adapted to the child's growth. If the usable length of the device is too short, the device will "dig into" the child's abdominal wall, causing pain and irritation. In addition, peristomal leakage is more likely because the stomach wall is squeezed against the abdomen. The correct length of the tract should be checked regularly (every 3–6 months in the growing child) and the tube upgraded as needed.

EDITOR'S NOTES

With the popularity and success of PEG and laparoscopic techniques, open Stamm gastrostomy is rarely performed as an isolated procedure, but continues to be executed in patients who require an open fundoplication and in some patients with atypical anatomy. The preoperative workup should include an upper gastrointestinal contrast study to evaluate gastric and esophageal anatomy and a pH probe study to quantitate the degree of reflux. The threshold to recommend a simultaneous fundoplication is usually lower in neurologically impaired children, especially when there is limited ability to protect the airway in the event of reflux. Although placement of feeding tubes is technical and routine for most pediatric surgeons, there are often significant emotional concerns for parents as they struggle with the decision whether to proceed with the operation and with the implications for the child's return to normalcy in the future. After a thoughtful discussion with a surgeon who is sensitive to these concerns, most parents understand that the proposed benefits outweigh the risks, both for the short term and long term.

The procedure described in this chapter is the standard technique. In the infant with a small stomach, two concentric purse-strings can sometimes incorporate too much of the anterior surface of the stomach. An alternative technique involves control of the mucosa with four fine straight hemostats and using an absorbable ligature to secure the mucosa circumferentially around the tube first, and then using a single purse-string suture to create a short gastric tube. Many surgeons also have switched to an absorbable suture for all suturing of the stomach, thus avoiding the foreign body reaction and possible granulation tissue that can result from the use of silk sutures. The traditional catheter to use is a Malecott or mushroom-tipped catheter, although a standard silicone gastrostomy tube with a balloon tip is not much more difficult to place and makes postoperative care of the child much easier. Buttons are somewhat more difficult to place and do not allow reliable postoperative decompression (venting) of the stomach, but are also placed primarily by many surgeons.

For laparoscopic gastrostomy, an alternative to using T-fasteners and a sequential Seldinger technique is to perform a Stamm gastrostomy directly through the gastrostomy site incision, which needs to be no longer than 1 cm in most cases. After an appropriate site is chosen by viewing through the umbilical camera port, the anterior wall of the stomach can be brought out through the incision. A standard purse-string is created around the gastrostomy tube and the stomach is tacked to the fascia in four quadrants. It is best to first place the four stitches in the stomach, leaving the needles on the sutures. The stomach is then placed back into the abdomen and the four stitches are placed in the fascia and tied. The anterior fascia and the skin are closed around the tube. This technique also works well through a 5-mm port site incision after laparoscopic fundoplication. There have been reports that the risk of site infection is higher in laparoscopically placed gastrostomies, although the reason for this is unclear. Fortunately, the infections are generally minor and easily treated with antibiotics and local care. Occasionally the incision needs to be opened and drained.

Granulation tissue can be a significant postoperative problem. Its cause is likely multifactorial, including foreign body reaction to the tube itself or the suture material, chronic irritation from gastric secretions and movement of the tube, and possibly colonization by microorganisms. Treatment consists of preventing chronic leakage and making sure the tube is of appropriate size and is relatively immobile. Sometimes multiple applications of silver nitrate are necessary. Most often, the problem resolves with time. We have had moderate success with application of Kenalog cream or an equivalent steroid preparation in resistant cases. In severely resistant cases, surgical excision of the tract can be performed in the operating room or under local anesthesia. Prolapsing gastric mucosa usually requires surgical excision.

Adolescents who have had a gastrostomy placed as infants often complain that their gastrostomy has "migrated" up against the costal margin, causing pain, leakage, and tube dysfunction, especially when they sit. This is due to disproportionate growth of the thoracic cage downward, rather than an actual migration of the gastrostomy. These patients benefit greatly from revision of the gastrostomy to a site farther from the costal margin.

Tube dislodgment is addressed fully in this chapter. My only comment is that old gastrostomy sites and tracts that have closed prematurely can usually be revived using a minimally invasive technique, including endoscopy (PEG), laparoscopic visualization, or needle localization under fluoroscopy and a sequential Seldinger technique.

–P.M.

SUGGESTED READINGS

Beasley SW, Catto-Smith AG, Davidson PM. How to avoid complications during percutaneous endoscopic gastrostomy. *J Pediatr Surg* 1995;30:671–673.

Gauderer M. Percutaneous endoscopic gastrostomy: a 10 year experience with 220 patients. *J Pediatr Surg* 1991;26:282–292.

Georgeson KE. Laparoscopic fundoplication and gastrostomy. *Semin Laparosc Surg* 1998;5:25–30.

Kutiyanawala MA, Hussain A, Johnstone JM, et al. Gastrostomy complications in infants and children. *Ann R Coll Surg Engl* 1998;80:240–243.

Nicholson L. Declogging small bore feeding tubes. *J Parenter Enter Nutr* 1987;11:6.

Tomacic JT, Luks FI, Shalon L, et al. Laparoscopic gastrostomy in infants and children. *Eur J Pediatr Surg* (in press).

SECTION

VII

COLON, RECTUM, AND ANUS

62

INTESTINAL POLYPS

FRAZIER W. FRANTZ

The significance of understanding the diagnostic and treatment approaches to intestinal polyps in children is twofold. First, they are the most common source of significant rectal bleeding in childhood beyond infancy. Second, they may occur as part of one of several familial polyposis syndromes that are associated with an increased risk for colorectal cancer. Identification of children with these hereditary syndromes allows aggressive surveillance and treatment to minimize morbidity and mortality to the child and to potentially affected family members.

Intestinal polyps can be broadly classified histologically as either neoplastic (adenomatous) or non-neoplastic (hamartomatous, hyperplastic, inflammatory, and lymphoid). All adenomatous polyps have malignant potential, and it is well accepted that essentially all colorectal cancers develop from adenomas through a progression from normal epithelium to adenoma to carcinoma. Natural history data from several studies supports an average time course of about 10 years for progression from a small adenoma to a clinical cancer.

For practical purposes, intestinal polyps in children that are of surgical import can be categorized as isolated juvenile polyps or polyps associated with inherited polyposis syndromes. In this latter group are included syndromes in which multiple intestinal hamartomatous polyps are found (familial juvenile polyposis and Peutz-Jeghers syndromes) as well as familial adenomatous polyposis (FAP). Although the great majority of polyps occur in the large intestine, these lesions, particularly when associated with polyposis syndromes, can be found anywhere in the gastrointestinal (GI) tract.

ISOLATED JUVENILE POLYPS

Juvenile polyps, also known as retention, inflammatory, or cystic polyps, account for nearly 90% of colorectal polyps in children, occurring in up to 1% of all preschool children. The peak incidence is at 4 years of age. They are hamartomas and have no malignant potential per se, although focal adenomatous changes rarely reported in these polyps may confer a small risk of carcinoma. Juvenile polyps were initially thought to be solitary and located predominantly in the rectum. However, as a result of more widespread use of colonoscopy over the past decade, they are now recognized to be multiple in 50% of cases and distributed proximal to the splenic flexure in 25%.

The most common clinical presentation of a juvenile polyp is asymptomatic hematochezia. The rectal bleeding is characteristically mild but can be profuse. Less common presenting symptoms include abdominal pain, prolapse of a rectal polyp, rectal prolapse, diarrhea, and tenesmus. In addition to juvenile polyps, disease processes that should be considered in children who present with rectal bleeding beyond infancy include intussusception, bleeding from a Meckel's diverticulum, anal fissure, rectal prolapse, infectious colitis, inflammatory bowel disease, intestinal duplications, and blood dyscrasias (Henoch-Schonlein purpura or hemolytic uremic syndrome).

The diagnosis of juvenile polyps requires a complete history, digital rectal examination, and sigmoidoscopy or colonoscopy. Rectal examination may allow palpation or visualization of a rectal polyp. Endoscopy allows for direct visualization of polyps, procurement of tissue for histopathologic analysis and confirmation of diagnosis, and simultaneous definitive treatment with polypectomy by snare electrocauterization.

I prefer colonoscopy to sigmoidoscopy in evaluating these children because it allows screening, removal, and analysis of all polyps from the entire colon. The total number and pathology of colonic polyps is important because multiple or recurrent polyps may indicate a polyposis disorder. If fewer that five polyps are encountered at colonoscopy, the more proximal polyps may be left in place, although removal of these would obviate the need for follow-up. If five or more are found, polypectomy is required because of the likelihood of an underlying polyposis syndrome, with the associated risk for malignant transformation. In the event that colonoscopy is not possible, either

F. W. Frantz: Department of Surgery, Division of Pediatric Surgery, Naval Medical Center, Portsmouth, Virginia.

for technical reasons or because of inadequate preparation, flexible sigmoidoscopy should be followed by an air-contrast barium enema in a well-prepared colon to detect polyps proximal to the splenic flexure.

Colonoscopy is facilitated by a mechanical bowel preparation consisting of polyethylene glycol (PEG) solution (40 mL/kg) given over 4 to 6 hours. Although this can be ingested orally, many children under 10 years of age require nasogastric administration to achieve adequate ingestion rates. To prevent dehydration, concurrent intravenous fluid should be administered. A normal saline enema (10 mL/kg) just prior to the procedure is a sufficient preparation for sigmoidoscopy. Colonoscopy can be safely performed under conscious sedation, but general anesthesia is more appropriate in younger children and when a prolonged or painful procedure is anticipated. From an equipment standpoint, a small-diameter colonoscope (11 mm) can be used for children beyond 2 years of age, whereas a small-diameter gastroscope (8 mm) may be required for infants.

Juvenile polyps located in the rectum and distal sigmoid colon can be safely removed via a transanal approach using a proctoscope/sigmoidoscope or with mechanical retraction of the anal canal. The polyps are grasped and drawn through the anus with subsequent removal by suture ligation of the stalk. One particular scenario to be wary of with transanal polypectomy involves polyps that have prolapsed into or through the anal canal from a stalk that is located proximal to the rectum. In this setting, amputation of the polyp transanally can be followed by prompt retraction of the stalk with subsequent hemorrhage and suboptimal visualization for further attempts at hemostasis. A technique that can help prevent this is to stabilize the bowel wall with tacking sutures adjacent to the polyp stalk prior to resecting the polyp and then suture ligate the stalk. Laparotomy with colotomy for removal of a juvenile polyp is rarely necessary.

Complications after endoscopic or open polypectomy are rare. After removal of isolated juvenile polyps, no further evaluation is necessary unless there is recurrence of rectal bleeding. In the event that proximal polyps have been left behind, testing for fecal occult blood and blood counts to detect microcytic anemia will be required periodically. Symptoms related to the polyps, anemia, or recurrent guaiac-positive stools would mandate colonoscopy with polypectomy.

INHERITED HAMARTOMATOUS POLYPOSIS SYNDROMES

Juvenile Polyposis Syndromes

Unlike isolated juvenile polyps of childhood, juvenile polyposis syndromes are uncommon and associated with an increased risk of GI malignancy. These rare familial syndromes include infantile juvenile polyposis, diffuse GI polyposis, and juvenile polyposis. Infantile juvenile polyposis presents within the first few months of life, usually without any family history, and is associated with diarrhea, rectal bleeding, protein-losing enteropathy, malnutrition, rectal prolapse, and intussusception. Polyps are frequently present throughout the GI tract. The effects of hemorrhage and protein losses in these young patients can be devastating and in many cases will result in death despite appropriate treatment.

Children with diffuse GI polyposis usually present between 6 months and 5 years of age with mild rectal bleeding and prolapse due to multiple polyps throughout the GI tract. Protein-losing enteropathy, malnutrition, and intussusception also can occur. The inheritance pattern for these affected children appears to be autosomal recessive. Juvenile polyposis, the most common of these syndromes, usually presents in the first decade of life with some combination of hematochezia, anemia, and rectal prolapse due to multiple colorectal polyps and is believed to have autosomal-dominant inheritance.

Histopathologic analysis of resected polyps from children with juvenile polyposis suggests a progression from juvenile polyps through adenomatous polyps to carcinoma. The cumulative lifetime risk of developing colorectal carcinoma is estimated at 50% in affected individuals, with the onset of cancer occurring before 40 years of age. Although colorectal cancer is the most frequently encountered malignancy in these patients, carcinomas of the stomach, pancreas, and small intestine have been reported. For these reasons, it is imperative that symptomatic children be appropriately evaluated and identified as having a polyposis syndrome so that long-term surveillance can be initiated. Asymptomatic children with positive family histories also must be screened. Both colonoscopy and upper endoscopy with polypectomy are required. The clinical criteria to diagnose juvenile polyposis include (a) five or more juvenile polyps in the colon and rectum, (b) juvenile polyps throughout the GI tract, or (c) any number of juvenile polyps in association with a positive family history of familial juvenile polyposis.

As a result of the small number of cases of children with juvenile polyposis syndromes reported in the literature, a consensus regarding appropriate therapy for this uncommon condition does not currently exist. At the center of the issue is the fact that there is considerable clinical variability of the disorder, which mandates individualized treatment. The current treatment options include long-term surveillance with polypectomy, subtotal colectomy with ileorectal anastomosis (IRA), and total proctocolectomy with ileal pouch–anal anastomosis (IPAA). Understanding that no consensus exists, a reasonable surveillance protocol would include colonoscopy with polypectomy annually and upper endoscopy with polypectomy every 3 years, with more frequent examinations for symptomatology (bleeding), adenomatous changes, or interval increases in polyp growth rates. The success of the long-term surveillance option is predicated on the essential requirement that periodic endoscopy and polypectomy can safely and accurately sample representative polyps and control the number and size of polyps present because these are the determinants that are most closely related to the risk of malignancy. If there are many large (>1 cm) polyps or too many polyps present to do this safely, colectomy is required.

As the natural history of this disorder unfolds, recommendations regarding timing of surgery and optimal surgical therapy are evolving. The decision of when to perform prophylactic colectomy is easier to make in symptomatic patients or in those in whom dysplastic polyps are found. In other patients with this syndrome, the timing is less clear. Historically, prophylactic subtotal colectomy with IRA at 20 years of age has been recommended. Because of the high rate of polyp recurrence in the rectum and the frequent need for further resection after this procedure, more recent reports have advocated total proctocolectomy with IPAA. At present, there are too few reported cases and too much clinical variability to declare one procedure uniformly superior, and surgical treatment should be individualized. The details of these procedures are discussed in the section on FAP. Although I have used total proctocolectomy with IPAA as the surgical procedure of choice in my practice, the children that I have treated have had extensive rectal involvement with polyps that were not amenable to regular endoscopic surveillance with polypectomy.

Additional pertinent recommendations regarding care of patients with juvenile polyposis are related to postsurgical surveillance and family screening practices. For patients with IRA, surveillance entails annual flexible sigmoidoscopy with polypectomy and upper endoscopy every 3 years until 40 years of age. Gastric polyps found to have dysplastic or carcinomatous changes may mandate gastric resection. For patients with IPAA, upper endoscopy will be required every 3 years. Although lower endoscopy has not been a typical part of routine surveillance for these patients, increasing reports of juvenile polyp recurrences in ileal reservoirs probably warrants evaluation every 3 years until the clinical significance of these lesions is better understood. All first-degree relatives of patients with juvenile polyposis should be screened because of the familial nature of the disease. This screening includes full colonoscopy and, if polyps are found, polypectomy and upper endoscopy to detect gastric polyps as well. If no evidence of colonic polyps is found, repeat screening may be accomplished at 3- to 5-year intervals until 40 years of age.

Peutz-Jeghers Syndrome

Peutz-Jeghers syndrome is an autosomal-dominant disorder consisting of an association of GI hamartomatous polyps (most commonly in the small intestine) and mucocutaneous melanin deposits in the lips and buccal mucosa. It is one tenth as common as FAP. The relative risk of a patient with Peutz-Jeghers syndrome developing a malignancy is 18 times greater than expected in the general population. Affected individuals are estimated to have a 50% chance of dying from cancer by 60 years of age. The interesting aspect of this increased cancer risk is that although malignancies have been reported in the stomach, small intestine, and colon, they also occur in extraintestinal sites such as the pancreas, breast, ovary, testicle, and cervix. Duodenal and gastric carcinomas account for about half of the GI cancers in these patients.

One third of individuals with Peutz-Jeghers syndrome are diagnosed during childhood and adolescence. Although the disease is detected in some of these children through screening programs based on family history, those that present with symptoms do so when the polyps become large enough to bleed, intussuscept, or cause intestinal obstruction. In general, surgery is not necessary for children with this syndrome. Most episodes of intussusception with partial intestinal obstruction resolve spontaneously with decompression of the GI tract and supportive care. Surgical intervention is indicated for persistent obstruction, prolonged or extensive GI bleeding, or frequent episodes of abdominal pain due to intussusception. At operation, reduction of intussusception and polypectomy usually provide adequate successful therapy. Intestinal resection should be avoided if feasible because of the recurrent nature of these polyps and the subsequent potential risk of short-gut syndrome.

Because of the significant risk of malignancy in patients with Peutz-Jeghers syndrome, a thorough surveillance protocol has been proposed. This includes upper endoscopy, colonoscopy, and upper GI series with small bowel follow-through every 2 to 3 years. At endoscopy, all polyps larger than 5 mm should be excised. Laparotomy with intraoperative enteroscopy should be used to remove all small intestinal polyps 15 mm or larger in diameter. Annual evaluations include fecal occult blood testing, complete blood count to detect anemia, breast and pelvic examinations (post-menarchal) with pelvic ultrasonography in girls, testicular examination with ultrasonography in boys, and pancreatic ultrasonography. Mammography also has been recommended beginning at 25 years of age. Presymptomatic screening in at-risk individuals should be initiated in the second decade of life and include fecal occult blood testing annually and flexible sigmoidoscopy every 3 years.

Familial Adenomatous Polyposis

Familial adenomatous polyposis is the most common genetic polyposis syndrome, occurring approximately once in every 8,000 births. It is typically characterized by the progressive development of hundreds of colorectal adenomas beginning in adolescence. Inheritance is autosomal dominant, although spontaneous mutations account for 25% to 30% of cases. If left untreated, all affected individuals will develop colorectal carcinoma, usually by the age of

40. In addition to colorectal polyps, polyps in the stomach and small intestine are found in over 90% of patients with FAP over the age of 18 years. Of these, duodenal polyps are the most worrisome because they are adenomatous and result in a 10% lifetime risk for duodenal or periampullary carcinoma. The gastric polyps are hamartomatous and harbor no malignant potential. Small intestinal polyps that occur distal to the duodenum are adenomatous but rarely undergo malignant transformation. Benign extraintestinal manifestations exhibited with this syndrome include cutaneous soft-tissue tumors, osteomas, supernumerary teeth, congenital hypertrophy of the retinal pigmentation epithelium, desmoid tumors, and mesenteric fibromatosis. Certain extraintestinal malignancies also occur more frequently in association with FAP, including central nervous system tumors, medullary thyroid carcinoma, adrenal tumors, and hepatoblastoma.

At the molecular level, FAP is caused by a germline mutation in the adenomatous polyposis coli (APC) gene, a tumor suppressor gene on the long arm of chromosome 5. Correlations appear to exist between the location of the mutations in the APC gene and the clinical presentation of FAP. For example, mutations located near the 5′ end of the APC gene or near the distal end of exon 15 generally result in an attenuated form of FAP with fewer adenomatous polyps and delayed cancer onset, whereas mutations located between codons 1250 and 1464 are associated with severe polyposis. Approximately 80% of FAP families have unique mutations of the APC gene, leading to considerable phenotypic differences in FAP related to these specific mutation sites. Identification of these mutation sites is useful in predicting the clinical manifestations of FAP in affected patients and the aggressiveness of polyp progression (i.e., age at onset, number of polyps, and subsequent risk of malignant transformation), and it may be useful as a guide to surgical therapy. Turcot's and Gardner's syndromes, both characterized by distinct clinical manifestations associated with adenomatous polyposis, are well-recognized variants of FAP and examples of the variable expression of mutations of the APC gene.

Early diagnosis of FAP is essential because of the inevitable risk of colorectal cancer. Until recently, screening for colonic adenomatous polyposis in all at-risk individuals (first- and second-degree relatives) was performed annually using flexible sigmoidoscopy beginning at 10 to 12 years of age. Today, genetic testing is the recommended approach to determine which family members have the disorder and require surveillance endoscopy. APC mutations can be directly detected in peripheral blood lymphocytes by protein truncation testing with 80% sensitivity and 100% specificity. In general, a germline APC mutation should be identified in a family with FAP before testing an asymptomatic family member. An alternative test for detection of APC mutation, linkage analysis, requires at least two additional family members and a pedigree. If the results of protein truncation testing are positive or uncertain (negative, but no affected family member has a positive result), the child will require annual flexible sigmoidoscopy. The frequency may be decreased to every 3 years after the age of 40. Screening for gastric, duodenal, and periampullary polyps should begin at the time of diagnosis of colonic polyposis and continue every 1 to 3 years thereafter. Although genetic testing is quite effective for identifying asymptomatic at-risk individuals who carry a mutant allele, considerable benefit is also gained by at-risk family members who test negative for APC mutations. These family members carry a cancer risk equal to that of the general population and can be relieved of the burden of annual examinations. Although it is somewhat controversial and may eventually prove unnecessary, a modified surveillance protocol is generally recommended for these "negative gene carriers" consisting of flexible sigmoidoscopy at ages 18, 25, and 35.

Most children with FAP are identified in early adolescence during routine sigmoidoscopic or genetic screening because of a positive family history. In those patients that are not identified by screening, presenting symptoms may include rectal bleeding, anemia, abdominal pain, or increased frequency of defecation. Once polyposis has been confirmed, colonoscopy is required to assess the distribution, number, and size of adenomatous polyps throughout the colon and to allow polypectomy with histopathologic analysis of large or worrisome lesions. This information will form the basis for subsequent treatment decisions.

SURGICAL MANAGEMENT

The treatment for FAP is surgical resection performed as a prophylactic procedure. The major decision points involve the timing of operation and the most appropriate operative procedure. With regard to timing, it is generally agreed that colectomy should be performed at the time of diagnosis in symptomatic patients. Prompt operation is also indicated when polyp density precludes safe endoscopic surveillance or when mucosal dysplasia is found. Because of the variable expression of this disorder related to different APC mutations, timing of prophylactic surgery must be individualized to some extent, but generally no later than 17 to 20 years of age. The complete spectrum of surgical options for these patients includes total proctocolectomy with end (Brooke) or continent ileostomy (Kock pouch), subtotal colectomy with IRA, and total proctocolectomy with IPAA. Although total proctocolectomy with permanent ileostomy is an effective procedure for removing all of the tissue at risk for development of carcinoma, its use in children is limited because it subjects the patient to a lifelong abdominal stoma. The Kock pouch has some advantages over end ileostomy in that the patient does not have to wear an ileostomy bag and can participate in most forms of physical activity without limitations. These advantages, however, are often outweighed by the high complication rate and technical complexity of the operation. The procedure is rarely used in children.

Both subtotal colectomy with IRA and total proctocolectomy with IPAA are effective treatment options for patients with FAP. Although I recommend the latter as the treatment of choice because it eradicates the risk of colorectal cancer by removing all at-risk mucosa, there are patients and families that are reluctant to undergo this procedure because of potential complications, such as impotence, incontinence, or pouch leak, especially if another family member has experienced these after IPAA. For these patients, subtotal colectomy with IRA can be used safely as long as two criteria are met. First, the child must have a limited number of rectal polyps that can be managed by endoscopic snare electrocauterization or fulguration. Second, the child and parents must understand the necessity for lifelong surveillance of the rectal remnant because of the persistent risk of carcinoma and the potential need for further surgical resection. Additional information to consider in determining the appropriateness of IRA for a particular patient involves the specific mutation site on the APC gene. Retrospective data have demonstrated much higher secondary proctectomy and rectal cancer rates after IRA in FAP patients with mutations located between codons 1250 and 1500 (severe polyposis phenotype). For these patients, total proctocolectomy with IPAA is likely a more appropriate choice.

The initial procedural details of subtotal colectomy with IRA and total proctocolectomy with IPAA share considerable common ground. Children are admitted the day before surgery for standard mechanical and antibiotic (erythromycin base 20 mg/kg/dose and neomycin sulfate 25 mg/kg/dose) bowel preparation and concomitant intravenous hydration. Patients in their middle to late teens may be candidates for outpatient bowel preparation with PEG solution (40 mL/kg) or a bottle of sodium phosphate solution and oral metronidazole. Broad-spectrum systemic antibiotics are administered perioperatively. The child is positioned on the operating table depending on the planned procedure: for IRA, modified semi-lithotomy, and for IPAA, lithotomy. Prior to incision, proctoscopy or sigmoidoscopy with minimal insufflation should be used to assess the adequacy of the bowel preparation and to ensure, for planned IRA, that any rectal polyps present are cleared. The rectum is then washed out with dilute betadine solution. Although a standard open midline approach is acceptable, both procedures are ideally suited for a laparoscopically assisted approach. Trocars are placed below the umbilicus and one each in the right and left upper and lower quadrants lateral to the rectus muscles. A 30-degree laparoscope is used to optimize visualization. The patient is placed in the Trendelenberg position and the operating table can be alternately rotated away from the side of the colon being mobilized to facilitate exposure. A total abdominal colectomy is then undertaken by first mobilizing the right and left colon along the peritoneal line with electrocautery and blunt dissection. Care should be taken to identify the ureters during this dissection. The omental attachments to the transverse colon and the avascular areas of mesocolon can be transected with the harmonic scalpel, whereas the mesocolic vessels should be ligated with endoclips. Once the colon is free from attachments, a limited abdominal incision is made to complete the procedure. I prefer a low midline incision, but a Pfannenstiel or transverse lower quadrant incision is certainly acceptable. For an ileorectal anastomosis, the ileum is transected as far distally as possible and further mobilized toward the pelvis by freeing its mesenteric attachments. The rectum is transected at or just below the peritoneal reflection. Because cancer has been reported to occur more frequently in the upper third of the retained rectum after ileorectal anastomosis, the rectal remnant should ideally be no longer than 10 cm from the anal verge. Intestinal continuity can be restored with a hand-sewn anastomosis or with an EEA stapler advanced transrectally. The postoperative care after IRA is relatively straightforward.

For IPAA, I prefer a two-stage approach with the first stage consisting of abdominal colectomy, rectal mucosectomy, endorectal IPAA, and diverting loop ileostomy. An alternative to mucosectomy with endorectal pull-through, the double-stapled ileoanal anastomosis, preserves the mucosa of the anal transition zone in an attempt to better preserve anorectal canal sensation and sphincter function. The second stage entails ileostomy closure approximately 8 to 12 weeks after the initial operation. After transection of the distal ileum and further mobilization of its mesentery to maximize length, the ability of the ileum to reach the anus without undue tension should be assessed. If additional length is required, the mesentery can be mobilized up to the third portion of the duodenum and, if necessary, the ileocolic vessels can be ligated at their origin, with care being taken to preserve the arcade vessels. Once adequate mesenteric length can be ensured, a J-pouch measuring 10 to 12 cm in length is fashioned with serial firings of the GIA stapler through an enterotomy at the apex of the pouch. Various pouch configurations (J, S, W, or lateral) can be used based on surgeon preference and ileal mesenteric length. I prefer the J-pouch because it is the simplest to construct and is historically associated with the fewest complications. Traction sutures are placed along the enterotomy in the pouch to facilitate eventual delivery of the pouch through the rectal cuff. At this point, the peritoneal reflection is circumferentially incised, and the proximal rectum is mobilized. The rectal mucosectomy is then initiated from the peritoneal approach, continued distally as far as possible, and completed from the perineal approach, if necessary, with removal of all mucosa down to the dentate line. Alternatively, the entire mucosectomy can be completed from the perineal approach, but this may require more aggressive stretching of the internal sphincter. The Lone Star retractor (Lone Star Medical Products, Houston, Texas) is particularly useful in optimizing exposure of this area while obviating the need for excessive stretching of the anal canal, which can damage the anal sphincters and impair fecal continence. Intestinal continuity is restored with a hand-sewn IPAA using interrupted absorbable sutures, with care being taken to avoid twisting of the ileal mesentery when the pouch is delivered through the rectal cuff. A temporary diverting loop ileostomy is then fashioned in the right lower quadrant approximately 20 to 25 cm from the pouch and matured in Turnbull fashion. Some surgeons feel that a protective ileostomy after this procedure in patients with FAP is unnecessary and have successfully performed total proctolectomy with IPAA using a double-stapled technique as a single-stage operation.

Postoperative convalescence after IPAA usually requires 6 to 7 days in the hospital and approximately 4 weeks to full activity. Most patients can be managed without a nasogastric tube, and oral intake is restarted once there is evidence of ileostomy function. After discharge, patients are examined in the clinic after 2 weeks, at which time anal dilation with Hegar dilators is initiated to prevent anastomotic stricture. Dilation is continued at least twice weekly until ileostomy closure. Between 6 and 8 weeks after surgery, a water-soluble contrast enema is given to ensure that the ileal pouch has no leaks. If everything appears to have healed properly, ileostomy closure is undertaken 8 to 12 weeks postoperatively. At the time of ileostomy closure, proctoscopy and ileoanal anastomotic dilation are performed.

ILEORECTAL ANASTOMOSIS VERSUS ILEAL POUCH–ANAL ANASTOMOSIS

The primary advantages of subtotal colectomy with IRA are (a) avoidance of an abdominal stoma; (b) avoidance of extensive pelvic dissection, thus reducing problems with postoperative sexual or urinary dysfunction; and (c) low morbidity rate because the procedure is technically less complex. Although fecal urgency, increased stool frequency (five stools per day), and gross fecal soiling (in 6% of patients) have been reported after this procedure, the bowel function profile of these patients compares favorably with that of IPAA patients. The main drawback of IRA, however, is that it leaves the patient at risk for developing carcinoma and requires long-term surveillance. The risk of developing carcinoma in the rectal segment after IRA has been reported between 12% and 20% at 20 years after surgery and up to 50% in patients over 60 years of age. Furthermore, even with lifelong surveillance, many of the cancers that develop in a rectal stump are already Dukes C lesions at diagnosis. Because of this significant risk, some clinicians have suggested conversion of the IRA with proctectomy and IPAA before 50 years of age. Unfortunately, conversion from ileorectal to ileoanal anastomosis in these patients can be complicated by the high rate of development of desmoid tumors, which can cause shortening of the mesentery that does not allow the terminal ileum to reach the anal canal.

Postsurgical surveillance after IRA should include regular proctoscopic examinations beginning at 6-month intervals with excision or fulguration of any rectal polyps that develop. Spontaneous regression of adenomatous rectal polyps after subtotal colectomy with IRA has been reported in 38% of cases, but, eventually, recurrence is common. However, if an increasing density of polyps is encountered, the surveillance interval may require shortening (to 3 months), and consideration should be given for conversion to IPAA. Conversion also should be undertaken as soon as moderate or severe mucosal dysplasia is found. Although enhanced polyp regression has been documented in response to treatment with sulindac, a reduction in cancer risk has not been proven, and polyps generally reappear after discontinuation of therapy. Thus, there is currently little indication for its use in the pediatric population. Surveillance for gastric and duodenal polyps with biopsies, polypectomy, and fulguration should be performed annually in patients with periampullary polyps and every 3 years in those without known polyps. Side-viewing endoscopy is recommended after routine upper GI endoscopy to optimize visualization of the ampulla of Vater and the periampullary region and to allow routine surveillance biopsies of this area. Periampullary polyps greater than 1 cm in diameter, rapid growth, induration, severe dysplasia, or villous changes suggest the need for more aggressive intervention.

The main advantage of total colectomy with IPAA is that all of the colorectal mucosa is excised and the previously significant risk for colorectal cancer in these patients is eliminated. The operation preserves the anorectal sphincter and maintains continence, and, with pelvic dissection confined to the endorectal plane, the incidence of postoperative impotence and urinary dysfunction are minimized. The overall complication rate of IPAA reported in a series of 187 patients with FAP from the Mayo Clinic was 24%. The most common complication reported was small bowel obstruction, 75% of which responded to nonoperative therapy. Pelvic sepsis due to anastomotic leaks occurred in 1.6% of patients. This diagnosis is most commonly established using a water-soluble contrast enema. With a protective ileostomy in place, the majority of these can be treated with antibiotics and percutaneous drainage under CT guidance (if a fluid collection is present) as long as the leak is confined to the pelvis and generalized peritonitis is not present. Pouchitis, diagnosed clinically, was reported in 3% of patients, much less frequent than the rates reported after IPAA for ulcerative colitis. This can usually be managed with oral metronidazole, 250 mg twice daily for 2 weeks. With regard to pouch function, the median number of stools per day was four (range, 1–12). Complete daytime continence was present in 84% of patients, with 12% experiencing fecal spotting and 4% fecal soiling. Nighttime continence was achieved in 74% of patients, with 22% having some spotting and 4% experiencing nocturnal soiling.

Effective medical therapy to help control stool output includes loperamide, 1 mg three times daily as needed, and supplementary fiber. Pouch failure requiring permanent diversion occurred in 4% of patients.

Two particular points of controversy regarding total colectomy with IPAA are (a) the optimal operative technique for ileoanal anastomosis (mucosectomy with hand-sewn anastomosis vs. double-stapled technique) and (b) the need for a proximal diverting ileostomy. Regarding anastomotic technique, there are conflicting reports in the literature of the functional outcome of either procedure, ranging from no difference between the two techniques to fecal incontinence and nocturnal soiling after mucosectomy with a hand-sewn anastomosis. My principal concerns are that the double-stapled ileoanal anastomosis requires more extensive pelvic dissection and risks leaving variable lengths of residual rectal mucosa at the anastomosis, exposing the patient to the risk for polyp progression and potential carcinoma.

The value of a temporary diverting loop ileostomy after IPAA is that it allows fecal diversion while the anastomosis heals, thus minimizing the risks for pouch leak, pelvic sepsis, and anastomotic dehiscence. Opponents of temporary ileostomy cite the potential complications of bowel obstruction, anastomotic leak after stoma closure, and dehydration with electrolyte imbalances associated with excessive stool output, in addition to the need for a second surgical procedure, as justifications to forego diversion. In general, although these risks are not trivial, they are highly preferable to the potentially catastrophic complications of pelvic sepsis and pouch failure that can result when a leak occurs without fecal diversion.

Historically, endoscopic surveillance in patients with FAP after IPAA was predominantly focused on the upper GI tract. However, reports of adenomatous polyps (in 40% of patients at 5-year follow-up) and rare adenocarcinomas in the ileal pouches of these patients after IPAA have prompted some surgeons to modify their surveillance regimens. At issue is the paucity of information available regarding the natural history of these postcolectomy ileal pouch polyps with regard to their potential for malignant transformation. Until this is better defined, the safest practice is to perform pouch surveillance every 3 years with removal or fulguration of polyps that are present. More frequent surveillance (6-month intervals) may be required in patients who have stapled anastomoses because of the increased risk for retained rectal mucosa and subsequent polyp formation. Surveillance for gastric and duodenal polyps after IPAA is identical to the post-IRA protocol.

Although thorough screening, surgical resection, and postsurgical surveillance in patients with FAP have markedly reduced the risk for colorectal cancer and increased survival, these patients still have more than a threefold increased risk for dying than the age-matched general population. The two leading causes of death after removal of the colon and rectum are periampullary cancer and desmoid tumors. Thorough and regular endoscopic surveillance with timely surgical intervention is designed to prevent mortality from periampullary cancer. When duodenal polyps increase in size or number or show premalignant features during surveillance, aggressive therapy is warranted to prevent cancer. Initial therapy may consist of endoscopic ablation of benign ampullary and duodenal adenomas, whereas large adenomas or malignant lesions will require surgical removal of the ampulla alone or of the duodenum by pancreas-sparing duodenectomy or pancreaticoduodenectomy. Desmoid tumors of the abdominal wall and small bowel mesentery can occur in up to 13% of these patients, typically within 6 to 30 months after surgery. These are aggressive benign tumors of fibroblasts that grow slowly and may compress or encase intraabdominal vessels, viscera, or ureters. Although simple local excision of abdominal wall desmoids is effective, operation to resect intraabdominal desmoids should be avoided. In the setting of intestinal obstruction due to desmoid tumors, bypass procedures are preferred. No ideal medical therapy for treating desmoids exists, but sulindac and tamoxifen have been successful in some patients.

SUGGESTED READINGS

Ambrose WL, Orangio GR, Lucas G. Surgical options for familial adenomatous polyposis. *Semin Surg Oncol* 1995;11:423–427.

Corredor J, Wambach J, Barnard J. Gastrointestinal polyps in children: advances in molecular genetics, diagnosis, and management. *J Pediatr* 2001;138:621–628.

Fox VL. High-risk, underappreciated, obscure, or preventable causes of gastrointestinal bleeding. *Gastroenterol Clin North Am* 2000; 29:37–66.

King JE, Dozois RR, Lindor NM, et al. Care of patients and their families with familial adenomatous polyposis. *Mayo Clin Proc* 2000;75:57–67.

Lynch HT, Smyrk T, Watson P, et al. Hereditary colorectal cancer. *Semin Oncol* 1991;18:337–366.

Markowitz AJ, Winawer SJ. Colorectal carcinoma: screening and surveillance for colorectal carcinoma. *Hematol Oncol Clin North Am* 1997;11:579–608.

Nyam DCNK, Brillant PT, Dozois RR, et al. Ileal pouch–anal canal anastomosis for familial adenomatous polyposis: early and late results. *Ann Surg* 1997;226:514–521.

Scott-Conner CEH, Hausman M, Hall TJ, et al. Familial juvenile polyposis: patterns of recurrence and implications for surgical management. *J Am Coll Surg* 1995;181:407–413.

Spigelman AD, Murday V, Phillips RK. Cancer and the Peutz-Jeghers syndrome. *Gut* 1989;30:1588–1590.

63

ULCERATIVE COLITIS

BRAD W. WARNER

Ulcerative colitis (UC) represents an important condition encountered in the pediatric population. Although most patients are in their teenage years, we have encountered several patients as young as 2 years with this disease. The major principles in dealing with this disease are the confirmation of the diagnosis and timing for surgery.

DIAGNOSTIC APPROACH

Before a definitive operation is performed for UC, it is critical that the diagnosis is secure. Surgical procedures designed for cure of UC typically are associated with unfavorable outcomes if the diagnosis ultimately turns out to be Crohn's disease. Despite the best preoperative evaluation, up to 20% of patients will have "indeterminate" colitis. Many of these patients demonstrate characteristics of Crohn's disease with less optimal outcomes.

Plain radiographs of the abdomen are useful to identify the presence or absence of megacolon, partial small bowel obstruction (which would suggest Crohn's disease), or, in extreme situations, free air. In addition, a thickened, edematous colon wall may assist in delineating the extent of inflammation and prevent a potentially harmful invasive test.

Colonoscopy is crucial to confirm that the inflammation begins in the distal rectum and extends proximally, that there are no skip lesions, and there is no extension of inflammation into the terminal ileum. Colonoscopic biopsies should demonstrate nonspecific inflammation with hemorrhage and without granulomas. The presence of granulomas on any biopsy sample is Crohn's disease until proven otherwise. Similarly, skip areas of inflammation throughout the colon as well as inflammation within the terminal ileum should raise a high index of suspicion for Crohn's disease.

Esophagogastroduodenoscopy is essential in the preoperative evaluation of a patient with UC. The main reason is to exclude any foregut inflammation or granulomas that would be diagnostic of Crohn's disease.

An upper gastrointestinal series with small bowel follow-through is important to exclude small intestinal abnormalities out of reach of upper and lower endoscopy. The presence of strictures, partial small bowel obstruction, or fistulas would all be highly suggestive of Crohn's disease.

Recently, serum levels of antineutrophil cytoplasmic antibody (ANCA) and anti-*Saccharomyces cerevisiae* antibody (ASCA) have assisted in distinguishing UC from Crohn's disease. Elevated levels of immunoglobulin A (IgA) or IgG ASCA antibodies would be most consistent with Crohn's disease. On the other hand, an elevated level of ANCA antibody with a specific perinuclear staining pattern (as opposed to pericytoplasmic) would be characteristic of UC. These tests may be useful in a patient with colitis that is histologically indeterminate.

PREOPERATIVE PREPARATION

The indications for definitive surgery in patients with UC are broad and include toxic megacolon, bleeding, failure of maximal medical management, complications of the immunosuppressive regimen, and concern for cancer. In comparison with adults, pediatric patients with UC tend to have a more progressive course of their disease. Nevertheless, many patients are managed medically for quite some time in anticipation of remission. Unfortunately, this management may be associated with growth retardation. Although unclear as to whether a result of the underlying disease or steroids, the development of growth retardation must be considered a strong indication for surgery. In addition, we have found that the combination of pancolonic involvement of UC in concert with steroid dependence (need for steroids for >3 months in the previous year) was

B. W. Warner: Department of Surgery, University of Cincinnati College of Medicine; and Division of Pediatric Surgery, Cincinnati Children's Hospital Medical Center, Cincinnati, Ohio.

associated with a significantly greater need for operative intervention.

In patients with toxic megacolon or significant hemorrhage, operation should be performed expediently. Broad-spectrum antibiotics should be given, and intravenous fluids and blood should be administered as necessary. Stress dosages of steroids should be administered (2 mg/kg hydrocortisone equivalent). There is no need for luminal antibiotics because the operation of choice in these patients would be a subtotal colectomy with terminal ileostomy.

In more elective situations, a full mechanical bowel preparation is performed. We routinely use a polyethylene glycol solution given at a dose of 40 mL/kg over 6 hours the afternoon before surgery. Sometimes a nasogastric tube is inserted to assure full intake of the preparation. In addition, luminal antibiotics are given as neomycin (20 mg/kg) and erythromycin base (20 mg/kg) at 1 P.M., 2 P.M., and 11 P.M. the day before surgery. Systemic antibiotics and stress levels of steroids are given the morning of surgery.

TECHNICAL APPROACH

There are multiple surgical options for the management of UC: (a) pancolectomy with a permanent ileostomy, continent ostomy (Kock pouch), or a double-stapled anastomosis at the top of the anal canal and an ileal pouch; (b) abdominal colectomy with ileorectal anastomosis; or (c) abdominal colectomy combined with a rectal mucosectomy, with or without the construction of an ileal reservoir. The standard approach at our institution has been a total abdominal colectomy, rectal mucosectomy, and construction of an ileal S-shaped pouch. I have always used a temporary protective ileostomy after the pouch construction.

For patients in whom the surgery is performed on an emergent basis (as for bleeding, toxic megacolon, etc.), I feel it is best to perform a subtotal colectomy with an ileostomy as the first stage. In the majority of cases, this results in rapid clinical improvement and allows the patient to wean from immunosuppressive medications. After several months of recovery, the rectal mucosectomy and ileal pouch are constructed as a second stage. The third stage involves closure of the ileostomy, which is done after a water-soluble contrast study has documented an intact pouch without leak or stricture. This is usually about 6 to 8 weeks later. This three-stage approach is also used for patients with requirements for high-dose immunosuppression (cyclosporine or azathioprine, or greater than 20 mg/day of prednisone) or if the anoscopy at the time of surgery reveals severe, active rectal disease. For all other cases, the definitive surgery is performed in two stages.

Intraoperative patient positioning is critical. Care must be taken to place the patient's legs in well-padded stirrups in a position that avoids ischemia to the calf muscles and compression of the peroneal nerve as it courses around the proximal head of the fibula. To prevent calf muscle ischemia, the weight of the legs must be directed to the heel, rather than the posterior calf. In addition, the time that the legs are elevated during the procedure must be minimized. This is facilitated by adjustable Allen stirrups (Allen Medical Systems, Bedford Heights, OH), in which the legs can be placed down during the abdominal portion of the procedure and elevated into a lithotomy position only during the perineal dissection. An additional advantage of the legs being down is that the intrapelvic dissection is facilitated. Prolonged leg elevation as well as lengthy compression of the calf musculature results in a compartment syndrome. If prolonged compression of the peroneal nerve occurs, the patient will have paresthesias and foot drop.

After positioning, a Foley catheter and a nasogastric tube are inserted. At this point, sigmoidoscopy is performed to assess the mucosa and verify that an endorectal mucosectomy is feasible. If so, a red rubber catheter is inserted and the sigmoid colon is lavaged with a half-strength povidone-iodine solution. The perineum is sprayed with a topical adhesive and the buttocks taped apart using cloth tape. The abdomen and perineum are then prepared in continuity.

The operation commences through a lower abdominal midline incision. Upon entering the peritoneal cavity, a general exploration is performed. Importantly, the entire small bowel is visualized to exclude Crohn's disease or other abnormalities. At this point, the colon is mobilized and resected. Removal of the omentum from the transverse colon will facilitate its removal. The proximal colon is transected with a stapler, with care taken to preserve a small cuff of cecum remaining attached to the terminal ileum. Transection of the bowel proximal to this point may prevent the ability of the pouch to reach the anus. The distal colon is similarly divided just above the peritoneal reflection, and the colon is submitted for gross pathologic confirmation of UC.

At this point, the rectum is mobilized from its circumferential peritoneal attachments. Posteriorly, the inferior mesenteric artery is doubly ligated and transected. This allows for a nice plane of rectal dissection posteriorly. Once this has been done and the rectum circumferentially mobilized for several centimeters, the rectal mucosectomy is started. This is carried as far distally as possible. I perform the majority of the rectal mucosectomy from inside the abdomen. Attention is then directed at the perineum. The legs are placed in a lithotomy position and a Lone-Star retractor (Lone Star Medical Products, Inc., Houston, TX) is placed in the anal canal. Using electrocautery, an endorectal dissection is then started at about 1 cm proximal to the top of the anal columns, thus preserving the transitional epithelium. When the dissection from below meets the dissection from above, the rectal mucosa is removed intact.

The ileal pouch is then constructed. It is important to first lengthen the mesentery of the terminal ileum by dissecting the root of the mesentery all the way to the inferior border of the pancreas. In addition, it is usually necessary to divide the ileal mesentery at several avascular points. It is sometimes useful to transilluminate the mesentery to identify major arterial branches. The ileocolic branch, as it comes off the superior mesenteric artery (SMA), may be transected close to the SMA to gain further length. This should be done after first test-occluding and monitoring the viability of the terminal ileum. Sufficient ileal length can usually be assured if the tip of the ileum reaches beyond the symphysis pubis.

The pouch is constructed in an S-shaped configuration with a hand-sewn technique using a monofilament, absorbable suture. The pouch should measure roughly 4 inches in length. The distal spout of the pouch should not extend longer than 1 cm away from the pouch because this may contribute to incomplete pouch emptying. Although this technique may take a little longer than a stapled J-shaped pouch, I am most comfortable with this particular method.

After the pouch is constructed, attention is directed to the perineum and the pouch is pulled through the rectal muscular cuff. A flat, malleable retractor should be used from the perineal side to facilitate the pull-through of the pouch. This will also help to prevent intussusception of the muscular cuff during pull-through. Three traction sutures are then placed to anchor the pouch in the endorectal canal. I use absorbable sutures placed at the 12, 3, and 9 o'clock positions between the pouch and the muscular sleeve of the rectum. Finally, the pouch–anal anastomosis is performed using interrupted, absorbable suture.

Prior to abdominal closure, a loop ileostomy is constructed in the right lower quadrant. After abdominal closure, the ostomy is matured in a Turnbull manner by cutting across the distal aspect of the antimesenteric loop at skin level. When the distal bowel is inverted, the proximal bowel projects slightly and fecal material is less likely to spill over into the distal bowel.

POSTOPERATIVE CARE

Postoperatively, a nasogastric tube is left in place until there is both gas and stool in the ileostomy bag. Neurovascular assessment of the lower extremities should be performed frequently during the first 24 hours after surgery. Stress-level steroids are maintained for 48 hours, and a rapid taper is then performed to the same preoperative level of steroids thereafter.

The ileostomy is closed least 6 to 8 weeks later. Prior to ostomy closure, a water-soluble contrast study is performed through the distal limb of the loop ileostomy. The integrity of the pouch should be evaluated and the pouch should empty without narrowing. Ostomy closure should be avoided if there are any areas of question with regard to a leak or fistula in the pouch. In this situation, the contrast study should be repeated after another 6 weeks.

After the ostomy is closed, I have found that the patients begin to pass stool very soon. I therefore do not feel that a postoperative nasogastric tube is necessary. It is not unusual for the patient to have frequent stools as well as episodes of incontinence for several weeks after the stoma is closed. In most cases, patients are totally continent and have about five to six bowel movements per day and one at night. The stool frequency is affected mostly by diet. The patient will have to learn which foods stimulate frequent bowel movements and make choices based on known consequences. In addition, avoiding frequent meals tends to avoid frequent stooling. For example, a large snack at bedtime will usually be rewarded with frequent stools through the night. I usually do not routinely use pharmacologic antimotility agents in the postoperative period. In extreme cases, loperamide is helpful to reduce the stooling frequency.

It is important that patients understand that the function of the colon is to absorb water and electrolytes. Without a colon, they are therefore more susceptible to dehydration and diarrhea. I find that the best means to monitor the degree of hydration is the urinary sodium. Urinary sodium of less than 10mEq/L is usually associated with volume contraction, and increasing the enteral fluids is necessary. In summer months or in patients who have vigorous exercise regimens, I recommend salt tablets as a means to maintain normal sodium status.

Pouchitis is always a concern and occurs in about 20% of patients. This presents clinically with crampy abdominal pain, fever, increased stool frequency, or blood in the stool. A recurrence of pouchitis warrants a pouch endoscopy with biopsy to exclude Crohn's disease. Pouchitis usually responds to a course of oral antibiotics such as metronidazole or ciprofloxacin. In addition, a rectal examination should be performed to rule out the presence of a stricture.

Continence is another important indicator of success with this operation. In our own experience, very young patients tend to have incontinence with a slightly greater frequency than do older patients. This tends to resolve over time. Persistent incontinence warrants further investigation, and studies should be performed to exclude muscular and neurologic injury.

Overall, the vast majority of patients are gratified with their operation and are able to resume normal, productive lives. Long-term follow-up of these patients is important.

SUGGESTED READINGS

Coran AG. A personal experience with 100 consecutive total colectomies and straight ileoanal endorectal pull-throughs for benign disease of the colon and rectum in children and adults. *Ann Surg* 1990;212:242–247.

Durno C, Sherman P, Harris K, et al. Outcome after ileoanal anastomosis in pediatric patients with ulcerative colitis. *J Pediatr Gastroenterol Nutr* 1998;27:501–507.

Falcone RA Jr, Lewis LG, Warner BW. Predicting the need for colectomy in pediatric patients with ulcerative colitis. *J Gastrointest Surg* 2000;4:201–206.

Fonkalsrud EW. Long-term results after colectomy and ileoanal pullthrough procedure in children. *Arch Surg* 1996;131:881–885.

Fonkalsrud EW, Loar N. Long-term results after colectomy and endorectal ileal pullthrough procedure in children. *Ann Surg* 1992;215:57–62.

Martin LW, Warner BW, Brockmeier M. Long-term evaluation of the endorectal Soave operation performed for ulcerative colitis or polyposis in the pediatric patient. *Surgery* 1993;114:893–896.

Ruemmele FM, Targan SR, Levy G, et al. Diagnostic accuracy of serological assays in pediatric inflammatory bowel disease. *Gastroenterology* 1998;115:822–829.

64

CONSTIPATION

KAREN M. KLING
CHARLES N. PAIDAS

CONSTIPATION

Constipation, although not the most glamorous topic for thought or publication, presents a problem for many children. Its proper treatment is essential for normal development, social acceptance, and, in extreme cases, to obviate colostomy. Constipation, by definition, is infrequent or difficult evacuation of feces. The word is derived from Latin *constipatus*, meaning "crowded together." It is most often self-limited and related to diet, environmental changes, or unrelated illness. Thus, the vast majority of cases are categorized as functional constipation. In the newborn period, however, constipation is always considered pathologic, often revealing congenital anatomic problems.

Etiology

The cause of constipation may be mechanical (anatomic), physiologic, or functional (behavioral). Although not exhaustive, Table 64.1 lists the most common causes of constipation. Anatomic causes most often present in the neonatal period. The most obvious anatomic cause is the spectrum of anorectal malformations (ARMs), from perineal fistulas to common cloaca. There is, particularly with low ARMs, almost uniform constipation, and 30% of patients have constipation severe enough to develop overflow incontinence in the postoperative period. Anal developmental anomalies also include anal stenosis, anteriorly displaced anus, Hirschsprung disease (HD), small left colon syndrome, meconium ileus, and meconium plug (associated with HD). In children with structural anal problems, even after repair, constipation should be anticipated. Presacral masses, such as those associated with anal stenosis and vertebral anomalies (Currarino triad), may present early or may be somewhat delayed in presentation, when dietary changes lead to stools of more solid consistency. Other masses, such as rectal duplications, rectal prolapse, intussusception, intestinal tumors (von Recklinghausen neurofibromas), and abdominal tumors, may obstruct the colon and rectum, causing constipation. Neurologic causes of constipation include spina bifida, myelomeningocele, and traumatic paraplegia. Constipation also can be due to atonic bowel caused by idiopathic reasons, or as a result of chronic functional constipation; in addition, decreased abdominal musculature, as one would see in prune belly syndrome, may make it difficult to generate intraabdominal pressures required for defecation.

Many physiologic factors contribute to constipation. Much of this is dietary in origin, with early introduction of cow's milk in babies or lack of appropriate fiber in older children. Drugs such as opiates, antidepressants, and antihistamines are also a frequent cause. Global metabolic conditions (sepsis in the newborn, hypothyroidism, maternal diabetes causing small left colon, hypoparathyroidism, and renal tubular acidosis), systemic neural impairments (multiple sclerosis and spasticity syndromes), and systemic illnesses (collagen vascular disease, inflammatory bowel disease, cystic fibrosis) can all be responsible for fecal impaction. Neuropsychiatric causes, such as retardation, depression, and psychosis, as well as toilet-training issues may cause constipation. Motility dysfunction may result from postischemic changes from necrotizing enterocolitis. In addition, postoperative neurovascular alterations may cause constipation from delayed transit and increased dehydration of stool. An important physiologic cause of constipation is ganglion cell-mediated dysfunction, such as HD, neuronal intestinal dysplasia (NID), and other neural crest disorders [pheochromocytoma, multiple endocrine neoplasia type 2B (MEN2B), Chagas disease] in which bouts of obstruction are common.

K. M. Kling and C. N. Paidas: Department of Pediatric Surgery, Johns Hopkins University School of Medicine and Johns Hopkins Hospital, Baltimore, Maryland.

TABLE 64.1. PARTIAL LIST OF CAUSES OF CONSTIPATION

Mechanical/anatomic
Anorectal malformation
Anal stenosis
Rectal duplication
Anterior displaced anus
Meconium plug syndrome
Small left colon syndrome
Presacral mass
Physiologic
Anorectal malformation after repair
Hirschsprung disease
"Neurogenic" rectum
Spina bifida
Myelomeningocele
Paraplegia
Neuronal intestinal dysplasia
Milk protein allergy
Drug-related
Opiates
Antidepressants
Antihistamines
Prune belly syndrome
Intestinal pseudoobstruction
Hypothyroidism
Hypoparathyroidism
Prematurity
Renal tubular acidosis
Cerebral palsy
Ischemic injury (e.g. after necrotizing enterocolitis)
Functional
Behavioral
Anal fissure (pain-related)

In contrast to the above organic causes of constipation, functional constipation, or constipation without identifiable cause, accounts for 95% of childhood constipation. It also can be environmental. Children may decrease stool frequency because they are uncomfortable outside of the home; they may be distracted and fail to fully evacuate; or they may have had anal fissures and recall painful defecation, which leads to voluntary decrease in bowel movements. Chronic constipation leads to accumulation of solid stool until defecation becomes difficult and perhaps painful. This serves to perpetuate the problem, and occasionally constipation is so severe that functional megacolon develops with the cycle of impaction, overflow incontinence, and encopresis.

Diagnosis

Evaluation should begin with a careful history and physical examination (Fig. 64.1). Pertinent questions include the time to first stool, stool caliber and consistency, history of anal or spinal cord anomalies, urinary retention, systemic illnesses, dietary customs, medications, and stool pattern of the parents. On physical examination, it is important to examine the position of the anus, degree of anal contraction, sphincter tone, contour of the buttocks and the presence of an anal fissure, posterior shelf, impacted fecal or abdominal mass, and palpable vertebral or spinal abnormalities. Likewise, rush of anal contents after digital examination should raise the possibility of HD, although this sign is highly unreliable. Suspicion for a spinal cause of constipation can be investigated using anteroposterior and lateral plain films of the lumbosacral spine as well as ultrasonography and magnetic resonance imaging (MRI) to evaluate the cord. These imaging studies are also useful in the diagnosis of presacral or intraabdominal masses contributing to constipation.

If the child has had a reconstruction for ARM, examination under anesthesia with sphincter stimulation is recommended after a Gastrografin (Shering Diagnostics, Berlin, Germany) enema (including postevacuation films). Meconium ileus requires a workup for cystic fibrosis, just as meconium plug and ileal or colonic atresias warrant evaluation for HD. Small left colon syndrome should prompt testing for maternal diabetes. Megacolon and impaction without evidence of another organic process suggest functional constipation. Especially important is the postevacuation film of the enema series, which may demonstrate radiologic evidence of HD, which should then be confirmed with rectal biopsy. In fact, if the workup is equivocal after radiographic studies, a rectal biopsy is mandatory. Absence of ganglion cells and increased acetylcholinesterase (AChE) are diagnostic of HD. Normal biopsy (presence of ganglion cells) must be reevaluated for AChE and the possibility of NID. These later studies require a fresh, nonfixed specimen. HD patients presenting with recurrence or increase in constipation postreconstruction should be evaluated with contrast enema, examination under anesthesia, and repeat biopsy to exclude retained aganglionic segment. Finally, if still no diagnosis is evident, upper gastrointestinal series may demonstrate a proximal intestinal obstruction. If the results are negative, endoscopy and biopsy can be used to obtain tissue for more obscure causes of constipation [e.g., inflammatory bowel disease (IBD), celiac disease, Chagas disease]. Motility studies using contrast or radiopaque markers can identify slow transit states. Manometry may detect ultra-short segment HD, demonstrating absent internal sphincter relaxation with distension of the rectum (rectoanal inhibitory reflex, or RAIR). However, we recommend rectal biopsy for the diagnosis of ultra-short HD. Some gastroenterologists feel that presence of RAIR should rule out HD. If there is any question, the single most reliable test for the diagnosis of HD is a full-thickness rectal biopsy. Increased rectal resting pressure and increased anal pressure with blunted urge to defecate are consistent with idiopathic constipation. Laboratory tests rarely play a role in the diagnosis of constipation. However, laboratory data can help assess some of the metabolic or systemic illnesses related to constipation.

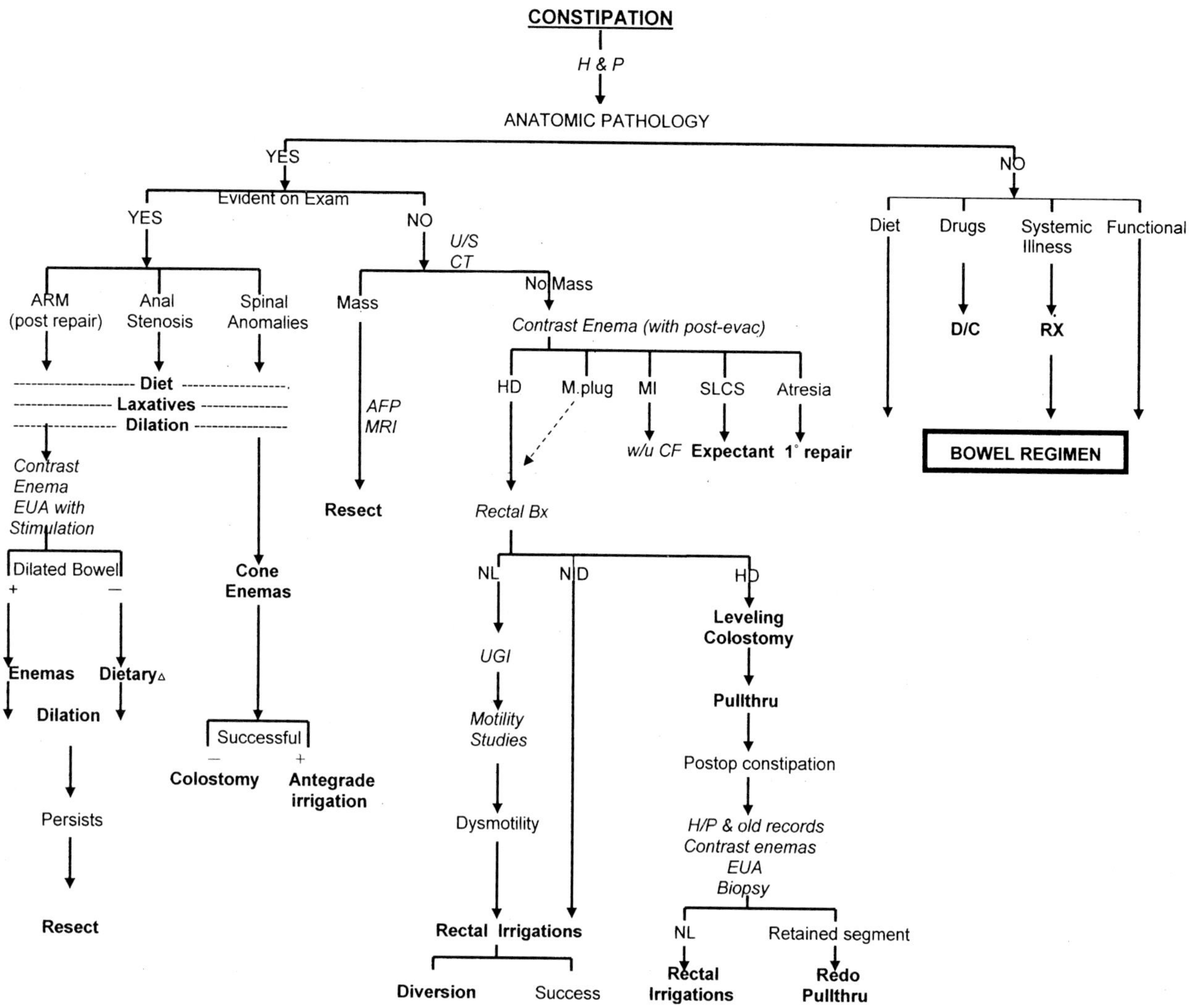

FIGURE 64.1. Algorithm for workup of constipation. Diagnostic tests are italicized and interventions are in bold. *M. plug,* meconium plug syndrome; *MI,* meconium ileus; *SLCS,* small left colon syndrome; *Bx,* biopsy; *NL,* normal.

Treatment

Treatment of functional constipation or that due to spinal problems should begin with initiation of a bowel regimen to empty the colon. Treatment should proceed in an organized, stepwise fashion, borrowing from cardiac physiology but in a slightly different sequence, first treating preload, then contractility, and finally afterload (Table 64.2).

Preload represents the volume and consistency of stool. Its management includes dietary modifications (increasing fluid intake, significantly reducing the intake of foods such as cheese, rice, bread, and nuts, introducing fruit juices, and increasing residue) and increasing activity level. It is also important to establish a daily routine for the child that facilitates evacuation. Defecation should be encouraged as a routine, shortly after meals, to take advantage of the brain–gut axis interaction. Stool softeners and sorbitol can draw in volume. Water-soluble fiber, such as Metamucil, adds bulk to the stool.

Contractility involves agents that promote increased motility and evacuation. These agents include laxatives (lactulose), prokinetic agents (metaclopramide), cathartics (e.g., Senokot, Purdue Frederick Co., Stanford, Connecticut), or stimulants to increase propulsion (caffeine). Other contractility agents such as polyethylene glycol and mineral oil mechanically move the stool along. Lactulose draws water into the colon, distending the bowel and stimulating propulsion. All of these agents may be useful to relieve impaction or intermittent severe constipation, but should be avoided for long-term routine use. For patients with decreased motility, prokinetic agents such as erythromycin, metaclopramide, and neostigmine may enhance evacuation.

Afterload reduction is a euphemism for rectal decompression and can be effected via digital examination, sup-

TABLE 64.2. BOWEL REGIMEN FOR CONSTIPATION

Preload	Fluid
	Fiber
	Sorbitol
	Prune juice
Contractility	Dulcolax
	Mineral oil
	Prokinetics
	Senekot
	Phosphosoda
	Magnesium citrate
	Golytely
	Miralax
	Lactulose
Afterload	Digital exam
	Suppositories
	Enemas
Reevaluation	History/physical
	Plain films
	Contrast enemas

Adapted from personal communication of Richard Katz, M.D.

pository, or enemas (tap water, soapsuds, mineral oil, or saline). Patients who have developed fecal impaction must be treated with enemas. Impaction may require manual disimpaction under anesthesia. Thereafter, routine enemas to keep the patient empty are necessary and can subsequently be weaned once regular bowel movements (independent of enemas) have occurred. Enemas become a significant part of the management scheme for children with spinal cord pathology; for example, cone enemas are particularly helpful in spina bifida patients. If enemas are successful, antegrade enemas (open appendicostomy or percutaneous cecostomy) should be useful, not as a panacea, but rather to improve quality of life. For patients in whom enemas are unsuccessful, colostomy should be recommended. The level of the colostomy is determined by intestinal manometry or by using radiopaque markers. This is not always straightforward.

For children in whom constipation is related to behavioral or psychiatric issues, the above measures may be necessary initially to bring constipation under control. However, behavioral modification may ultimately be necessary to treat the underlying cause appropriately, and only then would it be possible to withdraw any therapies. Occasionally, colonic inertia manifests such severe dilatation and poor motility that, in addition to the above measures, operative therapies have been recommended. We do not employ operative measures to treat colonic inertia, but rather rely on pharmacologic therapy. Myotomy to decompress proximal bowel pressure has been described, but has limited, if any, success. We do not recommend myotomy for management of colonic inertia. One particular role for resection involves the finding of chronically dilated and dysfunctional bowel (commonly, the rectosigmoid). Rectosigmoid resection frequently improves motility. Ileostomy may be indicated in recalcitrant cases. Rarely, total colectomy is necessary, and ileoproctostomy should be avoided because pharmacologic treatment for these conditions may be discovered in the future. Even when structural or physiologic problems causing constipation are properly diagnosed and remedied, such as obstructions, pelvic masses, and metabolic or septic causes, constipation often persists. These children may need a bowel regimen, regardless of the treatment plan.

The most common situations facing pediatric surgeons are ARM and HD. Both of these pathologies require aggressive and life-long bowel management and close physician follow-up. Constipation in the child with a low ARM should be anticipated, and treatment should begin immediately after reconstruction. Patients with high ARM may have postoperative constipation, pseudoincontinence from overflow, or true incontinence. Low ARM, defined as perineal fistulas, are treated with dilation and posterior sagittal anorectoplasty. These patients uniformly have some degree of constipation, which occurs days to weeks after colostomy closure. These children should be started on daily dilations 2 to 3 weeks postoperatively.

Evaluation of a new or worsening complaint of constipation in a child followed for ARM should begin with evaluation for anal stricture and verification that the anal opening has been positioned within the most concentric portion of the sphincter complex. Office dilation can be attempted and the home regimen reinforced, but more often than not dilation under anesthesia is necessary. Skilled professionals may have to be sent to the home if caregivers are unable to properly perform anal dilations. A contrast enema should also be performed. The degree of dilation will dictate whether daily enemas will be necessary in addition to routine dilations.

In children with postoperative constipation following repair of low imperforate anus, once adequate anoplasty has been verified, a bowel regimen should begin (Table 64.2). As with functional constipation, the use of dietary measures such as fruits, vegetables, and sorbitol-rich juices (pear nectar) may be sufficient to keep patients regular (preload). Following this, lactulose (contractility) and enemas (afterload reduction) can be used. Enemas may be tapered if and when the rectum is empty and a laxative regimen delivers daily full evacuation without accidents. Tap water, saline, sodium phosphate, soapsuds, or mineral oil enemas are all acceptable. In chronic, untreated constipation secondary to ARM, if a chronically dilated poorly propulsive sigmoid develops, resection is beneficial. Included in the spectrum of ARM is the anteriorly displaced anus, and this can be managed with diet and stool softeners. Anal stenosis requires dilations and dietary changes to keep stools soft.

The principle of treatment for HD is decompression, resection of the aganglionic bowel, and pull-through of normally innervated bowel. Some centers are performing primary pull-through for HD with good clinical results, but staged repair with decompression remains common and is imperative in those with enterocolitis. Two thirds of HD patients present by 3 months of age with the problem of difficulty evacuating. All patients with HD mandate full evacuation so that constipation and recurrent bouts of life-threatening enterocolitis do not occur. The longer the segment affected by disease, the more likely are motility and evacuation difficulties and diagnosis delayed. Again, the bowel regimen outlined above may be used, but these children are less likely to have problems with stool consistency that is remedied by diet and medication; their problems relate to aberrant motility, and they rely heavily on rectal irrigation, which in contrast to an enema uses a rectal tube placed high in the rectum. A schedule should be maintained to outline daily independent evacuation. If after examination of this stool pattern regular bowel movements without accidents are evident and the child is fully evacuated, then irrigations may be tapered to a schedule that maintains this state. The post-HD child that has success with frequent irrigations, but fails with any attempt to wean, may need irrigations indefinitely. Although appealing, the percutaneous antegrade method of irrigation alone will not overcome the external pressure required to evacuate the colon. These children typically have such low colonic pressure that they cannot overcome normal external anal sphincter to evacuate their colon without a tube in place.

In a postoperative HD patient who presents with constipation after a period of regular bowel movements, one should proceed from a food ingestion history and physical examination of the abdomen and anal anastomosis to reevaluation of their current bowel regimen. It is crucial to review old studies, operative notes, and biopsy results. We recommend performing examination under anesthesia and full-thickness biopsy to exclude any retained aganglionic segment or concomitant NID. A very short retained segment should be resected via a perineal or posterior sagittal approach. We do not recommend posterior myotomy for retained segment or ultra-short segment HD. Assessment via contrast enema is also necessary to determine the degree, if any, of dilatation. Dilated bowel must be treated with aggressive irrigation to effect adequate decompression. This is paramount before reoperation for retained segment so that proximally dilated bowel may recover and optimize its motility.

Treatment of chronic pseudoobstruction and NID can be challenging. Pseudoobstruction involves motor dysfunction of different sites and degrees in the gastrointestinal tract. It may be idiopathic or there may be myopathies, neurodegenerative issues, or ganglion cell abnormalities identifiable. NID specifically refers to hyperplasia of submucosal and myenteric plexuses with a moderate increase in AChE activity; mucosal inflammation also can be present. It may present in the neonatal period or at several years of age. NID manifests as a spectrum ranging from a self-limited several-month course to persistent dysmotility and feeding intolerance necessitating chronic parenteral nutrition and ileostomy. In short-segment NID, bowel resection can be curative. However, this is a difficult diagnosis to prove. For many patients, catheter bowel irrigation has been successful in treating NID. Often children are dependent on catheter irrigations for an extended period of time (months to years). In our experience, antegrade delivery of irrigations has not been a valuable adjunct to traditional rectal catheter irrigation, probably due to the poor propulsion in the diseased segment. This poor motility is diffuse, so delivery of irrigation higher than the rectal vault has yielded better results, and the catheter then also provides a route for egress of stool. Failure of the above strategies may require proximal stoma. The long-term follow-up of bowel management by a pediatric surgeon and staff cannot be overemphasized. Even in patients in whom treatment seems successful, constant reevaluation must be performed via history, physical examination, plain films, and contrast enemas to look for recurrent constipation. If one gets behind, a patient may spiral through bouts of constipation, enterocolitis, and develop a chronically dilated colon. This further perpetuates the cycle of evacuation difficulties.

INCONTINENCE

Incontinence is the inability to hold feces in the rectum due to failure of voluntary control over the anal sphincter, permitting untimely passage of stool and gas. Bowel control depends on successful coordination of many anatomic and physiologic elements. Socially acceptable behavior demands that every person, once bowel trained, must be able to distinguish between solid, liquid, and gas. Continence requires adequate function of the sphincter muscles (external striated voluntary sphincter and the levator mechanism and the internal involuntary smooth muscle sphincter) as well as adequate neurologic (local, psychiatric, and mental) function. Rectal distensibility, anal sensation, intestinal motility, stool volume, and the ability to fully evacuate together play significant roles in continence.

Etiology

Causes of incontinence are related to neuromuscular, anatomic, or physiologic causes. Neurologic causes include myelomeningocele, spinal cord tumors, tethered spinal cord, spina bifida, sacral dysgenesis syndromes, and trauma-related spinal cord or brain injury. Pertinent to our understanding of continence is the presence of the second through fourth sacral bones. However, the second and third sacral vertebrae may be all that are necessary for socially acceptable control of defecation. Trauma from obstetric injuries or sexual abuse may injure the internal and external sphincter complex and lead to incontinence. Prolapse, seen in some cystic fibrosis or spinal injured patients, may cause incontinence. Children with ARM are affected by a spectrum of continence problems from lack of adequate associated muscle, bone, and nerve. For example, in children with cloacal anomalies and high ARMs, sensory deficits distort proprioception, and dysmotility may yield rapid transit stools. Neuromuscular elements are often hypotrophic, leading to localized rectosigmoid dysfunction and thus decreased reservoir capability and downstream signaling to the anal reflexes in these children. ARM patients with the highest incidence of incontinence (25%) include the categories of males with rectal–bladder neck fistulas and girls with long channel (>3 cm) cloacal malformations. All patients with low ARMs must be monitored for constipation, which if inadequately treated may develop into overflow pseudoincontinence. Likewise, children with rectovestibular, prostatic urethral, and bulbar urethral anomalies also can suffer from overflow pseudoincontinence.

Physiologic causes of incontinence include indiscriminant use of laxatives and enemas, rapid transit states, and loose stools such as with short gut syndrome, IBD, or HD. Patients with IBD also may experience poor distensibility of the rectum and therefore decreased reservoir and sensation mechanisms necessary to signal a full rectal vault.

Diagnosis

One should distinguish between the inability to develop continence, as a milestone to becoming a toilet-trained child, from the child who is capable of having voluntary bowel movements (Fig. 64.2). Voluntary stooling is the most important determinant of potential for developing full continence. Presentation of the complaint of incontinence after a period of continence may be more common with physiologic, behavioral, or environmental causes. However, one must be sure there are no new spinal, neurologic, traumatic, or constipation-related causes.

Complete absence of continence should prompt the workup of sphincter muscle inadequacy and neurologic control mechanisms. Physical examination should, like the workup of constipation, mandate assessment of anal anatomy, contour of the buttock folds, sphincter tone and

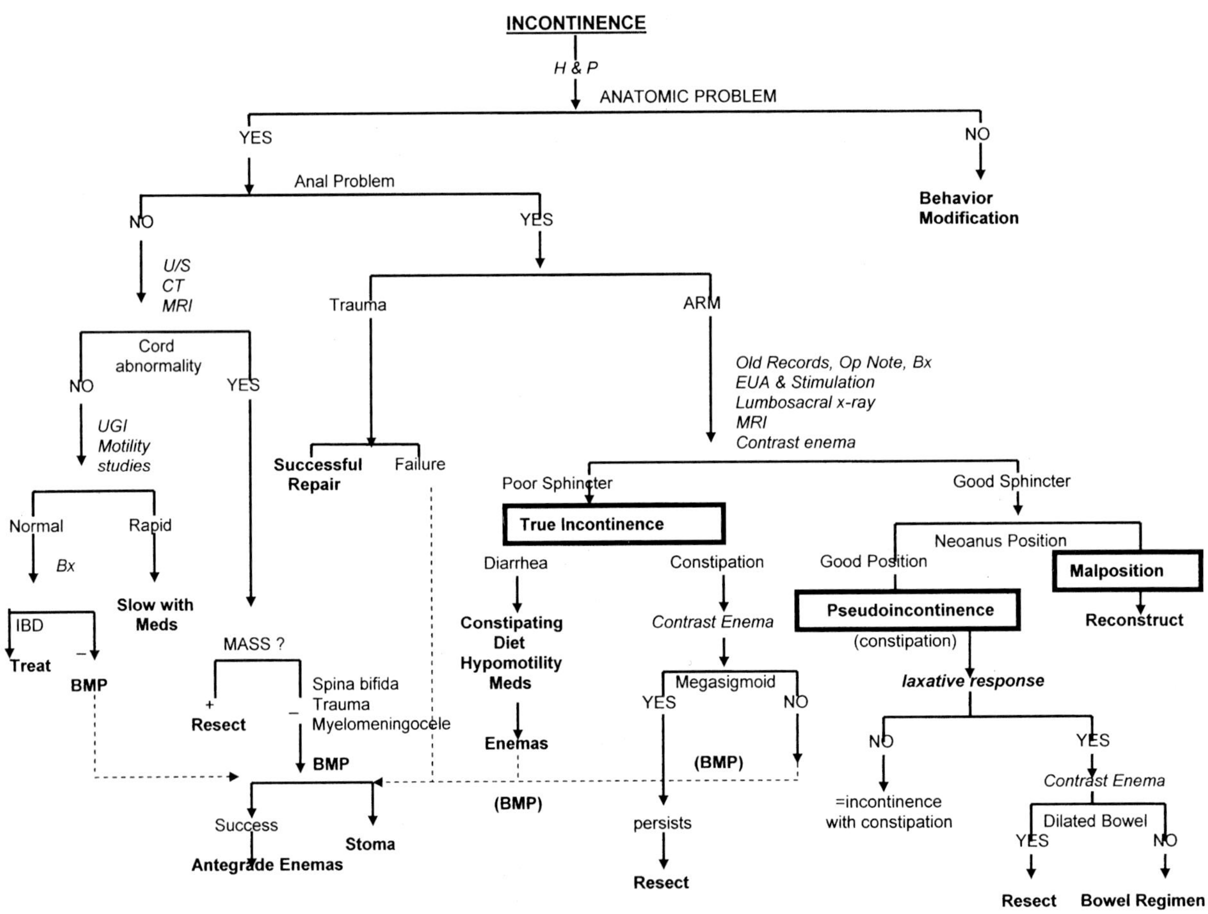

FIGURE 64.2. Algorithm for workup of incontinence. Diagnostic tests are italicized and interventions are in bold. *BMP,* bowel management program; *Bx,* biopsy.

evidence of trauma, presacral masses, or impaction. The child may have an obvious ARM, and workup should proceed with studies to assess an accurate classification of the defect (high or low). In addition, response to cutaneous nerve stimulation during an examination under anesthesia and studies to evaluate the genitourinary tract must be obtained. It is important, if the ARM patient presents with postoperative incontinence, to ascertain from old records, operative notes, radiographic studies, and biopsy results the type of anomaly and assess from those data the likelihood of continence. Examination under anesthesia with stimulation will be necessary to examine the relationship of the neoanus to the sphincter complex. MRI may be necessary to define the relationship between neoanus and striated muscle. If no structural spinal or anal problem is evident on physical examination, ultrasonography and MRI studies may demonstrate an occult lesion and define the neuromuscular anatomy.

Absence of sphincter problems or a neurologic cause would then lead to contrast enema to define the anatomy and look for findings such as a megasigmoid. Upper gastrointestinal series with follow-through may demonstrate motility problems or suggest IBD. Biopsy to evaluate more subtle neuromuscular pathology or IBD also may be helpful. Manometric studies may confirm or refute muscular abnormality, but often do not correlate well with degree of incontinence. Electromyography can test the integrity of innervation of the external sphincter.

Treatment

Treatment of incontinence is geared toward improvement in control and not necessarily cure. Basic principles include identifying and correcting anatomic irregularities, regularly emptying the rectosigmoid, improving the consistency of stools with bowel management, sometimes behavioral strategies, and finally providing realistic expectations about efficacy to the family. A bowel management program (BMP) as discussed in this chapter pertains specifically to a series of actions used to keep clean a child with permanent of temporary incontinence. Patients fall into three main categories: (a) truly incontinent patients with neuromuscular cause (ARMs of the upper tract or spinal anomalies); (b) patients with good potential for muscle function and control but a mislocated anus; and (c) pseudoincontinent patients who really have overflow incontinence as a result of overwhelming constipation.

True Incontinence

These patients have a neuromuscular cause for incontinence, and a significant number of these patients seen by the pediatric surgeon have high ARMs (e.g., bladder neck, long channel cloaca). These patients have no potential for bowel control, clinical and radiographic evidence of poor sphincters, poor sacral anatomy, and are therefore not candidates for operation. Poor prognosis is suggested by loss of more than two sacral vertebral bodies, poor gluteal definition, high ARMs with genitourinary fistula, attenuated muscle, and decreased intestinal length. The trick to keeping these children from soiling is to keep the colon empty and quiescent between scheduled evacuations through utilization of aggressive BMP.

In children identified as incontinent but with concomitant constipation, their hypomotility is used to an advantage and daily enemas are used for routine evacuations. Accidents here are usually due to failure to completely empty the rectosigmoid. In the incontinent child who also has increased motility or loose stool, bowel control is more challenging and necessitates the use of constipating foods or medications as well as enemas to maintain intestinal inactivity between scheduled evacuations. Failure in this subset of patients is usually due to inability to adequately slow the motility of the colon. BMP is usually successful (90%) within days; if BMP is successful, antegrade enemas via continent appendicostomy can be given for any age child. Those who fail bowel management with enemas should be advised that permanent colostomy will most likely be required for adequate lifestyle. The BMP described above for ARM also applies to those with irreversible neurologic compromise.

Anal Malposition

These patients have good sphincter complex, good sacral anatomy, and good bowel control potential. On anal stimulation, however, the neoanus is not within the most concentric area of sphincter complex and would therefore benefit from repositioning. The patient who has sphincter damage from trauma is another obvious candidate for reoperation. Reoperation for repositioning should yield continence in up to 80% of patients. If unsuccessful, an aggressive BMP will be needed.

Pseudoincontinence

Pseudoincontinent patients have the indicators of good bowel control but also have a properly located neoanus. They experience constipation and impaction, with or without a resultant megasigmoid, and their incontinence represents liquid stool overflow. It is imperative to make the distinction between pseudoincontinence secondary to fecal impaction versus the child who is in the constipated subgroup of true fecal incontinence. For this reason, their treatment should begin with disimpaction, laxatives, and enemas to clear the colon. Once the colon is clear, the proper dose of laxative to effect daily emptying is determined. Ninety-five percent should have relief with this treatment. Children with pseudoincontinence who respond to enemas and laxative treatment may have a megasigmoid colon as the cause of their problem. Resection of redundant sigmoid may be warranted. If laxative treatment does not remedy the problem, this is diagnostic of the fact that these children do not have impaction and pseudoincontinence but that they are truly incontinent and unable to have voluntary bowel movements. These children require a BMP (see section on True Incontinence).

FOLLOW-UP

For both patients with constipation and those with incontinence, close follow-up is mandatory, so that the majority of management can be preventive rather than management of cyclical complications. Of paramount importance is the proper recognition of which children are at risk for incontinence and which are likely to have constipation. Only then will the proper aggressive strategies to control these entities be used. A pitfall in the management of constipation or incontinence is related to making the incorrect diagnosis (e.g., true incontinence with constipation vs. overflow pseudoincontinence). Probable outcomes, dependent on the pathology, also should be discussed in detail with the child and parents so that expectations are realistic. A schedule of laxatives, enemas, voluntary bowel movements, induced bowel movements, and accidents should be kept on a calendar so that the adequacy of treatment can be judged. Once a plan has been implemented, its effectiveness must be ascertained. Frequent visits are necessary until patients and parents demonstrate an understanding of the methods selected and independence in using these protocols. Patients with ARMs and HD should be followed indefinitely to avoid the sequelae of inadequate bowel management. Meticulous follow-up of the stool pattern and telephone contact with the family to reinforce the treatment plan is necessary. Reevaluation of bowel habits and success of therapy must be evaluated by history, physical examination, contrast enemas, and sometimes biopsy. Early intervention when a patient deviates from a treatment algorithm is essential because persistent bowel dysfunction may become irreversible.

SUGGESTED READINGS

Loening-Baucke V. Functional constipation. *Semin Pediatr Surg* 1995;4:26–34.

Paidas CN. Fecal incontinence in children with anorectal malformations. *Semin Pediatr Surg* 1997;6:228–234.

Constipation, fecal incontinence, and proctologic conditions. In: Roy CC, Silverman A, Alagille D. *Pediatric clinical gastroenterology, 4th ed.* St. Louis: Mosby Year Book, 1995:494–521.

Paidas CN, Pena A. Rectum and anus. In: Oldham KT, Colombani PM, Foglia RP. eds. *Surgery of infants and children.* Philadelphia: Lippincott-Raven, 1997:1323–1362.

Pena A. Anorectal malformations. *Semin Pediatr Surg* 1995;4: 35–47. The Pull-thru Network, 2001. *www.pullthrough.org.*

Surgical Directives: Pediatric Surgery, edited by Peter Mattei. Lippincott Williams & Wilkins, Philadelphia © 2002

65

HIRSCHSPRUNG'S DISEASE

RICHARD R. RICKETTS

Hirschsprung's disease (congenital aganglionic megacolon) is the most common cause of intestinal obstruction in the neonate. It occurs in about 1 in 5,000 live births with a male:female ratio of 3.4:1. Total colon Hirschsprung's disease favors females 1.6:1. The transition zone is in the rectosigmoid in 75% of cases, but Hirschsprung's disease may involve the entire colon and terminal ileum in up to 8% of patients. The most common associated anomaly is Down's syndrome, occurring in 8% to 16% of patients. Approximately 5% of patients with Down's syndrome have Hirschsprung's disease.

Approximately 80% to 90% of patients are diagnosed during the newborn period. However, some patients present during infancy or as toddlers and some present during late childhood (or even as adults). It is useful clinically to approach patients according to the time of presentation because the workup and management within these three time periods vary.

THE NEWBORN WITH HIRSCHSPRUNG'S DISEASE

Diagnosis

Newborns present with a complete intestinal obstruction characterized by abdominal distension, emesis, and failure to pass meconium: 94% of normal full-term infants pass their meconium stool before 24 hours of age, whereas 94% of patients with Hirschsprung's disease do not. Family history is important because the risk for a sibling developing Hirschsprung's disease is 1% to 5% for short-segment disease and 9% to 33% for long-segment disease. Familial Hirschsprung's disease occurs in 4% to 8% of patients.

On physical examination, the abdomen is distended but relatively soft. Rectal examination may result in an explosive stool that temporarily relieves the obstruction.

R. R. Ricketts: Department of Surgery and Pediatrics, Emory Children's Center, Emory Children's Center; and Department of Surgery, Division of Pediatrics, Children's Healthcare of Atlanta at Egleston, Atlanta, Georgia.

The differential diagnosis includes other causes of a lower intestinal obstruction in newborns, including intestinal atresia, meconium ileus, meconium peritonitis, meconium plug, small left colon syndrome, and imperforate anus. Meconium peritonitis is characterized by calcifications seen on the plain abdominal film. Intestinal atresia and meconium ileus are associated with a microcolon, whereas Hirschsprung's disease is characterized by a normal colon or a megacolon. Small left colon syndrome is associated with maternal diabetes and is usually treated effectively with the contrast enema. Meconium plug syndrome is also treated effectively with the enema. In both of these conditions, the rectum has a greater diameter than the sigmoid colon. In Hirschsprung's disease, on the other hand, the rectum has a diameter smaller than the sigmoid colon. Failure to completely evacuate the barium on a 24-hour delayed film is also suggestive of Hirschsprung's disease. The barium enema has an error rate of 20% in newborns with Hirschsprung's disease. The diagnosis rests on the demonstration of aganglionosis and hypertrophy of the nerve trunks in a suction rectal biopsy. It is critical that the biopsy be performed at least 2 cm proximal to the mucocutaneous junction because the area distal to that point may have aganglionosis or hypoganglionosis in the normal infant. Manometry in the newborn cannot be used to reliably establish the diagnosis.

Preoperative Preparation

The initial goal of treatment is decompression. If one anticipates performing a primary pull-through procedure, initial decompression is achieved with rectal irrigations consisting of administering saline at a volume of 20 mL/kg three times daily via a large catheter located high in the rectum or descending colon. The irrigations can be performed for a few days or a few weeks prior to the definitive pull-through procedure. If the baby has other medical problems, or if the social situation is such that an irrigation program cannot be reliably executed, or if the baby presents with enterocolitis, then initial management should include a "leveling" colostomy. The level at which the colostomy is placed is determined by rapid frozen sections of seromuscular biopsies obtained from the colon during the operation. One must be assured that there are numerous normal ganglion cells at the site of the proposed colostomy. Although a loop colostomy will suffice, my preference is for a divided colostomy. Each limb of the colon comprising the colostomy is sutured to the abdominal wall fascia layer with several sutures to prevent prolapse or retraction. A budded stoma at least 1 cm in height is then created by primarily maturing the colostomy. The definitive pull-through procedure is delayed for 3 to 6 months or until the child weighs 5 to 10 kg.

With either a primary or a delayed pull-through, the baby receives neomycin 100 mg/kg/day in three or four divided doses on the day prior to surgery. The colon is then lavaged with a dilute betadine solution in the operating room immediately before the procedure.

Definitive Pull-Through Procedure

The type of definitive pull-through to be performed depends on the length of the aganglionosis: standard short-segment disease, long-segment disease involving bowel up to the transverse colon, or total colonic aganglionosis. Newborns and toddlers can be treated similarly for all three lengths of disease, whereas older children (and adults) are managed differently. For the standard short-segment disease, I prefer a primary laparoscopically assisted pull-through procedure as described by Georgeson. Three 3-mm ports and one 5-mm port are used. The camera is placed in the right upper quadrant, and the retraction port is in the left lower quadrant. One 5-mm port is placed to make use of the 5-mm stapling instrument, if required. A seromuscular biopsy sample is obtained from the suspected area of the transition zone and is sent for rapid frozen section analysis to confirm the presence of ganglion cells. I wait for the frozen section report before starting the perineal dissection to avoid "burning my bridges" if it turns out that the baby has long-segment disease instead of the suspected short-segment disease. The seromuscular biopsy site is used to mark the lowest area of the transition zone; the colon is divided well above this mark when performing the anastomosis. The bowel is dissected circumferentially from the site of the biopsy down to a level below the peritoneal reflection using the hook cautery. If the dissection is limited to the bowel wall, as in the Swenson procedure, it may not be necessary to use the clip applier during the procedure. Additionally, there will be no damage to the surrounding sympathetic and parasympathetic nerve fibers. After mobilizing the bowel down to a level below the peritoneal reflection, the submucosal transanal dissection, similar to a Soave procedure, is performed. Eight stay sutures are placed at the mucocutaneous junction to evert the anus to allow for an uncomplicated dissection. When the dissection from above is met by the dissection from below, the colon literally telescopes itself out through the anus. The remaining seromuscular layer is then divided, allowing one to pull the colon out through the anus to a site well beyond the original biopsy site. A single-layer anastomosis using absorbable suture is then made between the full thickness of the pulled-through bowel and the submucosal–mucosal layer of the everted anus. A diverting colostomy is not performed.

Newborns and toddlers with long-segment disease are treated initially with a leveling colostomy and subsequently with a Swenson pull-through procedure. The mesentery supplying the transverse and descending colon is divided in the standard way down to the level of the peritoneal reflection. At this point, the bowel is skeletonized circumferentially so that the remaining dissection from the level of the peritoneal reflection down to the anus stays on the bowel wall. Most of the dissection can be performed with electrocautery. Tension is placed on the vessels, which are subsequently cauterized as they enter the bowel wall. The dissection continues circumferentially all the way down until the rectum can be everted out of the anus, demonstrating a smooth transition between the anal skin and the mucosa of the bowel to be resected. It is essential that the bowel be mobilized sufficiently to allow it to be totally everted through the anus in order to accomplish the anastomosis 0.5 cm from the mucocutaneous junction anteriorly and 1 cm from the mucocutaneous junction posteriorly. The anastomosis is performed in two layers using silk for the seromuscular layer and absorbable sutures for the mucosal layer. When the last sutures are cut, the anus everts back into the pelvis and a digital examination confirms the presence of an adequate lumen with a circumferentially intact anastomosis. A diverting colostomy is not performed.

Newborns and toddlers with total colon Hirschsprung's disease are treated initially with a Kimura-type ileocolostomy. The ganglionated terminal ileum is anastomosed to the right colon with a 60- or 90-mm linear stapler depending on the size of the patient. This ileocolostomy is then brought out and primarily matured. The remaining colon down to the peritoneal reflection is resected. At a later date, when the nutritional status of the infant is satisfactory, a Swenson procedure is performed using the Kimura ileocolostomy. This definitive procedure may be delayed for 6 months to a year depending on the nutritional status of the infant. It should be delayed at least 2 to 3 months to allow for adequate collateralization of the blood supply between the ileum and the ascending colon, because the blood supply to the colon will by necessity be sacrificed during the pull-through procedure.

THE TODDLER WITH HIRSCHSPRUNG'S DISEASE

Diagnosis

Toddlers present with a history of chronic constipation. On careful questioning, one can usually determine that the baby did not in fact pass his or her first meconium stool within 24 hours of birth. The symptoms may have been delayed if the baby was being breast-fed because breast milk creates a softer stool, which the baby has less difficulty in passing. A clue to the diagnosis, then, is the onset of symptoms corresponding with the introduction of formula feedings. The toddler will typically have been managed with corn syrup, prune juice, or glycerin suppositories but will infrequently have stools on its own. Toddlers, as well as newborns, could present with an episode of acute Hirschsprung's-associated enterocolitis, which occurs in approximately 10% of patients. Enterocolitis is associated with abdominal distension, fever, emesis, and spontaneous diarrhea or an explosive diarrheal stool with gas during and following a rectal examination. Enterocolitis is treated with decompression of the rectum with a large catheter and with warm saline irrigations using 20 mL/kg three or four times a day, volume resuscitation, and administration of broad-spectrum antibiotics if signs of sepsis are present.

In toddlers, the barium enema is highly diagnostic for Hirschsprung's disease. The enema should be performed on an unprepared colon using a catheter without a balloon on it, which would artificially distend the rectum. Once the transition zone is identified, further instillation of barium is not necessary. Despite the reliability of the barium enema, the diagnosis must be absolutely established with a rectal biopsy. In toddlers, the suction biopsy sample may not be adequate because the mucosa is often too thick to allow for good sampling of the submucosa. Therefore, a full-thickness biopsy sample obtained in the operating room under general anesthesia is preferred. Manometry also can be diagnostic depending on the skill and experience of the person performing the test.

Preoperative Preparation

Toddlers with Hirschsprung's disease require an enema under anesthesia in order to fully evacuate the colon. The transverse or descending colon is typically of normal caliber and can be used for a primary pull-through procedure after the rectosigmoid has been completely evacuated. The toddler is kept in the hospital in order to receive colonic irrigations two to three times per day before proceeding with the pull-through procedure. The preoperative preparation with neomycin and dilute betadine irrigations and the definitive pull-through procedure are the same as those for newborns.

THE OLDER CHILD WITH HIRSCHSPRUNG'S DISEASE

Diagnosis

Children, teenagers, and even adults can present with Hirschsprung's disease. These patients present with chronic constipation, massive abdominal distension, and signs of poor nutrition with growth failure and wasting of the extremities. Most of these patients have short-segment disease. However, it is interesting that the length of aganglionosis does not correlate with clinical symptomatology. Therefore, patients presenting late could still have long-segment and even total colonic Hirschsprung's disease. These patients must be distinguished from those with chronic constipation without Hirschsprung's disease. Onset of Hirschsprung's disease normally occurs during the neonatal period, whereas symptoms of chronic constipation normally begin during the "potty training" period. Patients with Hirschsprung's disease have abdominal distension, whereas those with chronic constipation usually do not. Patients with Hirschsprung's disease do not typically soil their underwear, whereas patients with chronic constipation do. On rectal examination, patients with Hirschsprung's disease have an empty rectum, whereas those with chronic constipation have a large fecal impaction palpable just inside the anal sphincter. In patients with Hirschsprung's disease, the barium enema demonstrates a transition zone and the rectosigmoid diameter is larger than the rectal diameter; in patients with chronic constipation, no transition zone is identified. Manometry is useful in older children with Hirschsprung's disease. Among normal patients, distention of the rectal balloon causes relaxation of the internal anal sphincter. In patients with Hirschsprung's disease, there is failure of relaxation of the internal anal sphincter in response to inflation of the rectal balloon. Therefore, if one sees relaxation of the internal sphincter after rectal distension, the diagnosis of Hirschsprung's disease is excluded. Confirmatory evidence for the diagnosis still relies on a full-thickness rectal biopsy sample obtained in the operating room under general anesthesia. Once again, the biopsy sample must be taken at least 2 to 3 cm proximal to the mucocutaneous junction.

Preoperative Preparation

Older children, teenagers, or adults typically present with a massively dilated rectosigmoid colon with variable degrees of dilatation of the descending, transverse, and ascending colon. These patients require a vigorous enema under anesthesia using at least 6 L of saline in order to clean out the distal rectosigmoid. If the transverse or descending colon can be brought down to a relatively normal size with repeated irrigations, a primary pull-through can be accomplished. If not, these patients may require an ileostomy to achieve adequate decompression. A leveling colostomy in these patients typically results in a huge colostomy, which has a tendency to either prolapse or retract and to not adequately decompress the proximal bowel. An ileostomy to divert the fecal stream and a mucous fistula at the site of the ganglionated bowel may allow the bowel to decompress sufficiently to be used for a pull-through procedure later.

Definitive Pull-Through Procedure

Older children, teenagers, and adults present a different situation than newborns or toddlers. With standard short-segment disease, if the descending colon can be brought down to a normal size following enemas under anesthesia, a primary Swenson or Duhamel pull-through procedure is performed. The Swenson procedure in these patients is quite tedious and requires one to ligate several vessels rather than relying on electrocautery for hemostasis. The last 5 to 6 cm of the dissection are extremely difficult and require the use of a good headlight and long instruments. It is essential, as in the performance of all Swenson procedures, that the bowel be totally mobilized to allow it to be completely everted out through the anus to allow for a sufficiently low anastomosis. In large teenagers and adults, I have found that the Duhamel procedure is technically easier and has similar satisfactory results. The Martin modification of the Duhamel procedure should be used in order to prevent the formation of a fecaloma at the upper end of the rectum.

If the descending colon cannot be brought down to a normal size, a diverting ileostomy as well as a mucous fistula at the end of the ganglionated colon should be performed. Additionally, the massive rectosigmoid can be resected down to the level of the peritoneal reflection. After the transverse and descending colon have diminished in size sufficient to allow for a pull-through procedure, a Swenson or Duhamel procedure is performed. The ileostomy that remains following the procedure is closed at a later date.

For long-segment disease, a J-pouch ileo–anal pull-through procedure may be required because the right colon may be too large to be used for the pull-through. An ileostomy with resection of the colon down to the peritoneal reflection is performed first followed by a J-pouch ileoanal pull-through procedure with or without a protective ileostomy 6 to 8 weeks later.

For total colon Hirschsprung's disease in older children, teenagers, or adults, a Kimura ileocolostomy followed by a Swenson or Duhamel pull-through procedure or a J-pouch ileoanal pull-through procedure may be required, depending on the size of the colon and the ileum. Fortunately, most of these patients have short-segment disease and do not require such an extensive resection.

POSTOPERATIVE CARE

All patients are followed monthly for 3 months, then every 3 months for 1 year, then every 4 to 6 months for 2 years, and then every 6 to 12 months thereafter. Rectal examinations need to be performed frequently during their first several months of follow-up to detect any anastomotic strictures. If these are found, anal dilations must be used in order to help prevent problems with constipation. The family or the older patients themselves need to be schooled on the signs and symptoms of enterocolitis and should be told to seek medical attention immediately if the patient develops abdominal distention associated with obstipation or diarrhea. Many nonsurgeons are unfamiliar with Hirschsprung's-associated enterocolitis and may treat it as an episode of gastroenteritis with the potential for a fatal outcome. The families need to know the importance of contacting the surgeon directly should the patient develop any gastrointestinal symptoms.

COMPLICATIONS

The most common complication following treatment for Hirschsprung's disease, regardless of the type of pull-through procedure used, is constipation with or without "overflow" leakage of stool. It is difficult to render a patient with Hirschsprung's disease incontinent, but it is very easy to have one become constipated. A rectal examination should be performed to rule out anastomotic stricture. If mild laxatives and enemas are not sufficient to treat the constipation easily, a biopsy sample should be obtained to rule out a retained aganglionic segment. The pulled-through bowel may have had ganglion cells at the time of the procedure but may have lost them due to vascular compromise or other complications from the procedure. The most common cause for constipation is anal sphincter achalasia. The internal anal sphincter does not have ganglion cells and therefore does not relax normally in response to rectal distention. The internal sphincter is partially resected or destroyed with all of the pull-through procedures, but it may remain competent enough to cause constipation. Injection of botulinum toxin into the internal anal sphincter may temporarily paralyze it and allow the patient to resume normal bowel habits. If the toxin injection is successful, a myomectomy will likely provide a permanent solution to the problem of constipation. The toxin is used, in this instance, as a therapeutic trial.

Although rare, incontinence without associated constipation can occur following a pull-through procedure for Hirschsprung's disease. This can be effectively treated using biofeedback if the patient is old enough and is cooperative. With time, however, most of the incontinence resolves and the patient attains normal bowel function. According to all of the long-term results published, approximately 90% of patients ultimately achieve normal bowel function.

The most deadly complication associated with Hirschsprung's disease is Hirschsprung's-associated enterocolitis. Acute enterocolitis, characterized by abdominal distension, obstipation, or diarrhea, and an explosive, watery, foul-smelling stool following a rectal examination, can be treated with rectal irrigations and anal dilation. If the patient has signs of sepsis such as an elevated temperature and an elevated white blood cell count, intravenous antibiotics, including either metronidazole or vancomycin, should be given. It may be necessary to stretch the anus forcefully under anesthesia in the operating room two or three times in order to relieve repeated episodes of enterocolitis. Some patients develop repeated episodes of enterocolitis and do not respond to irrigations and forceful stretching of the anal sphincter. In these patients, it is particularly important to rule out a retained aganglionic segment, acquired postoperative aganglionosis, or intestinal neuronal dysplasia. In these cases, a repeat pull-through procedure may be required. Injection of botulinum toxin into the anal sphincter may help relieve chronic episodes of enterocolitis temporarily. Anal sphincter myomectomy will likely relieve the condition permanently. This is performed by making a transverse incision at the mucocutaneous junction, elevating the mocosa, resecting a strip of muscularis measuring about 0.5 cm in width by 4 to 5 cm in length. The bleeding is controlled with electrocautery. The mucosa is then resutured transversely to the skin with absorbable sutures. The patients receive one dose of antibiotics preoperatively and one to two doses postoperatively; the risk of infection is extremely low.

SUMMARY

Pediatric surgeons deal with patients with Hirschsprung's disease frequently, not only as an acute problem but for years thereafter. Patients tend to present in three distinct time periods: as newborns, as toddlers, or as older children or teenagers. The management of the patient in each of these time periods is somewhat different, although the underlying goal is the same: to remove the aganglionic bowel and to bring normal bowel down to the anus to restore normal bowel function. The pediatric surgeon must have at his or her disposal several different treatment options to manage patients who present at different ages and with a different set of problems and circumstances. Table 65.1 is a summary of my approach to Hirschsprung's disease in patients presenting in the various age groups.

EDITOR'S NOTE

There has been a recent trend toward primary pull-through for Hirschsprung's disease. Although there are still clear indications for a decompressive leveling colostomy (e.g., in infants with associated anomalies and in patients whose colons cannot be prepared adequately), sufficient intermediate-range data have been compiled to suggest that a primary pull-through approach should be the current standard of care for infants with classic, short-segment Hirschsprung's disease. The recent development of minimally invasive operations only adds to the elegance of the approach.

Although most pediatric surgeons develop a certain comfort level and a strong preference for one type of reconstruction or another, patients with Hirschsprung's disease present in many different varieties; to apply a single type of operation to every patient would be a mistake. Pediatric surgeons should have several types of reconstruction in their armamentarium and then carefully individualize their recommendation to the patient and family based on the age of the patient and the clinical circumstances at the time of presentation. This chapter nicely illustrates this thoughtful approach.

The workup for suspected Hirschsprung's disease is usually straightforward. A contrast enema can provide useful anatomic information and is critical to exclude other causes of bowel obstruction in the newborn, but it can only sug-

TABLE 65.1. MANAGEMENT OF HIRSCHSPRUNG'S DISEASE

	Newborn	Toddler	Older Child
Diagnosis	Barium enema (20% error) Suction rectal biopsy	Barium enema Full-thickness rectal biopsy	Barium enema Manometry Full-thickness rectal biopsy
Preoperative preparation	Rectal irrigations (20 mL/kg) Neomycin (100 mg/kg/day) Dilute Betadine irrigations in OR	Enema under anesthesia (EUA) Neomycin (100 mg/kg/day) Dilute Betadine irrigations in OR	EUA vs. ileostomy
Definitive pullthrough Standard	Primary Laparoscopically-assisted pullthrough	Primary Laparoscopically-assisted pullthrough	Primary Swenson or Duhamel vs. ileostomy with delayed pullthrough
Long-segment	Leveling colostomy Swenson pullthrough	Leveling colostomy Swenson pullthrough	J-pouch ileoanal pullthrough
Total colon	Kimura ileocolostomy; Swenson pullthrough	Kimura ileocolostomy; Swenson pullthrough	Kimura ileocolostomy; Swenson or Duhamel vs. J-pouch ileoanal pullthrough
Postoperative care	Follow-up every month three times, every 3 mo for 1 yr, every 4–6 mo for 2 yr, then every 6–12 mo R/O anastomotic stricture; expect delayed "potty-training"		
Complications	Constipation: R/O stricture, retained segment, intestinal neuronal dysplasia; Botox; myomectomy Incontinence: biofeedback, R/O constipation Enterocolitis: irrigations, anal stretching, with or without antibiotics Chronic enterocolitis: irrigations, anal stretching; Botox; myomectomy		

OR, operating room; R/O, rule out.

gest the diagnosis of Hirschsprung's disease. A rectal biopsy is mandatory to confirm the diagnosis. The decision whether to proceed with biopsy is based mostly on clinical grounds, so that a patient with a "negative" contrast enema may still need a biopsy if the level of suspicion remains high. Suction rectal biopsy is a safe and reliable approach in the newborn, but in toddlers and older children, an open rectal biopsy is usually required.

Premature infants with a clinical picture suggestive of Hirschsprung's disease can present a challenge. Despite studies that suggest that the incidence of Hirschsprung's disease in premature infants is the same as in full-term infants, there is a distinct clinical impression among pediatric surgeons that the disease occurs rarely, if ever, in these patients. In addition, many premature infants present with abdominal distension, feeding intolerance, or delayed passage of meconium that can usually be ascribed to immaturity of the bowel but that sometimes warrants consideration of another cause. The problem is compounded by the fact that both contrast enema and suction rectal biopsy have a much higher incidence of complications in premature infants. Contrast enema can result in hypothermia, apnea and bradycardia, or bowel perforation. Suction rectal biopsy can result in sepsis, hemorrhage, or full-thickness biopsy with perforation. Each have been associated with death and should therefore not be considered benign procedures. These patients require a thoughtful approach, with the avoidance of unnecessary tests and often a long period of careful observation before a workup is initiated.

Long-term follow-up of patients after operation is extremely important and is usually best carried out in the surgery department. A bowel management clinic staffed with experienced advance practice nurses and interested attending physicians can make the formidable task of closely following a large number of patients with Hirschsprung's disease and other anorectal anomalies somewhat easier. Postoperative constipation can be a challenging and frustrating problem and deserves a direct and honest approach like the one proposed by Dr. Ricketts. Although controversial, postoperative acquired aganglionosis, whether due to drop-out (or die-back) of ganglion cells or to lengthening of the distal cuff of native rectum, clearly does occur and can require reoperation. Paying special attention to the blood supply of the pull-through segment and careful handling of the distal end to prevent tissue trauma may help to prevent ischemia and subsequent loss of ganglion cells. Minimizing the length of the distal cuff of native rectum also may help prevent constipation. Some surgeons also have advocated routine myotomy or myomectomy at the time of the pull-through operation, which, given the apparently low rate of incontinence and other complications, seems like a reasonable way to prevent achalasia of the internal sphincter. A therapeutic trial of forced anal dilatation or botulinum toxin injection prior to recommending myomectomy is a common-sense approach that may increase the success rate of the procedure.

–P.M.

SUGGESTED READINGS

Bourdalat D, Vransky P, Pages R, et al. Duhamel operation 40 years after: a multicentric study. *Eur J Pediatr Surg* 1997;7:70–76.

Ikeda K, Goto S. Diagnosis and treatment of Hirschsprung's disease in Japan. An analysis of 1628 patients. *Ann Surg* 1984;199:400–405.

Kimura K, Nishijima E, Muraji T, et al. Extensive aganglionosis: further experience with the colonic patch graft procedure and long-term results. *J Pediatr Surg* 1988;23:52–56.

Langer JC, Birnhaum E. Preliminary experience with intrasphincteric botulinum toxin for persistent constipation after pull-through for Hirschsprung's disease. *J Pediatr Surg* 1997;32:1059–1062.

Ricketts RR. Hirschsprung's disease. In: *Oxford textbook of surgery, 2nd ed.* Morris PJ, Wood WC, eds. Oxford, England: Oxford University Press, 2000:2665–2672.

Ricketts RR, Pettitt BJ. Management of Hirschsprung's disease in adolescents. *Am Surg* 1989;55:219–225.

Sherman JO, Snyder ME, Weitzman JJ, et al. A 40-year multinational retrospective study of 880 Swenson procedures. *J Pediatr Surg* 1989;24:833–838.

Skinner MA. Hirschsprung's disease. *Curr Prob Surg* 1996;33: 389–468.

Wulkan ML, Georgeson KE. Primary laparoscopic endorectal pull-through for Hirschsprung's disease in infants and children. *Semin Laparosc Surg* 1998;5:9–13.

66

LONG-SEGMENT HIRSCHSPRUNG'S DISEASE

HARRY APPLEBAUM

Long-segment Hirschsprung's disease (LSHD) extends proximally into the right colon and beyond and requires consideration of relatively complex reconstructive operations. A functionally adequate procedure must provide means for the remaining bowel to compensate for a significant deficit of normal absorptive surface and reservoir capacity.

DIAGNOSIS

In its most common presentation, LSHD involves the entire colon and a relatively short segment of distal ileum, although longer segments of small intestine and even the entire foregut may be involved. In contrast to the overwhelmingly male preponderance in short-segment Hirschsprung's disease (HD), a female:male ratio of 2:1 is observed among patients with more extensive disease.

The substantial length of physiologically dysmotile bowel in these infants predisposes them to present with a high-grade obstruction early in the neonatal period. Surprisingly, however, up to a third can evacuate well enough to remain undiagnosed until 3 to 6 months of age.

Plain films of the abdomen typically display a large number of distended intestinal loops compatible with distal small bowel obstruction, with variability in this pattern dependent on the length of aganglionosis. A contrast enema characteristically exhibits spasm, spiculation, and shortening of the entire colon, with proximal small bowel dilatation, but is often nondiagnostic. A 24-hour film looking for delayed evacuation may be helpful.

H. Applebaum: Department of Surgery, University of California at Los Angeles, School of Medicine; and Division of Pediatric Surgery, Kaiser Permanente Medical Center, Los Angeles, California.

OPERATIVE DIAGNOSIS AND MANAGEMENT

As in all patients with suspected aganglionosis, rectal suction biopsy is usually confirmatory, but accurate determination of the extent of the abnormality requires multilevel biopsies. For this reason, a diagnosis of LSHD is often unanticipated prior to the initial operation. Laparotomy or laparoscopy allows for a direct examination of the bowel. If a probable zone of transition is visualized, biopsy samples taken distal and proximal to that area can be confirmatory. If none is obvious, biopsy excision should commence at the peritoneal reflection and progress proximally. Once aganglionosis is determined to extend proximal to the usual rectosigmoid area, the tedious biopsy and frozen section process can often be shortened by early removal of the appendix for examination. Aganglionosis of the appendix is usually accurate in confirming total colonic aganglionosis (TCA) and directs attention more proximally. A leveling stoma is followed by a delayed definitive procedure. Although some investigators have advocated waiting several months to several years before undertaking surgery, current experience shows that in the absence of extenuating circumstances, pull-through procedures can usually be safely performed after a short interval.

For the more typical forms of HD, the recent trend has been toward primary pull-through, either in the neonatal period or at the time of diagnosis, for infants who are not debilitated and do not present with enterocolitis. Operation via a transanal route, with or without laparoscopic assistance, has become popular. The question arises as to the appropriateness of applying these concepts to LSHD, because most procedures used for LSHD are derivatives of those developed for shorter segment disease. Although current experience is limited, there is probably little reason that one-stage procedures cannot be applied to some patients with LSHD, although some important caveats apply. First, bowel distension must be minimal following successful distal irrigations. This state will be difficult or impossible to achieve in many patients. Distension precludes insufflation for a laparoscopically assisted procedure, increases the difficulty of reconstruction via an open approach, and increases the risk of spillage and infection. Second, if attempting a transanal procedure, experience with bowel mobilization and biopsy via a laparoscopic approach is desirable. A circumumbilical mini-incision as an alternative to laparoscopy or conversion laparotomy has been described by Langer for use in this situation. This approach permits the entire colon and small bowel to be sequentially mobilized and biopsy samples taken through a small incision that is virtually invisible when healed.

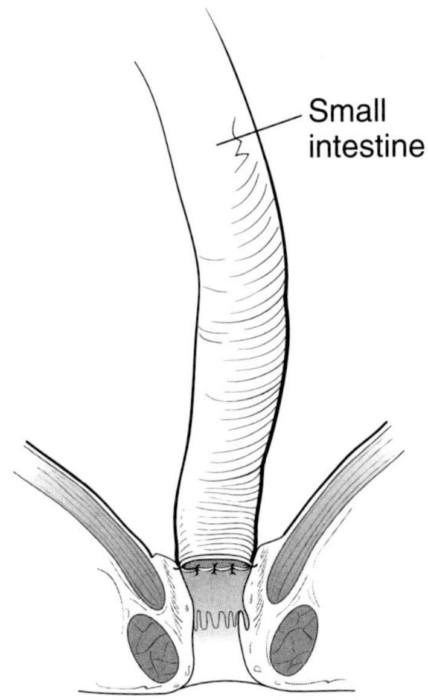

FIGURE 66.1. Swenson ileorectal pull-through.

DEFINITIVE PROCEDURES

Operations commonly used for relatively short-segment disease usually suffice for aganglionosis extending into the right colon. However, if most of the right colon must be discarded, there is little reason to preserve the cecum, because it provides minimal absorptive function and makes for a difficult anastomosis.

A number of small bowel pull-through procedures continue to be widely applied to LSHD, with none gaining even majority acceptance. Although the usual advice of proceeding with the type of procedure to which one is most accustomed probably still holds for LSHD, there is good evidence that reservoir procedures decrease the likelihood of significant short-term postoperative problems. The following procedural descriptions presume a typical TCA accompanied by a relatively short segment of aganglionic distal ileum.

Straight Ileal (Nonreservoir) Pull-Through Group

Swenson Procedure

Following removal of all aganglionic bowel, the operation is performed in the same manner as for shorter segment disease, with ileum anastomosed to very distal rectum. It can be relatively difficult to properly accomplish, with retained aganglionic bowel the most common residual problem (Fig. 66.1).

Ileoendorectal Pull-Through

The end of the ganglionic ileum may be used as a straight Soave-type endorectal pull-through after discarding the aganglionic bowel to the level of the distal rectum (Fig. 66.2).

Because neither of these procedures includes a reservoir or colonic absorptive surface, they are commonly associated with a high initial output and a relatively slow adaptive phase that may last a year or more.

Partially Aganglionic Reservoir Procedures

This group of procedures uses a retained segment of aganglionic colon applied side-to-side to a pull-through of ganglionic ileum to form a reservoir. One half of the pouch that

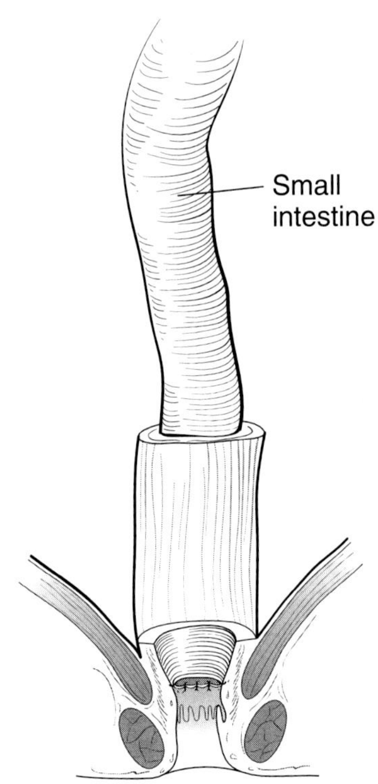

FIGURE 66.2. Soave ileoendorectal pull-through.

is formed is ganglionic, and the other aganglionic. The retained colon provides no motility, but absorbs water and slows evacuation to diminish diarrhea. The remaining aganglionic bowel is discarded.

Duhamel/Martin Procedure

In a variation on the Duhamel procedure, the ganglionic ileum is pulled down in the retrorectal (presacral) space. It is then stapled in a side-to-side manner to a segment of retained aganglionic rectum, sigmoid and left colon, using multiple GIA applications (Fig. 66.3). Endoscopic staplers provide a more comfortable fit for smaller infants. While Martin originally described retention of the entire left colon, a shorter length up to the level of the left colic artery is now recommended to minimize the associated complications of constipation, stasis, and enterocolitis.

Right Colon Onlay Patch Procedures

These procedures feature a pouch formed by an onlay patch of aganglionic right colon. The right rather than the left side is used because of its theoretically superior water-absorbing capability. Kimura described a multi-stage procedure. A leveling ileostomy is first formed. Subsequently, a 5- to 10-cm segment of right colon, with blood supply based on the right colic and ileocolic vessels, is anastomosed side-to-side to the distal portion of the ganglionic ileum. The next stage is performed approximately 6 weeks later to allow for the development of collateral blood supply from the ileum to the onlay patch. The stoma is taken down, the original blood supply to the onlay is transected, and the end of the ganglionic ileum is used as a Swenson, Soave, or Duhamel pull-through (Fig. 66.4).

Boley described a similar procedure that requires fewer stages by retaining the original vascular supply of the onlay. An initial leveling ileostomy is performed. As a second stage, a 5- to 10-cm segment of right colon with cecum removed, based on the preserved ileocolic and right colic vessels, is isolated and anastomosed in a side-to-side manner within 5 cm of the end of the ganglionic ileum. An endorectal pull-through concludes the operation. The orientation of the onlay patch is irrelevant in both procedures, because the aganglionic colon has no peristalsis. It should be applied in the manner best suited to preservation of its blood supply.

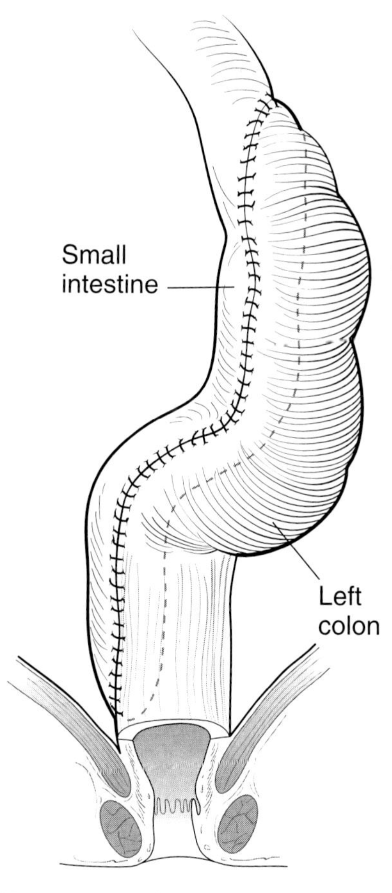

FIGURE 66.3. Duhamel/Martin procedure.

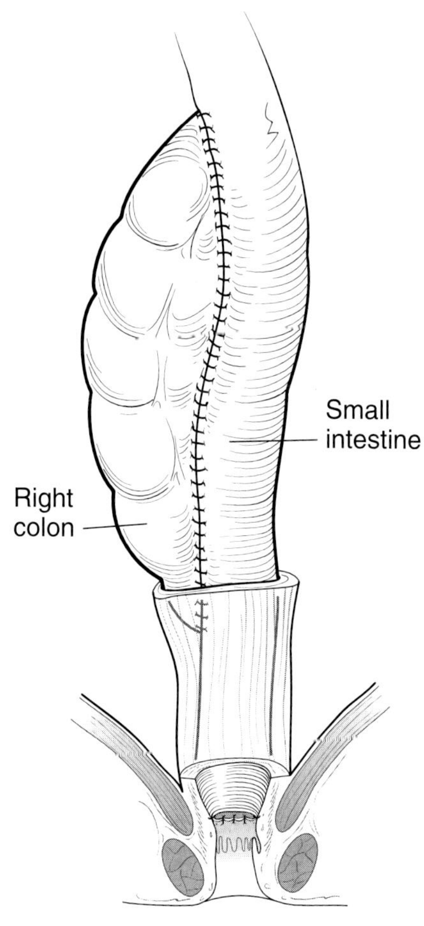

FIGURE 66.4. Kimura and Boley procedures.

Because of the technical ease and low complication rate associated with the Boley procedure, there appears to be little reason to use a multistage onlay/pull-through with this type of operation. Preservation of the original blood supply and lymphatics of the patch also may help it function more effectively by maintaining more normal fluid and electrolyte absorption and distensibility.

Onlay patch procedures have been criticized because they involve the retention of relatively large pieces of aganglionic bowel. Personal experience using them within a Soave pull-through has demonstrated that approximately 25% of patients with these procedures require an internal sphincterotomy to relieve constipation and distension.

Ganglionic Pouch Pull-Through

J-Pouch Pull-Through

This operation, with a long history of success in ulcerative colitis and familial polyposis, has been recently adapted for use in LSHD. It is a relatively simple procedure that discards all aganglionic bowel, yet provides the immediate advantages of a reservoir. A J-pouch is formed from the distal end of the ganglionic small bowel using one or two applications of a GIA stapler, with its length varying from 5 to 10 cm, depending on the size of the child. It is then used as an endorectal or Swenson-type pull-through. Achieving appropriate length while maintaining a good vascular supply is usually easier than with straight pull-throughs, because the curved end of the pouch, rather than the end of the small intestine, is used to reach the distal rectum. Ease of performance, coupled with both excellent short- and long-term results, makes this procedure my preferred method (Fig. 66.5).

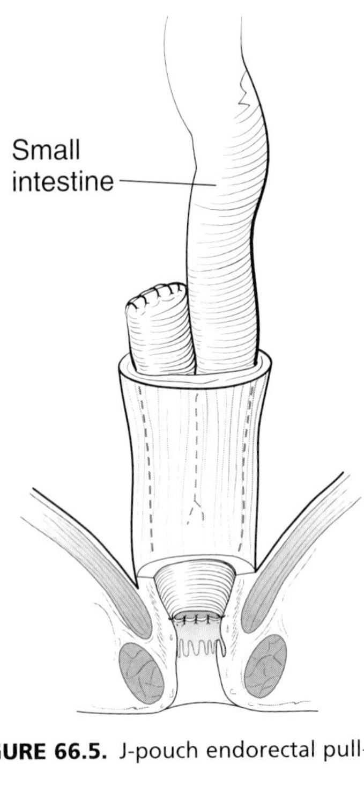

FIGURE 66.5. J-pouch endorectal pull-through.

Although usually unnecessary, discretionary diverting stomas may accompany any of the described pull-throughs. They are most appropriate in the presence of a tenuous anastomosis, and can also help avoid early debilitating diarrhea and perineal excoriation.

Short-Term Complications

Because of modern antibiotic coverage and improvement in technical skills, pelvic abscess formation has been steadily declining to the point where it is relatively uncommon. In contrast, frequent, loose stools and the fluid, electrolyte, and skin problems that result, remain problematic. As might be anticipated, favorable results are generally directly related to the original length of aganglionic bowel and the presence of a pouch, although there is great variability in the ultimate intestinal adaption of individual patients with similar bowel lengths and procedures. Meticulous, proactive skin care and medications commonly used for short-gut patients are of great benefit.

Long-Term Complications

Pouchitis, attributed to stool stasis, occurs in some reservoir patients. It is characterized by the new onset of frequent, loose, foul-smelling stools, and although *Clostridium difficile* is only occasionally cultured, the problem is usually managed effectively with a course of oral metronidazole. Rarely, repeated episodes may require surgically decreasing the size of the pouch. This problem can be minimized by initial formation of a pouch appropriately sized to the child, never greater than 10 cm in length, with its distal end near the end of the pull-through segment. In this configuration, it will lie deep in the pelvis at the level of the puborectalis sling and empty completely.

As in all patients undergoing a pull-through for aganglionosis, the remaining hypertonic anal sphincter may cause undue obstruction. Sphincterotomy or botulinum toxin injection will usually solve this problem. Incontinence can be an occasional issue after these procedures, although the symptoms must be differentiated from those of loose, frequent stools secondary to a short intestine.

Very Long Segment Disease

A major problem not amenable to any of the previously described procedures is very long segment aganglionosis that extends proximally well into the small bowel. Although a traditional leveling enterostomy will suffice for decompression, adequate enteral nutrition often cannot be achieved, particularly in patients with less than 40 cm of ganglionic intestine.

Ziegler Procedure

This concept has been of benefit to approximately 50% of these patients. A longitudinal 1-cm wide strip of muscularis

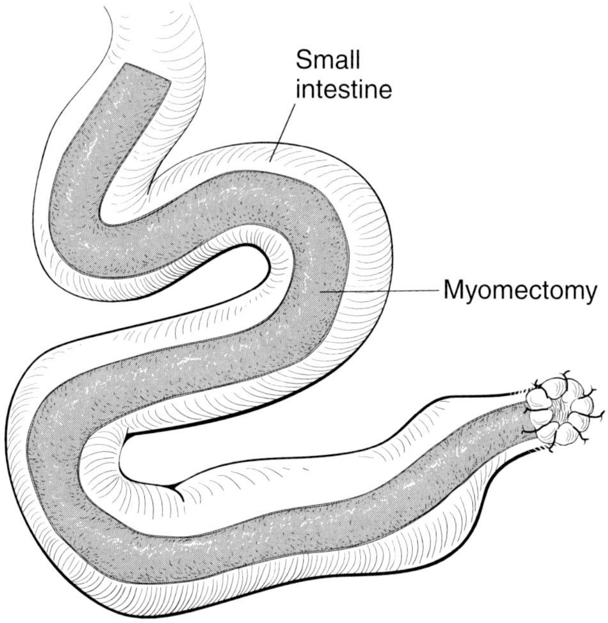

FIGURE 66.6. Ziegler procedure.

is removed from the aganglionic small bowel, commencing at the level of transition and proceeding distally, so as to allow for an adequate length of absorptive area (ideally 50–70 cm), but not so long as to cause an intestinal obstruction. The mucosa and submucosa are left intact, and an end-stoma is formed, with venting of the distal small bowel. If this arrangement functions well, the stoma can sometimes be advanced distally following removal of a muscular strip from the additional small intestine that is brought in-line (Fig. 66.6). The Bianchi bowel-lengthening procedure performed in the normally ganglionic bowel provides an alternative or conjunctive option. Intestinal transplantation has recently assumed an experimental role as an initial or final option to permit enteral nutrition in these patients.

SUGGESTED READINGS

Boley SJ. A new operative approach to total ganglionosis of the colon. *Surg Gynecol Obstet* 1984;159:481–484.

Cilley RE, Statter MB, Hirschl RB, et al. Definitive treatment of Hirschsprung's disease in the newborn with a one-stage procedure. *Surgery* 1994;115:551–556.

Curran TJ, Raffensperger JG. Laparoscopic Swenson's pullthrough: a comparison with the open procedure. *J Pediatr Surg* 1995;31: 1155–1157.

Emslie J, Krishnamoorthy M, Applebaum H. Long-term follow up of patients treated with ileoendorectal pull-through and right colon onlay patch for total colonic aganglionosis. *J Pediatr Surg* 1997; 32:1542–1544.

Hoehner JC, Ein SH, Shandling B, et al. Long-term morbidity in total colonic aganglionosis. *J Pediatr Surg* 1998;33:961–965.

Nishijima E, Kimura K, Tsugawa C, et al. The colon patch graft procedure for extensive aganglionosis: long-term follow-up. *J Pediatr Surg* 1998;33:215–219.

Langer JC, Seifert M, Minkes RK. One-stage pull-through for Hirschsprung's disease: a comparison of the transanal and open approaches. *J Pediatr Surg* 2000;35:820–822.

Martin LW. Surgical management of total colonic aganglionosis. *Ann Surg* 1972;176:343–346.

Saxton ML, Ein SH, Hoehner J, et al. Near-total intestinal aganglionosis: long-term follow-up of a morbid condition. *J Pediatr Surg* 2000;35:669–672.

Ziegler MM, Royal RE, Brandt J, et al. Extended myectomy-myotomy. A therapeutic alternative for total intestinal aganglionosis. *Ann Surg* 1993;218:504–509.

67

ENTEROCOLITIS ASSOCIATED WITH HIRSCHSPRUNG'S DISEASE

KATHLEEN GRAZIANO
ARNOLD G. CORAN
DANIEL H. TEITELBAUM

Despite major improvements in the understanding of the pathophysiology and genetics of Hirschsprung's disease, advancement has lagged in elucidating the etiology of Hirschsprung's-associated enterocolitis (HAEC). Despite the recognition of this process in Härald Hirschsprung's first description of the disease in 1886, little attention was focused on this disease process for the next 70 years. Swenson was the first to recognize the association of enterocolitis and Hirschsprung's disease. Over the past four decades, HAEC has been a major cause of morbidity and mortality in infants and children with Hirschsprung's disease. With an increased understanding of the mucosal defense mechanisms, a host of potential causative factors have been advanced to explain this process. This chapter reviews what is known clinically about this disorder and reviews the potential causes and therapy for HAEC.

DIAGNOSTIC APPROACH

Bill and Chapman were the first to accurately characterize the clinical aspects of HAEC. They speculated that the cause of this disorder was a partial mechanical obstruction similar to the colitis associated with other forms of bowel obstruction. Their description of the natural history of the process helped to alert physicians to the high risk of HAEC in patients with Hirschsprung's disease. The classic clinical manifestations that they described in HAEC include abdominal distension, fever, and foul-smelling stool. There is, however, a wide range of clinical presentations of HAEC. A compilation of symptoms from patients with HAEC, treated at our Children's Hospital, noted the following in decreasing frequency: abdominal distension, explosive diarrhea, vomiting, fever, lethargy, rectal bleeding, and shock. Many cases of diarrhea or abdominal distension may be mistakenly diagnosed as gastroenteritis or due to a persistently spastic internal sphincter after pull-through; however, most of these symptoms are mild in nature. To facilitate the diagnosis of HAEC, Elhalaby et al. developed a clinical grading system (Table 67.1) based on several clinical criteria. Another less common manner by which HAEC may present is that of a perforation of the bowel proximal to the aganglionic segment.

The timing of HAEC and the clinical course of Hirschsprung's disease shows that the two times an infant is at highest risk for the development of HAEC is before the diagnosis of Hirschsprung's disease has been made, and following the definitive pull-through. Although occasionally described, HAEC is distinctly uncommon in patients with a decompressing colostomy. The diagnosis of HAEC is usually based on the classic presentation of a neonate with a history of constipation starting in the newborn period, or after a pull-through procedure. The child typically has abdominal distension and liquid, foul-smelling stools. Examination shows a markedly distended abdomen that is hyperesonant to percussion. Rectal examination often results in an explosive discharge of gas and stool. Post-pull-through HAEC may present in a similar fashion and is typically seen days to weeks following the operation. Multiple episodes can occur over time, but the risk diminishes to zero after 1 to 2 years.

Abdominal radiographs are often quite helpful. The proximal colon is distended with an almost toxic megacolon appearance. An extremely useful finding is what we term a cut-off sign in the rectosigmoid region (Fig. 67.1A) with an absence of air distally. This sign was noted in 74% of patients during an HAEC episode compared with only

K. Graziano, A.G. Coran, and **D.H. Teitelbaum:** Department of Surgery, University of Michigan Medical School and the C.S. Mott Children's Hospital, Ann Arbor, Michigan.

TABLE 67.1. CLINICAL GRADING SYSTEM FOR HIRSCHSPRUNG'S-ASSOCIATED ENTEROCOLITIS

Grade	Clinical Symptoms
I	Mild explosive diarrhea, mild or moderate abdominal distension, and no systemic manifestations
II	Moderate explosive diarrhea, moderate to severe abdominal distention, mild systemic symptoms
III	Severe explosive diarrhea, marked abdominal distension, shock or impending shock

14% of the time between episodes of HAEC. Other common radiologic findings include small bowel dilatation in 74% and multiple air-fluid levels in 79%. Occasionally, pneumatosis intestinalis may be seen. A barium enema may show an irregular mucosal lining, with a resultant "saw-tooth" appearance (Fig. 67.1B). However, because of the risk for perforation, a contrast enema should be avoided when HAEC is suspected clinically.

Teitelbaum, Qualman, and Caniano showed that the diagnosis of Hirschsprung's disease after the first week of life places the neonate at a substantially higher risk for the development of HAEC. In this report, the mean age at diagnosis of neonates with Hirschsprung's disease was 16.6 days in those who developed HAEC and 4.6 days in those neonates without HAEC. Post-pull-through HAEC may be due to associated internal sphincter spasm, which can be seen with Hirschsprung's disease and may act to functionally obstruct the passage of stool. Although the course of enterocolitis is usually most severe in those infants who have not yet had the diagnosis of enterocolitis made, a recent report describes the death of five infants due to HAEC anywhere from 3 weeks to 20 months after their pull-through procedure.

INCIDENCE AND ASSOCIATED RISK FACTORS

The reported incidence of HAEC varies widely. Table 67.2 lists the incidence of HAEC in several large series. The mean incidence was 25%, but the range was quite broad (17%–50%) and may represent differences in the manner in which HAEC is diagnosed. This is perhaps most evident by the large variation in mortality rates in two of the largest series of Hirschsprung's disease

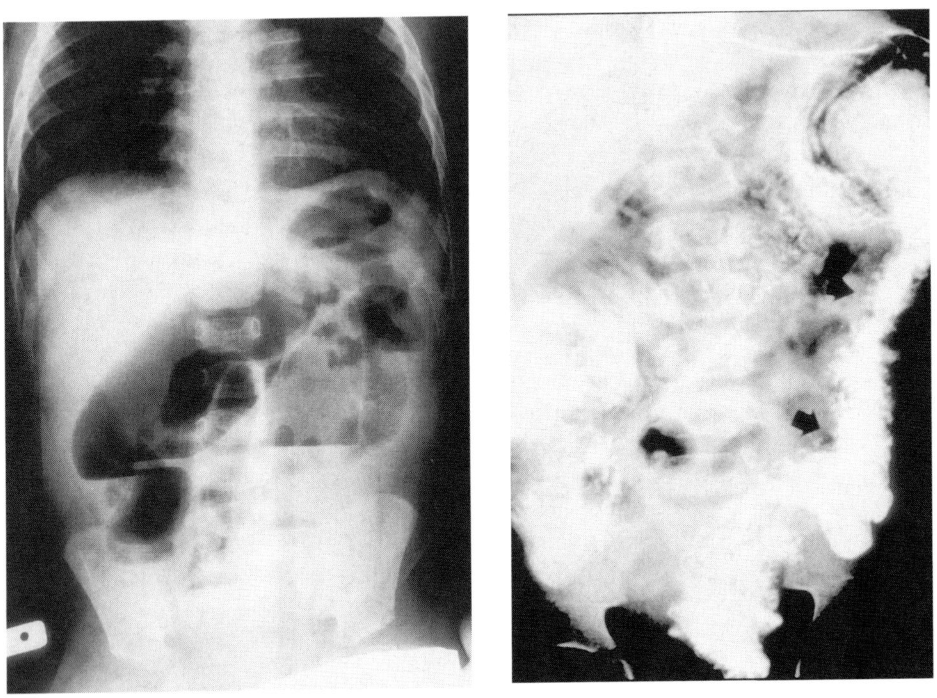

A B

FIGURE 67.1. Roentgenographic evidence of enterocolitis. **A:** Example of a cut-off sign on a plain radiograph, as demonstrated by the acute loss of air at the pelvic brim. **B:** Contrast enema in a child with enterocolitis. Note the irregular mucosal lining (*arrows*) consistent with edema and ulcerations of the mucosa.

TABLE 67.2. INCIDENCE OF ENTEROCOLITIS IN SEVERAL REPORTED SERIES OF HIRSCHSPRUNG'S DISEASE

Report	Overall	Trisomy 21	Long Segmetnt	Pre-Pullthrough	Mortality Rate[a]
Kleinhaus	18%	NS	25%	15%	30%
Ikeda	NS	NS	44.3%	29.2% (24.3–44.3)	1.8%–2.4%
Teitelbaum	24%	46%	29%	16%	16%
Elhalaby	33.9%	37.5%	55%	Not stated	0%
Rescorla	18%	26%	32%	6%	9%
Caneiro	32%	50%	Not different	16%	4%
Bill	50%	NS	66%	45%	33%
Foster	17%	NS	5%	10%	0%
Teitelbaum	44%	NS	—	—	—

[a]Mortality due to enterocolitis is based on the total number of infants with enterocolitis.
Data from Bill J, Chapman ND. The enterocolitis of Hirschsprung's disease: its natural history and treatment. *Am J Surg* 1962;103:70–74; Caneiro P, Brereton R, Drake D, et al. Enterocolitis in Hirschsprung's disease. *Pediatr Surg Int* 1992;7:356–360; Elhalaby EA, Coran AG, Blane CE, et al. Enterocolitis associated with Hirschsprung's disease: a clinical-radiological characterization based on 168 patients. *J Pediatr Surg* 1995;30:76–83; Foster P, Cowan G, Wrenn E, Jr. Twenty-five years' experience with Hirschsprung's disease. *J Pediatr Surg* 1990;25:531–534.

patients. In a review of the Surgical Section of the American Academy of Pediatrics, Kleinhaus reported a low rate of HAEC, but a high mortality rate. In contrast, in a review of Japanese cases of Hirschsprung's disease, Ikeda noted a high rate of HAEC, but a low mortality rate. With improved and more prompt diagnosis of the disease, a clear decline in the incidence has occurred over the past 40 years.

In addition to a delay in diagnosis of aganglionosis, several factors have been associated with an increased incidence of enterocolitis. Some have claimed that once an infant develops HAEC, he or she is at increased risk for developing other enterocolitic episodes in the future. Although some investigators have speculated that early development of HAEC may somehow alter the defense mechanisms of the intestine and predispose the patient to recurrent episodes of HAEC, many others have not found such a predisposition. Increased length of the aganglionic segment also has been associated with the development of HAEC. Although such an association appears intuitive, many have failed to find such an association. Infants with trisomy 21 appear to be at increased risk for developing HAEC, some studies suggesting that nearly half of infants with trisomy 21 and Hirschsprung's disease develop HAEC. This association is probably due to an immune deficiency, both humoral and cellular, that predisposes these infants to HAEC. Other associated anomalies may place the infant at risk for the development of enterocolitis. Caneiro found that 53% of infants with associated anomalies developed HAEC compared to 26% with Hirschsprung's disease alone. Elhalaby noted that 47% of infants with associated anomalies developed HAEC compared with 29% of those who had none.

POST-PULL-THROUGH ENTEROCOLITIS

Rates of post-pull-through enterocolitis vary widely among series, ranging from 2% to 27%. In some large clinical series, a significantly higher incidence of enterocolitis was noted in those patients undergoing the Swenson pull-through. This higher incidence was noted in Swenson's own review from 1975, and this may be due to the inclusion of several patients who underwent this pull-through in the earlier years of the Swenson procedure, prior to its being modified to a more distal anastomosis. Postoperative enterocolitis has been associated with a fairly high rate of mortality in several series. In fact, when examining deaths in children with Hirschsprung's disease, several series noted that approximately half the deaths resulted from complications directly related to an episode of enterocolitis.

PATHOLOGY

Like many other inflammatory disease processes of the intestine, HAEC is characterized histologically by the appearance of neutrophils within the crypts of the intestine. A careful histologic analysis of the natural progression of this disease process shows several discrete phases that can be used to grade the pathologic severity of the enterocolitic process. The ranking starts with a grade 0 for no pathologic abnormality, followed by grade I, which is characterized by a marked amount of mucus streaming from the crypts of the intestine (Fig. 67.2A). This mucin retention is a histopathologic process unique to only two diseases: Hirschsprung's and cystic fibrosis. In fact, the

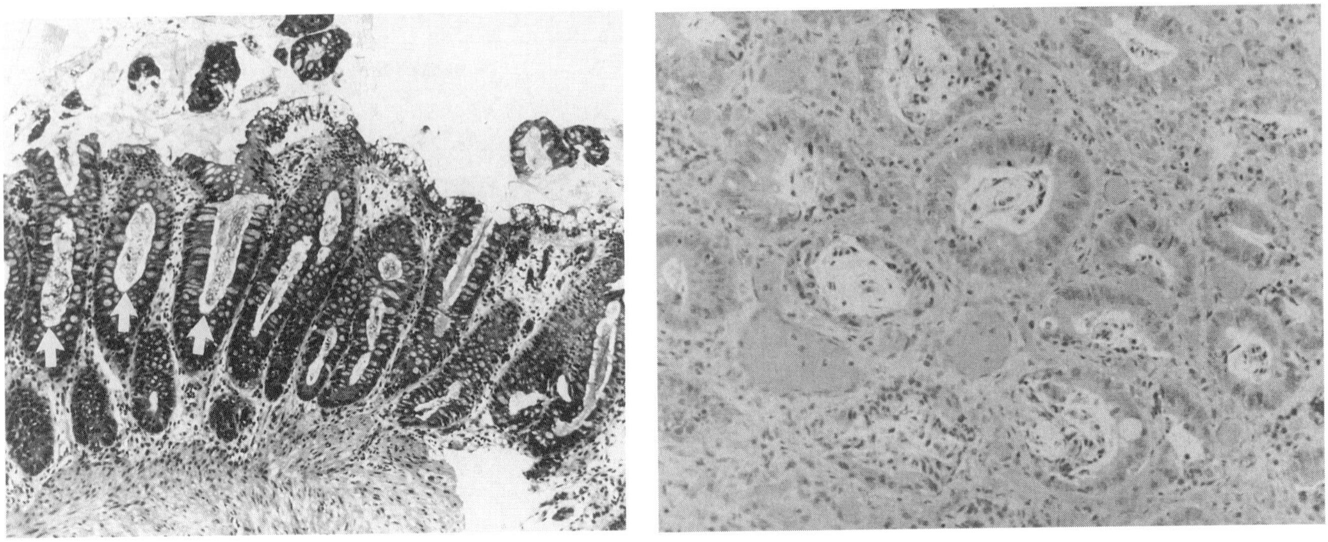

A B

FIGURE 67.2. Histologic appearance of Hirschsprung's-associated enterocolitis (HAEC). **A:** Histologic grade I HAEC. Note the mucin retention in the colonic crypts (*arrows*). **B:** Histologic grade III HAEC. Note the multiple crypt abscesses.

diagnosis of Hirschsprung's disease is strongly suggested based on this finding alone from a suction rectal biopsy. Subsequent grades of HAEC show a progressive increase in the number of crypt abscesses (Fig. 67.2B), followed by the destruction of the intestinal epithelium and eventual perforation of the bowel. The latter three grades look quite similar to ulcerative colitis, and the two processes may occasionally be difficult to differentiate in older patients.

MORBIDITY AND MORTALITY

The morbidity and mortality rates associated with the development of HAEC are quite high. Hospitalizations for many of these infants can be complicated and lengthy. Caneiro noted that hospitalizations ranged from 6 to 29 days (mean 13 days). The cost of caring for an infant with HAEC is over two and a half times as high as that for an infant with Hirschsprung's disease and no enterocolitis. In addition to morbidity, death also may occur. Although death is generally an uncommon outcome of HAEC, many series include reports of infants dying of the disease. In many published reports, such deaths comprise the majority of mortality with Hirschsprung's disease. Mortality rates range from 0% to 33%, again most likely reflecting differences in the way in which HAEC is diagnosed. Mortality rates also appear to be due to associated factors. In particular, trisomy 21 has a high association of death due to HAEC.

POTENTIAL CAUSES

An appreciation of the pathologic changes in HAEC allows for consideration of potential pathophysiologic processes that could cause this disease (Fig. 67.3). Historically, Swenson and Fisher postulated that the disorder was due to a defect in water and electrolyte metabolism. Subsequently, Swenson revised this concept and stated that improper fluid absorption was actually the result of chronic constipation. Several more recent theories on the cause of HAEC have since been proposed, including obstructive, infectious, alteration in the composition of mucus, increase in enteroinvasive organisms, and finally, alteration in immune function.

TECHNICAL APPROACH TO TREAT ENTEROCOLITIS

In 1964, Swenson suggested that the treatment of HAEC should be rectal tube decompression. Rectal washouts should be the initial approach in the care of a child, regardless of age, who presents with HAEC. The technique consists of the use of a soft red rubber catheter (at least 16 French) with multiple side holes cut to facilitate drainage. The catheter should be gently advanced (often as saline is flowing) above the aganglionic level. After catheter advancement, gas and stool should be aspirated, followed by repetitive irrigations of saline (generally up to 10 mL/kg per washout), followed by removal of the tube. The procedure should be repeated every 4 to 6 hours until the child is

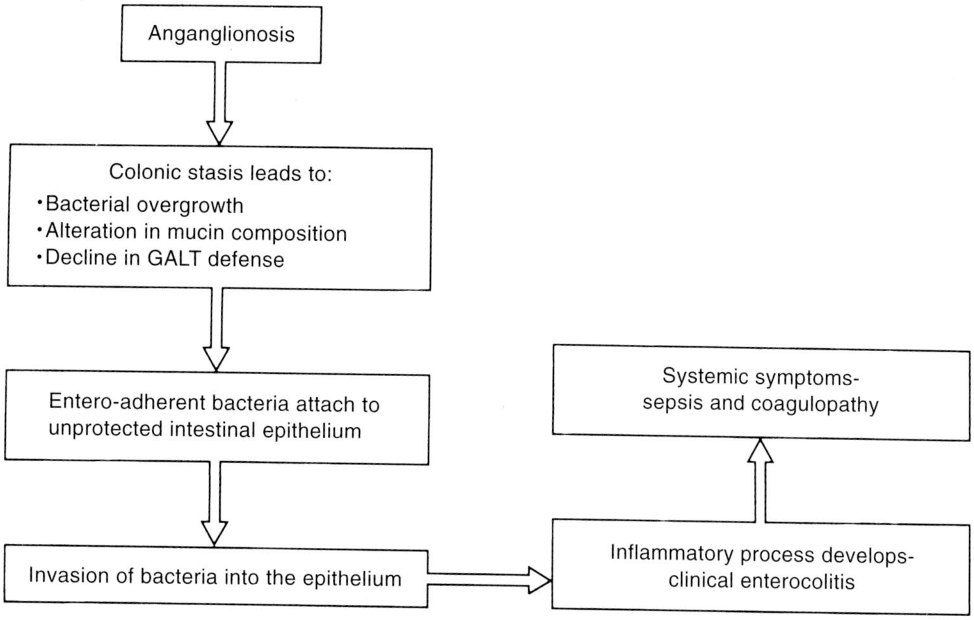

FIGURE 67.3. Schematic summary of the potential mechanisms involved in the development of Hirschsprung's-associated enterocolitis. *GALT,* gut-associated lymphoid tissue defense.

decompressed. Importantly, enemas without a decompressing tube should be avoided because they may worsen the enterocolitis. Not uncommonly, this treatment alone can often alleviate even a fairly high grade enterocolitis.

Along with washouts, intravenous antibiotics (ampicillin, gentamicin, and metronidazole) should be given for 3 to 7 days. In mild cases, oral metronidazole should suffice, and this drug also may be used once intravenous antibiotics are completed. Should the disease process fail to improve or if the infant deteriorates, consideration should be given to the performance of a decompressing colostomy. This typically occurs in infants with long-segment disease where rectal washouts cannot reach the dilated proximal bowel. The colostomy is ideally positioned just above the transition zone, which allows for a secondary pull-through and ostomy closure to be performed in the same procedure.

Recently, rectal irrigations have been used in a prophylactic fashion after the definitive pull-through procedure. In one report, a significant reduction in the number of patients who developed enterocolitis was noted. It is possible that the washouts serve to decompress the intestine for the first few months after the pull-through procedure; alternatively they may prevent colonic distension or wash out enteropathogenic organisms in the colonic lumen. In either case, this has become a routine in our center as well as others, and has proven itself to be a very useful way to decrease early episodes of HAEC.

If repeated bouts of enterocolitis persist after the definitive pull-through procedure, then an investigation into a mechanical cause should be undertaken. This should start with a contrast enema to ensure that there is no obstruction in the neorectum, a potentially correctable cause. If this is normal, a suction rectal biopsy should be performed to rule out retention of aganglionic bowel as well as other possible causes such as intestinal neuronal dysplasia (IND). Should these biopsies be normal, as is usually the case, consideration should be given to the performance of a posterior anal myotomy or myectomy. Published experience with this technique by several groups has demonstrated it to be safe, with an extremely low incidence of fecal incontinence. This more recent experience, however, is in contrast to a relatively poor experience with the procedure by Swenson, who felt it did not benefit many of his patients. Overall, results of these internal sphincterotomies are quite good; however, most surgeons advocate a significant period of conservative therapy, because many patients with post-pull-through enterocolitis will improve over time.

CONCLUSIONS

The development of enterocolitis in patients with Hirschsprung's disease remains a perplexing problem. Clearly, recognition of this problem is essential to both its prevention and for early intervention.

SUGGESTED READINGS

Caneiro P, Brereton R, Drake D, et al. Enterocolitis in Hirschsprung's disease. *Pediatr Surg Int* 1992;7:356–360.

Elhalaby EA, Coran AG, Blane CE, et al. Enterocolitis associated with Hirschsprung's disease: a clinical-radiological characterization based on 168 patients. *J Pediatr Surg* 1995;30:76–83.

Elhalaby EA, Teitelbaum DH, Coran AG, et al. Enterocolitis associated with Hirschsprung's disease: a clinical histopathological correlative study. *J Pediatr Surg* 1995;30:1023–1026; discussion 1026–1027.

Ikeda K, Goto S. Diagnosis and treatment of Hirschsprung's disease in Japan. An analysis of 1628 patients. *Ann Surg* 1984;199:400–405.

Kimura K, Inomata Y, Soper RT. Posterior sagittal rectal myectomy for persistent rectal achalasia after the Soave procedure for Hirschsprung's disease. *J Pediatr Surg* 1993;28:1200–1201.

Kleinhaus S, Boley SJ, Sheran M, et al. Hirschsprung's disease—a survey of the members of the Surgical Section of the American Academy of Pediatrics. *J Pediatr Surg* 1979;14:588–597.

Swenson O, Sherman J, Fisher J, et al. The treatment and postoperative complications of congenital megacolon: a 25 year follow-up. *Ann Surg* 1975;182:266–273.

Teitelbaum DH, Caniano DA, Qualman SJ. The pathophysiology of Hirschsprung's-associated enterocolitis: importance of histologic correlates. *J Pediatr Surg* 1989;24:1271–1277.

Teitelbaum DH, Qualman SJ, Caniano DA. Hirschsprung's disease. Identification of risk factors for enterocolitis. *Ann Surg* 1988;207:240–244.

Surgical Directives: Pediatric Surgery, edited by Peter Mattei. Lippincott Williams & Wilkins, Philadelphia © 2002

68

LAPAROSCOPIC PULL-THROUGH FOR HIRSCHSPRUNG'S DISEASE

TIMOTHY D. KANE
KEITH E. GEORGESON

DIAGNOSTIC APPROACH

Infants and children with a potential diagnosis of Hirschsprung's disease require biopsy-proven evidence of distal colonic aganglionosis prior to consideration for laparoscopically assisted endorectal colon pull-through. In the neonate, this consists of permanent pathology sections from specimens obtained by bedside suction rectal biopsy. Exclusion criteria for primary laparoscopic pull-through include severe enterocolitis or significant medical comorbidities that may contribute to the poor general condition of the patient. A barium enema is administered to assess for visual localization of the transition zone if present and for evidence of total colonic aganglionosis. A 24-hour follow-up radiograph is especially useful in identifying a transition zone in the neonate.

PREOPERATIVE PREPARATION

Decompression of the colon is achieved by frequent digital dilation of the anorectum or colonic irrigation with saline via a rectal tube if surgery is not performed immediately after the diagnosis. Two doses of antibiotic bowel preparation (erythromycin base) and neomycin are given by mouth 14 and 8 hours prior to surgery. Clear liquids are given orally for 24 hours preoperatively. Intravenous antibiotics (ampicillin and gentamicin) are administered on call to the operating room.

T. D. Kane: Department of Surgery, University of Pittsburgh School of Medicine; and Department of Pediatric Minimally Invasive Surgery, Children's Hospital of Pittsburgh, Pittsburgh, Pennsylvania.

K. D. Georgeson: Department of Surgery, Division of Pediatric Surgery, University of Alabama School of Medicine; and Department of Pediatric Surgery, Children's Hospital of Alabama, Birmingham, Alabama.

OPERATIVE APPROACH

Infants are placed transversely on the operating table, with the surgeons standing above the patient's head and right shoulder to perform the laparoscopic portion of the procedure. Older children are placed in stirrups with the surgeon standing to the right side of the patient. Video monitors are positioned at the foot of the operating table or at the patient's feet (Fig. 68.1). Infants are sterilely prepared from nipples to toes, whereas older children in stirrups are prepared from nipples to perineum. A urinary bladder catheter is placed in older children; in infants the bladder is emptied using the Credé's maneuver.

Pneumoperitoneum is achieved using a Veress needle through the umbilicus. Most infants have a natural umbilical defect that allows safe open access into the abdomen. Alternatively, if the umbilical cord is still present and considered less than optimal in terms of cleanliness, the umbilicus is avoided and the initial trocar is placed in the left midabdomen at the proposed site for the left trocar using the Veress needle technique. This can be done safely and avoids potential injury to the low-lying liver during access through the left upper quadrant. Depending on the size of the patient, 4- or 5-mm ports can be used. In neonates we typically use three trocars (one 5-mm and two 4-mm trocars), but a fourth trocar can be added in the suprapubic position to assist in retraction of the colon. Trocar placement is individualized according to patient size, but they usually are positioned as shown in Figure 68.2. Pressures of 12 cm H_20 are used for all groups. A 4-mm, 30 degree scope is used in infants and a 5-mm, 30 degree scope is used in older children.

Initially, three ports are placed to visualize the transition zone and to perform seromuscular biopsies with laparosopic scissors for histologic leveling. It is best to defer further dissection until the presence of ganglion cells is confirmed histologically above the transition zone. A window is then made between the colon and superior rectal vessels using

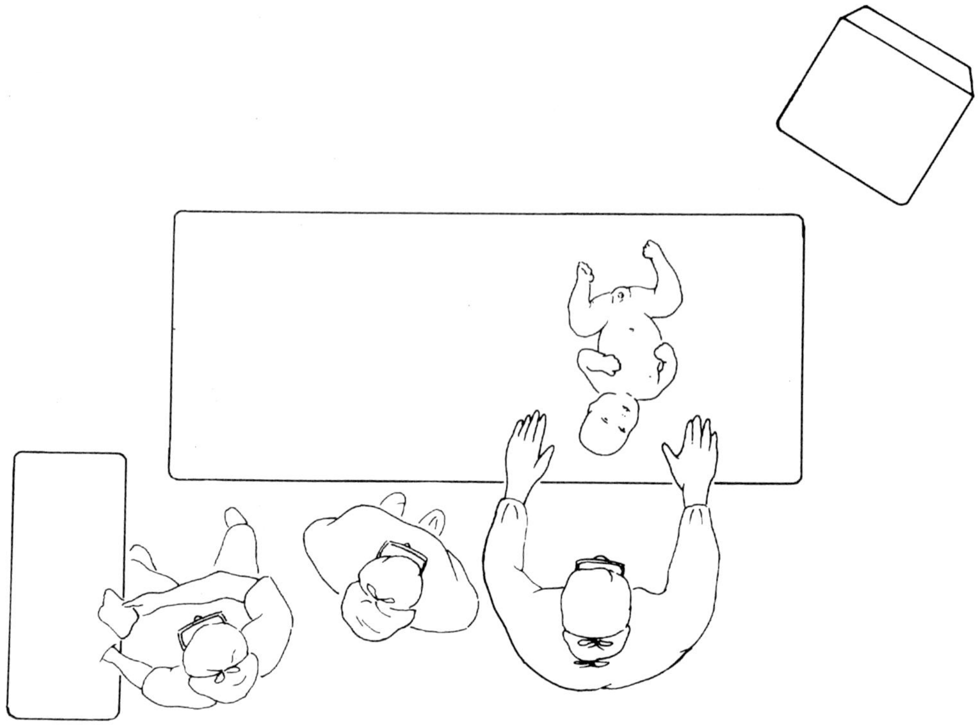

FIGURE 68.1. Operating room setup for an infant pull-through operation.

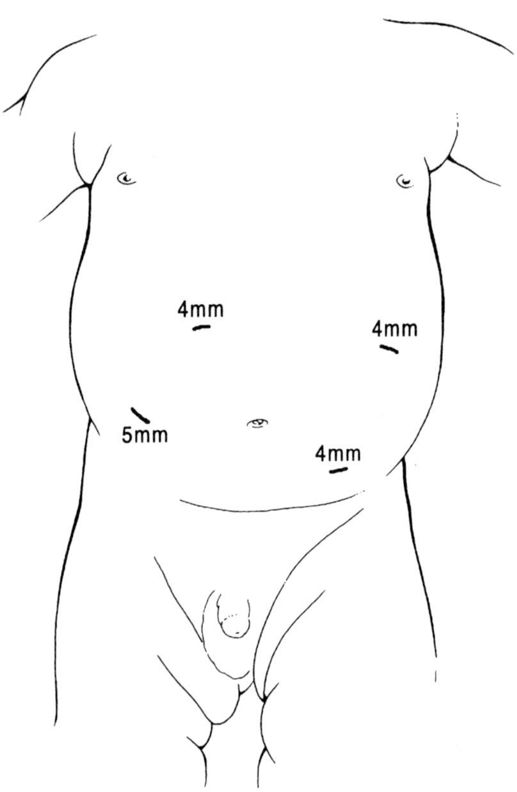

FIGURE 68.2. Position of trocar sites for laparoscopic pull-through with the optional left lower quadrant site shown.

hook cautery or the ultrasonic scalpel in older children. Distal dissection of the aganglionic colon is then performed circumferentially, keeping close to the colon wall, carefully preserving the mesenteric blood supply to the rectum. Blunt and sharp dissection of the avascular plane posterior to the rectum follows. Anteriorly, the rectum is dissected for about 1 to 2 cm below the peritoneal reflection. Care must be taken to avoid extensive lateral dissection or dissection too far anteriorly, where damage to the *nervi erigentes* can result in secondary impotence or bladder dysfunction. Hugging the rectal wall, circumferential dissection joins the anterior and posterior planes.

Proximal mesenteric dissection of the colon pedicle is performed using hook electrocautery or the ultrasonic scalpel with careful preservation of the marginal artery (Fig. 68.3). Dissection too close to the colon may cause ischemia to the pedicled colon with resultant stricture, dysfunction, or anastomotic disruption. Minimal proximal dissection is required in patients with low, rectosigmoid transition zones. Other patients require sigmoid colon mobilization or division of the lateral colonic fusion fascia up to the splenic flexure. Periodically, the colon pedicle is assessed for its ability to reach the deep pelvis without tension. For best complete functional results, the colon pedicle should be assessed for dysganglionosis, hypoganglionosis, and neuronal intestinal dysplasia, conditions that often

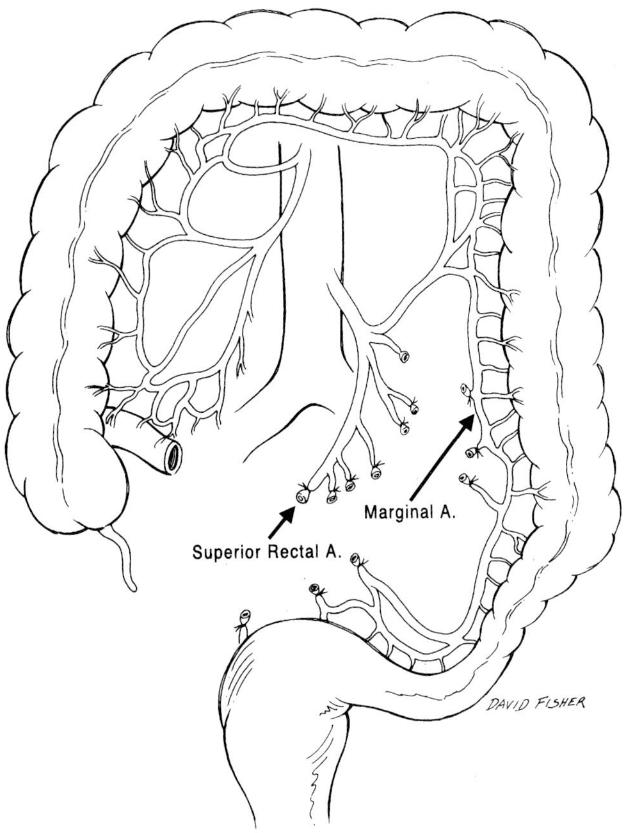

FIGURE 68.3. Division of the rectal and colonic mesentery to create the colon pedicle.

extend proximal to the aganglionic bowel in infants and children with Hirschsprung's disease.

After the endoscopic dissection of the colon and rectum has been completed, the pneumoperitoneum is released, the camera and instruments removed, and the perineal dissection started. The trocars are left in place for subsequent visualization following the pull-through. First, we place six to eight 2-0 silk traction sutures to evert the anus and expose the rectum. The mucosa is scored with electrocautery in a circular pattern 1 cm above the dentate line as shown in Figure 68.4. Silk sutures (3-0) are placed into the mucosal edges to provide traction for developing a circumferential submucosal plane. The plane is relatively avascular and can be developed by both sharp and blunt dissection. The submucosal plane is developed proximally until the colorectum begins to evert or prolapse, indicating that the transanal dissection has advanced to the level of the internal perirectal dissection (Fig. 68.5).

A malleable retractor is placed posteriorly between the muscular rectal sleeve and the submucosal plane of the colon. The rectal sleeve is then opened posteriorly with electrocautery to join the submucosal plane with the extramural

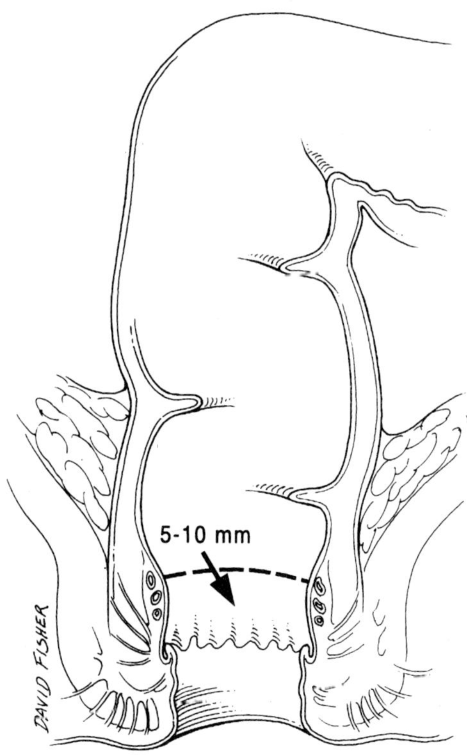

FIGURE 68.4. Mucosal incision 5 to 10 mm above dentate line marks the beginning of the transanal dissection.

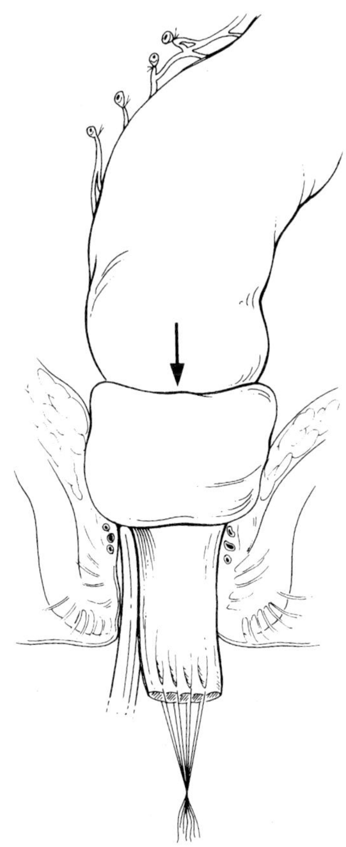

FIGURE 68.5. Silk traction sutures into the rectal mucosa and development of the submucosal dissection plane with blunt dissection.

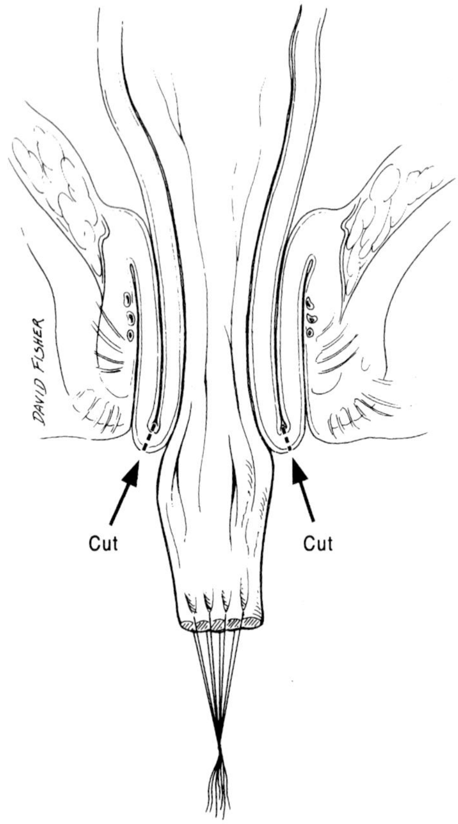

FIGURE 68.6. Transection of the rectal smooth muscular wall to join the intraperitoneal dissection. Transection should begin posteriorly to avoid injuring important anterior structures.

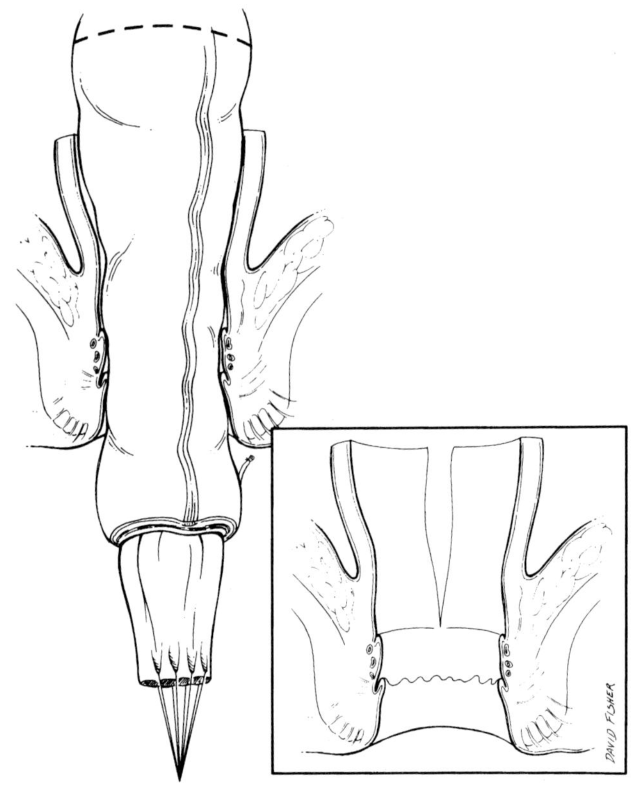

FIGURE 68.7. The remaining muscular sleeve is divided posteriorly from the proximal portion down to the level of the proposed anastomosis.

dissection from above (Fig. 68.6). The perineal and laparoscopic dissection planes are connected to leave a short muscular rectal cuff. At this point, we prefer to split the rectal cuff posteriorly within 1 cm of the proposed anastomosis to allow room for the developing neorectal reservoir (Fig. 68.7).

The colon and rectum are now pulled through the anus in continuity until the proximal ganglionated bowel appears at the anus. The most proximal biopsy site is pulled down beyond the point of the intended bowel anastomosis (Fig. 68.8). The anterior one third of the colon is transected and a circumferential single-layer anastomosis is created using absorbable suture. The remainder of the anastomosis is completed after transecting the posterior aspect of the pulled through colon.

Finally, reinsufflation for pneumoperitoneum is performed to inspect the colon pedicle for twisting or potential internal herniation. If necessary, interrupted sutures are used to reperitonealize the pelvis to close the potential internal hernia. The port sites are closed with fascial sutures and sterile strips and the entire procedure is usually accomplished in 2 to 3 hours.

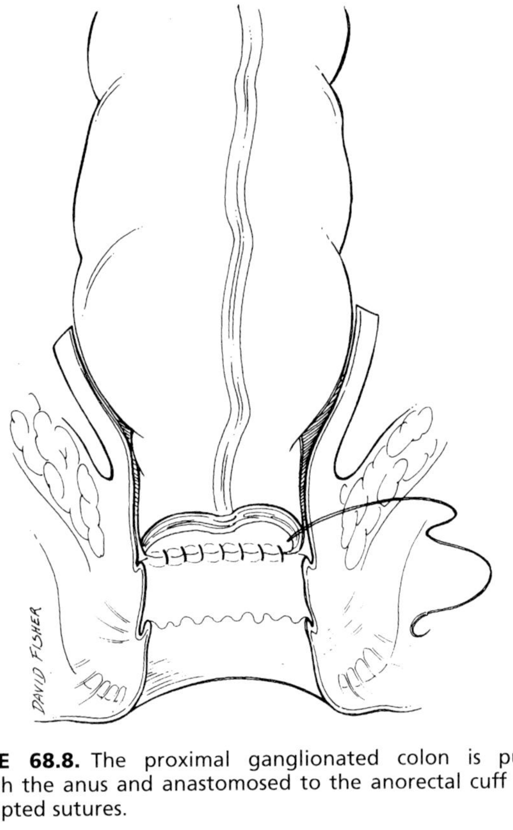

FIGURE 68.8. The proximal ganglionated colon is pulled through the anus and anastomosed to the anorectal cuff with interrupted sutures.

POSTOPERATIVE CARE

Nasogastric or orogastric decompression is used for 12 to 24 hours postsurgery. As soon as bowel function returns, an oral diet is initiated. This typically can begin on postoperative day 1 or 2. The patients remain on intravenous antibiotics for 24 hours postoperatively and are discharged when they can tolerate full oral feedings.

Rectal examination or dilation is performed 3 weeks following the surgical procedure. If necessary, parents can be taught to perform routine daily anorectal dilations. Routine daily rectal dilations do not seem to affect anorectal compliance over the long-term. Immediately following the pull-through operation, most patients have frequent stools, possibly due to the lack of a neorectal reservoir and to stretching and weakening of the internal sphincter.

The most frequent early complications after laparoscopically assisted endorectal pull-through have included enterocolitis and chronic diarrhea. These problems often respond to medical management, but proximal diversion may rarely be necessary in extreme cases. Other less frequent problems include anastomotic leak and bleeding, which are associated with technical error.

SUMMARY

There are three advantages of the minimal-access endorectal pull-through compared with the traditional open pull-through technique. First, mobilization of the colon pedicle laparoscopically minimizes peritoneal trauma. Second, the intraabdomininal colon is left intact, avoiding bacterial contamination of the peritoneal cavity. Third, transanal endorectal dissection minimizes peritoneal trauma. Despite the fact that many of the benefits of the pull-through procedure can be attained by transanal pull-through alone, significant advantages are realized by performing the laparoscopic dissection.

It is critical to verify the presence of ganglion cells in the proximal colon pedicle by laparoscopic seromuscular biopsy prior to proceeding with the irreversible step of endorectal dissection. In cases of total colonic aganglionosis, a different type of pull-through operation or ostomy may be considered. In addition, laparoscopic mobilization and devascularization of the intraabdominal aganglionic segment of rectosigmoid colon increases the mobility of the rectum and makes the endpoint of the endorectal dissection more definitive.

By facilitating the endorectal dissection with laparoscopic mobilization of the rectosigmoid colon, there is less potential for overdilating the internal anal sphincter mechanism, thereby weakening the patient's fecal continence mechanism during the transanal dissection. In patients with longer segments of aganglionosis, the laparoscopic approach affords the needed versatility in creating a ganglionated pedicle proximal to the aganglionic colon and allows for completion of the subsequent pull-through operation.

It has been our experience that the laparoscopically assisted colon pull-through for Hirschsprung's disease has resulted in a reduction in both the postoperative recovery time, as well as perioperative complications when compared with traditional open pull-through procedures.

SUGGESTED READINGS

Georgeson KE, Cohen RD, Hebra A, et al. Primary laparoscopic-assisted endorectal colon pull-through for Hirschsprung's disease—a new gold standard. *Ann Surg* 1999;229:678–683.

Georgeson KE, Fuenfer MM, Hardin WD. Primary laparoscopic pull-through for Hirschsprung's disease in infants and children. *J Pediatr Surg* 1995;30:1–7.

Teitelbaum DH, Coran AG., Weitzman JJ, et al. Hirschsprung's disease and related neuromuscular disorders of the intestine. In: O'Neill JA, Rowe MI, Grosfeld JL, et al., eds. *Pediatric surgery, 5th ed, vol 2.* St. Louis: Mosby-Year Book, 1998:1381–1424.

69

ACUTE APPENDICITIS

MARJORIE J. ARCA
DONNA A. CANIANO

Appendicitis continues to be the most common cause of acute abdominal pain requiring intraabdominal surgery in childhood. Patients with appendicitis present with a plethora of different clinical manifestations. The diagnosis of appendicitis continues to be suboptimal in children. Misdiagnosis rates range from 28% to 57% in children under 12 years of age and are close to 100% in patients under 2 years of age. Early and accurate diagnosis of appendicitis in infants and children can prevent perforation, abscess formation, and postoperative complications. Despite many advances in imaging and diagnostic modalities, appendicitis remains largely a clinical diagnosis; the history and physical examination allow the clinician to arrive at the diagnosis in the majority of cases. The goal of surgical management is to balance false-negative laparotomy and the development of perforation and peritonitis.

ANATOMY AND PATHOPHYSIOLOGY

The appendix is a long diverticulum located on the antimesenteric border of the end of the cecum. Its blood supply is derived from the appendiceal artery, which arises from the ileocolic branch of the superior mesenteric artery. The appendix is classically described as located at the McBurney's point, which is located one third of the distance from the right anterior superior iliac spine to the umbilicus. However, the appendix is more commonly found in a retrocecal (28%–68%) or intrapelvic (27%–53%) position. Other locations, in decreasing order of frequency, include right upper quadrant (4%), subcecal (2%), preileal (1%), left lower quadrant (1%), and left upper quadrant (<1%).

In the neonatal period, the average length of the appendix is 4 to 5 cm; its luminal opening is funnel-shaped, which theoretically accounts for the infrequency of acute appendicitis in infants. Inflammation of the appendix is usually precipitated by luminal obstruction from submucosal lymphoid follicles or a fecalith. Less commonly, parasites, neoplasms, or foreign bodies also can cause such an obstruction. The epithelial cells continue to secrete mucus, which distends the appendix. Transmural engorgement of the appendix ensues, which impedes venous and lymphatic flow initially, and subsequently arterial blood supply. Patches of appendiceal ischemia and necrosis occur. If the appendix is not removed, the area of ischemia thins out and perforates. This leads to abscess formation or frank peritoneal contamination. In children, the relatively short and thin omentum fails to contain a developing abscess and may therefore account for the higher incidence of peritonitis in this age group.

M. J. Arca and **D. A. Caniano:** Departments of Clinical Surgery and Pediatrics, Ohio State University College of Medicine and Public Health; and Departments of Surgery and Pediatrics, Children's Hospital, Columbus, Ohio.

EPIDEMIOLOGY

The lifetime risk of appendicitis is between 6% and 8%. Appendicitis is ultimately diagnosed in up to 8% of children presenting with acute abdominal pain in emergency rooms. There is a recognized seasonal variation in appendicitis, with an 11% increase in the May to August months compared with November to February. This increase parallels outbreaks in enteric infections caused by viral, bacterial, or parasitic pathogens.

AGE-SPECIFIC CLINICAL PRESENTATION

Abdominal pain is the most common symptom of appendicitis. The typical historical course of the pain is vague epigastric or periumbilical discomfort and subsequent localization of the pain to the right lower quadrant. However, this pattern is seen in only about half of adult patients, and even less commonly in children. The age of the patient often correlates with the symptomatology.

Neonates

Of the 122 neonatal cases of appendicitis cited in the literature, there is an associated mortality rate of 80%. Presenting symptoms in this age group are relatively nonspecific and include irritability/lethargy (22%), abdominal distension (60%–90%), and vomiting (60%). Other presenting symptoms are abdominal mass, abdominal wall erythema, hypotension, hypothermia, and respiratory distress. Interestingly, in this age group, classic luminal obstruction with an appendicolith has not been described. Instead, inflammation subsequent to distal obstruction (e.g., Hirschsprung's disease), hernia involvement, and vascular compromise are the most common causes of appendicitis in neonates. Prematurity is a risk factor for appendicitis of the newborn period.

Toddlers

In the child 2 years of age or younger, the most common presenting symptoms are vomiting, pain, diarrhea, and fever. A child in this age group also may present with irritability, grunting, respiratory symptoms, and right hip complaints (limp, stiffness). Diffuse abdominal tenderness is more often seen than localized right lower quadrant tenderness. On physical examination, fever, lethargy, abdominal distension, rigidity, and an abdominal or rectal mass may be seen. Toddlers have limited communication skills; therefore, there is a characteristic delay in diagnosis of about 4 to 5 days, which contributes to a high rate of perforation (82% to 92%) and bowel obstruction (about 80%).

Preschoolers (2 to 5 Years)

Typical symptoms in these children include abdominal pain, fever, anorexia, nausea, and vomiting. Unlike toddlers, preschoolers often have localized right lower quadrant pain and tenderness. One study concluded that fevers, involuntary guarding, and rebound tenderness are more often seen in patients with appendicitis compared to patients with other causes of abdominal pain. In this age group, vomiting often precedes abdominal pain.

School-Aged Children (6 to 12 Years)

These patients are better able to communicate their symptoms. Abdominal discomfort may be diffuse but is more often in the right lower quadrant. The pain is usually constant and made worse by movement; up to a third of these patients have intermittent pain. Clinically, the location of abdominal tenderness is largely dependent on the intraperitoneal position of the appendix. A retrocecal appendix most often presents with right flank or right upper quadrant pain. Vomiting, anorexia, diarrhea, constipation, and dysuria also may occur.

Children with acute appendicitis may have low-grade fever, rebound tenderness, and percussion tenderness. In adults, classically described signs of appendicitis include the Rovsing's sign, psoas sign, and obturator sign. No published studies have addressed the sensitivity or specificity of these physical signs in children.

Adolescents

The incidence of appendicitis peaks in early adolescence. The history and physical examination is reliable in this age group. Gynecologic diagnoses come into play in adolescent girls.

The symptom complex is usually present for less than 48 hours; beyond this, a ruptured appendix is more likely. A low-grade fever, typically below 38.5°C (101.5°F), is usually present. A higher temperature is suggestive of a perforated appendix.

LABORATORY ADJUNCTS

It is traditionally thought that the white blood cell (WBC) count is elevated in children with appendicitis. However, if symptoms have been present for less than 24 hours, an elevated WBC count (>15,000 for age <10 or >13,000 for age >10) is only 18% sensitive for appendicitis; this parameter increases in sensitivity to 90% if symptoms are present for longer than 48 hours. Neutrophilia is a more sensitive parameter than WBC count (95% vs. 18%) in children with symptoms that have been present for less than 24 hours. C-reactive protein is a nonspecific inflammatory protein that has been found, in limited studies, to be predictive of appendiceal rupture or abscess (>90% sensitivity).

RADIOLOGIC EVALUATION

Although plain abdominal radiographs are often taken in children with suspected appendicitis, recent studies have found that plain radiographs were normal or misleading in 77% of pediatric patients. The most specific finding in a plain film is an appendicolith, which is found in 13% to 22% of patients with appendicitis and in less than 2% of patients without appendicitis. An evidence-based clinical pathway designed by pediatric surgeons has advocated plain radiography in the context of suspected perforation, bowel obstruction, inflammatory mass, or a prior history of renal stones or gallstones.

Ultrasonography has a published sensitivity of 80% to 92% and specificity of 86% to 98%. Ultrasonograpic findings in acute appendicitis include diameter greater than 6 mm, "target sign," appendicolith, appendiceal distension, high periappendiceal echogenicity, and periappendiceal fluid. Because of patient obesity, superimposed air, an uncooperative patient, or abnormal location, the appendix is not visualized in many patients with appendicitis, contributing to most of the false negative study results.

Computed tomography (CT) is a modality that is frequently used as part of the diagnostic workup of abdominal pain in children. Prospective randomized trials were reported in combined pediatric and adult patients who either underwent laparotomy/laparoscopy or were followed clinically to exclude the diagnosis. The sensitivity of CT scanning to diagnose appendicitis was 87% to 99%, with specificity ranging from 83% to 97%. The highest sensitivity was seen in patients who underwent a focused appendiceal CT with combined oral and rectal contrast. In practical terms, a CT scan is most useful in a child who is suspected of a perforation or a patient whose clinical presentation may be less suspicious for appendicitis.

PREOPERATIVE PREPARATION

Children undergoing an appendectomy for acute appendicitis should be evaluated for dehydration and resuscitated accordingly. Intravenous antibiotics are also administered; a second-generation cephalosporin is usually adequate for cases of suspected acute appendicitis.

OPERATIVE APPROACH

After induction of general anesthesia, the child's abdomen is palpated for a mass. If a mass is found, the incision should be made in close proximity to the mass. A transverse right lower quadrant incision is created just below the level of the anterior superior iliac spine. The external oblique muscle is split along the direction of its fibers. The internal oblique and transverse muscles are split in the direction of their fibers. The peritoneum is opened. Free fluid should be aspirated.

The cecum and the appendix are delivered into the wound. The cecum is identified by the teniae coli, grasped anteriorly with a gauze pad, and delivered into the wound using a to-and-fro rocking motion. Often, the concomitant delivery of the appendix is impeded by its adhesions to surrounding bowel or omentum. A finger is inserted into the peritoneal cavity and the appendiceal adhesions are digitally lysed.

If the appendix cannot be delivered into the wound, other maneuvers that may be useful include the following: (a) dividing the lateral peritoneal attachments to the cecum; (b) laterally extending the skin and muscle incisions; and (c) medially extending the incision by opening the anterior and posterior rectus sheaths and dividing the inferior epigastric vessels between ligatures.

Once the appendix is delivered into the wound, the mesoappendix is divided between ligatures. The appendix is crushed with a straight clamp a few millimeters from its base. The clamp is applied slightly distal to this area, and a nonabsorbable suture is used to tie the appendiceal base. Inversion of the stump may be performed by dunking the ligated stump in the middle of a purse-string suture placed through the seromuscular layer of the cecum about a centimeter from the appendiceal base.

If the appendix has an inflamed wide base, it may be secured using interrupted seromuscular Lembert sutures or, alternatively, a surgical stapler. The cecum is carefully replaced into the peritoneal cavity. The right paracolic gutter and the pelvis are irrigated and aspirated until clear fluid returns. The internal oblique and transversalis muscles are closed with a running suture. The external oblique, Scarpa's fascia, and skin are closed individually with absorbable sutures.

COMPLICATIONS

The expected rate of wound infection is 1% to 2%. The risk for infection can be diminished by not allowing the inflamed appendix and omentum to touch the wound during dissection. Pelvic abscesses occur extremely rarely in patients with nonruptured appendicitis. Although rare, postoperative hemorrhage can occur and usually requires operative intervention.

Leaks from the appendiceal stump can present as gross abdominal peritonitis or persistent drainage from the wound. Gross abdominal peritoneal contamination may require operative intervention to clear the abdominal cavity of infected enteric material. If the leak is focal and presents as wound drainage, local fistula control using drains or stoma bags should be established in order to protect the skin. The patient should be given antibiotics. Nutritional status should be optimized. If the leakage persists for weeks, operative closure may be warranted. The surgeon should make certain that a fecalith was not left in the peritoneal cavity.

EDITOR'S NOTES

The diagnosis of acute appendicitis in children continues to be made predominantly on clinical grounds. Although many recent reports on the use of ultrasonography or CT suggest a diagnostic accuracy of greater than 90%, the fact remains that they are not 100% accurate and it has been difficult to demonstrate that their more liberal use has had any impact on the incidence of ruptured appendicitis or the negative appendectomy rate, even in adults. The history and physical examination are therefore the most important components of the workup for the child with abdominal pain. Nevertheless, the rate of ruptured appendicitis among children remains unacceptably high (one third to one half of all children with appendicitis) and a low but significant number of negative appendectomies are still being performed (up to 10% in some series).

The presentation is variable and depends on the age of the patient. Unfortunately, early appendicitis is essentially indistinguishable from other common causes of abdominal pain, including gastroenteritis, constipation, and mesenteric adenitis. It is often only after the suppurative process begins and the pain becomes localized that the possibility of appendicitis is even considered. The time between the start of this process and perforation can be quite brief, sometimes hours in very young children, thus accounting to some degree for the high rate of perforation. Most children will have abdominal pain, vomiting, and a low-grade fever. Most will have malaise and poor appetite, but the absence of either of these or both does not exclude appendicitis. (Likewise, the complaint of a painful car ride is common and nonspecific.) Pain localization and the complete clinical picture suggestive of appendicitis does not appear in most cases until after 12 to 24 hours. This is the basis for the period of hospitalization and observation that is sometimes recommended for patients with symptoms of early disease. In general, pain caused by viral illnesses, constipation, and mesenteric adenitis should resolve within 24 hours. If not, the diagnosis of appendicitis should be strongly considered.

Physical examination is the most important component of the diagnostic workup. Localized tenderness in a child is due to appendicitis unless proven otherwise. This is usually in the right lower quadrant (iliac fossa) but can be anywhere in the abdomen. Pain associated with signs of peritoneal irritation (guarding, percussion tenderness, or motion tenderness) is highly suggestive of a surgical process, which in children is nearly always attributable to appendicitis. Rebound tenderness is oversensitive, nonspecific, and associated with extreme pain in the presence of true peritonitis. Therefore, one should rarely need to test for it. An exception is the child in whom diffuse peritonitis is clearly not present and who might benefit from testing for rebound in the left lower quadrant, which, when it causes right lower quadrant pain, is highly suggestive of appendicitis (Rovsing's sign). A rectal examination rarely adds to the diagnostic assessment and should be avoided in most cases, except when the clinical findings suggest a pelvic abscess.

In most patients, the history and physical examination are sufficient to rule out appendicitis or suggest the need for an operation. The WBC count is elevated in 85% to 90% of patients with appendicitis but has a specificity of only about 50%. Therefore, once a clinical decision is made on the basis of the history and physical examination, the presence or absence of an elevated WBC count should rarely alter the ultimate recommendation. A left shift in the WBC count differential is more sensitive and specific. However, as with all laboratory analyses, it should be considered only in the context of the clinical findings. A urinalysis should be performed to rule out pyelonephritis as a cause of abdominal pain, however a few white cells and red cells per high-power field are often seen in cases of appendicitis, due to inflammation adjacent to the ureter or bladder. A plain radiograph of the abdomen may demonstrate a fecalith or an ileus, but is probably only necessary in cases of possible bowel obstruction.

Although laparoscopic appendectomy has proven to be safe and effective in children, for most young children who are thin, there is probably no advantage of the laparoscopic approach over the traditional open approach performed through a very small right lower quadrant muscle-splitting incision. There are several situations in which laparoscopy offers clear advantages, including treatment of an obese patient, cases of diagnostic uncertainty (especially when a gynecologic cause is suspected), and for interval appendectomy, where the extent of dissection might require a larger incision if done via laparotomy.

The incision needs to be large enough to accommodate the surgeon's finger and the appendix itself. In most children this need be no more than 2 or 3 cm. A muscle-splitting technique speeds recovery and minimizes postoperative discomfort. In most cases, the appendix can be mobilized safely with blunt finger dissection regardless of its location. This requires experience and a gentle technique. One must be certain not to mobilize the iliac artery or ureter by mistake—instances of both have been described. Once the appendix has been mobilized, it can be brought out through the incision. After careful division of the mesentery between ligatures, double ligation of the base with absorbable suture is all that is required. Dunking the stalk is usually unnecessary. The wound is closed in layers, and the skin can usually be closed with subcuticular sutures.

–P.M.

SUGGESTED READINGS

Birnbaum BA, Wilson SR. Appendicitis at the millennium. *Radiology* 2000;215:337–348.

Hardin J. Acute appendicitis: review and update. *Am Fam Physician* 1999;60:2027–2034.

Reynolds SL. Missed appendicitis in pediatric emergency department. *Pediatr Emerg Care* 1993;9:1–3.

Rothrock SG, Pagane J. Acute appendicitis in children: emergency department diagnosis and management. *Ann Emerg Med* 2000;36: 39–51.

Warner BW, Kulick RM, Stoops MM, et al. An evidence-based clinical pathway for acute appendicitis decreases hospital duration and cost. *J Pediatr Surg* 1998;33:1371–1375.

70

APPENDICEAL ABSCESS

THOMAS V. WHALEN

Children present with appendicitis having already perforated far more often than adults do, with the exception, perhaps, of the elderly. Treatment of perforated appendicitis varies somewhat, although prompt operative intervention is the predominant practice among surgeons operating on children. The approach varies somewhat, however, when there is a delayed presentation of a patient with perforated appendicitis. The child with a perforated appendix and the clear presence of diffuse peritonitis is viewed and treated differently from the child who has been ill for 7 to 10 days and who presents with fever, focal pain in the right lower quadrant, and the presence of a defined mass on physical examination.

DIAGNOSTIC APPROACH

Many surgeons have seen children with appendicitis without perforation despite several days of symptoms. Clearly the duration of symptoms cannot be the only factor considered when making decisions in these patients. The distribution and the duration of symptoms is a useful guide in determining the probability of perforation, but it is only a guide. Thus, the patient presenting with localized peritoneal signs after an appropriate history has been elicited coupled with other appropriate data (fever, leukocytosis, etc.) is almost always best handled by expeditious operative intervention for removal of the appendix.

It is important to approach the examination of any sick child, especially if there is the possibility of peritonitis, in a calm and compassionate manner. The average 4- to 10-year-old presenting with an appendiceal abscess already feels poorly and is in pain, and the surgeon is often one of many who have already examined him or her throughout the day. Any forceful technique of eliciting the presence or absence of rebound tenderness is doomed to failure. The clinician must attempt to gain the trust of the child, and often must use more subtle (and perhaps even sneaky) means of eliciting the presence and location of tenderness in the child's abdomen. The best known of these techniques is the use of the stethoscope for palpation with swift but smooth release of the instrument to judge the finding of rebound tenderness. Assessing for motion tenderness or percussion tenderness also might be useful and is often more humane than testing for true rebound.

Fever and leukocytosis are usually present. These findings are perhaps the best markers of early success or failure of nonoperative management of the child with an appendiceal abscess. A number of imaging modalities may be used to diagnose an appendiceal abscess. In the literature there are supporting and contrary data for each of the principal imaging modalities of ultrasonography, computed tomography (CT), and magnetic resonance imaging (MRI). To dispense with the last, the cost of MRI is too prohibitive, despite its accuracy, to be used as a routine diagnostic technique for this diagnosis. In addition, most children require sedation or anesthesia to undergo MRI, which adds to the cost and potential morbidity of the study. Ultrasonography is quick, economical, and highly accurate but is highly dependent on an experienced operator to perform and interpret the study. It is then perhaps by default that CT is considered the study of choice to assist the surgeon and others in delineating this process.

Computed tomography should be performed with enteral contrast, whereas intravenous contrast is not necessary (this is, of course, highly dependent on the preferences of the institution and the consulting radiologist). Such contrast has two paths to the cecum and surrounding intestine, oral or rectal. In the adult, CT is most often performed after rectal contrast instillation. The advantage here is one of time. Children are rarely cooperative enough to tolerate the enema necessary for this technique and, in addition, are not usually able to comply with the suggestion to retain the contrast within the colon and rectum until after the test is completed, creating both practical and aesthetic difficulties. On the other hand, there may be some degree of ileus or nausea and vomiting that can prevent orally ingested con-

T. V. Whalen: Departments of Surgery and Pediatrics, University of Medicine and Dentistry of New Jersey–Robert Wood Johnson Medical School, New Brunswick, New Jersey.

trast from reaching the distal ileum and cecum, making CT worthless. On balance, however, I have found that orally ingested contrast is the preferable pathway.

We are perhaps more frequently faced with the question of how to best manage the appendiceal abscess after an imaging study has clearly documented its presence, although there are certainly times when an appendiceal abscess is first identified in the operating room. This is usually seen in the case of a young child who clearly demonstrates the process of appendicitis by history and brief abdominal examination but in whom the actual phlegmon or abscess cannot be appreciated on examination. It would be inhumane to persist in trying to delineate such a mass in a child. In many pediatric emergency departments, the practice of administering narcotic pain relief, primarily out of compassion, accrues the added benefit of permitting a more thorough and revealing physical examination, but may complicate the decision-making process by masking important physical findings. There should be prompt operative exploration of such a child (after appropriate preparation, of course) without further delay. In defense of our pediatric emergency medicine colleagues, they are on the front line, seeing these patients when surgical consultation has been requested but is not always expeditiously available. If the surgeon can be at the bedside to evaluate the child within 30 minutes, then he or she has the right to insist that narcotics not be administered if such administration could change the physical findings. Conversely, with delayed availability, I feel that the surgeon abdicates decision-making power to some degree.

A child with a greater than 1-week history who is afebrile, has mild focal tenderness and has regained some appetite, regardless of whether or not a mass was detected during the physical examination, is probably better treated nonoperatively. In the adult experience, when there is a delayed presentation with an abdominal mass, a significant factor in the decision of immediate operation versus nonoperative therapy is whether the mass in the abdomen could represent a neoplasm rather than an appendiceal abscess or phlegmon. This concern is essentially nonexistent in the child, although the possibility of lymphoma in the adolescent cannot be ignored. The decision to manage the child with a "walled-off" abscess using a nonoperative approach is therefore one that can be made with confidence.

As an aside, many will suggest the use of the term *conservative* rather than *nonoperative* in such treatment of the patient with a right lower quadrant inflammatory process that is contained. I contend that there are many instances in which the "conservative" thing to do is to proceed expeditiously to the operating room rather than manage the case nonoperatively. This simply highlights the fact that the word *conservative* is subjective and should therefore be eschewed so as to avoid such a judgmental connotation imposing unnecessary constraint upon the decision-making physician.

One real consideration in the decision to manage a patient with appendiceal abscess nonoperatively must be the age of the patient. This is based on the fact that the omentum in a small child is different both anatomically and functionally than that of an older child or adult. The role of the omentum as the "guardian of the abdomen" is well established. The underdeveloped omentum of the 3- or 4-year-old simply cannot succeed in walling off the inflammatory process. One should therefore be hesitant to treat young children with appendiceal abscess nonoperatively. It follows in discussing the inadequacy of the omentum in this age range that many of these younger children present with physical examination characteristic of diffuse peritonitis and therefore, in my strategy of management, are not candidates for nonoperative management.

PREOPERATIVE PREPARATION

The preparation of a patient with acute appendicitis who has been ill for a short period of time is rapid and simple. The patient who clearly has perforated appendicitis and needs operative intervention need not be subjected to a prolonged delay, but will certainly require more time for resuscitation. It would be a mistake to bring a dehydrated patient to the operating room with some imperative to remove the perforated appendix. Likewise, it is mandatory that appropriate broad-spectrum antibiotic coverage be instituted before an operative procedure occurs. It is entirely prudent in some cases not to emergently operate on a patient with perforated appendicitis in the middle of the night. It must be emphasized that these decisions should be made only after a careful assessment of the individual patient and on the basis of mature judgment drawn from experience. As stated above, it may be difficult to distinguish a patient with perforated appendicitis from one with appendicitis that has yet to rupture, making generalizations in decision making potentially dangerous.

TECHNICAL APPROACH

The technical approach to the child with a perforated appendix and an abscess is determined by the treatment plan that has been chosen: nonoperative or operative. Children selected for nonoperative therapy should be free of signs of diffuse peritoneal irritation.

Appendiceal abscess is not the term that should be applied to the CT finding of the process that we are discussing; rather, *appendiceal phlegmon* is a more apt description of the pathophysiologic process. As such, percutaneous drainage is frequently not possible or even indicated. The child is started on broad-spectrum antibiotics. The traditional regimen is triple antibiotic therapy, including ampicillin, gentamicin, and metronidazole. The data clearly support the use of any reasonable broad-spectrum regimen, including monotherapy in some cases. As soon as possible, a percutaneously inserted central venous catheter is placed as a matter of convenience to the patient as well as to facilitate home care when the goals of inpatient management are met.

The goals of nonoperative therapy are simple: that the child be eating (or at the least drinking) well and afebrile. There should be a defined time line wherein one assesses the success or failure of this modality of treatment. One should allow 48 hours for signs of significant response of nonoperative management; if these are lacking, then the child should undergo surgery. Most children who appear to be responding to nonoperative management can be safely discharged to complete the course of antibiotics at home. The length of therapy is variable, depending on the size of the abscess, the duration of symptoms, and the overall clinical appearance of the child. A period of 10 to 14 days is typical, but depends on individual preferences as well. The end point of therapy also should be individualized. Some use only clinical criteria, whereas others use the presence of a benign examination and a normal white blood cell count as criteria for stopping antibiotics. In some cases, it may be reasonable to repeat the imaging studies, although inflammatory changes may persist for a long time and should not be confused with residual infection in the absence of clinical correlates.

A patient with a large phlegmon or who is more symptomatic (vomiting, pain, persistent fevers) should undergo drainage of the infected fluid, either by laparotomy or by a noninvasive technique. Many such fluid collections are immediately adjacent to the rectum and can be drained easily and safely using a transrectal approach. This usually requires the use of a general anesthetic and placement of a Penrose drain. Alternatively, an interventionalist may be asked to drain the fluid percutaneously, usually with the placement of a temporary drainage device. Many have found that adding noninvasive drainage to the nonoperative regimen can shorten the hospital stay and the ultimate course of therapy, in certain cases. However, it is my experience and that of others that for most patients the judicious use of antibiotic therapy alone is safe and adequate therapy, and that the insistence on drainage can sometimes only serve to increase morbidity and discomfort.

Operative management is not always embraced as a first-line therapy with an appendiceal abscess because of the risk for bowel injury and fistula formation, as well as the risk for inducing a more stormy infectious process by "stirring up" the partially or fully contained infectious process. Nonetheless, if operative management is indicated, then the process followed is in essence no different from that detailed elsewhere in this text on management of perforated appendicitis.

POSTOPERATIVE CARE

If nonoperative management is indeed successful, then the decision becomes whether or not one needs to perform an interval appendectomy: an elective removal of the appendix after a defined interval for resolution of the inflammation surrounding the appendix. The time-honored practice has been to remove the appendix within 2 to 3 months. Past studies, primarily in adolescents and adults, have shown that one may expect about a third of these patients to have recurrent problems with their appendix. Underscoring this number, however, is the fact that such "problems" are generally just appendicitis that may be treated by appendectomy. If a patient is likely to be in a remote location, isolated from standard medical care, then certainly the appendix should be removed. On the other hand, I personally give the parents the above data and then involve them in the decision. I have had multiple instances of success with this form of management.

71

CHRONIC APPENDICITIS AND APPENDICEAL COLIC

RICHARD J. STEVENSON

Chronic appendiceal pain may be divided into three categories: (a) chronic appendicitis as defined by a mononuclear cell infiltrate; (b) recurrent appendicitis documented by fibrosis, which indicates remote appendicitis; and (c) appendiceal colic.

In my opinion, *chronic appendicitis* is somewhat of a misnomer. The term is generally used in reference to any long-term appendiceal pain (relieved by appendectomy) whether inflammation is histopathologically documented or not. Probably, *chronic appendicitis* should be reserved for histopathologically proven cases of chronic appendicitis. Indeed, the overwhelming majority of appendiceal colic cases show no microscopic evidence of inflammation. In my experience, appendiceal colic is by far (>90%) the most common cause of chronic appendiceal pain.

Appendiceal colic is and always has been a controversial subject. The pain results from muscular contractions against a luminal obstruction. Obstructions may be extrinsic, intramural, or intraluminal. Commonly accepted causes of luminal obstruction include fibrosis, fecalomas, bands (adhesions), kinks (twists), foreign bodies (seeds), tumors (carcinoid), parasites (*Enterobius vermicularis*), and lymphoid hyperplasia. When the appendix attempts to evacuate mucus (secreted by the appendiceal mucosa) against an obstruction, colicky abdominal pain results.

The concept of appendiceal colic is straightforward. Appendiceal colic is to acute appendicitis as biliary colic is to acute cholecystitis. Careful observation of the patient with appendiceal colic usually shows that the patient's attitude is indistinguishable from that of patients suffering from colic secondary to other etiologies. Part of the problem is that surgeons are not encouraged during their training to view the appendix as a colic-producing structure, despite the fact that the initial periumbilical discomfort associated with the beginning evolution of acute appendicitis is generally considered to be secondary to appendiceal cramping. Why not prolonged or intermittent bouts of appendiceal colic without overt inflammation? The underlying problem is that it is exceptionally difficult to evaluate the appendiceal lumen. If the appendiceal lumen could be imaged as accurately as the biliary system, pancreatic duct, and ureters, there would be no controversy over the issue of appendiceal colic.

R. J. Stevenson: Department of Clinical Surgery, Division of Pediatric Surgery, University of Cincinnati, and Cincinnati Children's Hospital Medical Center, Cincinnati, Ohio.

INITIAL EXPERIENCE

My experience with chronic appendiceal pain began in 1983. I was asked to evaluate an 8-year-old girl with 6 months of right hip pain exacerbated with movement. Serial physical examinations documented mild McBurney point tenderness, but abdominal pain was a secondary complaint. Results of an extensive workup, including an orthopedic evaluation (bone scan and hip tap), were unremarkable. The patient was referred for a psychological workup. In desperation, an elective appendectomy was performed. The appendix was retrocecal, and although the structure looked normal, histopathology showed focal mild acute appendicitis. Long-term follow-up shows that the patient has remained free of abdominal and right hip pain.

The presentation and successful management of this patient sparked my curiosity. Consequently, I kept a log of all patients who presented with chronic right lower quadrant abdominal pain and subsequently underwent an elective appendectomy. Over the next 5 years there were 12 such encounters. In 1987, I had an emergency consultation for a 5-year-old boy who was felt to have a surgical abdomen. A barium enema the night before for presumed intussusception yielded unremarkable information. The appendix did not fill. The patient had an uneventful night on intravenous fluids, but breakfast the next morning exacerbated the same pain and vomiting within 5 minutes. My evaluation revealed a patient with colic as severe as I had seen with ureteral or biliary colic. Review of an abdominal radiograph taken in the morning just prior to consultation revealed an appendix filled with barium that outlined a large fecaloma. In retrospect, the patient had been experiencing intermittent colic for 3 months. An urgent appendectomy documented the fecaloma and relieved the pain.

Interestingly, later the same year this patient's mother brought his sister in to the office. She stated that her daughter's symptoms were the same as her brother's and her appendix should be removed. A thorough workup, including an upper gastrointestinal (GI) series with follow-through and barium enema—both with delayed films—failed to visualize the appendix. Elective appendectomy 1 month later documented a fecaloma and relieved the pain (follow-up 10 years). I'm certain that many surgeons identify with this scenario. What struck me as curious was how could this mother be so positive of the diagnosis? There must be a classic presentation for patients with appendiceal colic. The following summarizes what I have learned about this condition over the past 18 years, and my experience with over 400 patients.

ESTABLISHING THE DIAGNOSIS

The diagnosis of appendiceal colic is a clinical one. I use four steps to reach this diagnosis:

1. Verify that the pain has colic characteristics, thus confining possible causes to hollow muscular organs.
2. Confirm that there are autonomic manifestations secondary to the pain, suggesting that the pain is real.
3. Document the association of pain with eating, which indicates the likely organ system responsible is the GI tract.
4. Identify the point of maximal tenderness while the patient is experiencing pain—this will invariably locate the appendix if the patient has appendiceal colic.

HISTORY

The patient with acute appendicitis initially complains of periumbilical pain. This is generally felt to be secondary to appendiceal spasm; indeed, careful observation of such a patient early on will usually be suggestive of colicky discomfort. As the inflammation and necrosis progress, nerves die and the colic disappears.

In stark contrast to acute appendicitis when spreading infection and inflammation result in a still and quiet individual, the patient with appendiceal colic is usually uncomfortable. The child will be restless, writhing, and even screaming with pain (no problem taking a deep breath when there is no inflammation). The intensity, periodicity and frequency of the pain are variable and depend on the nature of the obstruction. For example, fecalomas (in contrast to fecaliths, which are calcified) may be extruded into the cecal lumen and lymphoid hyperplasia may vary with the inciting cause. As the obstruction increases, so does the pain. The reverse is also true. The patient with appendiceal colic complains of anorexia and usually nausea. Severe colic results in the expected reflexive vomiting.

Patients with significant appendiceal colic (as with all colic) experience an outpouring of catecholamines. Consequently, the patient's parents will usually have already noted facial pallor associated with the onset of the pain. This is suggestive that the pain is real and that the child is not malingering. Other notable associations include darkness below the eyes, glassy or sunken eyes, diaphoresis, and flushing over the zygomas. Mushy bowel movements (not diarrhea) secondary to rapid GI transit time are often reported. Painful episodes also may be associated with headaches, lightheadedness, and occasionally even syncopal attacks. Rarely, parents may note intense flushing, and in such cases their child will complain of hot flashes.

Virtually every article discussing appendiceal colic has failed to note a relationship between eating and the onset of pain. My experience has been exactly the opposite. Although not obvious at the outset of my experience, more patients and more careful questioning have established the link. In fact, a positive association of enteral intake and exacerbation of pain is exceptionally suggestive of appendiceal colic. On the other hand, negative history should make the practitioner wary that appendiceal colic may not be the diagnosis.

One might anticipate that anything stimulating GI tract peristalsis would also stimulate appendiceal contraction. Indeed, I have found this to be the case. Gallbladder contraction is rather delayed subsequent to a fatty meal (30 minutes to 2 hours). In contrast, appendiceal contraction occurs almost immediately after a meal. Anything resulting in gastric distention such as food or liquid (barium, soft drinks, water), fat or nonfat, will exacerbate peristalsis and appendiceal contraction, and very quickly at that, usually within 5 to 15 minutes. The patient or parents may not have recognized the association. Helpful questioning includes asking the patient when the last major attack was experienced and whether there was a meal just prior. Does the patient come to the table starved, take one bite, and push the plate away? Does the pain come on at school (when does the nurse call)? If so, how is it related to snacks or a meal? Central nervous stimulation also may exacerbate the pain. Does the pain start when the patient smells a steak cooking? Is the pain related to hunger? If so, it will usually be reported at bedtime or upon arising in the morning before breakfast. The pain may exacerbate as a result of anxiety just prior to an oral presentation or sporting event. Finally, I have had parents deny a relationship to eating yet report a 20 pound weight loss. Upon further questioning as to how they account for the weight loss, they invariably say,

"How do you expect him to keep his weight up when he won't eat anything?" Food fear is common in appendiceal colic patients. If all else fails, have the parents keep a log relating meals and snacks to pain. They will frequently report a positive correlation on the next visit. Although eating will not invariably result in pain, it generally happens often enough that the association is obvious.

PHYSICAL EXAMINATION

If the history is strongly suggestive of appendiceal colic, a positive physical examination almost invariably confirms the diagnosis. In contrast to acute appendicitis, when pressure in the right lower quadrant produces tenderness because of infection, pressure in the right lower quadrant in the case of appendiceal colic only produces pain when the appendix is actively cramping. Pressure on a cramping appendix increases the intensity of the cramp. In fact, unless the patient has already undergone an abdominal examination when experiencing pain, he or she may be unaware that the problem is in the right lower quadrant. Consequently, it is essential that the patient be examined during an acute painful episode. Conversely, pressure in the right lower quadrant when the patient is not experiencing pain almost invariably produces minimal to no tenderness. Results of the physical examination of a patient with appendiceal colic will most likely be unremarkable if the patient is not experiencing pain. Because eating may trigger the discomfort, one may try feeding the patient. If pain results, not only will the results of the physical examination be positive, but the point of maximal tenderness will locate the appendix. If eating does not trigger the pain, then arrangements will have to be adjusted to examine the patient when experiencing pain, no matter what the hour.

LABORATORY

Because there is generally no inflammation or infection associated with appendiceal colic, the white blood cell count is usually unremarkable, and there is no associated fever. Occasionally, with severe colic the white count may be markedly elevated. However, once the pain abates, the count plummets toward normal.

IMAGING STUDIES

The most popular imaging studies for the appendix are of virtually no value in diagnosing appendiceal colic. Because there is usually no inflammation present, ultrasonographic examination and computed tomography will document no pathology. If an appendix is seen, it is almost invariably regarded as normal.

Most physicians will concede that a fecalith documented on the abdominal radiograph in association with right lower quadrant tenderness will be virtually diagnostic of an appendiceal etiology. Unfortunately, most fecalomas (a leading cause of appendiceal luminal obstruction) are not radiopaque. Barium GI contrast studies are the imaging choice. In my experience, nonfilling or partial filling of the appendix proves nothing. However, a meniscus sign, filling defect, and delayed emptying are important diagnostic findings. The upper GI series with small bowel follow-through is by far the most patient friendly. Because barium may percolate through the vicinity of the appendix over a considerable period of time, there may be a better chance that it will fill. It is imperative that delayed films be obtained (12–24 hours). Even if a filling defect is suggested, there is a 20% to 32% false-positive rate. I have found GI contrast studies particularly useful for very young patients, for the mentally impaired, and in patients in whom there is a classic history for appendiceal colic but the point of maximal tenderness is somewhere other than at McBurney's point. The contrast study may prove that the cecum (or the appendix) is truly at the point of maximal tenderness. However, after the first 80 patients, it was clear that with a classic history and physical examination, GI contrast studies provided relatively little useful additional information. The patient was likely to have an appendectomy regardless of a normal study outcome. The advent of laparoscopy pretty much rendered ultrasonography obsolete because gynecologic structures would be visualized during the procedure. I currently use ultrasonography only if I am seriously concerned about alternative diagnoses.

LONG-TERM SEQUELAE

The consequences of missing the diagnosis of appendiceal colic may be very significant. The pain may continue for months or even years. School absenteeism increases, grades fall, athletics deteriorate, and social activities wane. After a multitude of laboratory and imaging studies fail to establish a diagnosis, consulting physicians and even the primary practitioner are at a loss to explain the problem. The parents are repeatedly reassured that nothing is wrong. They then usually assume their child is malingering. The child senses that no one believes she is truly having pain. When weight loss becomes an issue, the possibility of a psychiatric problem arises. Unfortunately, the psychiatrist usually assumes that all organic possibilities for the pain have been ruled out.

CLINICAL EXPERIENCE

My experience with appendiceal colic includes over 400 children and young adults ranging from 2 to 19 years of age. The first 225 patients have been evaluated. Fifteen patients were lost to follow-up at 1 year following elective appendectomy. Five patients experienced no relief of pain subsequent to appendectomy (all had a negative history for enteral exacerbation of pain). At 1 year follow-up, 205 patients remained pain free (98%). The duration of pain ranged from 1 day (patient presented with obvious colic) to 8 years. The mean was 11.2 months. The mean age was 9.9 years. Although 69% of the patients were female, it is interesting to note that if patients had experienced pain for less than 1 year 65% were female, but if they had experienced pain for greater than 1 year 77% were female.

The predominance of girls seems to be related to both a reluctance to refer adolescent females to surgeons and also a reluctance of surgeons to operate on them. This is illustrated by the fact that 95 patients had 75 prior emergency room visits and 65 admissions for the purpose of evaluating abdominal pain. The sign-in diagnosis was almost always "rule out appendicitis." Seventy-five percent of these patients were female, but if they had experienced pain for greater than 1 year, 86% were female. Figure 71.1 depicts the gender distribution of the 205 successfully managed patients. Clearly, there is a remarkable group of adolescent females successfully treated by elective appendectomy. Whatever the reason, there appears to be a significant reluctance to perform an elective appendectomy on these patients. Indeed, six patients had previously undergone surgical exploration, but the appendix was not removed. A second exploration with appendectomy finally resolved the issue.

There were 466 imaging or endoscopic studies (not including abdominal radiographs) performed on these 205 successfully managed patients. None provided useful information regarding the true etiology for the abdominal pain aside from 24 GI barium studies showing filling defects (n = 19) or delayed appendiceal emptying (n = 5).

The pathologic evaluation also suggests that appendiceal colic specimens comprise an unusual group. In my experience (also supported by the literature), the incidence of fecalomas in incidental appendectomies, acute appendicitis, and perforated appendicitis is 5%, 28%, and 54%, respectively. The incidence of fecalomas in this series of 205 patients was 34%. My incidence of fibrosis in incidental appendectomies (supported by the literature) was 5%. The incidence of fibrosis in this series was 16% (<1 year of pain = 12%, >1 year of pain = 23%). The incidence of microscopic focal inflammation was 9%. Totally normal appendectomies (according to pathology and surgeon) accounted for 12%. This emphasizes the fact that a grossly normal appendix may still be responsible for pain. I would suggest that if a patient's signs and symptoms are consistent with appendiceal colic, the appendix must be removed even if it appears totally normal.

Figure 71.2 shows my experience with 205 successfully managed patients over 18 years. In 1993, I presented my accumulated data to our gastroenterology division. Until that date, all patients were elective referrals (subsequently a small group of patients was identified in the emergency room). Most of the gastroenterologists were receptive to the concept of appendiceal colic. Indeed their subsequent referrals were tagged "rule out appendiceal colic." Of 35 referrals in this group of 225 patients, 32 were rendered free of pain (3 patients were pain free postoperatively but they were lost to long-term follow-up). In my opinion, the success of the gastroenterologists is not surprising in that other causes of right lower quadrant pain had been identified. In 1995, I presented my first 82 patients for pediatric grand rounds. Subsequent referrals by community physicians increased significantly. Gender of the patients, appendiceal pathology, and success in management has not changed appreciably. Patients referred to our division for appendiceal colic have remained stable since 1995 at approximately 50 to 60 cases per year. At the present time a careful history and physical examination remain the mainstay for diagnosis. Unnecessary laboratory work and imaging studies are intentionally held to a minimum. Laparoscopic appendectomy is the preferred technique in order to thoroughly evaluate the abdomen and pelvis.

I have witnessed many patients with pain and tenderness so impressive that they were misjudged to be suffering from appendicitis. The exploration and pathologic examination showed no evidence of inflammation (negative appendectomies), yet the patients were rendered free of pain over the

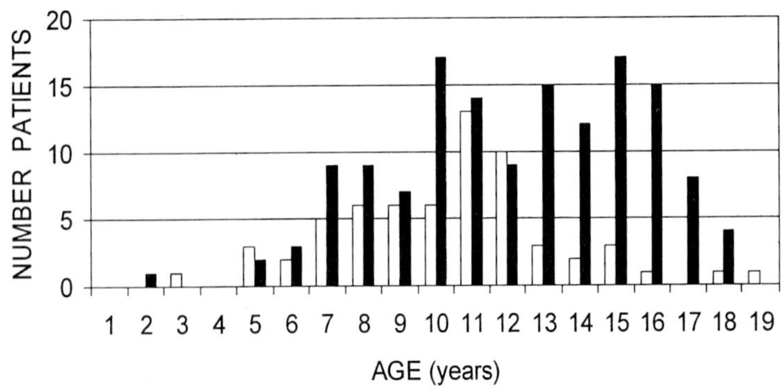

FIGURE 71.1. Successful elective appendectomies. (Light bar = male, dark bar = female.)

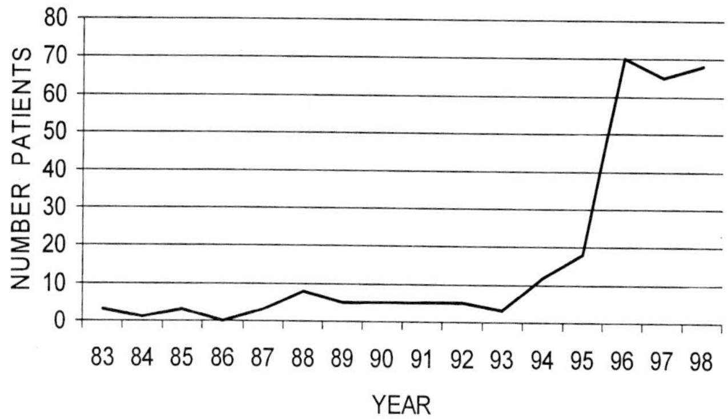

FIGURE 71.2. Successfully managed appendiceal colic.

long term. Upon chart review, at least one third of such patients actually had a long history of preceding intermittent abdominal pain. I suspect that a significant number of negative appendectomy patients are, in fact, suffering from appendiceal colic.

EDITOR'S NOTE

We have all seen children, often teenagers, with recurrent abdominal pain who undergo laparotomy or laparoscopy with incidental appendectomy despite an absence of other clinical findings to support a diagnosis of acute appendicitis but who nevertheless have complete resolution of their pain. We have also seen patients with what we believe, without a doubt, is acute appendicitis based on the history, physical examination, and our own clinical experience until that dreaded moment when the "lilly white" appendix is produced at operation for all to see. These patients also nearly always improve immediately upon removal of the appendix. The potential placebo effect of "sham" appendectomy notwithstanding, it is difficult to refute this collective, albeit anecdotal, experience that the appendix can be a source of abdominal pain without being acutely inflamed.

This continues to be a controversial view, however, and I applaud Dr. Stevenson's courage in presenting his data and discussing his experience at national meetings and in print. We are all taught as residents that the appendix produces symptoms only when acute appendicitis develops, or rarely when a chronic inflammatory process develops. For decades, standard pediatric surgical texts omitted or ignored the concepts of recurrent appendicitis and appendiceal colic, as though they could never occur. Many experienced surgeons scoff at the notion that these entities even exist. This might change over time as more clinical series are presented for discussion.

The sometimes vocal disdain for this stance is perhaps a result of the interesting history of "chronic and recurrent appendicitis." Shortly after appendectomy was first described in the late nineteenth century, it was for a time the most common surgical procedure performed in this country and some parts of Europe. The appendix was blamed for almost any abdominal complaint that had defied explanation at that time in medical history, including dyspepsia, reflux, and various types of abdominal pain. The indication for operation was often "chronic appendicitis," and for a time, general surgeons who offered the operation became quite popular—and wealthy. Over time it became clear that the operation was being performed much more often than necessary and surgeons who were proponents of the operation were then accused of quackery or fraud. Appendectomy for chronic appendicitis thus fell into disrepute and has not fully recovered to this day.

Nevertheless, it seems prudent to proceed cautiously in recommending the operation lest history repeat itself. I believe that Dr. Stevenson has contributed greatly to the care of patients with appendiceal colic by carefully compiling his astute clinical observations and proposing a rational approach to the problem. I also agree that laparoscopy has become a valuable adjunct in the care of these patients. My own approach is to recommend laparoscopy as a diagnostic tool with the aim to rule out unusual and otherwise difficult-to-diagnose pathology such as Crohn's disease, Meckel's diverticulum, endometriosis, or ovarian pathology, and to recommend incidental appendectomy if there is no evident pathology. If the patients are selected carefully, many will have relief of their pain using this approach. If they do not, at least we and the family can be assured that the complaints are being taken seriously and that everything possible is being done to find a cause and a cure for the child's pain.

–P.M.

SUGGESTED READINGS

Gorenstein A, Serour F, Katz R, et al. Appendiceal colic in children: a true clinical entity? *J Am Coll Surg* 1996;182:246–250.

Mattei P, Sola JE, Yeo CJ. Chronic and recurrent appendicitis: unusual entities often misdiagnosed. *J Am Coll Surg* 1994;178: 385–389.

Schisgall R. Appendiceal colic in childhood. The role of inspissated casts of stool within the appendix. *Ann Surg* 1980;192:687–693.

Stevenson R. Chronic right-lower-quadrant abdominal pain: is there a role for elective appendectomy? *J Pediatr Surg* 1999;34:950–954.

72

LAPAROSCOPIC APPENDECTOMY

MARJORIE J. ARCA
DONNA A. CANIANO

INDICATIONS

Since its first description by Semm in 1983, laparoscopic appendectomy has increasingly been used in managing appendicitis. Laparoscopic appendectomy should be considered in all children presenting with acute appendicitis, specifically in obese patients and adolescent girls. A laparoscopic appendectomy should be a routine part of diagnostic laparoscopy in a child with chronic abdominal pain (of >6 months duration), especially if the pain is primarily in the right lower quadrant. The laparoscopic approach is also the preferred method of performing an interval appendectomy.

TECHNICAL SUPPORT

Intravenous antibiotics are administered preoperatively. An orogastric tube is used. The patient's bladder is drained with a Foley or a red rubber catheter. The patient is placed in a supine position with a single monitor at the foot of the bed or two monitors on either side of the patient's hips. If possible, the patient's arms should be tucked; outstretched arms can interfere with the surgeon's or assistant's body position.

Usually three trocars are used: a 10- to 12-mm trocar in the umbilical position, a 5-mm trocar in the left lower quadrant, and a 5-mm trocar on the right side. The position of this last trocar should be modified according to the position of the appendix. It should be placed in such a fashion that the majority of the dissection is caudad to the trocar. For instance, in the case of a retrocecal appendix, the trocar should be placed more cephalad on the right side of the patient (Fig. 72.1).

Other options exist regarding trocar sizes and respective positions. Some surgeons find the linear cutter stapler expensive and cumbersome, opting instead for a pretied chromic loop (Fig. 72.2). A 12-mm trocar is not necessary in this instance. Other surgeons find that the 10- to 12-mm trocar is better placed in the left lower quadrant, because they feel that the postoperative pain with this incision is less than the pain of an umbilical incision. In older patients, some surgeons choose to forego the right-sided trocar and place a suprapubic one instead. Ultimately, surgeon's preference and the patient's anatomy determine the position of the trocars.

The patient is placed in a steep Trendelenberg position and the table is tilted right side up. This position allows the appendix to come into view. If the appendix looks grossly normal upon examination, a diagnostic exploration of the rest of the abdominal cavity is performed. If no other source is found, it is certainly reasonable to continue with the appendectomy.

The inflamed appendix is carefully grasped with atraumatic forceps. If it is gangrenous and necrotic, a pretied ligature can be used to manipulate the appendix to minimize the chances of intraoperative rupture. The base of the appendix is identified by following it to the cecum. How the appendix presents primarily determines whether the appendix or the mesoappendix is divided first. A window between the appendix and the mesoappendix is dissected out and an endoscopic stapler is used to control and divide the appendix and the appendiceal artery. The arterial branches may be secured using other methods, including clips, ultrasonic scalpel, or pretied suture ligatures.

Once freed, the appendix is grasped at the stapled end and brought into the largest port. The appendix and the trocar are removed together, protecting the incision from contamination. A bulky appendix should be placed in a specimen bag.

The trocar sites are closed with an absorbable suture at the fascial level, and the skin is closed with fine absorbable sutures.

M. J. Arca and **D. A. Caniano:** Departments of Clinical Surgery and Pediatrics, Ohio State University College of Medicine and Public Health; and Departments of Surgery and Pediatrics, Children's Hospital, Columbus, Ohio.

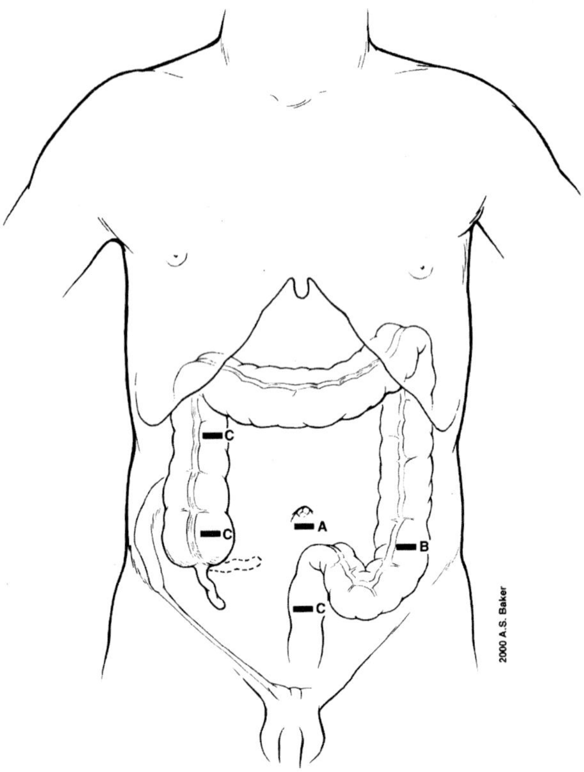

FIGURE 72.1. Trocar placement in laparoscopic appendectomy. The umbilical port (*A*) and the left lower quadrant port (*B*) are usually standard. The third port (*C*) may be placed in any of these sites, depending on the location of the appendix; right upper quadrant placement should be considered for retrocecal appendix. The mid-lower midline should be considered for older children.

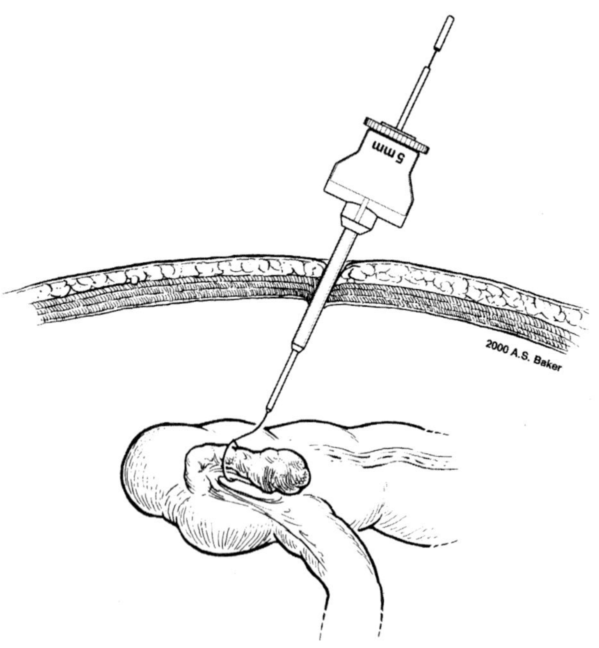

FIGURE 72.2. A commercially available pretied loop device may be placed through a 5-mm trocar site. The loop is placed circumferentially around the appendix at an area that is not necrotic. This allows manipulation of the appendix without touching the thin gangrenous area.

PITFALLS AND COMPLICATIONS

Bleeding can occur from the appendiceal stump, the mesoappendix, or the retroperitoneum during dissection. The bleeding area should be carefully irrigated and suctioned to maximize visualization, and a clip can be used to secure the bleeding. Earlier reports have described injury to the inferior epigastric vessels or even the iliac vessels. This can be prevented by using an open technique for the insertion of the first trocar and direct laparoscopic visualization when placing subsequent trocars.

Appendiceal perforation can certainly occur operatively when handling a tense, gangrenous appendix. Using a pretied loop may minimize the trauma when handling the appendix and prevent this complication. If rupture occurs, a suction/irrigator device should be used, removing the spilled pus and intestinal contents. If a fecalith falls out, this should be removed immediately because it is easily lost in the pelvis. The area of contamination should be copiously irrigated with 1 to 2 L of saline. Consideration should be given to administering extra doses of antibiotics postoperatively.

An incomplete appendectomy can occur when the appendix is not cut at its base. This leaves a stump, which can become inflamed, causing "recurrent appendicitis." It is therefore mandatory to identify the base of the cecum at the time of appendectomy.

POSTOPERATIVE CARE

The patient's incisions are infiltrated with long-acting local analgesia intraoperatively (bupivacaine). The patient is given acetaminophen in the recovery area, and if there are no contraindications, ketorolac is given. An antiemetic is often administered.

If the patient is awake and not nauseated, clear liquids are given a few hours after the operation. If this is tolerated, regular diet is initiated. Most patients are discharged the day after surgery. A few patients are discharged the same day of surgery. Patients and their parents are advised that the patient can return to "normal" activity when the patient feels comfortable with the activity in question. This usually takes 7 to 10 days. The patients are seen in the office 2 to 4 weeks after the operation for a wound check.

DISCUSSION AND CONTROVERSIES

In the pediatric population, the role of laparoscopic appendectomy has been challenged by clinicians who claim that the morbidity of appendicitis is determined by the disease process rather than the operative approach. Although it has been accepted and documented that the severity of the inflammatory process is the primary determinant of in-hospital stay and morbidity, laparoscopy is associated with decreased length of stay, better cosmesis, and earlier return to normal activity.

The literature cites two disadvantages of laparoscopy: longer operative times and a greater incidence of intraabdominal abscess formation postoperatively. The studies that cite longer operative times described operations performed in the mid-1990s. More recent descriptions of laparoscopic appendectomies cite an equivalent or shorter time compared with the standard technique, presumably reflecting the downslope of the learning curve.

A retrospective study by Horwitz et al. reported an increase in postoperative abscess formation in children who underwent laparoscopic appendectomies for gangrenous or perforated appendices. The authors postulated that a combination of factors might account for this finding: increased handling of the appendix during laparoscopy, impaired function of inflammatory cells within the peritoneal cavity, and increased bacterial entry into the lymphatics. Horwitz et al. ultimately suggested a conversion to an open procedure if a gangrenous or perforated appendix is encountered at laparoscopy. This study did not identify subgroups of gangrenous and perforated appendices within the laparoscopic or conventional groups. A perforated appendix is certainly more likely than a gangrenous one to develop a postoperative abscess. The findings of this study have not been replicated in a prospective randomized trial. Nevertheless, it should serve to make surgeons more careful in completely irrigating the peritoneal cavity during laparoscopy. Additionally, it may argue for a longer course of antibiotics in children with complicated appendicitis.

EDITOR'S NOTES

There continues to be some controversy regarding the appropriate use of laparoscopic appendectomy and whether complications such as intraabdominal abscess are more common using this approach. There are three clinical situations in which the laparoscopic approach is clearly superior: interval appendectomy; cases where there is diagnostic uncertainty, especially in teenage girls; and in patients who are very large or obese, in whom an open appendectomy incision might need to be rather large. It is in the more typical cases of appendicitis, especially in a healthy child who is thin and for whom an open appendectomy would require only a small right lower quadrant muscle-splitting incision, that the advantages of a minimally invasive approach are difficult to appreciate and perhaps harder to justify. On the other hand, unless (or until) cost issues become paramount, it seems inevitable that we as pediatric surgeons will be asked to justify why a procedure should be performed using an open technique when an acceptable minimally invasive approach is available. In the meantime, my preference is to use a standard open technique for routine cases of acute appendicitis when the patient is thin and the diagnosis seems certain.

There are many variations on the technique, the best being the one with which the surgeon is most comfortable. Port placement should be optimal for the dissection and manipulation of the appendix but should also be placed in locations that are cosmetically acceptable. The umbilicus, the low left lower quadrant, and the lateral right upper quadrant usually satisfy these requirements. Most appendices can be safely removed using three 5-mm ports, although occasionally an enlarged or friable appendix requires a 10-mm port to be removed safely. The appendiceal mesentery can be divided safely using a harmonic scalpel, clips, or linear stapler, or electrocautery of individual branches. The base of the appendix can be ligated with Vicryl endo-loops (Ethicon Endo-Surgery, Cincinnati, Ohio) or a linear stapling device. Although stapling can be somewhat quicker and arguably "cleaner," one must consider whether this outweighs the added cost and the need for at least one 12-mm port to accommodate the stapling device.

Lysis of adhesions or retroperitoneal attachments is generally straightforward to accomplish laparoscopically, making it the approach preferred by some surgeons for interval appendectomy or for dissection of a retrocecal appendix. A tense or gangrenous appendix mandates careful technique to avoid perforation and spillage of infected luminal material. In cases of diagnostic uncertainty, it is generally recommended that the appendix be removed regardless of a "normal" appearance. This allows histopathologic evaluation of the appendix, avoids future diagnostic uncertainty, and treats the rare case of appendiceal colic.

–P.M.

SUGGESTED READINGS

Blakely ML, Spurbeck WW, Lobe TE. Current status of laparoscopic appendectomy in children. *Semin Pediatr Surg* 1998;7:225–227.

Chung RS, Rowland DY, Li P, et al. A meta-analysis of randomized controlled trials of laparoscopic versus conventional appendectomy. *Am J Surg* 1999;177:250–256.

Foulds KA, Geasley SW, Maoate K. Factors that influence length of stay after appendicectomy in children. *Aust N Z J Surg* 2000;70:43–46.

Horwitz JR, Custer MD, May BH, et al. Should laparoscopic appendectomy be avoided for complicated appendicitis in children? *J Pediatr Surg* 1997;32:1601–1603.

Nguyen DB, Silen W, Hodin RA. Interval appendectomy in the laparoscopic era. *J Gastrointest Surg* 1999;3:189–193.

Semm K. Endoscopic appendectomy. *Endoscopy* 1983;15:59–64.

Stevenson RJ. Chronic right-lower-quadrant abdominal pain: is there a role for elective appendectomy? *J Pediatr Surg* 1999;34:950–954.

Stringel G, Berezin SH, Bostwick HE, et al. Laparoscopy in the management of children with chronic recurrent abdominal pain. *JSLS* 1999;3:215–219.

73

ANORECTAL MALFORMATIONS

ALBERTO PEÑA
ANDREW R. HONG

Anorectal malformation, or imperforate anus, is a class of congenital anomalies that is represented by a wide spectrum of defects. It may be relatively minor in appearance or quite severe. The most feared sequelae associated with the treatment of these defects is fecal incontinence. However, most patients do reasonably well. Roughly 75% can achieve a reasonably good degree of bowel control, provided they receive adequate treatment.

CLASSIFICATION AND TERMINOLOGY

Current terminology is based primarily on the location of the rectal fistula, which has prognostic and therapeutic implications. Terms such as *high, intermediate,* and *low* are confusing and inaccurate, and therefore should not be used.

Male Patients

Over 80% of male patients with imperforate anus have a fistulous connection between the rectum and the urinary tract. There are four main types: rectobulbar urethral fistulas, rectoprostatic urethral fistulas, recto bladder neck fistulas, and perineal fistulas, in which the rectal opening is onto the perineal skin and not to the urinary tract. Another unusual form is imperforate anus without fistula, in which the rectum ends blindly in the pelvis. Over 50% of these patients have Down's syndrome, and almost all patients with Down's syndrome and imperforate anus have imperforate anus with no fistula.

Female Patients

In females there are three main types of malformations: perineal fistulas, vestibular fistulas, and complex malformations called cloacas. In a perineal fistula, the rectum opens on the perineal skin, anterior to the anal dimple. In a vestibular fistula, the opening lies within the introitus, but outside of the hymen. A cloaca is a malformation in which the rectum, vagina, and urethra all open into a single channel, which subsequently opens onto the perineum. True rectovaginal fistulas are extremely rare. Unfortunately, this is a term that is grossly overused, and almost always inappropriately.

A. Peña and **A. R. Hong:** Departments of Surgery and Pediatrics, Albert Einstein College of Medicine, Bronx, New York; and Department of Pediatric Surgery, Schneider Children's Hospital, New Hyde Park, New York.

DIAGNOSTIC APPROACH

The initial diagnosis of imperforate anus is almost always made during the first newborn physical examination. The lack of an anal opening is fairly obvious. Occasionally, a mild perineal fistula will be missed. Two important questions must be answered in the first 24 hours of life in a newborn baby with an anorectal malformation. The first is whether a colostomy should be opened, deferring the repair of the defect until later in life, or to proceed with definitive repair during the newborn period without a protective colostomy. Physical examination, especially the perineal inspection, will provide enough clinical evidence to reach a decision about the need for a diverting colostomy in over 90% of patients. The second question is whether or not the patient has to receive urgent treatment for an associated defect that may threaten his or her life.

Physical Examination for Male Patients

The presence of a well developed midline groove between the buttocks, a prominent anal dimple, and meconium exiting through a small orifice located anterior to the sphincter in the midline of the perineum is evidence that the patient has a perineal fistula. Occasionally, one may see a prominent skin bridge over a tiny opening, with the appearance of a "bucket handle," or a midline raphe "black ribbon" of subepithelial meconium. These malformations can all be repaired via a perineal approach during the newborn period without a colostomy. On the other hand, a flat bottom, with no evidence of a perineal opening, and the presence of meconium in the urine are indications of a rectourethral fistula. Most surgeons will open a colostomy in these patients.

One should not be too hasty in ruling out a perineal fistula. It takes some time for the intraluminal pressure to increase enough to force the meconium past the pelvic musculature and out through a perineal or urinary fistula. This usually does not occur until after 16 hours of life. Unless meconium is definitely seen on the perineum or in the urine, one cannot conclude that the patient does not have a fistula before 16 to 24 hours. After this period, if the diagnosis is still in doubt, cross-table lateral radiography of the abdomen and pelvis with the infant in the prone position is indicated. The anal dimple is marked with a lead marker. This allows an estimation of the distance between the end of the dilated bowel and the skin. If the end is less than 1 cm from the skin, a primary repair can be attempted. If the distance is greater than 1 cm, we recommend that a colostomy be performed. This radiograph is necessary in less than 10% of male patients.

Physical Examination for Female Patients

The presence of a single perineal orifice at the place where the urethra is normally located in a female baby establishes the diagnosis of cloaca. All infants with cloaca require a colostomy.

In a girl with a normal urethra, the presence of a rectal orifice located within the vestibule of the female genitalia, but outside of the hymen, confirms the diagnosis of a rectovestibular fistula. In these cases, some surgeons simply dilate the fistula to allow stool to pass and alleviate the abdominal distension of the baby. Other surgeons prefer to open a colostomy and perform the repair at a later date. This is probably the safest way to treat these patients. Surgeons who are experienced in the treatment of this abnormality are now operating on these patients primarily without a protective colostomy. The decision should be made by the clinician depending on his or her experience and surrounding circumstances. This malformation is, by far, the most common defect seen in girls.

When the rectal orifice is located anterior to the center of the sphincter, but posterior to the vestibule of the genitalia in the area known as the perineal body, the diagnosis of perineal fistula is established. These babies can undergo a primary anoplasty without a protective colostomy. The absence of any of the above findings and the lack of meconium coming out through the genitalia after 16 hours of life indicate that the patient most likely has an imperforate anus without a fistula, particularly if the patient has Down's syndrome. The cross-table lateral radiograph in the prone position is used in girls in less than 5% of the cases.

A rectovaginal fistula is an *extremely rare defect*. Unfortunately, it is the most common *misdiagnosis* made on female babies born with anorectal malformations. True rectovaginal fistulas occur in less than 1% of all female patients.

Additional Workup

The waiting period of 16 to 24 hours can be used to answer the second question concerning associated defects. The higher the malformation, the more likely the chances that the patient has associated defects. As many as 90% of patients with cloacas have associated urologic defects, as do 40% of patients with vestibular fistulas. About 90% of male patients with recto–bladder neck fistulas have associated urologic defects, as do about 60% of patients with rectoprostatic fistulas and 30% of patients with rectobulbar urethral fistulas. Less than 20% of infants of either sex with perineal fistulas have urologic abnormalities. Thus, all patients must have an ultrasonographic study of the abdomen to rule out the presence of hydronephrosis.

A nasogastric tube should be passed to rule out esophageal atresia, which occurs in about 5% of all cases. The clinician should be alert for any signs of cardiac malfunction. About 10% of these patients have significant congenital cardiac malformations, such as tetralogy of Fallot, ventricular septal defects, or patent ductus arteriosus. In newborns with cloacas, abdominal ultrasonography must include the pelvis to rule out the presence of hydrocolpos or a distended bladder.

Ultrasonography of the spine is also important to rule out the presence of a tethered cord, which occurs in about 25% of all patients with anorectal malformations. This finding has important therapeutic and prognostic implications. A radiograph of the spine also must be taken. The presence of hemivertebra indicates an increased risk for associated urologic defects, and it also has negative prognostic implications for future bowel control. Anteroposterior and lateral radiographs of the sacrum must be taken. A poorly formed sacrum is associated with higher malformations and a bad prognosis. The presence of a hemisacrum or a split sacrum indicates that the patient has a mass behind the rectum. It is usually a dermoid, teratoma, lipoma, or anterior meningocele, or a mix of all or part of these.

During the diagnostic period, the baby needs intravenous fluids, administration of antibiotics, and a nasogastric tube to avert the possibilities of vomiting and aspiration.

The decision on whether to perform a primary repair or diverting colostomy should be made no later than 24 hours after birth because of the risk for colonic perforation.

TECHNICAL APPROACH

Colostomy

The ideal colostomy is created at the junction of the descending and sigmoid colon. By locating the proximal stoma at the distal descending colon, prolapse does not occur, because the colon is tethered to the lateral gutter. In addition, it assures that the distal colon will be long enough to allow the pull-through. The distal stoma, which is mobile, may prolapse, but to prevent this we recommend that the mucous fistula be made very small and that the colon be fixed to the lower abdominal wall. Both stomas should be exteriorized and completely separated. Loop colostomies are contraindicated, because they are frequently incompletely diverting, and overflow of stool into the distal limb exposes the patient to fecal contamination of the genitourinary tract. The two ends should be sufficiently separated to allow placement of an appliance around the proximal stoma without including the distal mucous fistula. Under no circumstances should the distal stoma be closed as a Hartman pouch. At the time of colostomy, one should gently irrigate the distal end with warm saline and a red rubber catheter to remove all of the meconium from the lumen. This prevents significant problems later on. A colostomy in a newborn is a delicate operation, and should be executed with meticulous care. Complications such as stenosis and prolapse are causes of significant morbidity, and must be avoided.

Hydrocolpos

If the baby has hydrocolpos, it must be drained during the initial operation. Sometimes, the vagina is so distended that it reaches the diaphragm. In this kind of giant hydrocolpos, the vagina can be easily exteriorized like a colostomy. At other times, a tense hydrocolpos is present, but the vagina is not larger than the bladder and cannot be anastomosed to the abdominal wall. In such situations, the hydrocolpos can be drained with a tube vaginostomy. An undrained hydrocolpos often causes ureterovesical obstruction and hydronephrosis. No treatment for the hydronephrosis should be considered until the hydrocolpos has been addressed. Once the vagina has been adequately drained, the hydronephrosis will most likely disappear. Even if there is no hydronephrosis, it is important to address the hydrocolpos, for an undrained vagina may become infected. This is known as pyocolpos and may lead to perforation, resulting in sepsis and possible loss of the vagina.

Anoplasty

In infants with a perineal fistula, we perform a formal anoplasty during the first several days of life. This is done without a protective colostomy. Broad-spectrum antibiotics are administered routinely. The operation uses a minimal posterior sagittal incision from the anal dimple to the rectal opening. Multiple 6-0 silk stitches are placed circumferentially around the rectal opening to allow significant, but uniform, traction. Circumferential dissection of the rectum is performed until enough length is gained and the rectum can be placed accurately within the limits of the sphincter. In male patients, one should keep in mind that the rectum and the urethra are intimately attached, and the operation should be performed with special care to avoid urethral injury. A Foley catheter should always be placed prior to anoplasty in a boy. If the baby is very sick, or significantly premature, or the anesthetic risk is extremely high, a simple cutback operation can be performed, which consists of making a posterior cut and subsequent suturing of the rectal mucosa to the skin. This allows the decompression of the rectum, although the cosmetic effect is unsatisfactory, and revision may be required later on. Interestingly, the type of initial treatment, whether dilations, a cutback, or a formal anoplasty, does not seem to affect the child's chances for bowel control. Almost all infants with this malformation have excellent bowel control, and the only patients who have fecal incontinence are those who undergo an overly aggressive operation that damages important anatomic structures necessary for bowel control.

If the operation is performed when the infant is still passing meconium, we keep the child on antibiotics and allow nothing by mouth for a minimum of 2 days, and then begin ad libitum feedings. When the operation is performed in babies who are already passing stool, full bowel preparation is necessary, and the patients are fasted for 5 days postoperatively, receiving parenteral nutrition.

Distal Colostogram

It is extremely important that the surgeon know the location of the fistula prior to the definitive repair. We perform an "augmented pressure distal colostogram" in all male patients who undergo a colostomy, and all female patients with a cloaca. The procedure is performed 2 to 4 weeks after the colostomy is opened, and it is the most valuable diagnostic study in the treatment of these patients. This study accurately shows the location of the fistula between the rectum and the genitourinary tract, the length of available colon from the colostomy to the fistula site, the distance from the rectum to the anal dimple, its relationship with the sacrum, the characteristics of the urethra in a male patient, the characteristics of the vagina in a female patient, and the presence or absence of vesicoureteral reflux. There is no other study that provides all this information in such an objective and accurate way. Eliminating this study prior to definitive repair has led to catastrophe in many of these patients.

The study should be performed by the surgeon in the fluoroscopy suite. It is begun with the patient in the supine position. An 8 French Foley catheter is introduced through the mucous fistula. The balloon is inflated with 1 to 2 mL of water. The catheter is pulled back firmly against the abdominal wall, occluding the lumen and allowing injection of contrast material under pressure. Only water-soluble contrast material should be used. *Barium is clearly con-*

traindicated. The injection is given by hand. With the patient in the supine position, the surgeon can see the length of bowel available for the pull-through. The patient is turned into the lateral position and the anal dimple is marked with a lead marker. As the injection is given, contrast material will usually stop progressing at the pubococcygeal line. This line represents the upper limit of the levator muscles. It requires a significant increase in hydrostatic pressure for the contrast material to progress beyond this point. A lack of understanding of this fact will lead to early termination of the study, and a report that the patient has a "high imperforate anus." This is why we always perform our own contrast studies. One can tell that it is levators, and not the end of the rectum, by the fact that the rectum ends in a transverse plane, as opposed to more of a cone shape. In a boy, the injection continues until the contrast material passes into the urethra. Usually the contrast material goes up into the bladder rather than toward the penis. The injection must continue until the bladder is full and the baby starts voiding. Radiographs are taken during the entire sequence, particularly during the voiding event. The surgeon can see the location of the fistula and its relationship to the bladder, bladder neck, and urethra. A distal colostogram is not necessary in patients who have vestibular fistulas, because the diagnosis is obvious just by inspection. In cloacas, this study is a little bit more complex. The contrast material usually passes into the reproductive tract, defining the vagina or frequently two hemivaginas. The contrast material usually does not go into the bladder. If necessary, one can complement the study by inserting a catheter into the perineal orifice and injecting contrast material to delineate the bladder and vagina. The goal of the study in patients with cloaca is to have images of the three crucial structures: the bladder, the vagina, and the rectum.

The information provided by the distal colostogram is extremely important. It allows the surgeon to estimate the prognosis of the patient and avoids false parental expectations. It allows for planning of the primary repair, including an estimation of the length of the operation and the best technical maneuvers applicable for each case. If the study shows the presence of a bladder neck fistula, the surgeon should know that the rectum cannot be reached posterior sagittally and a laparotomy will be necessary. If the surgeon fails to understand this important point, the result is a search for the rectum during the posterior sagittal approach, the consequences of which are frequently significant urologic injury and major morbidity. When the study shows a prostatic fistula, the surgeon knows that he or she should look for the rectum immediately below the coccyx during the posterior sagittal approach. The presence of a bulbar urethral fistula indicates that the rectum will be found easily, just deep to the levator muscles. In the case of an imperforate anus with no fistula, the surgeon will not spend time looking for the fistula site because he or she already knows that the patient has no fistula.

PRIMARY REPAIR

Male Patients

Posterior Sagittal Anorectoplasty

Patients born with a rectourethral fistula can be approached posterior sagittally. It is mandatory that a Foley catheter be placed prior to commencing the operation. The patient is placed into the prone position with the pelvis elevated. An incision is made in the midline from above the coccyx to below the anal dimple. Fine-needle tip cautery is used for the entire dissection. An electrical stimulator is used to determine the location of the sphincter mechanism. One must stay exactly in the midline, leaving an equal amount of muscle contraction on both sides of the incision. The incision is continued until the posterior wall of the rectum is located. The rectum is opened in the midline, and the sides of the walls are controlled with traction sutures. The incision is continued distally until one reaches the fistula site. The rectum is then separated from the urinary tract. This step is the most delicate part of the operation, because injury to the urinary tract can easily occur. The anterior wall of the distal rectum and the posterior wall of the urinary tract are intimately associated and there is no obvious plane of separation. We place multiple 6-0 silk mucosal stitches in a hemicircumferential manner just above the fistula to allow uniform traction on the rectum. The mucosa is incised between the silk stitches and the fistula. A submucosal dissection is performed for about 2 cm above the fistula until a more obvious plane of separation is reached. The fistula is then closed with fine long-term absorbable sutures. One should not attempt to open the urethra or see the Foley catheter. Maneuvers such as circumferential dissection around the rectum with a right-angle clamp should be avoided because the clamp may go around both the rectum and the urethra, resulting in urethral injury or even complete division of the urethra.

The dissection should be performed as close as possible to the rectal wall, while at the same time avoiding injury to it. The rectum has a characteristic pale white fascia that defines the plane of dissection. All of the extrinsic vessels of the rectum are divided and cauterized. Keeping the rectal wall intact guarantees that the intramural blood supply of the distal rectum is preserved. The dissection continues until enough rectal length has been gained so that an anastomosis between the rectum and the skin of the perineum can be created without tension. The electrical stimulator is used to determine the limits of the sphincter mechanism, and the edges are marked with silk sutures. The anterior portion of the incision is closed, and the rectum is placed within the limits of the sphincter. If the rectum is very dilated, the posterior wall should be tapered, in order to allow it to fit. The posterior edge of the levators are reapproximated behind the rectum. The posterior edge of the muscle complex is also sutured together in the midline, including a portion of the posterior rectal wall in order to anchor the rectum. Finally, the anoplasty is performed with 6-0 long-term absorbable sutures.

Posterior Sagittal Anorectoplasty and Laparotomy

Ten percent of all male patients with an anorectal malformation are born with a bladder neck fistula. This is the only group of patients that require a combined abdominal and posterior sagittal approach. These patients have a rather poor functional prognosis and an extremely high incidence of associated defects. At the time of the main repair, the colostomy is packed to avoid contamination and a total body preparation from the costal margins inferiorly is performed. This allows the entire lower half of the child to be in the field, and access to both the perineum and abdomen as required. The operation starts posterior sagittally, dividing the sphincter mechanism and creating a path that goes from the presacral space down to the anal dimple. The sphincter reconstruction is performed using a large rubber tube as a substitute for the rectum. Under no circumstances should the surgeon search for the rectum during the posterior approach. The patient is turned, the abdomen is opened, and the rectum is identified and separated from the bladder neck. This separation is a relatively easy maneuver because the rectum and bladder do not have a common wall. The dissection is performed as close as possible to the rectal wall to avoid injury to nerves, reproductive structures, and ureters. The rectum is separated from the urinary tract, tapered when necessary, anchored to the rubber tube, and pulled down to the perineum. It may be necessary to ligate one or more branches of the inferior mesenteric vessels in order to allow mobilization of the rectum down to the perineum. Careful inspection of the vasculature is necessary to determine which vessels may be divided while still preserving the blood supply to the rectum. Once adequate length has been achieved, the rectum is pulled through, the abdomen is closed, and the anoplasty is performed.

Female Patients

Posterior Sagittal Anorectoplasty

Perineal fistulas in female patients are repaired as described for male patients. Vestibular fistulas are repaired using a limited posterior sagittal incision. All pediatric surgeons should become adept at this repair because this malformation is the most common defect seen in girls. Furthermore, when properly treated, these patients have excellent bowel control; consequently, technical errors that lead to complications are considered unacceptable.

Multiple 6-0 silk stitches are placed circumferentially in the external orifice of the fistula to allow uniform traction on the rectum. The ability to place uniform traction on the rectum facilitates the creation of a dissection plane. It should be obvious by now to the reader that this is a universal principle that applies to all of the operations performed for the repair of anorectal malformations.

A posterior sagittal incision is made, dividing the entire sphincter mechanism, remaining exactly in the midline. The posterior rectal wall is identified by its characteristic whitish fascia, and the dissection is continued between this fascia and the rectal wall (as close as possible to the rectal wall). The dissection progresses laterally on both sides, always staying in the same plane. The dissection must continue in a circumferential manner in order to finally approach the most delicate part of the operation, the separation of the distal rectum from the vagina. These two structures have a thin, common wall with no true plane of separation. A submucosal plane in the rectum must be developed for the first 2 cm or so, until eventually a full-thickness plane can be developed and separation of both structures becomes relatively easy. This part of the procedure requires a meticulous and delicate technique. Once the rectum has been separated from the vagina, a circumferential dissection is performed until enough length is obtained that allows the creation of an anastomosis of the rectum to the skin without tension. If defects are created in the posterior vaginal wall or the anterior rectal wall during the dissection, the rectum is mobilized until it can be positioned in such a manner that sutures in the rectal wall are not located adjacent to sutures in the posterior vaginal wall, which would likely lead to formation of a true rectovaginal fistula. The perineal body is reconstructed using 5-0 long-term absorbable sutures bringing together the anterior limits of the sphincter. The rectum is placed within the limits of the sphincter. The levator muscle and the posterior edge of the muscle complex are sutured together in the midline, along with the posterior wall of the rectum. The wound is closed and the anoplasty is performed as previously described.

In the extraordinary event of a real rectovaginal fistula, the technique used is the same, except that the degree of exposure and dissection is greater than for vestibular fistulas.

Posterior Sagittal Anorectovaginourethroplasty for the Treatment of Cloacas

Cloacal malformations present as a wide spectrum of defects. The surgical repair of these malformations represents one of the most significant technical challenges in pediatric surgery.

Simple cloacas usually have a common channel shorter than 2.5 cm. Most of these can probably be safely repaired by general pediatric surgeons who have had adequate training in this procedure. However, at the other end of the spectrum, some malformations reach extreme degrees of complexity. The repair of these defects requires experience and a background training in urology.

At the time of primary repair, vaginoscopy and cystoscopy are performed. The length of the common channel is measured from the tip of the endoscope to the perineal skin when the scope is positioned at the urethral orifice. When the common channel is shorter than 2.5 cm, the surgeon may assume that he will be able to repair the entire malformation without opening the abdomen. In the author's experience, the abdomen has to be opened approximately 40% of the time. When endoscopy shows that the common channel is longer than 2.5 cm, it is better to prepare the patient with a total body preparation, in order to be able to turn the patient and open the abdomen if necessary. The operation starts posterior sagittally, dividing the entire sphincter mechanism in the midline. The incision continues anteriorly, until the surgeon reaches the single perineal orifice. The common channel, which is also known as the urogenital sinus, is opened. This usually results in clear exposure of the anatomy of the malformation. For the first 14 years of the senior author's experience, the repair of a cloaca consisted of separating all three structures, the rectum, the vagina, and the urethra from each other. The separation of the vagina from the urinary tract represented the most difficult portion of this operation, and frequent complications such as urethrovaginal fistulas, vaginal strictures, and acquired vaginal atresia were seen. During the past 5 years, a new technique that has significantly simplified the entire operation has been used. This maneuver, called total urogenital mobilization, allows the vagina and the urethra to be advanced down to the perineum as a single unit, and separation of the vagina from the urethra is not necessary. The rectum is then positioned within the sphincters as previously described. It is recommended that all surgeons contemplating a cloacal repair review this technique (see Recommended Readings). It usually provides about 2 to 3 cm of length, yet the tedious separation of the vagina from the urethra is avoided. About 50% of cloacas have a common channel shorter than 2.5 cm, and will be amenable to repair using this approach alone. Once the mobilization has been accomplished, the urethral orifice is sutured immediately behind the clitoris so as to create a normal anatomic arrangement. The vaginal edges are then sutured to the labia, creating an introitus with a remarkably normal appearance. If the patient has two hemivaginas, this is the time to remove the vaginal septum. The perineal body is reconstructed as described for a rectovestibular fistula, and the rectal component of the malformation is repaired as previously described.

When dealing with longer common channels, the total urogenital mobilization is still used, but frequently additional length is still necessary. The decision-making process that follows is complex, and requires a large experience in the management of these malformations. The separation of the vagina from the urinary tract is initiated posteriorly. The patient is then turned, the abdomen is opened, and the separation of the vagina from the urinary tract is completed from above. This is the most difficult part of the operation. Caution must be observed because both ureters usually run within the common wall that separates the vagina from the urinary tract. Prior to the separation of the vagina and bladder, it is recommended that the bladder be opened and catheters passed into the ureters to allow their identification and prevent injury. The surgeon must study the characteristics of the vagina. In the event of a small or high vagina, a vaginal replacement is necessary. We prefer colon tissue, but small bowel tissue can be used if colon is not available. On the other hand, if the patient has two large hemivaginas that are located up in the pelvis, a maneuver called "vaginal switch" can be used. This involves the complete separation of one hemivagina from the urinary tract, mobilizing the other side only partially in order to preserve its blood supply. The hemiuterus is resected from the mobilized vagina while preserving the ovary, the vaginal septum is resected, and both hemivaginas are tubularized into a single unit. This maneuver frequently allows the creation of a single vagina without the use of bowel. If the patient has a very dilated rectosigmoid colon, one can fabricate a neovagina by dividing the rectum longitudinally, and using the anterior portion for the vagina (see Recommended Readings). In patients with these complex malformations, a suprapubic cystostomy tube is inserted. In patients that undergo a repair without a laparotomy, a urethral catheter is left in position for 2 weeks.

POSTOPERATIVE CARE

After Colostomy

Complications after colostomy should be avoided, and a properly performed procedure is the first step in accomplishing this goal. In the newborn, broad-spectrum antibiotics are usually continued for 3 to 5 days. Once the colostomy is productive, the child is allowed to feed. A stoma therapist may teach the parents how to take care of the colostomy site. The mucous fistula is usually left exposed. If prolapse occurs, it is because the colostomy was opened in a mobile part of the colon. This can be prevented by fixing the mobile colonic segment to the inside of the anterior abdominal wall.

After Posterior Sagittal Anorectoplasty

Recovery after posterior sagittal anorectoplasty is usually rapid. Children appear to have surprisingly little pain. Patients can eat the same day of surgery. Broad-spectrum intravenous antibiotics are continued for 48 hours. The patient is then discharged, with a Foley catheter in place. For boys, the Foley catheter can usually come out 5 to 7 days after surgery. Neurogenic bladder and urinary retention in male patients should not occur and are almost uniformly due to poor surgical technique. Occasionally, the

Foley catheter accidentally comes out before the recommended time. If this occurs, we do not replace the catheter, since the overwhelming majority of patients are able to urinate, and the potential for injury during recatheterization is significant.

Anal Dilations

Two weeks after surgery, the anus is calibrated by the surgeon in the office. Hegar dilators are gently passed until mild resistance is noted. The infant should not have significant discomfort. This is the size that is used to begin the dilations. The parents are then taught by the surgeon how to dilate the anus. The dilator is gently passed through the anus into the rectum, and held in place for 30 seconds. The dilator is removed, and then passed again. The anus must be dilated twice per day. Every week the size is increased until the appropriate size for the patient's age is reached. A newborn baby will take a no. 12 Hegar dilator, a 1-year-old child takes a no. 15, a preschool child a no. 16, and older patients a no. 17. The dilation process must not be interrupted, or there is a high likelihood that a stricture will develop. Once the desired size is reached, the frequency of dilations is tapered to once a day for a month, then every other day for another month, to twice a week for a month, and once a week for another month. The colostomy can be closed anytime after the desired size has been reached.

Colostomy Closure

Colostomy closure is a standard, general surgical procedure. After the colostomy is closed, the patients develop multiple bowel movements that usually produce severe perianal excoriations. It may take some time for this to heal. If possible, the patient should receive a constipating diet, which helps decrease the number of bowel movements. Different creams and ointments are available that attempt to create a barrier between the skin and the stool, usually with variable success. The best treatment for the severe diaper rash is to avoid prolonged contact between the stool and the skin. It is helpful to avoid a diaper as much as possible. Instead, the parents are instructed to wash the perineum with mild soap and water every time stool appears. Soon after the colostomy closure, the number of bowel movements decreases, and the patients frequently develop constipation. Parents should be forewarned of this probability, so that they are alert for this change and are ready to treat it.

FOLLOW-UP

Constipation

Constipation is the most common sequela in patients with anorectal malformations. It is more severe in the benign group of malformations. The more complex malformations have a poorer prognosis in terms of bowel control, but lower chances for constipation. It is extremely important that constipation be treated aggressively. Constipated patients should understand that treatment is mandatory, and that prolonged use of laxatives is not contraindicated. Complications from prolonged constipation include soiling, overflow pseudoincontinence, and megarectum. Megarectum, in turn, provokes more constipation, and this provokes more megarectum, creating a vicious cycle. In order to avoid this, after the colostomy has been closed, the child must empty his or her rectum every day. This is achieved by consuming a high-fiber diet and laxatives if necessary, tailoring the dose to each individual patient.

Seventy-five percent of all patients with anorectal malformations enjoy voluntary bowel movements by the age of 3 when properly treated. However, about half of them still soil their underwear intermittently. This is usually related to the presence of constipation and can be avoided most of the time by adequate treatment of the constipation. If the soiling becomes significant, the patient should undergo bowel management.

Fecal Incontinence and Bowel Management

Globally, in the authors' series, 25% of all patients with anorectal malformations suffer from fecal incontinence. However, these patients can remain artificially completely clean without diapers 24 hours per day. We have developed a bowel management program that allows these patients to achieve that goal. Surgeons who operate on patients with anorectal malformations are morally obligated to follow and care for them after their operation. Consequently, one should have a good grasp of the concepts of bowel management, and be able to offer it to those patients that require it. It is necessary that one understand that the program is much more involved than just administering an enema every day. The program is tailored to the individual patient, and the volume and concentration of salt water enemas is manipulated until the colon remains clean for a total day. Prior to initiating the program, a contrast enema is obtained that shows the characteristics of the colon and allows an estimation of the volume of the enema that the patient will need. Parents are taught how to give the enema without causing significant discomfort to the child, and then a daily radiograph of the abdomen is taken to evaluate the results of the previous day's enema. Changes are made in concentration and volume until the colon is clean. A difficult concept for most surgeons to understand is that patients can be fecally incontinent and yet still have a tendency toward constipation. These patients typically still have their entire colon, and often have a megarectum. Most of these patients require large-volume enemas. Other patients have lost their distal colon, usually from some technical mishap during the operative repair. These patients are more difficult to successfully manage, because they have a hypermotile colon without a distal reservoir. Medication and diet are used to induce constipation. Any foods that have a laxative effect are avoided, and usually small-volume enemas are required.

Once it is demonstrated that the bowel management has been successful, the patient can be offered a procedure called a continent appendicostomy, or the Malone procedure. A small stoma is created in the deepest portion of the umbilicus, using the tip of the appendix. This allows the enemas to be given in an anterograde fashion. The cecum is plicated around the appendix to create a one-way valve that prevents stool from leaking back through the umbilicus. This operation is usually recommended when the patient wants to become more independent, for it allows the patient to administer the enema himself or herself without parental assistance. The Malone procedure should not be performed without demonstrating that bowel management has been successful. After all, the Malone procedure is just another way to administer an enema, and if the enema does not work through the rectum, it probably will not work through the umbilicus.

Urinary Incontinence

Boys with imperforate anus enjoy urinary control 99% of the time. An occasional patient with a myelomeningocele or a severe sacral abnormality may have urinary incontinence. We found that urinary incontinence in male patients, except in the above circumstances, is almost always due to iatrogenic problems.

On the other hand, female patients represent a completely different situation, particularly those who are born with cloacas. Approximately 56% of all patients with a cloaca who were treated by us have normal urinary control. Another 24% remain dry with intermittent catheterization and about 20% require a form of continent diversion.

Patients for Life

The management of patients with anorectal malformations is complex and requires an understanding of the multiple problems that these children have. Although it is extremely important for the surgeon to be able perform the operations without causing injury, technical mastery is clearly not sufficient. It is mandatory that the surgeon be able to manage the significant postoperative sequelae that many of these patients have. These are patients for life.

SUGGESTED READINGS

Levitt MA, Soffer SZ, Peña A. Continent appendicostomy in the bowel management of fecal incontinent children. *J Pediatr Surg* 1997;32:1630–1633.

Peña A. *Atlas of surgical management of anorectal malformations.* New York: Springer-Verlag, 1989:25–47.

Peña A. The surgical management of persistent cloacas. Results in 54 patients treated with the posterior sagittal approach. *J Pediatr Surg* 1989;24:590–598.

Peña A. Total urogenital mobilization—an easier way to repair cloacas. *J Pediatr Surg* 1997;32:263–268.

Peña A, Guardino K, Tovilla JM, et al. Bowel management for fecal incontinence in patients with anorectal malformations. *J Pediatr Surg* 1998;33:133–137.

Surgical Directives: Pediatric Surgery, edited by Peter Mattei. Lippincott Williams & Wilkins, Philadelphia © 2002

74

THE SURGICAL MANAGEMENT OF FECAL INCONTINENCE

H. WARNER WEBB
MICHAEL ERHARD

Fecal incontinence is a normal and expected fact of life in the infant and preschool child. After that age, however, the inability to control bowel movements becomes an increasing detriment to social, educational, and eventually vocational progress. Fecal incontinence may be functional or behavioral in origin and in these situations the term *encopresis* is used. Pediatric surgeons may be called upon to evaluate and manage such patients because of the frequent association of fecal retention and impaction and a suspicion of Hirschsprung's disease. Patients with Hirschsprung's disease, however, usually do not have soiling but do have longstanding histories of difficult or infrequent passage of stools. This may be accompanied by abdominal distension. The onset of functional encopresis is usually at a later stage of childhood, frequently after normal continence has already been established. On examination, children with encopresis have copious stool down to the anal level. This is an uncommon finding in Hirschsprung's disease. Children with encopresis frequently have other behavioral or neuropsychologic problems such as hyperactivity/attention deficit disorder or dyslexia. Encopresis is much more common in boys than girls. Conservative management of this disorder must focus on the associated behavioral aspects, and include training that takes advantage of the gastrocolic reflex. Family stress must be defused, and positive reinforcement applied. Ongoing family discord and inappropriate punishment may well perpetuate, or even cause, encopresis.

Fecal incontinence of organic origin may be the result of congenital abnormalities or conditions resulting in fecal incontinence acquired later in life. The most common congenital anomalies are spina bifida and myelodysplasia. Others in this group are children with high-level imperforate anus. Sometimes children are incontinent following surgical procedures, specifically for treatment of Hirschsprung's disease. Severe cerebral palsy also may be accompanied by fecal incontinence. Acquired fecal incontinence can be the result of either direct trauma to the rectum or perineal sphincter mechanisms, or secondary to neurologic injury to the spinal cord or sacral nerve roots. Naturally, treatment of the underlying clinical condition is of top priority, although fecal incontinence is a major hurdle in further rehabilitation.

Historically, the treatment of fecal incontinence has been nonsurgical. Sometimes, in extreme circumstances, a permanent diverting colostomy has been used as a last resort. This still remains a good option in those patients in whom all other measures have failed. First described in 1952, dynamic graciloplasty has been a reasonable solution for incontinence due to direct trauma to a well innervated anorectum.

MANAGEMENT

Nonsurgical measures for treating fecal incontinence include diet manipulation, stool softeners, laxatives, digital evacuation, and enemas. These measures, although effective to some degree, may not be a satisfactory answer for more intractable cases. Retrograde enemas are difficult for a disabled individual to administer, and retention of the enema is poor in those with neurologic deficits. Special enema catheters have helped to eliminate some of these hurdles but still may not offer a good solution for patient independence.

In 1991, Malone and his associates first described the use of the appendix as a conduit for the administration of antegrade colonic enemas. This practical concept overcomes the inherent disadvantages of retrograde enemas. The procedure as originally described consists of detaching the appendix from the cecum while retaining a small cecal cuff. It is then reversed 180 degrees on its pedicle, and the appendiceal tip is reanastomosed to the cecum, through a taenia, in a nonrefluxing manner. The cecal cuff is then brought out as a stoma in the right lower quadrant. It is now appar-

H. W. Webb: Department of Surgery, University of Florida; and Department of Children's Surgical Services, Wolfson Children's Hospital, Jacksonville, Florida.

M. Erhard: Department of Pediatric Urology, Nemours Children's Clinic; and Department of Urology, Mayo Medical School, Jacksonville, Florida.

ent that detachment with reversal is not necessary to achieve a nonrefluxing stoma. A simpler orthotopic appendicostomy consistently results in a continent stoma and decreases the complexity of the procedure. As long as the appendix is of normal length and caliber, it is generally not necessary to perform any additional nonrefluxing maneuvers at the appendicocecal junction.

In selected cases, an orthotopic appendicostomy can be constructed using minimally invasive laparoscopic techniques. A minimum of two ports is required: one umbilical port and one working port in the right lower quadrant at the site of the proposed stoma. The appendix is grasped through the working port and delivered to the skin for stomal construction. If the appendix is not readily accessible or cannot be mobilized through a single port, then an additional working port in the left lower quadrant may be required.

In construction of the stoma, the appendiceal tip is amputated, spatulated, and anastomosed to the skin in a noncircular fashion. Our preference is to use a V-shaped skin flap sutured into the spatulated appendiceal tip. We prefer placement of the stoma in the right lower quadrant low enough to be covered by underwear or a swimsuit. This position allows a more natural lie of the appendix, and prevents angulation.

One unfortunate complication we have experienced has been a volvulus of the right colon with the appendicostomy as the axis of the volvulus. For this reason we now look more closely at the anatomy of cecal attachment and, if necessary, carefully attach the cecum to the abdominal wall for stabilization.

Tougher technical problems arise when the appendix is absent or has been compromised by previous inflammation. Also, the appendix may have been used in the previous construction of a Mitrofanoff catheterizable urinary stoma. In these situations a neoappendix can be constructed from a short segment of ileum. We primarily use the technique described by Monti et al. A 2.5-cm (exact) segment of ileum is isolated, incised longitudinally on one side close to its mesentery, and then resutured transversely creating a tubular conduit that measures some 7 or 8 cm in length. The length of the original segment is the circumference of the tube and the circumference of the original ileal segment determines the length of the new conduit. In most situations this tube is of sufficient length to serve as a neoappendix, which is then attached in a nonrefluxing manner to a cecal taenia and the opposite end brought to the skin level for the stoma. The nonrefluxing anastomosis is created by developing a 2- to 3-cm tunnel longitudinally through the anterior cecal taenia. In some instances, such as in markedly obese patients, a longer tube can be constructed using a 4- to 5-cm segment of ileum. In these cases the ileal segment is partially divided down to the mesentery at the halfway point, creating two contiguous equal 2- to 2.5-cm segments based on one mesentery. Contralateral opposing incisions at the paramesenteric level allows unfurling of the segments in opposite directions. When tubularized, this creates a stomal limb approximately 15 cm in length. The mesentery is attached at the midpoint of the tube, which gives several centimeters of clearance at each end for reimplantation and stoma creation. Alternatively, two separate 2.5-cm ileal segments may be needed to create two 7-cm tubes, which when anastomosed together form a 14-cm conduit. We prefer the former method in which the two segments are not disconnected and are based on one mesentery. When carefully and meticulously constructed, these conduits should be easy to catheterize, and will remain continent.

Because fecal and urinary incontinence tend to occur together we strongly advocate performing the antegrade colonic enema (ACE) procedure concomitantly with any needed urologic procedure. If a Mitrofanoff stoma is planned, we feel it is best to leave the appendix in its orthotopic position for the ACE, constructing the urinary conduit from the ileum as previously described.

POSTOPERATIVE CARE

Regardless of which appendicostomy method is used, a stent is left indwelling for as long as 4 weeks. This allows complete maturation of the stoma, as indicated by healing of the mucosal–skin junction. The indwelling catheter is used for antegrade enema irrigations early postoperatively once normal intestinal activity has returned. After complete healing of the stoma, the stent is removed and the technique of catheterization is demonstrated to the patient or caregiver. We recommend that the irrigation program be performed every 3 days, although some variation can be made in this routine to suit patient convenience and to accommodate individual differences. The program is best scheduled for nighttime when ample time is available. In our experience the best irrigant is soapy water, although in some patients we recommend using a small phospho-soda enema prior to soapy water. This process may take from 30 to 90 minutes, depending on the patient's previous bowel capacity and motility.

Although simple in most patients, the appendicostomy procedure is more challenging in patients who are obese, or who have had extensive prior abdominal surgery. The dramatic improvement in quality of life brought about by eliminating fecal accidents well offsets the potential for complications. We have already noted the serious complication of volvulus associated with an appendicostomy. Other complications include perforation of the conduit, dehiscence of the ileal neoappendix, recurrent infection around the stoma leading to its removal, leakage from the stoma, and stricture formation making catheterization of the stoma difficult or impossible. Perforation, dehiscence, and significant infections, although serious, are fortunately uncommon. Leakage is usually minimal, but is increased with diarrhea and may in some instances require revision. Stricture formation is by far the most commonly reported complication. This most often occurs at the skin level. The V-flap stoma technique and prolonged postoperative stenting may help minimize this problem. Stomal stenosis can usually be overcome by dilatation under fluoroscopic guidance. In a few instances the stricture has required the placement of a gastrostomy button or Chait cecostomy button in order to preserve patency. We also have two patients in whom a gastrostomy button was placed as the procedure of choice because peritoneal adhesions were so severe that additional dissection and conduit construction were felt to be inadvisable. We have not used the technique of percutaneous placement under endoscopic guidance, but reports indicate a high degree of satisfaction with this procedure. We feel that it is better, if possible, to have a mucosal lined conduit that is catheterized rather than a permanent device, which would be difficult to change or replace.

There is no doubt that the appendicostomy procedure can offer a significant improvement in quality of life. The ability to access the proximal colon for enemas allows patients to have bowel elimination at the time and place of their own choosing and thereby be more involved in social and vocational activities.

SUGGESTED READINGS

Ellsworth PI, Webb HW, Crump JM, et al. The Malone antegrade colonic enema enhances the quality of life in children undergoing urological incontinence procedures. *J Urol* 1996;155:1416–1418.

Malone PS, Ransley PG, Kiely EM. Preliminary report: the antegrade continence enema. *Lancet* 1990;336:1217–1218.

Monti PR, Lara RC, Dutra MA, et al. New techniques for construction of efferent conduits based on the Mitrofanoff principle. *Urology* 1997;49:112–115.

Shandling B, Chait PG, Richards HF. Percutaneous cecostomy: a new technique in the management of fecal incontinence. *J Pediatr Surg* 1997;31:534–537.

Squire R, Kiely EM, Carr B, et al. The clinical application of the Malone antegrade colonic enema. *J Pediatr Surg* 1993;28:1012–1015.

Sugarman ID, Malone PS, Terry TR, et al. Transversely tubularized ileal segments for the Mitrofanoff or Malone antegrade colonic enema procedures: the Monti principle. *Br J Urol* 1997;81:253–256.

Webb HW, Barraza MA, Crump JM. Laparoscopic appendicostomy in the management of fecal incontinence. *J Pediatr Surg* 1997;33:457–458.

Webb HW, Barraza MA, Stevens PS, et al. Bowel dysfunction in spina bifida: an American experience with the ACE procedure. *Eur J Pediatr Surg* 1998;8:37–38.

75

PERIRECTAL ABSCESS AND FISTULA

GEORGE T. DRUGAS
WALTER PEGOLI, JR.

ABSCESS

Perianal infections and abscesses are common in infants and children. In infants under 1 year of age, boys and girls are affected equally, whereas in older children, boys are more likely to be afflicted. Staphylococcal or gram-negative enteric organisms associated with an infected diaper rash are the most common causes of superficial abscesses. The majority of anorectal suppurative disease results from infections of the anal glands. The prevailing cryptoglandular theory contends that the anal glands become obstructed, bacterial overgrowth of fecal and cutaneous flora ensues, and suppuration follows. These glands are located in the intersphincteric plane, traverse the internal sphincter, and empty into the anal crypts at the level of the dentate line. The *acute* phase of cryptoglandular infection results in formation of an abscess. If, following drainage, an infected tract persists, then the *chronic* phase of fistula-in-ano develops. Abscesses can spread either along the intersphincteric plane to the perianal space or extend through the external sphincter muscle to the ischiorectal fossa. Less frequently, the process ascends through the levator ani to the potential spaces surrounding the rectum. These more complicated infections result from enteric and anaerobic infections and are more likely to be seen with the less common causes of anorectal abscesses in children, including Crohn's disease, trauma, neoplasms, radiation, foreign bodies, human immunodeficiency virus (HIV) infection, tuberculosis, and actinomycosis.

Classification and Clinical Presentation

The classification, presentation, and treatment of anorectal abscess are dictated by the anatomic space involved by suppuration. Severe anal pain is the most frequent complaint. Fevers, chills, malaise, urinary retention, and life-threatening sepsis can occur. A tender, palpable, erythematous mass may be apparent in the perianal area or on digital examination of the rectum. There are five major types of abscesses (Fig. 75.1). *Superficial or perianal* abscess is the most common type. These abscesses develop at the anal verge as pus spreads caudally in the intersphincteric plane. Perianal abscesses are easily recognized as tender, erythematous, indurated, or fluctuant bulges adjacent to the anus. *Ischiorectal* abscesses form when suppuration extends through the external sphincter below the level of the puborectalis into the ischiorectal space. Early on, external signs of an ischiorectal abscess may be minimal. Ultimately, erythema, induration, or fluctuance develops a few centimeters from the anal verge. High fever is not uncommon. *Postanal space* abscesses result from transsphincteric extension in the posterior midline and frequently present with dull rectal pain radiating to the sacrum or coccyx. This space is difficult to examine, and unilateral or bilateral horseshoe extensions into the ischiorectal fossa are not uncommon. *Intersphincteric* abscesses arise when pus remains within the intersphincteric space. Rectal pain and focal tenderness on digital rectal examination characterize these infections. *Supralevator* abscesses are rare and form when an intersphincteric or ischiorectal abscess penetrates cephalad above the levators, lateral to the rectum, and below the peritoneal reflection.

Surgical Therapy

Once the diagnosis is established, perirectal abscesses should be treated by operative drainage. The role of antibiotics is limited unless there is extensive cellulitis, signs of systemic illness, or the patient is immunocompromised as in diabetes mellitus, leukemia, or HIV infection. Perianal and ischiorectal abscesses can usually be drained in an ambulatory setting. The child can be placed in an anterior lithotomy position, a prone jack-knife position, or a left lateral position depending on the surgeon's preference. Most children require some form of conscious sedation or deep

G. T. Drugas: Departments of Surgery and Pediatrics, University of Rochester School of Medicine; and Department of Surgery, Strong Memorial Hospital, Rochester, New York.

W. Pegoli, Jr.: Departments of Surgery and Pediatrics, University of Rochester School of Medicine and University of Rochester Medical Center, Rochester, New York.

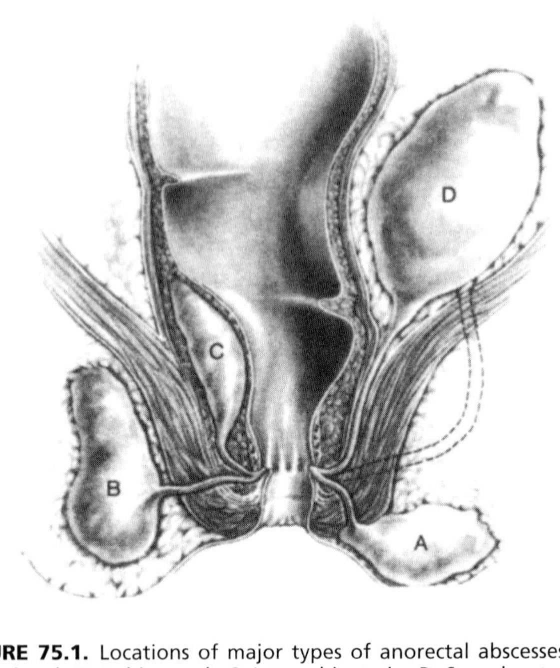

FIGURE 75.1. Locations of major types of anorectal abscesses. *A:* Perianal. *B:* Ischiorectal. *C:* Intersphincteric. *D:* Supralevator. (Reprinted from Corman M. *Colon and rectal surgery, 4th ed.* Philadelphia: Lippincott-Raven, 1998:225; with permission.)

sedation to perform the procedure. Local anesthetic agents are infiltrated in the skin overlying the abscess. A radial or cruciate incision proximate to the anus is made directly over the abscess. If a fistula develops, the resulting fistula tract is intentionally kept as short as possible. The abscess is evacuated, and loculations in the abscess cavity are disrupted digitally or with the tip of a hemostat. The wound is irrigated with saline and packed loosely with gauze. If the resultant cavity is particularly deep, the packing is removed in 24 to 48 hours and replaced as wet to dry gauze dressings twice daily. Superficial spaces may be treated with twice daily sitz baths following removal of the primary packing.

Postanal abscesses are bordered inferiorly by the external sphincter, superiorly by the levator ani, and bilaterally by the ischiorectal spaces. The anatomic limitations of the muscular boundaries often lead to delay in diagnosis because physical examination findings are frequently subtle. Diagnosis may be aided by computed tomographic (CT) imaging or careful digital examination under anesthesia. Needle aspiration during examination under anesthesia also may aid in localizing the abscess. If an internal opening is not identified on careful inspection of the anorectum, an incision is made posterior to the anus after splitting the external sphincter muscle fibers. If an opening is identified, then the abscess can be drained and a seton placed. Counterincisions can be used to drain any horseshoe extensions. Alternatively, the internal and external sphincters distal to the opening can be divided and the abscess can be drained into the distal anal canal with counterincisions placed to manage any horseshoe extensions.

Intersphincteric abscesses are frequently too painful to be examined without anesthesia. Confirmation of the diagnosis and treatment of these abscesses mandates an operating room setting with adequate anesthesia. A Hill-Ferguson retractor or similar instrument may be used to expose the area. The affected crypt is visualized and incised over the area of fluctuance. An internal sphincterotomy drains the abscess and destroys the infected crypt.

Supralevator abscesses are fortunately rare in children and may be diagnosed with CT imaging of the pelvis and occasionally can be appreciated on digital rectal examination. These abscesses may sometimes arise from a pelvic source such as diverticular disease, Crohn's disease, or pelvic inflammatory disease, in addition to the typical cryptoglandular infection. Supralevator abscesses should be drained transanally under general or spinal anesthesia in the operating room. If a pelvic source of infection is suspected, a CT scan or contrast examination of the gastrointestinal tract is appropriate for evaluation and further treatment.

FISTULA-IN-ANO

An anal fistula represents the chronic form of an anal cryptitis. The fistula is composed of the infected crypt and a tract extending to the site of previous abscess drainage. Fistulae also may develop in response to trauma, radiation, carcinoma, tuberculosis, actinomycosis, and Crohn's disease.

CLASSIFICATION AND CLINICAL PRESENTATION

The classification of fistulae parallels the classification of the abscesses from which they arise. Intersphincteric fistulae (Fig. 75.2) develop from perianal abscesses, transsphincteric fistulae (Fig. 75.3) from ischiorectal abscesses, and supralevator or extrasphincteric fistulae (Fig. 75.4) from supralevator abscesses. Suprasphincteric fistulae (Fig. 75.5) occur rarely (1%–3%) and originate in the intersphincteric plane, ascend to a supralevator location, and track between the puborectalis and levator ani muscles to terminate in the ischiorectal fossa. Occasionally, transsphincteric fistulae with supralevator extensions (Fig. 75.6) are encountered, particularly in individuals with inflammatory bowel disease. Fistulae generally present a variable time after drainage of an acute abscess. Persistent or recurrent purulent drainage from an external or internal opening is the sine qua non of a fistula-in-ano. Pain, swelling, and a palpable indurated tract may accompany the fistula. Fistulae in children generally extend radially from the external opening on the skin to the anal canal at the level of the involved crypt.

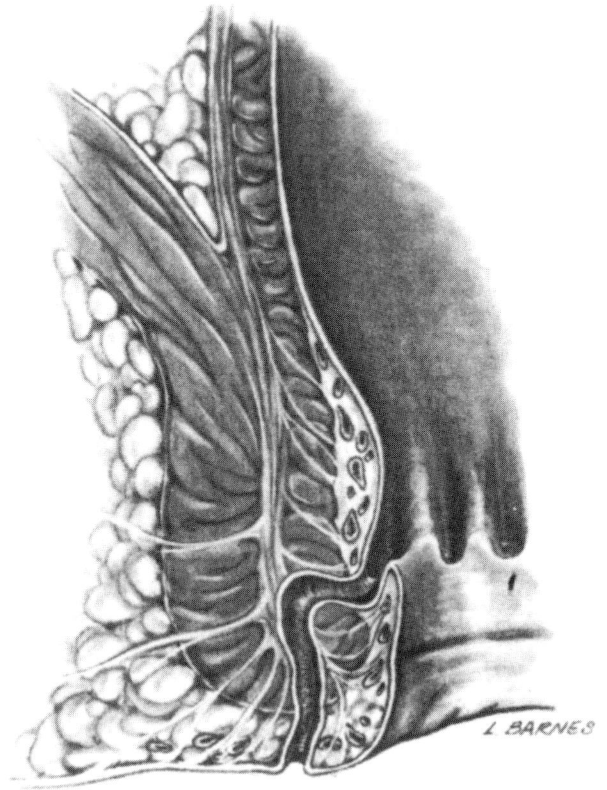

FIGURE 75.2. Intersphincteric fistula. The tract traverses the internal sphincter and the intersphincteric plane. (Reprinted from Corman ML. *Colon and rectal surgery, 4th ed.* Philadelphia: Lippincott-Raven, 1998:239; with permission.)

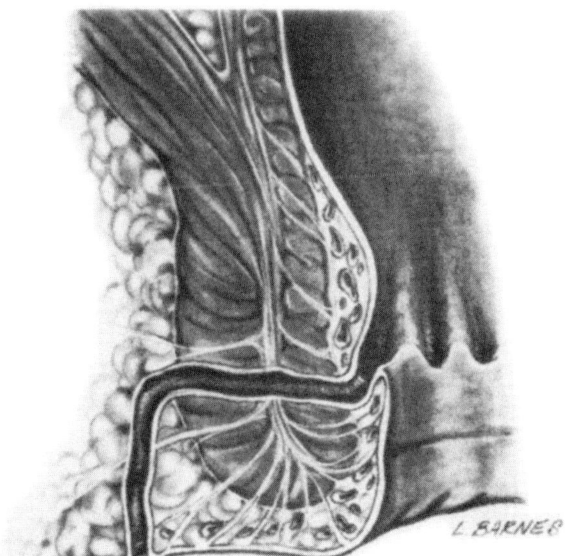

FIGURE 75.3. Transsphincteric fistula. The tract passes through the internal and external sphincters, into the ischiorectal fossa, and onto the skin. (Reprinted from Corman ML. *Colon and rectal surgery, 4th ed.* Philadelphia: Lippincott-Raven, 1998:239; with permission.)

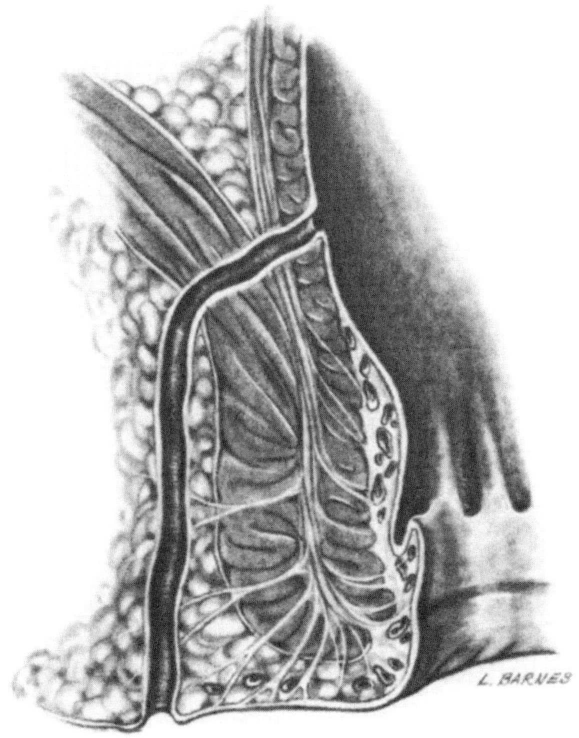

FIGURE 75.4. Extrasphincteric fistula. The internal opening of the tract is above the level of the levator ani muscles, and the tract passes to the skin outside of the external sphincter in the ischiorectal space. (Reprinted from Corman ML. *Colon and rectal surgery, 4th ed.* Philadelphia: Lippincott-Raven, 1998:240; with permission.)

Surgical Therapy

With few exceptions, the mainstay of therapy for anal fistulae is surgical. Most fistulae in children can be treated by fistulotomy. Under general anesthesia, the fistula tract is cannulated with a lacrimal duct probe and opened with electrocautery. The fistulous tract is excised with electrocautery or curettage, and the resultant wound is allowed to heal by secondary intention. Due caution should be exercised to avoid creating a false passage with forceful insertion of the probe. If the internal opening is inapparent, one can cannulate the external opening with an angiocath and inject a 1:1 mixture of hydrogen peroxide and methylene blue while looking for bubbles in the anal canal. If the fistula tract is well established with chronic granulation tissue, then a fistulotomy or fistulectomy (complete excision of the fistulous tract) can be performed over the probe. Antibiotics are unnecessary except in the setting of an immunocompromised host or when extensive cellulitis is present.

Intersphincteric and *transsphincteric* fistulae are usually amenable to fistulotomy, curettage, or cautery of the tract with healing by secondary intention. Success rates approach 95%, and continence is rarely impaired. *Supralevator* and

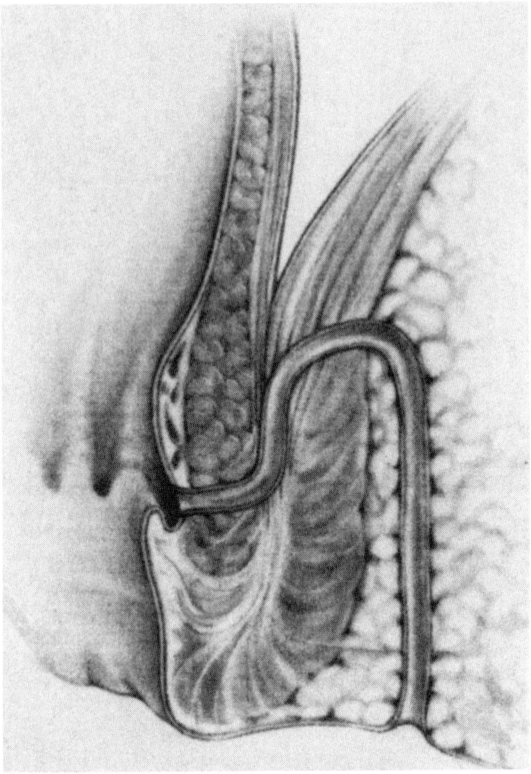

FIGURE 75.5. Suprasphincteric fistula. The tract begins in the intersphincteric plane, passes to a supralevator location, and traverses downward through the ischiorectal fossa to the skin. (Reprinted from Corman ML. *Colon and rectal surgery, 4th ed.* Philadelphia: Lippincott-Raven, 1998:240; with permission.)

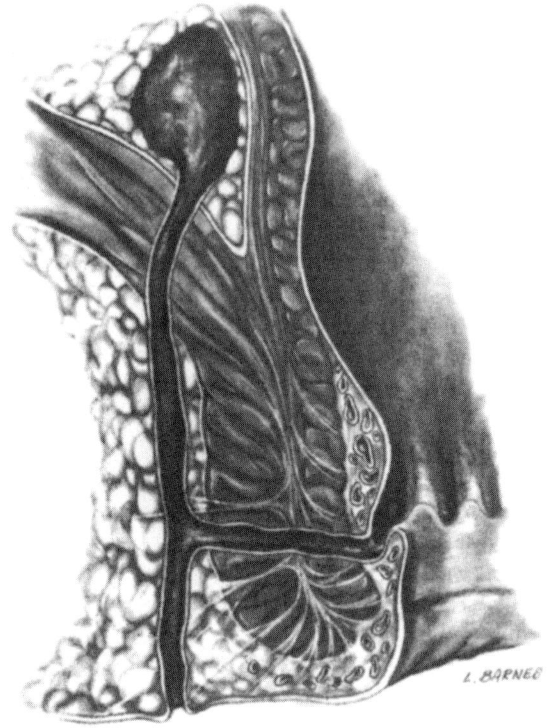

FIGURE 75.6. Transsphincteric fistula with supralevator extension. Drainage of the extension into the rectum is contraindicated. (Reprinted from Corman ML. *Colon and rectal surgery, 4th ed.* Philadelphia: Lippincott-Raven, 1998:240; with permission.)

extrasphincteric fistulae are not amenable to treatment with fistulotomy because a fistulotomy would result in division of the levator ani, leading to fecal incontinence. Fortunately, these fistulae are rare in children. These types of fistulae often develop in association with pelvic pathology (Crohn's disease, neoplasms, radiation, etc.) that must be defined and treated prior to addressing the fistula. Dynamic contrast-enhanced magnetic resonance imaging has emerged as a highly accurate diagnostic modality for characterization of these complex fistulae. Complicated fistulae should be treated either with a noncutting seton, fibrin glue injection, or primary drainage and use of an endorectal advancement flap. *Horseshoe* fistulae usually open internally at the posterior midline of the anus and extend anteriorly and laterally to the ischiorectal spaces from the postanal space. Incision and drainage are associated with high recurrence rates. Horseshoe abscesses and fistulae require incision and drainage of the postanal space and counterdrainage via separate incisions of the lateral ischiorectal extensions.

Alternative Treatments

Setons have been used in the treatment of fistulae for centuries. Setons are usually made of nonabsorbable material such as silk, silastic vascular tapes, or penrose drains. Cutting setons are placed through the fistula tract encompassing the anoderm, subcutaneous tissue, and sphincter muscle. The seton is secured tightly and allowed to cut through the muscle over time by pressure necrosis. Tightening of the seton may require several office visits to complete the process. Noncutting setons are used as adjuncts to the treatment of perianal sepsis. They are placed to prevent abscess formation until the fistula can be treated definitively. Noncutting setons may be particularly useful in perianal Crohn's disease complicated by multiple or deep fistulas.

Advancement flaps are used to treat complicated anterior fistulas, especially in women following obstetric-related trauma to the rectum. Mechanical bowel preparation is necessary prior to performing an advancement flap. Once the internal opening of the fistula tract is identified, a flap is made just beyond the internal opening by elevating rectal mucosa, submucosa, and circular muscle from the rectal wall. The internal opening is closed with an absorbable suture, and the flap is advanced beyond the internal opening and sutured to the anal canal with absorbable interrupted sutures. The external opening is enlarged and curetted to facilitate drainage away from the flap. Advancement flaps have a 70% to 80% success rate.

Fibrin glue has been used to treat fistulae with some success. In the operating room, the internal opening of the fistula must be identified. The fistula tract is curetted, and two syringes of a dual-chambered applicator are filled with thrombin and fibrinogen, respectively. The two syringes empty into a Y-connector attached to a catheter that is used to cannulate the fistula tract at the internal opening. The mixture (fibrin glue) is used to fill the fistula tract. A petrolatum gauze dressing is then applied over the external opening. Success rates of 55% to 65% are reported with fibrin sealant, with most treatment failures occurring in the first 3 months following the procedure.

Perianal Crohn's disease deserves special mention. Medical therapy with the antibiotic metronidazole, 5-aminosalicylic acid (Asacol, Proctor & Gamble, Cincinnati, Ohio), and cortisone as enemas or suppositories, and immunosuppressive agents such as azathioprine, 6-mercaptopurine, and cyclosporine have all been used to treat fistulae associated with Crohn's disease, sometimes with excellent results. The fistulae tend to recur once therapy has stopped, and the long-term effectiveness of these agents is further complicated by the intermittent nature of the disease. Infliximab (Remicade, Centocor, Malvern, Pennsylvania), a chimeric monoclonal antibody to human tumor necrosis factor-α, is the most recent promising medical advancement in the management of perianal Crohn's disease. Three parenteral doses of 5 mg/kg body weight given at 0, 2, and 6 weeks are associated with closure of the fistulae in approximately 60% of patients.

EDITOR'S NOTES

Most perianal disease in children is in the form of a perianal or superficial perirectal abscess that responds nicely to local care and drainage. Recurrent abscesses or persistent drainage suggest the presence of fistula-in-ano, which usually requires fistulotomy for definitive care. This procedure should be performed under general anesthesia in most cases, but recovery and healing are surprisingly well tolerated. Perianal abscesses are surprisingly common in infants under 6 months of age. Some infants present with tender nodules that respond to antibiotics and warm water baths, although some progress and require surgical drainage or fistulotomy. Recovery is typically uneventful, and sequelae are exceedingly rare.

Incision and drainage should be performed when there is a well-defined collection of infected fluid. Although the traditional approach was to pack the abscess cavity with gauze and then institute multiple dressing changes daily, many surgeons have found this to be extremely painful for the patient and unnecessary. Most perirectal abscesses can be simply drained and left open, with daily warm water baths and saline irrigations to maintain hygiene. The unusually large or complex abscess cavity will heal more quickly and painlessly if a small Penrose or silastic drain is placed at the time of operative drainage.

Most fistulae-in-ano are superficial to the musculature and are therefore best treated with formal fistulotomy and fistulectomy with the wound left open to heal by second intention. The rare fistula that travels deep to the sphincter complex is probably best treated with a seton to avoid injury to the musculature.

Most perianal disease in immunocompetent, otherwise healthy children respond well to standard forms of therapy such as incision and drainage, placement of drains, and fistulotomy/fistulectomy. A notable exception is perianal disease associated with Crohn's disease. In general, medical therapy directed against the Crohn's disease is the first line of therapy. Surgical management is conservative, with, at most, simple incision and drainage for pointing abscesses. More extensive procedures are frequently complicated by large, poorly healing wounds and recurrent fistulae. Supralevator abscesses can arise from affected bowel in the pelvis and therefore may respond to laparotomy and resection of the diseased segment. Perianal disease in patients with a highly localized segment of active disease elsewhere in the abdomen also sometimes responds to resection of that segment. Chronic draining sinuses and recurring fistulae are not generally considered indications for ileostomy or colostomy, because they do not consistently respond to diversion of the fecal stream; however, diversion might be considered if recurrent infectious complications such as large abscesses or sepsis occur.

–P.M.

SUGGESTED READINGS

Cintron JR, Park JJ, Orsay CP, et al. Repair of fistulas-in-ano using fibrin adhesive: long-term follow-up. *Dis Colon Rectum* 2000;43:944–949.

Corman ML. Anorectal abscess. Anal fistula. In: Corman ML, ed. *Colon and rectal surgery.* Philadelphia: Lippincott-Raven, 1998.

Festen C, van Harten H. Perianal abscess and fistula-in-ano in infants. *J Pediatr Surg* 1998;33:711–713.

Present DH, Rutgeerts P, Targan S, et al. Infliximab for the treatment of fistulas in patients with Crohn's disease. *N Engl J Med* 1999;340:1398–1405.

76

RECTAL PROLAPSE

SIGMUND H. EIN

PRIMARY RECTAL PROLAPSE

Rectal prolapse in children can be described as *primary* or *secondary* to a pull-through procedure. The *primary type* is a not uncommon presentation at a pediatric emergency department or general surgery clinic. Although I have seen this occur in newborns (usually a terminal event) and in a few older children (even into their teens), the vast majority occur in toddlers, especially at the time of toilet training, which combines with the all too common constipation to produce a handful of problems, one of which is rectal prolapse. Although it is most alarming to the parents when it first appears, it is not nearly as serious as it looks; in fact, it usually reduces spontaneously. When it does not reduce on its own, the rectal prolapse can almost always be easily reduced with steady pressure using a Vaseline gauze. I have never seen one that could not be reduced, nor have I ever seen one in which the prolapsed bowel had become necrotic.

The rare differential diagnosis that confuses the issue is a prolapsed anal, rectal, or sigmoid polyp, but to differentiate the two would be difficult to describe in words. I have seen an ileocolic intussusception actually prolapse out the rectum on a few occasions, but the history was always typical for that problem. The classic rectal prolapse is minimally symptomatic and happens suddenly.

Having reduced the rectal prolapse, I have never found taping the buttocks to be of any value in preventing it from happening again. Physical examination is always unremarkable. The pathologic abnormality for the pediatric prolapse is said to be the lack of curvature of the toddler's pelvis with possibly a loose attachment of the rectosigmoid, such that any increased intraabdominal pressure is easily transferred to the lowest exit point of the trunk in the form of a full-thickness bowel prograde prolapse through the anus.

The best way to treat this problem is to discuss the five common causes with the parents. In order of importance, these are: constipation, toilet training by having the child sit on the "potty" for too long, cystic fibrosis, paraplegia, and chronic diarrhea. Once they understand the two most common causes (by far) and take steps to treat them, the problem usually disappears. While the cause slowly comes under control, there will be more episodes of prolapse, almost always with a bowel movement (from occasionally to accompanying every bowel movement), but the parents, once they understand the problem, can quite easily deal with the prolapse. To the contrary, it is virtually impossible to get babysitters, teachers, and other caregivers to do the same, and this is what eventually prompts the family to request an operation. However, it should not be done unless the underlying cause has been successfully treated.

Even if there is not a history of chest infections or bulky stools that float, every child that has a rectal prolapse needs a sweat chloride test to rule out cystic fibrosis (CF). Much to my dismay, I have seen this disease on a few occasions present itself as a rectal prolapse in an otherwise well child. (The generation before mine always taught that the infants and children with CF who have a bad chest have a good gastrointestinal tract and vice versa.) The treatment is almost always nonoperative because this is usually a self-limiting problem. This is in contrast to children who are paralyzed and have rectal prolapse; they all require operative repair.

Operative treatment should not be considered until there has been an adequate trial of nonoperative management, which usually suffices. However, a small number of these children continue to prolapse despite adequate treatment, and the problem then becomes a major social problem for the child and his or her family. This small latter group will benefit from operative repair. All operations are relatively minor and can be performed on a same-day admit basis with a planned stay for a day or two until the patients have a normal bowel movement without the usual rectal prolapse. Only until then (and forever after) will the operation be deemed a success. I have observed or performed five different operations for this problem, each of which deserves brief description and some discussion.

I have seen sclerosing agents used with fair success, but have no personal experience with them. The second is

S. H. Ein: Department of Surgery, Division of General Surgery, Faculty of Medicine, University of Toronto; and Division of General Surgery, The Hospital for Sick Children, Toronto, Ontario, Canada.

called the Hospital for Sick Children (Great Ormond Street) or Lockhart-Mummery procedure in which a retrorectal packing is placed in the space behind the rectum and in front of the lower sacrum and coccyx. It is supposed to be left in place "until it smells" (usually 1 to 2 weeks) and then it is slowly removed over another week. It is almost always successful, because it sets up an inflammatory retrorectal reaction that scars the area, preventing the prolapse. Historically, the child has to spend all this time in the hospital, although I suspect that nowadays the entire postoperative course could be managed on an outpatient basis.

To this procedure is occasionally added the insertion of a Thiersch perianal subcutaneous wire (tied over an assistant's finger in the rectum), or the procedure can be executed *de novo*. It was always hard for me to understand the logic of placing a sphincter (which is designed to open and close) in a so-called fixed position, much like an antireflux operation, and expect it to work perfectly. However, it seems to work on many occasions, providing the child does not get impacted with stool, and the wire doesn't erode through the perianal tissues. I was always concerned about making a child incontinent if the wire severely damaged the internal sphincter, much like my concerns for injecting sclerosing agents into this area. For this reason, I tried a long-lasting dissolvable suture such as polyglycolic acid, which worked fairly well for a few months, until it dissolved. Erosion also occurs when nonabsorbable sutures of any kind (other than wire) are used. Overall, the perianal suture technique is at best only temporarily successful.

I have had the best success in the toddler age group with the Peña approach (for repair of the imperforate anus). Dr. Peña has alluded to the often-seen problem of anal prolapse (post-pull-through procedure for imperforate anus) and stated in passing that when closing the midline wound from the neoanus to the coccyx, one should grasp the tapered (or plicated) dilated pulled-through rectosigmoid and incorporate it into the midline muscle complex (levator sling) closure. Indeed, following this course has made quite a difference in the incidence of postoperative anal prolapse after imperforate anus surgery. Using this rationale and logic, and, in many ways, recreating the retrorectal fixation used in the retrorectal packing procedure from Great Ormond Street described above, the rectum, which has become dilated due to many previous rectal prolapses, is aggressively plicated using widely placed sutures to regain the normal rectal luminal caliber. This must be monitored stitch by stitch with repeated rectal examinations. Needless to say, the rectum must be washed out and prepared liberally at the time of surgery. Once the plication is completed, the Peña wound closure is performed, similarly grasping the rectum between plicating stitches and incorporating it into the muscle complex closure. The surgeon should not use nonabsorbable sutures on either suture line, and should use absorbable skin sutures.

This modification of Peña's posterior sagittal anorectoplasty should yield virtually 100% success in the toddler and younger child. However, in the older child it may fail because one cannot plicate the rectum down to normal size by this route: the hole is too deep and one cannot go wide enough. In these patients I have therefore resorted to a simple modification of another old-fashioned procedure for this situation called the Delorme procedure. This should be reserved for the older patient or rare recurrence of the modified Peña closure. The patient's legs are placed in stirrups, and the Lone-Star perianal retracting hooks (Lone Star Medical Products, Houston, Texas) are essential for good exposure. Once the anorectum is dilated, Babcock or Allis clamps are used to pull down the redundant rectum until it is quite taut, and this cobbled up rectal mucosa (and rectal wall) is sutured with big, interrupted, heavy silk sutures in a circumferential manner, so that at the end of this cobbling up, there is no more redundant rectum that can be pulled down and it feels like an anastomotic suture line about one inch up from the mucocutaneous (dentate) line. This suture line does not obstruct the rectal lumen and slowly diminishes in size in months. I have occasionally seen a small residual pseudopolyp of mucosa that caused some minor bleeding and that can be easily removed if necessary.

SECONDARY RECTAL PROLAPSE

The second category of rectal prolapse in the pediatric patient is the *prolapsed anal mucosa* after repair of the imperforate anus. This was so common after the old abdominoperineal pull-through procedure first described by Jonathan Rhoads in 1948 that at the time of closure of the colostomy a few months after the pull-through, it was often necessary to trim off some prolapsed anal mucosa. As mentioned above, this necessity has become much less common since the advent of the Peña posterior sagittal anorectoplasty, because the posterior pulled-through rectum is incorporated into the muscle complex closure. This anal prolapse is almost always one sided, which is good, because to excise a completely circular prolapse (which occurs in the rare caudal agenesis syndrome) invites the inevitable stricture.

I excise the one-sided mucosa (fortunately, it almost always needs to be done only once) whenever it becomes prominent, bleeds, or is cosmetically annoying to the parents or child. This usually occurs during infancy and only rarely in the older child. It usually requires a same-day admission with an overnight stay in the hospital. In the operating room the infant can have his or her legs taped up to an ether screen, whereas the older child will need stirrups. The prolapsed anal mucosa is grasped with a Babcock or Allis clamp and pulled out as far as possible (usually 2–3 cm), excised with electrocautery, and resewn to the skin edge with interrupted dissolvable sutures. I have had only one significant bleed from this simple procedure in 34 years.

I do not know how else to get around the problem of the rare complete circular anal mucosal prolapse other than to excise it in two stages. The alternative is to excise it completely in one stage, and if it heals with a stricture, correct this stricture with a one-sided diamond anoplasty, originally described by Kathryn Anderson. This latter anoplasty is a simple, clever operation, but we have learned several things about it. One seldom has to do more than one diamond anoplasty, although she described doing two (one on each side); the diamond must be cut bigger than desired (because it shrinks before your eyes); and there seems to be a significant number of wound dehiscences postoperatively after the children go home. Although they all eventually heal nicely, it is probably best to keep all anoplasty patients from sitting as much as possible for about 2 weeks postsurgery.

In summary, rectal prolapse is a relatively common pediatric surgical problem that rarely requires operative intervention. For primary rectal prolapse, which typically occurs in toddlers around the time of toilet training, treatment is initially nonoperative and includes treatment of underlying conditions, parental reassurance and education, and time. Operative intervention is recommended for patients in whom the rectal prolapse has failed to resolve in a reasonable amount of time or in the rare case of a symptomatic prolapse. Many operations have been described for primary rectal prolapse, including perirectal injection of sclerosants, subcutaneous wire sphincter, retrorectal packing, a modified posterior sagittal anorectoplasty (Peña) procedure, and a modified Delorme procedure. Rectal prolapse that occurs secondary to a pull-through procedure is treated with resection and reanastomosis, typically with good results, although occasionally supplemental procedures are required to prevent or treat subsequent strictures.

SUGGESTED READINGS

Anderson KD, Newman KD, Bone SJ, et al. Diamond flap anoplasty in infants and children with an intractable anal stricture. *J Pediatr Surg* 1994;29:1253–1257.

Jacobs LK, Lin YJ, Orkin BA. The best operation for rectal prolapse. *Surg Clin North Am* 1997;77:49–70.

Pearl RH, Ein SH, Churchill B. Posterior sagittal anorectoplasty for recurrent rectal prolapse. *J Pediatr Surg* 1989;24:1100–1102.

77

PILONIDAL SINUS DISEASE

STEPHEN A. ROWE
MARY E. FALLAT

It is unclear who first described pilonidal sinus disease. Credit has been given alternatively to Mayo, Anderson, and Hodges during the mid to late 1800s. Originally thought to be congenital in origin, pilonidal sinus is more likely acquired. Hair migrates through subcutaneous tissue, causing a chronically or acutely infected site involving dilated sebaceous and sweat glands. The etiology is important to understand, because it highlights the necessity of removing all hair from the cyst during definitive treatment.

Although classically described as a "cyst," pilonidal disease is perhaps better characterized as a chronically inflamed sinus tract with granulation tissue, chronic infection, and an exuberant foreign body reaction. It involves the superior aspect of the natal cleft and is always posterior to the coccyx. It most often presents in adolescence and is rarely seen after age 25 years. Although the typical patient is male, hirsute, and obese, the disease can affect anyone regardless of sex, race, or body habitus. Long periods of sitting, especially in the setting of poor hygiene and frequent movement, was felt to be a causal factor in the past ("truck drivers disease"), although most patients report no such unusual activities.

The clinical presentation is variable and the diagnosis is made by physical examination. Some present acutely with a tense, fluctuant mass that is typically exquisitely tender and sometimes spontaneously draining. The appearance is that of a typical subcutaneous abscess, involving the midline but rarely centered on the midline, with usually minimal cellulitis. Patients sometimes have fever and general malaise, but the process is more often localized. If the space between the coccyx and the anus is affected, it must be presumed that a perirectal abscess is involved, rather than a true pilonidal abscess.

Some patients present with subacute or chronic disease. Symptoms usually include pain or drainage. Subtle signs of quiescent disease include the presence of tiny midline pits, usually three to five in number, often with hairs protruding from them ("drill hairs") and sometimes associated with a slightly tender subcutaneous area of induration, representing granulation tissue. Other patients have a larger, more obvious opening lined with granulation tissue, with seropurulent drainage and hair at the base of the cavity. The hair is occasionally quite exuberant with long strands, suggesting a long-standing process.

Surgical intervention is indicated for all symptomatic patients. Some controversy remains as to how aggressive the management should be in those who are minimally symptomatic and have quiescent disease on examination. Given the morbidity of all forms of surgical intervention, most clinicians recommend patient education, good hygiene with or without hair removal, and close patient follow-up, with the goal being the avoidance of an acute infectious complication. Most clinicians also recommend surgical therapy for those who have been treated for an abscess with incision and drainage, although depending on the postdrainage appearance of the site, some patients might warrant a trial of nonoperative therapy. Treatment recommendations should be individualized and should include the needs and abilities of the patient and family.

SURGICAL MANAGEMENT

Management of pilonidal cysts depends on whether they are acutely infected at the time of presentation. There is significant controversy in the surgical literature about the best method of managing pilonidal sinus disease, because of the high incidence of recurrence and complications. This chapter first presents the way we manage pilonidal cysts, then follows with a summary of other methods outlined in the literature.

If a patient presents with an acutely infected pilonidal cyst or pilonidal abscess, we make no attempt at a definitive

S.A. Rowe: Department of Surgery, University of Louisville, Louisville, Kentucky.

M.E. Fallat: Department of Surgery, Division of Pediatric Surgery, University of Louisville; and Department of Surgery, Kosair Children's Hospital, Louisville, Kentucky.

excision during the first procedure. Initially, the abscess is drained in the operating room, and the patient is sent home for 2 to 3 weeks with normal saline or one-eighth strength Dakin's solution wet to dry dressing changes. Attempts to fully excise and then close an acutely infected pilonidal cyst invariably meet with failure. In addition to drainage, patients are given a course of antibiotics. *Staphylococcus* and *Bacteroides* species are most commonly cultured from infected pilonidal cysts, although mixed anaerobes and *Escherichia coli* also have been demonstrated. Either Unasyn (ampicillin/sulbactam, Pfizer, New York, New York) or cefuroxime are reasonable choices for antimicrobial monotherapy until all cellulitis is resolved. Because poor hygiene is often implicated in the development of pilonidal cysts, sitz baths also help during the postoperative period. The patient is hospitalized until pain can be managed with oral narcotics, wound care is taught, and all cellulitis is gone.

When the acute infection has resolved, patients undergo definitive treatment by excision and primary closure. Pilonidal cysts that present without acute infection are treated in a similar fashion. Preoperative antibiotics are given (usually cefazolin or clindamycin) and the patient is placed in the prone jackknife position. The buttocks are spread apart using wide tape and adhesive. Anesthesia can be general or spinal, depending on patient and physician preferences. An elliptical incision is made incorporating any visible sinus openings, and all affected tissue is removed down to the presacral fascia. If the cyst has not been previously incised and drained, care is taken not to enter the cyst. If the cyst is entered, the incidence of wound breakdown and infection increases considerably. Even pilonidal cysts that are not acutely infected harbor *Staphylococcus* or *Bacteroides* species 51% of the time. Following adequate excision and hemostasis, the wound is closed in multiple layers with absorbable suture. We use interrupted 00 Vicryl suture (Ethicon, Sommerville, New Jersey). The deepest layer incorporates a small amount of presacral fascia. If a lot of tension on the suture line is anticipated, the wound edges can be undermined at the fascial level prior to closure. The tape is released before placing and tying the sutures. The goal is to obliterate as much dead space as possible to avoid ensuing fluid collections and infections. Some clinicians advocate the use of closed suction drainage, but we do not routinely drain the wound. The skin is closed with monofilament interrupted vertical mattress sutures and the incision covered with a pressure dressing consisting of bacitracin ointment, sterile gauze, and a clear plastic bandage.

POSTOPERATIVE CARE

Postoperatively, two issues are paramount. First, adequate pain control must be assured. Second, the patient must limit his or her activity to avoid dehiscence of the wound, usually for at least 1 month after operation. Complications of primary closure after excision are infection (4%–13%), dehiscence (10%–20%), and uncontrolled pain (24%). Recurrence is reported to be as high as 10%. These numbers are balanced by the rapid healing of the wound that is not realized with open techniques. If a patient's wound dehisces or becomes infected, the treatment is to return to open dressing changes. Following complete wound healing, the patient should be instructed to use a depilatory monthly to help prevent future recurrences.

ALTERNATIVE APPROACHES

Because of the high recurrence and complication rate, many different approaches are advocated for treatment of pilonidal sinus disease. These approaches range from techniques less invasive than primary excision and closure to extensive operations involving musculocutaneous flap transposition.

Minimally invasive methods to treat pilonidal cysts take three basic approaches: (a) conservative treatment emphasizing hygiene and hair control, (b) open treatment of the wound, and (c) sclerosing the cyst by chemical or electricity.

Armstrong and Barcia reported a series of patients with pilonidal cyst disease who were managed by natal cleft shaving and improved hygiene. Drainage was only undertaken in a limited fashion in the event of acute abscess. They reported good results, but at a cost of prolonged hospital stay.

Open treatment of pilonidal sinus disease remains a popular approach. Marsupialization of the sinus, in which the edge of the cyst is approximated to the skin edge, continues to be performed with good results. Other open approaches that give good resolution are incision and curettage with removal of all chronically inflamed tissue, and excision with healing by secondary intention. There is disagreement whether the entire cyst needs to be excised, but several series using limited curettage demonstrated successful treatment without complete excision. Open approaches have the advantages of avoiding some of the postoperative pain and infection. However, wound healing is significantly delayed, and the patients must perform daily dressing changes.

Other efforts to minimize invasive treatment have involved attempts to sclerose the cyst cavity. Shafik describes a technique in which the cyst is electrocauterized under local anesthesia in the outpatient setting. Fifteen of eighteen patients were successfully treated. Schneider and Kockerling describe sclerotherapy of the cyst with phenol injections. Sixty percent of patients treated in this manner achieved resolution of their cysts.

Other surgeons have gone in the other direction, developing more extensive operations to treat pilonidal cysts. These techniques involve flap creation to decrease wound tension or to remove the incision from the midline.

Two of the simpler flap techniques are V-Y advancement flap and the rhomboid or Limberg flap. In both techniques, the cyst is entirely excised prior to closure. Advocates of these techniques cite decreased postoperative pain and minimal recurrences as the major advantages. V-Y plasty in particular involves minimal dissection. These techniques may be useful in the treatment of complex or recurrent pilonidal cysts.

Another popular flap technique is the Karydakis flap. This technique involves complete excision of the cyst through an eccentric elliptical incision. A thick flap is raised medially prior to closure. The resulting suture line is moved from the midline, decreasing recurrence. A recent series of 141 patients treated by the Karydakis procedure had only a 4% recurrence rate at 18 months. Proponents of this procedure feel that it not only removes the cyst, but also the factors leading to future sinus formation.

For recalcitrant disease, more extensive procedures have been described. Rosen and Davidson published a series of five patients who had chronic pilonidal disease for as long as 20 years. These patients were treated by excision and closure with gluteus maximus rotation flaps. This procedure resulted in cure for all patients. Follow-up was up to 40 months. The investigators concluded that this procedure is a good option for those patients who have repeatedly failed more conservative approaches.

Pilonidal disease remains a controversial subject, with many opinions on the best course of management. The method of primary excision and closure described above provides excellent results. However, knowledge of the breadth of procedures available may help in treating the recurrent or complicated patient.

SUGGESTED READINGS

Armstrong JH, Barcia PJ. Pilonidal sinus disease: the conservative approach. *Arch Surg* 1994;129:914–918.

Hyppolita da Silva J. Pilonidal cyst: cause and treatment. *Dis Colon Rect* 2000;43:1146–1156.

Khaira HS, Brown JH. Excision and primary suture of pilonidal sinus. *Ann R Coll Surg Engl* 1995;77:242–244.

Kitchen PRB. Pilonidal sinus: experience with the Karydakis flap. *Br J Surg* 1996;83:1452–1455.

Sondenaa K, Nesvik I, Andersen E, et al. Bacteriology and complications of chronic pilonidal sinus treated with excision and primary suture. *Int J Colorect Dis* 1995;10:161–166.

Surrell JA. Pilonidal disease. *Surg Clin North Am* 1994;74:1309–1315.

SECTION

VIII

THORAX AND MEDIASTINUM

78

PATENT DUCTUS ARTERIOSUS

JULIE R. GLASSON
SCOTT E. LANGENBURG

> As these two vessels are situated a little distance apart, their communication is effected by means of a third smaller one which forms a junction with each; this connecting vessel between the aorta and the vena arterialis, while all other parts of the body increase in size, not only stops growing but actually diminishes, becoming after a time completely shriveled and solidified.
>
> —Galen

The ductus arteriosus is a normal fetal structure that extends from the main or left pulmonary artery to the descending aorta near the origin of the left subclavian artery. During fetal life it diverts most of the ventricular output away from the lungs toward the lower limbs and placenta. In full-term newborns, the ductus closes within 24 to 48 hours after delivery, producing the ligamentum arteriosum. Persistent patency of the ductus may occur as an isolated lesion or may be associated with other congenital anomalies. In infants with complex congenital heart disease, pulmonary or systemic blood flow may be dependent on patency of the ductus, and decompensation occurs if the ductus closes. However, in preterm newborns without other cardiac lesions, the ductus frequently fails to close spontaneously. As a result, about 70% of preterm infants delivered before 28 weeks of gestation require either medical or surgical closure of a patent ductus arteriosus.

ANATOMY

Fetal cardiovascular development has an important impact on the configuration of the postnatal ductus arteriosus. The ductus is derived embryologically from the distal left sixth arch. In a normal fetal cardiovascular system, about 60% of the ventricular output is directed exclusively from the pulmonary artery to the aorta. Consequently, the ductus is usually equal in width to the descending aorta. It appears as a smooth extension of the pulmonary artery into the aorta. As a result, the proximal angle of the ductus is sharp, and the distal angle is obtuse. Such insertion characteristics allow the ductus to run almost parallel to the isthmus as it approaches the aorta.

Typically the ductus arises as a continuation of the main pulmonary artery or from the proximal portion of the left pulmonary artery. It continues on to connect to the descending aorta just distal to the origin of the left subclavian artery. The ductus, then, defines the distal end of the aortic isthmus. While the aortic end of the ductus is extrapericardial, the pulmonary end of the ductus is intrapericardial. The left recurrent laryngeal nerve passes around and under the aortic end of the ductus, just outside the pericardial reflection.

These sites of anatomic connection to the great vessels are usually consistent, especially in infants with an otherwise normal cardiovascular system. However, some anatomic variability does exist. The ductus is almost always a left-sided structure, but both right-sided and bilateral ductus can occur. Such anomalies are usually associated with abnormalities of the aortic arch, such as a right-sided arch, coarctation, or interruption. Rarely, a patent ductus inserts into the arch proximal to the left subclavian artery. With this arrangement, the recurrent laryngeal nerve is found passing under the arch itself, rather than under the ductus as expected. A large ductus with the nerve beneath it can create the illusion of this anatomically atypical ductus, and can result in misidentification of anatomy at the time of operation. Perception of a ductus with the left recurrent nerve under the arch should alert the surgeon to the presence of atypical variant anatomy so that all structures can be clearly identified prior to ligation.

HISTOLOGY

The histologic structure of the ductus arteriosus is unique. The wall thickness of the ductus approaches that of the

J. R. Glasson: Department of Pediatric Surgery, Children's Hospital of Michigan, Detroit, Michigan.

S. E. Langenburg: Department of Surgery, Wayne State University; and Department of Pediatric General and Thoracic Surgery, Children's Hospital of Michigan, Detroit, Michigan.

neonatal aorta and pulmonary artery. It contains an intact internal elastic lamina, as do other vessels in the neonate. However, the ductal intima is thicker than that of the nearby pulmonary artery and aorta. Also, the media lacks significant elastic fibers and instead contains layers of muscle cells arranged in a somewhat disorganized spiral pattern. This muscle layer gives the ductus a high level of intrinsic tone during fetal life. Importantly, the spiral muscle layer is less developed in preterm infants when compared with full-term infants. This histologic characteristic contributes to the persistence of patent ductus arteriosus in premature infants.

PATHOPHYSIOLOGY

In full-term infants, closure of the ductus occurs in two phases. First, smooth muscle constriction produces functional closure of the ductal lumen within hours after birth. Second, anatomic closure of the lumen occurs over the next several days secondary to extensive neointimal thickening and loss of smooth muscle cells from the media.

The first phase, smooth muscle constriction, occurs as a result of decreased prostaglandin levels after birth. In the fetus, ductal patency is maintained by locally produced prostaglandins (PGE_2, PGI_2), a significant source of which is the placenta. These prostaglandins induce active relaxation of the ductal musculature. After birth, absence of the placenta removes an important source of prostaglandins. Also, increased pulmonary blood flow results in metabolism of the prostaglandins, thereby reducing further circulating levels. Decreased prostaglandins result in less active ductal relaxation, thereby allowing the ductus to maintain its normally high intrinsic tone. Further ductal constriction is aided by the increase in partial pressure of oxygen in the blood circulating through the ductus. The oxygen stimulates active constriction of the smooth muscle within the ductus, leading to functional closure as the thickened intima bulges into the lumen. Over the next several days to weeks, fibrosis and degeneration of the subintimal layers result in permanent closure of the ductus, forming the ligamentum arteriosum.

In preterm infants, the ductus is less likely to constrict after birth than in full-term infants. The intrinsic tone of the ductus in infants delivered after less than 28 weeks of gestation is lower than it is in full-term infants. Additionally, the premature ductus is more sensitive to the vasodilating effects of prostaglandins. Finally, immature ductal tissue is much less reactive to oxygen, and postnatal ductal closure is less likely to occur. Consequently, most infants who ultimately require surgical ligation of a patent ductus arteriosus are premature.

NATURAL HISTORY AND DIAGNOSIS

Isolated patent ductus arteriosus occurs in approximately 1 in 2,500 to 1 in 5,000 live births. The incidence increases with prematurity and low birth weight. Isolated, untreated patent ductus arteriosus is associated with a high mortality rate, approaching 30%. Congestive heart failure is the leading cause of death, with pneumonia second. Patients surviving into late childhood and adulthood may develop severe pulmonary hypertension, right heart failure, and endocarditis.

Signs and symptoms resulting from patent ductus arteriosus depend on the size of the ductus, the pulmonary vascular resistance, the age at presentation, and associated anomalies. The ultimate clinical consequences of a patent ductus arteriosus are related to the degree of left-to-right shunting. Despite the ability in preterm infants of the left ventricle to augment cardiac output (by increases in heart rate), blood-flow distribution is altered secondary to decreased diastolic pressure and vasoconstriction. Such decreased organ perfusion has important consequences in terms of feeding intolerance, necrotizing enterocolitis, and decreased renal function.

The diagnosis of patent ductus arteriosus is often made by physical examination, which reveals a hyperdynamic circulation with a hyperactive precordium and bounding peripheral pulses. A continuous murmur in the pulmonary area heard on auscultation is a classic sign. Absence of a murmur, however, especially in premature infants, cannot rule out patent ductus arteriosus. Increasing need for ventilator support should raise suspicion for patent ductus arteriosus in a premature infant.

The chest radiograph may show an enlarged ascending aorta. Two-dimensional echocardiography is the most useful test for demonstrating a patent ductus arteriosus. It is essential for identification of any associated intracardiac lesions. Also, the flow characteristics of blood within the aorta beyond the ductus can provide an estimate of shunt size. Cardiac catheterization is reserved for older patients and those with atypical findings or pulmonary hypertension.

MANAGEMENT

Indications for Surgery

In full-term infants, the likelihood of spontaneous closure of a large patent ductus arteriosus is extremely small after the first few weeks of life. Intervention to accomplish closure is indicated because of the risk for endocarditis and increased mortality if left untreated. Most full-term infants do not respond to prostaglandin inhibition, and surgical closure is usually necessary. If symptoms are present, surgery should be performed immediately. If no symptoms are present, elective closure can be planned within the first 3 months of life.

In preterm infants, early closure of a patent ductus arteriosus is beneficial in reducing shunt and increasing peripheral perfusion, and may reduce the need for ventilator support. Primary medical management with indomethacin or ibuprofen may be attempted if no contraindications exist. Contraindications include thrombocytopenia, azotemia, evidence of gut ischemia, intraventricular hemorrhage, and sepsis. Surgical closure should be performed if contraindications to pharmacologic therapy exist, or if pharmacologic therapy fails.

Preoperative Preparation

Optimization of cardiovascular and pulmonary status is important; the operation should not be performed in the face of hemodynamic instability. Blood for transfusion should be available at the bedside at the time of operation. The procedure can be performed in the neonatal intensive care unit or the operating suite. It is important to keep the infants warm in an isolette and to maintain vigilance with respect to endotracheal tube position during transport and relocation to and from the operating suite.

Surgical Technique

Robert E. Gross, who performed the first successful surgical ligation of a patent ductus arteriosus in a child in 1938, recommended division and oversewing of both ends of the ductus. Alfred Blalock, in 1946, described the triple ligation technique for treatment of patent ductus arteriosus. Currently, the ductus can be closed by either suture or clip ligation, or by division with oversewing. Ligation is used most frequently; we prefer to close the patent ductus arteriosus with a heavy braided (silk) ligature.

Our surgical approach to the patent ductus arteriosus is through a left posterolateral thoracotomy. Oxygen saturation monitors are placed on the right upper extremity (preductal) and on either lower extremity (postductal). The infant is positioned in the right lateral decubitus position on a warming device. A transverse incision is made in the skin just inferior to the tip of the left scapula. The latissimus dorsi and serratus anterior muscles are divided, and the thoracic cavity is entered through the fourth intercostal space. A rib retractor is placed and the superior portion of the left lung is gently retracted anteriorly and caudad, exposing the mediastinum. The vagus and phrenic nerves are then clearly identified, and the pleura overlying the aortic isthmus is incised longitudinally, parallel to the vagus nerve, directly over the isthmus and descending aorta.

Sharp and blunt dissection is then carefully used to expose the aortic isthmus, descending aorta, distal aortic arch, left subclavian artery, ductus arteriosus, and recurrent laryngeal nerve (which passes around the ductus). It is imperative to clearly identify all of these structures before proceeding with ligation. A gentle test ligation of the identified ductus can be performed with a forceps. Confirmation of anatomy may be made during this test by listening for disappearance of the murmur, measuring equivalent blood pressure in the arm and leg, and ensuring stable oxygen saturation in the lower extremity. Should the murmur persist, or blood pressure and oxygen saturation vary between the arm and leg, further dissection should be performed to clearly identify the ductus prior to ligation.

Once the ductus is identified, it is exposed over most of its length using a fine hemostat. The dissection can be facilitated with the use of cotton-tipped applicators. A right-angle clamp is then used to bluntly clear a circumferential space around the ductus. Dissection is begun on the inferior side of the ductus in order to avoid injury to the recurrent laryngeal nerve. The instrument is passed around the ductus, through the areolar tissue several millimeters away from the ductus in order to avoid injury to its back wall. A heavy braided suture (2-0 silk) lubricated with glycerin or mineral oil is then used to centrally ligate the patent ductus arteriosus. Care is taken in tying the suture so as not to disrupt the friable ductal tissue, which is easily torn. In the event of hemorrhage, the ductus should be carefully grasped with a forceps, because proximal and distal control are impossible to obtain. Sutures or clips are then placed at the aorta and pulmonary artery junctions. After ligation, there should be loss of the cardiac murmur and an increase in pulse pressure, usually of about 10 mm Hg.

A 12 French chest tube is placed through a separate stab incision in the chest. The ribs are approximated with interrupted 3-0 braided absorbable suture followed by a layered closure of muscle with 3-0 braided absorbable suture. The skin is closed with running subcuticular 5-0 monofilament absorbable suture. The incision is covered with adhesive tape skin closures. The chest tube is placed on water seal. In most instances, the lung expands fully and the chest tube may be removed on the first postoperative day.

COMPLICATIONS

Potential complications after ligation of a patent ductus arteriosus include residual patent ductus arteriosus, vagus or recurrent laryngeal nerve injury, trauma to the lungs both with and without pneumothorax, chylothorax from thoracic duct injury, pneumonia, wound infection, and death. Also, inadvertent ligation of the wrong structure, including the aortic isthmus or left pulmonary artery, may occur, especially if anatomic variability is present.

CONCLUSIONS

Surgical ligation of a patent ductus arteriosus is a safe procedure and can be performed with little morbidity and a mortality rate that approaches zero, even in critically ill neonates. In premature infants, the degree of prematurity and associated illnesses (such as pulmonary disease and coexistent anomalies) have a significant influence on the ultimate survival of these patients.

EDITOR'S NOTES

Surgical ligation of a patent ductus arteriosus is an operation that continues to be performed safely by pediatric general surgeons in many centers, often in the neonatal intensive care setting. The ligation itself is elegant and usually uncomplicated, although there are significant potential pitfalls. The one major complication of the procedure, namely bleeding, can be difficult to manage and can result in the death of the patient.

Indications for surgery are well established, and there is usually consensus regarding the approach to treatment. I prefer to obtain a formal cardiology assessment and a complete two-dimensional echocardiogram less than 48 hours before the operation. In the absence of a contraindication, it is reasonable to attempt to induce closure of the ductus with medical therapy. Indomethacin seems to result in a ductus that is more friable and thus perhaps more susceptible to injury at operation. Likewise, the platelet dysfunction induced by nonsteroidal antiinflammatory agents may increase the risk of surgical bleeding. I do not consider either of these to be a contraindication to a trial of indomethacin, nor would I delay surgery in a baby who has been treated recently with the drug. Given the small but potentially devastating risk for bleeding (severe cases may require the equivalent of an exchange transfusion), packed red blood cells or whole blood need to be warm and immediately available (at least 80–100 mL/kg). I agree with the authors that a postductal pulse oximeter, blood pressure cuff, or arterial line should be in place to help avoid anatomic confusion and ligation of the wrong structure. The parents should be warned about the various potential complications, including vocal cord paralysis, effusion, bleeding, errant ligation, and death.

An extrapleural approach is especially easy to use in the neonate and has several advantages. The relevant structures are all much more easily dissected and visualized, a chest tube is not required, and there may be advantages to leaving the pleural space undisturbed. The importance of a clear understanding of the anatomy cannot be overemphasized. Confirming the relationship between the ductus, the vagus nerve, and the recurrent laryngeal nerve is especially helpful, but it is still important to accurately identify all adjacent structures, including the aortic arch, the descending aorta, and the subclavian artery. The lung should be gently retracted anteriorly to expose the mediastinal structures. Some infants will not tolerate lung retraction for the entire operation, in which case the lung may need to be released and ventilated intermittently throughout the case. Once the vagus and recurrent laryngeal nerves are carefully lifted off of the aorta and ductus, dissection of the ductus itself should proceed cautiously. The alveolar tissue above and below the ductus can be dissected sharply with fine tenotomy scissors. Dissecting around and behind the ductus must proceed with great caution and patience, because this friable structure can be easily disrupted. Bleeding can be profuse and startling. A calm and careful approach, with reliable suction and precise application of forceps, usually allows one to achieve proximal and distal control of the vessel with hemoclips. Once dissected completely, at least two heavy silk ligatures should be used to ligate the ductus. Others advocate only partial dissection and application of clips to obliterate the lumen. A test ligation with confirmation that the blood pressure in the lower extremities and oxygen saturation are being maintained should eliminate the likelihood of an errant ligation. If an extrapleural approach is used, a chest tube is not necessary.

It is important to realize (and to explain to the parents) that many infants will continue to be quite ill in the immediate postoperative period. With abrupt ligation of the ductus, they become relatively fluid overloaded and require ventilatory and sometimes hemodynamic support while they undergo a diuresis and adapt to their new anatomy. The majority of patients, however, begin to improve by the third or fourth postoperative day and most eventually do well.

–P.M.

SUGGESTED READINGS

Clyman RI. Ibuprofen and patent ductus arteriosus [Letter]. *N Engl J Med* 2000;343:728–729.

Fleming WH, Sarafian LB, Kugler JD, et al. Ligation of patent ductus arteriosus in premature infants: importance of accurate anatomic definition. *Pediatrics* 1983;71:373–375.

Gross RE. *The surgery of infancy and childhood.* Philadelphia: WB Saunders, 1953:806–827.

Gross RE. *An atlas of children's surgery.* Philadelphia: WB Saunders, 1970:122–125.

Gross RE, Hubbard JP. Surgical ligation of a patent ductus arteriosus. Report of first successful case. *JAMA* 1939;112:729.

Pontius RG, Danielson GK, Noonan JA, et al. Illusions leading to surgical closure of the distal left pulmonary artery instead of the ductus arteriosus. *J Thorac Cardiovasc Surg* 1981;82:107–113.

Van Overmeire B, Smets K, Lecoutere D, et al. A comparison of ibuprofen and indomethacin for closure of patent ductus arteriosus. *N Engl J Med* 2000;343:674–681.

79

VASCULAR COMPRESSION SYNDROMES

PETER B. MANNING

Vascular compression syndromes represent a mixed bag of anomalies that share the common feature of compromise of the esophagus or airway by adjacent arterial structures, be they systemic, pulmonary, or both. Although they may share similarities in clinical presentation and methods of diagnostic evaluation, their developmental embryology and treatment strategies may be markedly different. They are most easily segregated into three main groups: vascular rings, the innominate compression syndrome, and pulmonary arterial slings. Vascular rings include a number of anatomic variations of anomalous development of the aortic arch complex, resulting in vascular structures completely encircling both the trachea and esophagus. The innominate compression syndrome refers to tracheal compression by the adjacent, developmentally normal innominate artery, a problem more likely due to tracheomalacia as its primary pathology than to vascular malformation. Pulmonary artery sling refers to anomalous origin of the left pulmonary artery from the right pulmonary artery, coursing between the trachea and esophagus to the left hilum, and often associated with important tracheal stenosis or hypoplasia.

VASCULAR RINGS

The thoracic aorta originally develops as a series of arches with bilateral symmetry (Fig. 79.1A). By the end of the second month of gestation, components of the arch complex have regressed, leaving the typical anatomy of a left aortic arch with three arch branches (innominate, left common carotid, and left subclavian) and a left-sided ductus arteriosus from the proximal left pulmonary artery to the aorta in the general vicinity of the left subclavian artery origin (Fig. 79.1B). Vascular rings can virtually all be explained by anomalous regression or persistence of different components of the bilateral aortic arch complex (Fig. 79.2).

The two most common anatomic variants of true vascular rings, occurring in nearly equal frequency, are persistent double aortic arch and right aortic arch with anomalous origin of the left subclavian artery. In the latter, the left-sided ligamentum arteriosum completes the vascular ring as it passes from the left pulmonary artery to the left subclavian artery as it emerges from its retroesophageal course (Fig. 79.3). Occasionally a true vascular ring can be seen with a right aortic arch and normal "mirror image" branching if the ligamentum attaches to the proximal descending aorta instead of its typical position on the base of the left subclavian artery. In persistent double aortic arch (Fig. 79.4), the right-sided arch component is larger in the majority of cases; thus, for most vascular rings the surgical approach will be through a left thoracotomy.

The clinical presentations of a true vascular ring are varied. Symptoms may occasionally be noted in the newborn, but more often are recognized later. Many cases have been described with no or minimal symptoms attributed to the anomaly. When symptoms occur early in life they are most commonly airway related, typically stridor. Exacerbation of breathing difficulties with feeding or during upper respiratory infections may be described. Children with double aortic arch anomalies tend to present earlier than those with right aortic arch variants. Dysphagia is uncommon in the first months of life while children are on a liquid diet. Choking or swallowing difficulties are more common in older children as the presenting complaint. Occasionally a vascular ring is discovered during evaluation of a seemingly unrelated problem. Because of the variety of presentations described and the myriad of more common problems that may lead to feeding or respiratory problems in children, a high index of suspicion must be maintained to consider vascular rings in the evaluation of these complaints.

Physical examination should include careful characterization of noisy breathing. Distal airway problems such as reactive airway disease cause expiratory wheezes or noise. The more proximal in the airway an obstruction to flow is, the earlier the stridor becomes. Laryngotracheal obstructions typically cause both inspiratory and expiratory stridor, whereas supraglottic lesions result in predominantly inspi-

P. B. Manning: Department of Surgery, University of Cincinnati School of Medicine; and Department of Pediatric Cardiothoracic Surgery, Cincinnati Children's Hospital Medical Center, Cincinnati, Ohio.

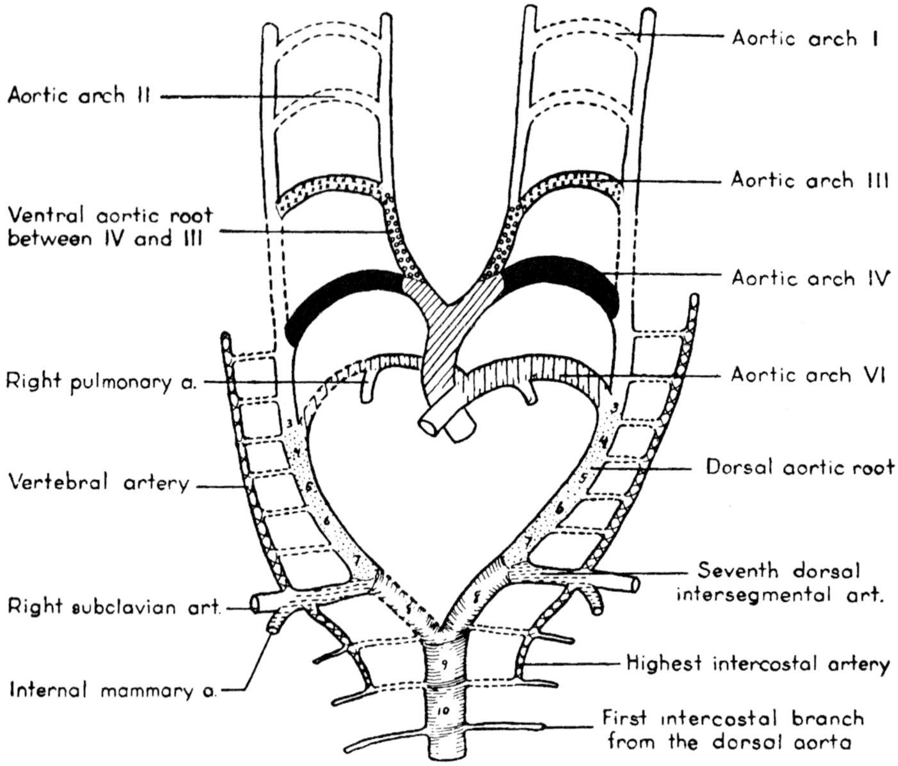

A

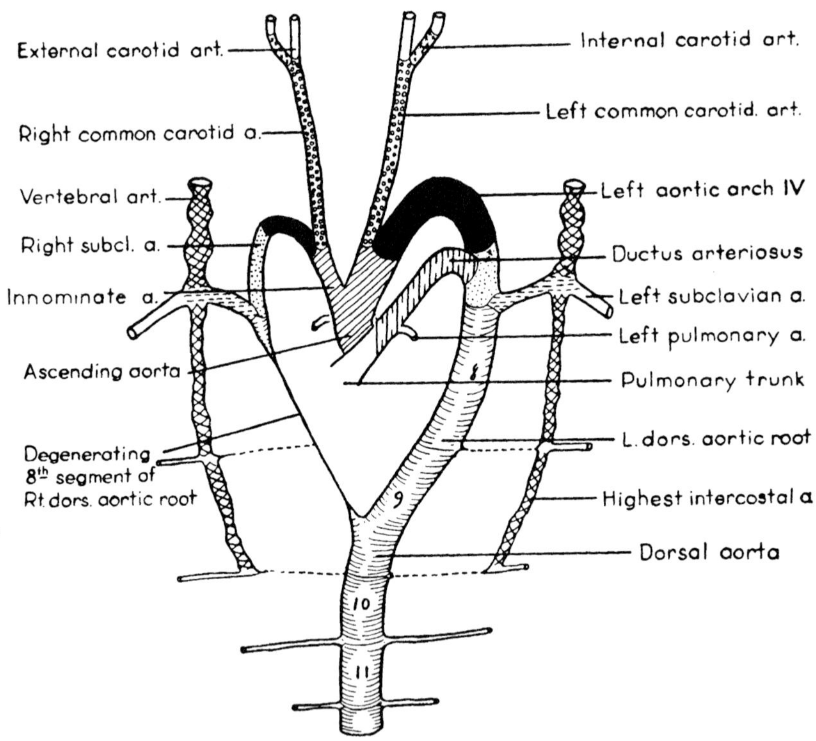

B

FIGURE 79.1. A: Schematic of the normal arch complex components in the fetus. **B:** Degeneration of the distal portion of the right arch occurring around the 17th week of gestation. (From Barry A. *Anat Rec* 1951;111:221–228, with permission.)

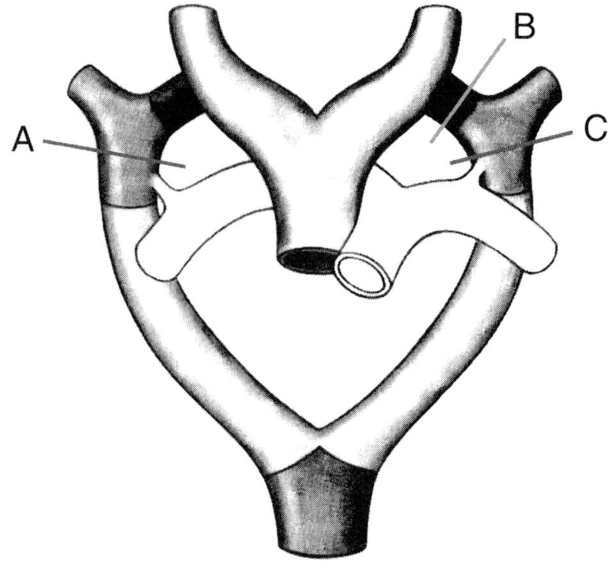

FIGURE 79.2. *A:* Site of regression of right arch in normal development. *B:* Site of regression in right aortic arch with aberrant left subclavian artery. *C:* Site of regression in right aortic arch, mirror image branching, and ligamentum to descending aorta/Kommerell's diverticulum. (Modified from Stark J, Deleval M, eds. *Surgery for congenital heart defects*, 2nd ed. Philadelphia: WB Saunders, 1994.)

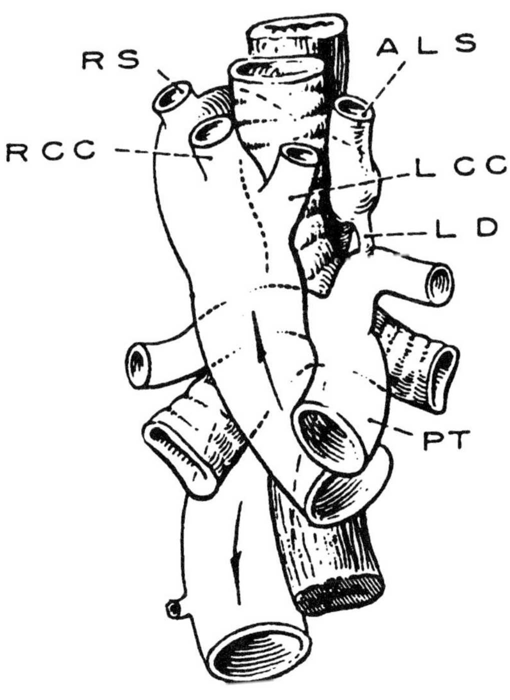

FIGURE 79.3. Right aortic arch with anomalous left subclavian artery. Vascular ring completed by the left-sided ligamentum arteriosum. (From Chun K, Colombani M, Dudgeon DL, et al. Diagnosis and management of congenital vascular rings: a 22-year experience. *Ann Thorac Surg* 1992;53:597–603, with permission.)

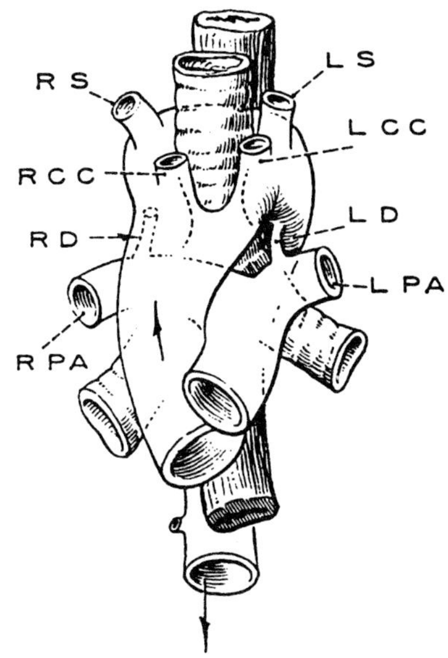

FIGURE 79.4. Persistent double aortic arch. (From Chun K, Colombani PM, Dudgeon DL, et al. Diagnosis and management of congenital vascular rings: a 22-year experience. *Ann Thorac Surg* 1992;53:597–603, with permission.)

ratory stridor. An examination of the pulses and blood pressure in all four extremities should be performed to rule out the rare case of a stenotic arch segment resulting in compromised flow to an arm, and for comparison with the postoperative examination. Auscultation of the chest for murmurs should be included to assess the need for more extensive evaluation for associated cardiac anomalies (which are uncommon).

Chest radiography is often performed as a part of the initial evaluation, and findings consistent with a right aortic arch should lead to suspicion of a vascular ring. The identification of the side of the aortic arch, though, may be particularly difficult in infants due to the size of the thymic shadow. Patients presenting with swallowing difficulties should undergo a barium swallow as part of the initial evaluation. This will typically demonstrate variable degrees of lateral compression on the anteroposterior views, and posterior indentation of the barium column on the lateral projections. A barium study demonstrating classic features of a vascular ring, coupled with a chest radiograph showing a right-sided aortic arch is generally all that is necessary to proceed with surgery. The demonstration of a dominant right arch on a plain film will dictate an operative approach via a left thoracotomy regardless of the specific anatomic variety of ring that exists. Chest computed tomography (CT) and magnetic resonance imaging (MRI) generally demonstrate the details of the arch anatomy extremely well and should be used routinely if the side of the aortic arch is unclear from plain radiography. These studies are limited in some cases when the ring is completed by the ligamentum arteriosum (right arch varieties), because this structure is not well seen with either of these modalities. When airway symptoms predominate, bronchoscopy may be performed, which often demonstrates extrinsic, sometimes pulsatile compression of the trachea.

Surgical intervention is indicated in all symptomatic cases. It may be argued that when the vascular ring anomaly is found incidentally, continued observation is appropriate. Although the symptoms that prompt the evaluation leading to the diagnosis may not be classic stridor or dysphagia, many clinicians feel that unusual presentations such as a barky cough or frequent upper respiratory infections may be associated with the vascular anomaly and constitute indications for surgery. Given the low risk associated with operative division of a vascular ring, it is difficult to recommend continued observation, particularly in younger patients.

The goal of surgical intervention for vascular rings should be conversion of a circumferential, closed ring into one that is open, realizing that there may still be a retroesophageal course of some of the vasculature. With the ring open in at least one direction, symptoms related to esophageal and tracheal compression will be relieved. It is also important to be cognizant of the effect of division of any vascular structure on the blood flow to the extremities. In all cases, pulse oximetry in both upper and one lower extremity as well as blood pressure in an upper and lower extremity should be monitored during operation. Test occlusion of the proposed site of ring division, particularly in double aortic arch should be accompanied by an assessment of its impact on four-extremity blood flow. Such monitoring also proves useful in cases where the anatomy appears unusual during surgical dissection. The identity of specific arch vessels may be made by temporary occlusion while observing for a loss of pulse oximeter sensing in the extremities.

A left, posterolateral, fourth-interspace thoracotomy is most frequently executed for vascular ring division because the sole or dominant component of the aortic arch is on the right in most cases. Because the descending aorta also may be on the right side, the only vascular structure immediately identifiable via this exposure is the left subclavian artery near the apex of the chest. Dissection should begin at this level working proximally, and ample dissection of enough of the anatomy should be performed to be absolutely certain of the identity of each structure. Care must be exercised to avoid injury to the vagus nerve, its recurrent laryngeal branch, and the esophagus, which may be distorted by the compressive vascular ring. In a double aortic arch with the right side dominant, the distal left arch is typically divided as it enters the descending aorta, distal to the origin of the left subclavian artery. Division of the ligamentum arteriosum is typically performed as well to allow further mobilization of the remaining proximal segment of the left arch. In vascular ring variants with a right aortic arch, division of the ligamentum arteriosum releases the compression. With anomalous origin of the left subclavian artery, the ligamentum courses from the left pulmonary artery to the left subclavian as it arises from its retroesophageal course. Often the segment of vessel attached to the ligamentum is quite dilated, a Kommerell's diverticulum, which may be resected to prevent posterior esophageal compression. This may not be feasible if doing so would compromise flow in the left subclavian artery. Occasionally in cases of a right aortic arch, the ligamentum attaches to the descending aorta (possibly to a Kommerell's diverticulum) despite the normal origin of the left subclavian artery. Division of the ligamentum and resection of the diverticulum is the appropriate treatment in this case as well.

Complete relief of symptoms may be noted immediately following operation, although persistence of some findings is not uncommon. In infants, there may be some degree of tracheomalacia associated with the vascular anomaly and persistence of some stridor, particularly during times of great activity or during upper respiratory infections. Depending on the specific anatomy, division of the ring may still leave either the subclavian artery or a segment of the aorta itself in a retroesophageal position. Improvement of swallowing symptoms in such cases may be seen only gradually.

INNOMINATE COMPRESSION SYNDROME

This syndrome typically presents in the first months of life with stridor, possibly associated with apnea or similar life-threatening event. Diagnosis is suggested by the finding of pulsatile anterior compression of the trachea, which may compromise the lumen by as much as 80% to 90%. Although some clinicians feel that the pathophysiology is caused by anomalous origin of the innominate artery farther to the left from the aorta causing it to drape across the trachea toward its bifurcation into the right common carotid and right subclavian arteries, it has been well demonstrated that the normal course of this vessel crosses the trachea from an origin slightly to the left of midline. The etiology of the stridor is virtually always multifactorial. Multiple structures must share a relatively limited space in the upper mediastinum/thoracic outlet region bounded by the rigid skeletal frame. The thymus is typically generous in these children, the innominate artery may be more prominent or follow a slightly more tortuous course, and most importantly, there is some degree of tracheomalacia present, resulting in a situation where the trachea is the most likely structure to be deprived of its domain. Analagous to what is seen in the case of gastroesophageal reflux, time favors spontaneous resolution of this syndrome. The thymus gradually regresses, the relationships of the airway and arteries gradually change, and most importantly, the airway enlarges and its cartilaginous support strengthens. When symptoms are not severe or life-threatening, observation is warranted. When apnea or life-threatening events are observed, or the tracheal lumen is compromised greater than 50%, operative intervention should be considered.

Bronchoscopy is important to characterize the degree and location of the tracheal compression. Barium swallow may be helpful to exclude vascular rings from the differential diagnosis. CT scan or MRI can likewise be helpful in ruling out arch anomalies, and demonstrating the spatial relationships of the thymus, innominate artery, and trachea.

Aortopexy, in which the aortic–innominate arterial junction is suspended to the posterior aspect of the sternum, is most frequently used when operation is recommended in this syndrome. Removal of one or both thymic lobes is an integral component of the operation. Avoiding any dissection between the vessels and trachea is crucial to allow the anterior displacement of the vessels to help suspend the floppy trachea open. The procedure can be performed through either a left or right thoracotomy, or with endoscopic guidance. A particularly useful method that I personally favor is via an anterior mediastinal approach through the bed of the resected second costal cartilage on the left. During the procedure, pulse oximetry or blood pressure monitoring of the right upper extremity should be used to ensure that flow in the innominate artery is not compromised during its suspension. Bronchoscopy immediately following the procedure should be performed to confirm adequacy of the relief of tracheal compression. Division and rightward translocation of the innominate artery via median sternotomy to a more proximal site on the aorta has been described, but this method should be reserved for exceptional cases.

Because most children have a significant component of tracheomalacia contributing to their stridor in this syndrome, and nothing is done directly to address this pathology, persistence of some stridor is often noted, especially with extreme agitation or during upper respiratory infections.

PULMONARY ARTERY SLING

Although not a complete vascular ring, this anomaly of pulmonary arterial development carries the highest risks for morbidity and mortality of the vascular compression syndromes due to the impact it may have on the development of the trachea. In pulmonary artery sling, the left pulmonary artery arises anomalously from the superoposterior aspect of the right pulmonary artery, courses between the trachea and esophagus forming a sling around the trachea, and ultimately reaches the pulmonary hilum in a nearly normal location (Fig. 79.5). There may be hypoplasia of the anomalous pulmonary artery itself or it may be quite large. Although the anomalous pulmonary artery may compress the adjacent trachea, resulting in airway-related symptoms similar to those seen in the other vascular compression syndromes, in 50% of cases there is associated tracheal stenosis. The stenosis is characterized by the absence of membranous trachea resulting in the presence of complete

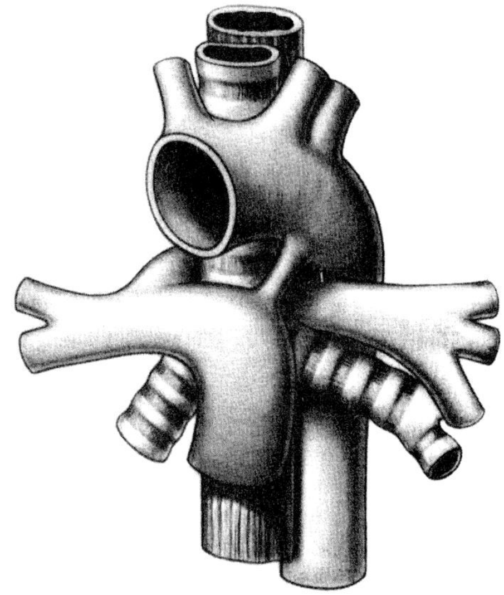

FIGURE 79.5. Pulmonary artery sling. (Modified from Stark J, Deleval M, eds. *Surgery for congenital heart defects*, 2nd ed. Philadelphia: WB Saunders, 1994.)

cartilaginous tracheal rings. In the most severe cases this may not only affect the distal trachea in the area of the sling, but may also result in long-segment tracheal stenosis.

Infants with pulmonary artery sling typically present with significant stridor in the first weeks to months of life. The time of onset and severity of the stridor is often largely dependent on the degree of tracheal stenosis. It is often surprising that an infant with significant tracheal stenosis may remain minimally symptomatic for a number of weeks only to rapidly deteriorate, often in the presence of a mild upper respiratory infection. Swallowing difficulties are not typically seen with this anomaly, and the pulmonary artery anomaly itself has little hemodynamic impact. Echocardiography demonstrates the vascular anatomy and is an important study to rule out the presence of other associated intracardiac anomalies, which have been reported to occur in up to 50% of cases. Angiography is rarely necessary in the initial evaluation. Careful bronchoscopy is crucial to delineate the tracheal anatomy, differentiating compression from true anatomic stenosis. This study may be particularly hazardous in the presence of important airway hypoplasia. Barium swallow is rarely helpful, but this study will differentiate a pulmonary artery sling from vascular ring anomalies by the anterior rather than posterior indentation of the esophageal contrast column.

Historically this anomaly was managed by mobilization and reimplantation of the left pulmonary artery via a left thoracotomy, although late occlusion of the reimplanted artery has been reported to be as high as 50%. This is felt to be due more to surgical technique than to associated hypoplasia of the artery seen in some cases. With modern cardiopulmonary support methods and vascular surgical techniques, the preferred approach is via sternotomy with bypass support. Division of the anomalous left pulmonary artery from its origin on the right, full mobilization to the pulmonary hilum, and reimplantation onto the main pulmonary artery results in excellent patency rates. Tracheal reconstruction should be performed simultaneously if associated tracheal stenosis is present. Short-segment stenosis can be addressed by resection and direct reanastomosis. When the tracheal pathology involves half or more of the tracheal length, more complex techniques such as patching or slide tracheoplasty must be used.

With current surgical management, late pulmonary stenosis is seen most commonly when hypoplasia of the left pulmonary artery has been present. Anastomotic stenosis is often not symptomatic, and its early detection requires regular cardiology follow-up. Virtually all of the mortality and major morbidity observed with a pulmonary artery sling is related to the associated tracheal pathology. Only small series have been reported describing combined repair of a pulmonary artery sling and tracheal stenosis, and good results have been described in many cases.

SUGGESTED READINGS

Adler SC, Isaacson G, Baksara RK. Innominate artery compression of the trachea: diagnosis and treatment by anterior suspension. A 25-year experience. *Ann Otol Rhinol Laryngol* 1995;104:924–927.

Backer CL, Ilbawi MN, Idriss FS, et al. Vascular anomalies causing tracheoesophageal compression. Review of experience in children. *J Thorac Cardiovasc Surg* 1989;97:725–731.

Backer CL, Mavroudis C. Vascular rings and pulmonary artery sling. In: Mavroudis C, Backer CL, eds. *Pediatric Cardiac Surgery, 2nd ed.* St. Louis: Mosby-Year Book, 1994:147–165.

Backer CL, Mavroudis C, Dunham ME, et al. Pulmonary artery sling: results with median sternotomy, cardiopulmonary bypass, and reimplantation. *Ann Thorac Surg* 1999;67:1738–1745.

Bullard KM, Adzick NS, Harrison MR. A mediastinal window approach to aortopexy. *J Pediatr Surg* 1997;32:680–681.

Chun K, Colombani PM, Dudgeon DL, et al. Diagnosis and management of congenital vascular rings: a 22-year experience. *Ann Thorac Surg* 1992;53:597–603.

Myer CM, Wiatrak BJ, Cotton RT, et al. Innominate compression of the trachea: current concepts. *Laryngoscope* 1989;99:1030–1034.

Van Son JAM, Hambsh J, Haas GS, et al. Pulmonary artery sling: reimplantation versus antetracheal translocation. *Ann Thorac Surg* 1999;68:989–994.

80

MEDIASTINAL MASSES

MILISSA A. McKEE
CHARLES N. PAIDAS

The diagnosis and management of mediastinal masses in children can be challenging. The etiology of these tumors encompasses a wide range of anomalies from congenital to acquired and benign to malignant tumors. These masses also may cause a variable degree of interference with cardiorespiratory physiology, given the confined space of the mediastinum and thoracic cavity. This physiologic derangement varies from minor to life-threatening depending on the size and location of the tumor. Urgent evaluation and treatment of these tumors is necessitated by the potential for airway obstruction and the high incidence of malignancy in children. Operative intervention may be required to obtain a tissue diagnosis or in some cases may be the primary treatment modality.

ANATOMIC DIVISIONS OF THE MEDIASTINUM

A working knowledge of the anatomy, divisions, and contents of the mediastinum serves as a basis for the initial evaluation and differential diagnosis of mediastinal tumors. The mediastinum is divided into three compartments: anterior, middle, and posterior (Table 80.1).

The anterior mediastinum is limited anteriorly by the sternum, posteriorly by the viscera (heart and great vessels), and superiorly by the thoracic inlet. The contents of the anterior mediastinum include the thymus, internal mammary vessels, lymph nodes, connective and adipose tissue, and occasionally thyroid or parathyroid tissue. Masses that arise in the anterior mediastinum include thymic masses, germ cell tumors, lymphomas, thyroid, lymphatic or vascular anomalies, lipomas, fibromas, and fibrosarcomas. The "four T's" traditionally describe the masses that arise most frequently in the anterior mediastinum: thyroid, thymus, teratomas, and terrible lymphomas.

The middle compartment of the mediastinum is located immediately posterior to the anterior mediastinum and extends posteriorly to the anterior surface of the vertebral bodies. Its contents are extensive and include the heart and great vessels as well as the tracheobronchial tree, esophagus, aorta, thoracic duct, vagus and phrenic nerves, and multiple extensive lymph node chains associated with the major visceral structures. Common tumors arising in this division include duplication, lymphomas, cysts, vascular masses, and, rarely, neuroendocrine tumors such as pheochromocytoma.

The posterior mediastinum consists of the paravertebral sulcus on each side and contains, most importantly, the ganglia of the sympathetic chain. The most common masses in the posterior mediastinum are tumors of neurogenic origin such as neuroblastoma, ganglioneuroma and primitive neuroectodermal tumor.

Tumors are typically derived from the anatomic structures that normally reside in a given compartment, but lymphomas, cystic hygromas, and vascular lesions may arise from and extend into any of the anatomic compartments.

EVALUATION AND DIAGNOSIS

Determining the etiology of a mass may be facilitated by a combination of the symptoms produced, age of the patient, location of the mass, and a basic understanding of the epidemiology of mediastinal masses. Presentation is variable. Anterior and middle mediastinal masses are usually symptomatic due to their large size and relationship to the tracheobronchial tree. As many as 80% are malignant, with lymphomas predominating. These tumors have a tendency to grow rapidly and surround vital structures.

Symptoms include cough, stridor, pain, and dyspnea. Dyspnea and especially orthopnea are ominous signs. In younger children, growth of these tumors is more often insidious; thus, symptoms may not appear until overt respi-

M.A. McKee: Departments of Surgery and Pediatrics, Yale University School of Medicine, New Haven, Connecticut.

C.N. Paidas: Department of Pediatric Surgery, Johns Hopkins University School of Medicine and Johns Hopkins Hospital, Baltimore, Maryland.

TABLE 80.1. CONTENTS AND TUMORS OF THE MEDIASTINUM

	Normal	Tumors
Anterior	Thymus	Thymomas, cysts
	Thyroid	Thyroid masses
	Lymphatic tissue	Lymphomas
	Connective tissue	Germ cell tumors
Middle	Heart, great vessels	Vascular masses
	Tracheobronchial tree	Cysts
	Lymph nodes	Lymphoma
	Esophagus	Duplications
	Nerves	Neurogenic tumors
Posterior	Sympathetic ganglia	Neuroblastoma, PNET

PNET, primitive neuroectodermal tumor.

ratory distress and cyanosis develop. Occasionally mediastinal masses are completely asymptomatic and identified incidentally during radiographic evaluation for other reasons. Systemic signs such as fever, fatigue, weight loss, and night sweats should be elicited in the history. These symptoms are typically associated with lymphomas. Physical examination should be directed to evaluation of general appearance (weight loss, pallor), cardiopulmonary examination (pulsus paradoxus), presence or absence of palpable masses or lymphadenopathy, and signs of venous obstruction (jugular venous distension, hepatomegaly).

Laboratory evaluation should be comprehensive, including a complete blood count with peripheral smear, chemistry profile, and, depending on the clinical suspicion, tumor markers such as vanillylmandelic acid (VMA), homovanillic acid (HVA), metanephrines, human chorionic gonadotropin (HCG), and α-fetoprotein (AFP). Specific tumor markers including VMA, HVA, and metanephrines may be elevated in the presence of neurogenic tumors. Germ cell tumors may cause elevations in HCG or AFP. Alkaline phosphatase and lactate dehydrogenase are nonspecific tumor markers. Cytopenia or abnormal cell types on peripheral smear may suggest the diagnosis of hematologic malignancy. Flow cytometry may in fact be adequate for specific diagnosis if the peripheral blood contains large numbers of lymphoblasts.

Radiographic evaluation is indicated in all cases. Plain posteroanterior and lateral chest radiographs should be obtained. Computed tomography with intravenous contrast administration should be performed for additional anatomic information and in many cases suggest a specific diagnosis. In addition, it is invaluable in the assessment of the degree of airway compromise. Magnetic resonance imaging (MRI) is less useful from a practical standpoint given the length of time needed to perform the examination and the need for sedation. MRI is indicated in cases of neurogenic tumors arising in the posterior mediastinum to evaluate for extension into the spinal canal. Nuclear medi-

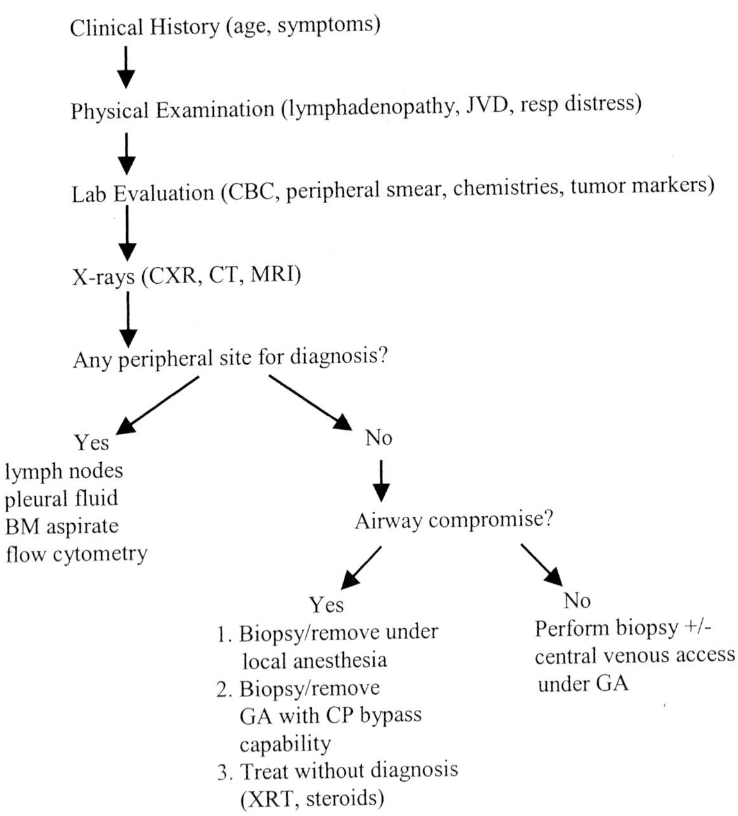

FIGURE 80.1. Algorithm for management.

cine scanning and angiography may be adjuncts in select cases, but are not typically necessary.

Obtaining a tissue diagnosis in cases of suspected malignancy is of paramount importance, but can be difficult or hazardous. The planned approach should minimize potential morbidity to the patient and take into account the relative risk of anesthesia in each individual situation. Because all patients with an anterior or middle mediastinal mass are assumed to have a critical or unstable airway, all alternatives to surgical biopsy should be considered, including flow cytometry from peripheral blood, bone marrow biopsy, cytologic analysis of pleural fluid, or peripheral lymph node biopsy. Transcutaneous biopsy under radiologic guidance is an alternative in cases in which no peripheral site can be accessed safely.

When all other routes have failed or are nondiagnostic, operative biopsy usually becomes necessary. This may involve mediastinoscopy, a Chamberlain procedure (anterior second intercostal space mini-thoracotomy), thoracoscopy, anterolateral or posterolateral thoracotomy, or median sternotomy. This is, of course, dependent on the ability to administer anesthesia to the patient, and decisions in these cases must be individualized. An algorithm for evaluation is presented in Fig. 80.1.

PREANESTHETIC

The preanesthetic evaluation of children with mediastinal masses is perhaps the single most important factor in the safe and effective treatment of these diseases. The potential for airway compromise with life-threatening implications has been well recognized. Ideally, the clinician would like to have the luxury of time as well as a definitive way of predicting which patients are at highest risk for airway obstruction. There have long been anecdotal reports warning of the danger of significant airway compromise. However, only within the past ten years has a more standardized approach to evaluation resulted in a practical way to prospectively evaluate these patients. This is done on the basis of a combination of pulmonary function testing and computed tomography. Pulmonary function testing may show obstructive or restrictive defects. The peak expiratory flow rate (PEFR) is the first component to show abnormality and is relatively easy to obtain. Reduction in the PEFR to less than 50% of predicted is cause for concern.

Computed tomography is the current mainstay of preoperative evaluation. CT scanning should be performed following a specific protocol, in which the cross-sectional area (CSA) of the trachea is evaluated with the CT window set at −450. It is important that the window be set correctly, because the CSA will vary if the window is changed. From this study, the measured tracheal CSA can be compared with norms for age. These predicted norms are available by graph for age and gender or may be calculated using the following formula: tracheal area = (age in years/9) + 0.035 cm^2 for boys and girls up to age 14. Tracheal compression of 50% or more of the area is associated with significant risk of airway compromise.

The Shamberger box is created by plotting the percentage of predicted values of PEFR versus tracheal CSA. Patients with both PEFR and CSA of greater than 50% of predicted are considered low risk and may safely undergo general anesthesia for any necessary procedure. At the other extreme, patients with both values less than 50% of predicted are high risk and should only receive local anesthesia. For the patients in the middle ground, where only one of the two predictors is low, the implications are not as clear. They should be considered moderate risk and general anesthesia avoided where possible. If they do require general anesthesia, it should be done with spontaneous ventilation only and paralysis avoided.

This section has focused on the obvious issue of airway compromise and evaluation, but it should not be forgotten that mediastinal masses may result in compression of cardiovascular structures as well. Echocardiography should be considered in the preoperative evaluation of patients in whom there is any concern, but especially if the mass is located in the anterior mediastinum. Following these guidelines will allow for the safe preoperative planning for nearly all patients.

OPERATIVE MANAGEMENT

After the appropriate preoperative evaluation is complete, operative intervention will be indicated in most patients. Commonly, biopsy is needed to confirm a tissue diagnosis. If a diagnosis of malignancy has been established, central venous access is usually required for the administration of chemotherapy. There will also be a significant number of patients for whom surgical excision is the primary treatment, such as those with neuroblastoma, germ cell tumors, teratomas, thyroid masses, and duplications of the aerodigestive tract.

The most straightforward way to establish tissue diagnosis is to perform open biopsy of a palpable mass or enlarged peripheral lymph node. This is usually easily accomplished under local anesthesia and monitored sedation, if the patient is at high risk for general anesthesia. As with most malignancies, children with mediastinal tumors require procedures for venous access. If they are in the low risk group for general anesthesia, central venous catheter placement can be performed in the usual manner. The CT scan obtained preoperatively should be evaluated critically for the possibility of venous compression prior to line placement. For patients with great vessel distortion or unacceptable anesthetic risk, venous access may be obtained using a peripheral central venous catheter. This will allow for the initiation of therapy and subsequent line placement after several weeks of therapy have resulted in tumor shrinkage.

Mediastinoscopy is an option for a patient with an anterior mediastinal mass or lymphadenopathy. It requires that the patient be under general anesthesia and is contraindicated for retrotracheal and hilar masses or nodes. Another option for biopsy of the anterior mediastinal mass is the Chamberlain procedure. A small transverse incision is made in a parasternal location over the second intercostal space. This allows for the incisional biopsy of masses in this location. It may be performed under local anesthesia if necessary, and a short segment of rib may be removed to improve access to the thoracic cavity. The dissection can be performed in an extrapleural fashion to prevent air entry into the pleural space. One also must be careful to avoid injury to the internal mammary artery and vein. From a technical standpoint, the procedure is usually easy to accomplish and allows for a rapid recovery. Chest tube placement is often not necessary. For patients with airway compromise it may be performed under local anesthesia and with the patient's head elevated to between 30 and 45 degrees, significantly improving their ability to tolerate the procedure from a respiratory standpoint.

Thoracoscopy is an alternative approach for the biopsy or excision of mediastinal masses and is gaining in popularity. The postoperative recovery is usually much quicker than that of a thoracotomy. However, this procedure does mandate general anesthesia, the availability of specialized instrumentation, and the operative expertise to execute the procedure in a minimally invasive fashion. Small masses, regardless of diagnosis, are frequently amenable to thoracoscopic resection, whereas large tumors continue to require more invasive methods. Teratomas, duplications, benign masses and neuroblastoma require operative removal and can be evaluated for either minimally invasive resection or open thoracotomy. Again, these decisions are at the discretion of the operating surgeon. In the case of advanced neuroblastoma extending into the spinal canal, initial tissue diagnosis may be needed to pretreat with chemotherapy prior to definitive resection.

There will remain a subset of patients in whom open thoracotomy is the only option. The open procedures may be accomplished via thoracotomy or median sternotomy, depending on the location of the tumor. This group of patients also includes those whose primary modality of indicated therapy is operative resection. The capability to immediately initiate cardiopulmonary bypass with the induction of anesthesia occasionally is required, such as in the case of massive tumor in the anterior mediastinum. Median sternotomy provides the additional benefit of allowing the surgeon to lift the tumor and directly relieve the compression of the underlying structures.

COMPLICATIONS

As with any intervention, there are risks associated with the diagnosis and treatment of mediastinal tumors. Infectious risks include wound infection, pneumonia, and empyema. These can usually be treated using standard protocols. Bleeding is potentially life threatening given the proximity of the great vessels and can be difficult to control when space and visualization are limited. As always, a thorough understanding of the relevant anatomy and the constant assessment of the potential for vascular injury are critical when dealing with these lesions. Injury to the thoracic duct may occur, resulting in a chylous effusion. Prolonged massive lymph leak can cause malnutrition and immunosuppression due to protein and lymphocyte losses. Most chyle leaks will stop with chest tube drainage and parenteral nutritional support. If enteral feeds are used, they should contain relatively high levels of medium-chain triglycerides to encourage direct absorption through the bowel wall. Somatostatin also has been used as an adjunct with variable success.

Several major nerves in the chest are in jeopardy, including the phrenic, vagus, and recurrent laryngeal nerves. Phrenic nerve injury results in paralysis and sometimes eventration of the diaphragm. Patients who are symptomatic or have an oxygen requirement may eventually require operative plication of the diaphragm. Unilateral recurrent laryngeal nerve injury may be temporary or permanent and results in significant morbidity for the patient.

Anesthetic risks such as loss of airway and cardiovascular collapse have been discussed at length. It is well known that patients who develop airway compromise in this setting are difficult to salvage. Attempts to position patients on their side to relieve the compression are rarely successful. Likewise, attempts to pass an endotracheal tube past the obstruction are usually futile. The best way to deal with these complications is to recognize their potential and avoid them.

Perioperative pain may be addressed with multimodality pain treatment such as an epidural catheter, intravenous narcotics, acetaminophen, and either Cox-2 inhibitors or nonsteroidal antiinflammatory drugs. Mortality in these patients is a significant risk given the potential for perioperative complications early on and the long-term risks of tumor treatment and recurrence.

SUMMARY

Mediastinal masses in the pediatric population represent a complex group of disorders requiring specialized multidisciplinary evaluation and treatment. Surgeons play an integral role in this process. Surgical intervention may be required for diagnosis, venous access, or as the primary mode of treatment. The majority of patients will be amenable to conventional diagnostic methods. Great care should be taken in the small but significant group of patients with airway compromise and no alternative to an invasive thoracic procedure to make a diagnosis. Using a thoughtful and individualized approach to evaluation and therapy will minimize morbidity and optimize the chance for a successful outcome in nearly all patients.

SUGGESTED READINGS

Azizkhan RG, Dudgeon DL, Buck JR, et al. Life-threatening airway obstruction as a complication to the management of mediastinal masses in children. *J Pediatr Surg* 1985;20:816–822.

Grosfeld JL, Shamberger RC, Esposito G, et al. Mediastinal tumors in children. *Semin Pediatr Surg* 1999;8:49–98.

Ricketts RR. Clinical management of anterior mediastinal tumors in children. *Semin Pediatr Surg* 2001;10:161–168.

Robie DK, Gursoy MH, Pokorny WJ. Mediastinal tumors—airway obstruction and management. *Semin Pediatr Surg* 1994;3:259–266.

81

LUNG INFECTIONS

MARY BRINDLE
IRENE W. Y. MA
R. LAWRENCE MOSS

Over the past 50 years, the spectrum of organisms encountered in pediatric pulmonary infections has radically changed. This change can be explained in part by the development of more effective antibiotics and the subsequent development of antibiotic-resistant organisms. Treatment options have broadened due to advancements in diagnostic and interventional radiology and bronchoscopic techniques. With these advances, the incidence of pulmonary abscess in children has decreased and the role of operation in the management of abscesses has assumed a less prominent role. Improvements in transplantation medicine and cancer therapy have created a population of immunosuppressed children who are vulnerable to opportunistic infections. Emerging opportunistic pathogens, especially fungi, necessitate the development of protocols to identify and combat these organisms.

LUNG ABSCESS

Historically, pulmonary abscesses are classified as either primary or secondary. Primary abscesses are those that develop in the absence of preexisting disease, whereas secondary abscesses occur in the setting of underlying medical illness. The clinical utility of this classification is limited, given the overlapping nature of the natural history, presentation, and microbiology.

A pulmonary abscess is an area of suppuration that has developed central necrosis and cavitation. These infected cavities are often multiple and polymicrobial, containing both aerobic and anaerobic bacteria. Pediatric pulmonary abscesses commonly form as a result of aspiration. Conditions that predispose to the development of aspiration, such as neurologic conditions that impair coughing and swallowing, are therefore risk factors for abscess formation. In Tan's 1995 study of pulmonary abscesses, 30% of affected patients had a significant neurologic disorder. Other factors predisposing to abscess formation include gastroesophageal reflux, septic emboli from bacterial endocarditis associated with congenital heart disease, and immunodeficiencies (congenital or acquired) (Table 81.1).

Abscesses tend to form in dependent regions of the lung, including the right upper lobe in the prone patient, the left lower lobe in the supine position, as well as the apical segments of both lower lobes. Because of the more vertical orientation of its bronchus, the right lung is most commonly involved.

In Tan's study of 34 patients, multiple organisms were cultured in every case. The most common *aerobic* organisms were

TABLE 81.1. FACTORS PREDISPOSING TO PULMONARY ABSCESS

Neurologic/neuromuscular
Impaired cough, gag, swallow
Sedation (including anesthetics)
Pulmonary
Pneumonia
Obstructing mass (including tumor, granuloma or foreign body)
Cystic lesion (bronchogenic cyst)
Chronic inflammation (cystic fibrosis)
Penetrating trauma (including surgical intervention)
Gastrointestinal
Increased gastroesophageal reflux
Impaired gastric emptying
Esophageal motility disorders
Tracheoesophageal fistula
Immune-related
Patients on immunosuppressive medications
Patients with neoplasia (especially hematologic)
Infectious spread
Hematogenous spread from bacteremia
Contiguous spread from other site (hepatic, splenic, subdural abscess, etc.)
Septic emboli (from congenital heart disease)

M. Brindle: Department of Surgery and Pediatrics, Stanford University Medical School; and Division of Pediatric Surgery, Lucile Packard Children's Hospital, Palo Alto, California.

I. W. Y. Ma: Department of Medicine, University of British Columbia, Vancouver, British Columbia, Canada.

R. L. Moss: Department of Surgery, Yale University School of Medicine; and Department of Surgery, Yale-New Haven Children's Hospital, New Haven, Connecticut.

Pseudomonas aeruginosa (n = 7), *Staphylococcus aureus* (n = 7), *Streptococcus pneumonia* (n = 4), and *Haemophilus influenza* (n = 4). The most common *anaerobic* organisms were *Bacteroides* species (n = 8). These numbers correspond with a 1979 study by Brook et al. in which a significant number of patients with pulmonary abscesses grew anaerobic organisms from abscess cultures. Studies performed prior to the mid-1970s did not assess for the presence of anaerobic bacteria. The growing recognition of the role of anaerobic bacteria in pulmonary abscesses has increased the success of treatment regimens and has improved understanding of abscess etiology.

Pediatric patients with pulmonary abscesses generally present with cough, fever, tachypnea, dyspnea, weight loss, and vomiting. They may occasionally present with pleuritic chest pain or shoulder-tip pain. Although sputum production is usually increased, it may not be clinically evident in these patients. Findings of decreased breath sounds over the involved lung and dullness to percussion are less common in pediatric patients.

The classical chest radiograph of a patient with a pulmonary abscess demonstrates an infiltrate with a cavity containing an air-fluid level. There are numerous conditions that may mimic this radiographic appearance, including bronchogenic cysts in the mediastinum, other congenital cystic structures, and pneumatoceles or sequestrations. A computed tomography (CT) scan will better define the nature of the pulmonary infiltrate in patients with less clear radiographic findings (Fig. 81.1).

Sputum culture results have gradually been replaced by more accurate methods of determining abscess flora. These methods include bronchoscopic alveolar lavage, transtracheal aspiration, and percutaneous transthoracic aspiration. Blood cultures, if positive, are helpful in identifying the pathogens involved.

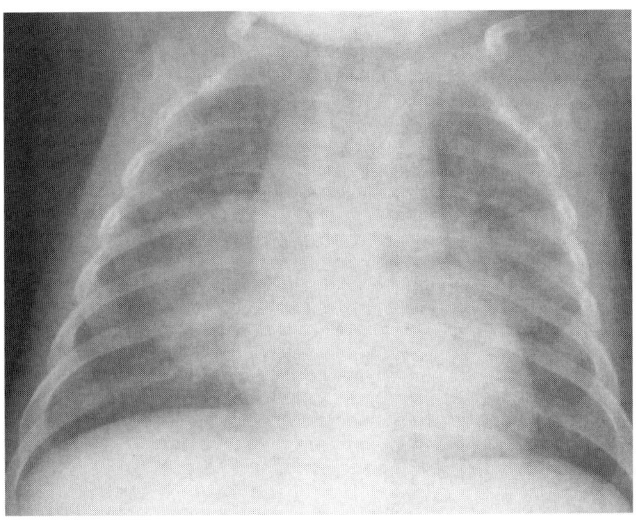
A

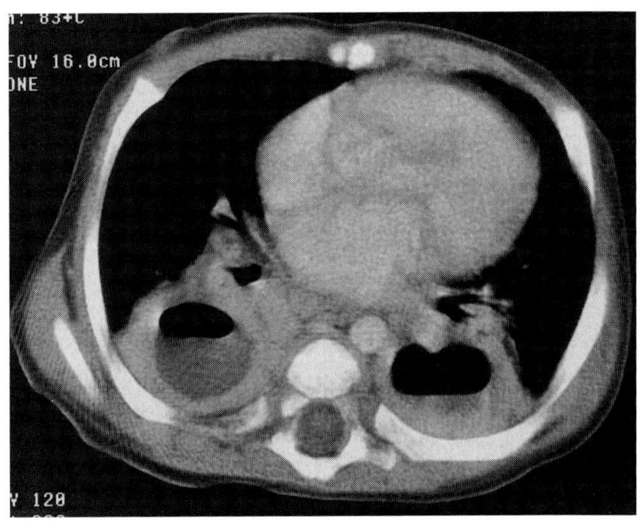
C

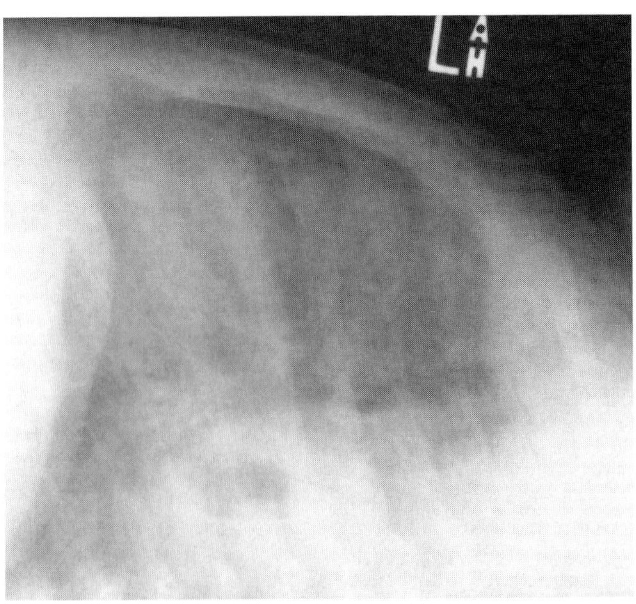
B

FIGURE 81.1 A: Chest radiograph of a 4-month-old infant with Kostmann neutropenia. The anteroposterior view shows evidence of a focal infiltrate behind the heart. **B:** A cross-table lateral chest radiograph more clearly demonstrates the abscess cavity with an air-fluid level. **C:** A cross-sectional computed tomography image of the same infant reveals bilateral lower lobe abscesses.

Antibiotics are now generally regarded as first-line therapy in the treatment of pediatric pulmonary abscesses. The principles of therapy are as follows:

1. Empiric antimicrobial therapy should be initiated, including a penicillinase-resistant agent as well as an agent that is active against *Streptococci* and anaerobes (e.g., clindamycin).
2. Specific at-risk populations should receive additional antibiotic coverage. Patients at high risk for aspiration or who are immunocompromised should receive gram-negative coverage. The antibiotic regimen for patients at risk for *Pseudomonas* infection (i.e., patients with cystic fibrosis) should include an aminoglycoside.
3. Therapy should be altered depending on culture and sensitivity results.
4. Parenteral antibiotics are administered for 2 to 3 weeks, followed by an oral antibiotic regimen for a total of 4 to 8 weeks.
5. Chest physiotherapy may be helpful, including postural drainage based on the anatomic location of the abscess. Bronchoscopy can be used, when necessary, not only to help facilitate drainage but to identify and treat obstructing elements.
6. If the patient is severely ill at the time of diagnosis or fails to improve after 7 to 10 days, drainage of the abscess cavity should be considered. Early intervention also should be considered in neonates and immunocompromised patients.
7. Regular clinical and radiographic evaluation over the course of treatment is valuable in determining response to treatment.

Pediatric patients are more likely than adults to require drainage of abscess cavities because of smaller airways and poor cough effort. This is especially true in children under 7 years of age. Percutaneous techniques guided by fluoroscopy, ultrasonography, or CT scan can be used to direct placement of a large catheter into the abscess cavity. Transbronchial catheter drainage is another method that has been used successfully. If smaller catheters are used, more frequent irrigation is necessary.

Surgical procedures are rarely required in the management of pulmonary abscesses. Open pneumonostomy, a technique developed prior to the antibiotic era, is still occasionally used today. This open drainage procedure still has a role in the management of acutely ill children with rapid progression of disease despite medical therapy. It is particularly useful in the treatment of large abscesses (4–8 cm). Other indications for surgical intervention include proximity of the abscess to the mediastinum and abscess cavities not amenable to percutaneous drainage. Preoperative radiographic localization is performed prior to surgery. A small incision is made directly over the abscess site. A short piece of the rib directly underlying the incision is then resected. The abscess is drained, and a large drainage tube is placed into the cavity. The wound is packed to prevent spillage of pus into the pleural space.

In rare patients with severe pulmonary infection unresponsive to therapy or with compressive symptoms related to abscess expansion, pulmonary resection is required. Wedge resections should be performed in order to minimize loss of healthy lung tissue. Resections can be performed through a thoracotomy or by using thoracoscopic techniques.

Adequate antibiotic therapy and prompt drainage of the abscess cavity results in cavity contraction and healing. In otherwise healthy children, there is minimal morbidity and mortality. Bronchopleural fistulas are uncommon in children because of their small airways. Chronic cavity formation is an infrequent complication that may result in abscess recurrence. Although hemoptysis can occur after drainage procedures, it is rarely significant. Immunocompromised pediatric patients are much less likely to respond to a conservative approach. The mortality rate associated with a pulmonary abscess in this patient population approaches 20%.

It is extremely important that every child with a lung abscess undergo follow-up radiographs of the chest until complete radiographic resolution has occurred. This may take up to 6 months. A small subset of patients will be found to have an underlying congenital lesion, such as a congenital cystic adenomatoid malformation or an intrapulmonary sequestration. During the acute phase of the infection, it is not possible to distinguish between an infected congenital lesion and a simple abscess. Only after the infection has been successfully treated will a chest radiograph or CT scan reveal the abnormality. The treatment of these congenital lesions is resection in order to prevent repeated episodes of infection and injury to adjacent normal lung.

After an abscess is successfully treated with antibiotics, it is common for children to develop cystic airspaces in the lung. These pneumatoceles are readily seen on the plain chest radiograph. Pneumatoceles typically resolve spontaneously over a 3- to 6-month period. Treatment is not necessary unless a recurrent abscess develops in a pneumatocele cavity.

PULMONARY INFECTIONS IN THE IMMUNOCOMPROMISED PATIENT

Advances in oncology, hematology, and transplant medicine have led to an increase in the population of children with impaired host defenses. Although bacteria cause most of the pulmonary infections in this population, these organisms are usually eliminated with antibiotic therapy. Fungal infections are becoming more frequent, occurring through inhalation of airborne fungal spores or progression from an upper airway fungal infection. These infections are challenging to diagnose and difficult to treat. Both medical and surgical therapies for deep-seated pulmonary fungal infections are imperfect and are, themselves, potentially harmful. *Aspergillus* is the most common and most lethal cause of fungal pneumonia, followed by *Candida*. Other pathogenic organisms include *Histoplasma* and *Coccidioides*.

ASPERGILLOSIS

Aspergillus species are ubiquitous fungi that are becoming increasingly common invasive pulmonary pathogens in the immunocompromised patient. Of the 150 species of *Aspergillus*, the 20 species that infect the human host include, most commonly, *A. flavus, A. fumigatus, A. terreus,* and *A. niger*. *Aspergillus* is an invasive organism that is frequently lethal in the immunocompromised host. In invasive pulmonary aspergillosis (IPA), the fungus spreads rapidly through lung parenchyma and invades blood vessels. Angioinvasion can result in life-threatening hemoptysis and also can provide a portal of entry for *Aspergillus* to spread and involve other organs such as the brain, liver, and kidneys. An aggressive approach to diagnosis and treatment is required.

Factors that predispose to invasive aspergillosis include: (a) neutropenia (polymorphonuclear cell count <500/μL), believed to be the greatest predisposing factor for fungal infection; (b) broad-spectrum antibiotic therapy; (c) concurrent chemotherapy; (d) concurrent steroid therapy; and (e) hospitalization in the month preceding.

The presentation of IPA is most frequently that of fever in a neutropenic patient. Symptoms such as cough, hemoptysis, dyspnea, and tachypnea may be present. A high degree of clinical suspicion for fungal infection is necessary in the febrile, neutropenic patient.

The characteristic chest radiograph findings of IPA include wedge-shaped, pleural-based densities or cavities. These findings generally occur late in the course of pulmonary infection. Earlier radiographic findings consist of nonspecific pulmonary infiltrates. More specific radiographic evidence can be found earlier in the course of the infection with the use of CT. One of the earliest findings is the halo sign, which occurs as a result of bleeding or edema surrounding an ischemic area and appears as an area of low attenuation around a pulmonary nodule. The halo sign has been found in up to 90% of patients with IPA at the time the patient presents with febrile neutropenia and pulmonary infiltrates on the chest radiograph. A later CT finding is the crescent sign, which occurs with contraction of infarcted tissue and appears as a crescent of air around the pulmonary nodule. The routine use of CT early in the evaluation of febrile neutropenic patients appears to shorten the length of time to diagnosis, allowing for earlier administration of antifungal therapy.

Aspergillus is part of normal flora of the airways. Therefore, sputum cultures demonstrating *Aspergillus* are of little value in the patient with normal host defenses. In immunocompromised patients, the positive predictive value of a positive culture is much greater, in fact as high as 80% to 90%. Bronchoalveolar lavage can increase the yield of a respiratory culture. There is little support for the use of transbronchial biopsies and brushings because these procedures have a high false-negative rate in high-risk groups. Although measurement of serial levels of antibodies to *Aspergillus* has been frequently used to monitor a known infection, particularly in the setting of noninvasive allergic bronchopulmonary aspergillosis, this test has little use in the diagnosis of IPA.

Definitive diagnosis of IPA requires a biopsy specimen. Lung tissue must demonstrate histopathologic evidence of septated, nonpigmented, acute-angle branching hyphae. Cultures from the lung (or a solid organ biopsy) also must grow *Aspergillus*. In order to make this diagnosis, it is often necessary to perform an open or thoracoscopic lung biopsy. A febrile, neutropenic child with a positive sputum culture and radiologic findings consistent with IPA should be promptly treated for presumed aspergillosis while attempts are made to confirm the diagnosis. There are some risks in treating a presumptive infection prior to establishing a diagnosis. These include the exposure to antifungal toxicity and the withholding of chemotherapy. It is therefore often necessary to perform invasive procedures in order to definitively establish the diagnosis.

The factor that has the greatest influence on patient recovery is the reversal of neutropenia or the return of graft function after bone marrow transplantation. In April 2000, the Infectious Diseases Society of America published a set of practice guidelines for diseases caused by *Aspergillus*. High-dose intravenous amphotericin B (1–1.5 mg/kg/day) is standard in the treatment of IPA. There is significant nephrotoxicity associated with the use of amphotericin B, which can be diminished with the use of lipid-based preparations. Lipid formulations are extremely expensive and require higher doses to achieve an equivalent effect. Currently, they can only be recommended in patients with marginal renal function or whose renal function deteriorates while receiving amphotericin.

Itraconazole has been found to have excellent response rates and offers an oral alternative to amphotericin. This obviously relies on patient compliance, normal gastrointestinal absorption, and the absence of interacting medications. Combination therapy with amphotericin and an azole or flucytosine has not demonstrated increased efficacy over amphotericin alone. In fact, antagonism, toxicity, and myelosuppression are all risks of combination therapy. A logical sequence would be intravenous amphotericin until disease progression is arrested, followed by oral therapy for prolonged treatment. Duration of treatment is highly dependent on patient response and is somewhat controversial.

Surgical therapy has a role in the management of aspergillus infections, sometimes on an urgent basis. The tropism of *Aspergillus* for the vascular wall puts patients at risk for pulmonary hemorrhage. Massive hemoptysis is a potentially lethal complication of IPA, and is an established indication for emergent pulmonary resection. Aggressive resuscitation is essential in these patients, followed by rapid and definitive treatment of the bleeding. Emergency bronchoscopy allows for lateralization and localization of the bleeding site. Once lateralization has been established, the patient should be placed with the affected side in a dependent position. Intubation of the unaffected lung may be performed. If the bleeding site is localized, a balloon-tip catheter, introduced through the bronchoscope, can tamponade the hemorrhagic artery. Contralateral lung intubation and balloon tamponade are temporizing measures to protect the unaffected lung from aspiration of blood.

Angioembolization has been performed, and its success in treating an acute pulmonary bleed is well documented. Embolization, however, is not always successful and is associated with potential complications. Moreover, this technique leaves behind the invasive *Aspergillus* lesion, which can progress and reinvade pulmonary vessels. Angioembolization remains a valuable method of controlling an acute pulmonary bleed prior to surgical intervention. In select patients who are not operative candidates, it may be the only option in the face of a catastrophic bleed.

The goal of emergency surgical resection of IPA is to remove only the angioinvasive lesion, preserving as much normal lung tissue as possible. At the outset of the operation, it is essential to establish rapid control of the main pulmonary artery at the mediastinum or in the pericardium. When the location of the lesion and its site of invasion have been established, it can be resected while vascular control is maintained. Lobectomy may be required for large lesions. Pneumonectomy is rarely required. Invasion of the main pulmonary artery may require sleeve resection and the use of pericardial flaps to repair injured adventitia.

There are diagnostic and therapeutic indications for elective resection of IPA. The most common indication for operation in patients with suspected fungal infection is the need to obtain diagnostic tissue. Pulmonary wedge resection, performed either thoracoscopically or through a thoracotomy, is commonly used. Thoracoscopy typically yields diagnostic tissue and is far less invasive in these already compromised patients.

The value of pulmonary resection as a form of treatment for IPA has not been established. Retrospective studies have demonstrated mixed results from aggressive pulmonary resection. At this time, surgical resection is recommended in patients with IPA unresponsive to aggressive medical therapy, who have adequate pulmonary function and are likely to tolerate a thoracotomy. Because of the dangers of catastrophic pulmonary hemorrhage associated with invasion of the pulmonary artery by *Aspergillus*, there is theoretical support for pulmonary resection to remove centrally located lesions. Therapeutic resections should attempt to achieve negative margins (at least macroscopically) and to remove all foci of IPA. Because of the frequency of microinvasion and multiple sites of infection, resection does not obviate the need for antifungal therapy. *Aspergillus* is an aggressive invasive organism. Lesions frequently cross lobar fissures and invade the chest wall, These features may preclude the use of thoracoscopic resection. Open thoracotomy is often necessary.

CANDIDA

As with *Aspergillus*, *Candida* is a ubiquitous organism that colonizes the pediatric airway. Pulmonary infections with *Candida* usually represent an extension of hematogenous disease in an immunocompromised patient. Biopsy may be required for diagnosis. *Candida* pneumonia is treated with fluconazole or intravenous amphotericin, depending on the species and sensitivity. Surgery does not have a role in the management of pulmonary candidiasis, except for providing a tissue diagnosis.

HISTOPLASMOSIS

Histoplasmosis capsulatum infections, previously rare in pediatric patients, have become more common with the increase of pediatric acquired immunodeficiency syndrome (AIDS). Histoplasmosis is endemic in Ohio, the Mississippi River valleys, Texas, Oklahoma, Kansas, Pennsylvania, Maryland, and Virginia. Most infected individuals develop asymptomatic and self-limited infections. Pediatric pulmonary infections usually occur in patients with AIDS who present with fever, cough, and adenopathy on chest radiography. Sputum cultures provide the diagnosis. Other diagnostic modalities, including skin test and antibody titers, do not provide sufficient evidence of acute infection. In patients who are ill, these pulmonary infections are treated with amphotericin B, although there are limited data regarding which antifungal agent to use in children.

COCCIDIOIDOMYCOSIS

As with histoplasmosis, *Coccidioides immitis* is an organism with a specific geographic distribution that generally follows a self-limited course. Most infected individuals live in the lower Sonoran Desert, central California, and northern Mexico. Inhalation of spores can cause localized infection with surrounding granuloma formation. In pediatric patients, there are reports of airway obstruction related to tracheal compression from mediastinal adenopathy. Progressive infection results in cavity formation. Infections also may disseminate, causing meningitis. Clinical presentation and radiographic findings may suggest the diagnosis, but to definitively demonstrate coccidioidomycosis, the organism must be isolated from a biopsy or sputum culture. Skin tests and antibody tests have little role in the diagnosis of pulmonary infection, although they may help monitor response to therapy. There is little information on the most appropriate antifungal medication to use in the pediatric population. With severe disease, amphotericin B is generally recommended. In milder disease, oral azole therapy may be substituted. These infections are generally responsive to medical therapy. Surgical resection of cavitary disease is recommended in patients who demonstrate progression of disease on maximum medical therapy or in the presence of severe or recurrent hemoptysis.

SUGGESTED READINGS

Abbasi S, Shenep JL, et al. Aspergillosis in children with cancer: a 34-year experience. *Clin Infect Dis* 1999;29:1210–1219.

Bernard A, Daillot D, et al. Surgical management of invasive pulmonary aspergillosis in neutropenic patients. *Ann Thorac Surg* 1997;64:1441–1447.

Brook I, Finegold SM. Bacteriology and therapy of lung abscess in children. *J Pediatr* 1979;94:10–12.

Donnelly LF, Klosterman LA. Pneumonia in children: decreased parenchymal contrast enhancement—CT sign of intense illness and impending cavitary necrosis. *Radiology* 1997;205:817–820.

Kosloske AM, Ball WS, Butler C, et al. Drainage of pediatric lung abscess by cough, catheter, or complete resection. *J Pediatr Surg* 1986;21:596–600.

Lacey SR, Kosloske AM. Pneumonostomy in the management of pediatric lung abscess. *J Pediatr Surg* 1983;18:625–627.

Salerno CT, Ouyang DW, et al. Surgical therapy for pulmonary aspergillosis in immunocompromised patients. *Ann Thorac Surg* 1998;65:1415–1419.

Stevens DA, Kan VL, Judson MA, et al. Practice guidelines for diseases caused by *Aspergillus*. *Clin Infect Dis* 2000;30:696–709.

Tan TQ, Seilheimer DK, Kaplan SL. Pediatric lung abscess: clinical management and outcome. *Pediatr Infect Dis J* 1995;14:51–55.

82

THORACOSCOPIC TECHNIQUES

THOM E LOBE

Thoracoscopy in pediatric surgery was first used by Rogers and others in the late 1970s, shortly after the development and ready availability of small endoscopes that used the Hopkins rod lens system. With improved video equipment and better instrumentation, we now use thoracoscopy regularly to perform most diagnostic and major operative intrathoracic procedures in infants and children.

In general, thoracoscopy is as effective as an open procedure for most conditions and is accompanied by less morbidity. Congenital disorders amenable to thoracoscopic correction are listed in Table 82.1. Other conditions in infancy and childhood for which thoracoscopy should be considered are listed in Table 82.2.

Most of the instrumentation we use for thoracoscopy in children is the same as that used in adults, particularly when considering older children and teenagers. In general, we prefer to use the smallest telescope that will suit our needs. Today, advances in video technology provide good images using scopes as small as 1 mm in diameter. Most of the 2.7- to 5-mm instruments that are now standard for endoscopic surgery can be used for thoracoscopy in children and are available with shorter shaft lengths. These include graspers, dissectors, scissors, and retractors, as well as special instruments such as Allis and Babcock clamps, suction-irrigation devices, and others. When endoscopic ligatures are required in small infants, we prefer the 5-mm single or multifire clip applicators.

Tissue extraction in cases for which the mass is too large to be removed through one of the trocar sites can be problematic. Large specimens can be removed using an automatic tissue morcellator after placing them in an endoscopic sac if the surgeon is experienced in using this device.

BASIC TECHNIQUES

Because of their small size, the airway in infants and young children will not accept standard double-lumen endotracheal tubes as will teenagers and adults. We use selective intubation with cuffed endotracheal tubes for most of our patients. Alternatively, a Fogarty catheter passed alongside a small-diameter endotracheal tube can be directed into the bronchus to be occluded as a bronchial blocker. A small flexible bronchoscope passed through the endotracheal tube lumen facilitates proper placement of this device.

When choosing an initial cannula, the surgeon must decide whether insufflation is needed. If insufflation with CO_2 is required, then a laparoscopic cannula with a gas-tight valve must be used. First we make a skin incision large enough to accept the cannula to be introduced. Blunt dissection with a mosquito hemostat can be helpful. The position of the first cannula depends on the procedure to be performed. Close communication with the anesthesiologist is essential to avoid a hemodynamically significant tension pneumothorax.

In some cases of infection and tumor we have noted that it is difficult to gain access to the chest because of the pleural adhesions. In these cases, we dissect through the muscles of the intercostal space bluntly, and make a sufficiently large hole to allow the introduction of a finger or telescope into the pleural space. We use blunt dissection with the finger (or the end of a thoracoscope using visual control), until a large enough space has been created that a trocar can be inserted safely. Occasionally, we use CO_2 insufflation to assist us with the pleural dissection. When the space is large enough to insert another instrument, we place a suction/irrigation device or a dissector into the pleural space to dissect the adhesions down bluntly, or we lyse the adhesions to make room to work. In rare instances it is impossible to gain access, and an open thoracotomy is indicated.

We rarely use instruments larger than 5 mm. The obvious exception is when an endoscopic stapler is required. When this instrument is used in small children, there must be at least 5 cm space in the chest cavity (from apex to diaphragm) to use the instrument. This obviates the use of the stapler in children much younger than 3 or 4 years of age.

The basic principle of creating a baseball diamond–like configuration is useful to keep in mind as we discuss spe-

T. E Lobe: Department of Pediatrics and Preventive Medicine, University of Tennessee; and LeBonheur Children's Medical Center, Memphis, Tennessee.

TABLE 82.1. CONGENITAL LESIONS AMENABLE TO THORACOSCOPIC REPAIR

Tracheoesophageal fistula
Esophageal atresia
Pulmonary sequestration
Lobar emphysema
Congenital cystic adenomatoid malformations
Patent ductus arteriosus
Vascular rings
Enteric duplications
Mediastinal cysts
Tracheomalacia

TABLE 82.2. ACQUIRED LESIONS AMENABLE TO THORACOSCOPIC MANAGEMENT

Mediastinal lymphadenopathy
Mediastinal mass
Empyema
Pulmonary interstitial infiltrate
Trauma
Pleural disease
Myasthenia gravis
Persistent pleural effusion
Pericardial effusion
Pulmonary metastases
Scoliosis
Infections
Emphysematous blebs

cific procedures. The lesion is surrounded with multiple access ports. This allows both the instruments and the telescope to change perspective to facilitate dissection.

BIOPSY OF A MEDIASTINAL OR PLEURAL LESION

Most mediastinal lesions can be easily sampled for biopsy via thoracoscopy. There are many instances in pediatrics for which biopsy of a mediastinal mass or lymph node is essential for diagnosis. Differentiating between infection and malignancy is usually the issue. Staging of a tumor or reevaluation after chemotherapy and radiation such as in patients with mediastinal lymphoma may be the impetus to perform the biopsy.

The position of the table depends on whether or not the lesion is in the superior or inferior mediastinum and whether it is anterior or posterior. We use the position that takes the greatest advantage of gravity, allowing the lung to fall dependently once it is collapsed.

Once the structure for biopsy is identified and its relationship to major vascular structures is clearly outlined, biopsy sampling can be performed using one of several techniques. A biopsy forceps can be used to take a bite out of the tissue. We wait for the pathologist to confirm that they have adequate tissue for diagnosis, markers (as in the case of lymphomas), or other biologic studies before we remove the instruments. Some bleeding may be encountered at the biopsy site. This can be controlled in most cases with tamponade, coagulation, or simply by aspirating the pneumothorax from the chest cavity, allowing the tissues to abut against each other.

EVACUATION OF A LOCULATED PLEURAL EFFUSION/EMPYEMA

Children occasionally develop persistent pleural effusions associated with pneumonia or frank empyema. In cases of loculated pleural effusion for which a chest tube may not adequately drain the fluid, or of an empyema that does not respond to antibiotics, it is helpful to perform an early thoracoscopy with drainage.

We position the patient laterally with the affected side up. The chest is entered through an intercostal space over the largest part of the fluid collection. One or two ports can be used, depending on how thick and tenacious one finds the substance in the pleural space. Chest tubes are placed until the drainage is minimal (<50 mL/day).

PLEURODESIS FOR MALIGNANT PLEURAL EFFUSION OR RECURRENT PNEUMOTHORAX

Recurrent pneumothoraces are frequent occurrences in some conditions of childhood, such as cystic fibrosis. Although pleural effusions are not as common in childhood cancer as in adults with this condition, when they do occur and the patient is symptomatic, it may be helpful to perform pleurodesis. This can be carried out using USP purified talc, caustic agents such as certain antibiotics or chemotherapeutic agents, or mechanical debridement using a disposable dissector or some sort of energy delivery device. Rarely, stripping the pleura from the chest wall will be necessary.

LUNG BIOPSY

The most commonly requested thoracic procedure in pediatric patients is a lung biopsy. Thoracoscopy allows the surgeon to select the area of biopsy by direct inspection, and permits the surgeon to obtain ample tissue with a minimum of morbidity. Childhood malignancies often present with pulmonary involvement. In these cases, biopsy becomes necessary to differentiate between granulomatous disease and metastatic disease. The differentiation is important for staging and prognosis. These biopsies for the diagnosis and staging of childhood tumors can be performed effectively using thoracoscopic techniques.

Biopsy of the lung using the linear stapler requires placement of a 12-mm cannula. We usually prefer to triangulate or surround the lesion by placing the thoracoscope, the stapler, and the grasping forceps at the apexes of a triangle, the center of which is the lesion to be sampled for biopsy.

After the stapler is fired and the lung has been adequately expanded, there are rarely air leaks. We refrain from routinely placing a chest tube, but instead prefer to obtain a postoperative radiograph to assure that there is no significant pneumothorax. If a pneumothorax is present but the patient is not in distress, we obtain a chest radiograph several hours later. If we discover an enlarging pneumothorax, we insert a chest tube through one of the trocar sites. In our extensive use with the linear stapler device, we have yet to place a chest tube after a segmental lung biopsy except in those cases on high positive pressure ventilation for which we place the tube prophylactically.

BLEBECTOMY

The resection of emphysematous blebs when they have ruptured and persist in leaking can be accomplished as easily as a lung biopsy. The apex of the upper lobe is grasped and the stapler is fired across the base of the portion that contains blebs, preferably through normal lung parenchyma. This procedure is usually combined with some form of mechanical or chemical pleurodesis. It is well tolerated, and in most patients bilateral resections can be performed during the same period of anesthesia.

LOBECTOMY

Lobectomy in children is rarely indicated except for infection or congenital anomalies such as pulmonary sequestration. When lobectomy is indicated, thoracoscopy may obviate the need for postoperative chest tubes and prolonged hospitalization.

Usually four or five cannulas are necessary to complete the procedure. We begin our dissection at the hilum, taking care to identify all structures carefully. Arteries and veins are clipped or ligated with a Ligasure (ValleyLab, Boulder, Colorado) device. In small children, clips may be adequate for the bronchus as well. Alternatively, once the tissue to the hilum is adequately dissected free, a vascular endoscopic stapler device may be applied across the hilum dividing the artery, vein, and bronchus in one application.

If the surgeon is adept at endoscopic suturing techniques, the individual hilar structures can be dissected free and then suture ligated. Extraction may require a small intercostal incision.

BRONCHOGENIC CYST

Cystic lesions of the mediastinum in children, such as bronchogenic cysts or duplications, can be easily excised thoracoscopically. If the lesion is likely to be next to the esophagus, an esophageal bougie should be passed for easier identification during dissection. In one of our cases, part of the cyst wall formed the posterior wall of a mainstem bronchus. The rent was closed with simple endoscopic sutures, and the patient did well.

LIGATION OF PATENT DUCTUS ARTERIOSUS

Although it may not be suitable for preterm or small infants, patients over six months of age who have no other cardiac defects and whose clinical condition warrants ligation of a patent ductus arteriosus are ideal candidates for a thoracoscopic approach.

A three-trocar technique is used with the patient placed prone with the left side elevated about 40 degrees. The first trocar is placed in the third left intercostal space, in the midaxillary line. The next two trocars are placed in the posterior axillary line in the second and fourth intercostal spaces. With collapse of the lung, either with a blocker, selective intubation, or simple insufflation, the descending aorta and the left subclavian artery can be seen through the pleura. An incision is made along the aorta, and the pleura is dissected free anteriorly to expose the ductus arteriosus and its junction with the pulmonary artery. This can be accomplished solely with a right-angled hook cautery. The goal is to encircle the ductus. Care should be taken so as not to injure the ductus or the recurrent laryngeal nerve that can be seen coursing around the structure. If possible, the ductus should be freed up for its entire length between the pulmonary artery and the aorta. A zero silk suture can then be passed around the ductus and tied extracorporeally. If the ductus is small enough, a couple of hemoclips can be applied. A chest tube usually is not necessary if the lung is reexpanded in the operating room. The complication rate is similar to ductus ligation performed using open thoracotomy

THYMECTOMY

Thymectomy for myasthenia gravis in childhood is easy to perform and has the advantage of a quicker recovery. A three-trocar technique similar to that described for ductus ligation is used, except that the patient is supine with the left side raised slightly. After cannula placement, insufflation, and telescope insertion, it is easy to visualize the thymus and distinguish thymic tissue from mediastinal fat and adjacent structures. An incision is made in the mediastinal pleura, anterior to the phrenic nerve. The inferior portion of the thymus, with any adjacent mediastinal fat, is swept off the pericardium. Dissection continues cephalad until the innominate vein is identified. Veins draining with thymus are ligated with endoscopic clips and divided. The arterial supply from the internal mammary vessels is also ligated and divided. All visible mediastinal fat should be removed from the neck to the apex of the heart because some of this fat may be remnants of thymic tissue.

The patient usually stays overnight due to concerns about postoperative weakness and the potential need for ventilator support.

AORTOPEXY

Aortopexy is a procedure of some controversy but is widely used by many pediatric surgeons whose patients have tracheomalacia secondary to esophageal atresia or vascular compression. Until recently, aortopexy was performed by placing several sutures into the adventitia of the aorta and innominate artery to suspend the aorta from the sternum. Recently, the technique of pericardial flap aortopexy has been described. This technique has become popular because it may be safer and is easier to perform. It is ideal for a thoracoscopic approach.

The patient is positioned and prepared as described above for a thymectomy. Bronchoscopy is performed first, as with the open procedure. If the decision to proceed is made, trocars are placed as for a thymectomy. Being careful to avoid the phrenic nerve, the thymus is dissected off the anterior pericardium. The left lobe of the thymus is then removed if it is in the way. Next, a 2 × 3 cm flap of pericardium is raised so that its base is at the aortic root. A small transverse incision is then made over the sternum and a pouch is made. A 2-0 nonabsorbable braided suture is passed through the anterior sternum and delivered into the operative field under direct thoracoscopic vision. This suture is then passed through a corner of the flap and subsequently passed back through the sternum near the first entry site. A second suture is passed in a similar manner so that the other corner of the flap is looped. While looking through the bronchoscope, tension is applied to the sutures until the aorta pulls the trachea sufficiently anterior. These sutures are then tied anterior to the sternum within the pouch and the sternal incision is closed. Alternatively, there is another percutaneous suturing technique that obviates the need for the incision over the sternum. When done, the pneumothorax is evacuated and the cannula sites are closed. A postoperative chest tube is not necessary.

SCOLIOSIS

Recently, pediatric orthopedists are involving us in the management of patients with spinal deformities, such as scoliosis. Thoracoscopy provides a minimally invasive approach to enucleating the desired disk spaces in order to facilitate a posterior fusion.

Patients are placed laterally on the table (or, as some surgeons prefer, prone so that they do not have to be repositioned). A telescope first is inserted into the chest cavity in the midaxillary line for inspection and selection of the disks for enucleation. Additional ports are placed as necessary for instrumentation. Typically, two other ports, one cephalad and one caudal to the telescope, are used for suction, hemostasis, and disk extraction at the desired levels. After the bone graft is placed in the empty disk spaces, if fusion is the goal, a chest tube is left for drainage for a few days. Most of these patients do quite well, and most of their discomfort seems to come from the spinal manipulation as opposed to the incision.

TRACHEOESOPHAGEAL FISTULA AND ESOPHAGEAL ATRESIA

We now have ample experience to recommend thoracoscopic repair of esophageal atresia with or without a tracheoesophageal fistula. The patient is positioned as for a ductus ligation, except the right side is exposed. This approach is transpleural, but otherwise follows the principles of the conventional extrapleural thoracotomy. The only other exception is that it is easier to ligate the fistula with clips, and the sutures are tied extracorporeally. To date, the results are comparable with open repair. The advantage of this approach is the postoperative appearance and the diminished risk of late, postthoracotomy scoliosis.

PITFALLS AND COMPLICATIONS

We have had relatively few complications of thoracoscopy in children. The complications can be grouped into two categories: access and operative. Early in our experience, one of our patients developed hemodynamic manifestations of what appeared to be an air embolism that occurred as air was being injected to establish a pneumothorax. On closer scrutiny, the patient had been selectively intubated and the lung on the affected side allowed to deflate. Without a pneumothorax, this maneuver results in elevation of the diaphragm. Our needle was inserted into the right fifth intercostal space, and thus had most likely passed through the elevated diaphragm into the liver. The air we injected caused an air embolism. The patient stabilized after several minutes and we continued with an uneventful thoracoscopy.

In one of our cases of a teenage boy who had undergone chemotherapy, a thoracotomy, and pulmonary radiation, we had difficulty establishing access because of the adhesions. Eventually, we discovered that our trocar had gone through the diaphragm and we were peering into the peritoneal cavity. We withdrew the trocar and had to perform a thoracotomy to rule out recurrent tumor arising from the diaphragm. There were no visceral injuries, the hole in the diaphragm was closed, and no tumor was discovered at thoracotomy.

There have been several cases of an apparent mediastinal mass or nodes as diagnosed by imaging techniques. Because it is difficult to feel in the mediastinum by palpation, we converted two cases to a thoracotomy when we could not find the suspected lesion. In both cases, no lesion was found. We no longer convert a thoracoscopic case to a thoracotomy if the suspected lesion cannot be identified, and we believe that an adequate thoracoscopic search has been performed. We converted one other case of a large subcranial mass to a thoracotomy when we discovered that the mass was intimately adherent to vital structures and we did not believe that we could adequately remove the mass thoracoscopically.

Although the instruments and techniques exist to obtain any amount of tissue desired, there is a temptation to get the smallest sample of tissue that will yield an answer to the diagnostic dilemma. This becomes a problem with some cases for which the diagnosis is not clear, despite multiple samples. When the pathologist cannot make a diagnosis, but we believe that we have sampled more than adequate material, we prefer to wait for the permanent sections to be interpreted and the cultures to be evaluated before we subject the child to an open procedure.

We have been so pleased with the airtight, hemostatic incision line generated by the endoscopic stapling devices that are available that we do not routinely use a postoperative chest tube in patients who do not require mechanical ventilation. We performed one such biopsy on a patient with severe interstitial lung disease who had a stormy postoperative course and who ultimately required ventilatory support. After several hours on the ventilator at high pressures, a tension pneumothorax developed on the side from which the biopsy sample was taken. Since then, we use postoperative chest tubes on all patients with severe parenchymal disease who are likely to require mechanical ventilation within 48 hours of biopsy sampling. We have had no postoperative hemorrhage or other significant problem requiring reoperation after thoracoscopy in our pediatric patients.

SUGGESTED READINGS

Chan W, Keyser-Gauvin E, Davis GM, et al. Empyema thoracis in children: a 26-year review of the Montreal Children's Hospital experience. *J Pediatr Surg* 1997;32:870–872.

Chen MK, Schropp KP, Lobe TE. The use of minimal access surgery in pediatric trauma: a preliminary report. *J Laparoendosc Surg* 1995;5:295–301.

Kercher KW, Attorri RJ, Hoover JD, et al. Thoracoscopic decortication as first-line therapy for pediatric parapneumonic empyema. A case series. *Chest* 2000;118:24–27.

Laborde F, Folliguet TA, Etienne PY, et al. Video-thoracoscopic surgical interruption of patent ductus arteriosus. Routine experience in 332 pediatric cases. *Eur J Cardiothorac Surg* 1997;11:1052–1055.

Lavoie J, Burrows FA, Hansen DD. Video-assisted thoracoscopic surgery for the treatment of congenital cardiac defects in the pediatric population [see comments]. *Anesth Analg* 1996;82:563–567.

Newton PO, Shea KG, Granlund KF. Defining the pediatric spinal thoracoscopy learning curve: sixty-five consecutive cases. *Spine* 2000;25:1028–1035.

Rao BN. Present day concepts of thoracoscopy as a modality in pediatric cancer management. *Int Surg* 1997;82:123–126.

Tobias JD. Thoracoscopy in the pediatric patient. *Anesthesiol Clin North Am* 2001;19:173–186.

Waldhausen JH, Tapper D, Sawin RS. Minimally invasive surgery and clinical decision-making for pediatric malignancy. *Surg Endosc* 2000;14:250–253.

83

EMPYEMA

CHRISTINE M. FINCK
SAMUEL D. SMITH

Empyema is a reactive infection of the pleural space, and primary bacterial processes in the lungs such as pneumonia are the cause in 60% of cases. Other causes include infections in the neck, chest wall, thoracic spine, mediastinal nodes, or following trauma. In addition, surgery on the esophagus, lung, or mediastinum accounts for 2% to 12% of cases. In children, approximately 0.6% of pneumonias are complicated by empyema, and the incidence of empyema in children ranges from 0.4 to 6 per 1,000 admissions.

In general, childhood empyema is secondary to direct spread of a pulmonary infection to a parapneumonic effusion. This pleural effusion may result from permeability changes secondary to inflammatory disease or infection. These fluid collections are a rich culture medium and are difficult areas for the body's defense system to function well.

Empyemas commonly develop in three stages. The acute or exudative phase (stage I) is characterized by thin, serous fluid with very little debris. In the transitional or fibrinopurulent phase (stage II), the fluid becomes turbid and thick with pleural fibrin deposition. At this stage, a peel starts to become evident and loculations may develop. In the last phase (stage III), organization occurs with a thick fibrous peel, fibroblast proliferation, and scar formation that may entrap the lung if allowed to progress. Empyema necessitans is a rare condition in which a chronic empyema erodes through the chest wall and manifests as a draining sinus or abscess.

Historically, the most common microorganisms associated with empyema in childhood included *Haemophilus influenzae*, *Staphylococcus aureus*, and *Streptococcus pneumoniae*. Since the introduction of routine vaccination of children against *H. influenzae*, most cases of empyema are now due to *Streptococcus pneumoniae* or *Staphylococcus aureus*. The majority of patients present after having been treated with antibiotics for a period of time. This may account for sterile cultures that are obtained at the time of definitive surgical drainage.

DIAGNOSTIC APPROACH

Patients with an empyema have symptoms that range from mild to severe. Fever, dyspnea, pleuritic chest pain, and a productive cough are common but are difficult to distinguish from the symptoms produced by the primary pneumonia. Tachypnea with retractions, diminished breath sounds, and dullness to percussion are often present, but are also not specific. Empyema should be suspected in any child with pneumonia who fails to improve with adequate antibiotics or whose symptoms begin to worsen after initial signs of improvement. High spiking fevers, hypoxia resulting in a supplemental oxygen requirement, and persistent white blood cell count elevation are all suggestive of an infected parapneumonic effusion or empyema.

Evidence of an empyema is usually identified first on a plain radiograph of the chest. Haziness or white-out of a portion of the hemithorax is suggestive of a fluid collection. Lateral decubitus films may show some layering of fluid if the empyema is still in its early stages. Ultrasonography is now the primary diagnostic modality we use in determining the stage of an empyema. The presence of loculations or debris indicates that the empyema is at an advanced stage (usually stage II–III) and is likely to require more than drainage or tube thoracostomy for treatment. Computed tomography (CT) is also used in some centers for evaluation of patients with possible empyema. CT has the added benefit of helping to define the extent of the underlying parenchymal disease, and can help determine if a lung abscess, pneumatocele, pulmonary necrosis, pneumothorax, or bronchopleural fistula is present.

TECHNICAL APPROACH

Parapneumonic empyema is an important source of morbidity in the pediatric population despite the development

C. M. Finck: Department of Pediatric Surgery, Arkansas Children's Hospital, Little Rock, Arkansas.

S. D. Smith: Department of Surgery, University of Arkansas for Medical Sciences; and Department of Pediatric Surgery, Arkansas Children's Hospital, Little Rock, Arkansas.

of more effective antibiotics and the trend toward earlier surgical drainage in patients in whom medical management has failed. Patients also typically present in a delayed fashion, and therefore conservative management often fails. Some surgeons recommend the use of antibiotics with tube thoracostomy alone in the treatment of empyema. In our experience, this is useful only in the management of an early (stage I) empyema. Several studies have documented success with chest tube drainage in advanced empyema, but this comes at the expense of prolonged hospital stay and the use of more than one chest tube. Hoff and colleagues reported a mean hospital stay of 20.7 days with this method, and McLaughlin et. al had an average hospital stay of 22.6 days. Meier et al. treated 27 children initially with tube thoracostomy and 25.9% of these children required more than two chest tubes. In addition, 63% of these children required general anesthesia or conscious sedation for placement of the chest tube. The question arises as to whether this is a safe procedure to be performed on a surgical ward as opposed to the operating room.

Tube thoracostomy with instillation of fibrinolytic agents has been described. Urokinase has been the most commonly used fibrinolytic, but has recently been removed from the market. Recombinant products are being investigated at present. Meier et al. reported on the use of fibrinolytic treatment with tube thoracostomy in 22 patients. The patients received a mean of 4.4 treatments, and 14.8% required salvage video-assisted thoracoscopic (VATS) surgery. This salvage surgery significantly increased the cost of treatment compared with initial VATS treatment alone. At the present time, tube thoracostomy with fibrinolytic therapy is not in wide practice.

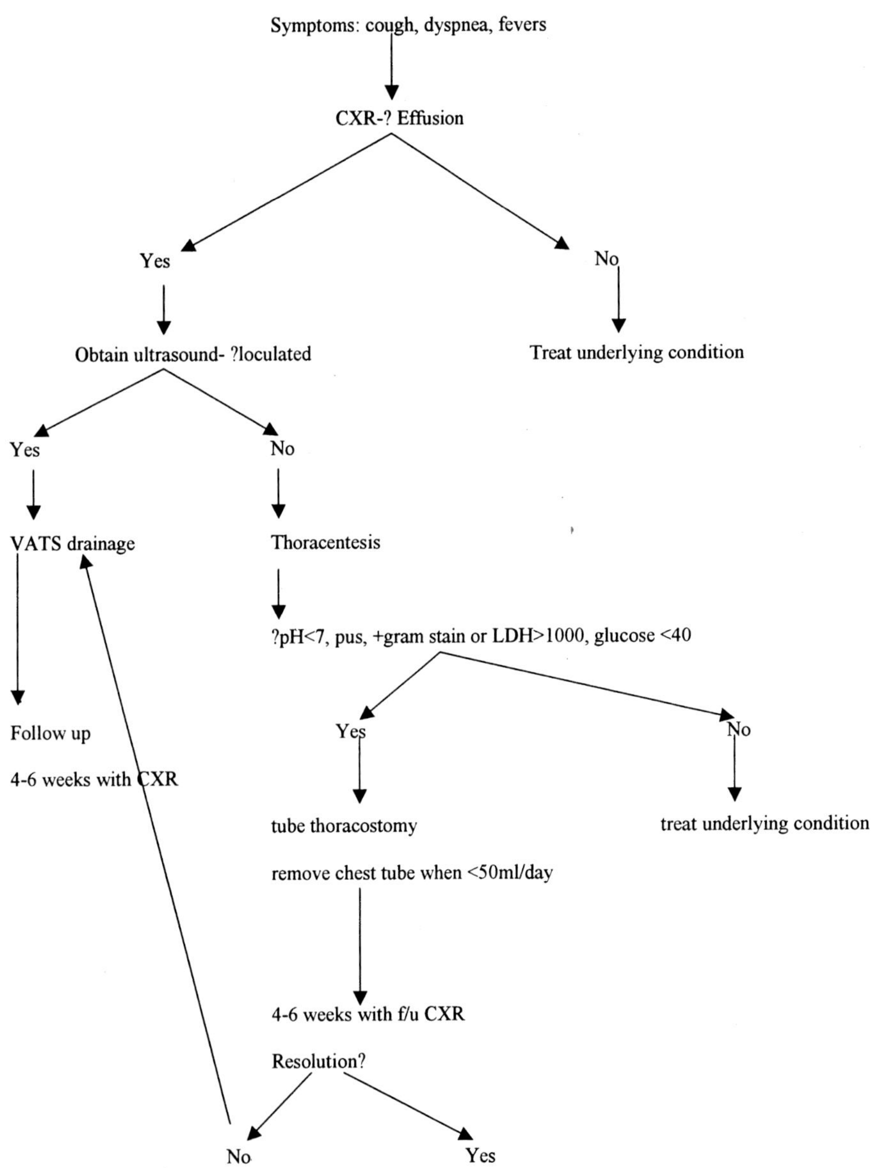

FIGURE 83.1. Algorithm for management of an empyema. *CXR,* chest x-ray.

In our opinion, the goal of treating an empyema is to drain and debride the pleural space, thus allowing the lung to expand and function normally. Figure 83.1 depicts our initial approach to the workup and management of a patient with an empyema. A patient with persistent or worsening fever, dyspnea, or cough undergoes chest radiography. If there is a parapneumonic effusion, chest ultrasonography is performed. If the effusion is loculated, the diagnosis of empyema is made and we recommend drainage and debridement by VATS surgery. If the effusion is free flowing and not loculated, we attempt to determine whether the fluid is infected or merely reactive by means of thoracentesis and analysis of the fluid. Fluid with a pH of less than 7, lactate dehydrogenase level of greater than 1,000 units/L glucose level of less than 40 mg/dL, many white cells, or a Gram stain showing bacteria is treated with tube thoracostomy. Patients treated with thoracostomy who fail to improve are then treated with operative debridement using VATS surgery (Fig. 83.1). We reported on 25 children treated with early VATS surgery and decortication as first-line treatment for empyema. Our postoperative length of stay using the above criterion was 4.9 ± 2.7 days. There were no postoperative complications, unplanned returns to the operating room, or deaths.

Open surgical drainage and decortication can be performed early in the course of the disease, usually within 3 to 5 days of hospitalization. Most children improve with this approach, but there are reports of increased morbidity, including wound infections, persistent air leaks, recurrent empyema, and bleeding causing increased lengths of stay. We feel that thoracotomy offers no significant advantage over the minimally invasive approach.

TECHNIQUE OF VIDEO-ASSISTED THORACOSCOPIC SURGERY

Video-assisted thoracoscopic surgery is performed under general anesthesia with a single-lumen endotracheal tube. Selective bronchial intubation is rarely necessary. We routinely use epidural anesthesia for postoperative pain relief. The patient is positioned in the lateral decubitus position with the involved side up. One laparoscopic trocar is used for the telescope and is placed in the sixth intercostal space in the midposterior axillary line. A 5- or 10-mm 0 degree telescope is used. Pleural fluid is aspirated and sent for Gram staining and culture. Carbon dioxide is insufflated, and additional incisions in the intercostal space are made under thoracoscopic visualization to allow placement of instruments directly into the thoracic cavity. All incisions should be made along a line that can be used for a thoracotomy if one becomes necessary. Curved, straight, ring, stone, and dressing forceps are used to debride the pleural cavity and remove the fibrinous peel. Then, under direct vision, the lung is expanded. If it does not expand completely, we perform a formal decortication, removing the visceral pleural peel. This can be done by using a sponge or peanut dissector. The cavity is irrigated with saline, hemostasis is verified, and a chest tube is placed through one of the trocar incisions.

Limitations of VATS surgery are related to the size of the patient. In general, children that are over 2 years of age are of adequate size to undergo the procedure with standard trocars, scopes, and instruments. Children under 1 year of age should be considered for open thoracotomy because the size of the camera and trocars are generally too large. The decision to perform VATS surgery in children who are 1 to 2 years of age is made on an individual basis.

POSTOPERATIVE CARE

For the majority of patients, postoperative recovery is on the pediatric surgery ward and not in the intensive care unit. Respiratory therapy is initiated on all patients and includes chest physiotherapy, deep breathing, and coughing exercises. Intravenous antibiotics are continued in the perioperative period and are modified according to culture results. We routinely use clindamycin and cefotaxime. In general, a chest tube is placed to water seal after 24 to 48 hours of suction. If drainage is minimal and chest radiography confirms expansion, the chest tube is removed. In our study, the average chest tube duration was 3.2 ± 2.2 days. In addition, we have found that the majority of postoperative chest radiographs do not show clearing for 4 to 6 weeks following decortication. For this reason, we use clinical criteria in determining when to discharge patients. In our study, the average length of stay for early VATS decortication was 4.9 days, patients were off supplemental oxygen in 2.3 ± 2 days, and all were afebrile prior to discharge. We frequently discharge our patients on a 7-day course of oral clindamycin, depending on culture results.

RESULTS AND FOLLOW-UP

Our patients are scheduled for a return visit in 4 to 6 weeks, at which time they have a repeat chest radiograph. We review symptoms, fevers, activity level, and appetite. The chest x-ray usually shows clearing of the empyema, although some still demonstrate residual opacification. In our study, follow-up data were available for 88% of the patients. In these children, symptoms had resolved and chest radiography showed clearing of previous radiographic abnormalities.

Complications from an empyema are rare and include anemia, osteomyelitis of the ribs or vertebrae, pericarditis, thrombocytopenia, mediastinal abscesses, scoliosis, and disseminated infections. Some pitfalls in treatment of patients with empyema include persistent pleural space infection, mistaking lung consolidation for effusion, development of pneumatoceles, and lung necrosis. In addition, follow-up radiographs may demonstrate restriction of the chest on the affected side with development of scoliosis. Clinically, if the patient is improved, observation and exercises are advised. In the majority of cases, radiographs demonstrate evidence of resolution of the process after another 6 weeks.

SUGGESTED READINGS

De Souza A, Offner PJ, Moore EE, et al. Optimal management of complicated empyema. *Am J Surg* 2000;180:507–511.

Grewal H, Jackson R, Wagner CW, et al. Early video-assisted thoracic surgery in the management of empyema. *Pediatrics* 1999;103:1–5.

Kercher KW, Attorri RJ, Hoover JD, et al. Thoracoscopic decortication as first line therapy for pediatric parapneumonic empyema: a case series. *Chest* 2000;118:24–27.

Meier AH, Smith B, Raghavan A, et al. Rational treatment of empyema in children. *Arch Surg* 2000;135:907–912.

Tuggle D. Acquired pulmonary and pleural disorders. In: Ashcraft KW et al., eds. *Pediatric surgery, 3rd ed.* Philadelphia: WB Saunders, 2000:287–289.

84

LUNG BIOPSY

WALTER PEGOLI, JR.
GEORGE T. DRUGAS

Lung biopsy is the most specific and sensitive procedure for diagnosing parenchymal lung disease in children or adults, whether it be infectious, neoplastic, or vasculitic. Most children with undiagnosed lung disease will have been seen by a multitude of pediatric subspecialists and will have undergone a battery of noninvasive radiographic studies to delineate the extent of their disease prior to consultation with a pediatric surgeon. In patients with interstitial lung disease of uncertain etiology, bronchoalveolar lavage and transbronchial biopsy are frequently performed to identify the underlying process. The diagnostic yield of bronchoalveolar lavage and transbronchial biopsy is moderate, establishing the diagnosis in well over half of patients. Complications using these techniques are uncommon. If the diagnosis remains uncertain, then lung biopsy is performed. Lung biopsy, performed as an open or minimally invasive procedure, provides adequate tissue for histologic and microbiologic examinations.

OPEN LUNG BIOPSY

Open lung biopsy in children is an invasive procedure requiring general anesthesia, thoracotomy, and partial lung excision. The site of biopsy is dictated by diagnostic imaging. Helical computed tomography (CT) scan is most often used to identify the pulmonary segment to be sampled for biopsy. In immunocompromised patients with an interstitial process of uncertain etiology, the disease is usually diffuse and bilateral. The lingula and the right middle lobe are the most accessible sites for biopsy. Anterolateral thoracotomy is the most common approach. The ipsilateral hemithorax is usually elevated to 30 to 45 degrees by placing a soft roll under the thorax. The fifth interspace is entered through a curvilinear skin incision at least one fingerbreadth below the nipple–areolar complex. Unless extensive exploration is necessary, the incision can be made quite small (2–4 cm in length) and still allow an adequate portion of lung to be brought out for inspection and biopsy. If pleural fluid is encountered, a sample is obtained and sent for appropriate cultures and cytology. The underlying lung parenchyma and pleural space are palpated. When the lesion in question is a nodule, the lesion should be excised with a margin of normal parenchyma. A variety of gastrointestinal and vascular stapling devices are well suited for this job. These devices fire a series of staples through the tissue that create a line of coaptation that is air and water tight.

In patients with interstitial pulmonary infiltrates, a representative portion of lung tissue is excised using the stapling device in a similar fashion. Some surgeons prefer using hand-sewn, overlapping, horizontal mattress sutures of monofilament nonabsorbable suture to close the underlying lung defect. The specimen is then submitted for appropriate histologic or microbiologic analysis. Most surgeons place a chest tube into the pleural space through a separate incision inferior to the primary incision. The chest tube is secured to the skin using a nonabsorbable monofilament suture. Prior to closure of the chest, saline is instilled into the pleural space and the lung is inflated to 40 cm water pressure. If an air leak is noted along the suture line, figure-of-eight sutures of monofilament absorbable suture or fibrin glue sealant are used to obliterate the leak. The ribs are then approximated using absorbable sutures. The chest wall musculature also is approximated in an anatomic fashion using absorbable sutures. The skin is approximated with running subcuticular suture or staples. The chest tube is placed to closed suction drainage and is removed in 24 to 48 hours if there is no air leak. Air leaks are usually self-limited and are more likely to occur in patients with severe parenchymal disease requiring significant mechanical ventilatory support.

W. Pegoli, Jr.: Departments of Surgery and Pediatrics, University of Rochester School of Medicine and University of Rochester Medical Center, Rochester, New York.

G. T. Drugas: Departments of Surgery and Pediatrics, University of Rochester School of Medicine; and Department of Surgery, Strong Memorial Hospital, Rochester, New York.

VIDEO-ASSISTED LUNG BIOPSY

The indications for video-assisted thoracoscopic (VATS) lung biopsy are similar to those for open lung biopsy. Compared with open lung biopsy, VATS lung biopsy affords better visualization and permits biopsy of any area of the lung. VATS surgery is performed using general endotracheal anesthesia. This technique requires creation and maintenance of a pneumothorax throughout the procedure to visualize the underlying parenchyma. A dual-lumen endotracheal tube is preferred. However, if there are size constraints and intubation with a double-lumen tube is not an option, then contralateral mainstem intubation with a bronchial blocker (Fogarty or Foley catheter) may be used to achieve single-lung ventilation. Flexible fiberoptic bronchoscopy facilitates endotracheal tube placement.

Positioning of the patient on the operating table is dependent on the anatomic site of the lesion. Therefore, preoperative evaluation using helical CT is a necessity. The straight lateral approach is most often used for apical lesions. The 30 degree posterolateral position is indicated for anterior lesions. The 30 degree anterolateral position may be used to sample posterior lesions for biopsy. Depending on patient size, a 5- or 10-mm, 0 degree or 30 degree thoracoscope is used. The primary strategy is to place the instruments and the videothoracoscope so that all are oriented in the same direction, facing the target disease within a 180 degree arc. The incisions should be placed widely distant from each other so that the instruments do not crowd each other. For most procedures, the anesthesiologist is asked to stop ventilating the ipsilateral lung so that the lung will be collapsed prior to insertion of the videothoracoscope into the pleural space. The videothoracoscope is typically inserted through a port placed in the midaxillary line at the level of the seventh or eighth intercostal space. Instruments are introduced through ports typically placed in the anterior axillary line of the fifth intercostal space and 2 to 3 cm away from the posterior border of the scapula (Fig. 84.1). Thoughtful placement should provide optimal retraction angles and a direct approach for biopsy. The endoscopic stapler requires 10-mm thoracoports to gain entry into the pleural space. Most endoscopic lung clamps require 5-mm thoracoports. Once the lesion is identified, it may be excised using single or multiple firings of the stapling device. For suspected malignancies, to prevent tumor implantation, small specimens can be removed via the thoracoport. Larger specimens are retrieved in a disposable plastic specimen retrieval bag. The pleural space is then irrigated to remove debris and evaluate hemostasis. Electrocautery may be used to coagulate sites of bleeding. Intercostal blocks can be performed under direct vision with a mediastinoscopy aspiration needle. The chest cavity may be filled with saline while the anesthesiologist reinflates the ipsilateral lung to evaluate for air leak. Most surgeons place a chest tube at this time. The chest tube is placed through one of the port sites and secured to the skin using a monofilament nonabsorbable suture. The remaining port sites are closed using absorbable suture. The skin is approximated using a subcuticular closure. Chest tube management is similar to that for the open technique.

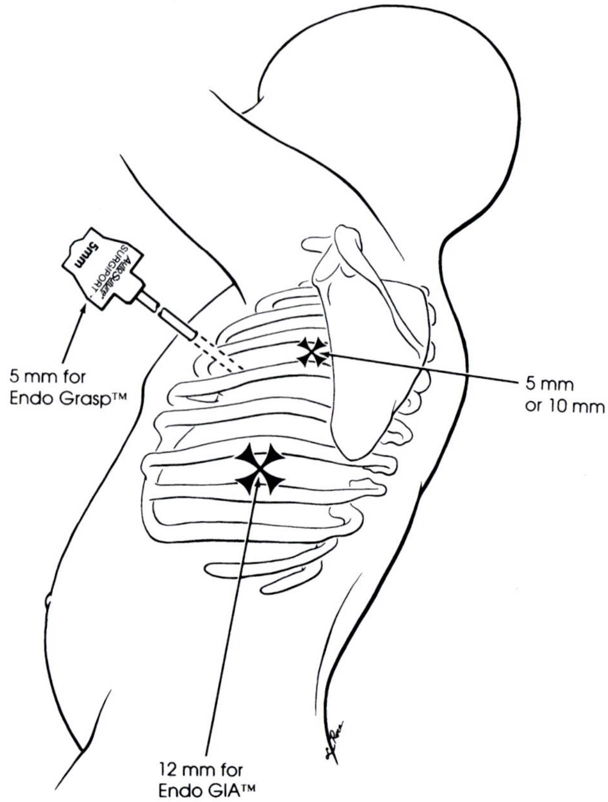

Figure 84.1. Typical trocar placement for video-assisted thoracoscopic lung biopsy using the triangular technique of trocar placement. Note that the Endo-GIA stapling device requires the use of a 12-mm port. (Reprinted from Lobe TL, Schropp KP. *Pediatric laparoscopy and thoracoscopy.* Philadelphia: WB Saunders, 1994:251; with permission.)

POSTOPERATIVE CARE

Procedure-related morbidity is low. Air leaks are common but the vast majority of them resolve spontaneously. Air leaks rarely impact respiratory status after the procedure. Only high-volume air leaks that more frequently reflect a failure of surgical pneumostasis rather than lung fragility per se may require reexploration and closure. Bleeding is rare, although more worrisome, with thoracoscopic biopsies. The use of vascular endoscopic staplers can often obviate this problem. Wound complications are minimal. Tumor seeding of a thoracoscopic incision by cancer has been reported with fatal outcome. A specimen bag should be used to protect the incision when removing a known or suspected malignancy. Prolonged drainage from the chest tube site is common. This problem is amenable to local wound care with wet to dry sterile dressings on an as-needed basis.

RESULTS

Lung biopsy in children is a useful diagnostic procedure that leads to significant changes in medical management and increases the diagnostic yield for infections, malignancies, and vasculitides. Complications are rare. The most serious complications, bleeding and persistent air leak, may necessitate open thoracotomy.

SUGGESTED READINGS

Korneckim A, Shemie SD. Open lung biopsy in children with respiratory failure. *Crit Care Med* 2001;29:1247–1250.

Lobe TE, Schropp KP, eds. *Pediatric laparoscopy and thoracoscopy.* Philadelphia: WB Saunders, 1994.

85

CHYLOTHORAX

SHERIF G.S. EMIL

Fluid in the pleural space is typically one of five entities: transudate, exudate, blood, pus, or chyle. Of these, chylous effusions are perhaps the easiest to diagnose but the most challenging to treat. Chylothorax is relatively common in the pediatric population. It is the most common cause of pleural effusion in the neonatal period, as well as during fetal life, if fetuses with hydrops fetalis are excluded. The pediatric surgeon is an important member of the team managing these patients, which often includes neonatologists, pulmonologists, pediatricians, cardiovascular surgeons, and dietitians. Early involvement is best, which allows the surgeon an accurate ongoing assessment of the patient's progress, the response to nonoperative management, and the need for surgical intervention.

Some general principles apply in the diagnosis and treatment of chylothorax in children of all ages. However, four discrete groups of patients can be identified based on pathophysiologic, therapeutic, and prognostic factors:

1. Fetuses with primary pleural effusions.
2. Neonates with congenital chylothorax.
3. Children with acquired chylothorax and absence of cardiac disease.
4. Children with acquired chylothorax after cardiac procedures.

DIAGNOSIS

Chylothorax is often suspected when a pleural effusion is discovered in the context of a clinical scenario that predisposes to its formation. If the chylothorax has increased rapidly in volume, or the effusion has gradually accumulated and reached a critical threshold of lung compression, patients present with respiratory embarrassment. Patients in intensive care units often have effusions identified on chest radiographs before symptoms have occurred.

S. G. S. Emil: Division of Pediatric Surgery, University of California, Irvine College of Medicine, Irvine, California; and Department of Pediatric Surgery, Miller's Children's Hospital, Long Beach, California.

In a symptomatic patient, tube thoracostomy is both diagnostic and therapeutic. A thoracentesis should be performed first in an asymptomatic or mildly symptomatic patient to establish the diagnosis. Some clinicians advocate repeated taps after the diagnosis is established. I do not advocate this approach. Thoracentesis in young children requires significant sedation and restraint. It has the potential of converting a chylothorax to a chylopneumothorax. Most importantly, placement of a tube thoracostomy begins the patient's treatment. It completely evacuates the effusion, permitting lung expansion and apposition of the visceral and parietal pleuras. Furthermore, it allows accurate documentation of the drainage amount, a key element in deciding further therapy. My approach is to use a catheter over needle device for the diagnostic thoracentesis and to aspirate as much fluid as possible the first time. If the effusion recurs, a tube thoracostomy should be performed. Suction is applied to the tube for the first 48 hours to optimize pleural apposition.

Chyle is generally milky with a yellowish hue. It is therefore often a visual diagnosis. This diagnosis is objectively confirmed by a differential cell count revealing more than 80% lymphocytes and a triglyceride level of more than 1.1 m*M* (100 mg/dL). If the patient has never been fed [e.g., after repair of esophageal atresia (EA) with distal tracheoesophageal fistula (TEF)], or has been fasted for several weeks, chyle may resemble a simple transudate in appearance and may not demonstrate a high triglyceride level. The lymphocyte count should still be elevated. However, if the diagnosis is uncertain, a standard diet or enteral formula may be used as a challenge to establish the character of the fluid.

MEDICAL TREATMENT

The vast majority of chylothoraces respond to nonoperative treatment. This treatment has three goals. The first is to externalize the chylous fistula through tube thoracostomy, avoiding recurrent accumulation of effusion and accurately documenting the output. This also helps to alleviate respiratory compromise.

The second goal is to counteract the effects of chyle loss. Chyle is rich in protein and lymphocytes. Chylothorax is therefore a source of protein loss. If the patient manifests continued net protein loss, the level of albumin and total protein in the effusion can be measured and used to guide parenteral or enteral nutritional therapy. In a few patients, particularly newborns and infants, a high-output chylothorax can constitute a significant volume loss. In these patients, replacement of the loss with 5% albumin is advisable. Because of the high lymphocyte count in chyle, the fluid has a bacteriostatic effect, generally rendering the effusion resistant to infection. It is commonly reported that this also leads to compromise of the patient's systemic immunity, but this only occurs if chyle loss is allowed to continue for several weeks. Routine antibiotics are probably not indicated.

The third goal of medical management is to decrease the chyle output by decreasing chyle production. A fistula is more likely to close if it has low output. Chyle production can be reduced either by completely resting the bowel and placing the patient on total parenteral nutrition (TPN) or by feeding the patient an enteral formula containing fat in the form of medium-chain triglycerides. TPN and complete bowel rest is the more aggressive form of nonoperative therapy. Some clinicians have advocated a week of enteral therapy before converting to TPN. A reasonable approach is to attempt enteral therapy (Vivonex, Novartis, New York, New York) for 48 hours. If there is no decrease in output, the patient should be switched to TPN. If the fistula demonstrates very high output from the beginning (>25 mL/kg/day), a trial of enteral nutrition is likely to fail.

A controversy is the duration of medical management before it is deemed a failure. Recommendations in the literature vary between 1 week and 3 months. Early intervention may result in unnecessary surgery, whereas late interventions may result in nutritional, and possibly immunologic, compromise. There is some evidence to suggest that the amount of drainage at 1 week is not predictive of success or failure. Therefore, most surgeons would be reluctant to intervene surgically before a 2-week period of maximal medical therapy has elapsed, unless there is profound lymphopenia or hypoalbuminemia. Some surgeons use a drainage amount of more than 10 mL/kg/day or 100 mL/year of age/day as a guideline. The pattern of drainage may be more important than the absolute amount. Drainage that does not progressively decrease over 2 weeks or that randomly fluctuates in amount, with periods of very high output, is unlikely to respond to medical measures within a reasonable time frame. If the amount of drainage is progressively decreasing, patience is almost always rewarded with resolution of the effusion.

High mean airway pressures and positive end-expiratory pressure have been used in the treatment of chylothorax, to decrease or equalize the normal abdomen-thorax pressure gradient. Successful use of somatostatin also has been reported.

SURGICAL TREATMENT

Multiple procedures have been suggested to treat chylothorax. These include identification and ligation of the leakage site, ligation of the thoracic duct above the diaphragm, pleurodesis, parietal pleurectomy, application of tissue adhesive, thoracoscopic approaches, and pleuroperitoneal shunting. Combinations of these procedures may be used because some are complementary. The choice also may be influenced by the cause of the chylothorax.

The patient should be prepared for surgery by optimizing respiratory and metabolic parameters. It would be convenient to have a road map of the thoracic duct and where the leak is occurring, but this is not always possible. It is often recommended to feed the patient cream preoperatively in an attempt to maximize fistula output and help identify it. The oral administration of iodine 123–labeled long-chain fatty acids may facilitate scintigraphic localization of leaks, but there is still limited experience in its use. It may be particularly worthwhile in cases of recurrence. Routine lymphangiography is not useful and is now rarely used.

Treatment of chylothorax lends itself nicely to a thoracoscopic approach, because visualization is excellent and minimal dissection is needed. Thoracoscopy is performed on the side of the chylothorax. Single-lung ventilation improves visualization greatly. In young children, temporary CO_2 insufflation to a pressure of 5 to 8 mm Hg also results in significant lung collapse.

Although the thoracic duct is variable in its position, its most predictable location is just superior to the aortic hiatus, through which it enters the chest. It can be found on the vertebral column a few millimeters medial to its right border. During operation for a right-sided chylothorax, the duct should be identified and traced upwards to identify the leakage point. Often the leakage is not in the duct proper but rather in a tributary or plexus of tributaries. If such a leakage is identified, the relevant tributaries should be clipped and treated with fibrin sealant. I also clip the duct above and below this point for added security. If no leakage point is identified, the duct is clipped as close to its origin as possible and a pleurodesis is performed. Finally, if neither the duct nor the leakage point can be identified, a pleurodesis alone should be performed. An effective thoracoscopic pleurodesis can be accomplished by insufflating 5 g of talc throughout the chest cavity. To accomplish this, place the talc in a trap and hook one end to the insufflator tubing and another end to a transparent silicone catheter. The catheter is then guided into all corners of the thoracic cavity using a grasper while the insufflator pressure is at 15 mm Hg. The resultant "snowstorm" distributes the talc throughout the thoracic cavity.

The thoracic duct crosses over to the left side at the level of the fifth thoracic vertebra. It is therefore seldom visualized on the left. Pleurodesis with ligation of the leak, if visualized, is the best option for left-sided chylothoraces.

Thoracoscopy can be used even after previous thoracotomy. The presence of the chyle prevents the visceral and parietal pleura from adhering and preserves free space within the chest cavity. The chest tube can be clamped for 48 hours prior to operation to allow chyle to build up, increasing the free space and facilitating open trocar placement. Thoracic adhesions after thoracotomy are typically thin and avascular. They can easily be taken down with endoscopic scissors.

Postoperatively, the chest tube is left on suction for 24 hours and then placed to water seal. It is removed when minimal serous drainage is seen, typically within 72 hours.

Pleuroperitoneal shunts have been successfully used to treat chylothorax. They essentially decompress the effusion into the abdomen and allow it to resolve over a long period of time. Although attractive in its simplicity, the procedure is associated with a significant incidence of shunt malfunction, infection, and abdominal wall hernias. It appears to be most successful when used as primary surgical therapy, not after other surgical approaches have failed.

FETAL CHYLOTHORAX

Fetal chylothorax, also called primary fetal hydrothorax, is diagnosed when a fetus has a significant pleural effusion in the absence of, or preceding the onset of, hydrops fetalis. The cause is unclear. It is frequently an isolated finding but also has been reported in association with Down's syndrome, Turner syndrome, and lymphatic malformations. Sonography may establish the diagnosis as early as 17 weeks' gestation. A large effusion can compress the lung and displace the mediastinum. Significant mediastinal compression can lead to hydrops and intrauterine demise. Polyhydramnios is common. The mortality rate in some series is as high as 50%. A good prognosis is associated with initial diagnosis after 33 weeks' gestation, delivery after 35 weeks' gestation, spontaneous resolution, the absence of hydrops, and unilaterality.

Diagnostic workup includes sonography, fetal echocardiography, and amniocentesis or cord blood sampling for cytogenetic analysis. Diagnostic thoracentesis is not recommended if the fetus is thriving, there is no hydrops, and the effusion is unilateral. It has significant risks and is unlikely to alter the management.

Treatment is dictated by the progress of the fetus and mother. If there is no hydrops and the effusion is small, observation and serial ultrasonography every 2 weeks suffice. If hydrops develops, the effusion should be decompressed. Repeated thoracenteses are associated with rapid fluid reaccumulation and poor results. Thoracoamniotic shunting appears to be the best option at this time. Hydrops developing at or near term is uncommon, but is best treated by delivery of the fetus. The presence of a large effusion without hydrops presents an interventional dilemma. Pulmonary hypoplasia is an inherent risk heightened by the threat of preterm delivery secondary to polyhydramnios. Close follow-up with ultrasonography is essential, and a thoracoamniotic shunt should be considered if the effusion continues to increase.

CONGENITAL CHYLOTHORAX

Congenital chylothorax does not always present immediately after birth. We recently treated a 6-week-old boy who presented with a right-sided chylothorax. The only pertinent history was the involvement of his mother in a motor vehicle accident 1 month before delivery. He responded very well to tube thoracostomy and dietary therapy. A history of traumatic delivery may be elicited in some cases.

Thoracoscopy is not a viable option in neonates and small infants. A mini-thoracotomy permits a reasonable exploration, in the rare cases where this becomes necessary. If chyle leaks are identified, they are ligated and treated with fibrin sealant. A parietal pleurectomy should be performed. The dissection is similar to the extrapleural approach to repair of an esophageal atresia.

ACQUIRED CHYLOTHORAX

Acquired chylothorax is usually the result of thoracic trauma or surgery. Any thoracic procedure, as well as any procedure that can injure the thoracic duct, can result in a chylothorax. It is seen after repair of esophageal atresia with distal TEF, CDH repair, and multiple attempts at placing a left subclavian venous line. The presentation of chylothorax can be delayed for up to 3 weeks after the injury. Superior vena cava thrombosis also may result in chylothorax. A child who acquires a chylothorax without an obvious predisposing factor should undergo computed tomography of the chest to look for lymphatic disorders, lymphomas, and inflammatory lesions, all of which can result in a chylothorax.

These patients usually respond to medical management. If operation is required, a discrete area of leakage usually can be identified.

CHYLOTHORAX AFTER CARDIAC SURGERY

These patients constitute the largest group in many series of pediatric chylothorax. The thoracic duct is vulnerable to injury during patent ductus arteriosus ligation and repair of aortic coarctation. A contributory factor is increased central venous pressure, which is transmitted to the thoracic duct and lymphatic tributaries. This pressure promotes leakage from injured lymphatics.

Treatment begins with attempts at prevention. The surgeon should be quite liberal in ligating lymphatics, because electrocautery is ineffective in sealing these vessels. Fibrin sealant should be used in any area that appears to have continued serous drainage at the end of the procedure. In this group of patients, medical treatment has the additional goal of optimizing cardiac function and preventing congestive heart failure. Most cardiac surgeons are extremely patient in treating this complication medically. Their patience is frequently rewarded, with few patients requiring reoperation.

Chyle leaks in these patients are typically diffuse and sometimes bilateral. Chemical pleurodesis and pleuroperitoneal shunting probably constitute the best alternatives. However, shunting may not be effective if right atrial pressure remains elevated above 20 mm Hg.

SUGGESTED READINGS

Alvarez JRF, Kalache KD, Grauel EL. Management of spontaneous congenital chylothorax: oral medium-chain triglycerides versus total parenteral nutrition. *Am J Perinatal* 1999;16:415–420.

Beghetti M, La Scala G, Belli D, et al. Etiology and management of pediatric chylothorax. *J Pediatr* 2000;136:653–658.

Buttiker V, Fanconi S, Burger R. Chylothorax in children: guidelines for diagnosis and management. *Chest* 1999;116:682–687.

Kettner BI, Aurisch R, Ruckert JC, et al. Scintigraphic localization of lymphatic leakage site after oral administration of iodine-123-IPPA. *J Nucl Med* 1998;39:2141–2144.

Laberge JM, Crombleholme TM, Longaker MT. The fetus with pleural effusions. In: Harrison MR, Golbus MS, Filly RA, eds. *The Unborn Patient, 2nd ed.* Philadelphia: WB Saunders, 1990: 314–319.

Wolff AB, Silen ML, Kokoska ER, et al. Treatment of refractory chylothorax with externalized pleuroperitoneal shunts in children. *Ann Thorac Surg* 1999;68:1053–1057.

Surgical Directives: Pediatric Surgery, edited by Peter Mattei. Lippincott Williams & Wilkins, Philadelphia © 2002

86

CONGENITAL LUNG ANOMALIES

TIPPI C. MACKENZIE
ALAN W. FLAKE

Congenital lung anomalies include congenital lobar emphysema, congenital cystic adenomatoid malformation, bronchopulmonary sequestration, and bronchogenic cysts. The presence of hybrid lesions containing elements of two or more of these anomalies has suggested a common embryologic basis of occurrence during the separation of the tracheobronchial tree from the primitive foregut. When there is a communication with the gastrointestinal tract, these lesions may be classified as communicating bronchopulmonary foregut malformations and lead to diverse clinical scenarios.

Many congenital lung anomalies are now diagnosed prenatally on routine ultrasonographic evaluation. Because there is a high incidence of coexisting anomalies, prenatal diagnosis should prompt a referral to a fetal diagnosis and treatment center with a full evaluation, including karyotype, ultrasonography, and, when necessary, ultrafast fetal magnetic resonance imaging (MRI). We have learned that the most important prognostic indicator with prenatally diagnosed pulmonary lesions is the size of the mass and its effects on normal physiology, rather than the histologic subtype. A large mass can cause mediastinal shift, lung hypoplasia from compression of normal lung, or polyhydramnios from compression of the esophagus. Most importantly, a large mass may compress the heart and great vessels, leading to cardiovascular compromise and hydrops. Fetuses with prenatally diagnosed lung anomalies should be followed closely for the development of hydrops, which is a harbinger of fetal or neonatal demise. Fetal intervention for such cases—by either lobectomy for predominantly solid lesions or thoracoamniotic shunting for lesions with a large cystic component—has been successful in select cases (Fig. 86.1). Although some lesions regress during fetal life, planned delivery at a tertiary care center with a thorough postnatal evaluation should be performed in all cases.

CONGENITAL LOBAR EMPHYSEMA

Congenital lobar emphysema (CLE) is defined as the abnormal inflation of an anatomically normal lung. It most commonly occurs secondary to an intrinsic defect in bronchial cartilage, which leads to airway collapse on expiration and progressive air trapping. However, extrinsic compression of bronchi from mediastinal masses (such as seen in congenital heart disease, bronchogenic cyst, etc.) or from long-term ventilation may lead to similar pathophysiology.

The most common site for CLE is the left upper lobe, followed by the right middle lobe and right upper lobe. Although babies may be asymptomatic immediately after birth, symptoms of respiratory distress and tachypnea develop within the first few days of life and progress quickly due to increased air trapping from crying. Rapid development of respiratory failure may require emergency thoracotomy.

The chest radiograph in CLE classically shows lobar hyperinflation, with mediastinal shift and flattening of the ipsilateral diaphragm. In newborns, the lesion may be radiopaque due to failure to clear lung liquid. The differential diagnosis includes pneumothorax or a congenital cystic adenomatoid malformation with a giant cyst. Further imaging with computed tomography (CT) may help to establish the correct diagnosis. In cases of CLE acquired from long-term positive pressure ventilation, a ventilation/perfusion scan may be useful to determine the portion of lung that is most severely affected (this would show poor perfusion and delayed uptake and clearance of radioisotope in the affected area).

Because CLE may be caused by extrinsic obstruction from abnormal mediastinal structures, it is crucial to exclude this preoperatively to avoid parenchymal resection of normal lung. This may be achieved by CT and preoperative bronchoscopy, as well as by mediastinal exploration at the time of surgery. Because patients with CLE have a high incidence of cardiac anomalies, echocardiography also

T. C. MacKenzie: Department of Surgery, Children's Hospital of Philadelphia, Philadelphia, Pennsylvania.

A. W. Flake: Department of Pediatric Surgery, University of Pennsylvania; and Department of Surgery, Children's Hospital of Philadelphia, Philadelphia, Pennsylvania.

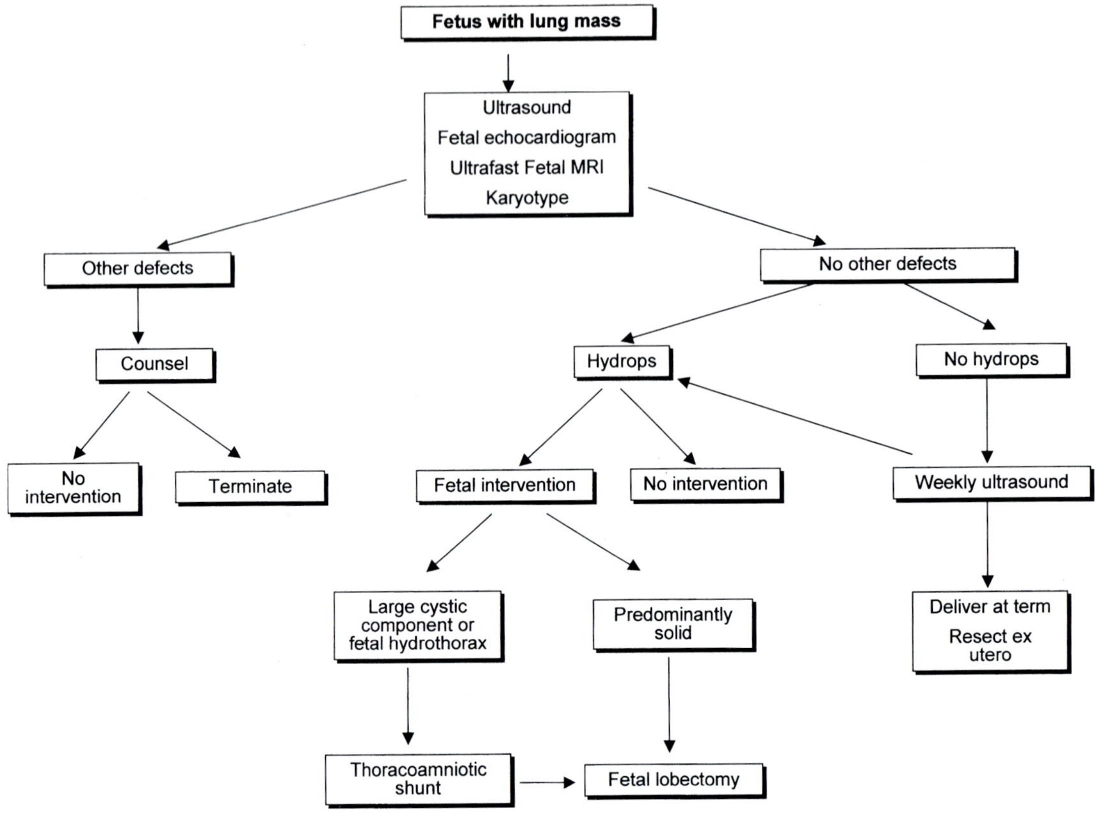

FIGURE 86.1. Algorithm for the management of prenatally diagnosed congenital lung lesions.

should be performed preoperatively. For patients who need ventilatory support preoperatively, high-frequency oscillatory ventilation should be used to avoid overexpansion of the lung. Positive pressure ventilation at the time of intubation for surgery may exacerbate air trapping, precipitating the need for emergent decompressive thoracotomy; it is therefore particularly important for the surgeon to be present during induction of anesthesia. The treatment of choice for CLE is lobectomy of the affected lung. Because there is a primary defect in cartilaginous support, bronchoplasty is not advocated.

CONGENITAL CYSTIC ADENOMATOID MALFORMATION

Congenital cystic adenomatoid malformation (CCAM) is characterized by abnormal overgrowth of bronchioles in one lobe of a lung, leading to disorganized cysts. Stocker has defined three types based on cyst size with varying prognoses. In patients who are prenatally diagnosed, a distinction is made between macrocystic lesions (with cysts >5 cm) and microcystic lesions (which appear echogenic on prenatal ultrasonography). Although the original classification assigned prognostic value to the histologic subtype, the outcome in prenatally diagnosed CCAM is more dependent on the size of the lesion and its effects on normal physiology. CCAM may be present in more than one lobe of the lung in 1% to 3% of cases.

Congenital cystic adenomatoid malformation is now commonly diagnosed prenatally by routine ultrasonography, especially when there is a large cyst. Although CCAM may be confused with a congenital diaphragmatic hernia on screening ultrasonography, detailed ultrasonography or ultrafast fetal MRI can be used to distinguish between these entities. Other possibilities in the differential diagnosis include bronchogenic cyst, foregut duplication cyst, congenital lobar emphysema, and mediastinal cystic teratoma. Patients who are not diagnosed prenatally may present as neonates with respiratory distress from a large lesion causing pulmonary hypoplasia, or with recurrent infections later in life from abnormal drainage of tracheobronchial secretions. Because there is a high incidence of associated anomalies (as high as 20%), it is important to do a thorough evaluation with echocardiography and karyotype.

It also has been noted that prenatally diagnosed lesions may regress spontaneously during gestation, resulting in an asymptomatic newborn with normal or minimal findings on chest radiography. It is our policy to perform postnatal CT on all of these infants to accurately document the

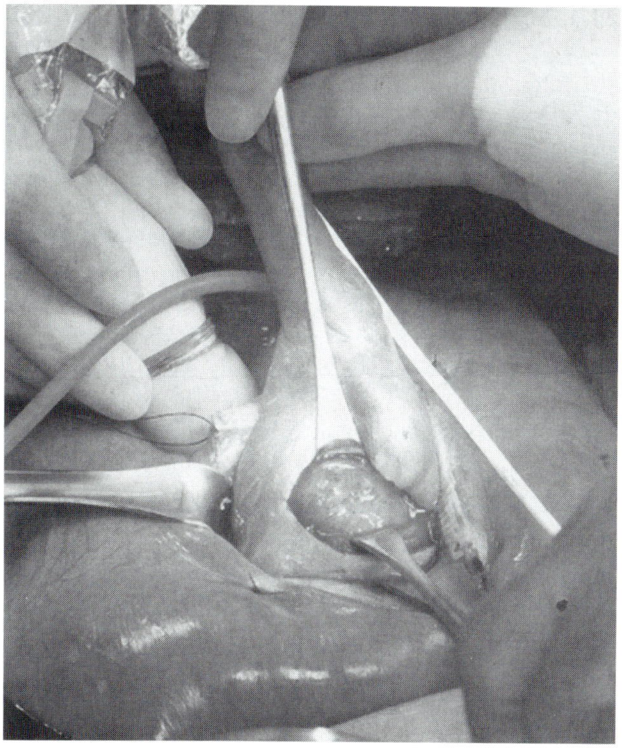

FIGURE 86.2. Intraoperative photograph of fetal lobectomy for a congenital cystic adenomatoid malformation. The fetal heart is monitored continuously by echocardiography during the operation.

extent of the residual CCAM. In our opinion, although controversial, all infants with residual macrocystic CCAM should undergo elective resection because of the known risks of infection, spontaneous pneumothorax, and the long-term risk for malignant degeneration (most commonly pulmonary blastoma and rhabdomyosarcoma). The presence of "hybrid" lesions with CCAM architecture and systemic blood supply is also recognized, further illustrating the close embryologic association between various congenital lung anomalies.

There is now considerable clinical data detailing the management and outcome of prenatally diagnosed CCAM. In our recent series of 134 cases of prenatally diagnosed CCAM, 101 were managed expectantly, with demise of all 25 fetuses who developed hydrops and were not treated *in utero.* In the fetal intervention category, 13 fetuses with hydrops underwent fetal lobectomy (Fig. 86.2), with 8 survivors, whereas 6 fetuses with giant cysts underwent thoracoamniotic shunting, with 5 survivors. This experience highlights the benefits of fetal intervention in select cases in which hydrops evolves, while illustrating that fetuses with large chest masses without hydrops can be managed expectantly by planned delivery and postnatal resection.

The treatment of choice is lobectomy of the involved segment. For patients who have had recurrent infections in that segment of lung, preoperative antibiotics should be used to reduce inflammation.

BRONCHOPULMONARY SEQUESTRATION

Bronchopulmonary sequestrations (BPS) are aberrant nonfunctional masses of normal lung tissue that do not communicate with the normal tracheobronchial tree. There are two types of sequestrations depending on whether the mass has its own pleural investment (extralobar) or exists within the normal pleura (intralobar). Extralobar sequestrations have a high incidence of associated anomalies, most commonly congenital diaphragmatic hernia. These are diagnosed earlier in life than intralobar sequestrations, because newborns often have respiratory distress or feeding intolerance. Extralobar sequestrations may be infradiaphragmatic and should be considered in the differential diagnosis of a retroperitoneal, suprarenal abdominal mass. Intralobar sequestrations, on the other hand, may be clinically silent until they present with recurrent pneumonias later in life. Associated anomalies are rare with this group of malformations. Sequestrations may be communicating with the gastrointestinal tract (communicating bronchopulmonary foregut malformations), confirming the close embryologic association between the two systems.

Many extralobar sequestrations are now diagnosed prenatally and may appear similar to microcystic CCAM on prenatal ultrasonography. Color Doppler imaging may demonstrate a systemic feeding vessel. In severe cases, the anomalous systemic blood supply may lead to arteriovenous fistula formation with high-output cardiac failure or hemorrhage. On plain film, extralobar lesions appear as posterior mediastinal masses, leading to a retrocardiac density on the anteroposterior view. Intralobar sequestrations that have been infected appear consolidated and may develop air-fluid levels. If there are clinical symptoms suggesting a communicating malformation, a gastrointestinal contrast study should be performed preoperatively.

Prenatally diagnosed BPS also may cause prenatal physiologic derangements, either from mass effect, as seen with large CCAMs, or more frequently from fluid exudation with development of tension hydrothorax. In our recent series of 41 prenatally diagnosed lesions, 3 fetuses developed tension hydrothorax from fluid or lymph secretion by the mass and needed fetal treatment with thoracoamniotic shunt or thoracentesis. Seven patients underwent postnatal resection with good survival and one patient with hydrops died after delivery despite postnatal ECMO. Twenty-eight of 41 lesions regressed in size during gestation, and no resection was required postnatally.

Extralobar sequestrations may be resected without disturbing the normal lung by either open thoracotomy or thoracoscopy. It is important to establish the blood supply to the lesion. Arterial supply is systemic, from the aorta, and may be infradiaphragmatic in 20% of cases. Venous drainage is usually to the azygous system for extralobar and to the pulmonary veins for intralobar sequestrations. The blood supply usually enters through the inferior pulmonary ligament, which should be suture ligated even if a feeder is not identified. Also, as many as 15% of sequestrations have more than one feeding vessel, which warrants caution even after the putative artery has been ligated.

Intralobar lesions should be resected using a formal lobectomy because segmental resection has a high risk for complications, especially if recurrent infection has distorted the normal architecture of the lung.

BRONCHOGENIC CYST

Bronchogenic cysts are mucus-filled cysts arising from the tracheobronchial tree and may occur proximally or distally. The main symptoms occur from compression of the normal lung or trachea, leading to respiratory distress, compression of the esophagus, leading to dysphagia, or from infection due to abnormal drainage of the secretions. Presentation can occur anytime in life depending on the size and location of the mass. The symptoms may be progressive as the cyst enlarges with continued secretion of mucus. Even if a lesion is not symptomatic at the time of diagnosis, excision is required due to the high lifetime risk for complications, including infection and malignant degeneration.

Although it is difficult to make a definitive diagnosis of a bronchogenic cyst prenatally, it should be considered in the differential diagnosis of a cystic chest lesion. Proximal bronchogenic cysts can cause respiratory distress from air trapping and may mimic congenital lobar emphysema. On chest radiography, they may appear as a smooth mass without calcifications or have an air-fluid level if they communicate with the airway or the gastrointestinal tract. Because the patient can present with an infection, seeing an air-fluid level in a patient with only a mild illness or after the illness has subsided suggests the diagnosis of bronchogenic cyst. Chest CT may help to make a definitive diagnosis if the cyst is not recognizable on plain films.

A bronchogenic cyst within the lung parenchyma may be excised by segmentectomy or lobectomy. Preoperative antibiotics may be required if the patient presented with a severe infection. Those in the mediastinum may be excised en masse, although if they have caused destruction of the airway due to inflammation, a more significant resection may be required to bypass damaged cartilage. A thoracoscopic approach may be used for excision of bronchogenic cysts, keeping in mind that mediastinal exploration may be required if the cyst is located beneath the mediastinal pleura.

GENERAL TECHNICAL CONSIDERATIONS

The technical approaches for segmental lung resection and lobectomy are considered in a number of surgical atlases. In general, major pulmonary resection is well tolerated by young children due to impressive compensatory lung growth following surgery, provided there is no significant immaturity or intrinsic lung disease. Access to the chest may be via standard posterior lateral thoracotomy, muscle-sparing thoracotomy, or, for upper lobe lesions, axillary thoracotomy. The presence of large CCAMs during development is often associated with fusion of the normal anatomic fissures, requiring careful division along the anatomic plane or division with a stapler. For small infants, the use of a stapling device close to the bronchus is not recommended because the staples are too large and may allow a bronchial air leak. We generally close the bronchus with a proximal ligature and distal suture ligation of fine nonabsorbable suture.

Rapid postoperative recovery is facilitated by the use of epidural anesthesia and careful intraoperative technique to avoid air leaks. The primary complication that delays discharge from the hospital is prolonged air leak. Other complications include recurrent infection, thoracotomy-related scoliosis, or, if an inadequate resection is performed (segmentectomy), recurrent disease.

CONCLUSION

Congenital lung anomalies are a diverse group of lesions of probably common embryologic origin with similar clinical presentations. Although many are now diagnosed prenatally, fetal intervention is warranted only in select cases in which the fetus develops hydrops. The main postnatal considerations are compression of the normal lung by the lesion (which leads to respiratory compromise or pulmonary hypoplasia), infection from failure of the lung to clear secretions normally, and the potential for malignant degeneration. Complete resection of the lesion is generally well tolerated even in the neonate and represents definitive therapy.

SUGGESTED READINGS

Adzick NS, Harrison MR, Crombleholme TM, et al. Fetal lung lesions: management and outcome. *Am J Obstet Gynecol* 1998; 179:884–889.

Kitano Y, Adzick NS. New developments in fetal lung surgery. *Curr Opin Pulmon Med* 1999;5:383–391.

Srikanth MS, Ford EG, Stanley P, et al. Communicating bronchopulmonary foregut malformation: classification and embryogenesis. *J Pediatr Surg* 1992;27:732–736.

87

PECTUS DEFORMITIES

ANDRÉ HEBRA

The spectrum of congenital chest wall malformations includes pectus deformities, Poland's syndrome, sternal defects, and chest dysplasias, as seen in diffuse skeletal disorders. The most common types of congenital chest wall deformities are pectus excavatum and pectus carinatum. Pectus excavatum is much more common than pectus carinatum by a 5:1 ratio. Both are seen more frequently in boys than girls (4:1). However, pectus excavatum is usually noticeable in the first year of life (in >90% of cases), while pectus carinatum is usually not appreciated until after the 11th birthday. Both deformities typically worsen significantly during puberty, leading most children to present for operative treatment as adolescents. The adage that a child will "grow out" of the pectus deformity is not true, and most children with this condition should be evaluated by a physician experienced in the field of congenital chest wall deformities for an early assessment and appropriate counseling. This chapter presents the most commonly used treatment modalities for the correction of pectus excavatum and carinatum. Treatment philosophies vary widely, and many pediatric surgeons believe that in most instances chest wall abnormalities produce cosmetic rather than physiologic problems. As a rule, corrective surgery to improve the appearance of the chest because the deformity interferes with the child's self-image and psychosocial well-being is indicated and appropriate.

The diagnosis is usually straightforward and based on the appearance of the patient's chest. The clinical presentation of pectus excavatum is characterized by the depressed middle and lower sternum ("caved-in" appearance), rounded, sloped shoulders, prominent potbelly, protrusion of the lower ribs at the costal margins, and classic abnormal breathing dynamics with retraction of the sternum on deep inspiration. Most patients with a pectus deformity develop the so-called "pectus posture," with slumped-over shoulders and excessive curvature of the spine, as if the patient had kyphosis. It is unclear if this is a result of the patient's subconscious attempt to hide the chest deformity or if it is associated with the underlying skeletal abnormality of the ribs and chest. It often resolves after operative correction of the defect, particularly if the patient is made aware of the issue. The symptomatology is quite variable, ranging from none to shortness of breath, palpitations, chest pain, rib discomfort, gastroesophageal reflux symptoms, reactive airway disease, and back pain. Most patients with pectus carinatum are asymptomatic, although some occasionally complain of chest pain and discomfort. The protrusion also can be asymmetric and limited to only one side of the sternum, with the costal cartilages producing a keel-like protrusion. A mixed deformity also occurs with both protrusion and depression components. The sternum is often rotated posteriorly toward the depressed side. The rarest form of pectus carinatum consists of a protrusion of the manubrium and the superior costal cartilages with a relative depression of the body of the sternum, also known as *pouter pigeon breast*. In such cases, the sternum may have a "Z" or "comma" shape, and it has been reported to be associated with an increased incidence of congenital heart disease.

Pectus deformities are sometimes associated with other musculoskeletal abnormalities (up to 20%) such as scoliosis, kyphosis, myopathy, Marfan's syndrome, Poland's syndrome, Pierre Robin syndrome, prune belly syndrome, neurofibromatosis, tuberous sclerosis, congenital diaphragmatic hernia, spondylometaphyseal dysplasia, and Ehlers-Danlos syndrome. Twenty to 30% of patients have a positive family history, suggesting a genetic predisposition. Patients with pectus excavatum often present with systolic murmurs or evidence of mitral valve prolapse. In some cases, the murmur is due to compression of the right ventricular outflow tract, but it also can represent an early finding seen in Marfan's syndrome, with aortic or mitral valve disease and aneurysmal dilatation of the ascending aorta. Any patient with suspected Marfan's disease should undergo preoperative computed tomography (CT) scan of the chest and consultation with a cardiologist and geneticist. In addition to the possible physiologic changes in cardiopulmonary function caused by the pectus deformity, one

A. Hebra: Minimally Invasive Pediatric Surgery Program, Department of Surgery, University of South Florida, and All Children's Hospital, St. Petersburg, Florida.

must give careful consideration to the psychological implications such as mood swings, depression, excessive shyness, poor self-image, emotional instability, and even suicidal thoughts. As previously mentioned, this may be the most important indication for corrective surgery.

PREOPERATIVE PREPARATION

Cardiology consultation, pulmonology consultation, pulmonary function tests, and complete blood count are not mandatory and are only obtained if indicated based on the medical history and physical examination findings. CT of the chest is useful in determining the CT index, which is derived by dividing the transverse chest diameter by the anteroposterior diameter. An index above 3.2 has been correlated with a severe deformity requiring surgery. Our experience at the Medical University of South Carolina suggests that the chest index also can be derived from plain anteroposterior and lateral chest radiographs; CT of the chest is used only in selected cases of asymmetric pectus excavatum or if significant cardiac displacement and rotation is suspected. In such cases, the CT scan can provide valuable information for planning the operative intervention. Prior to surgery, the chest is measured from the midaxillary line to midaxillary line in order to determine the approximate length of the bar required by subtracting one centimeter from that initial measurement. A gentle bowel preparation one day before surgery might be helpful in decreasing problems related to postoperative constipation. First-generation cephalosporin antibiotic (cefazolin) may be given approximately 1 hour prior to surgery. As a rule, patients can be admitted on the same day of surgery and there is no need for routine admission to a pediatric intensive care unit following surgery.

TECHNICAL APPROACH

The early technique for correction of pectus excavatum was based on the principle that the sternum should be raised by traction sutures through the skin and suspended above the patient's bed after partial resection of the rib ends along the sunken sternum. In 1939, Alton Ochsner, Sr. and Michael DeBakey discarded the then popular notion that pectus excavatum was caused by a short subxiphoid tendon that held the sternum posteriorly. They strongly advocated a new theory that the sternum was held in a posterior position by overgrown lengths of rib cartilage that would not allow the sternum to come forward (a change in the direction of rib growth would cause pectus carinatum). They believed it was important to elevate the sternum to relieve pressure on the heart and lungs and allow for normal growth and development. It was not until 1949 that there was a detailed description of the salient diagnostic features of pectus excavatum and a specific operative procedure for treatment of this condition was proposed. Mark Ravitch described an operation that is still used today to correct pectus deformities: subperichondrial costal cartilage resection, mobilization of the sternum with an osteotomy, and securing the sternum in an anterior position (which frequently requires the placement of a stainless-steel support bar).

The two most commonly used operations for repair of pectus deformities are described in this chapter. The modified Ravitch technique can be used for both pectus excavatum and carinatum, whereas the minimally invasive technique is limited to pectus excavatum.

Modified Ravitch Technique

It is important to emphasize that this technique for repair of pectus deformities should not be performed until children are at least beginning their pubertal growth spurt and the chest is more fully developed, thus minimizing the risk of recurrence and complications, such as acquired asphyxiating chest dystrophy.

An anterior transverse chest incision is used for this repair. Some surgeons prefer a midline incision similar to the one used for open-heart surgery. The transverse incision is cosmetically superior. The transverse incision is usually placed in the midportion of the sternal defect, to allow complete exposure of the entire deformed sternum and involved ribs (on the right and left sides of the sternum). The incision may be as long as 15 cm (extending from nipple to nipple) or shorter, depending on the degree of the deformity and the need for wide or limited exposure of the anterior chest wall. In girls, it might be possible to place the incision under the breast line in order to make it more cosmetically appealing. Skin flaps are created for exposure of the pectoralis muscles. The pectoralis muscles are then separated by incising in the midline. Pectoralis muscle flaps are raised on each side, exposing the involved ribs and sternum. One must be careful not to damage the muscles during this dissection and to avoid damage to the periosteum of the sternum or to the perichondrium around the cartilage. The use of blunt dissection technique combined with careful attention to tissue planes is important. Several small branching vessels between the pectoralis and the chest wall are cauterized in order to avoid bleeding from vessels that are cut and retract under the intercostal muscle plane. The flaps should be wide enough to allow for complete exposure of the cartilages to be resected. Subperichondrial resection of the costal cartilages is performed by incising the perichondrium longitudinally. The perichondrium is then dissected away from the costal cartilage in a bloodless plane. This allows for complete removal of the cartilage leaving the growth plate. It is frequently necessary to divide the cartilage in the middle so that the proximal and distal pieces can be elevated for better exposure of the posterior plane between the cartilage and the perichondrium. At this point the perichondrium can be pushed bluntly away from the cartilage by the operating surgeon's finger and gauze. Next the cartilages are divided at the point of junction of the sternum and divided at the level of the costochondral junction. It is important to remove all rib cartilages that are deformed, including the lower ones next to the xiphoid. Typically, three to six cartilages are removed on each side. This process is tedious but must be accomplished without injury to the perichondrium or growth plate. It is also necessary to separate the attachments of the rectus muscles to the lower sternum by dividing the xiphoid attachment to the sternum. This maneuver is necessary in patients with pectus excavatum, in order to facilitate the anterior elevation of the sternum and to allow entry into the retrosternal space. It is usually not necessary during the correction of pectus carinatum.

The surgical approach to the sternum is the main difference between the modified Ravitch technique for pectus excavatum and carinatum. In patients with pectus excavatum, a sternal wedge osteotomy is created above the last deformed cartilage at the point of posterior angulation of the sternum. This is generally around the insertion of the second or third cartilage. The osteotomy can be created using an electrical or air drill, or it can be created using a mallet and chisel. The osteotomy can be created obliquely if the sternum is twisted as well as depressed. The posterior sternal plate is preserved. It is frequently necessary to add a second or even a third wedge osteotomy in order to achieve the best possible correction to the deformed sternum. Finger blunt dissection is used behind the sternum, through the retrosternal space created by separating the xiphoid. This is done carefully in order to avoid entry into the pleural cavity. The finger can lift the sternum to a more normal position by applying pressure behind the sternum. There is some controversy as to the next step, fixation of the sternum in its new elevated position. This can be accomplished by the use of internal metallic struts or suture fixation. Metallic strut fixation was popularized by Rehbein, Adkins, and Jensen. The most commonly used technique in North America involves the placement of a single stainless-steel bar (Adkins strut) behind the sternum, which is secured to the lateral ribs and maintains the sternum in its new position. The suture closure technique is accomplished by placing strong sutures through the anterior sternal plate, over the osteotomy sites, in order to keep the wedge resection site closed, keeping the sternum moved up and forward. Surgeons in Japan have used the "turnover" technique, in which the sternum and costal cartilages are completely separated from the chest wall and flipped over, with reattachment of the avascular graft to the chest wall. This technique has not been well accepted in North America. If a strut is used, it is fixed with pericostal sutures at each end to prevent migration. The strut can be removed as early as six months after surgery. Figure 87.1 illustrates the technique described above.

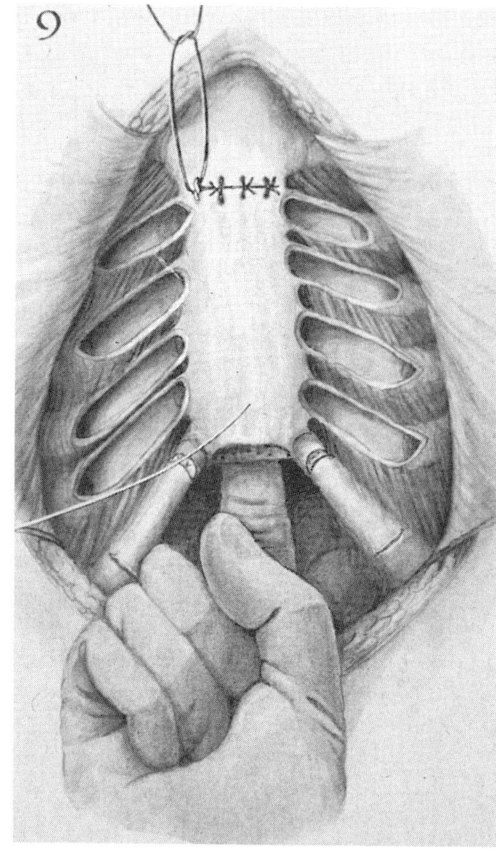

FIGURE 87.1. Open modified Ravitch technique for repair of pectus excavatum. The involved cartilages are resected with preservation of the perichondrium. Sternal osteotomy is necessary to allow for the forward displacement of the sternum by the surgeon's index finger. Note that the xiphoid was separated from the lower sternum in order to allow for sternal mobilization. A small metal strut is used to keep the sternum in its new position (not shown).

For patients with pectus carinatum, the technique is modified. The sternal osteotomies are created as previously described, but it is not necessary to perform wedge resection of the anterior sternal plate at the osteotomy site. As with pectus excavatum, it is frequently necessary to have more than one osteotomy. The sternum is then bent down until the desired correction is obtained. Typically, suture fixation is enough for keeping the sternum in its new position. Some surgeons also have used metallic strut fixation in such cases, but this is not usually necessary.

The final step is to close the perichondrial spaces. This should be carefully performed in order to provide the best appearance to the newly shaped anterior chest. Interrupted silk sutures are used for that purpose. Some surgeons advocate mincing the resected cartilage and placing pieces within the perichondrial space to serve as a graft, which may improve healing and rib remodeling. Chest tubes are only necessary if the pleural space was entered during the procedure. Small drains are typically placed under the muscle flap and under the skin flap. Placement of a small 7 French drain that runs from under the skin flap to under the muscle flap and out through a lateral stab wound is very effective in preventing the formation of postoperative seromas. The pectoralis muscle is reapproximated on the midline with absorbable sutures, and the xiphoid is reattached. The skin is reapproximated with absorbable subcuticular suture. The average operative time is 3 to 4 hours. A chest radiograph should be obtained after surgery to rule out a pneumothorax.

Minimally Invasive Technique for Repair of Pectus Excavatum

The clinical observations that provide the rationale for developing a less invasive operation for correction of pectus excavatum are numerous. First, children have a soft and malleable chest. Second, the phenomenon of chest remodeling is well known in adult patients with emphysema, who develop a barrel-shaped chest. If the chest wall can be reconfigured in older adults, the same should be possible for children and teenagers, given the increased malleability of their anterior chest wall. Third, the use of braces and internal fixating devices has allowed orthopedic surgeons and orthodontists to correct skeletal anomalies such as scoliosis, clubfoot, and maxillomandibular malocclusion. The anterior chest wall, being quite malleable, is therefore ideal for this type of correction. Such observations led to the concept that placement of a convex steel bar under the sternum through a small lateral thoracic incision could correct the condition known as funnel chest. Thus, thanks to Donald Nuss, the minimally invasive repair of pectus excavatum (MIRPE), also known as the Nuss technique, was developed.

The ideal age for candidates of MIRPE is 8 to 12 years. The operation can be safely performed in teenagers and young adults, but they are more likely to experience increased discomfort in the first few days after surgery when compared with younger patients. The surgical technique for MIRPE is described here in detail:

1. The patient is positioned supine with both arms abducted at the shoulders to allow access to the lateral chest walls.
2. The patient is prepared and draped such that the entire anterior chest is exposed.
3. The chest is marked with a sterile marking pen in the following areas: the deepest portion of the pectus, making sure that it is not inferior to the lower end of the sternum; the corresponding intercostal spaces on the right and left sides where the bar will be inserted, usually on the midaxillary line, and the points on the pectus ridge that correspond to the horizontal plane from the deepest point of the pectus to the lateral chest wall incisions (usually at the midclavicular line).
4. At this time the measurement of the Lorenz pectus bar (Walter-Lorenz Co., Jacksonville, FL) is reconfirmed using the marks made on the chest.
5. The bar is then curved from the center out to either end, making small gradual bends, using a bar-bender instrument. The curvature (convexity) of the bar is shaped in such way that it will conform to the patient's chest. It may be necessary to exaggerate the curvature slightly to allow for the anterior chest wall pressure that may alter the original configuration of the bar. The bar must fit snugly over the chest.
6. A transverse 2-cm skin incision is made on the midaxillary line at the level of the skin marks in line with the deepest point of the depression on the right and left sides.
7. A skin tunnel is raised anteriorly from both incisions to the top of the pectus ridge at the previously selected intercostal space; the skin pocket also should be extended posteriorly to allow for the distal end of the pectus bar to hug the chest wall posterior to the midaxillary line.
8. At this point a thoracoscope should be inserted. A 5-mm trocar is placed one or two intercostal spaces below the space that has been chosen for the pectus bar on the patient's right side. A 30 degree thoracoscope provides excellent visualization of the pleural cavity, lung, and mediastinal structures. If necessary, a scope can be used bilaterally. Only rarely is it necessary to insufflate the pleural cavity with CO_2; in most cases, controlled ventilation by the anesthesiologist with small tidal volumes will result in limited lung expansion and good thoracoscopic visualization of vital structures.
9. Using a thin, deep retractor, the skin incisions are elevated and the intercostal space previously marked is identified. A long instrument, such as a 15-inch Crawford vascular clamp or a Lorenz pectus introducer, is inserted through the appropriate right intercostal space at the top of the pectus ridge, in line with the point that corresponds to the deepest depression of the sternum. Figure 87.2 illustrates the steps described here. The clamp or introducer is carefully advanced across the anterior mediastinal space immediately under the sternum with videoscopic guidance. The point of the instrument should always be facing anteriorly and in contact with the sternum. The sternum is forcefully lifted as the instrument is passed to the contralateral side. Monitoring for cardiac ectopy is important to assure that the instrument is not in close contact with the heart or pericardial sac.
10. Once the instrument is passed behind the sternum, the tip is pushed through the intercostal space at the top of the pectus ridge on the left side and brought out through the left skin incision. Thoracoscopy on the left side is not usually necessary unless there is uncertainty as to the position of the instrument in the left chest.

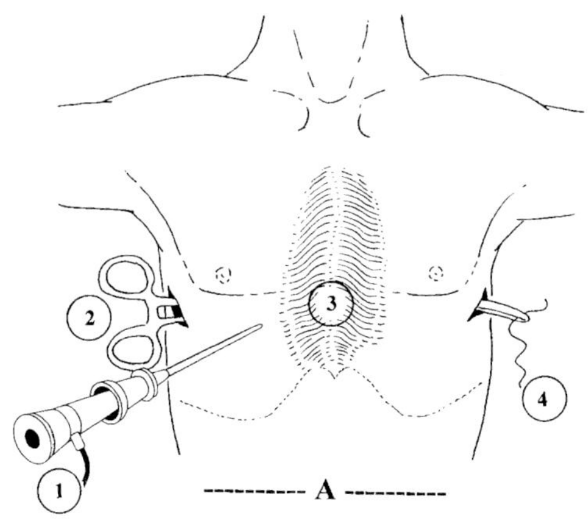

A

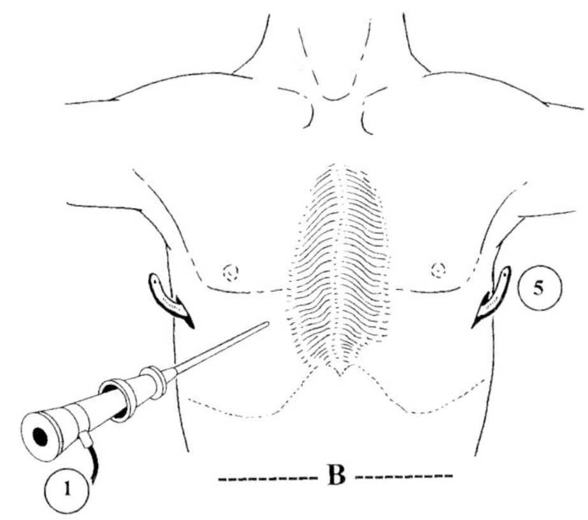

B

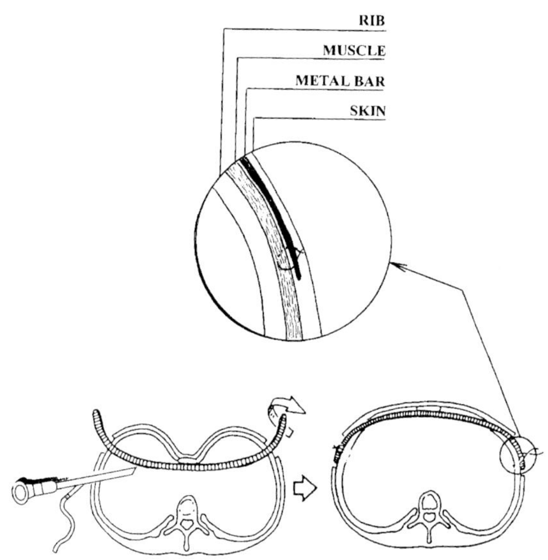

C

FIGURE 87.2. Minimally invasive technique for repair of pectus excavatum. **A:** Under thoracoscopic guidance (*1*), a long curved instrument (*2*) is passed behind the sternum in the anterior mediastinal space at the point of maximal depression of the pectus deformity (*3*). The instrument is brought out on the contralateral side, and umbilical tape (*4*) is grasped and passed back through the same tract. **B:** Still under thoracoscopic visualization, the tape is used to guide the stainless-steel metal bar that is passed behind the sternum with its convexity facing down (*5*). **C:** Once in place, the bar is rotated 180 degrees, and the sternum is pushed forward, correcting the deformity. Adequate fixation is obtained by suturing the metal bar to the muscle layer of the anterior chest, as illustrated in the insert diagram. (Reprinted from Hebra A. Minimally invasive pectus surgery. *Chest Surg Clin North Am* 2000;10:329–339; with permission.)

11. When using the Crawford clamp, it should be advanced such that the tunnel space created is enlarged; if using the Lorenz pectus introducer, it is not necessary to further dilate the space. The Lorenz pectus introducer comes in two sizes: a short one for younger patients with a small chest, ages 4 to 12, and a longer one for older and larger patients, ages 13 to 20.
12. Using the clamp or the introducer, two strands of umbilical tape are pulled through the tunnel; one tape is used as a spare.
13. One of the tapes is used to guide the previously prepared pectus bar through the tunnel and anterior mediastinal space using traction on the tape and concomitant thoracoscopic visualization. The bar is inserted with the convexity facing posteriorly.
14. Using a Lorenz pectus bar rotational instrument (bar flipper) the bar is turned over such that the concave part now faces posteriorly (to the mediastinum) and the convex part faces anteriorly. The ends of the bar are placed in the subcutaneous tissue, anterior to the muscle fascia (not under it and not within the muscle tissue). It is important that the shape of the bar is done in such a way that it will gently conform to the contour of the rib cage, so that the ends of it do not protrude under the skin pocket. However, one must note that the bar should not hug the chest too tightly, in order to avoid postoperative pain and discomfort from chronic pressure against the ribs. If after flipping the bar the correction of the pectus excavatum is not ideal (either undercorrected or overcorrected), then the bar should be flipped back, pulled back out, and bent again to fit the patient's chest to achieve the best possible correction of the deformity. If pressure has caused the bar to straighten out, it should be turned over and, using small hand-held benders, the curvature can be increased as appropriate. This can be repeated as many times as necessary. Typically only one bar is necessary to correct the deformity, but occasionally a second bar

may be necessary, and it can be placed above or below the first one. The thoracoscope and trocar are removed at this point.

15. Once the bar is in place, it is imperative to determine its stability. Such assessment will dictate the need for placement of a stabilizing bar. The stabilizer serves to limit rotation of the pectus bar, and it is sutured around the bar (with stainless-steel suture) and to the muscle after being properly fitted on the end of the pectus bar. Teenagers usually require one stabilizer bar that can be placed on either side of the pectus bar. Occasionally two stabilizers are necessary, one on each end of the pectus bar.
16. With the bar properly placed and stabilized, figure-of-eight sutures are placed to the lateral chest wall musculature. Heavy nonabsorbable sutures are placed on one side and absorbable sutures are place on the opposite side.
17. At this point, the anesthesiologist should place the patient in the Trendelenburg position, and large tidal volumes are used in combination with positive end-expiratory pressure such that any residual pneumothorax is eliminated. A chest tube is rarely needed. The subcutaneous tissue and skin are reapproximated with absorbable sutures. A radiograph of the chest is obtained as soon as possible to confirm good lung expansion and to show the final positioning of the bar.
18. The patient is extubated deep in order to minimize any movement or agitation since this may result in bar displacement if the patient thrashes about.

One of the most common complications following MIRPE is bar displacement. An additional technical step used by many pediatric surgeons to minimize the occurrence of such problem is the placement of a third point of fixation for the pectus bar. After the pectus bar is passed, rotated, and positioned in the anterior mediastinal space, a nonabsorbable suture is placed under thoracoscopic guidance around a rib and around the bar on the anterior chest, to the right of the sternum, as illustrated in Fig. 87.3. The location for the third point of fixation is easily determined by placing the thoracoscope next to the bar and against the anterior chest wall, such that the light from the scope will transilluminate through the chest wall. Typically, the third point of fixation is to the right of the lateral sternal margin at a point where the pectus bar crosses a rib cartilage, away from the internal mammary vessels. A 3-mm skin incision is made at the point where the bar and one rib overlap, on the anterior chest, lateral to the sternum. Through this skin opening, an 18-gauge spinal needle is introduced into the right pleural cavity, above or below a rib, as close as possible to the pectus bar, under thoracoscopic guidance. With the needle in place, a 0 polypropylene suture is passed through the needle into the chest. The needle is than removed, leaving the suture in place. Using the same skin incision, a 3 mm laparoscopic grasper is passed, this time

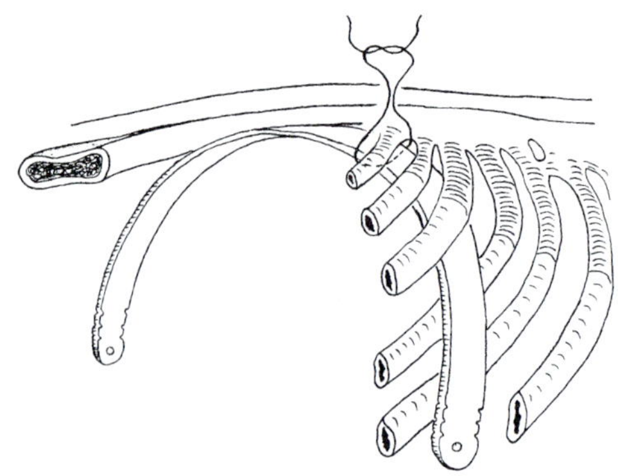

FIGURE 87.3. Third point of fixation for stabilization of the Lorenz pectus bar. A Prolene suture is placed percutaneously around the bar and around a rib next to the sternum, under thoracoscopic guidance. (Reprinted from Hebra A, Swoveland B, Egbert M, et al. Outcome analysis of minimally invasive repair of pectus excavatum: review of 251 cases. *J Pediatr Surg* 2000;35:252–257; with permission.)

over the opposite margin of the rib (opposite margin where the suture was introduced), again as close as possible to the pectus bar. Under thoracoscopic visualization, the grasper is used to grab the suture and bring it back to the outside. The suture is tightened and several knots are placed and buried under the skin. The small skin incision is closed with absorbable subcuticular suture. It is important to note that this technique does not preclude the use of a lateral stabilizer if additional reinforcement to the fixation of the bar is felt to be necessary (particularly recommended for teenaged patients).

The combination of general endotracheal anesthesia and a thoracic epidural block is considered ideal for both the modified Ravitch operation and MIRPE. However, many surgeons do not use the thoracic epidural block when performing the Ravitch repair. If used, the epidural catheter is left in placed up to 3 or 4 days following the operation. This is particularly important for patients who undergo MIRPE. It is important that patients and families understand that although the technique is considered minimally invasive, postoperative pain and discomfort can be significant due to the forceful bending of the sternum and cartilage. An indwelling Foley catheter is also placed due to the common occurrence of urinary retention with thoracic epidural blocks. Orogastric tube decompression of the stomach is recommended during the operation. Hemodynamic monitoring by the anesthesiologist does not necessitate central venous or arterial lines, unless the patient has significant underlying cardiac compromise.

POSTOPERATIVE CARE

The management of pain typically calls for keeping the patient well sedated for the first few days to prevent bar displacement. This is particularly true after MIRPE. Medications and therapies depend on the patient's response to pain and may include the use of the epidural catheter, intravenous narcotics for breakthrough pain, patient-controlled analgesia, and nonsteroidal antiinflammatory drugs. After MIRPE, we use the following protocol. In the first postoperative day the patient is kept supine and flat with only a small pillow. Mobilization is permitted on the second postoperative day by flexing the bed at the hip level, keeping the back straight. Waist bending, twisting, and logrolling are not permitted. The patient should be discouraged from sitting in the bed with the thoracic spine flexed. The patient will need assistance in getting out of bed at first. The epidural catheter is removed on the third or fourth postoperative day and the patient should be fully ambulatory after that point. Patients are discharged when they are able to walk without assistance.

The average length of stay is between 4 and 7 days for both MIRPE and the open repair. Good posture with a straight back is important even after discharge. Again, no bending at the hip and no slouching are allowed for the first month. Regular activity is permitted as pain decreases and mobility increases. Heavy lifting is not permitted for 1 month following surgery, and contact sports are to be avoided for at least 3 months. After open repair, patients should be particularly careful in the first 3 months after surgery, because of the unstable nature of the chest following removal of the affected cartilages. The pectus bar will generally remain in place for 2 years following MIRPE and for 6 months following open repair. The removal of the Lorenz bar or of the Adkins strut is accomplished by a straightforward 20- to 40-minute outpatient procedure under general anesthesia.

COMPLICATIONS

The overall complication rate for the open and minimally invasive technique for repair of pectus deformities is quite acceptable. However, because the MIRPE technique has not been in use as long as the modified Ravitch operation, early reports with the minimally invasive technique have demonstrated more numerous complications than expected, primarily due to the steep learning curve associated with the use of any new operative technique. Two large series have been reported that looked at complications and outcomes of MIRPE. In those reports, patient and family satisfaction was found to be good, with excellent and good results reported at 93% and 96%, respectively. However, the only multiinstitutional study, which reviewed 251 cases of MIRPE, demonstrated a significant rate of complications. By far the most common complication requiring reoperation was displacement of the support bar. Such displacement can be a 90 degree rotation, 180 degree rotation, or migration. Teenaged patients are at higher risk, probably because of the increased stress on the bar generated by a larger chest and more rigid chest cage.

As the overall surgeon experience with MIRPE continues to increase nationwide, the occurrence of complications should decrease. Table 87.1 illustrates the possible complications following minimally invasive repair of pectus excavatum.

The open surgical repair of pectus excavatum has evolved from the 1950s to the status of a safe procedure with good long-term results. Interestingly, no comprehensive studies focusing on the complications and outcomes are available. Table 87.2 lists the complications of the open procedure. Complications are relatively uncommon and limited to few case reports in the medical literature.

One of the most dreaded complications following the modified Ravitch operation, more common in young children, is the acquired Jeune's syndrome, or chest wall restriction (reported by Haller and associates in 1996). Such patients experience severe symptoms of respiratory distress with exercise, primarily due to failure of chest wall growth, resulting in restrictive lung disease. Most patients with this problem had undergone removal of five or more cartilages on each side, and all had undergone surgery before 5 years of age. These patients become symptomatic as older children and adolescents, with progressive exercise intolerance and dyspnea. Several of the patients had repeated bouts of severe pneumonia. They are found to have a small, immovable anterior chest wall, a long torso, abdominal respiration, very little movement of the downward displaced diaphragm, and, interestingly, no evidence of recurrence of the pectus deformity. The patient's appearance is similar to the congenital abnormality known as asphyxiating thoracic chondrodystrophy, or Jeune's syndrome. Such patients can be treated by an operation using Rehbein metal splints to

TABLE 87.1. COMPLICATIONS FOLLOWING MINIMALLY INVASIVE REPAIR OF PECTUS EXCAVATUM

Common complications (reported incidence of 1%–9%)
Pectus bar displacement requiring reoperation
Pneumothorax requiring tube thoracostomy
Epidural catheter complications
Infectious complications (wound infection, pneumonia)
Pleural effusion
Postoperative ileus
Constipation
Weight loss
Rare complications (reported incidence of <1%)
Thoracic outlet syndrome
Pericarditis
Empyema
Sepsis
Blood loss requiring transfusion
Cardiac injury
Sternal erosion of the bar
Arterial or venous injury
Gastroduodenal stress ulceration
Pectus excavatum recurrence
Death

TABLE 87.2. COMPLICATIONS OF THE MODIFIED RAVITCH PROCEDURE

Early complications
Bleeding
Pneumothorax
Strut displacement with injury to lungs and great vessels
Hemothorax
Atelectasis
Wound infection
Mediastinitis
Pneumonia
Pleural effusion
Pericardial effusion
Skin flap necrosis
Death
Late complications
Strut displacement
Floating sternum
Hemopericardium
Strut erosion into mediastinum
Chest constriction (acquired Jeune syndrome)
Pectus excavatum recurrence

support the sternum in a much elevated position, after making rib-relaxing incisions with resection of the abnormal costal cartilage.

A floating sternum is defined as a sternum in which the only bony attachment to the chest wall is via the manubrium. Lateral bony nonunion characterized by fibrous bands and scar tissue is present. Presumably due to excessive resection of the costal cartilages and perichondrium and failure of regrowth and reattachment of new cartilage to the sternum, such morbid phenomena may manifest many years after the original repair of pectus. It can cause significant sternal pain, chest wall instability, and respiratory dysfunction, which are also the indications for correction. The operative repair consists of mobilizing the lateral and inferior edges of the sternum, detaching the fibrous perichondrium, performing anterior sternal osteotomies, and supporting the sternum with substernal Adkins struts.

FOLLOW-UP

It is advisable to have patients enrolled in a physical fitness program, under the guidance of a certified physical therapist, to develop a progressive weight-lifting program that focuses on the build-up of pectoralis, deltoid, rectus, and latissimus muscles. This will promote normal remodeling of the chest and development of a healthy muscle mass. Early during the fitness program, patients may complain of being aware of the bar, particularly after MIRPE. This typically resolves completely 2 to 3 months after the operation. Following MIRPE, patients should be followed at 6-month intervals to monitor the appearance of the chest. There have been two patients who developed a variant of pectus carinatum within 1 year after MIRPE, probably due to overcompensation of the pectus excavatum deformity by the pectus bar. The pectus bar generally remains implanted for 2 years following MIRPE and for 6 months following open repair. The removal of the Lorenz bar or of the Adkins strut is performed as an outpatient procedure. Long-term follow-up (after bar removal) is recommended for all patients, particularly after the modified Ravitch operation, in order to monitor for the development of a floating sternum or acquired Jeune's syndrome.

SUGGESTED READINGS

Fonkalsrud EW, Bustorff-Silva J. Repair of pectus excavatum and carinatum in adults. *Am J Surg* 1999;177:121–124.

Haller JA Jr, Colombani PM, Humphries CT, et al. Chest wall constriction after too extensive and too early operations for pectus excavatum. *Ann Thorac Surg* 1996;61:1618–1624.

Haller JA Jr, Kramer SS, Lietman SA. Use of CT scans in selection of patients for pectus excavatum surgery: a preliminary report. *J Pediatr Surg* 1987;22:904–908.

Haller JA Jr, Scherer LR, Turner CS, et al. Evolving management of pectus excavatum based on a single institutional experience of 664 patients. *Ann Surg* 1989;209:578–582.

Hebra A. Minimally invasive pectus surgery. *Chest Surg Clin North Am* 2000;10:329–339.

Hebra A, Swoveland B, Egbert M, et al. Outcome analysis of minimally invasive repair of pectus excavatum: review of 251 cases. *J Pediatr Surg* 2000;35:252–257.

Moss RL, Albanese CT, Reynolds M. Major complications after minimally invasive repair of pectus excavatum: case reports. *J Pediatr Surg* 2001;36:155–158.

Nuss D, Kelly RE Jr, Croitoru DP, et al. A 10-year review of a minimally invasive technique for correction of pectus excavatum. *J Pediatr Surg* 1998;33:545–552.

Nuss D, Kelly RE Jr, Croitoru DP, et al. Repair of pectus excavatum. *Pediatr Endosurg Innov Techniques* 1998;2:205–221.

Ravitch MM. The operative treatment of pectus excavatum. *Ann Surg* 1949;129:429–444.

88

PNEUMOTHORAX

BRADLEY M. RODGERS

Pneumothorax refers to the abnormal collection of air in the pleural space, from disruption of either the parietal or visceral pleura. When the air accumulates under pressure and causes a shift in the mediastinal structures, it is referred to as a tension pneumothorax. The causes of pneumothorax are generally considered to be posttraumatic, iatrogenic, or spontaneous. Spontaneous pneumothoraces are further categorized as primary and secondary (Table 88.1). Primary spontaneous pneumothorax (PSP) occurs in the absence of obvious underlying lung disease. It is seen most commonly in young males with a lean body habitus. Secondary spontaneous pneumothorax (SSP) occurs with a background of chronic pulmonary disease, such as chronic obstructive pulmonary disease, emphysema, asthma, or cystic fibrosis. SSP is more common in older individuals and maintains a male predominance. Smoking is a risk factor for both PSP and SSP.

The pathophysiology of the patient's response to a pneumothorax relates to diminished tidal volume secondary to collapse of the ipsilateral lung. There also may be a ventilation perfusion mismatch. With tension pneumothorax there is a shift of the mediastinum to the contralateral side, with compromise of the tidal volume of both lungs as well as diminished venous return to the heart and diminished cardiac output. Symptoms of a pneumothorax usually include the sudden onset of ipsilateral chest pain. The degree of respiratory compromise may be quite variable and is usually most severe in those patients with posttraumatic pneumothorax and SSP. The diagnosis of a pneumothorax can be made by a review of the clinical history and a careful physical examination. The patient generally appears uncomfortable, with pleuritic chest pain, and might be in respiratory distress. Breath sounds in the ipsilateral hemithorax are absent or diminished when compared with the other side. Patients with a tension pneumothorax have an expansion of the ipsilateral hemithorax. A most important physical finding is the position of the trachea in the suprasternal notch. In patients with a tension pneumothorax, the trachea is displaced from the midline to the contralateral side.

B. M. Rodgers: Department of Surgery, Division of Pediatric Surgery, University of Virginia Health System, Charlottesville, Virginia.

DIAGNOSIS

The diagnosis is confirmed with chest radiographs, demonstrating a collapse of the lung with or without mediastinal shift. In many patients with SSP, the pneumothorax may be difficult to identify on plain radiographs because of the cystic changes in the underlying lung. Chest computed tomography may help to define the pneumothorax in these situations and to evaluate its magnitude. Patients with posttraumatic pneumothorax and SSP are initially treated by tube thoracostomy. We prefer to connect the chest tube to underwater seal with approximately 20 cm of water suction until the ipsilateral lung is fully expanded and the air leak has ceased. At that time, the suction can be eliminated from the system. If the lung remains fully inflated after 12 to 24 hours, the chest tube may be removed. Patients with the first PSP may be considered for less aggressive treatment. Those patients who are asymptomatic and with less than a 20% pneumothorax may be safely observed without placement of a chest tube. In these patients, the addition of supplemental oxygen by facemask may accelerate absorption of the pneumothorax by increasing the gradient for nitrogen absorption. Patients with a small PSP who are minimally symptomatic may undergo aspiration of the air from the chest with a 20-gauge angiocatheter. These patients are followed closely with subsequent radiographs to detect any recurrence of the pneumothorax, which would be an indication for a chest tube. Patients with larger PSPs, with or without symptoms, should be treated immediately with tube thoracostomy.

Patients who have recovered from their first spontaneous pneumothorax have a 30% to 75% chance of experiencing an ipsilateral recurrence. They also have approximately a 50% chance of having a contralateral pneumothorax. The generally accepted indications for surgical treatment in patients with a pneumothorax are (a) a recurrent pneumothorax, (b) occurrence of bilateral pneumothoraces, (c) persistent (>7 days) air leak, (d) severe symptoms with the initial pneumothorax, (e) living a great distance from medical care, and (f) a high-risk occupation such as diving or flying. We have tended to be quite aggressive in recom-

TABLE 88.1. PNEUMOTHORAX ETIOLOGY

Postoperative
Traumatic
Iatrogenic
Spontaneous
Primary (PSP)
Secondary (SSP)

mending surgical treatment in children with SSP, particularly cystic fibrosis patients. Pneumothorax is the cause for some mortality in these patients and tends to have a high likelihood of recurrence.

TREATMENT

The definitive surgical treatment of all forms of pneumothorax is creation of a pleurodesis, combined with resection of subpleural blebs or attempts at closure of visceral pleural leaks. A pleurodesis may be created by one of several different techniques. Perhaps the most commonly performed technique is a mechanical abrasion of the visceral and parietal pleura, to stimulate the formation of inflammatory adhesions. Because most PSPs occur following rupture of apical subpleural blebs, many surgeons prefer an apical parietal pleurectomy for treatment of this form of pneumothorax. Another method of producing pleural adhesions is performance of a chemical pleurodesis. A variety of agents have been used for chemical pleurodesis, including doxycycline, bleomycin, doxorubicin, and USP pure talc (Table 88.2). Of these agents, the use of talc has been associated with the lowest recurrence rate in all reported series, averaging about 5%. Regardless of the method selected, at the time of pleurodesis, a careful inspection of the pulmonary surface should be made to identify blebs or other causes of air leak, which can be individually managed. The traditional surgical approach for treatment of spontaneous pneumothorax has been through a transaxillary thoracotomy, with pulmonary bleb resection and a mechanical pleurodesis. An apical pleurectomy also may be performed through this approach. The recurrence rate after transaxillary thoracotomy and pleurodesis for spontaneous pneumothorax is approximately 3% to 5%.

TABLE 88.2. PNEUMOTHORAX PLEURODESIS

Mechanical (abrasion)
Apical pleurectomy
Chemical
Doxycycline
Bleomycin
Doxorubicin
USP pure talc

All of the techniques used for creation of a pleurodesis may be performed by thoracoscopy, a minimally invasive surgical procedure. In the past 10 years there has been considerable interest and experience in using this technique for patients with spontaneous pneumothorax. The entire pulmonary surface can be evaluated nicely with the thoracoscope, and blebs may be resected or rents in the visceral pleura may be closed with an endoscopic stapling instrument. Many surgeons prefer to use mechanical pleurodesis in these patients, usually using either a small piece of polypropylene mesh or a piece of the disposable cautery scratch pad to abrade the parietal pleura. We prefer to use a talc pleurodesis in these patients, feeling that it gives the lowest incidence of recurrence. Dry, sterile, USP pure talc is insufflated with a pneumatic device, covering the entire visceral pleural surface. Approximately 2 g of talc are required for this procedure, which may be performed under regional anesthesia with an intercostal rib block. A thoracoscopic talc pleurodesis is easier to perform than an apical pleurectomy and can be performed more rapidly than a pleural abrasion. The results appear to be superior to pleural abrasion and at least comparable with apical pleurectomy in terms of eliminating recurrent pneumothorax.

Postoperatively, all of these patients are managed with a chest tube connected to underwater seal and 10 to 20 cm of water suction until the ipsilateral lung is fully expanded and the air leak has ceased. At this point, the tube is placed to underwater seal, without suction, for 12 to 24 hours, and complete expansion of the lung is confirmed by chest radiography. The tube is then removed and the patients may be discharged from the hospital immediately thereafter. Our average postoperative hospitalization for pediatric patients with PSP and SSP has been 4 to 5 days. In the past 15 years, we have treated all of the pediatric patients with spontaneous pneumothorax who met the criteria for pleurodesis with thoracoscopic techniques. We have had no mortality and only a single significant complication, bleeding from a pleural adhesion in a patient who had undergone a previous mechanical pleurodesis at another institution. This was controlled by thoracoscopic cauterization. We have experienced two small recurrent pneumothoraces (7%), both in patients with SSP with underlying cystic fibrosis. In both of these patients, the initial therapy had been by thoracoscopic pleural abrasion. Although we had initially treated all of our cystic fibrosis patients with SSP with thoracoscopic talc pleurodesis, with the increasing use of pulmonary transplantation in these patients, we had thought that a mechanical pleurodesis would be less troublesome for the transplant surgeon. Having experienced these recurrences, we have now returned to the use of talc in these patients and have not experienced another recurrence. Our current approach is to perform a thoracoscopic talc pleurodesis in all patients with SSP. This procedure may be performed with either regional anesthetic techniques or general anesthesia, depending on the clinical condition of the patient.

Pneumothorax remains a relatively common condition encountered in a pediatric surgical practice. Treatment strategies have undergone significant evolution in the past decade, in an attempt to establish a cost-effective and reliable treatment algorithm. The introduction of the minimally invasive technique of thoracoscopy has stimulated a somewhat more aggressive surgical approach to these patients and has significantly reduced the incidence of ipsilateral recurrent pneumothorax. At the present time, these patients can be treated with a variety of techniques with an acceptably low incidence of recurrence.

SUGGESTED READINGS

Cardillo G, Facciolo F, Giunti R, et al. Videothoracoscopic treatment of primary spontaneous pneumothorax: a 6-year experience. *Ann Thorac Surg* 2000;69:357–362.

Light RW. Management of specimen pneumothorax. *Am Rev Respir Dis* 1993;148:245–248.

Liu HP, Yim APC, Izzat MB, et al. Thoracoscopic surgery for spontaneous pneumothorax. *World J Surg* 1999;23:1133–1136.

Stringel G, Amen NS, Dozor AJ. Video-assisted thoracoscopy in the management of recurrent spontaneous pneumothorax in the pediatric population. *J Soc Laparoendosc Surgeons* 1999;3: 113–116.

Weissberg D, Refaely Y. Pneumothorax: experience with 1199 patients. *Chest* 2000;117:1279–1285.

89

ACCESS TO THE ANTERIOR SPINE

JOSEPH S. JANIK

Access to the anterior spine was introduced and popularized by Hogdson in 1956 for treatment of Pott's disease of the spine. This technique has been extended to the correction of spinal deformities and the resection of tumors. The primary indication for this surgical approach in pediatrics is the correction of spinal deformities secondary to congenital disease (i.e., scoliosis, kyphosis, lordosis) and neuromuscular disease (myelodysplasia, cerebral palsy, spastic quadriplegia, etc.).

PREOPERATIVE PREPARATION

In general, a comprehensive review of all medications, including aspirin, nonsteroidal antiinflammatory drugs, and valproic acid, should be undertaken preoperatively to prevent excessive bleeding. If possible, autologous or directed donor blood should be available. All thoracic and high thoracoabdominal (TA) exposures, and certain forms of instrumentation require a collapsed lung on the operative side. This can be accomplished with bronchial blockade using a Fogarty catheter in a small child, and a double-lumen endotracheal tube in the preadolescent and adolescent. All patients with normal neurologic function should have the benefit of stimulated evoked potential (SEP) monitoring during the procedure. SEP monitoring is especially sensitive to drugs, drug-induced hypotension, hemorrhage, transection of vessels, distraction of the cord, and malpositioning of retractors (especially on the genitofemoral nerve). Due to the length of these procedures, positioning of the child with a beanbag device and extensive padding with pillows and sheepskin is mandatory.

J.S. Janik: Department of Pediatric Surgery, University of Colorado Health Sciences Center, School of Medicine; and Department of Pediatric Surgery, The Children's Hospital, Denver, Colorado.

POSITION AND EXPOSURE BASICS

Choosing the appropriate body position is essential for the smooth conduct of the orthopedic procedure. A major point needs to be made here. General surgeons are accustomed to seeing radiographs taken in a posteroanterior direction and place them on a view-box with the heart on the surgeon's right side; spine surgeons are accustomed to looking at radiographs taken in an anteroposterior direction and place them on a view-box with the heart on the surgeon's left side. Therefore, before positioning the child for any of these procedures, it is of paramount importance to be sure where the heart shadow is located, where the gastric bubble is located, where the convex portion of the curve is located, and where the radiography technician's marker is located. The surgeon should not proceed until this point has been clearly resolved in everyone's mind. Once all of the landmarks have been identified, scoliotic curves must be positioned with the convex part of the curve upward. The disc spaces are wider on the convex side and much easier to incise and curette in this position. The vertebral bodies can be distracted with less force than from the concave position. Kyphotic curves can be positioned on either side, although the right side seems to be most popular. Lordotic curves usually require supine positioning, but in select cases may be approached from an oblique direction.

In all cases it is important to discuss the exposure with the orthopedic surgeon. Preoperatively several issues require resolution. Which levels will be exposed? Which curve is of primary surgical interest? Which side is the convex side of the scoliotic curve? Do the segmental vessels require division? Does the diaphragm require incision? Will subperiosteal rib excision be required? Will a second thoracotomy without rib excision be necessary to allow instrument placement? Will additional lateral osteotomies of adjacent ribs be helpful? Will thoracoplasty be performed? Will bone be harvested from the iliac crest? Answers to these questions will dictate patient position, incision location, extent of skin preparation, actual size of torso opening, number and site of thoracic wall openings, stability of thoracic wall upon completion of the procedure, need for tube thoracostomy, and need for nasogastric decompression. As a general rule, the segmental vessels at the same vertebral level should not be divided on both sides, either simultaneously or sequentially. The segmental vessels provide some and occasionally all of the nourishment to the cord at a given level. Two-sided division in any chronologic sequence risks damage to the cord. This obviously does not apply to the cord that has been previously impaired.

EXTENT OF EXPOSURE

The extent of the spinal exposure can range from the first thoracic vertebral body (T1) to the first sacral vertebra (S1) in a variety of combinations. These combinations can include a single vertebral body or multiple vertebral bodies, in one region to several regions simultaneously. They can be performed all at the same time or in a planned or unplanned staged fashion, and can even be performed for recurrent disease. For the sake of simplicity, T1 through T4 can be exposed via a posterolateral thoracotomy with the posterior end of the incision curving upward midway between the scapula and the spinous processes to allow the shoulder to slide forward. T4 through T12 curves can be exposed via a standard thoracotomy. T4 through S1 combination curves can be exposed via a TA transdiaphragmatic retroperitoneal approach through a single or double incision with a single or double thoracotomy. L1 through S1 curves can be exposed via an oblique flank retroperitoneal approach. The lumbosacral junction can be exposed via an oblique flank retroperitoneal approach for simple anterolateral vertebra exposure, or a low midline or Pfannenstiel transperitoneal approach for a true anterior double-sided vertebra exposure.

THORACIC EXPOSURE (T1–T12)

As a general rule the child is placed on a beanbag in the thoracotomy position with ample padding and an axillary roll. The incision is placed over the rib originating at, or one vertebra above the highest vertebra to be exposed (T6—T12). Limited anterior spinal surgery can be performed via a simple thoracotomy without subperiosteal rib excision. However the majority of anterior spinal instrumentation requires more expansive access. Exposure can be enhanced with single- or double-rib excision, single or double thoracotomy, or with single-rib excision coupled with two to four posterolateral excisional osteotomies. Generally double thoracotomy does not require a second incision. The second thoracotomy can be made above or below the primary skin incision by sliding under the chest wall muscles. High thoracic exposures (T1–T5) require the incision to be located over the seventh rib with posterior extension upward between the medial edge of the scapula and the spinous processes. In this situation the shoulder slides forward exposing the thoracic wall. Remember that multiple rib excision or osteotomy is limited in the high thoracic region (T1–T4). Preferentially the shoulder girdle requires the support of at least two intact ribs (1 and 4, 2 and 3, 2 and 4, etc.).

The harvested ribs are removed subperiosteally and put aside for the orthopedic surgeon. The bed of the periosteum is preserved and opened in the midline. The pleura over the vertebrae is opened longitudinally. The discs appear as bulges and the vertebral bodies appear as depressions with the segmental vessels overlying them. At this point the segmental vessels are looped and preserved or tied and divided depending on the orthopedic surgeon's needs. When segmental vessel division is required they are divided near the aorta and far from the intervertebral foramina. In questionable situations, temporarily clamping the segmental vessels and waiting 5 or more minutes before dividing may be of value. This allows changes in the SEP monitoring to develop and prevents harmful division of blood supply to the cord. Thoracic exposures that require visualization of the T12–L1 disc space or the top of L1 usually do not require full division of the diaphragm. Instead the spinal hiatus can be widened bluntly or sharply, allowing enough space for discectomy. Placement of instrumentation in T12 occasionally requires more extensive diaphragmatic division; instrumentation of L1 always requires more extensive diaphragmatic division. Closure of the chest and placement of a tube thoracostomy is per standard protocol. Closure of the pleura significantly controls postoperative chest tube drainage, even if this requires the use of hemostatic materials to complete the closure. Areas of multiple osteotomy must be stabilized to adjacent intact ribs.

THORACOABDOMINAL EXPOSURE (T1–S1)

This exposure requires an incision placed over ribs 8, 9, 10, 11, or 12 and curved downward over the costal margin along the lateral aspect of the rectus sheath. The upper and the lower extent of the incision are dictated by the vertebrae involved and follow the principles enumerated above under thoracic exposures. Extremely long exposures (e.g., T2–S1) are best accomplished via a high thoracic exposure with rib excision coupled with a lower TA exposure with rib excision. For a routine TA exposure, the surgeon should enter the thorax first, divide the external and internal oblique muscles next, and then slowly dissect through the transverse abdominus at the costal margin. The first sign of fat signals the peritoneal sac. At this point the peritoneum is swept bluntly from the underside of the diaphragm, the medial and lateral abdominal muscles, and off the iliopsoas. It is easy to incorrectly dissect between the iliacus and the psoas, but should be avoided. The genitofemoral nerve lies on the surface of these muscles and is in harm's way of retractor blades and reckless dissection. The surgeon should stay anterior to these muscles and proceed to the spine medially. The ureter is swept anteriorly with the peritoneal sac. The diaphragm is divided circumferentially 2 to 4 cm from the thoracic wall down to the spinal hiatus. Radial division of the diaphragm results in diaphragmatic paralysis. Caution should be taken when exposing the great vessels. In particular, the iliolumbar vein over L4 is generous in size and flow, even in the smallest child. It can be mistaken for the iliac vein. Patients who have had significant and prolonged discitis in this area will have dense inflammation between the vessels, discs, and anterior longitudinal ligament. It is better to dissect between the anterior longitudinal ligament and vertebrae and leave a piece of the anterior longitudinal ligament with the back wall of the vessel, rather than risk creating a hole in the posterior aspect of the vessels. Finally, the iliac vein has multiple posterior branches. These can be torn during dissection and manipulation. Rents in the peritoneal sac can occur at any time and should be repaired primarily with absorbable suture. Free air on initial postoperative radiographs may be seen.

Closure and tube thoracostomy follow the principles enumerated above in thoracic exposures. The retroperitoneum does not require drainage like the thorax. Small chyle leaks will seal under the weight of the peritoneal sac. The surgeon should avoid penetrating the peritoneal sac and its visceral contents during abdominal muscle closure. Diaphragmatic contraction makes the diaphragm appear longer on one side during repair. Diaphragmatic suturing should compensate for this visual disparity. Vessel injuries from dissection or orthopedic misadventures can and should be repaired primarily following standard vascular surgery techniques. Vascular bypass grafting is rarely necessary. Postoperative ileus requiring nasogastric decompression is often necessary and prolonged. Postoperative superior mesenteric artery (SMA) syndrome secondary to weight loss or changing the position of the SMA and the duodenum is a recognized occurrence. SMA syndrome is more common and more severe in neuromuscular scoliosis, and most postoperative SMA syndromes resolve with supportive intravenous or tube enteral feeding.

RETROPERITONEAL EXPOSURE (L1–S1)

Exposure of the vertebrae and the disc spaces from L2 to S1 can be accomplished simply with an oblique incision and a retroperitoneal approach. The incision begins halfway between the 12th rib and the iliac crest, extends medially to the edge of the rectus sheath, and downward to just above the pubic bone for L2–S1 exposure. This incision can be modified to expose fewer vertebral bodies. For L2–L3 exposure, the medial end of the incision should be curved to end above the umbilicus, for L3–L4 exposure just below the umbilicus, and for L4–L5 exposure half way between the umbilicus and the pubic bone. In all retroperitoneal exposures the retroperitoneum is entered, the peritoneal sac is dissected anteriorly, and the vertebrae and vessels exposed as noted above. Exposure of T12–L1 disc space, the body of L1, and in many cases the L1–L2 disc space cannot be exposed simply in this manner. Instrumentation of these areas always requires a TA approach as described above with the incision placed over the 10th, 11th, or 12th rib. If instrumentation is not required and avoidance or minimization of diaphragmatic division is necessary, then the oblique incision retroperitoneal flank approach can be modified. With the child at a 45 degree angle, an oblique incision is made over the 12th rib. The incision is extended downward depending on the number of lower vertebrae to be exposed. The retroperitoneum is entered as described above but at a distance from the 12th rib. Once in the retroperitoneum, the dissection is carried upward to the region of the 12th rib and then downward to the spine, fully exposing the underside of the diaphragm and the spine. At this point the surgeon must ascertain whether the desired superior disc space and vertebrae are exposed. If more exposure is necessary, the diaphragm may be opened starting at the spinal hiatus outward. The diaphragmatic incision should be curtailed when the exposure is adequate. Closure and precautions are similar to that for TA exposure. Tube thoracostomy may not be necessary.

LUMBOSACRAL/TRANSPERITONEAL EXPOSURE (L5–S1)

The choice of incision for isolated exposure of the lumbosacral junction is dependent on whether the orthopedic surgeon needs to work on both sides of the L5–S1 disc space (transperitoneal exposure), or just from the anterolateral aspect (lumbosacral exposure). A transperitoneal exposure requires an approach via a low midline incision or a Pfannenstiel incision. The bowel is packing away in all directions, and the peritoneum over the bifurcation of the great vessels is opened. The median sacral vessels are divided, the tissues over the L5–S1 disc are cleared, and the iliacs are dissected off the lateral aspect of the disc. The surgeon should be careful to avoid damage to the posterior branches of the iliac veins. The medial edge of the left iliac vein is always innocently disguised under the tissue in the bifurcation directly over the left lateral L5–S1 disc. One should clear away only what is necessary to visualize the disc. Extensive dissection inferior to the L5–S1 disc can damage the hypogastric plexus and interfere with ejaculation in males.

When anterolateral exposure of L5–S1 (lumbosacral exposure) is necessary, an oblique incision with a retroperitoneal approach should be used. The child is positioned at a 45 degree angle. The incision begins midway between the 12th rib and the iliac crest. It proceeds anteriorly and downward along the edge of the rectus sheath, stopping half way between the level of the umbilicus and the pubic bone. The retroperitoneum is entered as described above. In this situation the lateral branches of the aorta, cava, and iliacs on one side can be divided to enhance exposure. The posterior branches of the iliacs and the space below the bifurcation should be handled as noted above. Principles for closure of these exposures are as noted in previous sections.

ENDOSCOPIC EXPOSURES

Thoracoscopy and laparoscopy have been used extensively in thoracic and transperitoneal exposures in adults, and in thoracic exposures in children. Laparoscopic lumbar exposures have been hindered by difficulties with vascular control, adequacy of discectomy, and inability to insert spinal instrumentation. Thorascopically assisted thoracic exposure in children is primarily used to provide visualization of discectomy for scoliosis from T5 to T12. The scapula prevents discectomy at higher levels. Thorascopically assisted placement of intricate correction systems has not been accomplished on a large enough scale to claim that the technique is efficacious. However, placement of small bars and screws over short distances (two to three vertebrae) for fractures, hemivertebrae, and very limited scoliotic curves has been accomplished with great satisfaction. Single lung ventilation is of paramount importance. The pleura can be incised longitudinally over the full course of the spine involved, or it can be incised transversely over each disc. Usually the former is closed with a running suture; the latter is left open, although this is usually followed by more postoperative chest tube drainage. Ideally, discectomy is most successful when the end of the thorascope and the disc removal instruments are positioned directly over the disc. At the very least this requires multiple mini-thoracostomies. Because of depth-of-field limitations and the angle of the curve in relationship to the rib interspaces, full complete discectomy cannot always be assured except for the disc at, and possibly the two discs immediately adjacent to, the apex of a scoliotic curve.

EDITOR'S NOTE

Providing exposure to the anterior spine for our orthopedic colleagues should be considered more than the sum of making an incision and closing an incision. Rather, we become important members of a surgical team who provide a valuable service to the patient in the form of anatomic and technical expertise and an organized approach to tissue dissection. Dr. Janik has contributed a great deal over the years to help raise this class of procedures almost to the level of an art form.

The location of the incision is based on the level of the repair as well as on the number of vertebrae that are involved, and what needs to be done at those levels (discectomy or instrumentation). One should use a thoughtful approach that will minimize the length of the incision and the extent of dissection, while providing sufficient space for the safe completion of the procedure. One should also anticipate that the incision may need to be lengthened if an additional number of adjacent levels must be addressed. For example, for thoracic procedures, a thoracotomy position is required, but if there is the possibility of abdominal extension, the abdomen needs to be prepared into the field. The incision also should be made in such a way that extension results in adequate exposure and a cosmetically acceptable scar.

Positioning for thoracotomy should include an axillary roll with a diameter that approximates that of the patient's upper arm, and all pressure points should be padded. A beanbag may be used according to local custom, although well-placed rolled towels are often sufficient and do not usually limit available exposure. Although for most pediatric thoracic surgical procedures removal of a rib is rarely necessary, it should be considered in most orthopedic access cases for several reasons: it increases exposure considerably, it may be more comfortable for the patient postoperatively, and it provides autogenous bone graft material if a fusion is planned. The thorax is entered through the bed of the rib and the periosteum is preserved so that some replacement of bone may occur. Exposure of T12–L1 is usually possible by enlarging the diaphragmatic hiatus or making a short incision in the slip of muscle that overlies the spine at this level. At the completion of the procedure, closure of the pleura helps with hemostasis and minimizes the amount of drainage from the chest tube. For the TA approach, it should be emphasized that the diaphragm is incised circumferentially near the chest wall to preserve the innervation of the diaphragm but that attention should be directed to the course and insertion of the phrenic nerve medially to preserve its central branches. Radial incisions can result in denervation and eventration of the diaphragm.

Thoracoscopy can provide excellent exposure for discectomy and fusion in most patients. Single lung ventilation is critical to the success of this approach, which can limit its application in this patient population due to their frequently distorted mediastinal anatomy. Fortunately, the major mediastinal vascular structures typically stay in a more medial position despite the exaggerated curvature of the vertebral column and therefore stay out of harm's way. An angled lens is also important, although 30 or 45 degrees is usually adequate. Also, only one or two disc spaces can be addressed through a given thoracoscopy incision, especially at the extremes of the curve, so multiple incisions are usually required. The incisions are placed in the midaxillary line and usually need to be 10 mm or greater to accommodate the orthopedic instruments. Nevertheless, patients seem to tolerate the procedure well and recover more quickly than they do with a thoracotomy incision.

Access to the anterior lumbar spine requires a careful retroperitoneal approach with attention to anatomic detail to prevent injury to important structures such as the ureter and genitofemoral nerve. This is outlined nicely in the chapter. Suffice it to say that intimate knowledge of the anatomy and anticipation of having to deal with anatomic variants is very important. Careful attention to hemostasis is important because patients can lose a huge volume of blood into the retroperitoneum before it becomes clinically evident, and even stable retroperitoneal hematomas can result in significant morbidity.

–P.M.

SUGGESTED READINGS

Janik JS, Burrington JD, Janik JE, et al. Anterior exposure of spinal deformities and tumors: a 20-year experience. *J Pediatr Surg* 1997; 32:852–859.

Regan JJ, ed. *Atlas of endoscopic spine surgery.* St. Louis: Quality Medical, 1995.

Watkins RG, ed. *Surgical approaches to the spine.* New York: Springer-Verlag, 1983.

SECTION IX

ABDOMINAL WALL, PERITONEUM, AND DIAPHRAGM

90

ASCITES

ANNE C. FISCHER

ETIOLOGY

Ascites is the pathologic accumulation of peritoneal fluid manifested by a wide variety of disorders. Ascites can occur prenatally or at any age, and a limited number of causes, such as liver or renal disease, account for the majority of cases in children (Table 90.1). Hepatic causes include hepatocellular disease, hepatorenal syndrome, biliary tract perforation, or failed surgical portoenterostomy. Nonhepatic causes include congenital cardiovascular disease with failure, congenital lymphatic disorders, urinary obstruction, and gastrointestinal or gynecologic conditions. In contrast, the most common causes of ascites in adults are parenchymal liver disease with cirrhosis, alcoholic hepatitis, and malignancy.

Fetal ascites distinct from hydrops fetalis is unusual and can resolve prior to birth. The causes of fetal ascites are of the same spectrum as that of neonatal ascites (Table 90.2). Hydrops fetalis, however, is characterized by the prenatal appearance of scalp edema, pleural effusions, polyhydramnios and placentomegaly at two sites on the fetus. The underlying cause of hydrops fetalis is often systemic and life threatening, varying from inborn metabolic errors, chromosomal abnormalities (trisomies, Turner's syndrome), isoimmunization, and nonimmune high-output cardiac failure. Cytomegalovirus is the most common infection causing fetal ascites and hepatocellular disease. Intrauterine meconium peritonitis is a sterile peritonitis caused by prenatal bowel perforation. Genitourinary causes of fetal ascites are common and necessitate early evaluation and potential fetal intervention to prevent progressive renal parenchymal destruction from obstructive uropathy and pulmonary hypoplasia.

Increased hydrostatic pressure in the setting of decreased oncotic pressure from hypoalbuminemia causes ascites. These factors alter the Starling forces and result in the movement of intravascular fluid to the extravascular space. When hepatic lymphatic drainage is exceeded by the production of extravascular fluid, then peritoneal fluid accumulates as ascites. Two theories attempt to account for the pathogenesis of ascites. The accumulation of ascites in the peritoneal cavity as a result of altered hydrostatic pressure and Starling forces is the *underfill* theory. Increased hydrostatic pressure can be caused by congestive heart failure or intrahepatic venous obstruction from intrahepatic scarring. The increased pressure in conjunction with low oncotic pressure from decreased hepatic synthesis, malnutrition, and protein-losing enteropathy causes low intravascular volume. Contracted blood volume results in decreased renal perfusion, secondarily stimulating salt and water retention. The *overflow* theory explains the presentation of patients with high cardiac output and hypervolemia. The initiating cause is attributed to renal sodium retention and plasma volume expansion via a hepatorenal mechanism; increased intravascular volume increases hydrostatic pressure and further fluid extravasation.

Peripheral vasodilation from decreased hepatic inactivation of endogenous vasodilators does diminish effective blood volume, leading to activation of the renin–angiotensin–aldosterone system and the sympathetic nervous system. This activation increases renal vascular resistance and promotes proximal and distal tubular sodium reabsorption, augmenting effective blood volume.

DIAGNOSIS

Abdominal distention and recent weight gain are the *sine qua non* of ascites. A history of liver disease is usually associated with physical signs of chronic liver disease: jaundice, large hemorrhoids, umbilical collateral veins (caput medusa), spider angiomas, and peripheral edema. Massive ascites is quite dramatic on physical examination, with marked distention, umbilical herniation, and scrotal swelling, and is associated with a resting tachypnea from compromised diaphragmatic breathing. In less obvious cases, ascites may be difficult to detect. Clinical features include a distended abdomen, bulging flanks, and dullness

A. C. Fischer: Department of Surgery, Division of Pediatric Surgery, Johns Hopkins Hospital, Baltimore, Maryland.

TABLE 90.1. DIFFERENTIAL DIAGNOSIS OF ASCITES

Serous ascites
Portal hypertension
Prehepatic (portal vein thrombosis)
Hepatic (cirrhosis, fibrosis)
Posthepatic (Budd-Chiari syndrome, congenital heart failure)
Hypoalbuminemia
Nephrotic syndrome
Protein-losing enteropathy
Malnutrition
Metabolic
α_1-Antitrypsin
Lysosomal storage disorders
Hypothyroidism
Postsurgical
Ventriculoperitoneal (V-P shunts)
Peritoneal dialysis
Gynecologic
Ruptured cyst
Hydrometrocolpos
Urinary ascites
Urinary obstruction/perforation
Posterior urethral valves
Ureterocele
Neurogenic bladder
Acute pancreatitis
Biliary ascites
Biliary atresia/perforation
Neonatal hepatitis
Cytomegalovirus infection
Failed portoenterostomy
Chylous ascites
Malrotation with volvulus
Lymphangiectasia/lymphangioma
Bowel obstruction (hernia)
Trauma
Pancreatic ascites
Pseudocyst
Acute pancreatitis
Malignant ascites
Pseudoascites

TABLE 90.2. CAUSES OF NEONATAL AND FETAL ASCITES

Structural abnormalities
Urinary obstruction
Congenital heart disease
Lymphatic obstruction
Biliary perforations
Ovarian cyst or hydrometrocolpos
Malrotation
Pulmonary malformation (CCAM, sequestration)
Hydrops fetalis
Isoimmunization
Twin–twin transfusion
High-output cardiac failure
Gastrointestinal
Meconium peritonitis
Cystic fibrosis
Atresias
Metabolic
α_1-Antitrypsin deficiency
Lysosomal storage disorder
Infection
Toxoplasmosis
Viruses (cytomegalovirus, parvoviruses)
Syphilis
Hemochromatosis/Thalassemia
Iatrogenic
Central venous hyperalimentation
Umbilical catheter injury

to percussion. Three signs can detect ascites more accurately on physical examination. Flank dullness is dull percussion at the level of the ascites-filled flanks in contrast to the tympanic sounds at the umbilicus reflecting gas-filled loops. Shifting dullness is the movement of dull percussion to the dependent side as the patient is placed in a lateral decubitus position. A fluid wave is a transmitted wave on the contralateral side when one side of the abdomen is percussed.

Classic radiographic findings on plain films include abdominal haziness, indistinct psoas muscle shadows, and obliteration of the lower lateral hepatic angle. An increased distance (>2 mm) between the right colon and the properitoneal fat stripe, the flank stripe sign, is suggestive. Ultrasonography is very sensitive. Real-time sonography can detect 10 mL or less in the most dependent spaces: the Morrison's pouch (hepatorenal recess) and the pelvic cul de sac. Identification of free-flowing ascites versus a loculated collection can differentiate true ascites from pseudoascites, such as omental and mesenteric cysts or intestinal duplications. If a diagnostic paracentesis is inconclusive, comprehensive imaging should include abdominal computed tomography (CT) or magnetic resonance imaging (MRI), echocardiogram (ECHO), and voiding cystourethrography. Diagnostic paracentesis initiates the evaluation of the ascitic fluid for biochemical and microbiologic characteristics (Table 90.3). The traditional classification of ascites was to distinguish transudative from exudative categories by examining the ratio of fluid to serum total protein and lactate dehydrogenase. Typical serous ascites from increased hydrostatic pressure is a straw-colored fluid with a low total protein concentration (<2.5 g/dL) and a low leukocyte count (<250–500 cells/mm^3). Exudative ascites, secondary to an inflammatory peritoneal process, can be turbid, with an elevated protein content (>3 g/dL) and elevated leukocyte count. The caveat is that the protein concentration and leukocyte count can be affected by diuretic therapy, impairing the classification based on these ratios. The serum: ascites albumin gradient is a more accurate and reliable evaluation. The albumin in the serum and ascites needs to be measured simultaneously. A high gradient defines a transudative ascites and a low gradient defines exudative ascites

TABLE 90.3. CLASSIFICATION OF ASCITES

Type of Ascites	Color	pH	Albumin	Characteristic Feature
Serous	Straw colored	7.35	~2 g/dL	Less than half plasma protein
Biliary	Dark gold	>7.4	~3 g/dL	Two to three times serum bilirubin
Urinary	Yellowish	<7.0	<1 g/dL	Five to ten times serum creatinine, urea
Chylous	Milky turbid	7.5	<3 g/dL	≥1,000 mg/dL triglyceride, leukocytosis
Pancreatic	Turbid or bloody	>7.4	Serum	>500 U/mL amylase Elevated lipase

(Table 90.4). A serum: ascites albumin gradient exceeding 1.1 g/dL is 97% accurate in identifying ascites from portal hypertension. The best predictor of peritonitis is a neutrophil count greater than 250 cells/mm^3 because the overall leukocyte count is commonly elevated and nonspecific. A low ascitic fluid pH, less than 7.31, is associated with a high mortality rate. A Gram stain and a direct inoculation of ascites into blood culture bottles should always be performed.

Diagnostic paracentesis, directed by a clinical suspicion, typically identifies a category for the causative pathology. Biliary ascites is dark gold as in patients with cholestasis but has elevated total and direct bilirubin. Urinary ascites has elevated creatinine and urea with markedly decreased levels of sodium and chloride. Serous ascites has a low protein content. The color of pancreatic ascites varies from milky turbidity to hemorrhagic discoloration. Amylase is elevated, unless the ascitic fluid is from an infant (amylase deficient), in whom lipase is elevated. Chylous ascites is characterized by a milky appearance, leukocytosis (1,000–5,000 cells/mm^3), and high triglyceride count. The lipid and protein content exceed that of plasma. In unfed infants the fluid is clear and the fat content varies with ingestion of fat. Fat globules can be detected microscopically as chylomicrons with Sudan stain.

TABLE 90.4. SERUM ASCITES CONCENTRATION GRADIENT

High Gradient (≥1.1 g/dL)	Low Gradient (<1.1 g/dL)
Portal hypertension	Infected peritonitis
Cirrhosis	Peritoneal carcinomatosis
Portal vein thrombosis	Biliary ascites
Cardiac heart failure	Nephrotic syndrome
Massive hepatic metastases	Chylous ascites
Hypothyroidism	Pancreatic ascites
Venoocclusive disease	Serositis, lupus
Budd-Chiari syndrome	

Modified from Runyon BA. Ascites and spontaneous bacterial peritonitis. In: Sleisenger, Fortran, eds. *Gastrointestinal and Liver Disease;* with permission.

MANAGEMENT

Therapy should be directed at the underlying pathology. Ascites can cause secondary complications such as respiratory and cardiovascular compromise, early satiety, and malnutrition.

Serous Ascites

For serous ascites, initial therapy should be salt restriction. Sodium should be restricted to 1 to 2 mEq/kg/day even in combination with diuretic therapy. Inadequate salt restriction is a reason for ascites to be refractory. Excessive fluid intake should be discouraged, and fluid restriction should be implemented when the serum sodium is below 130 mEq/L. Spironolactone is the first-line diuretic therapy (2–3 mg/kg/day) and inhibits aldosterone, preventing sodium reabsorption in the distal and collecting renal tubules. The dose can be doubled up to a maximum of 400 mg/day. Potential complications include hyperkalemia metabolic acidosis due to inhibition of renal hydrogen secretion and gynecomastia (antiandrogenic effect).

Furosemide (1–2 mg/kg/day) is a second-line therapy to work in concert with spironolactone therapy. Furosemide inhibits sodium absorption proximally in the loop of Henle, and spironolactone prevents sodium absorption downstream in the collecting tubules. Furosemide is a potent natriuretic drug and can cause a hypokalemia metabolic alkalosis from kaliureses and azotemia. Patients with ascites in the absence of edema should be made to lose approximately 300 to 500 mL/day of urine. Aggressive diuresis can elicit hypovolemia and can initiate the hepatorenal syndrome. Nutritional management in these patients is essential because the hypoalbuminemia causes an edematous intestinal tract and malabsorption. Patients with hepatocellular disease malabsorb fat and fat-soluble vitamins. Patients with diuretic-resistant ascites are refractory to medical therapy and should consider surgical options. Large-volume paracentesis (4–6 L/day) can be performed in a hemodynamically stable fashion, if an intravenous infusion of salt-poor albumin is given concurrently (8 g/L of ascitic fluid). Large-volume therapeutic paracentesis is the treatment of choice for symptomatic relief in tense ascites.

Surgical palliation is appropriate for a refractory underlying condition. Peritoneovenous shunting and transjugular intrahepatic portosystemic shunting for intractable ascites as a bridge for transplantation have been applied to infants and children. The Leveen shunt has a perforated end that is placed in the peritoneum and a silicone catheter that can be tunneled subcutaneously for internal jugular venous placement. The Leveen shunt has a one-way pressure-sensitive valve so that fluid flows into the vascular compartment when a pressure gradient exceeds 3 cm H_2O. The Denver shunt has an additional bulb such that additional fluid can be pumped intravascularly as it fills the bulb. Other shunts, customized for neonatal sizes, have used a reversed ventriculoperitoneal shunt or a newborn peritoneal dialysis catheter. Complications of shunts include infection, intravascular coagulation as the ascitic fibrin split products are delivered directly into the venous system, and shunt occlusion (25% by 5 years). Contraindications include liver failure, severe coagulopathy, bacterial peritonitis, and variceal hemorrhage.

Transjugular intrahepatic portosystemic shunts lower portal pressures, prevent rebleeding from variceal hemorrhage, and provide effective control of ascites in patients refractory to conventional therapy. They also cause a delayed natriuresis, improved hemodynamic central blood volume, and renin–angiotensin–aldosterone activity. In patients with a clear anatomic abnormality such as a suprahepatic web as in Budd Chiari, interventional radiology has used innovative techniques with balloon dilatation and stents to restore normal blood flow (Figs. 90.1 and 90.2).

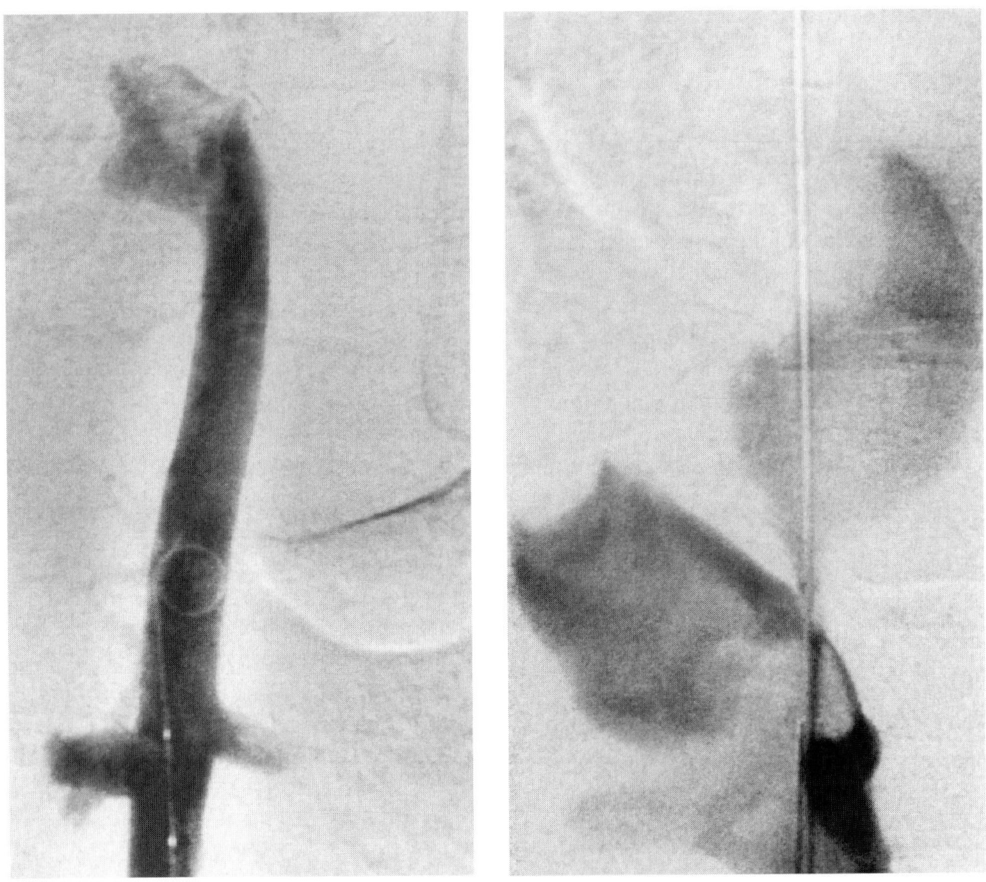

FIGURE 90.1. A venocavagram in a patient with Budd-Chiari syndrome. Ultrasonography and magnetic resonance venography (MRV) demonstrated reversal of flow in the intrahepatic inferior vena cava. The inferior vena cava venocavagram pictured here is narrowed above the origin of the hepatic veins to the level of the right atrium. The acute narrowing above the origin of the hepatic veins is diverting all the venacaval flow into the right hepatic vein.

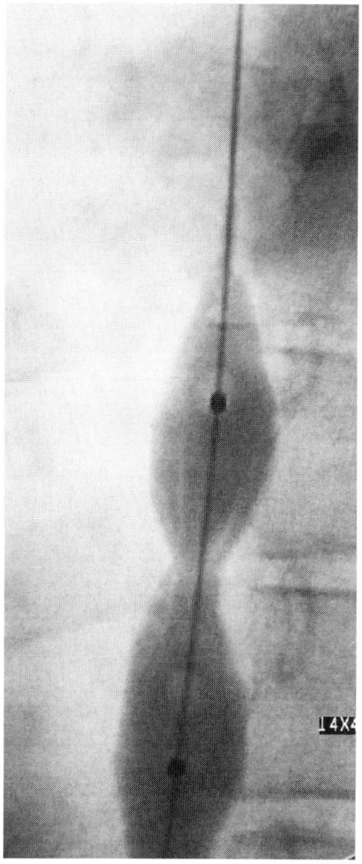

FIGURE 90.2. A percutaneous venoplasty was performed and the inferior vena caval web was balloon dilated. The waist of the balloon demonstrates the constriction of the web.

Pancreatic Ascites

Pancreatic ascites is usually related to a traumatic injury in children. In the absence of an anatomic lesion such as a duct injury, pancreatic ascites typically resolves without specific therapy. Most cases are associated with the development of a pancreatic pseudocyst, of which more than half resolve spontaneously. Simple ultrasound- or CT-directed aspiration is an initial option that is associated with a 30% or greater recurrence rate and possible infection of the cyst, which would then necessitate catheter drainage. A conservative approach entails hyperalimentation, avoidance of oral intake, and waiting 6 weeks for the wall of the pseudocyst to mature into a fibrous capsule. Ductal anatomy is important, and a communication can be bridged via endoscopic pancreatic stents or operative management. Formal internal drainage surgically drains the pseudocyst via cystogastrostomy or cystojejunostomy, depending on the location of the cyst.

Biliary Ascites

Typically ascites occurs at a young age, under 12 weeks, and less frequently in older children. The common causes can be spontaneous perforation, neonatal hepatitis, or a failed portoenterostomy. Spontaneous perforation of the biliary tree is idiopathic and occurs in the newborn period. Infants present with ascites, jaundice, and acholic stools. A technetium 99m DISIDA scan can demonstrate the leak from a perforation, typically at the juncture of the common bile duct and the cystic duct. Cystic fibrosis also can present with biliary tract obstruction. Treatment for biliary ascites is surgical, and laparotomy, cholecystostomy to image the ductal anatomy, and external biliary tract drainage are performed. Biliary tract repair is not essential because with adequate drainage over 80% of patients recover in 3 weeks on hyperalimentation, bowel rest, and antibiotics. Complex biliary tract reconstruction is hazardous and fraught with difficulty. Traumatic or iatrogenic injuries in older children usually necessitate ductal repair as well as drainage.

Urinary Ascites

Urinary ascites is a common cause of ascites in the newborn and has been associated with a high mortality in the past. Boys are predominantly affected, with a 7:1 incidence. Urinary ascites occurs in fetuses and neonates with complex urogenital malformations such as hydrometrocolpos, prune belly syndrome (abdominal wall laxity, megacystis, megaureters, and cryptorchism), or Potter's syndrome (renal insufficiency, oligohydramnios, and pulmonary hypoplasia). Mechanical obstruction from posterior urethral valves accounts for 70% of cases. Hyponatremia, metabolic acidosis, and elevated serum blood urea nitrogen reflect peritoneal absorption of urine. Ultrasonography, voiding cystourethrography, and intravenous urography demonstrate the obstruction and site of extravasation. Resuscitation, antibiotics, correction of electrolytes, and urinary drainage are essential, whereas actual repair of the perforation is rarely necessary. Urinary drainage can relieve the obstructive uropathy and can be accomplished using a Foley catheter, valve ablation, percutaneous nephrostomy, or a vesicostomy.

Meconium Peritonitis

Isolated ascites is often caused by a gastrointestinal pathology such as meconium peritonitis, which can be due to a prenatal obstruction such as an atresia or volvulus, concretions from cystic fibrosis, or intrauterine viral infections from parvovirus B19, CMV, or hepatitis A. The free spillage of meconium initiates a sterile chemical peritonitis and intrabdominal calcifications. Asymptomatic neonates without concurrent bowel compromise do not require surgery for this prenatal event.

Chylous Ascites

In children chylous ascites is more frequent in infants and results more commonly from congenital abnormalities (40%) than malignant causes (3%). There may be an anatomic lesion in the case of a lymphoma, lymphangiectasia, or trauma that requires surgical correction. Both lymphoscintigraphy and lymphangiography can localize the anatomic pathology and lymphatic leak. Nonoperative therapy resolves 50% to 75% of non-neoplastic cases. Bowel rest with total parenteral nutrition and enteral feeds with specialized formula that is high in medium-chain triglycerides are two acceptable options. Short- and medium-chain fatty acids (12 carbons) are directly transported to the portal system and bypass the lymphatic system, unlike long-chain fatty acids. Failure of nonoperative therapy after 4 to 6 weeks may require preoperative imaging with lymphangiography or MRI and then surgery for exploration and possible ligation of the cisterna chyli. Preoperative feedings of cream or lipophilic dye can best demonstrate the leak intraoperatively. Other therapies need to be directed toward the various underlying pathologies such as lymphoma, tuberculosis, and parasitic infection. The overall mortality rate in children with chylous ascites is 21% due to the complications with malnutrition, immunosuppression, and infection. The underlying cause in adults is often neoplasia, and consequently ascites in this setting is associated with a high mortality rate (>80%). Peritoneovenous shunts used in serous ascites can be quite useful for recalcitrant chylous ascites in both traumatic cases and postsurgical ascites.

SUGGESTED READINGS

Abbas BS, et al. Idiopathic perforation of the extrahepatic bile duct in infancy; pathogenesis, diagnosis, and management. *J Pediatr Surg* 1993;28:950–952.

Beal AL, Gormley CM, Gordon DL, et al. Chylous ascites: a manifestation of blunt abdominal trauma in an infant. *J Pediatr Surg* 1998;33:650–652.

Cao S, Monge H, Sembe C, et al. Emergency transjugular intrahepatic portosystemic shunt (TIPS) in an infant: a case report. *J Pediatr Surg* 1997;32:125–127.

Machin GA. Diseases causing fetal and neonatal ascites. *Pediatr Pathol* 1985;4:195–211.

Pettitt BJ. Use of a modified Denver peritoneovenous shunt in a newborn with intractable ascites. *J Pediatr Surg* 1992;27:108–109.

Runyon BA, Montano AA, Akriviadis EA, et al. The serum-ascites albumin gradient in the differential of ascites is superior to the exudate/transudate concept. *Ann Intern Med* 1992;117:215–220.

Zelop C, Bencerrat BR. The causes and natural history of fetal ascites. *Prenat Diagn* 1994;14:941–946.

91

GASTROSCHISIS

GEORGE B. MYCHALISKA
MICHAEL D. KLEIN

Gastroschisis is a congenital defect of the abdominal wall in which there is a small defect (usually <4 cm in diameter) to the right of the umbilical cord, through which the entire midgut is herniated. Frequently, the stomach, small intestine, and colon are eviscerated, but never the liver. The defect is occasionally separated from the cord by a strip of skin. There is no sac or membrane covering the midgut. These features distinguish gastroschisis from omphalocele (midline defect, sac present, liver in the defect) and umbilical cord hernia (essentially a very small omphalocele). In the 1950s and 1960s gastroschisis was thought to be an uncommon defect related embryologically to a failure of formation of the abdominal wall. It is now the most common of the congenital abdominal wall defects, and probably is related to a failure of formation of the umbilical coelom. As the midgut elongates, beginning at 5 or 6 weeks, it has no space into which to herniate. Although the peritoneal cavity is hypoplastic, the abdominal musculature is normal. The intestine then comes out of the abdominal cavity to the right of the umbilical cord, because the right umbilical vein has resorbed and the abdominal wall is relatively unsupported there.

All babies with gastroschisis have malrotation. There is a 10% to 15% incidence of intestinal tract atresia; there are seldom other associated anomalies. Children with gastroschisis are frequently premature or small for gestational age. Their mothers are often young, with poor prenatal care and lower socioeconomic status. Gastroschisis can usually be diagnosed with antenatal ultrasonography, and it is associated with increased maternal serum alpha-fetoprotein.

The bowel and its mesentery are usually thickened, edematous, foreshortened, and covered with a fibrinous peel. This is felt to be responsible for the prolonged failure to tolerate enteral feedings. The lack of peristalsis and slow return of bowel function often lasts 20 to 30 days. Some have attributed this injury to the change in the electrolyte composition of the amniotic fluid, which occurs after the fetal kidney begins to function, and for this reason have argued for the early delivery of children with an antenatal diagnosis of gastroschisis. We have noted that in most cases this characteristic bowel injury is often not present immediately at birth, but only develops in the first 5 to 20 minutes following birth. We believe that it is due primarily to venous obstruction by the mass of the bowel hanging out over the abdominal wall and being exposed to the drying effect of air. There is transudation of fluid and edema formation in the bowel wall. It is our opinion that immediate operation in the delivery room may minimize this bowel injury and lead to early restoration of gastrointestinal function.

DIAGNOSIS

The diagnosis is easy to make if one keeps in mind the characteristic features of gastroschisis: small defect to the right of midline with no sac. Other congenital abdominal wall defects include omphalocele, umbilical cord hernia, cloacal exstrophy (infraumbilical omphalocele, exstrophy of the bladder, imperforate anus), and Cantrell's pentalogy (supraumbilical omphalocele, sternal cleft, intracardiac anomaly, defect in diaphragm, and defect in pericardium). Antenatal diagnosis with ultrasonography allows for counseling of families and for the medical team to prepare for early operation following delivery.

PREOPERATIVE PREPARATION

Cesarean section has not been shown to confer any special benefit over vaginal delivery. In some institutions it allows for more expeditious repair, although a baby born vaginally can be carried directly to the operating room just as swiftly. Some surgeons have argued for early delivery of these children at preterm gestational age to avoid the bowel damage that they presume is due to the change in amniotic fluid

G. B. Mychaliska: Department of Pediatric General Surgery, Children's Hospital of Michigan, Detroit, Michigan.

M. D. Klein: Department of Surgery, Wayne State University; and Department of Surgery, Children's Hospital of Michigan, Detroit, Michigan.

electrolyte composition. Having observed scores of babies with gastroschisis in the delivery room with our program of immediate repair, we are convinced that there is seldom bowel damage present at birth. Early delivery only adds the complications of prematurity to a child who must already face many challenges.

Delivery should occur at a facility with a level III nursery and expertise in pediatric surgery. Attention should be directed to keeping the patient warm, and the bowel moist and decompressed. A Replogle nasogastric (NG) tube should be placed immediately and placed on low continuous suction. The baby should then be placed in a bowel bag used commonly in adult surgery. This is a transparent plastic bag with an umbilical tape drawstring. The entire lower half of the baby can be placed in it, and the drawstring is pulled snugly around the chest at the level of the axilla. A few drops of water in the bag will keep the atmosphere inside moist. Placing moist gauze on the bowel increases evaporative heat loss, can abrade the bowel, and prevents visual assessment of the color and viability of the bowel.

Upper extremity intravenous lines are preferable because primary closure may embarrass venous return from the lower extremities. If the foot is needed for a peripheral intravenous line, a small hole can be made in the bag and the foot brought out of the bag. A Foley catheter is placed to monitor urine output. Blood is drawn for hemoglobin and other studies as indicated by the child's concomitant problems, which may include prematurity and respiratory distress. We routinely give ampicillin and cefotaxime intravenously.

Children with gastroschisis have a fluid requirement of 200 to 300 mL/kg in the first 24 hours. A fluid bolus of D5LR at 20 mL/kg is given, and then urine output and tissue perfusion guide fluid administration, usually starting at 200 mL/kg/24 hours.

Spontaneous ventilation is certainly best. Bag and mask ventilation should be avoided in favor of early intubation to prevent intestinal distention.

OPERATIVE THERAPY

We prefer to take the patient to the operating room only moments after delivery. There is no need to go first to the neonatal intensive care unit (NICU). The patient should receive preoperative antibiotics, an NG tube, and a Foley catheter. The baby must be kept warm during the procedure. We use muscle paralysis and assume that patients will go to the NICU intubated on a ventilator following the operation, although not all require this. While the anesthesiologist is starting an intravenous line and intubating the patient, prior to attempting to reduce the bowel, we try to create more space by placing a finger in the abdomen through the defect and massaging laterally and upward to literally stretch the abdominal wall. We do a rectal examination to evacuate meconium and begin reducing the bowel under clean circumstances. This reduction is performed without exploration or particular attention to what each loop of bowel represents. Sometimes the bowel content may be pressed out of the bowel through the rectum or milked proximally and aspirated. There are occasionally adhesions of the bowel to the skin in the abdominal wall, which must be lysed prior to attempts at reduction. Often the entire mass of intestine is reduced prior to the skin preparation.

At this point we prepare and drape the patient. The rim of skin and scar is excised circumferentially around the defect. The umbilical arteries and the umbilical vein, as well as the urachus, are ligated and divided with 3-0 absorbable ties. We do not translocate the umbilical vein and catheterize it, preferring to use an external jugular central venous catheter at a later date, if central venous access is required. In premature babies, it may be wise to place an umbilical artery catheter and translocate that lateral to the midline for blood gas monitoring.

The abdominal wall defect may be enlarged longitudinally to facilitate primary closure. This enlargement is also helpful if a silo is placed, because it prevents the creation of a narrow base and eases reduction of bowel. Skin flaps are then developed widely, and an attempt is made to close the fascia with interrupted simple and mattress sutures of 2-0 absorbable suture. If this cannot be done, or if doing so results in unacceptably high ventilatory pressures (>35 cm H_2O), an attempt is made to dissect the skin flaps further and obtain a skin closure with the acceptance of a ventral hernia. In this case, the skin is closed with running 3-0 nylon or polypropylene. With primary closure, an attempt at umbilicoplasty is often made using a purse-string technique. Alternatively, if one uses a running skin suture and draws it tight, by 1 year of age the contracted scar will often be as cosmetically acceptable as one constructed with a formal umbilicoplasty.

A tight primary abdominal closure can result in ventilatory compromise, impeded venous return, and compression of small bowel mesentery leading to intestinal ischemia. If primary closure is impossible, we use a silo of Dacron-reinforced Silastic (0.007 inches thick, Dow Corning, Midland, MI). We suture one piece to each side with running 3-0 polypropylene. The stitches are placed so that the knots are on the outside, and the Silastic and fascial edge evert. We then use running 3.0 polypropylene sutures up each side and choose a comfortable height where we can continue the 3.0 polypropylene across the top before cutting off excess Silastic. The configuration of the silo is important. It should be constructed as a cylinder or trapezoid with no narrowing of the silo at the base. At the conclusion of the procedure, we do not use tape or dressings, but cover the incision and sutures with povidone-iodine solution ointment. The patient is then taken to the NICU. Throughout this procedure, and postoperatively, we use morphine and midazolam for pain and sedation along with pancuronium for paralysis.

POSTOPERATIVE CARE

We use pressure-controlled ventilation, and often the peak inspiratory pressure (PIP) is as high as 30 or 35 mm Hg soon after reduction, especially in primarily closed patients. Weaning is guided by oxygenation/ventilation as assessed by blood gases, and by the need for paralysis and sedation. If a silo was placed, the babies are not extubated prior to abdominal wall closure. Fluid management is crucial during the first 2 to 3 days. The babies remain on D5/0.45 normal saline with 20 mEq KCl/L for the first 12 to 24 hours and then are changed to D5/0.2 normal saline with 20 mEq KCl/L at a rate of 150 to 200 mL/kg/day. Fluid status is carefully monitored with urine output, specific gravity, tissue perfusion, and central venous pressure. On the second or third postoperative day, total parenteral nutrition (TPN) is initiated with a caloric goal of 120 kcal/kg/day. A central venous catheter or peripherally inserted central catheter (PICC) line is used for TPN.

Return of bowel function is notoriously slow, and many infants require TPN and bowel rest for 2 to 4 weeks. An NG tube is kept on low continuous suction until the appearance of bowel function. After return of bowel function, enteral feeds are initiated and advanced as tolerated to goal. We remove the sutures at 3 weeks. After 3 weeks, if there has been no evidence of bowel function, we do a contrast study. Seldom does one find a real anatomic obstruction from adhesions, stenosis, or atresia. Continued observation on TPN for another several days to weeks is usually all that is required. A few children with gastroschisis go on to develop chronic intestinal pseudoobstruction and the need for long-term TPN.

Whether the babies are closed primarily or have a silo, one must be alert to the possibility of an abdominal compartment syndrome, which is heralded by a tense abdomen, difficulty with ventilation, increased peak inspiratory pressures, and decreased urine output.

MANAGEMENT OF THE SILO

Various techniques of reducing the silo have been described. We prefer to simply reduce the bowel content with gloved hands, and then apply a bowel clamp directly above the intestines. The clamp can be left in place or sutures can be run across the top of the clamp. Once the bowel has been completely reduced, the patient is ready to go to the operating room for removal of the silo and closure of the abdominal wall.

When Samuel Schuster introduced the prosthetic staged repair of abdominal wall defects, reduction would take place every 3 days in the operating room. Several investigators have studied the intraabdominal pressure that can be tolerated during reduction. This pressure can be measured through a gastrostomy tube, through an NG tube, or by attaching a water manometer to the Foley catheter. The lesson learned is that intraabdominal pressure of less than 20 cm H_2O is well tolerated. More importantly, if one does monitor intraabdominal pressure, one reduces the intestinal contents much more frequently. In fact, we seldom measure pressures, but using the information from these studies, we reduce the intestinal content at least once a day. It is important to have the contents reduced and the silo removed by 2 weeks (ideally in less than 1 week) because the silo separates if left on too long, and infectious complications are more likely.

When the silo is removed in the operating room, the skin flaps will need to be elevated again. An attempt at fascial closure can be made. If this is done, one must be careful to place the sutures (2-0 absorbable suture) only through the fascia and rectus muscle on each side. It is tempting to place the stitches through the fascia only, which seems tough, but this will often result in a ventral hernia that will require repair later. A Gore-Tex soft tissue patch (A.L. Gore & Associates, Newark, Delaware) can be used at this point to try to obtain a definitive closure, however, it must be covered by healthy skin. In general, we do not use this technique. If we cannot get a fascial closure, we perform a skin closure at this time and repair the resulting ventral hernia at 1 year of age. We have a few patients who have not required a repair but somehow have developed a very solid abdominal wall. Most patients require repair of this ventral hernia, and even the largest seem to do well at 1 to 2 years of age. We admit the patient to the hospital at the time of ventral hernia repair and use an NG tube postoperatively.

Many surgeons have found success using a new preformed silo that has a spring-wound open lower end. This can be placed even at the bedside with the spring-wound lower end going inside the abdomen and being self-securing. We have found that as one increases the pressure by reducing the silo, the spring can pop out, requiring a trip to the operating room, either for closure or replacement of the device. When we use this device, we usually use it in the operating room, and we suture the wire component of the ring to the abdominal wall fascia after it has been introduced.

FOLLOW-UP

Most children transition to enteral feeding and can be discharged from the hospital 3 to 6 weeks following birth. We usually follow the patients carefully in the office up to 1 year of age to be sure that they are gaining weight and growing appropriately.

COMPLICATIONS

The most significant pitfall is overaggressive attempts at primary closure at any stage in the operative therapy. Patients with a taut abdomen, low urine output, persistent acidosis, and high peak ventilatory pressures may need to go back to the operating room for placement of a silo or to have more bowel exteriorized into their silo. Other complications include sepsis, abdominal wall cellulitis, necrotizing enterocolitis, and TPN-related cholestasis. Absorption of carbohydrates, protein, and fat may be abnormal in the first few months, but usually returns to normal by 6 months of age. On rare occasions, intestinal atresia is missed, and this is diagnosed by an inability to tolerate enteral feedings or upper gastrointestinal with small bowel follow-through after 3 to 4 weeks of a prolonged ileus.

CONCLUSIONS

The overall outcome for babies with gastroschisis is good. The mortality rate is 10% and is related to sepsis or complications secondary to intestinal atresias or short-bowel syndrome. With advances in neonatal critical care, TPN, and surgical technique, the majority of these babies can lead healthy and productive lives.

EDITOR'S NOTES

Reduction and repair of a gastroschisis defect often challenge the judgment and skill of the pediatric surgeon, yet the result is usually gratifying, at least from the technical standpoint. On the other hand, the postoperative care and management of complications that often arise can be vexing and extremely frustrating. It is telling that although these infants are typically otherwise healthy, with rare associated anomalies, and with what should be a relatively simple problem to address surgically, they have only an 85% to 90% survival rate in most large series. These infants are at risk for a myriad of unusual complications, including necrotizing enterocolitis, unexplained sepsis, venous thrombosis, and short bowel syndrome, as well as the morbidity associated with prolonged parenteral nutrition, such as hepatic dysfunction, access issues, and line complications.

The approach suggested in this chapter by Drs. Mychaliska and Klein is interesting but somewhat controversial. The idea that reducing the bowel into the abdomen as quickly as possible after birth to avoid further injury certainly makes sense and is supported by their very good results; however, some find it logistically challenging, and debate continues as to its relative benefit. Nevertheless, most of us would agree that rapid reduction is best and should be the goal in all cases.

There should also be a low threshold to use staged repair with a silo. Although considered by some to be an extraordinary maneuver, experience with the technique has shown it to be well tolerated, with surprisingly few complications, and with results comparable to those of primary repair. It is certainly preferable to a very tight closure with abdominal compartment syndrome and the persistent concern about bowel ischemia. If a reasonable attempt at primary repair results in a PIP of greater than 25 mm Hg, then staged repair should probably be considered without delay. Some technical points are worth emphasizing. The silo should be secured to the fascia with a running monofilament suture, with a good purchase of fascia with each bite, and with care not to cinch the suture too tight so as to strangulate the tissue or to excessively narrow the base of the silo. It is critical that the silo be created in such a way that the base is broader than the top; otherwise, attempts at reduction will be difficult and disruption of the fascial suture line may occur. The silo is constructed by rolling a rectangular piece of reinforced Silastic into a tube. Because the silo is round at the bottom and flat at the top, it will be broader at the top unless the side is trimmed as well (Fig. 91.1). Reduction of the silo can be performed daily or every other day, depending on surgeon's preference, with the goal to effect complete reduction within 7 to 10 days. Beyond this time, the risks of sepsis and suture line disruption are far greater. I find that every-other-day reduction allows about half of the bowel to be reduced each time, so that by the third attempt, reduction is complete and the fascia is starting to come together. Most patients can return to the operating room for removal of the silo and closure of the fascia by the 7th or 8th day.

The goal at each operation should be to work quickly and return the infant to the NICU as soon as possible. No attempt should be made to lyse adhesions, debride the peel, or deal with an atresia. These maneuvers only serve to prolong the case and increase the risk of hemorrhage and perforation. Gross perforations can be gently approximated in a single layer with simple or figure-of-eight sutures. Resec-

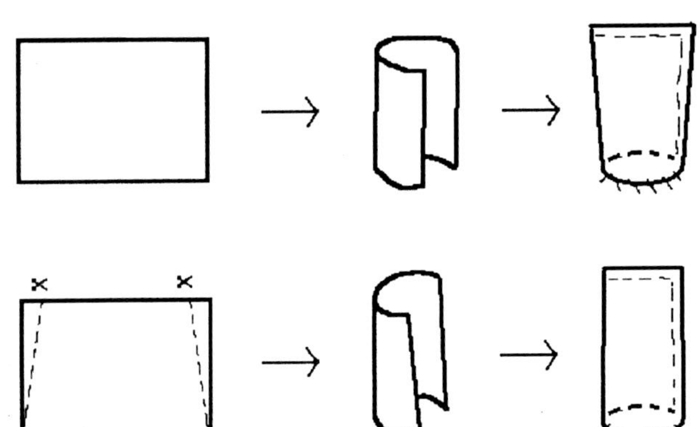

FIGURE 91.1. Creation of a silo from a rectangular piece of Silastic requires that the sides be trimmed so as to prevent an inverted-pyramid configuration. The result is a silo with straight or slightly tapered sides that allows for easier and safer bowel reduction.

tion and reanastomosis is inadvisable and likely to fail. Stomas are considered acceptable but are almost never necessary. It is usually best to reduce the bowel and address the obstruction after 4 to 6 weeks have passed and the acute inflammation has subsided.

Infants with gastroschisis often develop a prolonged ileus that is thought to be due to the injury associated with exposure to amniotic fluid. There is not always a correlation, however, between the visible extent of bowel injury and time to return of bowel function. Another possibility is that babies with gastroschisis have a primary motility disorder that causes both the gastroschisis and the prolonged ileus. Whatever the cause, this is a period of anxiety and uncertainty for the parents and the caregivers. The point at which it is time to consider the possibility of a bowel obstruction is also debatable. Most would probably agree that if after 4 to 6 weeks the child is not advancing adequately on feedings, then an obstruction needs to be ruled out. An upper gastrointestinal contrast study can sometimes show dilated loops of bowel or other evidence of an obstruction, but a laparotomy needs to be considered when the study is equivocal in the setting of high clinical suspicion.

–P.M.

SUGGESTED READINGS

Coughlin JP, Drucker DE, Jewell MR, et al. Delivery room repair of gastroschisis. *Surgery* 1993;114:822–827.

Drongowski RA, Smith RK, Coran AG, et al. Contribution of demographic and environmental factors to the etiology of gastroschisis: a hypothesis. *Fetal Diagn Ther* 1991;6:14–27.

Dunn JC, Fonkalsrud EW, Atkinson JB. The influence of gestational age and mode of delivery on infants with gastroschisis. *J Pediatr Surg* 1999;34:1393–1395.

How HY, Harris BJ, Pietrantoni M, et al. Is vaginal delivery preferable to elective cesarean delivery in fetuses with a known ventral wall defect? *Am J Obstet Gynaecol* 2000;182:1527–1534.

Minkes RK, Langer JC, Massiotti MV, et al. Routine insertion of a Silastic spring-loaded silo for infants with gastroschisis. *J Pediatr Surg* 2000;35:843–846.

Snyder CL. Outcome analysis for gastroschisis. *J Pediatr Surg* 1999; 34:1253–1256.

92

OMPHALOCELE

LISA P. ABRAMSON
SUSAN R. LUCK
ROBERT M. ARENSMAN

An omphalocele is a persistent opening in the abdominal wall that results from incomplete fetal growth and fusion of the cephalic, lateral, and caudal tissue folds (Fig. 92.1). The umbilical ring remains open and the viscera are covered by a thin sheet of fused amnion and peritoneum contiguous with the base of the umbilical cord. During normal fetal development, the midgut grows and elongates outside of the embryonic coelom beginning at approximately 4 weeks' gestation. During the 10th week, the midgut should assume an intraabdominal position, undergoing counterclockwise rotation with retroperitoneal fixation of the right and left colon. If intestinal herniation into the sac persists after the 10th gestational week, some form of nonrotation will result and the midgut will not assume a normal intraabdominal position with fixation of the mesenteric base. This lack of fixation and a narrow mesentery can predispose to midgut volvulus.

The incidence of omphalocele is approximately 1 in 5,000 live births, with a slight male predominance. The umbilical defect and overlying sac can range in size from 4 to 12 cm. Visceroabdominal disproportion (VAD) is defined as the volume mismatch between the hernia contents and the size of the abdominal cavity. The degree of VAD is useful in determining treatment strategies for each infant. Giant omphaloceles have a massive sac herniating through fascial defects greater than 8 cm and contain most of the abdominal viscera, including the liver (Fig. 92.2). This occurs in approximately 10% of omphaloceles, and these children have special considerations secondary to small, underdeveloped peritoneal cavities. The combination of high VAD, absent or decreased muscle tissue, and pulmonary hypoplasia makes primary closure impossible. Reduction of the eviscerated liver may compromise the drainage of the main hepatic veins, leading to infarction. A review of chest radiographs in these infants shows smaller chest widths and lung areas, resulting in pulmonary hypoplasia. Pulmonary hypoplasia, in combination with tight abdominal closures, can lead to prolonged need for mechanical ventilation and poor outcomes for these babies. The lack of intraabdominal visceral fixation may result in a deficiency of chest wall expansion and contribute to the pulmonary dysfunction.

More than half the infants with omphaloceles have associated anomalies that involve the cardiovascular, alimentary, genitourinary, musculoskeletal, or central nervous systems (Table 92.1). The two most common cardiac defects are tetralogy of Fallot and atrial septal defects. Others may be affected by genetic syndromes such as trisomy 13 to 15, 18, and 21 and Beckwith-Wiedemann syndrome (umbilical defects, macroglossia, hyperinsulinism, visceromegaly), which results from an abnormality on chromosome 11. This syndrome is found in approximately 12% of cases, although the associated omphalocele is usually small.

PRENATAL DIAGNOSIS AND TREATMENT

The prenatal diagnosis of omphalocele can be established by ultrasonography during the second trimester. Insertion of the umbilical cord into the sac overlying the herniated viscera differentiates this condition from gastroschisis. Prenatal counseling facilitates optimal planning for delivery and immediate access to a tertiary care hospital with a neonatal intensive care unit and pediatric surgical expertise. On the other hand, in the EUROCAT study published in 1995, 33% of fetuses diagnosed prenatally with omphalocele were aborted electively. Maternal serum alpha-fetoprotein (MSAFP) measured during the second trimester is another screening tool and may be elevated in both patients with omphaloceles and those with gastroschisis. A two-fold increase in MSAFP from the median level is 78% predictive

S. R. Luck and R. M. Arensman: Departments of Surgery and Pediatrics, Northwestern University Medical School; and Department of Pediatric General Surgery, Children's Memorial Hospital, Chicago, Illinois.

L. P. Abramson: Department of Surgery, University of California, Davis, Sacramento, California; and Department of Pediatric General Surgery, Children's Memorial Hospital, Chicago, Illinois.

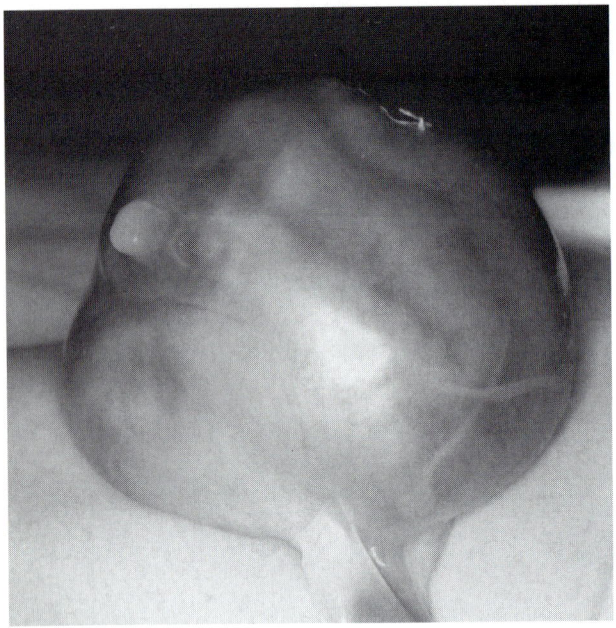

FIGURE 92.1. Typical omphalocele with the umbilical cord inserting on the sac.

of omphalocele and 99% predictive of gastroschisis. Amniocentesis with chromosomal analysis is recommended. Despite ongoing debate, recent studies indicate that cesarean section should be performed for obstetric reasons only.

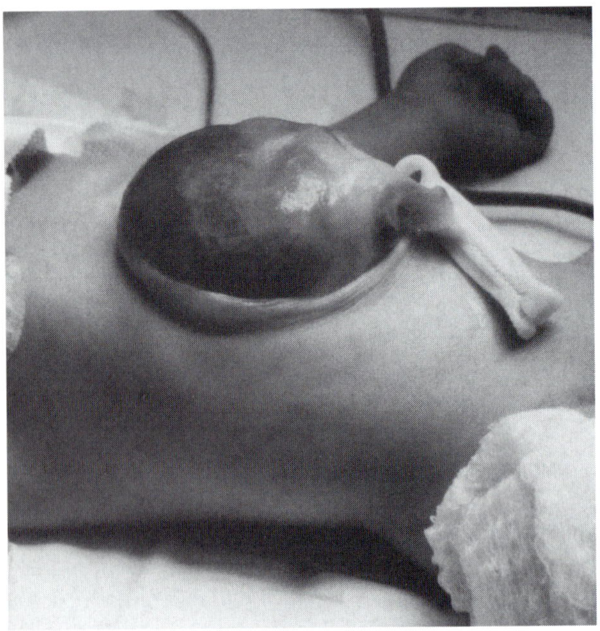

FIGURE 92.2. Giant omphalocele. Note the liver contained within the hernia sac.

TABLE 92.1. ANOMALIES ASSOCIATED WITH OMPHALOCELE

Associated Anomalies
Cardiac defects
Malrotation
Beckwith-Wiedemann syndrome
Trisomy 13 to 15, 18, 21
Bladder or cloacal extrophy
Sacral vertebral anomalies
Diaphragmatic hernia
Meningomyelocele
Reiger syndrome
Prune-belly syndrome
Pentalogy of Cantrell
Meckel diverticulum
Cleft palate
Cryptorchidism

POSTNATAL CARE

Treatment at birth begins with the immediate insertion of an orogastric or nasogastric tube to decompress the stomach and prevent vomiting, aspiration, and bowel distention. The intact sac is covered with a moist dressing or plastic intestinal bag, and the baby is transferred to a thermoneutral environment. Baseline laboratory studies should include an immediate serum glucose analysis. Severe hypoglycemia is associated with Beckwith-Wiedemann syndrome and if untreated, can result in brain injury and mental retardation. If the viscera are contained in an intact sac, insensible losses are not extensive. However, approximately 10% of neonates will have sustained a prenatal sac rupture and have increased fluid losses requiring urgent intestinal coverage. Small tears of the sac may be sutured closed or tied at bedside. A short course of broad-spectrum antibiotics is administered to cover the expected contamination from delivery and may include ampicillin 100 mg/kg/day and gentamycin 5 mg/kg/day. Initial evaluation includes a complete physical examination, chest radiography, renal ultrasonography, and cardiac echocardiography to search for associated anomalies.

OPERATIVE MANAGEMENT

Surgical treatment varies depending on the size of the defect, the degree of VAD, the degree of associated pulmonary hypoplasia, and the congenital malformations present. Approximately 60% to 70% of omphaloceles can be closed primarily. The goal of any surgical technique for omphalocele repair is coverage of the eviscerated intestine without creating an abdominal compartment syndrome or compromising hepatic venous return. Intraabdominal pressure greater than 20 mm Hg causes reduction in renal and splanchnic blood flow, decreased cardiac output, compromised respiratory function, and decreased venous return. Ideally, the abdominal wall is closed primarily to decrease infection and allow earlier return of bowel function and enteral feedings. However, primary operative closure is not recommended in infants with minimal tissue for coverage, severe pulmonary hypoplasia, and a high degree of VAD resulting in a tight closure.

A fascial defect smaller than 4 cm can be closed primarily in all cases. The baby is prepared and draped from neck to pubis. A central venous access catheter should be considered, especially when the defect is large. A 5-mm incision is made in the midline at the superior and inferior edges of the abdominal wall defect. A subcutaneous tunnel is developed from the xiphoid to the pubis. The abdominal wall may need manual stretching with one or two fingers from inside the abdomen along the abdominal wall. The sac is excised, and care is taken to avoid injury to the liver because the sac is often adherent and may cause significant hemorrhage. In some cases it may be safer to leave a portion of the sac in place. The intestines are carefully inspected for abnormalities and then reduced through the defect, making sure that the mesentery is not kinked. Skin, fascia, or both are then closed depending on the hemodynamic and respiratory status of the infant. Fascia is closed in an interrupted single layer, and the skin is closed with sterile strips. Creation of an umbilicus is performed by elevating the skin and subcutaneous tissue off of the fascia for 1.5 cm around the defect before closure.

We have adopted a nonoperative strategy to treat infants with large defects that cannot be closed primarily. Dilute povidone-iodine solution (0.1%), silver sulfadiazine, or plain saline is used to paint the omphalocele sac. A stable eschar subsequently forms over a period of 2 to 3 months. The hernia sac eventually scars and contracts, creating a smaller defect over time. Elective ventral hernia repair is then planned when the child reaches 20 pounds or 1 year of age. This technique minimizes the need for mechanical ventilatory support necessitated by operative elevation of intraabdominal pressure. In comparison with silo treatment, nonoperative therapy results in earlier enteral feedings and decreased length of hospitalization. We apply the same technique to low-birth-weight infants, defined in a recent study from our institution as less than 1,500 g. The clinical status of the neonate and the amount of pulmonary hypoplasia are important considerations when trying to determine whether an operative or nonoperative approach is appropriate in very small babies.

Some surgeons use a prosthetic silo to perform a staged surgical closure in moderate to giant defects that cannot be closed primarily. Gentle daily reduction of the viscera at the bedside often allows reduction in 3 to 6 days. Once reduction is complete, definitive fascial repair or skin closure is performed in the operating room. The use of the silo technique has frequent complications, including delay in enteral feedings and a higher incidence of systemic sepsis, wound infection, dehiscence, and intestinal fistula.

POSTOPERATIVE CARE

Close hemodynamic monitoring is warranted for the first 24 to 48 hours after repair in the intensive care unit. The following parameters have been predictors of poor outcomes: central venous pressure elevations of greater than 2 mm Hg, bladder or gastric pressures of greater than 20 mm Hg measured by Foley catheter or orogastric tube, and airway resistance of greater than 25 mm Hg. Enteral feedings are begun several days after fascial closure once resolution of the postoperative ileus occurs. Prolonged ileus is uncommon after closure of omphaloceles, in contrast to babies with gastroschisis, who often have a 3- to 4-week ileus, presumably due to severe inflammation and edema of the bowel. The need for postoperative ventilatory support and paralysis is an indication that the primary closure is too tight or that significant pulmonary hypoplasia is present.

COMPLICATIONS AND OUTCOMES

It should be emphasized that most early and late complications occur secondary to high intraabdominal pressures after closure. The resultant increased intraabdominal pressure may cause a baby with borderline pulmonary hypoplasia to require chronic ventilatory support. The most commonly encountered complications seen in the initial postoperative period include wound dehiscence, bowel infarction, bowel obstruction, enteric fistulas, renal failure, and respiratory distress (Table 92.2). Wound infection, dehiscence, and systemic sepsis are more often seen after primary surgical closure or with staged repairs. Liver and bowel infarction has been reported secondary to kinking of

TABLE 92.2. EARLY VERSUS LATE COMPLICATIONS FOLLOWING OMPHALOCELE REPAIR

Early	Late
Respiratory failure	Ventral hernia
Sepsis	Gastroesophageal reflux
Wound dehiscence	Esophagitis
Necrotizing enterocolitis	Inguinal hernia
Bowel infarction	Growth delay
Bowel obstruction	Low IQ
Renal failure	Cryptorchidism
Hypovolemia	Intestinal obstruction
Ileus	Midgut volvulus
Wound infection	
Enterocutaneous fistula	
Hepatic hematoma	
Hepatic infarction	
Midgut volvulus	

the venous return upon reduction of the eviscerated segment. Pulmonary insufficiency is usually the result of pulmonary hypoplasia in combination with a tight abdominal closure. This can result in chronic ventilatory dependence and is a major cause of mortality in these infants.

Late complications also appear to be caused by increased intraabdominal pressures at the time of primary or staged closure (Table 92.2). These include ventral hernias, large inguinal hernias, and gastroesophageal reflux disease (GERD). One series reported the presence of GERD in 43% of patients after omphalocele repair. Malrotation with obstruction or bowel necrosis can occur at any time. Growth delay and low IQ are also seen in these patients and reflect the prolonged hospitalization and degree of prematurity. Outcome is dependent on associated malformations, with overall survival ranging from 70% to 90%. Most deaths are secondary to respiratory failure and concomitant congenital defects.

PENTALOGY OF CANTRELL

Pentalogy of Cantrell consists of an upper abdominal wall omphalocele, shortened or bifid lower sternum, pericardial and anterior diaphragmatic defects, and congenital heart malformation. This syndrome is thought to result from developmental failure of the lateral mesoderm between days 14 and 18. The omphalocele repair is delayed if the sac has not ruptured, because avoidance of high abdominal and intrathoracic pressures is critical in the presence of severe cardiac malformations. Sometimes a one-staged surgical repair with the cardiac and pediatric surgeons is possible depending on the severity of the defects. Overall survival is poor.

SUGGESTED READINGS

Calzolari E, Bianchi F, Dolk H, et al. Omphalocele and gastroschisis in Europe: a survey of 3 million births 1980–1990. *Am J Med Genet* 1995;58:187–194.

Hershenson MB, Brouillette RT, Klemka L, et al. Respiratory insufficiency in newborns with abdominal wall defects. *J Pediatr Surg* 1985;20:348–353.

How HY, Harris BJ, Pietrantoni M, et al. Is vaginal delivery preferable to elective cesarean delivery in fetuses with a known ventral wall defect? *Am J Obstet Gynecol* 2000;182:1527–1534.

James CY, Fonkalsrud EW. Improved survival of infants with omphalocele. *Am J Surg* 1997;73:284–287.

Koivusalo A, Rintala R, Lindahl H. Gastroesophageal reflux in children with a congenital abdominal wall defect. *J Pediatr Surg* 1999;34:1127–1129.

Nuchtern JG, Baxter R, Hatch EI, Jr. Nonoperative initial management versus silon chimney for treatment of giant omphalocele. *J Pediatr Surg* 1995;30:771–776.

Reynolds M. Abdominal wall defects in infants with very low birth weight. *Semin Pediatr Surg* 2000;9:88–90.

Wakhlu A, Wakhlu AK. The management of exomphalos. *J Pediatr Surg* 2000;35:73–76.

Yaster M, Scherer LR, Stone MM, et al. Prediction of successful primary closure of congenital abdominal wall defects using intraoperative measurements. *J Pediatr Surg* 1989;24:1217–1220.

93

INGUINAL HERNIA

PHILIP J. WOLFSON

Robert Gross claimed, "There is nothing as interesting as an inguinal hernia." Indeed, although inguinal hernia repair is the most commonly performed operation by pediatric surgeons, several surveys of senior surgeons have demonstrated a remarkable lack of consensus on many basic aspects of inguinal hernia management. In addition, although the operation is considered to be technically straightforward and therefore a junior resident level procedure, inguinal hernia repair can be extremely challenging in small infants or when the hernia is incarcerated, and the sac can have the consistency of wet tissue paper. Postoperative complications, which are not infrequent or insignificant, are almost always technical in nature and therefore preventable, and attest to the requirement for the utmost in gentleness and skill on the part of the surgeon. I consider inguinal hernia repair to be among the most difficult of operations to guide residents and fellows through, and find that their performance is an excellent indicator of their surgical expertise.

CLINICAL MANIFESTATIONS

All inguinal hernias in children can be assumed to be indirect, because direct hernias are rare in this age group. They occur in approximately 3% of children overall. The incidence may increase to 30% in very premature infants and is also higher in conditions associated with increased intraabdominal pressure or connective tissue disorders (e.g., ventriculoperitoneal shunts and Ehlers-Danlos syndrome). Boys are affected 6 to 10 times more frequently than are girls. Inguinal hernias involve the right side twice as often as the left, presumably because the right testicle descends later embryologically and is therefore more likely to have a persistently patent processus vaginalis. Approximately half of inguinal hernias in childhood appear before 1 year of age, and most of these are manifest within the first 6 months.

P. J. Wolfson: Department of Surgery, Thomas Jefferson University, Philadelphia, Pennsylvania; and Division of General Surgery, Alfred I. duPont Hospital for Children, Wilmington, Delaware.

An inguinal hernia is usually first noticed either by the parents or the primary care physician as an intermittent mass in the groin, often extending into the scrotum or labium, which is especially evident when the child cries or strains. Unlike in adults where one may feel an impulse through an enlarged ring, in children the only certain sign that a hernia is present is to palpate it and reduce it when it is out. Nothing else feels quite like a hernia. In children who are old enough, I first examine them in a standing position. If it is not obvious, the child can be asked to jump up and down, perform a Valsalva maneuver, or blow up a balloon, depending on his or her level of cooperation. Infants should be examined from the right side of the table with someone preferably holding their legs extended to keep them still. If the hernia is not visible, I apply suprapubic pressure or hold the arms extended over their head (which causes them to attempt to struggle free) in order to increase the intraabdominal pressure. It is always crucial to verify that both testes are in the scrotum, as a retractile testicle in the groin can easily be mistaken for an inguinal hernia.

Sometimes, despite a suggestive history, no amount of effort can elicit the hernia during the examination. If I am certain that the hernia has been witnessed by a reliable observer, I will schedule surgery even if I do not visualize it myself. If a parent reports a significant mass that comes and goes abruptly, especially with crying or straining, a hernia is very likely; if they add that it "gurgles" or feels "squishy," there is no doubt. If the referring physician has felt the hernia, then a phone call can also be confirmatory. Suggestive signs of a hernia include palpating the spermatic cord where it crosses the public tubercle and encountering a sliding sensation (the silk glove sign) or more commonly feeling a thickened cord due to the presence of a hernia sac. These findings are only circumstantial evidence and may add credence to the history, but are not incontrovertible evidence. If doubt still exists, it is always reasonable to have the child return for a reexamination, with clear instructions for the parents to watch the area closely. They may even be able to obtain a photograph when the hernia is out. In girls, a history of intermittent swelling in the labia can rarely be anything other than a hernia, because there is no testicle that can retract and hydroceles are very rare. Using the above guidelines I have only twice operated and found no hernia present.

A scrotal hydrocele can almost always be distinguished from a hernia by examination, because a hydrocele does not usually extend upward into the inguinal canal, is more mobile, and does not reduce. In contrast, a hydrocele of the spermatic cord is often misdiagnosed as an incarcerated inguinal hernia (especially by the primary physician), because both are manifested by an irreducible mass above the testicle. Even before I examine the child, I can predict that if he is happy, playful, and eating normally, he will have a hydrocele. Unlike a hernia, a hydrocele of the cord is spherical, movable, does not extend upward, and is nontender. Most pediatric surgeons find transillumination to be useless, because air-filled bowel will transilluminate as readily as will fluid. Inguinal lymphadenopathy also may be confused with a hernia but has a different consistency, is usually more lateral in the groin, may be multiple, and may be associated with infections involving the lower extremity. The swelling and tenderness in testicular torsion is usually confined to the scrotum. If there is still doubt about the diagnosis of an incarcerated hernia, radiography (if it shows air below the inguinal ligament) or ultrasonography (demonstrating peristalsis) may sometimes be useful, but often is not sufficiently diagnostic. Rarely, an operation may be the only means by which to make the diagnosis.

TREATMENT

All inguinal hernias need to be repaired, because they never resolve spontaneously. Children who are otherwise healthy require no additional testing, and surgery can be scheduled as an outpatient at a time that is convenient for the family and the surgeon, within a reasonable time interval. If the family asks whether it is safe for the operation to be delayed, I am usually willing to wait several weeks, but not for many months. I am not aware of evidence that activity will precipitate incarceration, and therefore do not restrict the child prior to hernia repair, unless a given activity produces discomfort. I do warn the parents that if there is any evidence of incarceration (pain, vomiting, or skin redness) they should contact me immediately, and I document this instruction in the chart. In obtaining informed consent, I mention the small possibility of a minor wound infection and the unlikely chance of damage to the vas deferens or testicle. I tell them the chance for recurrence is almost but not quite zero. (I have inadvertently divided the vas deferens once and have had two known recurrences in 20 years.)

Surgeons are divided on the timing of surgery in the very young and especially the premature infant who presents with an inguinal hernia. In this circumstance, the operation is more difficult technically and has a higher reported incidence of complications such as recurrence and damage to the spermatic vessels and vas deferens. Respiratory complications, such as postanesthesia apnea and prolonged ventilator dependence in babies with bronchopulmonary dysplasia, also may occur (although apnea occurring beyond several hours following surgery has been questioned). However, if surgery is delayed, the risk of incarceration is also highest in these small infants. My view is to individualize. I discuss the advantages of waiting until the child is 52 postconceptual weeks of age (an arbitrary time, but the age at which our hospital will permit surgery to be performed as an outpatient). Parents must know they can call at any time with questions or concerns. If the hernia has incarcerated or is otherwise a problem for the parents (i.e., they live far away, feel the hernia is making the child irritable, or are uncomfortable with monitoring the hernia at home), it is reasonable to repair the hernia earlier, so long as the facilities offer full pediatric surgical expertise, and then monitor the child postoperatively in the hospital overnight.

An incarcerated hernia is a true emergency, not only because of the risk of strangulation to the intestine, but because the testicle or ovary may infarct. An incarcerated hernia can almost always be reduced, which is advantageous because the complication rate of emergency surgery is much higher than that for elective repair. The child's legs are held (preferably by someone other than the parents) and pressure is applied with the first three fingers of each hand to the mass, squeezing it upward into the internal ring. If reduction cannot be accomplished, the child may be sedated with 0.05 to 0.1 mg/kg intravenous midazolam, and/or 0.1 mg/kg intravenous morphine. Infants must be carefully monitored, with resuscitation equipment and expertise readily available. I do not use ice (which may provoke more crying and even render a small child hypothermic). I then position them supine with their head slightly lowered. After 30 minutes an incarcerated hernia frequently reduces itself, or at least can be easily pushed back. Necrotic viscera almost never reduce, and my only contraindications to attempting reduction are discoloration or edema of the overlying skin and overt peritonitis. Following successful reduction, hernia repair is delayed for 24 to 48 hours for edema of the sac to subside. If the child has required sedation, I admit them, but if the hernia has reduced fairly easily and the parents are reliable, they may be sent home. If reduction fails, surgery must be performed without delay.

An exception to the emergency treatment of an incarcerated hernia is the asymptomatic girl with an irreducible but movable and nontender ovary. Surgeons differ in their opinions as to the risk of strangulation and the urgency of repair. I schedule these patients for urgent but not emergent surgery within the next several days, so long as they remain asymptomatic.

An unresolved question is whether to explore the contralateral side when a child presents with a unilateral inguinal hernia. There is less tendency to routinely explore the opposite side than in the past, but surgeons are still divided. A contralateral patent processus vaginalis, which may be found in up to 50% of these children, does not predict that an actual hernia will develop, and most studies indicate a 10% to 15% incidence of future hernias. The dilemma is more philosophic than medical—whether it is preferable to explore the asymptomatic side unnecessarily in 9 out of 10 children in order to avoid a 10% chance of requiring an additional operative procedure. The age and gender of the child do not seem to influence the likelihood of the subsequent development of a hernia, but prematurity, increased intraabdominal pressure, connective tissue disorders, and cystic fibrosis are associated with an increased risk. My approach is to discuss the situation with the parents and recommend contralateral exploration in boys less than 1 year of age who are premature and in all girls who are under 4 (since there is no danger of damaging a vas deferens or spermatic vessels), as well as in individuals with chronic ascites, ventriculoperitoneal shunts, Ehlers-Danlos syndrome, Marfan's syndrome, cystic fibrosis, a strong family history of bilateral inguinal hernias, and in children for whom another general anesthesia will be particularly hazardous. When parents specifically request that the contralateral side be explored, it is also reasonable to do so. Laparoscopy has been used to examine the internal ring on the asymptomatic side, but I believe that the risk of a negative exploration is so low in experienced hands that if contralateral exploration is elected, it is preferable to just perform it through a small groin incision.

OPERATIVE TECHNIQUE

There are as many variations in the technical details of inguinal hernia repair as there are surgeons who perform these procedures. They all have as a common goal the high ligation of the sac at the internal ring, without damaging any other structures. The child should be in optimal condition; there is no excuse for proceeding with an elective operation on a patient with a cold or a significant diaper rash. If the surgery is to be performed on an inpatient in the nursery, we prefer to wait until the infant is ready to go home and is therefore as large and healthy as possible. General anesthesia is always used, but I leave to the anesthesiologist the choice of airway (an endotracheal tube, a laryngotracheal mask, or a face mask). Although there has been some enthusiasm for operating on infants with severe bronchopulmonary dysplasia under spinal anesthesia, I am not convinced there is a significant advantage, and if the child cries or strains it can make the operation more formidable.

It is always advisable to examine the child's groin area after the induction of anesthesia, because if the hernia has popped out, reducing it will simplify the operative procedure. The scrotum is prepared into the field, because it may need to be manipulated during the operation.

A 2- to 3-cm transverse incision is made slightly above and extending laterally from the pubic tubercle, where there is often a skin crease. The surgeon and assistant each grasp the skin edges with tissue forceps, nick the subcutaneous fat with scissors, and then spread first in the direction of the incision and then at right angles to it. Subcutaneous veins do not need to be divided, but can be retracted to either side. The Scarpa's fascia, which is surprisingly well developed in young children, is grasped on either side and similarly cut and spread. Small retractors are inserted, exposing the external oblique aponeurosis. There may be some areolar tissue overlying it, which needs to be cleared so that the fibers of the aponeurosis can be clearly seen. The shelving edge of the Poupart's ligament is visualized by spreading at the lateral-most edge of the external oblique parallel to the direction of its fibers. By bluntly dissecting with the scissors inferomedially along the shelving edge, the external ring is encountered. It may be dilated by the hernia and readily seen, or may be identified only as an area where the fibers become more vertically oriented.

It is unnecessary to open the external oblique in young children, because the inguinal canal is quite short, and the external and internal rings are almost superimposed. The dissection of the cord can proceed where it emerges from the external ring; when the sac is ligated proximally, it will essentially be at the internal ring. For older children (over 7 or 8 years of age) or when the hernia is very large or incarcerated and additional exposure is needed, I open the external oblique in the direction of its fibers through the external ring. Both edges of the external oblique are held with hemostats, and the undersurfaces are dissected free with a small peanut. Whether or not the external oblique has been opened, the next step is to grasp the most superficial fibers of the spermatic cord between two blunt tissue forceps and split the cremasteric fibers longitudinally. The underlying cord is grasped with one of the forceps through the opening created and lifted upward, while the other forceps is used to dissect the cremasteric fibers off to either side. The cord should be able to be elevated toward the wound, or the tissue grasped is probably not really the spermatic cord. When the bottom of the cord is visualized on both sides, a curved mosquito is inserted under the cord from lateral to medial (I find the curve of the hemostat is much superior to using a forceps for this step), and is then replaced by a closed Allis placed from medial to lateral by the assistant and held slightly open, exposing the length of the cord.

The next step is to identify the sac and separate it from the spermatic vessels and vas deferens; all these structures are encased within the internal spermatic fascia. The surgeon uses two smooth forceps, one to grasp the cord medially (where the sac will be located) and the other to carefully peel off the internal spermatic fascia laterally. As more sac is exposed, the first forceps should be adjusted to regrasp the newly exposed sac ever more laterally, so that the traction and countertraction exerted by the two forceps are in close proximity. The spermatic vessels will appear, and by grasping the tissue immediately adjacent to them can be separated from the sac, and held laterally with a retractor. There is often a small quantity of adipose tissue visible between the sac and the vessels, and if this yellowish tissue is dissected away from the sac, the vessels will invariably accompany it. The vas deferens will be found deeper, between the vessels and the sac. The vas deferens must never be grasped directly with a forceps or a hemostat, because its patency can be permanently compromised; instead, the tissue immediately next to the vas deferens is peeled away, pulling the vas deferens along with it. The vas deferens is then placed on the same retractor as the vessels.

If the hernia sac ends at this level, that end is grasped with a hemostat. More commonly the sac continues toward the scrotum, and it is then cross-clamped after identifying its edges (it is best to include as little extraneous tissue as possible in the hemostats other than the sac). It is always good policy to confirm that the vas deferens is safely retracted away before clamping and cutting the sac; palpating its cordlike consistency will further assure that a large vessel is not being mistaken for the vas deferens. The Allis is removed from beneath the cord. The surgeon exerts traction on the hemostat holding the sac while the assistant applies gentle countertraction on the vas deferens and vessels. The spermatic fascia is then dissected proximally, separating the sac from the vas deferens and vessels up to the ring. At times the spermatic fascia is particularly strong and does not come off easily with blunt dissection. In this situation, a useful maneuver is to insert one blade of a small tenotomy scissors into this fascial layer behind the vas deferens and vessels; the spermatic fascia can be safely cut proximally, releasing the vas deferens and vessels from the sac. I then insert a second retractor into the external ring (or internal ring if the external oblique has been opened) to assure a high ligation, and maintaining the sac on traction, have the assistant push the vas deferens and vessels away from the sac with a small peanut. I then doubly suture ligate the sac at the ring with 3-0 Vicryl and transect the sac distally. Some surgeons twist the sac prior to ligating it to give it more substance and reduce any structures within it, but I am concerned that the vas deferens or vessels might become incorporated into the twist. I also never narrow the internal ring, even when is quite dilated from a large hernia (unless there is clearly an associated direct hernia), and have not seen any recurrences as a result.

If there is a distal sac, it is not necessary to dissect it, because bleeding or injury to the cord structures may needlessly occur—the sac is simply left open. The testicle, which has often been pulled upward by the traction on the cord, is manipulated back down to the scrotum. A single absorbable stitch is placed in the Scarpa's fascia, the skin is closed with absorbable subcuticular sutures, and a drop of collodion is placed on the wound edges.

In girls the procedure is similar and usually simpler, because there are no spermatic vessels or vas deferens to contend with. The round ligament is the analogue of the spermatic cord and is usually dissected and ligated along with the hernia sac, to which it strongly adheres. Once the sac and round ligament have been circumscribed, their distal attachments toward the labia are divided. There is often a vessel in this vicinity that may need to be coagulated. The sac is dissected to the ring, suture ligated, and excised. The main pitfall here is the high incidence of sliding hernias in girls, in which the Fallopian tube or ovary forms a portion of the sac wall. I do not routinely open the sac in girls if it is clear that there are no structures within it. If there is any doubt, the sac must be opened and its contents inspected. The easiest way to deal with a sliding hernia in girls is to suture ligate the sac just distal to the sliding component. The sac is then invaginated through the internal ring, which is sutured closed.

There are several special considerations to consider. If a thin sac should start to tear, the edges may be approximated and held together with a small hemostat in order to prevent the sac opening from extending toward the ring, where it may be difficult to control. Similarly, if the sac is intentionally opened to inspect or reduce any herniated structures within it, the cut edges can again be held together with a hemostat. It may at times be difficult to circumscribe the cord in a small infant with a very large hernia. In this case, I always open the external oblique through the external ring. Once the cord structures have been dissected off the undersurfaces of the external oblique, the peanut that has been used is pushed down along the inner aspect of the lateral edge of the external oblique toward its shelving edge. As the spermatic cord is elevated with a smooth forceps, the peanut is pushed down and medially against the superior ramus of the pubis, under the cord. The end of the peanut is then directed upward and more medially, and it will emerge on the medial side of the spermatic cord, having gone under it without creating a hole in the sac. If a hernia sac becomes very shredded and all its edges cannot be easily retrieved, it is acceptable to repair the hernia with an absorbable purse-string suture through the internal ring, being careful to avoid the vas deferens and vessels.

If an indirect hernia sac that would account for the patient's clinical findings cannot be found, it is important to examine the floor of the inguinal canal. If it appears that there is a direct hernia, suturing the transversalis fascia to the shelving edge of the inguinal ligament suffices. Mesh or plugs have not been used in children.

Sometimes the anesthesiologist performs a caudal block during induction, which lowers the requirement for anesthesia during the procedure and provides pain relief postoperatively. If not, I administer a local block. Prior to closing the Scarpa's fascia, I inject 0.25% or 0.5% bupivacaine with epinephrine (maximum dose 0.4 mL/kg of the 0.5% solution) just below the external oblique laterally and medially to block the ilioinguinal and iliohypogastric nerves, respectively, and also inject subcutaneously.

For incarcerated hernias I begin with an inguinal approach but with a somewhat longer than usual incision, and always open the external oblique. The sac is opened, and if the bowel or ovary are viable, they can usually be reduced through the internal ring with blunt tissue forceps (the ring may be dilated with a hemostat if necessary). Sometimes the viscera will have reduced spontaneously, and if there is no hemorrhagic or foul-smelling fluid, the hernia repair may proceed. If a resection and anastomosis are necessary, it is usually easiest to perform it through a separate laparotomy incision.

RESULTS AND COMPLICATIONS

Children recover rapidly following hernia repair, and I try to minimize the postoperative instructions. I do not place any arbitrary restrictions on their activities, telling parents that children will limit their own activity. (I have had only one minor problem, when an 8-year-old boy felt so good the first evening that he went out on his bicycle, and later was very sore.) I allow patients to bathe in 48 hours, at which time the incision is epithelialized. Young children require only Tylenol or Advil for analgesia, in addition to the ilioinguinal block they have received; for children over 7 or 8 years of age, I prescribe Tylenol with codeine.

Although some surgeons have eliminated the postoperative office visit altogether, I prefer to see the child in 2 to 4 weeks to verify that the wound is healing well and confirm that both testes remain descended, as well as to reassure the parents that everything is fine. If all is well, they do not need to return again.

Postoperative swelling around the testicle or along the spermatic cord is common, especially if the hernia repair has been difficult or the sac dissected down to the testicle. When anticipated, it is helpful to warn parents in advance, so that they do not become alarmed that the hernia has recurred.

Recurrence of a nonincarcerated indirect hernia should be extremely uncommon (reports vary from 0.1%–2.8%), and is almost always due to technical errors (missing the sac, a not high enough ligation of the sac, a tear in the sac above the ligature, or a severe infection) but can also occur in association with connective tissue disorders. A direct hernia following the repair of an indirect hernia is either due to a concomitant one that was missed or injury to the floor of the inguinal canal during the indirect repair.

A noncommunicating hydrocele may occasionally result postoperatively from trapped fluid distally and will usually resolve. I observe these for 6 months and if they persist, aspirate them in the office with a no. 23 butterfly needle as many as three times. I have only once had to subsequently perform an operative excision.

Cryptorchidism following inguinal hernia repair may result if the testicle has not been replaced into the scrotum at the conclusion of the operation, although sometimes the testis also may retract spontaneously. Operative orchidopexy is usually necessary.

A smaller testicle on the hernia repair side has been reported in 2.5% and atrophy in 1%, presumably caused by damage to the spermatic vessels either operatively or by the hernia itself. Injury to the vas deferens is difficult to quantitate, but segments of the vas deferens have been detected histologically in the excised sac in 0% to 2%. Small glandular inclusions in the sac from müllerian duct remnants are common and not significant, and probably account for at least some of these cases. It has been suggested, and I agree, that in this era of cost containment, routine histologic examination of excised hernia sacs is not justified, unless the surgeon is concerned about injury to the reproductive structures in a given patient. Men do not seem to have subsequent diminished fertility rates following inguinal hernia repair in childhood.

The incidence of most complications is significantly higher after the emergency repair of incarcerated inguinal hernias. The recurrence rate is up to 20% and the incidence of testicular atrophy is reported to be 5%.

SUGGESTED READINGS

Allen GS, Cox CS Jr, White N, et al. Postoperative respiratory complications in ex-premature infants after inguinal herniorrhaphy. *J Pediatr Surg* 1998;33:1095–1098.

Grosfeld JL, Minnick K, Shedd F, et al. Inguinal hernia in children: factors affecting recurrence in 62 cases. *J Pediatr Surg* 1991;26:283–287.

Kemmotsu H, Oshima Y, Joe K, et al. The features of contralateral manifestations after the repair of unilateral inguinal hernia. *J Pediatr Surg* 1998;33:1099–1103.

Langer JC, Shandling B, Rosenberg M. Intraoperative bupivacaine during outpatient hernia repair in children: a randomized double blind trial. *J Pediatr Surg* 1987;22:267–270.

Patrick DA, Bensard DD, Karrer FM, et al. Is routine pathological evaluation of pediatric hernia sacs justified? *J Pediatr Surg* 1998;33:1090–1094.

Phelps S, Agrawal M. Morbidity after neonatal inguinal herniotomy. *J Pediatr Surg* 1997;32:445–447.

Wiener ES, Touloukian RJ, Rodgers BM, et al. Hernia survey of the section of the American Academy of Pediatrics. *J Pediatr Surg* 1996;31:1166–1169.

94

EVENTRATION OF THE DIAPHRAGM

SAMUEL Z. SOFFER
CHARLES J.H. STOLAR

Eventration of the diaphragm constitutes an abnormal elevation of one or both hemidiaphragms resulting from a congenital or acquired palsy. Congenital eventration is more rare and results from the development of an intact but abnormal diaphragmatic muscle. The muscle may be severely thinned in areas that are normally very muscular. The etiology of congenital eventration is unknown, although it may be associated with fetal rubella or cytomegalovirus infection. There is no familial predisposition for congenital eventration. Acquired eventration of the diaphragm most often follows intrathoracic surgery or trauma during birth, both of which may result in injury to the phrenic nerve. In these instances the diaphragmatic muscle itself is normal. In addition, eventration of the diaphragm is associated with spinal muscle atrophy (Werdnig-Hoffman syndrome), in which a generalized progressive loss of neurologic function leads to eventration.

Eventration may be associated with other congenital abnormalities, including congenital heart disease, cerebral agenesis, and chromosomal anomalies. It is also seen with pulmonary hypoplasia. Physiologically, altered diaphragmatic function causes a restrictive deficit manifested by reduced lung volume, decreased tidal volume, and increased work of breathing leading to respiratory compromise, which may require mechanical ventilation.

CLINICAL PRESENTATION

Eventration of the diaphragm may be asymptomatic in some patients and is discovered only incidentally. Other patients may experience respiratory collapse at birth or following intrathoracic surgery with injury to the phrenic nerve. Asymptomatic patients may be treated conservatively with periodic follow-up, whereas most symptomatic patients require surgical correction. With severe congenital eventration the baby may develop respiratory distress soon after birth, requiring mechanical ventilation and hemodynamic resuscitation. Alternatively, the baby may have persistent or recurrent respiratory infections, chronic bronchitis, or pneumonias unresponsive to conventional treatment. The most common presentation of acquired diaphragmatic eventration is postoperative respiratory failure following an intrathoracic procedure. Gastrointestinal symptoms are most commonly seen with left-sided eventrations and include intermittent vomiting, postprandial pain, bloating, and failure to thrive.

DIAGNOSIS

Unilateral eventration is diagnosed by chest radiography when the right hemidiaphragm is more than two rib levels higher than the left, or the left hemidiaphragm is at least one rib level higher than the right. Bilateral eventration (usually congenital) is rarely suspected when both hemidiaphragms are elevated. Ultrasonography provides an even better assessment of the diaphragm because dynamic function can be assessed during respiration. Absent or paradoxic diaphragmatic movements during inspiration are suggestive of eventration. Fluoroscopic evaluation of the diaphragm also can show paradoxic movements, but the ease of ultrasonography has supplanted fluoroscopy as the diagnostic test of choice.

PREOPERATIVE CARE

Preoperative preparation for congenital eventrations must include a thorough workup for chromosomal abnormalities and congenital cardiac defects. An echocardiogram should be performed to rule out associated structural cardiac anomalies. Children who have evidence of eventration following an intrathoracic procedure (acquired eventration) or even following birth should be allowed a period of conservative management because phrenic nerve function may sometimes improve with time. Those children who do not

S. Z. Soffer and C. J. H. Stolar: Department of Surgery, Division of Pediatric Surgery, Columbia University College of Physicians and Surgeons; and Children's Hospital of New York, New York, New York.

improve require an operation. Intraoperative assessment of the diaphragm can reveal the cause of the eventration, which affects the type of repair that is undertaken.

SURGICAL REPAIR

Diaphragmatic eventration can be repaired with either a thoracic or abdominal approach. Unilateral eventration should be approached via a seventh intercostal space thoracotomy. Thoracotomy allows for optimal visualization of the phrenic nerve and its branches as they course into the diaphragm. This helps protect the phrenic nerve from injury during the operation.

Transthoracic repair of a *congenital* eventration involves excising the thinned portion of the hemidiaphragm (usually centrally located) and approximating the edges with nonabsorbable pledgeted mattress sutures. The goal is to bring muscularized diaphragm together without excessive tension. Rarely, a prosthetic patch may be required. Transthoracic repair of an acquired eventration involves plicating redundant areas of diaphragm to create a taut closure. This involves grasping the central portion of the affected hemidiaphragm with a noncrushing clamp and marking the extent of the plication with a surgical marker. The plication should be oriented in an anteromedial to posterolateral configuration. Again, nonabsorbable pledgeted mattress sutures are used and care must be taken to avoid incorporating any abdominal viscera in the repair with an overly aggressive bite.

Bilateral eventration is best approached via a transverse upper abdominal incision, which allows for the best exposure of the complete diaphragm. Eventrations presenting with gastrointestinal symptoms or cases of suspected malrotation should also be approached abdominally. The liver, stomach, and spleen are carefully retracted. Plicating sutures are oriented in the same manner as a transthoracic approach, and care must be directed to avoiding the phrenic nerve based on its expected location.

POSTOPERATIVE CARE AND OUTCOME

Most children can be weaned from the ventilator within 1 week of surgery. Intrapleural drainage is maintained for several days following the transthoracic approach. Outcome related to the surgery itself is usually excellent, with dramatic improvement in respiratory function. Recurrent eventration requiring reoperation is rare. Children with bilateral eventrations do not seem to do as well as unilateral eventrations due to severe pulmonary hypoplasia. In contrast, there is potential for lung growth following repair of significant unilateral diaphragmatic eventration. This may be responsible for the overall favorable prognosis in these patients if other associated anomalies, such as cardiac defects, can be adequately addressed.

SUGGESTED READINGS

Jawad AJ, al-Sammarai AY, al-Rabeeh A. Eventration of the diaphragm in children. *J R Coll Surg Edinb* 1991;36:222–224.

Kizilcan F, Tanyel FC, Hicsonmez A. The long term results of diaphragmatic plication. *J Pediatr Surg* 1993;28:42–44.

Langer JC. Phrenic nerve palsy. In: Fallis JC, Filler RM, Lemoine G, eds. *Pediatric thoracic surgery.* New York: Elsevier, 1991:210–214.

Stokes KB. Unusual varieties of diaphragmatic herniae. *Prog Pediatr Surg* 1991;27:127–147.

95

CONGENITAL DIAPHRAGMATIC HERNIA

NICOLA A. LEWIS
BRUCE A. HOLM
PHILIP L. GLICK

Congenital diaphragmatic hernia (CDH) occurs once in every 3,500 live births in the United States. The estimated survival rate for fetuses delivered alive is 70% to 80%. Previous studies suggested a mortality rate of up to 88% in fetuses diagnosed antenatally. However, many of these deaths were due to associated anomalies, and a more favorable outcome is anticipated for the fetus with an isolated CDH. CDH accounts for approximately 4% to 10% of deaths that are secondary to congenital anomalies.

The majority of diaphragmatic defects are posterolateral, with 85% to 90% of these occurring on the left. Anterior defects (Morgagni) and pars-sternalis defects are rare. Herniation of abdominal viscera into the thoracic cavity is a dynamic process, and there is a variable amount of intestine in the chest at any given time. It occurs prior to the fixation of the intestine to the posterior abdomen and therefore results in malrotation in nearly all cases. In 10% to 20% of cases, the hernia is associated with a hernia sac.

The pathophysiology of CDH involves pulmonary hypoplasia, pulmonary hypertension, and a surfactant deficiency. Because of bowel herniation into the chest during crucial stages of lung development, airway divisions are limited to the 12th to 14th generation on the ipsilateral side and to the 16th to 18th generation on the contralateral side. Normal airway development results in 23 to 35 divisions. Because airspace development follows airway development, alveolarization is similarly reduced. In CDH there is a demonstrable decrease in surfactant phospholipids, surfactant proteins A and B, and surfactant function. Pulmonary hypoplasia and associated impairment of the surfactant-producing system result in atelectasis, decreased functional residual capacity, a decrease in the capillary–air interface, and increased dead space in patients with CDH. In infants with CDH, there is also impairment of the pulmonary antioxidant enzyme system and a higher susceptibility to oxygen toxicity, barotrauma, and volutrauma.

Development of the pulmonary arterial system also parallels development of the bronchial tree; therefore, fewer arterial branches are seen in CDH. Abnormal medial muscular hypertrophy is seen as far distally as the acinar arterioles, and the pulmonary vessels are more sensitive to stimuli of vasoconstriction. Pulmonary hypertension resulting from these arterial anomalies leads to right-to-left shunting at the atrial and ductal levels. This persistent fetal circulation leads to right-sided heart strain or failure and the vicious cycle of progressive hypoxemia, hypercarbia, and acidosis seen in the neonatal period. In addition, a left ventricular hypoplasia is seen in CDH. This is thought to arise from decreased blood flow to the left ventricle during development, mechanical compression by the herniated viscera similar to that seen in the lungs, and a primary yet unidentified developmental defect that results in diaphragmatic hernia and pulmonary and cardiac hypoplasia.

DIAGNOSIS

Congenital diaphragmatic hernia is being detected more frequently prior to the 25th week of gestation by ultrasonographic examination. Features suggestive of CDH include an absent intraabdominal gastric bubble or identification of an intrathoracic gastric bubble and mediastinal shift. Polyhydramnios and hydrops fetalis also can occur. Nearly half of patients with diaphragmatic hernia have associated anomalies, which frequently contribute to morbidity and mortality. Frequently associated anomalies include chromo-

N. A. Lewis: Departments of Surgery and Pediatrics, The State University of New York at Buffalo; and Department of Surgery, The Children's Hospital of Buffalo, Buffalo, New York.

B. A. Holm: Office of the Provost, The State University of New York at Buffalo; and Department of Pediatrics/OB-GYN, The Children's Hospital of Buffalo, Buffalo, New York.

P. L. Glick: Departments of Surgery, Pediatrics & OB-GYN, The State University of New York at Buffalo; and Department of Pediatric Surgery Services, The Children's Hospital of Buffalo, Buffalo, New York.

somal anomalies (trisomy 21, 18, and 13), cardiac defects, ventricular hypoplasia, renal anomalies, urogenital anomalies and neural tube defects. Amniocentesis for karyotype analysis and a search for other anomalies should accompany a diagnosis of CHD. In addition to level III fetal ultrasonography, computed tomography, magnetic resonance imaging, amniography, and fetoscopy are additional techniques that have been used to image the fetus and to identify prognostic indicators.

Herniation of the stomach into the chest is associated with a high mortality rate (71% vs. 7%). The fetus with a chromosomal anomaly has a prognosis consistent with that anomaly. The presence of a cardiac defect, low left ventricular mass, and a contralateral lung to thoracic transverse area ratio of less than 0.5 are each associated with a poor outcome. A contralateral lung to head circumference ratio of less than 0.6 is also associated with a poor prognosis.

Standard care of the pregnant patient with a CDH fetus should involve a multidisciplinary team consisting of social workers, ethicists, obstetricians, perinatal specialists, genetic counselors, neonatologists, and pediatric surgeons. The multidisciplinary team should be involved in counseling the family about the prognosis and anticipated care in the prenatal, perinatal, and postnatal periods. The continuation of the pregnancy, availability of antenatal therapies, and transfer to a tertiary care center can be discussed and informed decisions made.

ANTENATAL THERAPY

Potential antenatal therapies for CDH are being explored in experimental animal models and small clinical trials. Neonates with CDH have a surfactant deficiency similar to that encountered in the neonate with respiratory distress syndrome. Theoretically, fetuses with CDH should benefit from antenatally administered corticosteroids. In the fetal lamb model, administering corticosteroids at 24 and 48 hours prior to delivery was associated with significant increases in lung compliance. Further investigation is required to determine optimal timing and dosage of corticosteroids.

Experimental fetal surgery has been expanding rapidly over the past two decades. The fetus most likely to benefit from *in utero* intervention has lethal pulmonary hypoplasia and no coexisting lethal congenital anomalies. To date, no prenatal parameter has been able to reliably predict the occurrence of lethal pulmonary hypoplasia. Selection criteria for antenatal intervention therefore remains controversial.

Formal antenatal repair can be performed using the "two step" technique. The viscera are reduced, the diaphragm is reconstructed with a Gore-Tex patch, and the abdominal cavity is enlarged. This results in compensatory lung growth, but the benefit of this procedure in the fetus without liver herniation has yet to be proved.

The fetal lung produces fluid, which exits the trachea and enters the amniotic fluid during fetal breathing movements. Tracheal occlusion (using external clips or an internal plug) has been shown to reverse pulmonary hypoplasia and the pulmonary vascular anomalies in the CDH lamb model. However, experimental studies show that the surfactant deficiency and impaired antioxidant enzyme system persist in these lungs.

POSTNATAL MANAGEMENT

In contrast to historical management patterns that focused on the actual repair of the diaphragmatic hernia, the contemporary management of CDH places emphasis on the management of pulmonary hypoplasia, pulmonary vascular abnormalities, and surfactant deficiency. Current management uses a variety of gentle alveolar recruitment strategies, and a nonurgent approach to the operative treatment of CDH. Immediately following delivery, the infant is intubated (bag and mask ventilation is avoided). Our protocol includes the administration of exogenous surfactant therapy (100 mg/kg of Infasurf) prior to the first breath. Surfactants containing surfactant proteins A, B, or C are more efficacious. It must be noted that the use of rescue surfactant therapy is not as effective as prophylactic surfactant therapy in CDH. During resuscitation, care must be taken to minimize known stimulants of pulmonary vasoconstriction: hypothermia, acidosis, and hypoxia.

A nasogastric tube is passed to decompress the stomach and to prevent bowel distension. Umbilical artery and central venous lines are placed. Adequate assessment includes continuous cardiac monitoring, arterial blood gas and systemic pressure measurements, urinary catheterization to monitor fluid resuscitation, and both preductal and postductal pulse oximetry. An early chest radiograph is obtained to confirm the diagnosis of CDH. Findings include loops of bowel in the chest, mediastinal shift, and paucity of bowel gas in the abdomen. Further investigations should include echocardiography to detect cardiac defects, to determine left ventricular mass and function, and the degree and level of right-to-left shunting. Repeated echocardiography is recommended to measure changes in the pulmonary artery pressure, left-to-right shunt fraction, and flow across the ductus arteriosus.

Pressure-limited ventilation should be used, allowing the lowest airway pressures compatible with staying on the steep side of the pressure volume loop, and to maintain preductal oxygen saturations above 90%. Peak inspiratory pressures (PIPs) should be less than 30 cm H_2O. This reduces lung injury associated with barotrauma and volutrauma. Hypercarbia is permitted as long as the pH can be maintained above 7.20 with bicarbonate therapy. The use of muscle relaxants and sedation with intravenous narcotic infusion is recommended to help control ventilation and reduce airway pressures.

With conventional ventilation, some neonates develop severe respiratory distress. The primary cause is persistent high pulmonary vascular resistance, and right-to-left shunting across the foramen ovale and patent ductus arteriosus (persistent fetal circulation). Alternative means of support should be considered for the patient who fails to stabilize on conventional ventilation.

We use high-frequency oscillatory ventilation (HFOV) for infants with hypercarbia and hypoxemia resistant to conventional ventilation or requiring high PIP (>30 cm H_2O). HFOV uses an oscillating diaphragm to create a sinusoidal column of air within the airways. The diaphragm oscillates at a high frequency and improves gas exchange without increased ventilatory pressures. Increased gas exchange leads to elimination of CO_2, which decreases the stimulus for pulmonary vasoconstriction and subsequent pulmonary hypertension.

Inhaled nitric oxide (iNO) is a highly selective pulmonary vasodilator, and is used as rescue therapy in infants with persistent pulmonary hypertension (PPHN). By producing pulmonary vasodilatation, iNO decreases the ventilation-perfusion mismatch and reverses the ductal shunting seen in PPHN. It has been used with limited success in infants with CDH. We hypothesize that this is secondary to poor delivery of nitric oxide to the surfactant-deficient lung in CDH and have demonstrated an improved efficacy of iNO following surfactant therapy in the lamb model of CDH.

The selection criteria for extracorporeal membrane oxygenation (ECMO) eligibility in CDH are the standard criteria used for other neonates with respiratory failure: a pH less than 7.15, oxygenation index greater than 40, and failure to respond to maximal medical treatment. ECMO therapy also should be considered when complications related to barotrauma occur, for example, pneumothorax. ECMO should be reserved for patients who fail to respond to the alternative therapies, if the extent of pulmonary hypoplasia is not considered lethal, and when acute deterioration occurs in the postoperative period. ECMO in these cases provides respiratory support without additional barotrauma or oxygen toxicity. It allows time for the transition from fetal circulation, as well as the maturation of the surfactant and NO systems.

SURGICAL REPAIR

There is no ideal time for repair of CDH, but we suggest that the window of opportunity lies within 24 to 48 hours of achieving normal pulmonary arterial pressures and satisfactory oxygenation and ventilation on minimal ventilator settings.

Following measures to prevent hypothermia, the patient is placed supine on the operating table with a small roll placed under the back at the level of the 12th rib. The patient is prepared and draped widely. A right subcostal or transverse incision is made. The abdominal viscera are examined and reduced by gentle traction. Following careful dissection of the posterior leaf of the diaphragm, primary repair can be accomplished in a single layer using interrupted nonabsorbable sutures. If the diaphragmatic defect is large enough to preclude primary closure, a Gore-Tex patch can be used. A hernia sac is sought and must be excised if found. If the patient is stable, a formal Ladd procedure should be performed. If abdominal closure interferes with chest wall and diaphragmatic compliance or leads to a concern about an abdominal compartment syndrome, then a Silastic silo is created with planned delayed primary closure of the fascia. Alternatively, some surgeons advocate closure of the skin only, with elective repair of the fascial defect 6 months to a year later. A chest tube is usually placed prior to closure, but some surgeons feel it is not routinely necessary.

The patient with a right-sided defect and an intrathoracic liver presents a unique challenge. The neonatal liver is extremely friable, and kinking of the hepatic veins and the inferior vena cava can accompany the return of the liver to the abdomen. Careful manipulation of the liver into the abdomen must be accompanied by hemodynamic monitoring. Occasionally a thoracoabdominal approach may be necessary to reduce the liver safely.

Surgical repair while the patient is on ECMO may be associated with an increased mortality rate, surgical site hemorrhage, and intracranial hemorrhage. To decrease the hemostatic complications associated with ECMO, the platelet count is maintained above 100,000/mm^3 and the activated clotting time is decreased to 170 to 180 seconds. Intraoperative and postoperative blood loss can be decreased by minimizing the use of blunt and sharp dissection, judicious use of electrocautery, use of Gore-Tex patch repair, and application of topical thrombin to the suture line.

Repairing the diaphragmatic hernia after decannulation from ECMO avoids the hemostatic complications associated with ECMO. This can lead to recurrent pulmonary hypertension in some patients. However, we have found that even neonates who did not respond to iNO prior to the initiation of ECMO will often respond following decannulation. In rare cases, a second run of ECMO should be considered.

COMPLICATIONS

Complications seen in the early postoperative period can be technical or result from the unique physiology of infants with CDH. Technical complications should be rare but include hemorrhage, disruption of the suture line with recurrent hernia, and the development of an abdominal compartment syndrome. Each may require reexploration.

As is typical for most reexplorations for bleeding, a distinct bleeding site is rarely found. Disruption can sometimes be repaired with additional sutures, but consideration should be given to the use of a patch if the repair is under a great deal of tension. Release of abdominal pressure with the use of a patch or silo may be necessary in the rare instance of abdominal compartment syndrome. Chylothorax can occur but usually responds to standard conservative measures. Infection of the patch material mandates removal of the foreign material. If this occurs as a late complication, a primary repair is often possible using available tissues. In rare cases, consideration must be given to the use of a latissimus dorsi or other local muscle flap to effect a tension-free repair of the diaphragm. Patients are also at risk for adhesive small bowel obstruction and for midgut volvulus, although the latter appears to be a rare occurrence. Nevertheless, the diagnosis should be considered in any patient who presents with bilious emesis or other signs of obstruction.

Infants with CDH are at risk for a variety of physiologic complications. The majority have significant gastroesophageal reflux, and some eventually require an antireflux operation. Feeding difficulties secondary to reflux or ongoing pulmonary difficulties are also relatively common. Some patients will therefore require placement of a gastrostomy tube for feeding access. The principal long-term source of disability for these infants is persistent pulmonary dysfunction. This may vary from a mild oxygen requirement to a long-standing need for mechanical ventilation. Early tracheostomy should be considered, although the outlook for infants with such severe pulmonary hypoplasia is poor.

RESULTS

Overall, infants with CDH who survive do well. However, with improved survival in CDH, significant morbidity is seen among newborns who would have otherwise died as recently as 5 to 10 years ago. Failure to thrive is often seen despite apparently optimal feeding regimens. Functional and anatomic esophageal abnormalities in survivors are sometimes associated with gastroesophageal reflux requiring surgical management. The use of ECMO, hyperventilation treatment, and ototoxic medication places this population at a higher risk for sensorineural hearing loss and neurodevelopmental abnormalities, including cognitive and developmental delay, cerebral palsy, seizure disorders, and impaired vision. Those who require ECMO therapy and those with associated anomalies, especially cardiac defects, are at higher risk for poor neurodevelopmental outcome. Altered musculoskeletal development results in thoracic scoliosis, pectus deformities, and a decreased thoracic cavity on the affected side.

NEW DEVELOPMENTS

Liquid ventilation uses perfluorocarbon, which is an inert compound with low surface tension and greater solubility for respiratory gases than blood. In partial liquid ventilation (PLV), the lungs are filled with perfluorocarbon to the functional residual capacity, and conventional ventilation is superimposed. PLV is associated with improved oxygenation and decreased PIP requirements. This may be due to recruitment of atelectatic lungs and decreased ventilation/perfusion mismatch. Theoretically, PLV would decrease the requirements for ventilation and so decrease barotrauma and hyperoxia-induced pulmonary injury in CDH.

There is growing interest in the role of antenatal or postnatal therapy with growth factors in the acceleration of lung development. This would potentially decrease the need for respiratory support and the morbidity and mortality associated with pulmonary hypoplasia.

Tracheal occlusion can be performed using video-assisted fetal endoscopy in animal models. This is of potential benefit if a less invasive procedure decreases the premature onset of labor and fetal loss associated with open fetal surgery and if clear guidelines for fetal intervention can be implemented.

SUGGESTED READINGS

Glick PL, Irish MS, Holm B, eds. New insight into the pathophysiology of congenital diaphragmatic hernia. *Clin Perinatol* 1996.

Glick PL, Leach CL, Besner GE, et al. Pathophysiology of congenital diaphragmatic hernia. III: Exogenous surfactant therapy for the high-risk neonate with CDH. *J Pediatr Surg* 1992;27:866–869.

Kapur P, Holm B, Irish MS, et al. Lung physiology and metabolic changes in lambs with congenital CDH after administration of prenatal maternal corticosteroids. *J Pediatr Surg* 1999;34:354–356.

Karamanoukian HL, Glick PL, Wilcox DT, et al. Pathophysiology of congenital diaphragmatic hernia. VIII: Inhaled nitric oxide requires exogenous surfactant therapy in the lamb model of congenital diaphragmatic hernia. *J Pediatr Surg* 1995;1:1–4.

Karamanoukian HL, O'Toole SJ, Glick PL, et al. "State of the art" management strategies for the fetus and neonate with congenital diaphragmatic hernia. *J Perinatol* 1996;16(suppl):40–47.

Ting A, Glick PL, Wilcox DT, et al. Alveolar vascularization of the lung in a lamb model of congenital diaphragmatic hernia. *Am J Respir Crit Care Med* 1998;157:31–34.

Wilcox DT, Glick PL, Karamanoukian HL, et al. Pathophysiology of CDH. XII: Amniotic fluid L/S ratio and phosphatidylglycerol concentrations do not predict surfactant status in congenital diaphragmatic hernia. *J Pediatr Surg* 1995;30:410–412.

SECTION

X

LIVER, BILIARY TREE, PANCREAS, AND SPLEEN

96

NEONATAL JAUNDICE

JOHN F. POHL
WILLIAM F. BALISTRERI

The approach to the workup of the jaundiced neonate is initially more of a medical rather than a surgical issue. A detailed patient and maternal history and a careful physical examination often lead to a prompt diagnosis of the nature of the cholestasis before an extensive laboratory and radiographic evaluation becomes necessary. Although the differential list of jaundice in the neonate is large (Table 96.1), a thoughtful approach focused on the most likely causes will prevent the "shotgun approach" of ordering more tests than necessary and delaying the diagnosis.

The appearance of jaundice during the neonatal period is extremely common. Approximately 60% of full-term infants and 80% of preterm infants exhibit jaundice, which is usually due to the accumulation of unconjugated, nonpolar, lipid-soluble bilirubin pigment in serum. This form of bilirubin is formed from the metabolism of hemoglobin catalyzed by heme oxygenase and biliverdin reductase in the reticuloendothelial cells. Jaundice also can occur after the bilirubin pigment is converted to a conjugated, polar, water-soluble glucuronide ester by uridine diphosphoglucuronic acid glucuronyl transferase in the hepatocyte microsomal system. Although an elevation of conjugated bilirubin in serum is benign in itself (unlike unconjugated bilirubin, which has neurotoxic effects in high concentration), its presence is suggestive of cholestasis. Although, strictly speaking, a conjugated bilirubin level that is greater than 2 mg/dL or over 15% of the total bilirubin concentration warrants an evaluation for cholestasis, the detection of any amount of conjugated bilirubin is abnormal. Any neonate who remains jaundiced beyond 2 weeks of age also deserves careful analysis for possible hepatobiliary disease.

J. F. Pohl: Department of Pediatrics, Section of Pediatric Gastroenterology, Scott and White Hospital, Texas A&M Health Science Center, Temple, Texas.

W. F. Balistreri: Department of Pediatrics, University of Cincinnati; and Departments of Pediatrics, Gastroenterology, Hepatology, and Nutrition, Cincinnati Children's Hospital Medical Center, Cincinnati, Ohio.

IATROGENIC CONSIDERATIONS

Neonatal exposure to certain drugs can lead to cholestasis, and a careful review of medications is essential. Transplacental delivery of medications such as flecainide acetate (used in the treatment of fetal tachycardia) can lead to neonatal cholestasis. Vanishing bile duct syndrome, a presumed autoimmune phenomenon caused by drug exposure, is a rare cause of cholestasis. Several agents have been implicated in this disorder, including amoxicillin-clavulanic acid, ibuprofen, and trimethoprim-sulfamethoxazole.

Parenteral nutrition (PN), although an essential form of nutrition for the preterm infant, is one of the most common causes of conjugated hyperbilirubinemia in the newborn intensive care unit. Nearly half of all infants receiving PN for more than 2 weeks develop cholestasis. The etiology is multifold and includes immaturity of bile secretion, decreased enterohepatic circulation, sepsis, and inherent hepatotoxic properties of PN. Advancement of enteral feeds is essential for resolution of the cholestasis. Prolonged PN in the neonatal period also can lead to biliary stasis, sludging, and cholelithiasis, especially in situations where bile acid transit and recycling are impaired, such as congenital duodenal or jejunal atresia, diaphragmatic hernia, gastroschisis, or loss of the ileocecal valve.

Extracorporeal membrane oxygenation (ECMO) has been associated with cholestasis. Although the underlying primary disease leading to ECMO may predispose to cholestasis through hypoxia, hypotension, and acidosis, ECMO itself may be causative through complement activation, loss of pulsatile blood flow, hemolysis, and the toxic effects of plastic circuit agents.

INFECTIOUS CAUSES OF CHOLESTASIS

Various infectious agents can cause cholestasis via direct hepatocyte infection or by production of hepatotoxins. An obstetric history and screening serologies may reveal exposure to many of the well-described congenital infections known to

TABLE 96.1. CAUSES OF NEONATAL JAUNDICE

Iatrogenic
Fetal/neonatal drug exposure
Parenteral nutrition
Extracorporeal membrane oxygenation
Infectious diseases
Bacterial sepsis
Viral causes: congenital rubella, herpes simplex virus, cytomegalovirus, parvovirus B19
Neonatal syphilis
Leptospirosis
Inherited/metabolic diseases
Endocrine abnormalities: hypothyroidism, panhypopituitarism
Chromosomal disorders: trisomy 18, trisomy 21
Cystic fibrosis
α_1-Antitrypsin deficiency
Alagille's syndrome (arteriohepatic dysplasia)
Forms of progressive familial intrahepatic cholestasis: PFIC-1 or Byler syndrome (*FIC1* mutation), PFIC-2 (*BSEP* mutation), PFIC-3 (*MDR3* mutation)
Defects of bile acid synthesis
Disorders of amino acid metabolism: tyrosinemia
Disorders of carbohydrate metabolism: galactosemia, fructosemia
Disorders of lipid metabolism: Niemann-Pick disease (sphingomyelinase deficiency), cholesterol ester storage disease or Wolman disease (acid lipase deficiency), Gaucher disease (glucocerebrosidase deficiency)
Neonatal iron storage disease
Peroxisomal disorders: Zellweger syndrome (cerebrohepatorenal syndrome)
Obstructive diseases
Biliary atresia
Inspissated bile plug syndrome
Cholelithiasis
Choledochal cysts
Sclerosing cholangitis
Idiopathic bile duct perforation
Miscellaneous
Hemophagocytic lymphohistiocytosis
Navajo neurohepatopathy

cause cholestasis such as toxoplasmosis, syphilis, and rubella. Hepatosplenomegaly, rashes, thrombocytopenia, and seizures are common manifestations in such infants. Neonatal syphilis also can present with metaphyseal abnormalities and endocrine disorders such as hypoglycemia or hypopituitarism. Leptospirosis is a rare cause of neonatal cholestasis and should be considered if exposure is suspected.

Cholestasis is present in up to 10% of neonates with sepsis. Most of these patients are infected with gram-negative bacteria, and it has been proposed that the lipid A moiety of endotoxin may interfere with excretion of conjugated bilirubin into the bile canaliculi by inhibition of parenchymal cell Na^+, K^+ adenosine triphosphatase. Other bacteria such as *Staphylococcus aureus*, *Staphylococcus epidermidis*, *Streptococcus* species, and *Enterobacter* species have been implicated as well.

Viral causes of neonatal cholestasis include rubella, herpes simplex virus, and cytomegalovirus. A maternal history of exposure to these agents can clarify the diagnosis. Cytomegalovirus infection, commonly seen in the premature infant, can cause bile duct destruction and leads to characteristic cytomegalovirus inclusions on liver biopsy. Congenital parvovirus infection (specifically, parvovirus B19) has been described to cause a congenital syndrome of cholestasis, hepatomegaly, hydrops fetalis, and bone marrow suppression. Hepatitis B virus, hepatitis C virus, and human immunodeficiency virus are transmitted vertically but rarely present with hepatic disease in the neonatal period.

INHERITED AND METABOLIC CAUSES OF CHOLESTASIS

Abnormalities of the endocrine system such as congenital hypothyroidism or hypopituitarism can cause cholestasis. Septooptic dysplasia (De Morsier syndrome) presents with optic nerve hypoplasia and dysgenesis of the septum pellucidum. These patients have visual field defects ("wandering" nystagmus) often with hypothalamic–pituitary dysfunction. Chromosomal disorders, including trisomy 18 and 21, are associated with neonatal cholestasis. Cystic fibrosis is a rare cause of neonatal cholestasis that can present as an inspissated bile syndrome or ductal atresia. Cystic fibrosis can resemble biliary atresia and may lead to exploratory laparotomy. Kasai hepatoportoenterostomy should be avoided in the patient with cystic fibrosis. The diagnosis of cystic fibrosis should be considered if other associated abnormalities are present, such as meconium ileus or intestinal atresia. Diagnosis can be established by measuring sweat chloride concentration, measuring nasal transepithelial potential, or evaluating for known mutations of the *CFTR* gene.

Disorders of amino acid, carbohydrate, and lipid metabolism can lead to cholestasis, and prompt diagnosis is essential so that appropriate dietary therapy can begin. Tyrosinemia is an autosomal-recessive disease due to a deficiency of fumarylacetoacetate hydrolase, an enzyme required in the degradation of tyrosine. Toxic metabolites from altered tyrosine metabolism lead to both hepatic and renal disease in the neonate. Detection of succinylacetone, an intermediate metabolite, from urine and blood is essential for the diagnosis of tyrosinemia. Treatment consists of dietary elimination of tyrosine and phenylalanine, although the disease progresses, making hepatic transplantation necessary. Recently, use of 2-[nitro-4-trifluoromethylbenzoyl]-1, 3-cyclohexanedione, or NTBC (an inhibitor of 4-hydroxyphenylpyruvate dioxygenase) has shown promise as a medical therapy for this disorder. Galactosemia, a disorder of galactose metabolism, is due to a deficiency of galactose-1-phosphate uridyltransferase and leads to cholestasis as well as fatty infiltration of the liver with cholangiocyte proliferation. Infants with galactosemia present with vomiting, diarrhea, and anorexia immediately upon exposure to galactose, and often these infants have a history of *Escherichia coli* sepsis. Treatment requires galactose elimination from the diet. Hereditary fructose intolerance, like galactosemia, can present with vomiting, hepatomegaly, and cholestasis upon exposure to fructose. A deficiency of fructose-1-phosphate aldolase can lead to symptoms, and diagnosis depends on direct measurement of this enzyme from hepatic or small intestinal tissue. Treatment consists of dietary elimination of fructose. Various disorders of lipid metabolism such as Niemann-Pick disease (sphingomyelinase deficiency), cholesterol ester storage disease or Wolman's disease (both with acid lipase deficiency), and Gaucher's disease (glucocerebrosidase deficiency) can present with neonatal cholestasis as well. The diagnosis of these rare disorders requires specific enzyme analysis from hepatocytes, leukocytes, or fibroblasts while electron microscopy of liver tissue may demonstrate abnormal lysosomal inclusions.

Neonatal iron storage disease (NISD) presents with fulminant liver disease in the first few days of life. This disorder is characterized by both hepatocellular and extrahepatic siderosis sparing reticuloendothelial cells. NISD may be caused by either a primary hepatic iron metabolism disorder or abnormal placental iron metabolism leading to subsequent fetal liver disease. Testing usually reveals an elevated ferritin level with normal serum iron and low to normal iron-binding capacity. Diagnosis is one of exclusion and requires demonstration of extrahepatic siderosis via lip biopsy or abdominal magnetic resonance imaging. Although liver transplantation has been described as a successful therapy, most patients die of liver failure and coagulopathy in the first few days of life. Aggressive antioxidant therapy using a combination of deferoxamine, vitamin E, N-acetylcysteine, selenium, and prostaglandin E_1 has been used as supportive management in this disorder, although results have been discouraging.

Peroxisomal disorders, particularly Zellweger syndrome (cerebrohepatorenal syndrome), can lead to neonatal cholestasis. Peroxisomes are involved in β oxidation of fatty acids, and disordered metabolism of very long chain fatty acids may lead to abnormalities of neurologic, hepatic, and renal systems. Zellweger syndrome presents with a typical phenotype in the neonatal period consisting of craniofacial dysmorphism, cortical hypoplasia with retinopathy and impaired hearing, hypotonia, epiphyseal stippling, renal cysts, and liver disease. The prognosis is invariably poor, with most patients dying of respiratory failure.

Alpha-1-antitrypsin deficiency can present as neonatal cholestasis in infancy or emphysematous lung disease in adulthood. Alpha-1-antitrypsin is a protease inhibitor of leukocyte elastase as well as trypsin, plasmin, and thrombin. The lack of this inhibitor leads to cellular damage through production of superoxide radicals by proteases. We routinely order an α_1-antitrypsin phenotype in any infant with cholestasis. Approximately 5% to 10% of individuals with the homozygous phenotype, PiZZ, present with infantile cholestasis as well as adult pulmonary emphysema. Heterozygous phenotypes (PiMZ and PiMS) also can lead to disease, although this is much more rare. Liver biopsy in these patients is essential to confirm the diagnosis. In most cases, cholestasis resolves by 1 year of age, although chronic hepatic failure requiring transplantation can occur.

Alagille's syndrome (arteriohepatic dysplasia) is a syndrome consisting of interlobular bile duct paucity, pulmonary artery stenosis or other cardiovascular anomalies, butterfly-like vertebrae, posterior embryotoxon on ophthalmologic examination, and a characteristic facies. The syndrome is due to a mutation of the *JAGGED1* gene on chromosome 20, which is involved in organ differentiation. Infants with this syndrome present with cholestasis and can slowly progress to cirrhosis. The diagnosis of Alagille's syndrome is made by the clinical demonstration of the above-mentioned organ abnormalities, although not all affected individuals demonstrate all of these criteria. Indications for liver transplantation include end-stage liver disease or intractable pruritus. Other progressive familial intrahepatic cholestatic (PFIC) syndromes have recently been characterized. PFIC-1 (or Byler's syndrome) has been described in the Amish population and is characterized by chronic cholestasis and progressive liver disease despite a normal biliary tree and no evidence of abnormalities of other organ systems (Table 96.2).

Defects in bile acid synthesis have become increasingly understood as a cause of neonatal cholestasis, and histologically, these disorders can appear similar to neonatal hepatitis. Indeed, perhaps up to 2% of neonatal cholestasis cases

TABLE 96.2. INTRAHEPATIC CHOLESTATIC SYNDROMES

Syndrome	Pruritus	Serum γ-GTP	Serum Bile Acid Concentration	Gene Defect
Alagille syndrome	Present	High	High	*JAGGED1, 20p*
Byler disease (PFIC-1)	Present	Low	High	*FIC1, 18q*
BSEP deficiency (PFIC-2)	Present	Low/normal	High	*BSEP, 2q*
MDR3 deficiency (PFIC-3)	Present	High	High	*MDR3*

GTP, guanosine triphosphate; BSEP, bile salt export pump.

may be due to such synthetic defects. Multiple enzyme defects in the synthetic pathway of bile acids have been described, and diagnosis is made by fast atom bombardment ionization–mass spectrometry as well as by gas chromatography–mass spectrometry of both urine and serum specimens. Treatment often consists of dietary addition of substitute bile acids.

Other rare causes of neonatal cholestasis should be considered in certain clinical scenarios. Hemophagocytic lymphohistiocytosis (HLH disease) presents with hepatosplenomegaly, jaundice, and bone marrow failure due to histiocyte infiltration. Ethnic considerations can be helpful in the diagnosis of neonatal cholestasis when considering extremely rare disorders such as Navajo neurohepatopathy.

EXTRAHEPATIC CHOLESTATIC SYNDROMES

Biliary atresia is characterized by progressive obliteration of both extra- and intrahepatic ducts leading to obstruction of bile flow, cirrhosis, and hepatic failure. Biliary atresia accounts for 30% of cases of neonatal cholestasis, with an incidence range of 1 in 10,000 to 1 in 20,000 births. It is often seen as an obliterative lesion of the extrahepatic biliary tree, which suggests an infectious or autoimmune process. However, biliary atresia may be associated with other anomalies, such as duodenal atresia, polysplenia, and malrotation. Infants born with biliary atresia are usually healthy until approximately 3 to 6 weeks of age, when they present with jaundice and acholic stools. Serum transaminases and conjugated (direct) bilirubin levels are elevated. A percutaneous liver biopsy demonstrating cholestasis, bile duct proliferation, and fibrosis is necessary for diagnosis. Prompt diagnosis of this disorder is essential because the Kasai hepatoportoenterostomy is most effective prior to 3 months of age.

Inspissated bile plug syndrome causes obstructive jaundice and is due to a variety of conditions, including neonatal hemolysis from ABO or Rh blood group incompatibility, prolonged PN, delayed enteral nutrition, and diuretic usage. Cystic fibrosis should be considered in this clinical scenario. Cholelithiasis, although extremely rare, also can occur in the jaundiced neonate in association with PN, abdominal surgery, hemolytic disease, malabsorption, sepsis, and necrotizing enterocolitis.

Other lesions of the external biliary tract are less common; however, they must be considered if obstructive disease is present. Choledochal cysts are dilatations of the biliary tree that are divided into five variants, although the most common presentation is the type I cyst, or diffuse enlargement of the common bile duct. The classic triad of jaundice, pain, and presence of an abdominal mass occurs in less that 20% of pediatric patients. Prompt excision of the cyst is necessary to prevent hepatic fibrosis or perforation of the cyst. Removal of the cyst is important because choledochal cysts carry a significant risk of malignancy.

Sclerosing cholangitis can occur in the neonatal period and often is associated with other underlying conditions such as inflammatory bowel disease, acquired or congenital immunodeficiency, or Langerhans cell histiocytosis. Neonatal sclerosing cholangitis usually presents with conjugated hyperbilirubinemia in early infancy and resolves by 3 to 6 months of age. The jaundice recurs in later childhood, often in association with hepatosplenomegaly. Neonatal sclerosing cholangitis in the neonatal period has been identified as an autoimmune phenomenon with elevated anti-smooth muscle antibody titers.

Idiopathic bile duct perforation is another cause of jaundice in the neonate. Although it is an extremely rare condition, it is a common cause of jaundice necessitating surgical evaluation. Patients are born generally healthy but soon develop poor weight gain, jaundice, and ascites. Often these infants are misdiagnosed with biliary atresia or a choledochal cyst.

LABORATORY EVALUATION OF NEONATAL CHOLESTASIS

After a careful history and physical examination are performed, it is imperative for the examiner to decide if the cholestatic process is intrahepatic or extrahepatic. Fractionation of serum bilirubin by spectrophotometry is essential to determine if the hyperbilirubinemia is conjugated (or from the hepatobiliary system). An elevation of serum transaminase level can indicate hepatocellular damage. Alkaline phosphatase is elevated during a child's growth because of osteoblastic activity, and it often is not helpful in diagnosing an obstructive pattern. However, elevation of γ-glutamyltransferase can be used to indicate obstructive disease because this enzyme is located on smooth endoplasmic reticulum of biliary epithelium and is not present in bone. Hepatic synthetic function can be ascertained by determining serum albumin and prothrombin time. Elevation of serum bile acids also is helpful for diagnosing hepatic disease, although serum bile acid levels can be normal in bile acid synthetic defects or in conjunction with intestinal losses of bile salts as seen with the loss of the ileocecal valve.

Infectious causes of neonatal cholestasis can be identified by obtaining cultures (blood, urine, and cerebrospinal fluid) and viral titers, and by performing a Venereal Disease Research Laboratory (VDRL) test series. Laboratory testing for metabolic or genetic conditions depends on the clinical scenario, although a good screening evaluation would include a thyroid screen, α_1-antitrypsin phenotype, urine for reducing substances, urine succinylacetone, urine organic acids/serum amino acids, and a sweat chloride evaluation (Table 96.3).

TABLE 96.3. REQUIRED TESTING FOR EVALUATION OF THE JAUNDICED NEONATE

Serum bilirubin with fractionation into conjugated and unconjugated components
Serum aminotransferase levels, alkaline phosphatase, γ-glutamyltransferase
Serum albumin
Prothrombin time
Serum bile acid level (conventional assay)
Cultures (blood, urine, cerebrospinal fluid) if indicated
VDRL if indicated
Thyroid function tests: thyroxine, thyroid-stimulating hormone
α_1-Antitrypsin phenotype
Urine for reducing substances
Urine succinylacetone
Urine organic acids/serum amino acids
Sweat chloride determination
Ultrasonography of the hepatobiliary system
Percutaneous liver biopsy

VDRL, Venereal Disease Research Laboratory (test).

RADIOGRAPHIC EVALUATION OF NEONATAL CHOLESTASIS

Multiple radiographic techniques are available for assistance in the evaluation of neonatal cholestasis in which an obstructive cause is likely. Ultrasonography has a role in the evaluation of biliary anatomy, and advantages include its relative ease of performing as well as lack of patient exposure to radiation. Cholelithiasis, inspissated bile plug syndrome, and choledochal cysts can all be demonstrated by this technique. Measuring a fasted gallbladder length along its longitudinal axis can be helpful in diagnosing biliary atresia, although the presence of a normal-appearing gallbladder is seen in situations where there is obliteration of the hepatic ducts with preservation of the cystic and common bile ducts. Demonstration of the triangular cord sign, an echogenic density representing the fibrotic remnant of the duct at the porta hepatis, by high-resolution ultrasonography has been shown to be helpful in the diagnosis of biliary atresia. However, ultrasonography is not helpful in diagnosing the early stages of biliary atresia where the porta hepatis has not yet become fibrotic.

Hepatobiliary scintigraphy also been used in the evaluation of neonatal cholestasis using technetium 99m–labeled iminodiacetic acid (IDA) as well as analogues such as ^{99m}Tc-trimethylbromo-iminodiacetic acid (TBIDA or mebrofenin). Although excretion of this tracer into the intestinal lumen eliminates the possibility of biliary atresia, lack of excretion does not rule out other conditions associated with poor hepatocyte clearance of labeling agents, such as Alagille's syndrome, idiopathic neonatal hepatitis, and α_1-antitrypsin deficiency.

Magnetic resonance cholangiography (MR cholangiography) is a new diagnostic modality that has recently been used for diagnosis of biliary disorders in infants and children. MR cholangiography is effective at demonstrating both a normal extrahepatic biliary tree and anatomic abnormalities such as a dilated common bile duct or choledochal cyst; however, the usefulness of MR cholangiography in diagnosing biliary atresia has yet to be determined. The demonstration of the extrahepatic duct excludes biliary atresia, while the presence of a high-intensity signal on T2-weighted images at the porta hepatis is consistent with periportal fibrosis seen in biliary atresia. False-positive findings for biliary atresia can occur, because neonatal sclerosing cholangitis looks similar on MR cholangiography. This imaging technique has much potential, although improvements in spatial resolution and signal-to-noise ratio are needed.

Endoscopic retrograde cholangiopancreatography (ERCP) has recently arisen as a potential diagnostic procedure for neonatal cholestasis. Smaller endoscopes for infants are now available that have adequate channel size for cannulation of the major papilla. The success rate of cannulation in neonates has ranged from 86% to 88%, and ERCP has not been useful in diagnosing biliary atresia when a complete study cannot be performed. More experience is needed in this technique before it can qualify as a useful diagnostic tool.

LIVER BIOPSY

The percutaneous liver biopsy described by Menghini is currently the best method for diagnosing the cause of cholestasis in the neonate. Contraindications to percutaneous liver biopsy include coagulopathy, ascites, presence of focal hepatic lesions such as an abscess or vascular anomaly, or concurrent right lung pathology (pneumonia, empyema, etc.). In situations where a percutaneous biopsy is not indicated, liver tissue may be obtained by a transjugular approach or laparotomy. For the initial biopsy of every infant, enough tissue must be obtained for formalin fixation, frozen preparation in aluminum foil, and electron microscopy. Once an extrahepatic obstructive cause of neonatal jaundice is determined, an exploratory laparotomy with intraoperative cholangiography is imperative (see Table 96.4 for histologic differences between neonatal hepatitis and biliary atresia).

TABLE 96.4. HISTOLOGIC DIFFERENCES BETWEEN NEONATAL HEPATITIS AND BILIARY ATRESIA

Histologic Features	Neonatal Hepatitis	Biliary Atresia
Bile duct proliferation	Absent	Present
Bile plugs	Absent	Present
Portal/perilobular fibrosis	Absent	Present
Portal/perilobular edema	Absent	Present
Lobular architecture	Panlobular disarray	Intact
Inflammatory cell infiltrate	Present	Absent
Hepatocellular necrosis	Present	Absent
Giant cell transformation	Present or absent	Present or absent

MEDICAL THERAPY FOR NEONATAL CHOLESTASIS

Nutritional therapy is essential in neonatal cholestasis to ensure adequate growth and development. All neonates have an increased caloric requirement compared with adults, and caloric needs are greatly increased in the presence of cholestatic disease. In addition, fat malabsorption occurs in the cholestatic patient due to decreased excretion of bile salts with resultant steatorrhea. Malabsorption of essential fatty acids and fat-soluble vitamins are especially problematic. Energy intake should be increased to 125% to 200% of the recommended daily allowance, and increased formula caloric density as well as continuous supplemental nasogastric tube feedings should be considered. Medium-chain triglycerides (MCTs) are less dependent on bile acids for absorption and should make up 50% to 70% of dietary fat; however, essential fatty acids are lacking in MCTs and should be supplemented. The fat-soluble vitamins also should be supplemented at two to four times the recommended daily allowance, and periodic measurement of serum vitamin A, 25(OH) vitamin D, vitamin E, and prothrombin time are helpful in monitoring effective levels.

Pruritus can be a significant problem even during the neonatal period. The etiology of pruritus may be caused by abnormal stimulation of opioid receptors by bile acids or increased release of endogenous opioids. Rifampin, an antibiotic mainly used in treatment of tuberculosis, has been used successfully to treat pruritis in children with Alagille's syndrome, progressive intrahepatic cholestasis, and biliary atresia. Its antipruritic mechanism may enhance the hepatic oxidase system, which, in turn, decreases the bioavailability of toxic bile aids. Naloxone, an opiate antagonist, also has been used to decrease pruritis, possibly through inhibition of centrally mediated opioid receptors.

Ursodeoxycholic acid (UDCA) is a standard treatment for neonatal cholestatic syndromes and functions through multiple mechanisms, including inhibition of intestinal absorption of bile acids. UDCA has a protective effect on hepatocytes through membrane stabilization and increased canalicular bile flow. The decreased toxic bile acids also cause UDCA to have an antipruritic action. UDCA lowers serum cholesterol through inhibition of intestinal cholesterol absorption as well as increasing conversion of cholesterol to bile acids, and this effect is helpful in decreasing xanthoma size in conditions associated with hypercholesterolemia, such as Alagille's syndrome.

Progressive cholestatic liver disease manifested by poor weight gain, portal hypertension, ascites, and variceal hemorrhage requires surgical intervention. Although endoscopic therapy (variceal sclerotherapy, variceal banding) or portosystemic shunting can provide temporary relief of bleeding tendencies, pediatric patients with end-stage liver disease should be considered for orthotopic liver transplantation. New therapies such as liver-related donor transplantation and hepatocyte transplantation are currently available and may increase donor organ pool availability for these patients.

EDITOR'S NOTE

When a neonate presents with jaundice, there is an important distinction to be made between "indirect" and "direct" hyperbilirubinemia. Indirect bilirubin is the unconjugated, lipid-soluble form that, when present in high concentrations, can cause significant neurologic injury in the infant. The direct component of the total bilirubin level represents bilirubin that has been conjugated by hepatic enzymes. It is water-soluble and is not harmful to developing neural tissues. Although less toxic, an elevated direct bilirubin has potentially grave significance depending on the age of the child and the clinical circumstances. A direct bilirubin level that is greater than 2 mg/dL, is more than 15% of the total bilirubin level, or is present to any degree after 2 weeks of age mandates further workup.

The most common cause of direct hyperbilirubinemia is probably cholestasis due to PN. This is especially common in premature infants. Other common causes include infectious agents, metabolic disorders, and cholestasis secondary to sepsis or drugs. It should be kept in mind that the "surgical" causes of direct hyperbilirubinemia are relatively rare: biliary atresia, choledochal cysts, congenital anomalies of the biliary tree, and perforation of the common bile duct. A potential surgical cause usually is considered after an extensive metabolic and infectious workup has been performed by the neonatologists.

The workup should proceed systematically and without delay. The results of Kasai portoenterostomy for correction of biliary atresia are best when performed early—preferably before 8 weeks of age, ideally before 6 weeks. The diagnostic algorithm will vary somewhat based on institutional preference, but generally begins with ultrasonography of the liver and biliary system. Although not usually diagnostic for biliary atresia, ultrasonography is useful to rule out certain conditions such as a choledochal cyst and cholestasis due to stones or extrinsic compression of the bile duct. A small, shrunken gallbladder, especially if there is evidence of fibrosis of the extrahepatic biliary system, suggests that the diagnosis of biliary atresia needs to be considered strongly. A *HIDA scan* that shows bile excretion, on the other hand, suggests that biliary atresia is not the cause of the jaundice. Most infants being evaluated in this way have little or no excretion of bile by hepatobiliary IDA, which unfortunately is a nonspecific finding. *MRI* (or MR cholangiopancreatography) may soon become the imaging study of choice in infants with suspected biliary atresia, but it is not considered standard in most centers at this time. The next step is usually percutaneous *liver biopsy*. This is usually useful to rule out idiopathic neonatal hepatitis, Alagille's disease, or other hepatopathies while evidence of bile duct proliferation supports the diagnosis of biliary atresia. The definitive study is *laparotomy and cholangiography* with plans for portoenterostomy at the same operation. This is addressed in more detail in the chapter on biliary atresia.

Although rarely primarily responsible for the workup of hyperbilirubinemia, the pediatric surgeon should be familiar with the differential diagnosis and the diagnostic approach to these infants, and should be prepared to facilitate the workup for biliary atresia if clinically indicated.

–P.M.

SUGGESTED READINGS

Balistreri WF. Inborn errors of bile acid biosynthesis and transport. Novel forms of metabolic liver disease. *Gastroenterol Clin North Am* 1999;28:145–172.

Bove KE, Daugherty CC, Tyson W, et al. Bile acid synthetic defects and liver disease. *Pediatr Dev Pathol* 2000;2:1–16.

Greenholz SK, Krishnadasan B, Marr C, et al. Biliary obstruction in infants with cystic fibrosis requiring Kasai portoenterostomy. *J Pediatr Surg* 1997;32:175–179.

Hoffman AF. Pharmacology of ursodeoxycholic acid, an enterohepatic drug. *Scand J Gastroenterol* 1994;29(suppl 204):1–15.

Iinuma Y, Narisawa R, Iwafuchi M, et al. The role of endoscopic retrograde cholangiopancreatography in infants with cholestasis. *J Pediatr Surg* 2000;35:545–549.

Jaw T, Kuo Y, Liu G, et al. MR cholangiography in the evaluation of neonatal cholestasis. *Radiology* 1999;212:249–256.

Kim MJ, Park YN, Han SJ, et al. Biliary atresia in neonates and infants: triangular area of high signal intensity in the porta hepatis at T2-weighted MR cholangiography with US and histopathologic correlation. *Radiology* 2000;215:395–401.

Pittschieler K. Liver disease and heterozygous alpha-1-antitrypsin deficiency. *Acta Paediatr Scand* 1991;80:323–327.

Postemma RR, Hazebroek FW. Choledochal cysts in children: a review of 28 years of treatment in a Dutch children's hospital. *Eur J Surg* 1999;165:1159–1161.

Roberts EA. Primary sclerosing cholangitis in children. *J Gastroenterol Hepatol* 1999;14:588–593.

97

BILIARY ATRESIA

DEBORAH A. NEIGUT
FRANCISCO G. CIGARROA

Biliary atresia is a liver disease of infants characterized by progressive obliteration of extra- and intrahepatic bile ducts. The cause is unknown and the incidence in the United States has been estimated to be approximately 1 in 15,000 live births. Successful treatment requires early diagnosis and biliary reconstruction by hepatico portoenterostomy. There is no medical therapy to reverse this obliterative process. Patients with untreated biliary atresia progress to biliary cirrhosis, portal hypertension, and death at 6 to 12 months of age. Liver transplantation is the only option for survival in children who fail to improve following hepaticoportoenterostomy.

ETIOLOGY AND PATHOGENESIS

During the third week of embryogenesis the liver primordium appears as a ventral outgrowth of the foregut. The hepatic diverticulum consists of the pars cranialis (hepatica), from which the liver parenchyma arises, and the pars caudalis (cystica). The pars cystica forms the extrahepatic biliary ductal system, including the gallbladder, during the fourth week. There is a period during which elongation and rapid epithelial proliferation of the bile ducts occurs, causing temporary obliteration of the lumen. During the 6th week the ducts recanalize, beginning with the common hepatic duct and proceeding distally. Hepatocyte precursor cells give rise to the intrahepatic biliary system, which then joins the extrahepatic biliary bud at the hilum. Biliary atresia may result if the extrahepatic bile ducts fail to recanalize, but this is not felt to be a common cause of biliary atresia. Few stillborn and newborn infants have been identified with atretic bile ducts.

The etiology of biliary atresia remains unknown. The likelihood that it occurs as the result of a postnatal insult is supported by the fact that it is a progressive disease characterized by acute and chronic inflammation within the portal triads. Landing believes that "infantile obliterative cholangiopathy" is an underlying disorder that evolves into either neonatal hepatitis or biliary atresia. It has been observed that mice infected with reovirus-3 developed obliterative inflammation of the extrahepatic ducts, but there is no proven association between the virus and biliary atresia in humans. Hepatobiliary defects similar to biliary atresia can be elicited in animal models subjected to mechanical obstruction of the bile ducts, ligation of fetal arteries supplying the biliary tree, and chemical exposure *in utero.* Vascular accidents may cause some cases of biliary atresia, particularly when it is associated with intestinal atresia. Other theories include cell-mediated immunologic bile duct injury, and bile duct regression secondary to an imbalance of paracrine growth factors. There exists a 20% incidence of associated anomalies with biliary atresia, which supports a prenatal cause. These anomalies include cardiac and genitourinary malformations, preduodenal portal vein, intestinal malrotation, and polysplenia. It is not believed that biliary atresia is an inherited disorder. Biliary atresia is probably the final common outcome of various insults occurring at different periods during gestation and infancy.

Pathology

There are several variants of biliary atresia. In the first type, the proximal extrahepatic ducts are patent and the distal ducts are fibrosed. In the second type, the proximal ducts are obliterated and the gallbladder, cystic duct, and common bile duct are patent. In the third type, the proximal and distal bile ducts are obliterated.

The liver histology in biliary atresia is characterized by bile duct proliferation with an associated inflammatory cell infiltrate and prominent cholestasis (Fig. 97.1). Over time, these changes progress to fibrosis with end-stage cirrhosis if bile flow is not restored (Fig. 97.2). The histology is often

D. A. Neigut: Department of Pediatrics, The University of Texas Health Science Center at San Antonio, San Antonio, Texas.

F. G. Cigarroa: Offices of the President, The University of Texas Health Science Center at San Antonio; and Department of Surgery, University Hospital, San Antonio, Texas

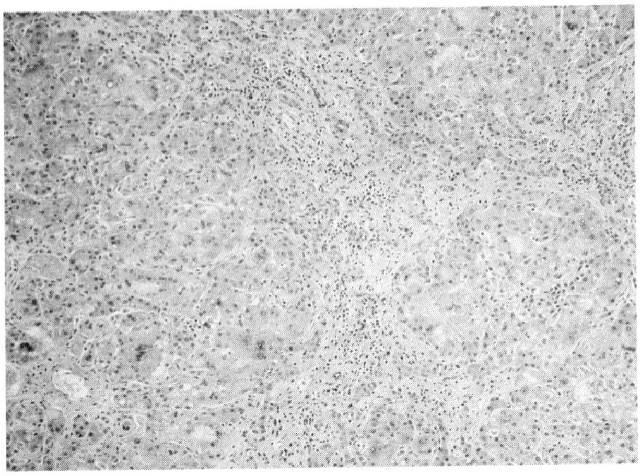

FIGURE 97.1. Liver biopsy in an infant with biliary atresia demonstrating expanded portal areas, bile stasis, early bile ductular proliferation, and mixed inflammatory infiltrate (hematoxylin and eosin, original magnification ×40; courtesy of Josefine M. Heim-Hall, M.D., University of Texas Health Science Center, San Antonio).

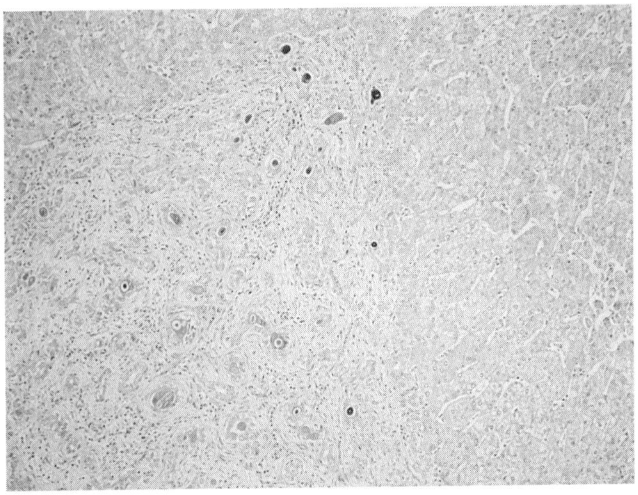

FIGURE 97.2. Liver biopsy demonstrating progression to biliary cirrhosis with broad bands of fibrosis, marked bile stasis, and extensive ductular proliferation (hematoxylin and eosin, original magnification ×40; courtesy of Josefine M. Heim-Hall, M.D., University of Texas Health Science Center, San Antonio).

similar in neonatal hepatitis and biliary atresia, although giant cell transformation and hepatocellular necrosis are more common in idiopathic neonatal hepatitis. Likewise, the histology of α_1-antitrypsin deficiency may mimic biliary atresia, except that this metabolic disease can be distinguished by the presence of periodic acid-Schiff-positive diastase-resistant granules.

DIAGNOSIS

Clinical Presentation

Jaundice in infants that persists after the 2nd week of life should be evaluated. Conjugated hyperbilirubinemia, in which more than 15% of the total bilirubin is conjugated, is always indicative of a pathologic condition. The differential diagnosis of conjugated hyperbilirubinemia in infants is broad, and includes infections, metabolic disorders, idiopathic neonatal hepatitis, biliary hypoplasia (either secondary to Alagille's syndrome or nonsyndromic bile duct paucity), choledochal cyst, and extrinsic compression of the biliary tree.

Infants with biliary atresia are usually active and initially appear well nourished; they generally do not appear ill. Physical examination of an infant with biliary atresia often reveals a jaundiced but otherwise well-appearing child. Hepatosplenomegaly is frequently present early, but the signs of chronic liver disease are not seen. Stools are usually acholic.

Appropriate Workup

Serologic studies should be obtained for toxoplasmosis, rubella, syphilis, cytomegalovirus (CMV), herpes, and hepatitis B. Immunoglobulin M (IgM) titers are preferable because IgG is transferred across the placenta. Urine should be cultured for bacteria and CMV. A serum α_1-antitrypsin level and phenotype, and thyroxine assay should be done. Assays for urine and plasma amino acids should be performed. The urine should be tested for reducing substances

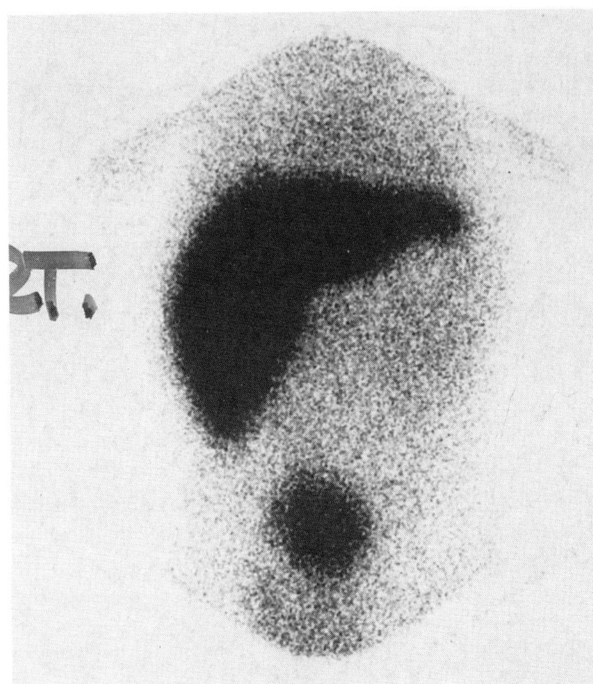

FIGURE 97.3. Technetium 99m diisopropyl iminodiacetic acid scan demonstrating good hepatic uptake, but no excretion of the tracer into the intestine is seen at 24 hours.

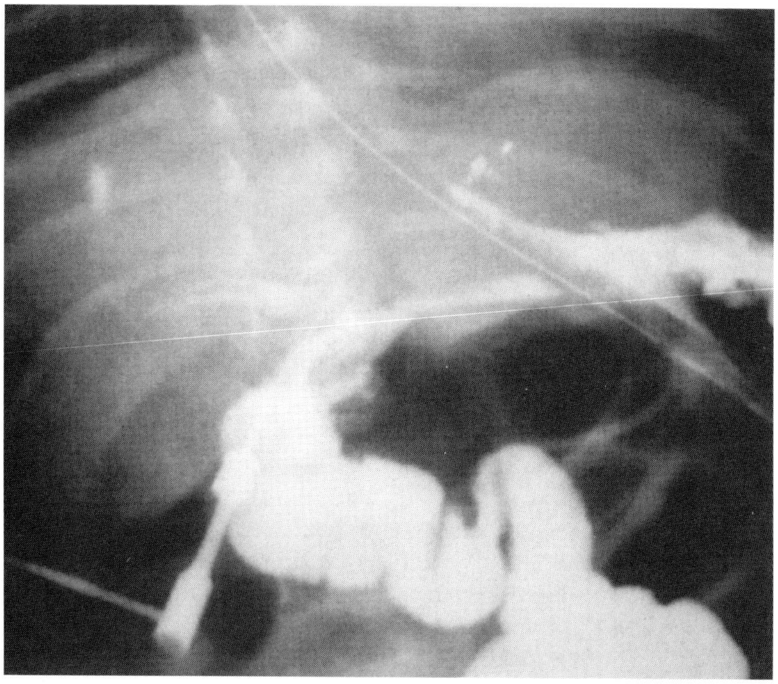

FIGURE 97.4. Intraoperative cholangiogram demonstrating good excretion into the duodenum, but with a paucity of intrahepatic biliary branches. (courtesy of Melvin D. Smith, M.D.)

to rule out galactosemia (if the formula contains lactose or if the infant is breast-fed) or fructose intolerance (if the formula contains sucrose). A sweat chloride test should be performed to rule out cystic fibrosis.

Ultrasonography of the liver and gallbladder should be performed to rule out any cause of obstructive jaundice such as a choledochal cyst or a mass impinging on the portal triad, resulting in bile duct dilatation. Patients with biliary atresia generally have a shrunken or absent gallbladder without visible extrahepatic bile ducts.

If no etiology of the cholestasis is identified, a nuclear hepatobiliary scan is performed to evaluate the patency of the biliary system. Derivatives of iminodiacetic acid—technetium 99m–labeled diisopropyl iminodiacetic acid and ^{99m}Tc-labeled mebrofenin—have excellent uptake and excretion by the liver. Phenobarbital is used to enhance the accuracy of the study because it upregulates hepatic enzymes, facilitating bilirubin conjugation and excretion as well as improving the uptake and excretion of the ^{99m}Tc– iminodiacetic acid (IDA) tracer. The infant is administered 5 mg/kg of phenobarbital in two divided doses for 5 consecutive days before intravenous administration of ^{99m}Tc-IDA tracer. After the injection, images are obtained every 10 minutes for 1 hour, and delayed images are obtained at 6 and 24 hours (Fig. 97.3). The diagnosis of biliary atresia is excluded if the hepatobiliary scan demonstrates the presence of radiotracer in the bowel. When there is no activity detected within the bowel, this study is unable to distinguish between biliary atresia and other causes of cholestasis. At this juncture, there are two possible next steps. A routine recommendation at this point is to perform a percutaneous liver biopsy if the coagulation parameters are within safe limits (platelet count >50,000/mm^3, prothrombin time <1.4 times control). However, if there is a high index of suspicion that the infant does have biliary atresia, or if the patient has a significant coagulopathy, some surgeons prefer to perform an open biopsy and an intraoperative cholangiogram at the same time. If a needle biopsy is performed first and the histologic features are consistent with biliary atresia, exploratory laparotomy with intraoperative cholangiography is indicated and should be performed as expeditiously as possible. Therefore, some surgeons prefer to forgo the initial needle biopsy in infants who are strongly suspected of having biliary atresia. Cholangiography is performed via the gallbladder (Fig. 97.4). The visualization of the intrahepatic ducts and the passage of contrast into the duodenum exclude the diagnosis of biliary atresia. It should be noted, however, that unexplained persistence or progression of jaundice for weeks following the diagnosis of neonatal hepatitis might signal the progression of "hepatitis" to biliary atresia, and reexploration might be indicated.

MANAGEMENT

The success of surgical correction of patients with biliary atresia is directly dependent on the infant's age. Ohi et al. reported a 10-year survival rate of 73% for infants undergoing surgery before 61 days of age, 35% at 61 to 71 days, 23% at 71 to 90 days, and only 13% when surgery was performed on patients over 90 days of age. Timing is critical. The entire evaluation of an infant with conjugated hyperbilirubinemia should take no longer than a week, and prompt surgical correction of obstructive jaundice should be undertaken.

Surgical Correction

In 1959 Kasai and Suzuki introduced hepaticoportoenterostomy for the treatment of biliary atresia. They understood that biliary atresia was not a static process and that there was progressive fibrosis of the extrahepatic biliary tree. Kasai recommended an early surgical approach with high transection of the extrahepatic bile ducts at the level of the portal vein bifurcation, thereby maximizing the potential for exposing patent intrahepatic bile ducts. Cross-sections through the bile duct demonstrate a marked decrease in the diameter of the lumen (Fig. 97.5). More than 50% of the infants who underwent surgery before 2 months of age achieved bile drainage. Less than 7% of the infants achieved bile drainage if hepaticoportoenterostomy was delayed beyond 4 months of age.

Preoperatively, the patient's prothrombin time should be measured. If prolonged, vitamin K (2 mg intramuscularly) should be administered and the prothrombin time repeated 12 to 24 hours later to establish normalization. Fresh-frozen plasma should be available to correct the child's coagulopathy if it is unresponsive to vitamin K administration.

The initial goal of surgery is to confirm the diagnosis, and a right subcostal incision is recommended to allow visual assessment of the gallbladder and the extrahepatic biliary tree. Intraoperative cholangiography is performed via the gallbladder to define duct patency and options for surgical reconstruction (Fig. 97.6). If the gallbladder, cystic duct, and common bile duct are patent, the gallbladder can be used as a conduit for reconstruction as a hepatic portocholecystostomy. If the gall bladder is fibrotic and these ducts are obliterated, a Roux-en-Y hepaticoportoenterostomy is the only option available for reconstruction. A significant number of patients will have complete obliteration of the gallbladder lumen, making performance of cholangiography impossible.

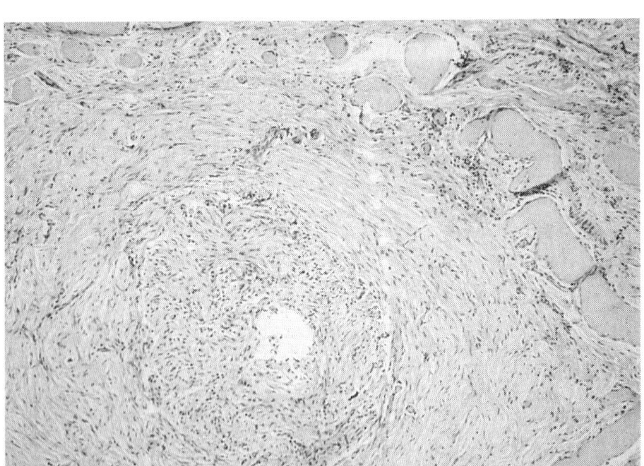

FIGURE 97.5. Cross-section of the extrahepatic bile duct in biliary atresia, demonstrating fibrous obliteration and chronic inflammation. Note the dramatic reduction of the luminal diameter. (Courtesy of Mark R. Matthews, M.D., Austin Pathology Associates.)

In the Kasai procedure, the gallbladder, cystic duct, and extrahepatic duct remnants are gently mobilized. The common duct is divided distally and mobilized toward the liver hilum up to the bifurcation of the portal vein. In this area the common hepatic duct broadens into a cone of fibrous tissue, which is transected flush with the liver parenchyma. This tissue historically has been sent for frozen section analysis to define patency of intrahepatic ducts, dictating a more proximal dissection and reexcision of the porta hepatis if ducts are not patent. Generally this is no longer done, and bile duct dissection is performed at the level of the hepatic plate–parenchymal junction. The operation is completed by directly anastomosing to this area a Roux-en-Y limb of jejunum 30 to 40 cm in length, hence the term *hepaticoportoenterostomy*. There is no clear correlation between the ductule size and outcome, but historically it was believed that the chance of long-term effective bile drainage is negligible if the intrahepatic ducts measure less than 100 μm in diameter.

The major postoperative complication of the Kasai procedure is cholangitis as a result of bile stasis and bacterial contamination from the intestinal conduit. Cholangitis is a significant clinical problem because recurrent inflammation of the bile ducts can lead to sclerosis, with decreased bile drainage. Several operative options have been devised to decrease bacterial contamination via the intestinal conduit.

Infants with a patent gallbladder, cystic duct, and common bile duct can undergo reconstruction via a portocholecystotomy. The incidence of cholangitis with this procedure is decreased, most likely related to the sphincter of Oddi preventing reflux of intestinal contents. Tube decompression of the gallbladder is recommended postoperatively for approximately 4 to 6 weeks to prevent rupture of the small gallbladder and cystic duct. This approach has not been popular among some pediatric surgeons because of the inadequacy of the gallbladder as a conduit and technical problems related to kinking of the cystic duct.

When the gallbladder cannot be used for reconstruction, other options have been used in an attempt to decrease the incidence of cholangitis. These methods all use the principle of exteriorizing the conduit in order to decrease intraluminal pressure and thereby diminish resistance to bile flow. The double-barreled hepaticoportoenterostomy is known as the Surgura I procedure. The Surgura II procedure uses a subcutaneous enterostomy for the distal jejunal limb with the insertion of a jejunal tube, in the hope that the intestinal flora is completely diverted from the biliary anastomosis. Kasai later recommended a double Roux-en-Y hepaticoportoenterostomy. The most recent technical modification in an

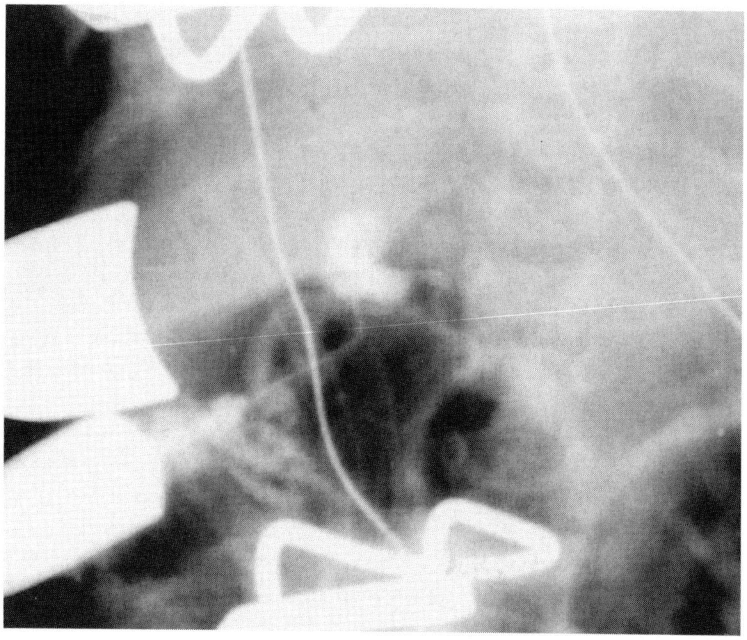

FIGURE 97.6. Intraoperative cholangiogram demonstrating a lack of contrast seen within the intestine after injection (courtesy of Melvin D. Smith, M.D.).

attempt to further decrease the chance of bacterial contamination from enteric flora has been the construction of an intussuscepted antireflux valve in the distal intestinal conduit. There is no evidence that these procedures significantly improve the rate of cholangitis, progression of liver disease, or death, and generally are not currently used. Intestinal stomas created at the time of surgery should be closed when bile flow reaches a steady state, because progression to portal hypertension can lead to significant life-threatening bleeding from peristomal varices.

The evidence is not clear that exteriorization of the Roux-en-Y portoenterostomy reliably diminishes the frequency of cholangitis. Exteriorization, however, permits precise measurement of bile output and treatment of declining bile output. It is the authors' preference to perform the Kasai portoenterostomy without external drainage.

RESULTS

Kasai Procedure

Successful bile drainage can be achieved in more than 70% of infants with biliary atresia if portoenterostomy is performed prior to 10 weeks of age. Portoenterostomy is considered curative for one third of patients with biliary atresia. One third of patients will have minimal bile flow following reconstruction and will experience rapid development of biliary cirrhosis. The other one third of patients who undergo portoenterostomy achieve moderate bile drainage, but will have gradual but progressive biliary cirrhosis and portal hypertension, ultimately requiring liver transplantation, probably during school-age or adolescent years.

Postoperative Management

Ursodeoxycholic acid is a bile salt and a potent choleretic agent that increases bile flow, and is given at a dose of 15 to 30 mg/kg/day postoperatively. Methylprednisolone is used for its antiinflammatory effect in the immediate postoperative period. Trimethoprim sulfamethoxazole is used for long-term bacterial prophylaxis to decrease the incidence of cholangitis.

Cholangitis is a serious but common problem following portoenterostomy. Cholangitis damages the existing bile ducts, causing decreased bile flow and an increased rate of fibrosis. Unfortunately, the incidence of cholangitis has not been reliably decreased by the administration of prophylactic antibiotics or choleretic agents.

Following a surgical procedure for biliary atresia, cholangitis is suspected in a child who has fever, increasing serum bilirubin and amino transferase levels, and tender hepatomegaly. The child should be promptly evaluated and aggressively treated. Recommended therapy includes hospitalization, hydration, broad-spectrum intravenous antibiotics, pulse steroids, and, at times, surgical exploration of the portoenterostomy. The use of pulse steroids in this clinical setting is controversial. Steroids act by decreasing the inflammatory reaction in the bile ducts and thereby promoting bile flow. However, they should not be used if the child has evidence of sepsis. The portoenterostomy should be explored only in patients who have an abrupt cessation of normal bile flow. In these patients, inspissated sludge or granulation tissue may block the portoenterostomy, and removal of the obstructing material may result in resumption of bile flow and salvage of the portoenterostomy. The disadvantage of reexploration is that it may make eventual liver transplantation more difficult technically. For this reason, indications for reexploration are few, and repeated reexploration should be avoided.

Two thirds of children treated with a Kasai procedure will have progressive hepatic fibrosis with resultant portal hypertension. Infants who never establish adequate bile flow have a rapid onset of cirrhosis and sequelae of portal hypertension. The remainder develop complications of portal hypertension over several years, including malnutrition, hypersplenism, ascites, and esophageal varices. Ascites can often be managed with salt restriction and spironolactone or furosemide. Esophageal varices may be controlled with sclerotherapy or banding. Portosystemic shunting procedures should be used in select circumstances where liver transplantation is contraindicated. Aggressive medical management should be continued if hepatic function is stable and the child is able to maintain normal growth parameters.

Nutrition

Infants with biliary atresia have deficient enterohepatic circulation of bile salts, with resultant malnutrition and inefficient absorption of fat and fat-soluble vitamins. In children who do not drain significant amounts of bile through their portoenterostomy, these deficits may become severe and symptomatic. All children with biliary atresia should be given supplemental vitamins A, D, E, and K. Nutritional supplementation should also include formulas that provide the majority of fat calories as medium-chain triglycerides, because they can be directly absorbed without bile salt–dependent micellar stabilization. Fat malabsorption can result in significant malnutrition and impaired linear growth. Vitamin D deficiency can result in rickets, and children should be supplemented with 5 to 7 µg/kg/day of 25-hydroxyvitamin D. Ataxic neuromyopathy results from vitamin E deficiency, and 15 to 25 IU/kg/day should be given as tocopherol polyethylene glycol succinate, which is a more water-soluble form. Vitamin K deficiency results in coagulopathy secondary to decreased levels of factors II, VII, and IX, and 5 to 15 mg/day of vitamin K should be given orally. In some instances intermittent injections of vitamin K are required. Inadequate levels of vitamin A can result in dermatitis, night blindness, keratomalacia, and xerophthalmia. It is recommended that infants with biliary atresia be given 5,000 to 15,000 IU/day of water-miscible vitamin A.

Transplantation

Infants who fail to drain bile after portoenterostomy should be referred for early transplantation. Patients who do well initially but whose growth curves become inadequate or whose hepatic function deteriorates also should be considered for liver transplantation. Because portoenterostomy has little to no effect after the child is 4 months of age, an infant this age at the time of diagnosis should be referred for liver transplantation, rather than subjected to a portoenterostomy.

The advent of immunosuppressants, cyclosporine A, and tacrolimus has made liver transplantation successful in children; 5-year survival rates approach 85% in most centers. The importance of timely referral cannot be overemphasized. Transplantation should be performed before the child has progressed to end-stage liver failure, because the mortality of transplantation is substantially increased at that point. A significant problem to date, however, remains a shortage of organs for children. The inability to obtain adequate donor organs has been responsible for the death of many children awaiting transplantation. This serious problem has led to the development of reduced-size liver transplants from cadavers, and living-related liver transplants.

The advent of more selective immunosuppressants has allowed improvement in the management of rejection. Early tapering of steroids reduces the susceptibility to infection and improves linear growth. It is now possible for many children to live active and productive lives following liver transplantation, but there must be a commitment by both patient and physician for long-term follow-up. A team approach with involvement of the surgeons, general pediatricians, hepatologists, psychiatrists, social workers, and nutritionists is essential in the development of a successful pediatric transplantation program.

CONCLUSIONS

Biliary atresia occurs in only 1 in 15,000 live births in the United States. The etiology remains unknown, although several theories have been proposed. Patients can be grouped into three broad anatomic categories. The differential diagnosis of neonatal conjugated hyperbilirubinemia is large. As a result, the workup may be extensive, but it should take no longer than a week because timing of surgical correction is critical. The results of Roux-en-Y portoenterostomy (Kasai procedure) are best when the operation is performed before 2 months of age. Modifications of the Kasai procedure designed to prevent cholangitis have been described; however, objective data documenting fewer problems with cholangitis are not available. Management of nutritional deficits is important before and after surgery. Revision of a portoenterostomy is now rarely indicated because the results of liver transplantation have improved. In most centers the 5-year survival rate after transplantation for biliary atresia is around 85%.

ACKNOWLEDGMENTS

The authors would like to thank Dr. Barry R. Cofer in the Department of Surgery and Dr. Josefine Heim-Hall in the Department of Pathology, at the University of Texas Health Science Center, San Antonio, for their advice, photographs, and critical review. We are grateful to Juanita Sherfield for her assistance in the preparation of this manuscript.

SUGGESTED READINGS

Cigarroa FG, Schwarz KB, Colombani PM. Biliary atresia. In: Pitt HA, Carr-Locke DL, Ferrucci JT, eds. *Hepatobiliary and pancreatic disease.* Boston: Little, Brown, 1995.

Holmes JB. Congenital obliteration of the bile ducts: diagnosis and suggestions for treatment. *Am J Dis Child* 1916;11:405–431.

Kasai M. Details of operative techniques of hepatic portoenterostomy [Abstract]. Presented to the Pacific Association of Pediatric Surgeons, Fukuoka, Japan, May 15, 1983.

Kasai M, Suzuki S. A new operation for non-correctable biliary atresia-hepatic portoenterostomy. *Shujutsu* 1959;13:733–739.

Ladd WE. Congenital atresia and stenosis of the bile ducts. *JAMA* 1928; 91:1082–1085.

Landing BH. Considerations of the pathogenesis of neonatal hepatitis, biliary atresia, and choledochal cysts—the concepts of infantile obstructive cholangiopathy. *Progr Pediatr Surg* 1974;6:113–139.

Matory YL, Miyano T, Suruga K. Hepaticoportoenterostomy for biliary atresia. *Surg Gynecol Obstet* 1985;161:541–545.

Miyano T, Suruga K, Suda K. Abnormal choledochopancreatico-ductal junction related to etiology of infantile obstructive jaundice diseases. *J Pediatr Surg* 1979;14:16–26.

Ohi R, Nio M, Chiba T, et al. Long term follow up after surgery of patients with biliary atresia. *J Pediatr Surg* 1990;25:442–445.

Swenson O, Fisher JH. Utilization of cholangiogram during exploration for biliary atresia. *N Engl J Med* 1952;247–249.

Thaler MM, Gellis SS. Studies in neonatal hepatitis and biliary atresia. II. The effect of diagnostic laparotomy on long term prognosis of neonatal hepatitis. *Am J Dis Child* 1968;116:262–270.

98

CHOLECYSTITIS AND CHOLELITHIASIS

MOHAMMAD A. EMRAN
RICCARDO A. SUPERINA
ROBERT M. ARENSMAN

Due to improved survival in children with serious illnesses and more accurate radiologic capabilities, the incidence of cholelithiasis and cholecystitis in children is increasing. This overview focuses on the clinical presentation of biliary calculi in children, disorders associated with cholelithiasis, indications for surgery, and some of the newer methods to treat these children.

Making the diagnosis of biliary tract disease solely on clinical grounds is difficult in children. Pain patterns are atypical, and children are often unable to communicate effectively with the examiner. Children are also more difficult to examine than a cooperative older person. When assessing a child with abdominal pain, the possibility of biliary tract disease is always kept in mind, particularly if any predisposing conditions are present. Of all cholecystectomies performed in pediatric patients 80% to 90% are for cholelithiasis, 10% to 15% are for biliary dyskinesia or acalculous cholecystitis, and 2% are for sludge or polyps.

PATHOGENESIS

The presentation of cholecystitis and cholelithiasis differs in children from adults primarily due to the underlying etiologies. Acalculous cholecystitis is more common in children than adults. Two thirds of these cases occur in the postoperative period or are associated with trauma, burns, shock, sepsis, or parenteral nutrition. Boys have a higher incidence of acalculous cholecystitis than do girls.

Numerous hematologic or metabolic conditions can predispose a child to biliary disease and are always sought when gallstones are present. Underlying disorders that cause hemolysis include spherocytosis, thalassemia, and sickle cell disease. These hemolytic diseases and hemoglobinopathies are eliminated first, because they are the most common and carry well-known surgical risks. Although these disorders produce pigmented stones, cholesterol stones are more common; therefore, other factors should be considered. Fasting serum cholesterol and triglycerides are measured. Additional conditions or disorders associated with cholelithiasis include major prior bowel resections or short bowel syndrome, malabsorption, Crohn's disease, cystic fibrosis with pancreatic insufficiency, choledochal cysts, transplantation, recent weight loss, obesity, and ethnicity.

As in adults, children of Pima, Hopi, or Navajo Indian origin and those of Hispanic descent have a higher incidence of cholesterol stones. More rarely, certain inborn errors of metabolism predispose to biliary disease. Examples are conditions that impair bile salt metabolism or cholesterol biosynthesis, hyperlipidemia syndromes, or lipoprotein receptor defects.

CLINICAL PRESENTATION

Abdominal pain associated with biliary disease is often described as "colicky." If biliary tract disease is suspected, a history should be obtained that focuses on the perinatal history for hemolytic diseases of the newborn, prematurity, or

M. A. Emran: Departments of Pediatric Surgery and Cancer Biology, Northwestern University Medical School, and Children's Memorial Hospital.

R. A. Superina: Department of Surgery, Northwestern University Medical School; and Department of Transplant Surgery, Children's Memorial Hospital, Chicago, Illinois.

R. M. Arensman: Departments of Surgery and Pediatrics, Northwestern University Medical School; and Department of Pediatric General Surgery, Children's Memorial Hospital, Chicago, Illinois.

a prolonged period of parenteral nutrition. A pattern of pain occurring with meals or after the ingestion of fatty foods with spontaneous resolution should be sought. Other clues to the presence of biliary stones may be found in a family history of hemolytic diseases, hyperlipidemia, or parental gallbladder disease.

The majority of gallstones (60%–80%) in children are asymptomatic. Symptoms are generally associated with stones passing through the cystic or common duct, or the impaction of a stone near the biliary ampulla. Pain, nausea, and vomiting are the most common symptoms. Physical signs include right upper quadrant tenderness and guarding, or signs of peritoneal irritation when inflammation of the parietal peritoneum occurs secondary to cholecystitis or pancreatitis. Approximately 5% to 10% of children with gallbladder disorders develop jaundice, and 10% to 15% develop gallstone pancreatitis. Although common duct stones should be considered in all patients with jaundice, the cause is often unclear.

Cholangitis with bacteremia, fever, and chills sometimes follows biliary obstruction. The most common bacteria associated with cholangitis and biliary sepsis include *Escherichia coli, Enterobacter, Klebsiella, Bacteroides,* and group D streptococci. In diabetic patients *Clostridium* species may cause cholecystitis and progress to emphysematous cholecystitis. Therefore, the appropriate selection of antibiotics includes an evaluation of the underlying susceptibility of the host to unusual pathogens. It is important to note that opportunistic pathogens may play a role in the evolution of cholecystitis in immunosuppressed patients such as those infected with human immunodeficiency virus or those taking immunosuppressive medications. Cryptosporidiosis and cytomegalovirus are two of the most commonly seen biliary pathogens in immunocompromised hosts, although they are rarely encountered in children.

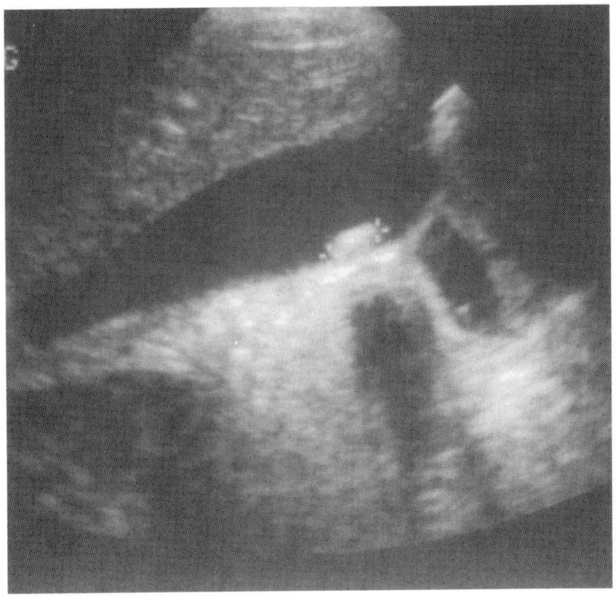

FIGURE 98.1. Ultrasound of the gallbladder in an 11-year-old boy demonstrating cholelithiasis. Notice the hyperechoic stone with acoustic shadow beneath.

INVESTIGATION

The evaluation of a child with abdominal pain often includes plain films of the abdomen. One or more opacities in the right upper quadrant suggest gallstones. Air in the biliary tree or following the outline of the gallbladder may represent cholangitis or emphysematous cholecystitis. Ultrasonographic examination of the abdomen has become the most popular and least invasive method of evaluating the bile ducts, liver, and pancreas in children. Gallbladder wall thickening, pericholecystic edema, cholelithiasis (Fig. 98.1), choledocholithiasis (Fig. 98.2A), common duct distension (Fig. 98.2B), biliary gas, pancreatitis, sludge, and polyps are radiologic signs of biliary disease. Because abdominal ultrasonographic examination has become a more commonly used modality for the evaluation of a wide variety of intestinal, biliary, and urologic conditions, asymptomatic gallstones are diagnosed with increasing frequency. It is not uncommon for gallbladder stones to be found in the neonatal period or even *in utero.*

Computed tomography is not used for routine screening of biliary tract disease but may be used in more complex cases to clarify questions of anatomy such as pancreatic anomalies or intrahepatic lesions. Radionucleotide hepatobiliary scanning is also used as an ancillary diagnostic method, particularly to diagnose cholecystitis. This test, however, has limited use in cases where jaundice is present and is not performed if the bilirubin is greater than 6 to 8

FIGURE 98.2. A: Ultrasonogram of the common bile duct (*three small arrows*) in a 12-year-old girl demonstrating choledocholithiasis (*large arrow*). **B:** Common duct dilation to 42 mm in the same patient with the common duct stone. **C:** Endoscopic retrograde cholangiopancreatography of the same patient with common duct stone clearly defining the extent of common duct and hepatic duct dilation.

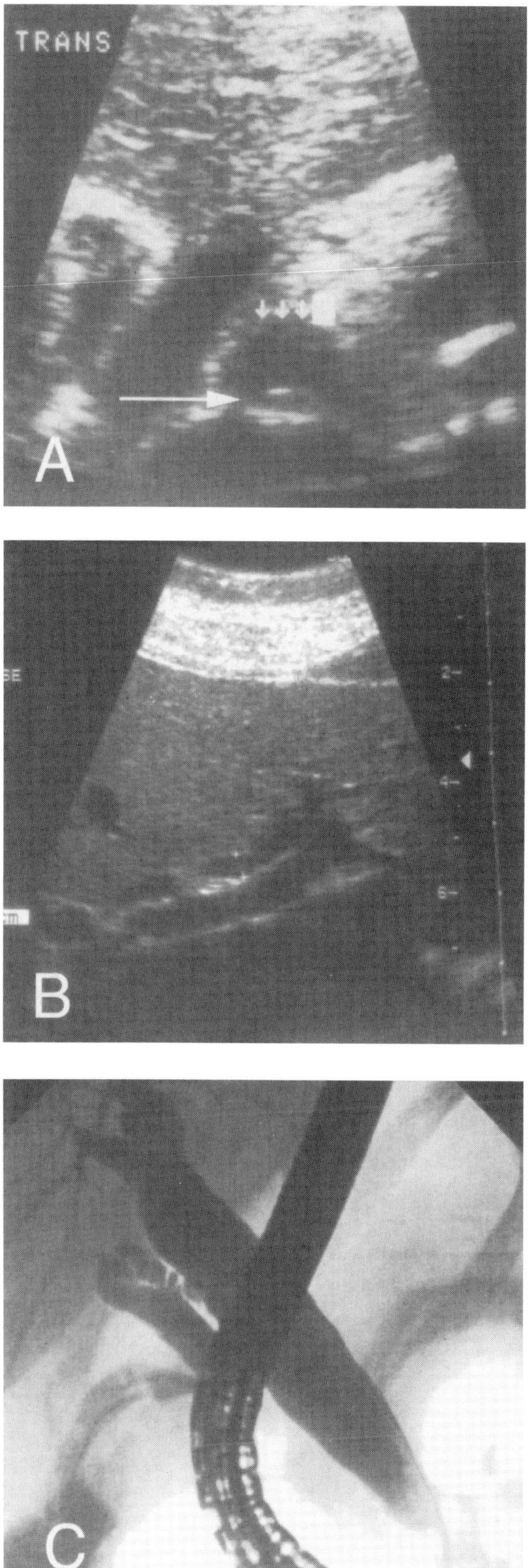

mg/dL. Abnormal measures of gallbladder emptying (<40%–50%) by scintigraphy or ultrasonography after cholecystokinin injection is also suggestive of biliary dyskinesia.

Endoscopic retrograde cholangiopancreatography (ERCP) (Fig. 98.2C) or transhepatic cholangiography (Fig. 98.3) is used to directly visualize the extrahepatic biliary tree and parts of the intrahepatic biliary tree. These tests also may visualize the pancreatic duct. ERCP is used therapeutically to perform sphincterotomy for the treatment of common duct stones, ampullary stenosis, or sphincter of Oddi dysfunction. In infants and babies, operative cholangiograms (Fig. 98.4) may be the most accurate means of diagnosing biliary tract abnormalities and also may be curative when the biliary obstruction is caused by sludge as in "inspissated bile syndrome."

Laboratory tests to exclude hemolysis as the underlying etiology of the gallstones include osmotic fragility testing, red cell smear, serum haptoglobins and hemoglobin electrophoresis. Liver function tests, including conjugated and unconjugated bilirubin, alkaline phosphatase, serum transaminases, amylase, calcium, and fasting cholesterol and triglycerides are also useful adjuncts in assessing the

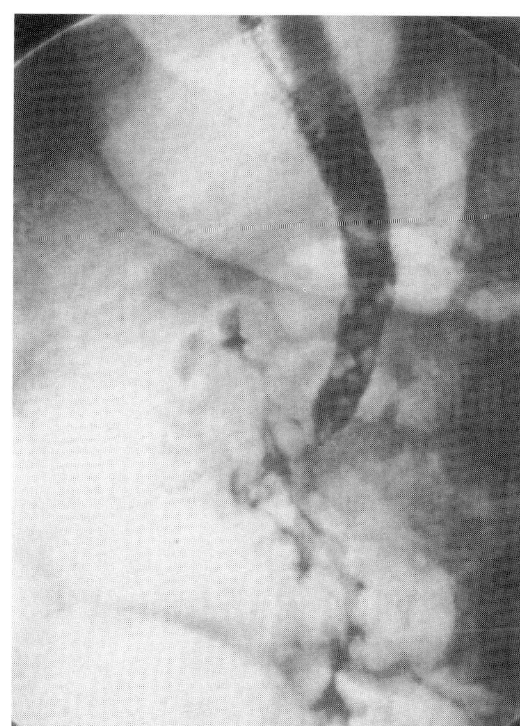

FIGURE 98.3. Transhepatic cholangiogram displaying numerous common duct stones.

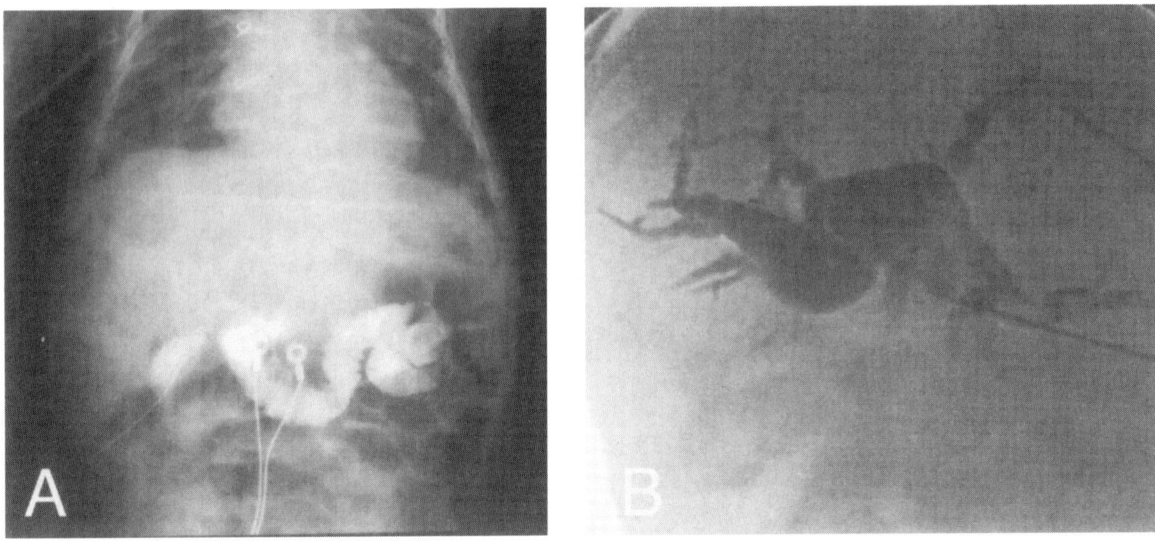

FIGURE 98.4. A: Operative cholangiogram demonstrating normal biliary anatomy, with drainage of contrast into the small intestine. **B:** Operative cholangiogram with markedly dilated ducts secondary to obstruction. Drainage of contrast into the duodenum cannot be clearly defined.

severity of the disease process, the presence of possible underlying disorders, and charting the treatment algorithm.

TREATMENT

After determining the nature of the biliary tract disease, the site of calculi, and complicating features, treatment options are considered. Restoring normal fluid balance by adequate intravenous hydration and treatment of sepsis in cases of cholecystitis or cholangitis take priority over operative intervention. Preoperative antibiotics are given for wound prophylaxis when acute infection is not present prior to surgery. Cholecystectomy ensues during the acute episode or may be deferred until all symptoms have improved with conservative measures. Laparoscopic cholecystectomy has become the standard of care in most children requiring a cholecystectomy. Currently, 71% or more of cases are completed laparoscopically.

When considering the diagnosis of acalculous cholecystitis, choose patients for surgery carefully because a high percentage of patients have persistent symptoms after cholecystectomy. Patients with dyspeptic symptoms (abdominal discomfort, belching, bloating, heartburn, indigestion, and specific food intolerance) have a higher rate of persistent symptoms after cholecystectomy. Differentiation of these patients is made by obtaining a thorough history. Without a clear indication for cholecystectomy such as classic biliary attacks or complications of stones, patients are investigated for other causes of abdominal pain before proceeding with surgery. The treatment of acalculous cholecystitis includes supportive measures such as hydration, treatment of infection, and treatment of any underlying predisposing conditions in addition to cholecystectomy.

Patients with asymptomatic gallstones generally require only close observation. Cholecystectomy is considered in patients at high risk for developing cholecystitis or those with conditions that are characterized by frequent and episodic abdominal pain such as sickle cell disease. Transplant patients with asymptomatic stones are considered for prophylactic cholecystectomy. Patients with underlying hematologic disorders causing hemolysis and biliary calculi may benefit from simultaneous splenectomy and cholecystectomy.

SUMMARY

The incidence of cholelithiasis in children is increasing, in part due to our ability to detect stones that are asymptomatic. The management of children with this disease takes into account the natural history of the disease process, the age of the child, the location of the stones, and the symptoms. Of particular interest is the management of cholelithiasis in the newborn period and even in the unborn fetus. It is becoming clearer that the majority of stones in these patients resolve spontaneously, but surgery may be needed on occasion. In addition, laparoscopic cholecystectomy has made removal of the gallbladder less traumatic for the average child, with less postoperative pain and a shorter hospital stay.

SUGGESTED READINGS

Debray D, Pariente D, Gauthier F, et al. Cholelithiasis in infancy: a study of 40 cases. *J Pediatr* 1993;122:385–391.

Gholson CF, Grier JF, Ibach MB, et al. Sequential endoscopic/laparoscopic management of sickle hemoglobinopathy-associated cholelithiasis and suspected choledocholithiasis. *South Med J* 1995;88: 1131–1135.

Gholson CF, Sittig K, McDonald JC. Recent advances in the management of gallstones. *Am J Med Sci* 1994;307:293–304.

Grosfeld JL, Rescorla FJ, Skinner MA, et al. The spectrum of biliary tract disorders in infants and children. Experience with 300 cases. *Arch Surg* 1994;129:513–518; discussion 518–520.

Ishitani MB, Shaul DB, Padua EA, et al. Choledocholithiasis in a premature neonate. *J Pediatr* 1996;128:853–855.

Strasberg SM, Clavien PA. Overview of therapeutic modalities for the treatment of gallstone diseases. *Am J Surg* 1993;165: 420–426.

Stringer MD, Lim P, Cave M, et al. Fetal gallstones. *J Pediatr Surg* 1996;31:1589–1591.

99

LAPAROSCOPIC CHOLECYSTECTOMY

THOM E LOBE

Cholecystitis and cholelithiasis now are recognized with increasing frequency in infancy, childhood, and adolescence. Most cases can be managed laparoscopically, regardless of the patient's age.

Congenital anomalies of the gallbladder, while rare, often can be associated with cholelithiasis. Agenesis, duplication, a bilobed gallbladder, and ectopic location are the most frequently encountered malformations. Otherwise, the incidence of gallstones is reported to be between 0.15% and 0.22%. Any disturbance in the concentration of lecithin, bile salts, or cholesterol renders the bile lithogenic and predisposes the child to form cholesterol stones that probably result from poor solubilization of cholesterol, stasis, and nucleating factors.

Pigmented stones can be black or earthy brown. Black pigmented stones usually are associated with a hemolytic process, after ileal resection, or in patients receiving total parenteral nutrition (TPN) and are also more common among those of Far Eastern Asian descent. Earthy calcium bilirubinate stones develop in patients with infected bile or biliary strictures. Biliary sludge develops in gallbladders with impaired contractility and in patients on TPN. The gallstones in children with short-bowel syndrome or inflammatory bowel disease maintained on TPN are predominantly pigmented stones.

In the absence of an underlying hematologic disorder, most gallstones are associated with obesity, adolescent pregnancy, a positive family history for cholelithiasis, the use of oral contraceptives, chronic illnesses such as cystic fibrosis, spinal cord disease, intestinal pseudoobstruction after correction of congenital duodenal atresia or stenosis, and as a complication of choledochal cyst. An increased risk of cholelithiasis also has been documented in children receiving treatment for Wilms' tumor, neuroblastoma, and Hodgkin's and non-Hodgkin's lymphoma. In addition to the chemotherapeutic agents, there is a high correlation between abdominal tumor resection (63%) and abdominal irradiation (50%) and cholelithiasis in these patients. Despite these known risk factors, the origin of gallstones in approximately 80% of pediatric patients remains unknown. Although there is no sex predilection, girls begin to predominate in adolescence with a ratio of 11:1 to 22:1, probably due to the influence of estrogen.

DIAGNOSIS

Symptomatology and associated medical history are more important in diagnosing cholelithiasis than are laboratory tests. Jaundice is the most common symptom in children under 1 year of age, being present in greater than 90% of symptomatic patients. Overall, the most common symptom is vomiting (60%). Right upper quadrant pain in the absence of vomiting does not appear to be a common finding.

Most children with acute cholecystitis present with abdominal pain, nausea, and vomiting. The pain is less well localized in younger children and is often confused with that of appendicitis. Chronic cholecystitis is commonly characterized by recurrent bouts of right upper quadrant pain associated with meals. The pain usually is much less specific and rarely is associated with fatty food intolerance.

Acalculous cholecystitis tends to occur as a complication of severe illness, a result of prior surgery, a severe burn, multisystem trauma, massive blood transfusion, and various infections, including pneumonia, generalized sepsis, typhoid, *Salmonella,* otitis media with meningitis, giardiasis, and Kawasaki disease. The underlying features involved in the pathogenesis include dehydration, adynamic ileus, gallbladder stasis, treatment with TPN, and hemolysis from multiple transfusions. Acute acalculous cholecystitis accounts for 2% to 15% of all cases of acute cholecystitis, and the incidence of acute acalculous cholecystitis may be as high as 32% in children undergoing cholecystectomy.

In smaller children, the symptoms of acalculous cholecystitis include fever, right upper quadrant pain, nausea, vomiting, and occasionally diarrhea when the underlying

T. E Lobe: Departments of Surgery, Pediatrics, and Preventive Medicine, University of Tennessee, and LeBonheur Children's Medical Center, Memphis, Tennessee.

infection is caused by a pathogenic intestinal organism. Tenderness to palpation and muscle guarding are noted on physical examination. A right upper quadrant mass is sometimes palpable and must be distinguished from acute hydrops. Leukocytosis and jaundice are often observed, and an elevated serum amylase level signifying associated pancreatitis has been noted in some patients. The diagnosis is confirmed by ultrasonography.

On physical examination children with acute cholecystitis may demonstrate fever, right upper quadrant abdominal tenderness, and guarding. A right upper quadrant mass occasionally is present. Although jaundice may indicate choledocholithiasis, more often it is simply due to hemolysis. In patients with chronic cholecystitis and cholelithiasis, the physical examination is often normal.

Laboratory tests in instances of acute cholecystitis may demonstrate an elevated white blood cell count and left shift on the differential smear. With choledocholithiasis, elevation of serum direct bilirubin, alkaline phosphatase, and γ-glutamyl transferase levels can be observed. The serum amylase level may be elevated with associated pancreatitis.

The most accurate and useful diagnostic test is the ultrasonographic examination, which has an accuracy of approximately 96%. Cholescintigraphy with technetium 99m–labeled iminodiacetic acid compounds is the most useful test to assess the patency or obstruction of the cystic duct and is the procedure of choice to diagnose acute cholecystitis. This test has a sensitivity near 100% and a specificity of 95%. Cholescintigraphy is also useful in detecting common bile duct obstruction or a choledochal cyst.

Spiral computed tomographic cholangiography is a relatively new imaging technique that results in biliary opacification and three-dimensional reconstruction. This study, as well as magnetic resonance cholangiography, proves useful in complicated cases of obstruction or pancreatitis and often obviates the need for endoscopic retrograde cholangiopancreatography (ERCP) or other forms of cholangiography.

The topic of biliary dyskinesia is a controversial one. Some children, typically preteens or adolescents, present with postprandial epigastric or right upper quadrant pain, often associated with nausea, but have morphologically normal gallbladders by ultrasonography and no evidence of cholelithiasis. There is sometimes a clear association with fatty foods. Some of these patients benefit from cholecystectomy, although some do not, and distinguishing the two groups prior to surgery can be difficult. Some clinicians use a nuclear medicine scan to calculate gallbladder ejection fraction after intravenous bolus administration of cholecystokinin, although the lower limit of normal for gallbladder ejection fraction is somewhat unclear. Pain precipitated by cholecystokinin injection can suggest the diagnosis as well, although many individuals with normal gallbladder function have pain after being given the drug, and young children may not be able to distinguish it from the pain they have been having. Some surgeons require that two hepatic iminodiacetic acid (HIDA) scans be performed, both demonstrating an ejection fraction of less than 35%, before recommending an operation. Nevertheless, others argue that the entity simply does not exist, and patients and their families need to understand that regardless of the clinical and laboratory findings, the symptoms may not be relieved with cholecystectomy.

TREATMENT

Spontaneous resolution of gallstones in some neonates and infants up to age 3 with cholelithiasis has been observed on serial ultrasonographic examinations. Children with gallstones and typical symptoms of right upper quadrant or epigastric pain with food intolerance should undergo cholecystectomy. Eighty-two percent of children with cholelithiasis and atypical symptoms had improvement with dietary manipulation. Pediatric patients with gallstones that are asymptomatic or associated with atypical symptoms can be safely followed without complications.

If choledocholithiasis with obstructive jaundice occurs, ERCP and endoscopic sphincterotomy with stone removal can be used to clear the common bile duct. This technique is now possible in infants. If gallstones remain after clearing the common bile duct, a formal cholecystectomy should be performed, because recurrent complications are likely. If endoscopic sphincterotomy is unsuccessful or if the child is too small for ERCP, a procedure with irrigation of the common bile duct through the cystic duct or a transduodenal sphincterotomy may be helpful. If bile duct perforation has occurred, early peritoneal irrigation and drainage usually provide effective treatment.

For children with sickle cell anemia and gallstones, elective cholecystectomy (or perhaps cholelithotripsy) can reduce the high morbidity caused by infection. As many as 50% of previously asymptomatic patients require operation within 3 years because of significant complications or symptoms of acute cholecystitis.

Cholecystectomy is recommended for all symptomatic patients with thalassemia or spherocytosis as well as those undergoing splenectomy in whom a preoperative ultrasonographic examination demonstrates gallstones. Some surgeons, however, prefer simple cholecystotomy with removal of stones at the time of splenectomy for spherocytosis.

Davidoff et al. were among the first to describe the technique of laparoscopic cholecystectomy in children. They noted that the benefits of laparoscopic cholecystectomy include decreased pain and ileus after surgery, shortened hospitalization, and improved cosmesis and concluded that laparoscopic cholecystectomy is safe and efficacious in children, and it compares favorably with traditional cholecystectomy in children. This technique is of particular value in the obese child, for cholecystitis in pregnancy, and in managing the biliary complications of heart transplant patients.

The role of intraoperative cholangiography is somewhat controversial. Although some surgeons believe that the procedure should be performed routinely, the majority recommend selective studies.

In 10 of our cases, common duct stones were known to exist. In these cases, we made an incision in the cystic duct and dilated this sufficiently large with a balloon catheter to insert another endoscope into the bile duct. For a "pediatric choledochoscope," we have found it convenient to use a pediatric cystoscope. This allows for good visualization and provides access for irrigation and instrumentation (e.g., passage of a stone basket). A second camera can be attached to this choledochoscope so that the surgeon can see intraductal and extraductal anatomy simultaneously. Usually, after the endoscope is removed from the duct, the cystic duct stump can be ligated in the standard fashion. This approach also has been found to be safe in adult patients.

Holcomb et al. looked at their experience with 100 consecutive laparoscopic cholecystectomies. The patients ranged in age from 25 to 230 months, with a mean of 105 months. Only 19 patients had hemolytic disease as the cause of their cholelithiasis. Two patients had biliary dyskinesia. Seventy-eight patients underwent an elective operation. Twenty-two children required urgent hospitalization because of complications from their cholelithiasis: acute cholecystitis (n = 7), jaundice and pain (n = 6), gallstone pancreatitis (n = 5), and acute biliary colic (n = 4). All 6 patients who presented with jaundice underwent ERCP before their laparoscopic cholecystectomy. Two patients required laparoscopic choledochal exploration. The operating time and postoperative hospitalization were significantly longer in the complicated group when compared with the elective patients. Significant complications, such as the need for reoperation, injury to the common bile duct or to other viscera, bile leak, or retained common duct stone, did not occur.

Most of our own cases have been for symptomatic cholelithiasis in children with sickle cell disease. In these patients who present with recurrent abdominal pain, we usually remove the appendix concurrently. Of interest is the finding of pathology in 50% of the appendices removed from these children. The pathology was mixed, demonstrating scarring in some and inflammation in others.

Lugo-Vicente recently studied infants and children requiring cholecystectomy. Their mean age was 15 years. Females (76%) with classic biliary symptoms predominated; 12% of the patients developed gallstone pancreatitis and 7% jaundice. Abnormal liver chemistry values, obesity, and elevated triglyceride levels comprised the most significant predisposing factors. Indications for surgery were cholelithiasis in 86%, biliary dyskinesia in 12%, and sludge/polyp in 2%. Fifty-nine cholecystectomies (71%) were performed laparoscopically and 29% of them were performed using an open method. Choledocholithiasis in 7% was managed by open extraction with t-tube placement or endoscopic papillotomy followed by laparoscopic cholecystectomy. No major ductal complication was identified. The predominant pathologic finding was chronic cholecystitis, including among the subgroup with biliary dyskinesia. Statistical comparison showed that laparoscopic cholecystectomy is superior to open cholecystectomy in regard to length of stay, diet resumption, use of pain medication, operating time, and cosmetic results.

PROCEDURE

Laparoscopic cholecystectomy can be performed either in a supine position or "French style," with the surgeon standing between the patient's legs. In either situation, the patient should be positioned on the bed to facilitate operative cholangiography if that is deemed necessary. After administering the general anesthetic, the stomach and bladder are emptied with tube decompression or a Credé maneuver on the bladder.

We prefer to use a 10-mm trocar in the umbilicus for gallbladder extraction and clip application, even though we will use a 3- or 5-mm telescope through this port. In an infant, a 5-mm umbilical trocar should suffice. Pneumoperitoneum is performed using an open (Hasson) technique or by using a Veress needle, depending on the surgeon's preference. If the patient has had abdominal surgery before, then we prefer to use the open technique.

Three additional trocars are inserted. These can be 3-mm trocars in most cases, but occasionally 5-mm trocars may be necessary in large or obese patients. The first of these trocars is placed in the right anterior axillary line between the level of the umbilicus and just above the iliac crest. This is used to retract the dome of the gallbladder cephalad and anteriorly. The next trocar is placed near the midclavicular line, below the costal margin, and is for retraction of the neck of the gallbladder. The final trocar is placed either in the midline (in larger patients) or toward the left midclavicular line (in smaller patients), and is used for dissection.

After inserting the trocars, the fundus of the gallbladder is retracted as described, the neck of the gallbladder is retracted caudally, slightly posteriorly, and to the patient's left to best display the cystic duct and vascular elements. The peritoneum is incised to expose these structures after disrupting any adhesions.

A Maryland-style dissector is useful to expose the cystic duct and artery, and the junction of the cystic duct with the common bile duct. Making certain of the anatomy is essential before any structures are divided, so that damage to the ducts is avoided. Once the anatomy is clear, the cystic artery and duct can be clipped and divided.

If a cholangiogram is necessary to clarify the anatomy or because of suspected stone disease, this should be done before any structures are clipped and divided. There are many techniques and devices designed for cholangiography. We prefer simply to clip the distal cystic duct, make a nick in the cystic duct near the clip, and introduce a cholangiogram catheter percutaneously so that it can be guided into the nick in the duct. If using a balloon-tipped catheter, inflation of the balloon will secure the catheter in place for the image. Otherwise, a clip can be placed across the duct with the catheter in place to prevent a leak.

After any imaging or duct exploration (a flexible endoscope can be used for this or, in small children, a pediatric cystoscope can be passed through a trocar site), the ductal structures and vessels are clipped and divided using 5-mm endoscopic clips applied through the umbilical trocar (the telescope is moved to another port for this).

The gallbladder then is removed from its bed using electrocautery or an ultrasonic dissector. It is noteworthy that before this step, the use of any energy delivery device is avoided so as not to cause injury to the delicate structures.

The gallbladder is then extracted through the umbilical port, spreading the facial incision as necessary. If there are numerous stones preventing you from extracting the gallbladder, then a stone forceps or similar instrument is used to extract the stones from inside the gallbladder to make it easier to extract the gallbladder itself.

The liver bed then is inspected for hemorrhage, the abdomen is lavaged if necessary, the instruments are all withdrawn, and the wounds are closed. We inject the wounds with a local analgesic to make the immediate postoperative recovery easier on the patient.

POSTOPERATIVE CARE

Postoperatively, patients are offered diet as tolerated and are discharged to home later the same day or the next morning, depending on the patient's disease and condition. Perioperative antibiotics can be used if preferred, and analgesic use is minimal. Most patients can resume usual activities immediately and more strenuous activities as tolerated.

COMPLICATIONS

Complications are rare. Ductal injuries are the most serious and often are recognized at operation. Any postoperative fever or jaundice should be investigated. Ultrasonography is sometimes used to demonstrate a collection of fluid or a dilated biliary tree, but the best test is generally a nuclear medicine study. It will demonstrate an obstruction if one is present and is sensitive enough to show all but the smallest bile leaks. Treatment of a common bile duct injury generally involves a major open reconstructive procedure, the discussion of which is beyond the scope of this chapter.

The risk of major bile duct injuries should be exceedingly low as the collective and personal experience with laparoscopic cholecystectomy increases. The key is proper visualization and attention to technical detail. The dissection of the cystic duct should begin close to the antrum of the gallbladder. The cystic duct should be visualized as it enters the gallbladder before it is clipped and divided. Traction of the infundibulum of the gallbladder with the surgeon's left hand grasper should be directed away from and perpendicular to the liver bed. This exaggerates the Y-configuration of the cystic duct–common duct junction and avoids making the common duct appear to be an extension of the cystic duct. The cystic duct should be clipped and divided close to the gallbladder. When in doubt, a cholecytogram should be performed to better delineate the anatomy. In difficult cases, the gallbladder can be removed in a "top-down" fashion or converted to an open procedure. Bile leaks from the liver bed or accessory bile ducts appear to be exceptionally rare in children.

Bleeding is a rare complication but can be an indication for conversion to an open procedure. Bleeding from the cystic artery rarely occurs and can usually be controlled easily with clips or cautery. The cystic artery should be seen to be entering the gallbladder to avoid inadvertent injury to the right hepatic artery, which sometimes travels parallel and very close to the cystic artery and the posterior aspect of the gallbladder. After division of the cystic duct and artery, all further dissection close to the gallbladder itself should be possible with electrocautery. Encountering large structures that appear to require control with clips should give one pause to consider whether the plane of dissection is incorrect and if the structure should be preserved. Bleeding from the liver bed can be controlled in most cases with precise application of electrocautery.

Injury to adjacent viscera from instruments or electrocautery burns are unusual but should be prevented by using meticulous technique. Trocar incisions 5 mm or greater should be closed at the level of the fascia in all infants and children to avoid the rare port-site hernia. Postoperative pulmonary problems are occasionally seen in patients with sickle cell disease and can be a source of significant morbidity or even mortality in these patients.

Cholecystectomy is being performed with increasing frequency in the pediatric age group. Laparoscopy is safe and is currently the standard approach for removal of the gallbladder in children, as it is in adults. With attention to proper technique and careful anatomic dissection, the risk for significant complications in experienced hands is low. The procedure is well tolerated in the majority of patients and the return to normal activities is generally rapid.

SUGGESTED READINGS

Davidoff AM, Branum GD, Murray EA, et al. The technique of laparoscopic cholecystectomy in children. *Ann Surg* 1992;215:186–191.

Grosfeld JL, Rescorla FJ, Skinner MA, et al. The spectrum of biliary tract disorders in infants and children. Experience with 300 cases. *Arch Surg* 1994;129:513–518; discussion 518–520.

Holcomb GW 3rd, Morgan WM 3rd, Neblett WW 3rd, et al. Laparoscopic cholecystectomy in children: lessons learned from the first 100 patients. *J Pediatr Surg* 1999;34:1236–1240.

Kasirajan K, Obermeyer RJ, Kehris J, et al. Microinvasive laparoscopic cholecystectomy in pediatric patients. *J Laparoendosc Adv Surg Techniques [A]* 1998;8:131–135.

Lugo-Vicente HL. Trends in management of gallbladder disorders in children. *Pediatr Surg Int* 1997;12:348–352.

Waldhausen JH, Graham DD, Tapper D. Routine intraoperative cholangiography during laparoscopic cholecystectomy minimizes unnecessary endoscopic retrograde cholangiopancreatography in children. *J Pediatr Surg* 2001;36:881–884.

100

CHOLEDOCHAL CYST

GARRETT ZALLEN
FREDERICK M. KARRER

Choledochal cysts are diagnosed in Western countries in one in 150,000 live births, and more frequently in Asian countries. Choledochal cysts can cause severe and occasionally fatal complications such as cholangitis, stone formation, and malignant degeneration. The first description of a fusiform dilation of the common bile duct was in 1723 by Vater. It was not until over 100 years later that Douglas realized that this dilation was of congenital origin. Alonzo-Lej published his seminal article in 1959 wherein he described a case series of choledochal cysts and provided the first classification system to describe the different types of cysts (Fig. 100.1). In his classification system, type I malformations, which represent 80% to 90% of patients, are cystic dilations of only the common bile duct. Type II cysts are characterized by a diverticular outpouching of the common bile duct. Type III malformations, also known as choledochoceles, are cysts isolated to the intrapancreatic portion of the common duct and often involve the ampulla. The second most common lesion is type IV, which involves dilation of the common bile duct as well as intrahepatic duct cysts. Finally, type V choledochal cysts, originally described by Caroli, involve the intrahepatic bile ducts without involvement of the extrahepatic ducts. In 1977, Todani proposed a modification to the original classification scheme by adding a subclassification to the type IV cysts. Type IVa deformities have multiple cysts of both the intra- and extrahepatic ducts, and type IVb deformities have multiple cysts in the extrahepatic ducts only.

The pathophysiology of choledochal cysts remains poorly understood. One theory holds that anomalous pancreaticobiliary ductal anatomy leads to reflux of pancreatic digestive enzymes into the bile ducts, resulting in damage to the developing ducts and subsequent dilation. Work by Babbitt in 1969 and Todani in 1984 demonstrated the common occurrence of ductal anomalies of the pancreaticobiliary system. They found that 65% to 80% of patients with choledochal cysts had abnormal entry of the pancreatic duct, resulting in a long common channel, which may result in the reflux of pancreatic secretions into the biliary system. More recent studies involving endoscopic retrograde cholangiopancreatography (ERCP) have demonstrated that choledochal cysts are associated with intrapancreatic ductal anomalies as well. Koshinaga found that almost half of the patients he studied had either an ansa pancreatica, loop, or a divisum type anatomy to their pancreatic ducts. These anomalies may contribute to pancreatitis seen in patients with choledochal cysts. Another theory of the development of choledochal cysts is the presence of a distal duct obstruction. Spitz produced cystic dilation of the common bile duct by ligating the distal duct in newborn lambs, but ligation in adult sheep failed to produce the same dilation. It was concluded that obstruction of an immature duct produces the type of dilation seen in types I and IV, but did not produce the other types of anomalies observed in humans. Clearly there is more to the development of choledochal cysts than distal obstruction, but these factors have not been elucidated.

DIAGNOSIS

Choledochal cysts can produce symptoms in any age group, but most cysts present within the first decade of life. Infants usually present with persistent asymptomatic jaundice. Children can present with jaundice, cholangitis, or pancreatitis. Pancreatitis in a child should always warrant a workup for choledochal cysts. Adult patients tend to present in a more insidious fashion. It is not unusual for older patients to present with choledocholithiasis, cholangitis, and cirrhosis that have progressed to include portal hypertension. Malignant degeneration (cholangiocarcinoma) is also found in up to 16% of adults with choledochal cysts.

The diagnostic workup should consist of routine laboratory work, including analysis of conjugated bilirubin and

G. Zallen: Department of Pediatric Surgery, Children's Hospital of Buffalo, Buffalo, New York.

F. M. Karrer: Department of Surgery, University of Colorado, School of Medicine; and Department of Pediatric Surgery, The Children's Hospital, Denver, Colorado.

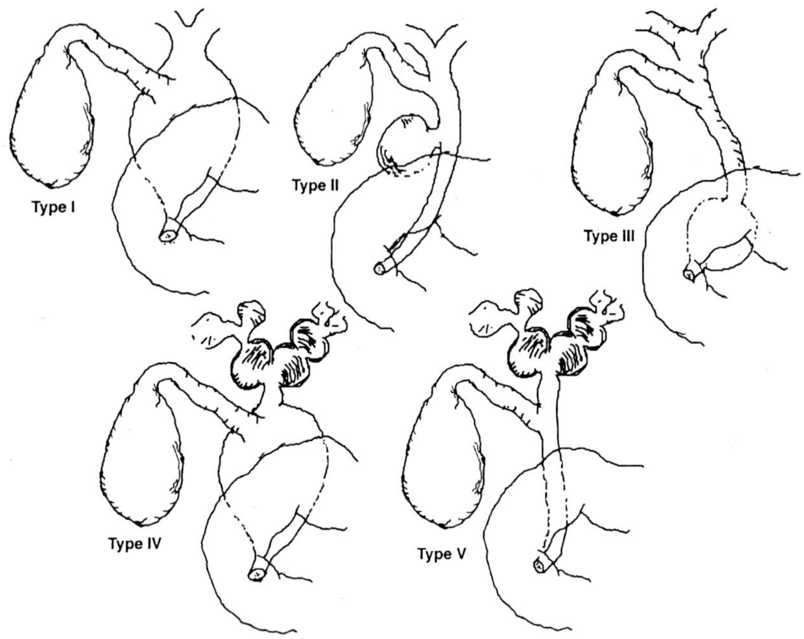

FIGURE 100.1. Standard Alonzo-Lej classification system of choledochal cysts.

alkaline phosphatase, both of which may be elevated. The most useful diagnostic tool remains ultrasonography. Although reports of magnetic resonance cholangiopancreatography and intraluminal endoscopy can be found in the literature, there has been no benefit demonstrated to these types of imaging. In children, no further preoperative imaging is absolutely necessary once dilation of the extrahepatic biliary ducts has been demonstrated by ultrasonography. However, the use of preoperative ERCP may provide further information about biliary and pancreatic ductal anatomy that may aid in the preoperative decision making. Finally, hepatobiliary scintigraphy may help provide additional information, especially when biliary atresia is suspected.

SURGICAL THERAPY

Historical attempts at medical therapy met with disastrous results and mortality rates as high as 97%. Surgical therapy initially consisted of marsupialization of the cyst, but development of external fistulas and excessive fluid loss led to an unacceptable rate of complications. The definitive therapy of complete cyst excision and internal drainage with hepatoduodenostomy was performed by McWhorter in 1924. Unfortunately, this procedure did not become practical until advances in perioperative care made the mortality rate acceptable. In the meantime, internal drainage with choledochocyst-duodenostomy without cyst excision became accepted therapy, but anastomotic strictures leading to cholangitis produced a long-term mortality rate that approached 50%. To remedy this problem, Roux-en-Y cyst-jejunostomy was tried, but similar complications occurred and drainage did not prevent the malignant progression in these cysts.

Total cyst excision with Roux-en-Y hepaticojejunostomy with or without a valved intestinal conduit is now standard therapy. If pericystic inflammation makes complete cyst excision hazardous, then mucosectomy as described by Lilly provides a safe alternative. The choice of surgical technique depends on the type of cyst encountered. There have been isolated reports of laparoscopic excision of type II lesions, but these are rare malformations, and laparoscopic removal has not become a standard approach. Type IV cysts may require a lateral hilar dissection with opening of the lowermost intrahepatic cysts and subsequent large ostial anastomosis for drainage. Cysts that are isolated to the liver (type V) may best be treated with liver transplantation, unless they are isolated to a single lobe, in which case an anatomic resection might be reasonable. Caroli's disease involving both lobes can only be palliated with transhepatic drainage or U-tubes until a transplant can be performed.

After the anatomy and extent of disease has been clearly delineated by diagnostic imaging studies, standard preoperative preparation is undertaken, including assessment of coagulation. Prophylactic antibiotics are administered and the patient is positioned supine on a fluoro-ready table with a roll placed transversely under the upper abdomen. A transverse, midline or right upper quadrant oblique incision can be used. We prefer a right subcostal incision with slight extension across the midline. Use of a self-retaining retractor aids in exposure. Unless preoperative ERCP was performed, the gallbladder is used for intraoperative cholangiography once the abdomen is entered. This is easily performed by placing a small intravenous cannula into the fundus of the gallbladder and securing it with a purse-string suture. A short segment of intravenous tubing is connected to a three-way stopcock and half-strength intravenous contrast is injected slowly under live fluoroscopic visualization. Forceful injection should be avoided because of the small risk of inducing pancreatitis. The goal is to provide an anatomic roadmap of the biliary system with visualization of the cyst itself, the distal common bile duct, and, most importantly, the hepatic duct and its bifurcation, where the anastomosis will eventually be made.

In the most common variant, type I, the gallbladder is dissected from the gallbladder fossa and the cystic artery is ligated. The hepatic flexure of the colon may be mobilized to aid in exposure of the distal cyst. A Kocher maneuver with division of the lateral aspect of the gastrohepatic ligament will help expose the distal aspect of the cyst. If the degree of pericystic inflammation permits a safe dissection of the posterior cyst wall from the portal vein, the cyst is circumferentially dissected. Usually medial reflection of the gallbladder with traction on the cystic duct reveals the posterior plane of dissection. If the cyst is densely adherent to the portal structures posteriorly, then the technique of intramural mucosectomy may be used. Once the cyst is encircled, the dissection is carried distally toward the head of the pancreas. Care must be taken not to injure the pancreatic duct at this level. Stay sutures are placed at the distal neck of the cyst, the cyst is transected, and the stump is oversewn with a monofilament, absorbable suture. Once the distal duct has been divided, the cyst is reflected cephalad and the posterior dissection is continued until the bifurcation of the hepatic duct is encountered. Normally the hepatic ducts are mildly dilated or of normal caliber, but if the cystic dilation continues proximally, then longitudinal incision of the lowermost portion of the dilated intrahepatic ducts is recommended to promote adequate drainage. Stay sutures are placed laterally in the proximal duct, and the diseased portion of the extrahepatic duct is transected and removed.

Construction of the Roux-en-Y jejunal conduit is performed by selecting a 40-cm length of jejunum. The limb is brought to the hilum in a retrocolic fashion. The proximal end should lie easily and without tension against the porta hepatis. To complete the Roux-en-Y, an end-to-side jejunojejunostomy is performed using a two-layer closure, and the mesenteric defect is closed. The hepaticojejunostomy is performed in an end-to-end fashion. An end-to-side anastomosis also may be performed. The anastomosis is constructed using full-thickness, single-layer, running monofilament absorbable sutures. A closed suction drain is placed in the subhepatic space and brought out through a separate incision. Perioperative antibiotics are administered for a short course, and the drain is removed if there is no bilious drainage following the resumption of a regular diet.

If pericystic inflammation makes the posterior dissection dangerous, then intramural dissection may be performed as described by Lilly. Once the cyst is exposed anteriorly, it is incised transversely in the midportion of the cyst. The contents are evacuated and stay sutures are placed in quadrants for exposure. An intramural plane is dissected laterally and then carried posteriorly. A bridging incision is then made within the cyst wall and the dissection is executed both caudad and cephalad until normal duct is encountered. The intramural portion of the cyst can then usually be transected proximally and distally without having to remove the entire cyst. The standard Roux-en-Y reconstruction can now be performed.

Type II cysts are rarely seen. The operative approach is generally the same as described above. The diverticulum can occasionally be excised at its base with minimal manipulation of the common bile duct, but this is only possible when the base is narrow, when the common duct is clearly normal, and when the cyst wall is not adjacent to the duct causing regional inflammation and fibrosis. More often the base is broad, and at minimum some form of ductoplasty is required. Because primary closure of an incision in the common duct is likely to result in a stricture, and although in some cases one might consider leaving a T-tube in place, it is usually more prudent to resect the common bile duct and perform a hepaticojejunostomy as described above.

Type III choledochal cysts are actually intramural duodenal choledochoceles. These can be treated using a transduodenal approach, as for a sphincterotomy. The cyst is unroofed and the lining is carefully excised. The ampulla is typically involved, and both the common bile duct and the pancreatic duct must be visualized and examined for evidence of injury or stricture. The cyst may then be marsupialized so as to freely drain into the duodenum.

RESULTS

The largest study of outcomes comes from Japan, where Miyano reviewed 180 cases of choledochal cysts. In this series, there was no mortality and, interestingly, there were no malignancies found at the time of operation. Hepaticojejunostomy was performed in 169 of 174 patients. There were four cases of postoperative intrahepatic stones, and three of these patients developed cholangitis. All four had anastomotic strictures and underwent successful revision without further complications. There were no cases of cholangitis without concomitant stones, and there were no cases of postoperative pancreatitis. Subgroup analysis demonstrated that if a patient undergoes surgery before the age of 5 years, there was a zero incidence of postoperative stone formation. It would appear that young patients identified before the development of irreversible intrinsic liver disease can expect excellent long-term results with a Roux-en-Y hepaticojejunostomy.

SUGGESTED READINGS

Alonso-Lej F, Rever WB, Pessagno DJ. Congenital choledochal cysts, with a report of two and an analysis of 94 cases. *Int Abstr Surg* 1959;108:1–30.

Babbitt DP. Congenital choledochal cysts: new etiological concept based on anomalous relationships of the common bile duct and pancreatic bulb. *Ann Radiol (Paris)* 1969;12:231–240.

Caroli J, Soupalt R, Kossakiwski J, et al. La dilatation polykystique congenitale des voies biliares intrahepatiques. Essai de classification. *Semin Hop Paris* 1958;34:488–495.

Komi N, Tamura T, Miyoshi Y, et al. Nationwide survey of cases of choledochal cyst. Analysis of coexistent anomalies, complications and surgical treatment in 645 cases. *Surg Gastroenterol* 1984;3: 69–73.

Koshinaga T, Fukuzawa M. Pancreatic ductal morphological pattern and dilation in postoperative abdominal pain in patients with congenital choledochal cyst: an analysis of postoperative pancreatograms. *Scand J Gastroenterol* 2000;35:1324–1329.

Lilly JR. The surgical treatment of choledochal cysts. *Surg Gynecol Obstet* 1979;149:36–42.

Miyano T,Yamataka A, Ohshiro K, et al. Complications after cyst excision with hepaticoenterostomy for choledochal cysts and their surgical management in children versus adults. *J Pediatr Surg* 1997;32:1097–1102.

Spitz L. Experimental production of cystic dilatation of the common bile duct in neonatal lambs. *J Pediatr Surg* 1977;12:39–42.

Todani T, Watanabe Y, Fujii T, et al. Anomalous arrangement of the pancreatobiliary ductal system in patients with a choledochal cyst. *Am J Surg* 1984;147:672–676.

Todani T, Watanabe Y, Narusue M, et al. Congenital bile duct cysts: classification, operative procedures and review of thirty-seven cases including cancer arising from choledochal cyst. *Am J Surg* 1977;134:263–269.

101

BENIGN HEPATIC TUMORS

ANDREW M. DAVIDOFF

Primary tumors of the liver occur in fewer than three per million children in the United States per year. Of these neoplasms, more than two thirds are malignant, making benign hepatic tumors rare in infants and children. Nevertheless, establishing the correct diagnosis of a hepatic tumor promptly and safely is important because a number of benign entities, especially vascular tumors, often do not require surgical resection unless they become symptomatic.

Most infants and children with hepatic tumors present with abdominal distension, with or without a palpable mass. Ultrasonography is useful as the initial investigative modality. It can confirm the presence of a hepatic lesion, as well as determine if the lesion is solid or cystic, if there are multiple lesions, and whether or not it is vascular. Computed tomography (CT) and magnetic resonance imaging (MRI) provide more information, helpful in formulating a differential diagnosis and demonstrating anatomic detail that may be useful when considering a surgical resection. Many consider MRI to be the best modality and the ability to perform MR angiography can provide critical preoperative information and obviate the need for conventional angiography, a study that can sometimes be problematic in small children. However, although CT or MRI can often suggest a specific diagnosis or at least whether a lesion is benign or malignant, this usually does not obviate the need for a tissue diagnosis.

All patients should have a serum alpha-fetoprotein (AFP) determination as part of their initial evaluation. More than 90% of children with hepatoblastoma and approximately 60% of children with hepatocellular carcinoma (excluding those adolescents with the fibrolamellar variant) have elevated serum AFP levels, whereas those with benign liver tumors usually do not. One must be aware of the normal age-specific range for AFP; these levels are normally high in the newborn and decline to a stable low level (<10 ng/mL) in infants by 8 months of age. Liver function studies and coagulation profiles are generally not helpful in the initial evaluation of children with liver masses because the uninvolved liver is typically normal and, even with large tumors, provides normal synthetic function. A complete blood count is important because several types of benign liver tumors can present with thrombocytopenia or anemia.

A. M. Davidoff: Departments of Surgery and Pediatrics, University of Tennessee, Memphis, School of Medicine; and Department of Surgery, St. Jude Children's Research Hospital, Memphis, Tennessee.

HISTOLOGIES

Vascular Tumors

The most common benign tumors of the liver in infants and children are hemangiomas, of which there are two types: cavernous hemangiomas and hemangioendotheliomas. These tumors vary greatly in size, from small and asymptomatic to very large and life threatening. Cavernous hemangiomas are usually asymptomatic and may be associated with cutaneous hemangiomas. Patients may present with abdominal pain or a full sensation in the upper abdomen, and an abdominal mass or hepatomegaly may be noted on physical examination. Cavernous hemangiomas are usually solitary lesions or have a dominant mass, although diffuse hemangiomatosis of the liver has been reported. Histologically, these are large blood-filled, endothelium-lined sinuses separated by fibrous septae.

The natural progression of these lesions is that of spontaneous involution with fibrosis or thrombosis and calcification, although rare cases of rupture (usually following trauma), biliary obstruction and liver failure have each been described. Surgery is rarely indicated, except in the relatively unusual circumstance where a biopsy is needed to confirm the diagnosis. Biopsy of these highly vascular lesions under direct vision is recommended, either with an open procedure or via a laparoscopic approach, both because of the potential for significant bleeding and because the need for a biopsy may be obviated if a lesion with the characteristic red-purple appearance is encountered. Percutaneous biopsy of these lesions is not advised.

Most often, the diagnosis can be made with appropriate imaging studies. The finding of a homogeneously echogenic, well-defined, highly vascular mass on ultrasonography suggests the diagnosis of hemangioma that can be confirmed by dynamic CT obtained during rapid intravenous contrast injection. This often demonstrates the characteristic peripheral enhancement of the lesion initially, followed by delayed central filling. Rarely, a hypervascular malignancy cannot be excluded and a biopsy must be performed. Selective hepatic artery embolization may hasten the process of involution of very large lesions. Surgical resection is reserved for cases in which symptoms such as pain or fever persist, or rupture has occurred or the lesion is large enough to be at high risk for traumatic rupture.

Infantile hemangioendotheliomas are capillary hemangiomas that usually are diagnosed in infancy, more often in girls (>2:1). These lesions are composed of many small vascular channels lined by one or more layers of endothelial cells. Although most infants present with asymptomatic abdominal distension and, occasionally, cutaneous hemangiomas, nearly half have symptoms of high-output cardiac failure secondary to arteriovenous shunting within the liver. This can result in significant mortality (>65%) for untreated infants.

Generally, the younger the patient at presentation, the worse is the prognosis. Medical treatment of congestive heart failure with digitalis and diuretics should begin promptly, and radiologic embolization or surgical ligation of the principle feeding hepatic artery should be attempted. Thrombocytopenia associated with platelet sequestration and consumptive coagulopathy (Kasabach-Merritt syndrome) are other potential significant complications of infantile hemangioendotheliomas. Tumor rupture and malignant transformation to angiosarcoma have been reported but are rare.

These lesions also tend to involute spontaneously, although infants often need prompt treatment to resolve the complications of the lesions. In addition to the treatment of congestive heart failure and physical occlusion of feeding vessels, a variety of drugs have been used for infants with symptomatic hemangioendotheliomas. The administration of high-dose corticosteroids is still considered first-line medical therapy in most centers. Prednisone is given at 1 to 4 mg/kg/day. Alternatives include cyclophosphamide or α-interferon (1–3 mU/m^2/day), which also can be combined with steroid therapy. All forms of medical therapy may take several weeks to elicit a response, however. Therapy may be limited by adverse effects of the drugs. The potential complications of corticosteroids and cyclophosphamide are well known. The use of α-interferon in these young patients can cause a characteristic syndrome of lower extremity neurologic injury, spastic diplegia, which can be irreversible and often limits therapy. Radiation therapy is very rarely used for these lesions. Indications for surgical excision include symptomatic lesions that do not respond to medical therapy or in patients whose therapy is limited by side effects. Rarely, surgery is recommended due to concerns about the potential for traumatic rupture. Liver transplantation has been used in rare cases of extremely large or multiple tumors.

Nonvascular Tumors

Benign tumors of the hepatic parenchyma are extremely rare in children. The most common histologic types are adenomas and focal nodular hyperplasia (FNH). Hepatic adenomas are usually solitary, although hepatic adenomatosis has been described. Hepatic adenomas are usually asymptomatic and are often incidental findings on radiologic examinations. MRI is probably the best modality for defining the lesions, although there are no clear diagnostic characteristics. Grossly, these lesions are yellow or tan with areas of necrosis or hemorrhage. Histologically, they are characterized by a uniform mass of benign-appearing hepatocytes without ducts or portal triads. These tumors appear to have a small risk of rupture and hemorrhage, and may contain foci of malignancy or undergo malignant transformation; therefore, surgical resection is recommended both for diagnosis and treatment. An association has been observed between the use of oral contraceptives or anabolic steroids and hepatic adenomas. An association has also been observed between these agents and a variety of other conditions in children, including glycogen storage disease types I and IV, Fanconi's anemia, Hurler's disease, galactosemia, and familial adenomatous polyposis.

Focal nodular hyperplasia is another benign hepatic lesion. It almost always occurs in young women, although it can occur in children of any age. A causative link with oral contraceptive use has not been proved. FNH usually occurs as a small, asymptomatic, nonencapsulated mass, although approximately 10% of affected patients have multiple lesions. Grossly, these lesions appear as a nodule of hyperplastic liver tissue, generally paler than the surrounding normal parenchyma. They have a characteristic stellate central scar that histologically contains biliary ductules, infiltrating lymphocytes, and blood vessels. In fact, it has been hypothesized that the proliferation of hepatocytes is secondary to a preexisting vascular malformation. Imaging with CT or MRI may demonstrate the central scar, but often a biopsy is required to confirm the diagnosis. Because this lesion is not considered to be premalignant and rupture is rare, surgical resection is not required.

Mesenchymal hamartomas are rare nonvascular hepatic tumors that are generally detected in infants. These lesions are felt to represent embryologic maldevelopment of the liver with subsequent degenerative changes. Lesions detected *in utero* and followed with serial ultrasonography have suggested that this lesion progresses from a solid phase to a cystic one. The lesions eventually consist of multiple cysts containing gelatinous fluid, separated by primitive mesenchyme together with hepatic parenchyma and biliary epithelium. Degeneration of this primitive stroma creates the cystic spaces. The lesions can expand due to increasing accumulation of fluid within the cysts. CT or MRI demonstrates a multicystic lesion with variable amounts of intervening solid tissue. Although spontaneous resolution of mesenchymal hamartomas has been observed, because of rare reports of undifferentiated sarcoma arising from these lesions, surgical resection is recommended.

Adenomas and hamartomas of the liver tend to be smaller than malignant tumors or benign vascular lesions of the liver and therefore limited wedge resection is usually possible. Although resection is curative for benign hepatic tumors, one should consider that their prognosis is extremely favorable, with morbidity being more likely caused by treatment than growth of the tumor. Other benign hepatic lesions have been reported rarely in children. These are of little clinical significance except to be distinguished from malignancy.

SUGGESTED READINGS

Boechat MI, Kangarloo H, Ortega J, et al. Primary liver tumors in children: comparison of CT and MR imaging. *Radiology* 1988; 169:727–732.

Daller JA, Bueno J, Gutierrez J, et al. Hepatic hemangioendothelioma: clinical experience and management strategy. *J Pediatr Surg* 1999;34:98–106.

Dehner LP, Parker ME, Franciosi RA, et al. Focal nodular hyperplasia and adenoma of the liver. A pediatric experience. *Am J Pediatr Med Oncol* 1979;1:85–93.

Dehner LP. Hepatic tumors in the pediatric age group: a distinctive clinicopathologic spectrum. *Perspect Pediatr Pathol* 1998;4:217–268.

Luks R, Yazbeck S, Brandt M, et al. Benign liver tumors in children: a 25-year experience. *J Pediatr Surg* 1991;26:1326–1330.

Meyers WC, Jones RS. Neoplasms of the liver: benign tumors. In: Meyers WC, Jones RS, eds. *Textbook of liver and biliary surgery.* Philadelphia: JB Lippincott, 1990:93–104.

Murray JD, Ricketts RR. Mesenchymal hamartoma of the liver. *Am Surg* 1998;64:1097–1103.

Reynolds M. Pediatric liver tumors. *Semin Surg Oncol* 1999;16: 159–172.

Stringer MD. Liver tumors. *Semin Pediatr Surg* 2000;9:196–208.

Weinberg AC, Finegold MJ. Primary hepatic tumors in childhood. In: Finegold MJ, ed. *Pathology of neoplasia in children and adolescents.* Philadelphia: WB Saunders, 1986:333–372.

Wu JT, Book L, Sudar K. Serum alpha fetoprotein (AFP) levels in normal infants. *Pediatr Res* 1981;15:50–52.

102

HEPATIC RESECTION

NICHOLAS A. SHORTER
MICHAEL P. LA QUAGLIA

The principles of liver resection are based on the segmental anatomy of the liver, as described by Couinaud and others. Safe, successful liver resection depends on a thorough knowledge of this anatomy and of the common biliary and vascular anatomic variants that may be encountered (Fig. 102.1). The liver is divided into eight segments (I–VIII), each supplied by a portal triad containing a branch of the portal vein, a branch of the hepatic artery, and a tributary of either the right or left hepatic duct, and each having separate drainage into the hepatic veins (with the exception of segment I, the caudate lobe, which drains directly into the inferior vena cava) (Figs. 102.2 and 102.3). This vascular and biliary arrangement allows each segment to be removed individually, if necessary, but more commonly, specific groups of segments are removed together. The standard liver resections are listed in Table 102.1. In addition, we have successfully used a central resection (segments IV, V, and VIII) in several cases, which allows resection of centrally located tumors while preserving more normal parenchyma than would be possible with a standard resection. For detailed descriptions of the general and segmental anatomy of the liver and for the specific anatomic and technical details of each of the major resections, readers are referred to the suggested readings. This discussion will deal with generalities applicable to the topic of hepatic resection as a whole.

INDICATIONS

Hepatic resection may be indicated for either benign or malignant disease. The regenerative capacity of the liver is considerable, and up to 85% of a normal liver can be removed without fear of hepatic insufficiency. On the other hand, preexisting disease, such as cirrhosis, may limit what can be removed and has a profound effect on rates of morbidity and mortality. Severe liver disease makes a patient inoperable, even when the lesion is anatomically resectable. Fortunately, in the West, most childhood tumors, both benign and malignant, do not occur in the setting of preexisting liver disease. On the other hand, many patients with malignant tumors, particularly hepatoblastoma, now come to resection following multiple courses of chemotherapy, the effects of which may significantly complicate the intraoperative and postoperative course. What data exist indicate as much as a three- to fourfold increase in complications (but no difference in mortality) in patients who are resected following chemotherapy compared with those undergoing primary resection. Although these figures were not based on a prospective randomized trial and, therefore, the difference is likely to have been inflated somewhat by patient selection, the general point appears to be a valid one. Preoperative chemotherapy does not appear to have a significant effect on postoperative hepatic regeneration.

The need for resection is clear with primary malignant tumors of the liver because cure is not yet possible without surgical resection. The decision may be more difficult in the case of benign lesions, because many of these can safely be observed. Factors that enter into the decision in either instance were nicely summarized by Dr. James Foster in 1989: "Whether a patient should have an operation on the liver depends on the nature of the lesion and its symptoms, on the geography of the lesion in relation to the inflow and outflow vessels, on the condition of the rest of the liver, and on the general condition of the patient."

With recent improvements in diagnostic imaging of the liver, resectability can usually be determined from a combination of ultrasonography, computed tomography, and magnetic resonance imaging. These can accurately demonstrate the relationships between the tumor mass and the main vascular and biliary structures. Arteriography, once an important part of the evaluation of liver tumors, is now

N. A. Shorter and M. P. La Quaglia: Department of Surgery, Weill-Cornell University Medical School; and Department of Pediatric Surgery, Memorial Sloan-Kettering Cancer Center, New York, New York.

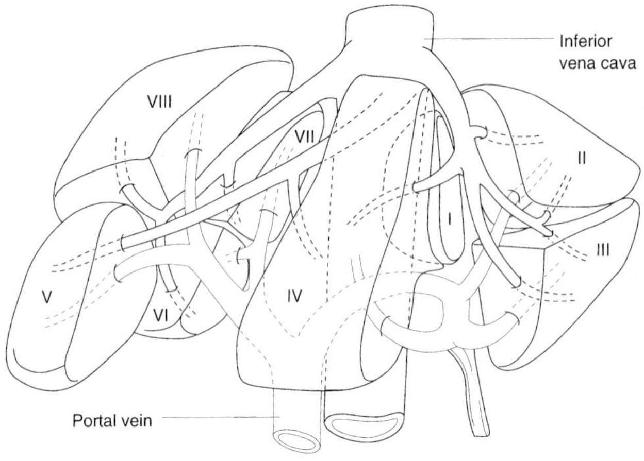

FIGURE 102.1. Functional division of the liver and liver segments according to Couinaud's nomenclature. (Reprinted from Byrd DR. Hepatobiliary anatomy. In: Greenfield LJ, Mulholland MW, Oldham KT, et al., eds. *Surgery: scientific principles and practice, 3rd ed.* Philadelphia: Lippincott Williams & Wilkins, 2001:917; with permission.)

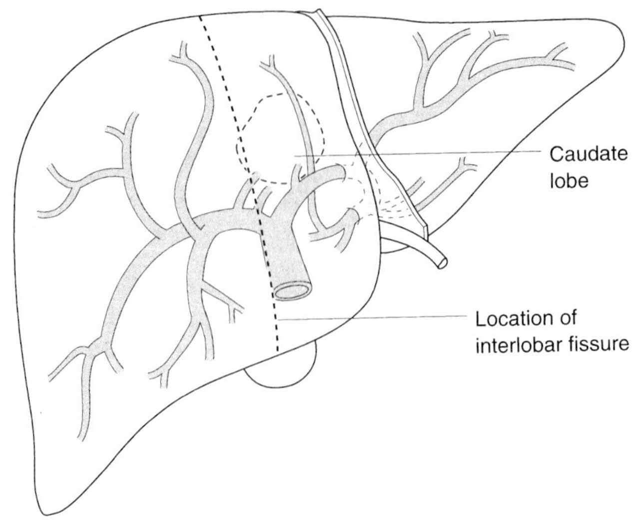

FIGURE 102.3. Intrahepatic divisions of the portal vein. (Reprinted from Byrd DR. Hepatobiliary anatomy. In: Greenfield LJ, Mulholland MW, Oldham KT, et al., eds. *Surgery: scientific principles and practice, 3rd ed.* Philadelphia: Lippincott Williams & Wilkins, 2001:918; with permission.)

rarely necessary. If, at the time of resection, there are still questions about resectability, intraoperative ultrasonography is often helpful. It also may be useful in determining the proper plane of parenchymal transection in those cases where the tumor mass is known to be close to the margin of resection.

Although generally successful resection of liver tumors requires a margin of normal liver, narrower margins are acceptable for hepatoblastoma, and, in fact, a positive microscopic margin may still be compatible with survival, which is not the case with hepatocellular carcinoma. Similarly, although metastatic disease, both to distant sites and to regional nodes, would argue strongly against hepatic resection in cases of hepatocellular carcinoma, these are not necessarily contraindications in children with hepatoblastoma. When resectability is questionable, it is best to err on the side of caution when dealing with hepatoblastoma, which is likely to shrink in response to preoperative chemotherapy, and to take the opposite approach with hepatocellular carcinoma, which is unlikely to do so.

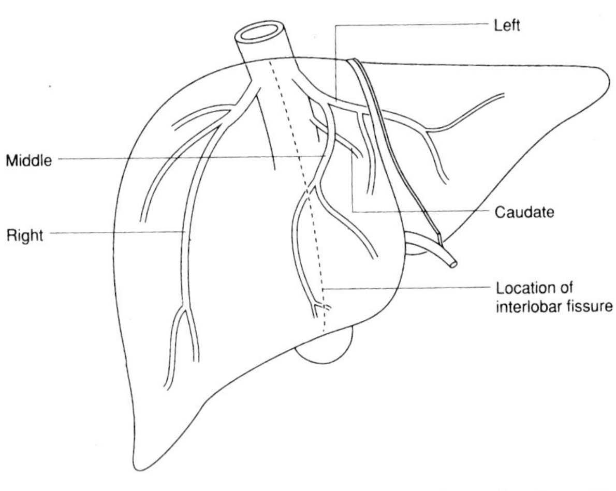

FIGURE 102.2. Three major hepatic veins drain the liver. The caudate segment of the liver usually drains directly into the inferior vena cava. (Reprinted from Byrd DR. Hepatobiliary anatomy. In: Greenfield LJ, Mulholland MW, Oldham KT, et al., eds. *Surgery: scientific principles and practice, 3rd ed.* Philadelphia: Lippincott Williams & Wilkins, 2001:918; with permission.)

SURGICAL TECHNIQUES

The key to successful liver resection is adequate exposure. We usually use a bilateral subcostal incision, to which, if necessary, can be added a vertical midline extension (which can be extended to a median sternotomy, if intrapericardial control of the inferior vena cava is needed) or an extension into the right chest, dividing the costal margin and the diaphragm (Fig. 102.4). In a few cases a

TABLE 102.1. STANDARD LIVER RESECTIONS

Procedure	Segments Removed
Right hepatic lobectomy	V, VI, VII, VIII
Left hepatic lobectomy	II, III, IV
Extended right hepatic lobectomy (right trisegmentectomy)	IV, V, VI, VII, VIII, sometimes I
Left lateral segmentectomy	II, III
Extended left hepatic lobectomy (left trisegmentectomy)	II, III, IV, V, VIII sometimes I

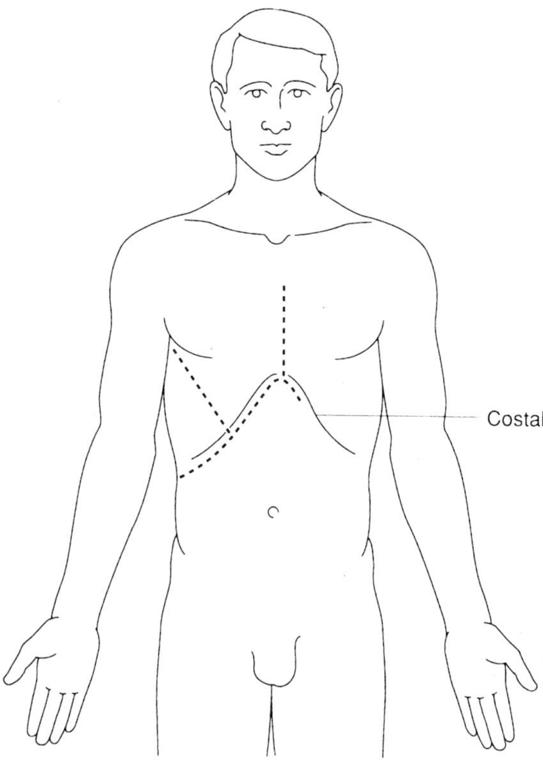

FIGURE 102.4. Incisions commonly used for hepatic resection. (Reprinted from Byrd DR. Hepatobiliary anatomy. In: Greenfield LJ, Mulholland MW, Oldham KT, et al., eds. *Surgery: scientific principles and practice, 3rd ed.* Philadelphia: Lippincott Williams & Wilkins, 2001:924; with permission.)

standard thoracoabdominal incision may be appropriate. The following steps are then applicable to all major liver resections:

1. Mobilization of the portion of the liver to be removed, by dividing the ligamentous attachments
2. Control of the vascular inflow and outflow and the biliary drainage of the segments to be removed, with preservation of the same for the segments being preserved
3. Division of the liver parenchyma, with control of the vessels and bile ducts along the plane of resection
4. Efforts to ensure hemostasis and prevent bile leaks along the transected surface

Some surgeons advocate total vascular exclusion for all hepatic resections, but in our experience this is rarely necessary. It has generally been our practice to ligate the appropriate vessels and ducts at the hilum. The resulting color demarcation within the liver then makes the proper plane of transection easy to identify. We also prefer, when possible, to ligate the hepatic veins outside the liver substance, and to do this prior to parenchymal transection, because doing so decreases bleeding and lessens the risk of accidentally tearing the vein during manipulation. In some cases, however, it is safer or technically necessary to find the applicable veins within the liver parenchyma, and some surgeons favor this approach in all cases. Damage to the hepatic veins is the most common cause of massive blood loss during liver resection. In some instances, safety requires gaining control of the inferior vena cava above and below the liver. When working on the hepatic veins, the patient should be placed in a 15 degree, head-down position, to reduce potential blood loss and to minimize the risk of air embolus. It is also important to keep the child's central venous pressure below 5 mm Hg. Several separate, smaller veins drain into the inferior vena cava from the posterior surface of the liver, and some of these must also be ligated and divided during the course of most resections.

Once inflow and outflow are controlled, parenchymal transection is performed. A Pringle maneuver can be used at this point, although it is not absolutely necessary if the specific inflow vessels have been ligated at the hilum. When it is used, the normothermic liver will tolerate inflow occlusion for up to an hour, if necessary, but it is safer to maintain it for intervals of 5 to 10 minutes, releasing it for short periods in between. Numerous techniques have been advocated for division of the parenchyma. The simplest and our preferred method is, after scoring the liver capsule, to crush the liver tissue with a Kelly clamp along the plane of resection. The exposed bridging vessels and ducts are then clipped or suture ligated. An endoscopic stapler can also be used in some situations. The transection should be performed as quickly as possible, while maintaining safety. Blood loss can be significant during this step, and if it is not adequately replaced, hypovolemia can easily develop, particularly in an infant or small child. Following removal of the specimen, final hemostasis is secured using a combination of sutures and the argon beam coagulator. The best available data indicate that drainage is not necessary unless a biliary reconstruction has been performed.

The current mortality rate for liver resection in children and adolescents is 1% to 3%. Morbidity ranges from 8% to 25% or more, depending on patient selection. The most important potential intraoperative complications are hemorrhage, air embolism, tumor embolism, and injury to vascular or biliary structures within the hilum of the liver. By far the most common is hemorrhage. Postoperatively, potential complications include hemorrhage, bile leak, abscess formation, pulmonary complications and wound complications. Not surprisingly, the most significant predictor of problems postoperatively is intraoperative hemorrhage and attendant massive transfusion, with or without hypotension, which leads to coagulopathy and hypothermia and puts the patient at risk for respiratory distress syndrome, liver failure, and renal failure. If significant intraoperative hemorrhage does occur, it should initially and immediately be controlled temporarily, with pressure for venous bleeding and a Pringle maneuver combined with pressure for arterial hemorrhage. This then allows time for full resuscitation of the patient, for acquiring additional exposure and additional help if necessary, and for planning the next steps.

POSTOPERATIVE CARE

Admission to the intensive care unit is mandatory postoperatively. In the immediate postoperative period, patients are at risk for hypoglycemia. Fever is not uncommon, due to small areas of devitalized liver tissue. Hypoalbuminemia commonly develops and may take several weeks to resolve. Administration of albumin often makes overall fluid management easier. Close attention must be directed to maintaining a normal coagulation profile over the first few days, and support with vitamin K and clotting factors is often necessary. Transient hyperbilirubinemia often occurs. Bowel function returns quickly in uncomplicated cases. Bile leaks are usually from the transected surface and almost always close spontaneously after catheter drainage. Liver regeneration occurs rapidly and is usually complete within 90 days. With large tumors, which have replaced all or most of one lobe, hypertrophy of the other lobe has often already occurred preoperatively.

SUGGESTED READINGS

Blumgart LH. liver resection for benign disease and for liver and biliary tumors. In: Blumgart LH, Fong Y, eds. *Surgery of the liver and biliary tract, 3rd ed.* Philadelphia: WB Saunders, 2000:1639–1695.

Foster JH. Liver resection techniques. *Surg Oncol Clin North Am* 1989;69:235–249.

Goldsmith NA, Woodburne RT. The surgical anatomy pertaining to liver resection. *Surg Gynecol Obstet* 1957;105:310–318.

Gray SW, Skandalakis JE, Colborn GL, et al. Surgical anatomy of the liver and associated extrahepatic structures, parts 1–5. *Contemp Surg* 1987;30:37–47, 26–38, 15–23; 31:25–36, 27–39.

103

PORTAL HYPERTENSION

FREDERICK C. RYCKMAN
MARIA H. ALONSO

The survival of children with portal hypertension has improved over the past decade. This has been the result of (a) progress in the pharmacologic control of acute portal hypertensive hemorrhage; (b) improved efficacy and safety of endoscopic methods to treat acute esophageal variceal hemorrhage, which also reduce the risk of rebleeding; (c) recognition of the role for advanced surgical therapy (portocaval shunts); and (d) improved success with pediatric liver transplantation as a definitive treatment for children with end-stage liver disease. This review will examine the role each of these treatment modalities plays in the management of portal hypertension in children.

DEFINITION AND ETIOLOGY

Portal hypertension is defined as an elevation of the portal pressure above 10 to 12 mm Hg. In healthy children, portal pressure rarely exceeds 7 mm Hg. Increased pressure within the portal circulation leads to the formation of collateral circulatory pathways connecting the high-pressure portal vasculature to the low-pressure systemic venous system. The most common and potentially dangerous communications occur within the esophageal wall, connecting the coronary and short gastric veins to the esophageal venous plexus. Less threatening collateral communications can develop between the recanalized umbilical vein and abdominal wall veins (caput medusa), the inferior rectal veins as hemorrhoids, and in the retroperitoneum. In addition, any surgical union between the portal and systemic venous circulation, such as occurs with intestinal stomas, is a possible, and often problematic, site of variceal development. Favorable collateral vessels developing within the tissues surrounding the pancreas, duodenum, and left kidney form "spontaneous" splenorenal shunts.

F. C. Ryckman and M. H. Alonso: Department of Surgery, Division of Pediatric Surgery, University of Cincinnati, and Cincinnati Children's Hospital Medical Center, Cincinnati, Ohio.

The progressive development of collateral vessels connecting the portal and systemic circulation has the beneficial effect of decreasing portal pressure. However, this effect is diminished by the concurrent development of a hyperdynamic circulatory state. Portal hypertension has been associated with the presence of autonomic nervous system dysfunction, as well as an excess of circulating cytokines, leading to tachycardia, decreased systemic and splanchnic vascular resistance secondary to vasodilatation, plasma volume expansion, increased cardiac output, and subsequently increased portal inflow.

The combination of increased portal inflow, venous outflow obstruction, and the remarkable collateral circulation that develops account for many of the complications associated with portal hypertension. Superficial submucosal collateral vessels, especially those in the esophagus and stomach, and to a lesser extent those in the duodenum, colon, or rectum, are prone to rupture and bleeding. In addition, submucosal arteriovenous communications between the muscularis mucosa and dilated precapillaries and veins within the stomach result in vascular ectasia or congestive hypertensive gastropathy, significantly contributing to the risk for hemorrhage from the stomach.

Each of the causes of elevated portal pressure shares the common mechanism of increased resistance to blood flow from the visceral/splanchnic portal circulation to the right atrium. In children, the location of this increased resistance can be (a) *prehepatic (or presinusoidal)*, usually within the portal vein and its primary feeding branches; (b) *intrahepatic*, which may be secondary to presinusoidal obstructions (congenital hepatic fibrosis, congenital or acquired arterioportal fistula, or schistosomiasis), postsinusoidal cirrhosis, or venoocclusive disease; or (c) *posthepatic*, secondary to hepatic vein obstruction. The primary factor influencing the prognosis and treatment algorithm is the intrinsic functional status of the liver. Presinusoidal obstruction does not result in impairment of hepatic synthetic function; therefore, coagulopathy is absent. Treatment should be directed toward the prevention of hemorrhage through palliative interventional procedures while

TABLE 103.1. DISEASES ASSOCIATED WITH PORTAL HYPERTENSION IN CHILDREN

Presinusoidal
Venous obstructions
Portal vein thrombosis/cavernous transformation
Splenic vein thrombosis
Portal vein malformation (congenital)
Congenital hepatic fibrosis
Arteriovenous fistula
Schistosomiasis
Hepatoportal sclerosis
Sinusoidal
Hepatocellular disease
Autoimmune hepatitis
Hepatitis B, C
Wilson disease
α_1-Antitrypsin deficiency
Glycogen storage disease type IV
Toxins and drugs
Histiocytosis X
Gaucher's disease
Peliosis
Biliary tract disease
Biliary atresia
Cystic fibrosis
Choledochal cyst
Intrahepatic cholestasis syndromes
Sclerosing cholangitis
Sinusoidal venoocclusive disease
Postsinusoidal
Budd-Chiari syndrome
Inferior vena cava obstructions
Chronic congestive heart failure
Venoocclusive disease (s/p bone marrow transplantation)
Prothrombotic disease

spontaneous collateral venous channels develop. In contrast, postsinusoidal obstruction is characterized by hepatic synthetic compromise, coagulopathy, and progressive hepatic failure. Although intervention to prevent or treat potentially fatal complications may be necessary, definitive correction with liver transplantation is often required. Table 103.1 reviews the diseases associated with portal hypertension in children.

PRESINUSOIDAL OBSTRUCTION

The most common type of presinusoidal obstruction is extrahepatic portal vein obstruction (EPVO) at any level of the portal vein. Umbilical vein infection in infancy or similar infections in older children, such as perforated appendicitis, primary peritonitis, and inflammatory bowel disease, have been identified as predisposing factors, as have primary biliary tract infections and cholangitis. Inherited abnormalities predisposing to hypercoagulability, such as factor V Leiden mutation, protein C, protein S, and antithrombin III deficiencies, as well as hyperviscosity/polycythemia in infancy or umbilical venous catheterization, can all lead to secondary thrombosis, especially when accompanied by neonatal dehydration or systemic infection and phlebitis. Embryologic malformations such as tortuous, poorly developed portal veins, webs, or diaphragms also can be a primary cause for EPVO or predispose to an increased risk of thrombosis. Presinusoidal obstruction also can result from congenital hepatic fibrosis, schistosomiasis, and hepatoportal sclerosis. Presinusoidal portal hypertension can occur in the absence of portal vein obstruction in rare cases where increased portal blood flow is attributed to congenital or acquired arteriovenous fistula within the portal system. Despite thorough evaluation, over half of reported EPVO cases have no identifiable cause.

POSTSINUSOIDAL OBSTRUCTION

Postsinusoidal obstruction to the portal venous system is caused by intrinsic liver disease, secondary to cirrhosis, or obstruction to the hepatic vein outflow from the liver. Cirrhosis resulting from primary liver diseases is the most common cause of postsinusoidal portal hypertension, with venous obstruction arising secondary to intrahepatic scarring. The numerous causes of cirrhosis include recognized disorders such as extrahepatic biliary atresia, metabolic liver diseases such as α_1-antitrypsin deficiency, Wilson's disease, glycogen storage disease type IV, hereditary fructose intolerance, and cystic fibrosis. When hepatic synthetic failure is not present or only slowly progressive, direct treatment of portal hypertension or its complications is indicated. Because many of these conditions are associated with progressive liver failure, the primary treatment in most cases is liver transplantation.

Hepatic vein obstruction (Budd-Chiari syndrome) can occur secondary to obstruction to the hepatic veins at any point from the sinusoids to the entry of the hepatic veins into the right atrium/inferior vena cava (IVC). Although a specific etiology is often not found, thrombosis can complicate neoplasms, collagen vascular disease, infection, trauma, or hypercoagulability states. Venoocclusive disease also has emerged as one of the most frequent causes of hepatic vein obstruction in children. Most cases occur after total body irradiation with or without cytotoxic drug therapy associated with bone marrow transplantation. This condition also has occurred after the ingestion of herbal remedies containing the pyrrolizidine alkaloids, which are sometimes taken as medicinal teas.

DIAGNOSIS AND EVALUATION

Clinical history and examination should concentrate on identifying factors that predispose to the development of cirrhosis, including a family history of inherited metabolic disease and possible exposure to viral or toxic pathogens. Clinical examination findings suggesting underlying liver disease (ascites, liver size/contour, nutritional status), hypersplenism (splenomegaly, bruising), or hepatopulmonary syndrome (spider angiomas, clubbing, cyanosis) contribute to diagnostic evaluation and therapeutic planning. Hypercoagulability and its complications should be evaluated in both the patient and family members due to the inherited basis for these protein abnormalities.

Imaging tests are essential to confirm the presence of portal hypertension, define the portal venous anatomy, and formulate options for therapy. Initial screening with ultrasonography can suggest the presence of chronic liver disease and should determine portal venous patency. Doppler examination can depict both the direction of portal flow and the degree of hepatopetal flow, which correlates with the risk of variceal hemorrhage. The branches of the portal venous system are examined to exclude splenic vein thrombosis or widespread portal system thrombosis. Magnetic resonance angiography or contrast-enhanced computed topography has replaced mesenteric angiography when further definition of portal anatomy is necessary, such as when liver transplantation or portosystemic shunt procedures are planned.

Upper gastrointestinal endoscopy is the most accurate and reliable method for detecting esophageal varices and for detecting the source of acute gastrointestinal hemorrhage. This is especially valuable in the presence of acute hemorrhage, where up to one third of patients with known varices may have bleeding from sources other than esophageal varices, such as portal hypertensive gastropathy or gastric/duodenal ulcerations. In addition, endoscopy can identify features associated with an increased risk for hemorrhage, such as large varices, "red spots" apparent over varices representing fragile telangiectasis within the shallow submucosa, and portal hypertensive gastropathy. Endoscopy is also used to initiate treatment when acute bleeding varices are identified.

Liver biopsy may be helpful in determining the etiology of intrinsic liver disease and in defining further therapy or need for transplantation.

TREATMENT OF PORTAL HYPERTENSIVE COMPLICATIONS

The decision to undertake pharmacologic, endoscopic, or surgical treatment for portal hypertension must be based on the natural history of the disease and the possibility of life-threatening complications. The prognosis is related to the primary etiology of the portal hypertension. It has been generally accepted in patients with portal hypertension due to EPVO that the risk of acute variceal bleeding decreases with age, concurrent with the development of spontaneous portosystemic collateral vessels. This postulated natural history has been the primary argument supporting conservative management of hemorrhage in these patients, using endoscopic therapy to obliterate esophageal varices while awaiting the development of favorable retroperitoneal and peripancreatic collateral vessels. Children who have experienced bleeding complications prior to age 12 and those with grade II or III varices remain at a higher risk for further hemorrhage at a later age.

In patients with intrinsic liver disease, therapeutic choices are influenced by the probability of progression of their disease and their potential need for liver transplantation in the future. A significant number of these patients require temporizing endoscopy or surgical portosystemic shunt therapy to treat complications or maintain stability prior to undergoing liver replacement.

The most common portal hypertensive complication is gastrointestinal bleeding. Regardless of the site and mechanism, initial therapy is directed toward fluid resuscitation and, when necessary, blood replacement. A nasogastric tube should be placed to confirm the upper gastrointestinal tract as the source of bleeding, and for evacuation of blood from the stomach. A histamine receptor blocker or proton pump inhibitor should be administered to decrease the risk of further bleeding from gastric erosions. In patients with hepatic synthetic dysfunction and coagulopathy, administration of vitamin K, fresh frozen plasma or cryoprecipitate, and platelets when thrombocytopenia is present also may be necessary. Adequate volume resuscitation is essential; however, volume overload from excessive transfusion or crystaloid administration is counterproductive, because this leads to a further increase in portal pressure and continued hemorrhage.

PHARMACOLOGIC TREATMENT

Pharmacologic intervention to decrease portal pressure may be considered in patients with continued bleeding. A variety of options are now available when intervention is required.

Vasopressin

Vasopressin increases splanchnic vascular tone, decreasing splanchnic arterial inflow, thus decreasing portal venous pressure. It is administered as an initial bolus of 0.3 units/kg over 20 minutes followed by a continuous infusion of 0.002 to 0.005 units/kg/min. Intraarterial infusion into the superior mesenteric artery has no advantage over intravenous routes. Although vasopressin infusion has been associated with control of variceal hemorrhage in 53% to 85% of cases in children, its use has been limited by systemic effects such as vasoconstriction to the heart, bowel, and kidneys, impaired cardiac function, and fluid retention. Nitroglycerin has been used to augment the decrease in portal pressure and ameliorate the untoward systemic effects, but is inappropriate when systemic blood pressure is low or unstable.

Octreotide

Somatostatin, a 14–amino acid peptide, also reduces splanchnic blood flow by selective mesenteric vascular smooth muscle constriction. Its short half-life complicates treatment, which led to the development of octreotide, an 8–amino acid synthetic somatostatin analogue. Octreotide can be administered subcutaneously, but is best used as a continuous intravenous drip (25–50 $\mu g/m^2/h$, or 1.0 $\mu g/kg/h$). In adult studies, both somatostatin and octreotide have achieved excellent results in controlling acute variceal hemorrhage. Its use and efficacy in children can only be inferred.

Beta Blockers

Beta blockers have no role in the treatment of acute variceal hemorrhage. They have been used in an effort to prevent variceal hemorrhage in high-risk patients, decreasing portal pressure by decreasing the heart rate by 25%, thereby decreasing cardiac output, portal inflow, and perhaps blocking β receptor–mediated vasodilatation, allowing unopposed α stimulation within the mesenteric arterioles.

Efficacy has been evaluated in two groups: (a) patients with documented varices who underwent β-blocker treatment in an attempt to prevent the first episode of bleeding (primary prophylaxis); and (b) patients treated following the initial hemorrhage in an attempt to prevent recurrent bleeding (secondary prevention). The efficacy of therapy differs with the indication.

In adult patients treated for primary prophylaxis, β blockers were associated with significantly lower rates of bleeding and death from bleeding. Combined treatment using nadolol and isosorbide mononitrate further decreased the risk for first variceal hemorrhage by more that half in comparison with nadolol alone.

The results of β blockade for secondary prevention of recurrent variceal hemorrhage are more controversial. In 11 randomized controlled trials including 755 adult patients, rebleeding was reduced in all trials and the death rate was reduced. In low-risk patients (Childs class A), the risk of rebleeding has been reported to be as low as 3%. This advantage seems to be lost in class B and C patients, where the reported risk for recurrent bleeding is 46% to 72%.

Fewer studies have been performed in children. Because of the presence of extrahepatic portal hypertension in up to half of all children who are candidates for treatment, pediatric results may not correlate directly with adult patients, nearly all of whom have intrinsic liver disease. However, several investigators have confirmed the safety of propranolol administration to pediatric patients. Similar to the adult experience, dosage must be adjusted to achieve a reduction of 25% in resting heart rate to achieve a therapeutic result. Beta blocker treatment is recommended for primary prophylaxis in all patient groups, but may have limited benefit for secondary prevention in high-risk patients.

MECHANICAL TAMPONADE

Mechanical tamponade using balloon catheter tubes (Sengstaken-Blakemore or Minnesota tubes) provides mechanical compression of esophageal and gastric fundal varices. Although balloon tamponade is usually successful in stopping refractory hemorrhage, the effect is often transient, and recurrence following removal is common. This high rate of complications and the success of octreotide infusions for acute hemorrhage have limited their use to emergency control until other measures or surgical intervention can be instituted.

ENDOSCOPIC INTERVENTION FOR ESOPHAGEAL VARICES

In most cases, variceal hemorrhage can be controlled with fluid resuscitation, correction of coagulation, and pharmacologic support. However, the risk of recurrent hemorrhage and the need for accurate diagnosis of the site of hemorrhage often mandate endoscopy during the early posthemorrhage period. When variceal hemorrhage is confirmed or strongly suspected, variceal sclerotherapy or variceal band ligation can be used to eradicate the present or future sites of bleeding.

Endoscopic sclerotherapy (EST) has been widely used as the primary treatment for refractory variceal bleeding due to its high success rate (>90%) and the ability to institute initial treatment at the time of diagnostic endoscopy. The procedure is successful using both intravariceal and perivariceal injection techniques. In children, 5% ethanolamine, 1% to 1.5% tetradecyl sulfate, or 5% sodium morrhuate have all been successfully used. Most patients require three to six sessions at intervals of 2 to 4 weeks to eradicate esophageal varicies. Minor early complications, which occur in almost all patients, include retrosternal pain, fever, and transient dysphagia. Esophageal ulceration at the site of injection, a direct consequence of the procedure, is seen in 70% to 80% of patients and can be the source of recurrent bleeding. Serious complications such as esophageal strictures, esophageal perforation, or mediastinitis occur in 10% to 20% of patients.

In an attempt to overcome these complications but preserve the treatment success of EST, esophageal band ligation (EBL) of varices has been developed, using techniques similar to those for banding internal hemorrhoids. Band ligation has the advantage of ligating only the submucosal venous varices, without harming the submucosal lining. Initial variceal obliteration was achieved by EBL in 73% to 100% of children with rebleeding prior to completion of obliteration less common than with EST; however, recurrence of varices was seen in 75% of patients with intrahepatic disease. In addition, the small size of the child's esophagus limits the number of bands that can be placed at one treatment session. The thinner esophageal wall of small (<1-year-old) children makes full-thickness ligation a risk, precluding EBL below this age.

Both EST and EBL have been used for the primary prophylaxis of variceal hemorrhage. Prophylactic EST decreased the incidence of bleeding in children from 42% to 6%, but 16% developed congestive hypertensive gastropathy and 38% bled from this lesion. This was in contrast to the control group, in which only 6% had congestive hypertensive gastropathy, with no gastropathy-associated bleeding episodes. Prophylactic EST did not alter patient survival compared with the control group. We feel that EST or EBL is an acceptable and occasionally life-saving measure when esophageal variceal hemorrhage is refractory to octreotide infusion therapy. The risk of accelerated formation of gastric varices may overshadow any prophylactic benefit for either EST or EBL and thus we do not use these treatment modalities for primary prophylaxis.

PORTOSYSTEMIC SHUNTS

Numerous surgical procedures have been devised to divert portal blood into the low-pressure systemic venous circulation, thereby decreasing the portal venous pressure. Enthusiasm for the use of portosystemic shunting in children was limited by early reports suggesting that children under 8 years of age, and those with vessels for the shunt anastomosis of less than 8 to 10 mm, would be unsuitable candidates due to the high risk for shunt thrombosis. In addition, Voorhees et al. suggested a high incidence of neuropsychiatric disturbances following nonselective shunts in children. Recent experience in centers skilled in pediatric vascular reconstruction has established that a high rate of success can be achieved with minimal complications, even in small pediatric patients. To achieve these goals, we have found that the following principles should be followed: (a) anastomosis should be constructed using fine (6.0–7.0) monofilament sutures with a provision for growth; (b) sufficient mobilization and modification of the vessels is necessary to prevent kinking or twisting of the shunt after the viscera are returned to their normal location; (c) postreconstructive venography should be performed in order to ensure division of all collateral vessels, anastomotic quality, and adequate shunt flow; (d) selective postoperative intravenous anticoagulation should be undertaken in high-risk patients; (e) antiplatelet drugs administered to all patients for a minimum of three postoperative months; and (f) the surgical team should be skilled at pediatric vascular reconstruction.

In general, portosystemic shunts can be classified into two groups: nonselective and selective. *Nonselective shunts* are constructed to communicate with the entire portal venous system, and therefore have the potential to divert blood from the normal antegrade perfusion to the liver. Historically, the mesocaval shunt (Clatworthy shunt) was used. The distal IVC is ligated and divided, and its proximal portion is then anastomosed to the side of the superior mesenteric vein (SMV). We now construct an H-graft shunt when a nonselective procedure is indicated, using a short segment of internal jugular vein to connect the SMV and the IVC (Fig. 103.1). The limited intraabdominal dissection needed to complete the H-graft shunt contributes to its technical ease, and if liver transplantation is needed, the shunt can be easily occluded at that time. Other nonselective shunts have significant disadvantages in children due to the need for splenectomy (proximal splenorenal) or dissection of the main portal vein, which compromises liver transplantation (end-to-side, side-to-side portocaval shunts).

Selective shunts are constructed to divert the gastrosplenic portion of the portal venous flow into a systemic vein, most frequently the left renal vein or the immediately adjacent

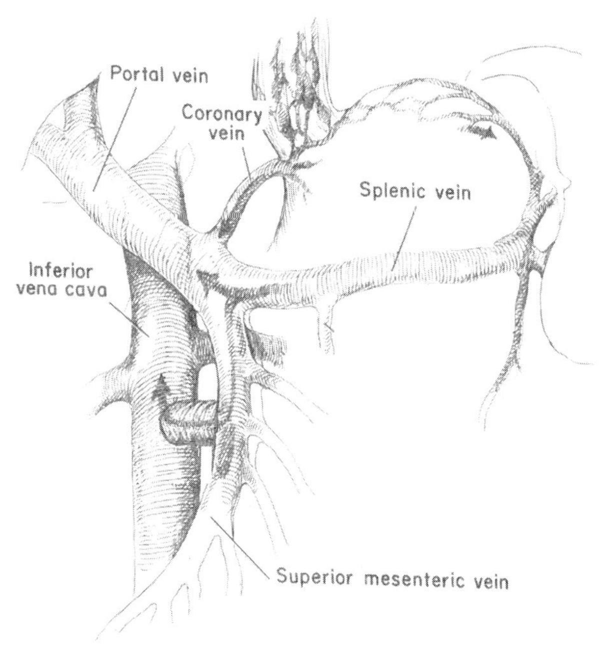

FIGURE 103.1. Interposition H-graft mesocaval shunt, a nonselective shunt using either internal jugular vein harvested from the patient, or polytetrafluoroethylene vascular graft material. This shunt allows the superior mesenteric vein to communicate with the infrarenal inferior vena cava. (Modified from Zollinger RM, Zollinger RM. *Atlas of surgical operations, 4th ed.* New York: Macmillan, 1975; with permission.)

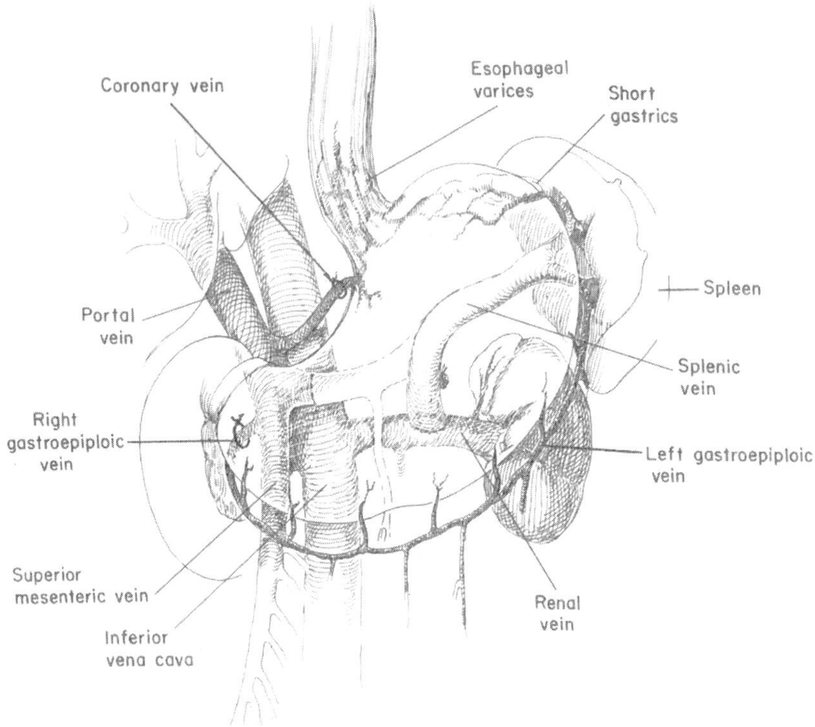

FIGURE 103.2. Distal splenorenal shunt, a selective shunt allowing communication between the splenic vein and the left renal vein. The esophagogastric venous complex communicates via the short gastric veins, decompressing esophageal varicies without decreasing perfusion through the mesenteric portal system to the liver. (Reprinted from Zollinger RM, Zollinger RM. *Atlas of surgical operations, 4th ed.* New York: Macmillan, 1975; with permission.)

IVC. Communication between the central mesenteric portal circulation, which perfuses the liver, and the gastrosplenic portal circulation is severed by dividing the gastroepiploic veins, the coronary vein termination at the portal vein, and the retroperitoneal pancreatic collateral vessels. The most common selective shunt, the distal splenorenal shunt (DSRS) or Warren shunt, preserves antegrade perfusion to the liver within the mesenteric portion of the portal circulation, while decompressing the esophageal venous plexus through the short gastric veins and splenic vein (Fig. 103.2). This theoretical selective advantage can unfortunately be lost over time as the high-pressure mesenteric component progressively decompresses into the lower pressure gastrosplenic compartment. Complete isolation of the pancreas from the splenic vein decreases the frequency and rapidity of this change. Despite this potential for progressive loss of selectivity, we use this shunt as our primary shunt option in children. When the adrenal vein is appropriately located and dilated, it serves as an alternative anastomotic site to access the left renal vein.

When performed in centers experienced in complex vascular reconstruction of the portal system, shunt patency has ranged from 83% to 100%. When shunt patency is maintained, recurrence of variceal bleeding is uncommon, although decompressed varices may still be identifiable on endoscopy. Encephalopathy is uncommon in children following successful portosystemic shunting, even in patients with intrinsic liver disease. In these children, this can be controlled with lactulose and dietary intervention.

Methods to directly reconstruct the portal circulation in patients with EPVO into the left branch of the portal vein have been described and represent ideal solutions. This mesentericoportal shunt (REX shunt) reestablishes normal portal inflow into the intrahepatic portal vein, using either an interposition jugular venous graft or the dilated coronary vein (Fig. 103.3). The procedure is unique in that it restores hepatopetal portal perfusion and the inflow of hepatatrophic substances to the liver. Candidates for this procedure must fulfill three conditions: (a) the liver parenchyma must be normal, (b) they must not have a hypercoagulable state, and (c) the umbilical portion of the left hepatic vein must be accessible and patent. Doppler ultrasonography and direct portography suggest that approximately two thirds of children with EPVO have sufficient left portal vein patency to undergo this procedure. In the reported experience (16 cases), all shunts have maintained initial patency, although three required revision secondary to stenosis and one shunt occluded at 7 months. Hypertensive gastropathy resolved, and variceal bleeding did not recur. In these selected patients, this option should be considered despite the more complex technical challenge it presents.

We now consider the following children to be candidates for portosystemic shunting: (a) children with documented variceal hemorrhage who have progressive or continued

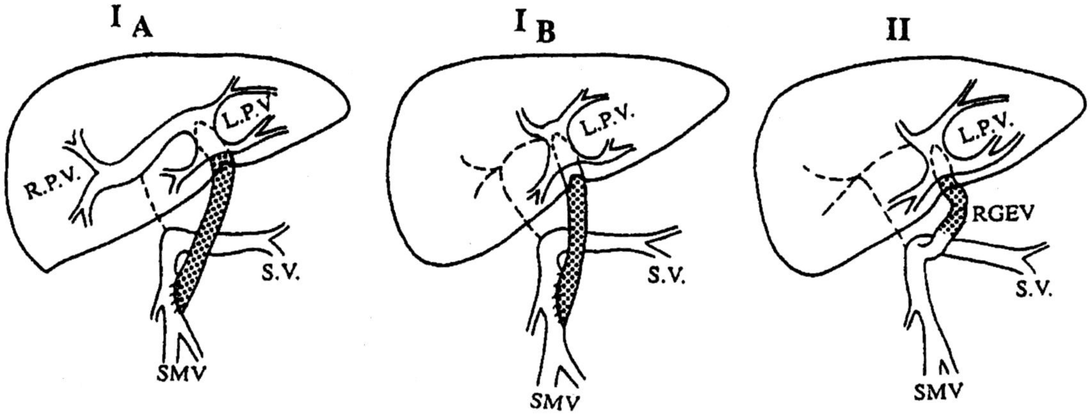

FIGURE 103.3. Mesentericoportal shunt to restore portal blood flow to the left branch of the intrahepatic portal vein. This shunt returns portal blood flow directly to the hepatic portal circulation, and is useful only in patients with extrahepatic portal vein obstruction and a patent intrahepatic portal venous system. An interposition jugular venous graft (*stippled*) is often required. (Reprinted from de Ville deGrote J, Alberti D, Clapuyt P, et al. Direct bypassing of extrahepatic portal venous obstruction in children: a new technique for combined hepatic portal revascularization and treatment of extrahepatic portal hypertension. *J Pediatr Surg* 1998;33:597–601; with permission.)

esophageal variceal bleeding despite endoscopic intervention and who have preserved hepatic synthetic function; (b) children who fail endoscopic treatment and have intrinsic liver disease, but have adequate liver synthetic function to predict that liver transplantation will not be needed for several years (selective shunt only); (c) severe portal hypertension in patients with cystic fibrosis and variceal hemorrhage whose microbiologic flora compromise liver transplant survival; (d) children with severe portal hypertension who reside a great distance from emergency medical care endangering their survival should significant hemorrhage occur; and (e) children with EPVO and uncontrolled hypersplenism.

TRANSJUGULAR INTRAHEPATIC PORTOSYSTEMIC SHUNT

The introduction of the transjugular intrahepatic portosystemic shunt (TIPS) has added another therapeutic option for the patient with complex portal hypertension. This procedure uses interventional radiographic techniques to place an intrahepatic expandable metallic shunt between a portal vein branch and the hepatic vein, forming a central nonselective portocaval shunt. Technical difficulties in establishing a safe but large enough tract for sufficient shunt flow limit the usefulness of this procedure in infants. In children with biliary atresia, the close proximity of the biliary Roux-en-Y conduit to the portal vein and the often diminutive size of the portal vein increase the risk of stent perforation, malposition, or perforation. The two principal long-term complications of TIPS are encephalopathy and shunt occlusion

Pediatric experience with TIPS is still limited, primarily due to a lack of appropriate candidates for the procedure. The majority of children with biliary atresia and an ineffective portoenterostomy develop end-stage cirrhosis within their first 2 years of life. These patients are poor candidates both by virtue of their size and the frequency of portal vein abnormalities within this population. The majority of experience is in children over 5 years of age. Success rates appear to approximate the adult experience, with 75% to 90% initial success following TIPS placement. Postprocedural encephalopathy seems to be less common in children, although limited clinical experience and the difficulties in diagnosing subtle encephalopathy in children makes this observation tentative. The complications of shunt stenosis are equally problematic, and patient growth over time may cause the initial shunt to be too short, requiring revision or restenting to maintain access to both the portal and hepatic venous circulation. These limitations and risks make TIPS a reasonable and suitable treatment for acute unresponsive variceal hemorrhage in older children with established intrinsic liver disease. It is particularly helpful when used as a bridge to achieve stability by controlling refractory hemorrhage in patients awaiting liver transplantation. Long-term decompression is better achieved through surgical shunts at the present time, and TIPS is not indicated in patients with extrahepatic portal vein occlusion.

NONSHUNT PROCEDURES FOR PORTAL HYPERTENSION

The use of nonshunt surgical procedures for the management of portal hypertension does not offer the same success as shunt therapy. These operations have included both direct variceal ligation through a transthoracic or abdominal approach, gastroesophageal devascularization procedures (*Sugiura procedure*), or, rarely, translocation of the spleen into the thorax. In general, these procedures have been abandoned except in cases where widespread thrombosis of the mesenteric venous vasculature makes shunt therapy or transplantation poor alternatives.

The *Sugiura procedure* has been used with the most success in children (Fig. 103.4). This procedure includes devascularization of the upper two thirds of the greater and lesser curvatures of the stomach, and ligation of the left gastroepiploic, short gastric, and left gastric vessels. Ligation of all retrogastric collateral vessels, transhiatal devascularization of the lower esophagus, and esophageal transection with fundoplication and pyloroplasty if the vagus nerves are damaged complete the operative procedure. Splenectomy was advocated in the original descriptions of this procedure as well, but splenectomy has been associated with a greater risk of intraoperative bleeding, need for intraoperative blood transfusions, and postoperative portal vein thrombosis. Because of these risks and the known increased potential for postoperative infectious complications of splenectomy, we do not routinely perform splenectomy in children. Following extensive devascularization to achieve portoazygous disconnection, rebleeding rates of 5% to 10% can be achieved during long-term follow-up. Survival has been reported to be 88% at 5 years and 80% at 10 years. This is a safe alternative for variceal control in patients with anatomy unsuitable for shunting, or when the expertise for emergency portocaval shunt or liver transplantation is not available.

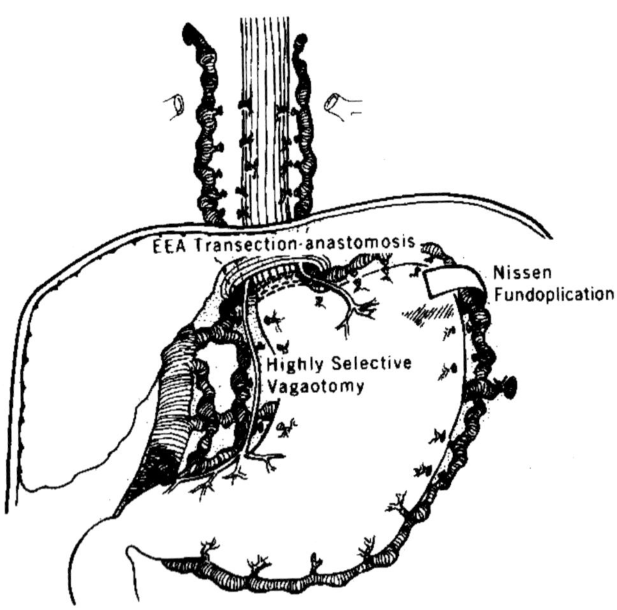

FIGURE 103.4. Sugiura procedure for gastroesophageal devascularization, modified for pediatric patients to include division of the short gastric veins without splenectomy. (Reprinted from Superina RA, Weber JL, Shandling B. A modified Sugiura operation for bleeding varices in children. *J Surg* 1983;18:794–799; with permission.)

LIVER TRANSPLANTATION

The progressive improvement in both the operative techniques and the immunosuppression management of children who have undergone liver transplantation has led to 1-year survival rates approaching 90% in many centers, with 5-year survival rates of 85%. Regardless of the primary etiology of portal hypertension, liver transplantation successfully reverses the portal flow obstruction and allows the resolution of hypersplenism and hypertensive portal gastropathy. The introduction of innovative surgical procedures to allow transplantation of liver segments and reduced-size grafts has increased donor availability and donor access for children of all ages. However, the use of primary transplantation as a treatment modality for portal hypertension is limited by the availability of suitable donor organs and the long-term risks of immunosuppression, opportunistic infections, and lymphoproliferative disease. When children have progressive intrinsic hepatic disease, the course of their progression and the amount of hepatic functional reserve should determine the use of primary transplantation compared with temporizing treatments such as sclerotherapy or surgical shunts. At present, primary transplantation is recommended for children who have significant portal hypertensive complications such as bleeding, hypersplenism, or hepatopulmonary syndrome, and those who have progressive hepatic synthetic failure. Children with intrinsic liver disease but preserved hepatic synthetic function, who may not require transplantation for several years will achieve excellent palliation with selective DSRS. TIPS is reserved for patients who have unresponsive variceal bleeding as a therapeutic bridge to transplantation, allowing them to achieve suitable stability while awaiting transplant donor organ availability.

PULMONARY SYNDROMES ASSOCIATED WITH PORTAL HYPERTENSION

Hepatopulmonary syndrome, characterized by hepatic dysfunction, hypoxemia, and pulmonary vascular dilatations, typically occurs in children with long-standing liver disease and portal hypertension. This constellation of symptoms is thought to be secondary to the effects on the pulmonary vasculature of vasoactive substances that are normally inactivated in the liver. Although this syndrome is usually seen in patients with portal hypertension and spontaneous portosystemic communications, it has been reported following surgical portosystemic shunting as well. Progressive hypoxemia, which is exacerbated by the horizontal position (orthodeoxia and platypnea), is commonly seen on evaluation. Hypoxemia does not correct with 100% oxygen ventilation, confirming the presence of intrapulmonary shunts contributing to the alveolar perfusion abnormalities. Abnormal extrapulmonary (brain) uptake of technetium 99m macroaggregated albumin after lung perfusion scanning, or the presence of early microbubble perfusion on echocardiography, are diagnostic and predictive of morbidity with general anesthesia or liver transplantation. Present experience suggests that these abnormalities are reversible following successful liver transplantation.

Pulmonary hypertension is associated with severe liver disease and portal hypertension in 1% to 2% of patients. In the presence of spontaneous or surgically created portosystemic communication, pulmonary vasoconstrictive substances can pass directly into the systemic circulation, bypassing hepatic metabolism. Possible agents include histamine, serotonin, purine, pyrimidine, neuropeptide-Y, and thromboxanes. Symptoms of dyspnea, exercise intolerance, and palpitation occur; however, many patients remain asymptomatic until late in the course of their disease. Initial treatment with oxygen and vasodilators is occasionally helpful. The pathologic lesion, plexogenic pulmonary arteriopathy, results in increased smooth muscle, increased thickness of the media, concentric luminal fibrosis, and eventually fibrinoid necrosis. Case reports suggest that liver transplantation may assist in reversal, provided diagnosis and transplantation are undertaken at the early stages of pathologic evolution. In later stages, resolution cannot be anticipated.

SUMMARY

Therapeutic options for children with portal hypertension now include a broad range of pharmacologic, endoscopic, and surgical procedures. Thoughtful application of all of these options can improve quality of life by decreasing the complications of portal hypertension, and decrease mortality by preventing the consequences of variceal hemorrhage. The development of portal hypertensive gastropathy following palliative procedures such as endoscopic sclerotherapy and band ligation may limit their long-term success in children. The excellent results now obtained with selective portosystemic shunts and liver transplantation assure that definitive surgical treatments will continue to be a critical component in the treatment of children with portal hypertensive complications or progressive liver disease. Evolving procedures, such as TIPS, represent excellent short-term life-preserving techniques to stabilize critical patients while awaiting liver transplantation. Their role in the future long-term management of children is yet to be defined.

SUGGESTED READINGS

Alonso MH, Ryckman FC. Current concepts in pediatric liver transplant. *Semin Liver Dis* 1998;18:295–307.

Balistreri WF. Transplantation for childhood liver disease: an overview. *Liver Transplant Surg* 1998;4(suppl):18–23.

D'Amico G, Pagliaro L, Bosch J. The treatment of portal hypertension: a meta-analytic review. *Hepatology* 1995;22:332–354.

de Ville deGrote, Alberti D, Clapuyt P, et al. Direct bypassing of extrahepatic portal venous obstruction in children: a new technique for combined hepatic portal revascularization and treatment of extrahepatic portal hypertension. *J Pediatr Surg* 1998;33:597–601.

Gauthier F, de Dreuzy O, Valayer J, et al. H-type shunt with an autologous venous graft for treatment of portal hypertension in children. *J Pediatr Surg* 1989;24:1041–1043.

Karrer FM, Narkewicz MR. Esophageal varices: current management in children. *Semin Pediatr Surg* 1999;8:193–201.

Maksoud JG, Goncalves ME. Treatment of portal hypertension in children. *World J Surg* 1994;18:251–258.

Orloff MJ, Orloff MS, Rambotti M. Treatment of bleeding esophagogastric varices due to extrahepatic portal hypertension: results of portal-systemic shunts during 35 years. *J Pediatr Surg* 1994;29:142–151.

Ryckman FC, Alonso MH. Causes and management of portal hypertension in the pediatric population. *Clin Liver Dis* 2001;5:789-818.

Schneider BL, Groszmann RJ. Portal hypertension. In: Suchy FJ, ed. *Liver disease in children*. St. Louis: CV Mosby, 1994:249–266.

104

ACUTE AND CHRONIC PANCREATITIS AND EXOCRINE PANCREATIC TUMORS

REBECKA L. MEYERS
MARK O. McCOLLUM

The predominant causes of acute pancreatitis in children are trauma, viral infection, and drugs. The predominant cause of chronic pancreatitis is familial.

Numerous classifications have been published over the years. The most recent Marseilles-Rome classification defines *acute pancreatitis* as a "group of pancreatic and peripancreatic lesions generally considered to be reversible: edema, necrosis, hemorrhagic necrosis, and fat necrosis." The causes of acute pancreatitis are usually extrapancreatic, such as gallstones, viral infections, drugs, surgery, endoscopy, hyperlipoproteinemia, and so forth. The severity of the acute inflammation varies from mild and self-limiting to severe and necrotizing. Once these episodes of acute inflammation completely resolve, they may recur, and the term *acute relapsing pancreatitis* is used. If, however, the inflammatory changes do not completely resolve, there may be a progression to chronic pancreatitis.

Chronic pancreatitis is defined as "the presence of chronic inflammatory lesions characterized by the destruction of exocrine parenchyma and fibrosis and at least in the later stages, the destruction of endocrine parenchyma." The two different types of chronic pancreatitis distinguished in the Marseilles-Rome classification are chronic obstructive pancreatitis and chronic calcifying pancreatitis. *Chronic obstructive pancreatitis* is uniform, not patchy, and localized distal to the site of the obstruction. Examples include posttraumatic strictures and other obstructive processes such as pancreas divisum, enteric duplications, choledochal cyst, and tumors. *Chronic calcifying pancreatitis* is patchy, with atrophic duct epithelium, and is dominated by intraductal stones composed of calcium salts or protein plugs. Familial pancreatitis and alcoholic pancreatitis are two of several subtypes of chronic calcifying pancreatitis.

R. L. Meyers and M. O. McCollum: Department of Surgery, Division of Pediatric Surgery, University of Utah School of Medicine, and Primary Children's Medical Center, Salt Lake City, Utah.

ACUTE PANCREATITIS

Acute pancreatitis presents a great variety of morphologic and clinical manifestations, which range from mild transitory illness to fatal disease. The most common causes of acute pancreatitis in children are trauma, viral infection, or drugs. The myriad other potential inciting factors are listed in Table 104.1. The final common physiologic pathway resulting in tissue damage seems to be activation of pancreatic digestive enzymes within the parenchyma. The exact cellular mechanism leading to this autodigestion is not completely understood, although theories include intraductal zymogen activation, intracellular zymogen activation, reflux of activated proteases from the duodenum, and pancreatic duct hypertension leading to increased duct permeability.

When compared with adults, children usually recover more quickly and tend to have fewer complications; yet the clinical course is often unpredictable and can progress rapidly. The most frequent complaint at presentation is midepigastric pain, which ranges from mild to severe. The pain is not colicky, but sharp and steady. It may radiate through to the back, although back pain seems to be less common in children than adults. Associated symptoms include anorexia, nausea, and vomiting. A history of trauma should increase suspicion of possible associated pancreatic parenchymal disruption. Physical findings include epigastric tenderness, abdominal distension, and increased tympany due to associated ileus, and in severe cases there may be peritoneal signs, sepsis, and shock. In the case of associated hemorrhage, the Gray-Turner's or Cullen's sign may be present. Serum amylase and lipase are elevated. The urinary amylase:creatinine ratio is increased due to increased renal tubular reabsorption of amylase. Electrolyte abnormalities may suggest dehydration, acidosis, and hypocalcemia. Other serum values may point to an underlying etiology such as elevation of biliary canalicular enzymes, drug levels, or hyperlipidemia.

TABLE 104.1. CAUSATIVE FACTORS IN ACUTE PANCREATITIS

Trauma
- Blunt abdominal
- Abuse
- Surgical manipulation

Biliary tract disease
- Cholelithiasis
- Choledocholithiasis
- Choledochal cyst
- Ductal anomalies

Systemic disease
- Reye syndrome
- Collagen vascular disease
- Henoch-Schoenlein purpura
- Inflammatory bowel disease
- Transplantation

Metabolic abnormalities
- Cystic fibrosis
- Hypercalcemia
- Hyperlipidemia
- Organic acidemias

Infectious disease
- Viral infection
- Sepsis/shock

Drugs
- Azathioprine
- Chlorothiazides
- Furosemide
- L-asparaginase
- Steroids
- Sulfonamides
- Tetracycline
- Valproic acid

Abdominal radiographs are usually of limited value, but may show a nonspecific ileus or a sentinel loop, and can be used to rule out other catastrophic causes of abdominal pain such as a perforated viscus. Ultrasonography may show pancreatic edema and can be used to investigate the possibility of biliary tract disease or extrapancreatic fluid collections. Although less useful in children due to the relative absence of retroperitoneal fat, abdominal computed tomography (CT) can provide more detailed information than ultrasonography regarding grading and severity of the pancreatic inflammation and is especially helpful in evaluating pancreatic injury due to trauma. Although endoscopic retrograde cholangiopancreatography (ERCP) and magnetic resonance cholangiopancreatography (MRCP) have clear and indispensable roles in the evaluation of pancreatic and biliary anatomy in chronic pancreatitis, they are rarely needed in acute pancreatitis unless one needs to rule out a major traumatic ductal injury.

There is no pediatric equivalent to the adult predictive criteria of Ranson. Clinical features associated with a poor prognosis include progressive hypovolemic shock, respiratory decompensation, renal failure, and hypocalcemia. CT anatomic grading of severity also follows adult guidelines and is based on the severity of pancreatic edema, the presence or absence of extrapancreatic fluid or phlegmonous collections, nonperfused parenchyma suggestive of necrosis, and possible associated infection (Table 104.2).

Most patients with acute pancreatitis are managed nonoperatively. The cornerstone of medical management is intravenous fluid resuscitation aimed at restoration of intravascular volume. Care also must include correction of acid-base and electrolyte abnormalities, adequate pain management, and respiratory support if necessary. Although the child should definitely be allowed nothing by mouth to decrease pancreatic stimulation, the use of a nasogastric tube is controversial. In the absence of uncontrollable vomiting, nasogastric decompression is probably not necessary. Somatostatin pancreatic suppression has been studied in adults, with some studies showing a small decrease in mortality. There have been no similar studies in children. Adult studies of acid suppression with histamine or proton pump blockers have shown that they do not consistently decrease the duration or severity of the illness. A growing body of literature in adults suggests that early enteral nasojejunal tube feeds may be preferable to intravenous hyperalimentation if they can be tolerated. Although the use of prophylactic antibiotics has historically been controversial, several recent adult prospective studies have shown a significant reduction in mortality when broad-spectrum antibiotics (e.g., imipenem) are used to treat CT evidence of nonperfused pancreatic tissue or necrosis.

Surgical intervention is needed in a few specific circumstances: (a) to treat the underlying biliary tract disease in cases of biliary pancreatitis; (b) to debride infected pancreatic necrosis; and (c) to address the occasional major ductal injury or a posttraumatic pseudocyst that remains symptomatic despite initial treatment with pancreatic rest. In the first case, cholecystectomy is generally performed after the acute pan-

TABLE 104.2. COMPUTED TOMOGRAPHIC ANATOMIC CLASSIFICATIONS OF ACUTE PANCREATITIS

Severity of acute pancreatitis
- Edematous or interstitial pancreatitis: radiographic enhancement of entire gland by contrast media
- Necrotizing pancreatitis: failure of enhancement of portions of the gland is indicative of tissue necrosis

Classification of traumatic pancreatic injury
- Class I: contusion or laceration without duct injury
- Class II: distal transection or parenchymal injury with ductal involvement
- Class III: proximal transection or parenchymal injury with probable duct injury
- Class IV: combined pancreatic and duodenal injury

creatic inflammation has resolved. Rarely, sphincterotomy or common duct exploration is needed if an obstructing stone fails to pass spontaneously. In the second case, once necrotic pancreatic tissue shows clear signs of infection and abscess, the infected tissue should be debrided and externally drained. Although controversial, recent adult studies show that the aggressive, multiple trips to the operating room for the open-abdomen, "zipper" debridements commonly undertaken in the 1980s are so fraught with secondary complications that in the clinically stable patient debridement can often be performed more safely once the abscess progresses to an encapsulated phase. Finally, it has been traditional to treat traumatic distal pancreatic injury with distal pancreatectomy and pseudocysts with drainage. There is a growing body of literature to support much less aggressive management of all grades of isolated pancreatic injury. Although children with a ductal injury frequently develop pseudocysts and less frequently pancreatic fistulas, many of these can be managed safely with observation, pancreatic rest, and judicious use of percutaneous drainage. Prospective studies have not shown increased risk of complications with nonoperative management, and outcomes are similar, including length of hospital stay. In the case of pseudocysts, neither internal nor external drainage appears mandatory unless the child is symptomatic. Many of these cysts spontaneously resolve with careful expectant management.

CHRONIC PANCREATITIS

Unlike acute pancreatitis, chronic pancreatitis is generally a progressive and irreversible disease. Initially manifest by recurrent attacks of inflammation and intermittent pain, progressive glandular destruction leads to both exocrine insufficiency (steatorrhea) and endocrine insufficiency (diabetes). In its advanced stage the acute pancreatic attacks decrease or disappear, amylase and lipase are often normal, and a chronic unrelenting pain that may lead to narcotic dependence replaces intermittent pain. Chronic pancreatitis is broadly categorized into two main types: *obstructive* and *calcifying*. In *chronic obstructive pancreatitis* the main cause is a fixed obstruction such as a scar from a previous attack of acute pancreatitis or trauma, papillary stenosis occasionally associated with pancreas divisum, and, rarely, extrinsic compression from choledochal or duplication cysts or tumors. Inflammation proximal to the obstruction is uniform, not patchy, the ductile epithelium is preserved, and calcified stones are not found. The "familial" or "hereditary" subtype of *chronic calcifying pancreatitis* is the most common form seen in children. This and other forms of calcifying pancreatitis (nutritional, alcoholic, tropical, and hypercalcemic) are categorized by the biochemical composition of the pathognomonic stones, variably composed of calcium carbonate (calcite), pancreatic stone proteins (PSP, PSP-S, PSP-S1), and other amorphous nonfibrillar proteins. Even in its earliest stages, before there is any apparent damage to the pancreatic parenchyma, chronic calcifying pancreatitis seems to be a lithiasis.

Chronic pancreatitis has not historically been considered a surgical disease. The traditional belief was that once the pancreas is sufficiently destroyed, the pain would improve. This approach was probably flawed for several reasons. Not only will the process of pancreatic burnout take many years, but the pain may never be completely alleviated, extrapancreatic complications such as pseudocysts, splenic vein thrombosis, and biliary obstruction may develop, and there will be an inevitable progression toward exocrine insufficiency and diabetes. Based on the pioneering work of Nealon, there is an ever-increasing body of literature suggesting that early operation is not only effective in ameliorating the pain and reducing narcotic dependence, but also may slow the development of exocrine and endocrine insufficiency.

Surgical therapy should be considered when standard medical therapy, including non-narcotic analgesia and enzyme replacement, has failed to relieve the pain. When the physician reaches the point where he or she considers prescribing narcotics for pain relief, he or she should screen the patient with regard to suitability for surgery. A multidisciplinary team approach is mandatory and should include surgeons, gastroenterologists, radiologists, and occasionally psychiatrists and endocrinologists. Ideally, surgical options will be considered before the patient has become addicted to narcotics, become diabetic, suffered significant nutritional impairment, or become severely depressed.

Surgical strategy revolves around the anatomy of the pancreatic duct. Consequently, ERCP, and in some cases MRCP (Fig. 104.1), is critical in determining whether the patient is a good surgical candidate and in tailoring the operation to the patient's specific needs. The site of strictures may influence whether a proximal or distal resection is appropriate or where the Roux-en-Y limb should be placed. Obstructive pancreatitis implies a single site of obstruction from a stricture or tumor, whereas calcifying pancreatitis implies multiple "chain-of-lakes," or "string of beads" strictures throughout the gland. Anomalies of the ductal system such as pancreas divisum or ampullary strictures may be amenable to stricturoplasty. A bulky thickened pancreatic head may represent the chronic fibrosis of calcific disease or perhaps a tumor and necessitates some sort of resection or biopsy. With pseudocysts or a fistula, the exact size, location, and point of communication with the main duct must be defined. The presence and severity of intrapancreatic bile duct obstruction determines the potential need for concomitant biliary drainage.

Because the pathologic features in all cases of pancreatitis are not uniform, no one operation can be rigidly applied in all cases. Ultimately the procedure should (a) correct all

A 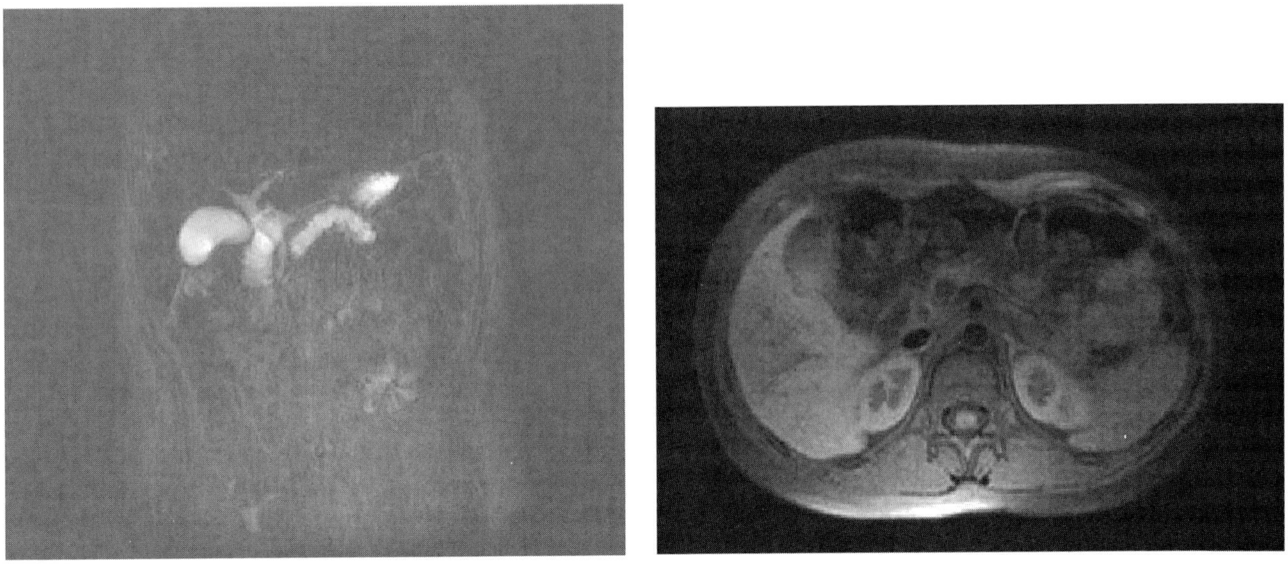 B

FIGURE 104.1. MRCP from a 12-year-old girl with chronic calcifying pancreatitis. Note the dilated string of beads appearance of the pancreatic duct. **A:** Magnetic resonance cholangiopancreatography (MRCP) sagittal image. **B:** MRCP axial image.

structural abnormalities; (b) relieve pain; (c) have acceptable morbidity and mortality rates; (d) acknowledge the likelihood of compliance with drug abstention; and (e) minimize exocrine and endocrine insufficiency postoperatively. In an attempt to meet these goals, two broad surgical principles have been applied: drainage (either endoscopic or surgical) and resection. A variety of *endoscopic drainage techniques* have been introduced and can be effective in selected cases of chronic obstructive pancreatitis where the pathology is confined to the main pancreatic duct. However, stent occlusion, stent dislocation, pancreatic duct obstruction by stone fragments, and the need for multiple repeat procedures limit their utility in most children. In cases of discrete obstruction, such as papillary stenosis in pancreatic divisum, *sphincterotomy* of the stenotic minor papilla is often, but not always, curative.

In patients with a hypertensive pancreatic duct, an adequate pancreaticojejunostomy relieves pain with little or no impairment of exocrine or endocrine function. Options include the longitudinal pancreaticojejunostomy (*modified Peustow procedure*) and local resection of the head of the pancreas combined with longitudinal pancreaticojejunostomy (*Frey procedure*). Because many reports have attributed surgical treatment failures after the modified Peustow procedure to recurrent disease in the head of the gland, we now prefer the Frey procedure for most eligible patients (Fig. 104.2). In either case, surgeons differ on what duct size makes these operations technically feasible. Some surgeons do not perform a duct decompression with ducts less than 8 to 10 mm in diameter, but like many others, we have found that by sewing to the capsule of the pancreas rather than the duct, these operations are reliable with ducts as small as 4 to 5 mm in diameter.

Like the Frey procedure, the duodenum-preserving *Beger procedure* involves resection of the head of the pancreas, although in the latter the resection is more extensive. The body and tail of the gland are preserved and drained end to end to a Roux-en-Y pancreaticojejunostomy, with a second anastomosis to the preserved portion of pancreas along the inner aspect of the duodenum associated with the intrapancreatic portion of the common bile duct. A prospective randomized trial found that both the Beger and Frey procedures had excellent and comparable results with regard to pain relief, overall quality of life, and preservation of endocrine and exocrine function, but found the Beger procedure to be somewhat more technically challenging with a higher perioperative morbidity.

Some advocate a *Whipple procedure* or pancreaticoduodenectomy, again because the changes of chronic pancreatitis often begin and are most dominant in the head and uncinate process. If other alternatives exist, we hesitate to recommend the operation for benign disease because of its increased operative morbidity. We have used it successfully in a unique patient with obstructive chronic pancreatitis secondary to an extensive duodenal duplication. More extensive pancreatic resection procedures (80% distal pancreatectomy, or *Child procedure*, and *total pancreatectomy*) have the major drawback of the inevitable development of insulin-dependent diabetes and pancreatic exocrine insufficiency. *Autotransplantation of islet cells* has been advocated to reduce the severity of postoperative diabetes, but the long-term viability of these autografts is not yet known and

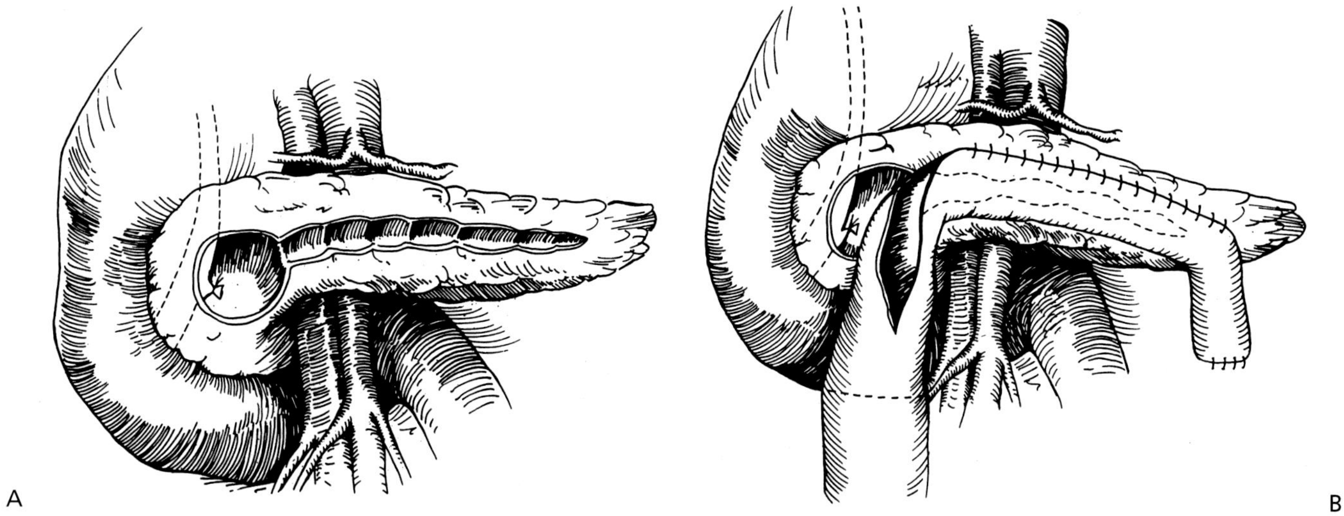

Figure 104.2. Frey procedure for chronic pancreatitis. **A:** The main pancreatic duct is opened throughout its length in the body and tail of the pancreas and then carried as far as possible to the duodenum. After location of the superior mesenteric vein and portal vein to avoid injury to these structures, the anterior head of the pancreas is cored out to remove retention cysts, areas of necrosis, and impacted calculi. If the position of the common bile duct cannot be determined readily, a dilator or catheter can be passed distally through the cystic duct stump to identify its course. **B:** A Roux-en-Y limb is used to drain the main pancreatic duct in the head, body, and tail of the pancreas by means of a two-layer, side-to-side pancreaticojejunostomy. (Reprinted from Frey CF, et al. Pancreatic resection for chronic pancreatitis. Surg Clin North Am 1989;3:499-528; with permission.)

even in the short term some degree of insulin dependence is present in most of these patients. Although techniques are improving, the number of cells that can be harvested from a fibrotic inflamed pancreas is often insufficient to keep the patient euglycemic. Exocrine insufficiency remains inevitable and is treated with pancreatic enzymes.

Prospective, controlled adult series show that 65% to 85% of patients undergoing duct drainage or pancreatic resection have substantial pain relief. Comparable studies in children do not exist, although retrospective series of the modified Peustow procedure have shown comparable results. Although it is controversial, some investigators report that pancreatic resection is rarely successful in relieving pain that has continued after pancreatic duct drainage.

PANCREATIC EXOCRINE TUMORS

Tumors arising from the pancreatic exocrine tissue include cystic tumors, papillary cystic tumors, pancreatoblastomas, and pancreatic adenocarcinomas. Cystic tumors range from congenital cysts to neoplastic cysts, including serous and mucinous cystadenomas. *Congenital cysts* are most often discovered incidentally, although rarely they may become large enough to cause compressive symptoms and be felt on physical examination. Preoperative differentiation from the pseudocystic disease of pancreatitis, or neoplastic cystic disease, may be difficult. Fortunately, most of these cysts are located in the body and tail of the gland and are amenable to simple resection. Examination of the cloudy straw-colored cyst fluid shows normal levels of pancreatic enzymes, indicating a lack of communication with the pancreatic ductal system. Both serous and mucinous cystadenomas have a histologically identifiable epithelial cyst lining. *Serous cystadenomas* are often microcystic, and although historically they have not been considered to have malignant potential, there have been recent case reports of malignant transformation. *Mucinous cystadenomas and mucinous cystadenocarcinomas* are macrocystic and filled with thick mucoid fluid. Although their radiographic appearance may resemble a pseudocyst, histologic examination of the cyst wall will confirm an epithelial lining, indicating the need for complete excision. *Papillary cystic tumors* are seen in adolescent girls and are often confused with pseudocystic disease. Although benign, they commonly reach large size and when causing compressive symptoms they should be completely resected.

Although pancreatic adenocarcinoma and pancreaticoblastoma are rare in children, they are seen with sufficient frequency that the pediatric surgeon must be aware of the appropriate treatment strategies. In adults, *pancreatic adenocarcinoma* typically arises from the ductal cells, whereas in children adenocarcinoma more commonly arises from the acinar cell. Improved survival has been reported in children; therefore, aggressive surgical resection with pancreaticoduodenectomy, even sometimes in the setting of venous invasion, is recommended. *Pancreaticoblastoma* is a tumor of infants and young children thought to arise from embryologically immature duct cells. Again, the prognosis is better than in adult adenocarcinoma, and aggressive surgical resection is recommended.

SUGGESTED READINGS

Frey C. The surgical management of chronic pancreatitis: the Frey procedure. *Adv Surg* 1999;32:41–85.

Hirohashi S, Hirohashi R, Uchida H, et al. Pancreatitis: evaluation with MR cholangiopancreatography in children. *Radiology* 1997; 203:411–415.

Jobst M, Canty T, Lynch F. Management of pancreatic injury in pediatric blunt abdominal trauma. *J Pediatr Surg* 1999;34: 818–824.

Lerner A, Branski D, Lebenthal E. Pancreatic diseases in children. *Pediatr Clin North Am* 1996;43:125–156.

Peterson C, Goetz A, Burger D, et al. Surgical therapy and follow-up of pancreatitis in children. *J Pediatr Gastroenteral Nutr* 1997;25: 204–209.

Shilyansky J, Sena L, Kreller M, et al. Nonoperative management of pancreatic injuries in children. *J Pediatr Surg* 1998;33: 342–349.

Tagge E, Tarnasky P, Chandler J, et al. Multidisciplinary approach to the treatment of pediatric pancreaticobiliary disorders. *J Pediatr Surg* 1997;32:158–165.

105

NEONATAL PANCREATIC ENDOCRINE DISEASE

MARSHALL Z. SCHWARTZ

The pancreas is a complex organ that serves both digestive and endocrine functions. Although abnormalities in development of both functions can occur, the most devastating and life-threatening problems are those affecting the endocrine function of the pancreas. The endocrine function of the pancreas is centered in the cells of the islets of Langerhans. These cells are believed to arise from pleuropotential periductular cells. Interestingly, there appear to be two generations of islets that develop, with the first generation undergoing regression after the 5th month of gestation. Although the islet cells make up only approximately 2% of the pancreatic mass, they play a vital physiologic role. There are four major types of cells within the islets, and each type secretes a specific peptide hormone. The most common, comprising 70% of the total islet cell mass, is the insulin-secreting β cell.

Abnormalities involving the β cells result in hypoglycemia, the most common pancreatic endocrine disorder in neonates. The relationship between hypoglycemia and hyperinsulinemia is well established, but the etiology of the hyperinsulinemia remains poorly understood. It appears that the glucose-mediated feedback inhibition of insulin release is lost or disrupted. A family history of hyperinsulinism can be found in 10% to 25% of infants with this disorder, and it has been suggested that it is transmitted as an autosomal-recessive disorder. Chromosomal studies have shown a defect on the short arm of chromosome 11. Further studies have demonstrated mutations resulting in alterations in the adenosine triphosphate–binding domain of the sulfonylurea receptor gene responsible for the familial syndrome.

Preceding the availability of detailed and sophisticated chromosomal and gene studies, the resected specimen was the focus of evaluation in neonates with hyperinsulinemia. The initial hypothesis was that hyperplasia of the β cells led to hyperinsulinemia. The term *nesidioblastosis* was coined to suggest β cell hyperplasia. However, extensive pathologic studies have shown a variety of abnormalities, including focal or diffuse nesidioblastosis, islet cell hyperplasia, islet cell nuclear hyperplasia, dysplasia, and adenomatosis. It is important to note that frequently no pathologic alterations are identified. As a reflection of the many hypotheses regarding its cause, numerous terms have been used to describe clinical hyperinsulinemia in the neonatal period, including β cell adenomatosis, nesidioblastosis, and islet cell dysplasia. More recently, a more generalized term has been used: persistent hyperinsulinemic hypoglycemia of the neonate (PHHN).

CLINICAL PRESENTATION

Infants with PHHN are typically large (95th to 99th percentile for weight). Symptoms and signs of hypoglycemia are nonspecific and include hypotonia, irritability, pallor, poor feeding, and tachycardia. Unfortunately, the first manifestation may be seizures and coma as a result of severe hypoglycemia. Conversely, infants with mild hyperinsulinemia may be asymptomatic until they develop an illness that results in diminished caloric intake. It is customary in most nurseries to monitor blood glucose levels frequently in newborns, but the diagnosis of hypoglycemia needs to be considered and urgently excluded in infants showing any of these signs or symptoms.

DIAGNOSIS

There are numerous causes of hypoglycemia in the neonate that are not related to pancreatic endocrine dysfunction. Metabolic disorders such as glycogen storage disease, other hormone abnormalities such as adrenocorticotropic hormone deficiency, and maternal abnormali-

M. Z. Schwartz: Department of Surgery, Thomas Jefferson University, Philadelphia, Pennsylvania; and Department of Surgery, A.I. duPont Hospital for Children, Wilmington, Delaware.

ties such as maternal diabetes can result in hypoglycemia. True hyperinsulinism is based on the following criteria: (a) inappropriately elevated plasma insulin levels in relation to blood glucose levels obtained at varying postprandial and fasting times; (b) the need for a glucose infusion rate of more than 10 mg/kg/min to maintain a blood glucose level above 35 mg/dL; (c) low plasma concentration of free fatty acids and blood ketone bodies; and (d) an increase in blood glucose levels in response to glucagon. The diagnosis is confirmed by simultaneously comparing blood glucose levels to insulin levels. Infants with hypoglycemia should have little or no detectable serum insulin. When insulin levels are detectable or elevated, in the presence of low blood sugar, the diagnosis of hyperinsulinemia is confirmed. In the past, imaging studies of the pancreas were routinely obtained. The only endocrine abnormality detectable by imaging is an insulinoma, which is a rare entity in the neonate.

MEDICAL MANAGEMENT

The obvious goal of medical management for patients with PHHN is to stabilize the serum glucose level. Because this might require 15% or 20% glucose infusion, a central venous catheter is appropriate. In addition, frequent oral feedings are indicated. Fortunately, the availability of several pharmacologic agents has significantly improved the management and outcome in these infants. These agents include glucagon, diazoxide, and the long-acting somatostatin analogue octreotide. In the majority of patients, these agents can stabilize blood glucose levels.

Because pharmacologic management can be effective on a short-term basis, some clinicians have advocated its long-term use. Octreotide is the mainstay of this management and is administered subcutaneously or intravenously. Frequent feedings are also necessary, often requiring placement of a gastrostomy tube. It is important to point out that although hyperinsulinism can be self-limited, it is difficult to predict in which infants this will occur. Long-term medical management is a reasonable approach in those infants in whom the hypoglycemia is relatively easy to control. If this is not the case, the infant is at significant risk of permanent neurologic impairment as a result of severe hypoglycemia, and surgical management is therefore indicated.

SURGICAL MANAGEMENT

The surgical management of patients with hypoglycemia secondary to hyperinsulinism has been somewhat controversial. There should not be a sense of urgency to proceed to the operating room. It is critical that control of the patient's blood sugar and overall metabolic status be accomplished. If glucose homeostasis is not achieved, there is a significant risk for wide swings in blood sugar and potentially severe neurologic impairment.

The controversial aspect to the surgical management of PHHN is the question of how much of the pancreas should be removed (Fig. 105.1). The ideal resection would remove enough to allow normalization of blood sugar levels but would retain enough to avoid exocrine insufficiency or diabetes. In 1953, Dr. Robert Gross reported that a 75% to 80% pancreatic resection was adequate to achieve these goals. Since then, there has been a tendency to recommend a higher percentage of resection, based on the desire to avoid further pancreatic resection for persistent hypo-

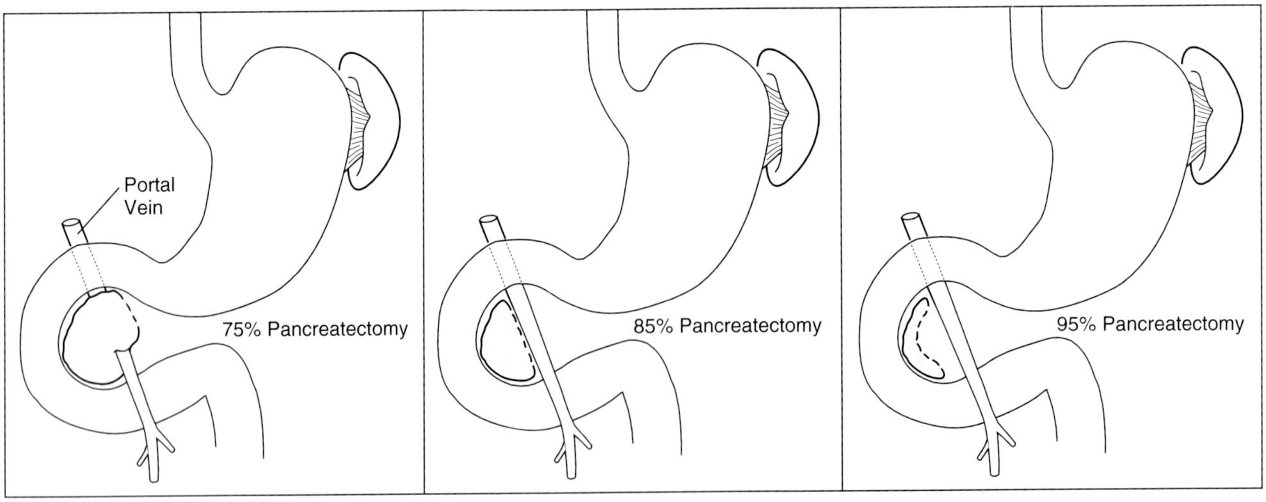

FIGURE 105.1. Recommended percentages of pancreatectomy.

glycemia. For the past 10 to 15 years, the consensus seems to be that a 95% pancreatic resection is best. Nonetheless, it has been my bias over the past 25 years to perform an 85% pancreatectomy. I have not wavered from this approach for the following reasons: (a) it is successful in treating the hypoglycemia and eliminating the need for medical management in most patients; (b) it does not result in exocrine dysfunction; (c) sufficient islets remain so that insulin insufficiency and diabetes occur infrequently; and (d) if further resection is necessary, it is not a difficult surgical procedure.

Following glucose and metabolic stabilization of the patient and placement of a central venous catheter (for vascular access for blood sampling as well as infusion of glucose), the abdomen is entered through a transverse left upper quadrant incision. In infants, it is not necessary to make a large incision, and it has been my practice to incise only over the width of the left rectus muscle. Although mobilization of the spleen facilitates the dissection of the tail of the pancreas, this is not necessary. The procedure is begun by entering the lesser sac and exposing the anterior surface of the pancreas. The inferior edge of the pancreas is mobilized, exposing the posterior surface. Starting at the tail of the pancreas, the small branches arising from the splenic artery and vein can be defined and ligated. These vessels are quite small and very short. If ligation is not practical, small hemoclips can be used. As the dissection proceeds toward the midline, care must be taken to avoid injury to the portal vein and superior mesenteric artery. Dissection of the pancreas along its superior border continues up to the medial border of the portal vein. It should be noted that at the beginning of the mobilization and periodically throughout the dissection, visual inspection and palpation of the gland should be undertaken to determine the rare presence of an insulinoma as the etiology of the hyperinsulinemia.

Once the dissection to the medial border of the portal vein is complete, the pancreas can be transected. It is my preference to use a gastrointestinal stapling device, although in some cases it is best to apply a vascular clamp, transect the pancreas, and oversew it with absorbable monofilament suture. The main pancreatic duct is typically found in the superior posterior aspect of the gland, but identification of the duct itself can be very difficult. It has been my approach to attempt to identify the duct, but if this is not possible, then I place a "U" stitch through the gland at the expected location of the duct. Although I initially left a drain at the site of the pancreatic transection, over the past 15 years I have not done so and this has not led to morbidity.

POSTOPERATIVE CARE

Postoperatively, it is important to monitor blood sugar levels in these patients carefully, avoiding both hypoglycemia and hyperglycemia. Hyperglycemia is more common, but I have been reluctant to use insulin in these patients unless their blood sugar exceeds 300 mg/dL. Ketosis is rare when the glucose level is below 300 mg/dL. It can be difficult to determine the correct insulin dose in these infants, thus creating the risk for significant hypoglycemia and permanent neurologic sequelae. In the postoperative period, reoperation is indicated if the infant remains hypoglycemic and requires significant amounts of intravenous glucose or significant pharmacologic management to maintain adequate blood sugar levels. I have preferred a 95% pancreatectomy in these circumstances. This involves the resection of most of the head of the pancreas, leaving a 0.5 to 1 cm rim of pancreas on the duodenum. Although it has been reported, it is rare to require further pancreatic resection as a third intervention.

FOLLOW-UP

Several recent publications have reviewed the results of a primary 95% pancreatectomy. Unfortunately, the long-term follow-up data have demonstrated that most if not all children who have undergone a 95% pancreatectomy are diabetic by 14 years of age. Many of these patients were found to be diabetic starting as early as 4 years of age. Thus, there has been a shift back to performing a 75% pancreatectomy. This was the recommendation made by Dr. Robert Gross more than 50 years ago. It remains my bias to continue to perform an approximate 85% pancreatectomy because this reduces the incidence of reoperation as well as the development of diabetes in the long term.

UNUSUAL PEPTIDE-SECRETING TUMORS OF THE PANCREAS

In addition to β cells, the islets of Langerhans contain α cells that secrete glucagon, δ cells that secrete somatostatin, and G cells that can secrete gastrin. Each of these cells has been the source of a benign or malignant tumor secreting their respective peptide. A tumor of the G cells (gastrinoma) is the only non–β cell pancreatic tumor that can present in the neonatal period. The presentation is that of gastric acid hypersecretion with secondary peptic ulceration. The excessive gastric hypersecretion also results in diarrhea, and this symptomatology is known as the Zollinger-Ellison syndrome. The diagnosis is made by determination of serum gastrin levels under a fasting state. Once a diagnosis is made, the difficult problem is identifying the site of the gastrinoma. Frequently, these tumors are within the pancreas. However, they also may be in the wall of the duodenum or jejunum. Because these tumors may be small (frequently <1 cm) they may be difficult to visualize by magnetic resonance imaging or computed tomography.

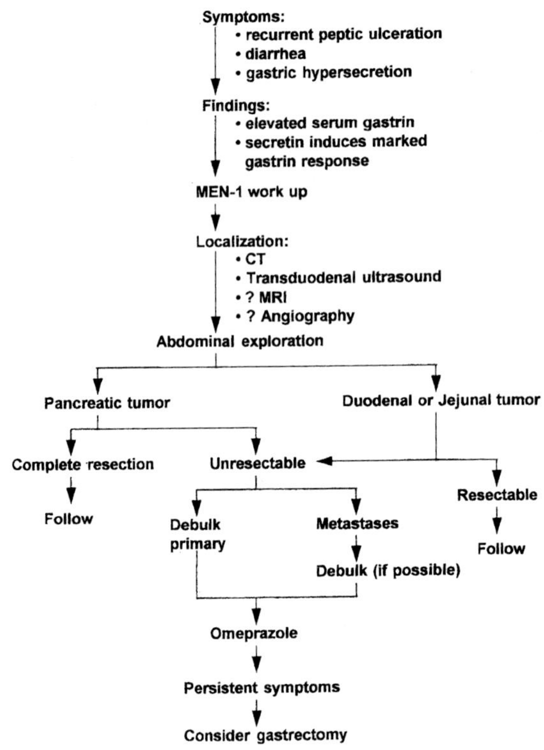

FIGURE 105.2. Workup and management of the child suspected of having a gastrinoma. (Reprinted from Schwartz MZ. Unusual peptide-secreting tumors in adolescents and children. *Semin Pediatr Surg* 1997;6:143; with permission.)

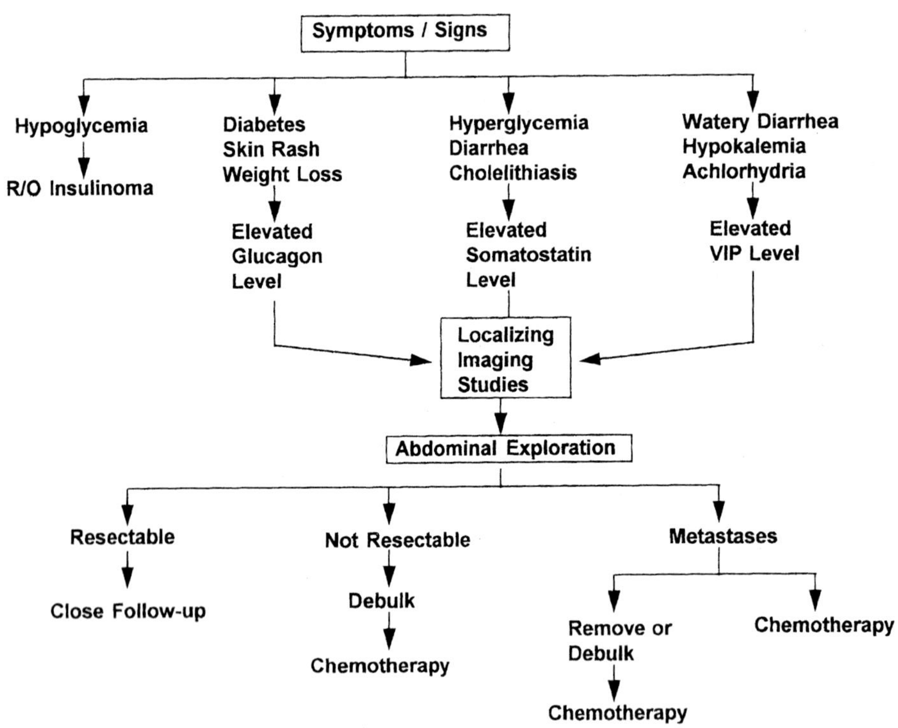

FIGURE 105.3. An algorithm using clinical presentation to help identify and treat some of the more common pediatric endocrine tumors of the pancreas. (Reprinted from Schwartz MZ. Unusual peptide-secreting tumors in adolescents and children. *Semin Pediatr Surg* 1997;6:142; with permission.)

The optimum treatment is resection of the tumor, which cures the hypersecretion (Fig. 105.2). Prior to the availability of agents that can significantly block acid secretion (histamine blockade, proton pump inhibition) the next step in management was subtotal or total gastrectomy to remove the source of the gastric hypersecretion. Because medical management can be effective in the absence of identifying the primary tumor, it is the treatment of choice at the present time, and major gastric resection should be avoided. A treatment algorithm that applies to the common endocrine tumors of the pancreas is depicted in Fig. 105.3.

In summary, although abnormalities of the endocrine portion of the pancreas are rare, they can be life threatening. The diagnosis can be made by identification of the hormone that is being hypersecreted. Prompt diagnosis and treatment are critical to a successful outcome.

SUGGESTED READINGS

Gross RE. *The surgery of infancy and childhood.* Philadelphia: WB Saunders, 1953:580–587.

Miyano T. The pancreas. In: O'Neill J, et al., eds. *Pediatric surgery, 5th ed.* St. Louis: CV Mosby, 1998:1535–1538.

Schwartz MZ. Unusual peptide secreting tumors in adolescents and children. *Semin Pediatr Surg* 1997;6:141–146.

Shilyansky J, Cutz E, Filler RM. Endogenous hyperinsulinism: diagnosis, management and long-term follow-up. *Semin Pediatr Surg* 1997;6:115–120.

Thomas CJ, Cuenca RE, Azizkhan RG, et al. Changing concepts of islet cell dysplasia in neonatal and infantile hyperinsulinism. *World J Surg* 1988;12:598–609.

106

SPLENECTOMY

MARK L. WULKAN

Splenectomy is performed for several hematologic and surgical conditions. The most common indication for splenectomy in children has shifted from trauma to hematologic disorders since nonoperative management of splenic trauma has become the standard of care. This chapter will be limited to the discussion of elective splenectomy, primarily for hematologic disorders.

DIAGNOSTIC APPROACH

The indications for splenectomy are related to the underlying disorder. In many hematologic disorders that require splenectomy, the primary symptom is splenic sequestration or destruction of red blood cells (e.g., hereditary spherocytosis) or platelets (e.g., idiopathic thrombocytopenic purpura). It is useful to consider the common disease entities individually.

All patients should be immunized against *Streptococcus pneumoniae*, *Neisseria meningitidis*, and *Haemophilus influenzae* prior to splenectomy to minimize the risk of postsplenectomy sepsis.

Hereditary Spherocytosis

Hereditary spherocytosis is an autosomal-dominant hemolytic anemia in which the red blood cells are trapped and destroyed in the spleen. Patients usually have chronic anemia that may require transfusion. Due to constant hemolysis, these patients also may have elevated bilirubin levels and develop bilirubinate gallstones. Hereditary spherocytosis is generally a chronic condition; however, patients may have acute crises that result in dramatic decreases in hematocrit. Crises are usually treated with transfusion. Splenectomy is the primary treatment of hereditary spherocytosis.

Splenectomy is usually deferred until the patient is at least 5 years old due to the risk of postsplenectomy sepsis. Occasionally, splenectomy may be necessary at a younger age due to high transfusion requirements and frequent crises. The risk:benefit ratio should be weighed on a case-by-case basis.

Idiopathic Thrombocytopenic Purpura

Idiopathic thrombocytopenic purpura (ITP) is an autoimmune cause of thrombocytopenia. Circulating antibodies bind to platelets that are destroyed in the spleen. Many patients (about 75%) undergo spontaneous remission after the acute episode. Chronic ITP is defined as persistent thrombocytopenia beyond 6 months. Many patients with chronic ITP are treated with steroids and intravenous γ globulin. Indications for surgery are failure of medical management with persistent thrombocytopenia.

Sickle Cell Disease

Occasionally we are asked to perform splenectomy for sickle cell disease and splenic sequestration. Splenic sequestration crisis is the most common indication for splenectomy in children with sickle cell disease. Splenectomy may be performed for either minor recurrent splenic sequestration crises or major splenic sequestration crises. Most patients are offered splenectomy after either two episodes of minor recurrent splenic sequestration or one episode of major splenic sequestration. Most of the patients have splenomegaly. This group of patients must be prepared for surgery with intravenous hydration and transfusion if necessary. The patients must be watched postoperatively for approximately 72 hours for acute chest syndrome, which can be life threatening. Aggressive mobilization, pain management, and pulmonary toilet are necessary to prevent acute chest syndrome. Sickle cell patients are monitored in the hospital on intravenous fluids for approximately 72 hours.

Other Hemoglobinopathies

Splenectomy also may be undertaken for other hemoglobinopathies, such as the thalassemias. A splenectomy is

M. L. Wulkan: Department of Surgery, Division of Pediatric Surgery, Emory Children's Center; and Department of Pediatric Surgery, Children's Healthcare of Atlanta at Egleston, Atlanta, Georgia.

indicated in these patients when their need for blood transfusion greatly increases, or when their reticulocyte count exceeds 10% consistently. Some of these children also may develop hypersplenism and massive splenomegaly.

Other Indications for Splenectomy

Other reasons for splenectomy include Gaucher's disease, which is an inherited lipoidosis. The disease is caused by a β-glucosidase deficiency. The splenectomy is indicated for hypersplenism. Other reasons for splenectomy include malignancy such as Hodgkin's disease, for which a staging laparotomy or laparoscopy may be performed. The indication for staging laparotomy or laparoscopy has been markedly reduced by the use of chemotherapy alone or in combination with radiation therapy as the primary treatment modality. Splenectomy also may be undertaken for other rare tumors of the spleen such as angiosarcoma or lymphomas. The general indications for splenectomy are symptoms of hypersplenism. Occasionally splenic abscess or splenic cysts may necessitate operations of the spleen. The most common type of cyst is a posttraumatic pseudocyst. These can be easily managed using laparoscopic techniques and unroofing the cyst.

TECHNIQUE

Splenectomy may be accomplished using either open or laparoscopic techniques. In general, most surgeons approach splenectomy using a minimally invasive philosophy. That is, either a small incision through which the spleen can be removed or laparoscopic methods. There are several studies suggesting that patients who undergo laparoscopic splenectomy have a shorter recovery time and less pain. They also have better cosmesis. The operative time is generally longer than with the open technique.

I prefer the laparoscopic technique for splenectomy. The patient is placed supine with a rolled sheet under the left side of the body. This sheet tilts the body approximately 30 degrees. This is done so that when the operating table is tilted to the left, the patient is essentially flat, and when the operating table is tilted to the right, the patient is in a lateral decubitus position (Fig. 106.1). A rolled sheet also may be placed in the position of a kidney rest on the right side to open the angle between the costal margin and the iliac crest. The operation is started with the patient in the flat position. A Veress needle is placed in the umbilicus, and the abdomen is insufflated. A 10-mm trocar is placed in the umbilicus. The remaining trocars are placed under direct visualization. If the patient has gallstones and the gallbladder needs to be removed, trocars are placed for that procedure at this time. The details of that procedure will not be covered in this chapter. For the splenectomy, a 5-mm trocar is placed in the left upper quadrant and a 3.5- or 5-mm trocar is placed in the midline approximately halfway between the xiphoid process and the umbilicus. These two ports constitute the working ports for the operating surgeon. A retractor port is placed either subxiphoid or at the left anterior axillary line at about the level of the costal margin. Occasionally, ports need to be placed in both locations for adequate retraction (Fig. 106.2). Generally, four trocars are used.

After the trocars are placed, the table is placed in the tilt right position so that the patient is now in a lateral decubitus position. The lateral attachments of the spleen provide stabilization of the spleen and allow gravity to retract the stomach and liver medially for exposure. The abdomen is explored for any accessory spleens in the omentum or the splenic hilum. If any are found, they may be removed easily. The dissection is begun at the inferior pole of the spleen where the gastrolienal ligament is divided with hook electrocautery. The dissection is continued up along the greater curvature of the stomach until all of the short gastric vessels are divided. We typically use hook electrocautery. The ultrasonic scalpel also may be used. Once the short gastric vessels are divided, attention is then directed to the splenic flexure. The lienocolic ligament is divided using electrocautery. At this point, the splenic hilum may be approached. If the surgeon desires, the splenic artery may be identified in the lesser sac and dissected free and clipped prior to approaching the hilum of the spleen. This may facilitate the splenic dissection as well as somewhat shrink a large spleen if venous drainage is allowed to continue.

The splenic hilum is then approached close to the spleen from inferior to superior. The vessels may be clipped, tied, or divided with the LigaSure (Valleylab, Boulder, CO) electrocautery device. Alternatively, the anterior and posterior aspect of the hilum may be dissected free so that an endoscopic vascular stapling device can be used to divide the hilum. Care is taken to protect the pancreas during this portion of the dissection. Once the hilum is divided, the lateral attachments of the spleen are taken down and the spleen should be completely free. A bag is then introduced into the abdomen. We have found that the easiest way to place the spleen in the bag is to move the spleen out of the left upper quadrant and place the bag in the left upper quadrant. Some irrigation fluid may be put in the bag to help stabilize it. The spleen is grasped by the hilar vessels and placed in the bag. Then the spleen is brought out piecemeal using an instrument fracture technique to remove the spleen through the umbilical incision.

Postoperative pain control is maintained with a combination of morphine injections or patient-controlled analgesia (PCA), acetaminophen, and ketorolac. The patients are started on a liquid diet the evening of surgery and advanced as tolerated to a regular diet. Most patients are discharged home on the first postoperative day.

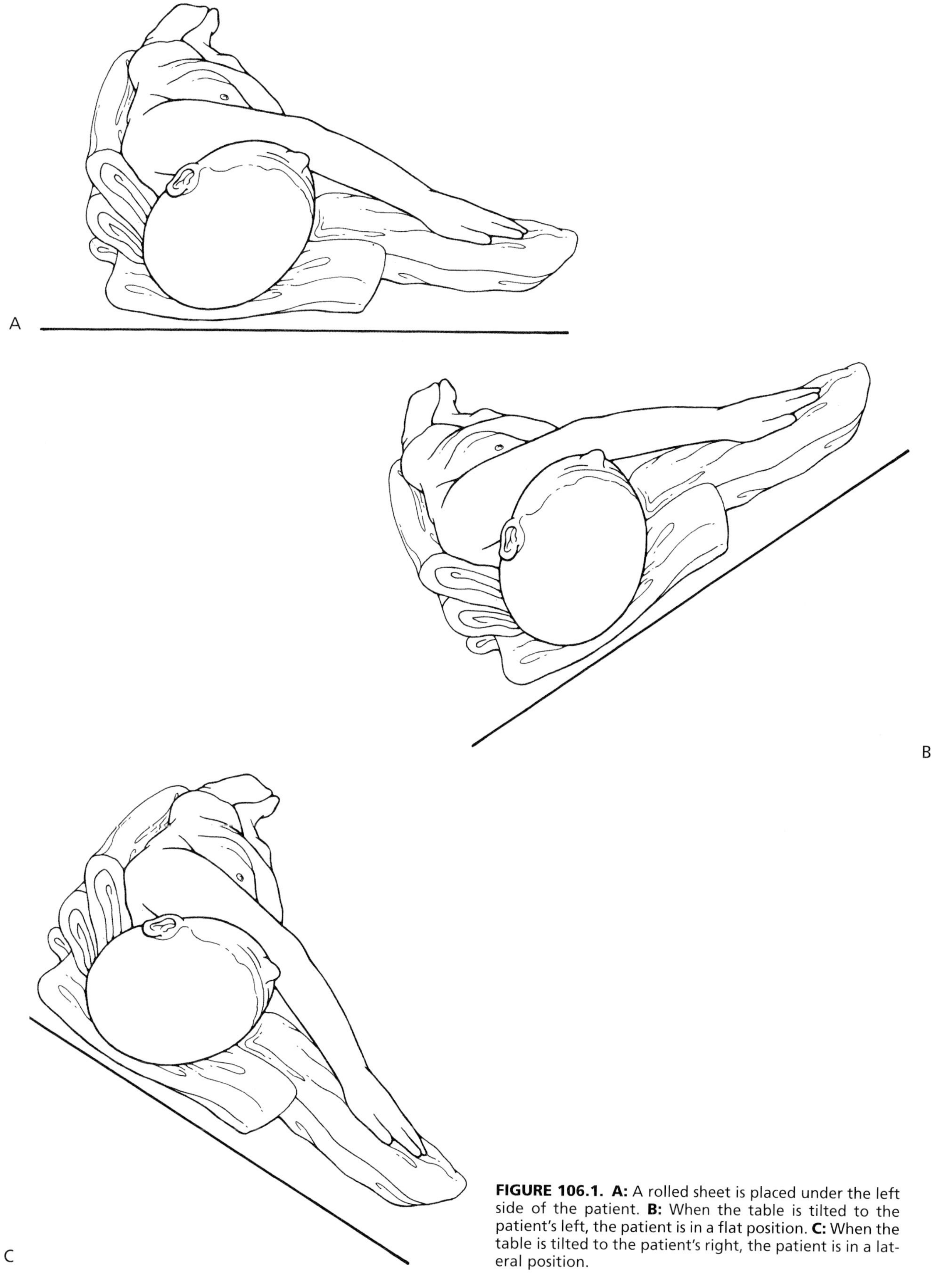

FIGURE 106.1. **A:** A rolled sheet is placed under the left side of the patient. **B:** When the table is tilted to the patient's left, the patient is in a flat position. **C:** When the table is tilted to the patient's right, the patient is in a lateral position.

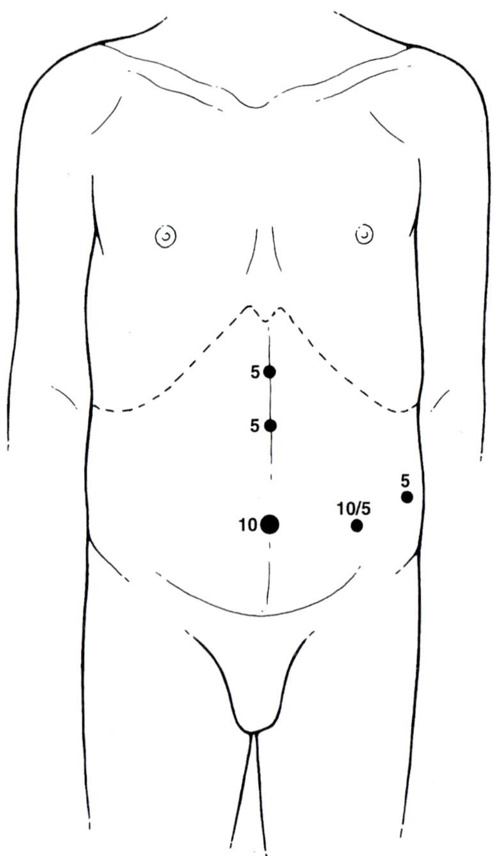

FIGURE 106.2. Location of primary and optional port sites for laparoscopic splenectomy.

PARTIAL SPLENECTOMY

Several surgeons have suggested that partial splenectomy is adequate to treat many hematologic diseases while reducing the risk of postsplenectomy sepsis. There is currently no long-term data to support this assertion. This technique has been reported primarily with an open technique.

POSTOPERATIVE CONSIDERATIONS

Splenectomy puts patients at risk for overwhelming postsplenectomy sepsis. The risk is increased with younger age. The most common organism responsible for postsplenectomy sepsis is *Streptococcus pneumoniae.* Other encapsulated organisms such as *Neisseria meningitidis* and *Haemophilus influenzae* are common causes of postsplenectomy sepsis. The remaining causes are other organisms such as gram-negative species. As stated earlier, all patients undergoing elective splenectomy should receive vaccination against *Streptococcus pneumoniae, Neisseria meningitidis,* and *Haemophilus influenzae.* Patients are also placed on long-term prophylactic penicillin. In addition, it is important to educate patients and their parents about postsplenectomy sepsis. Patients are instructed to seek medical attention at the onset of any febrile illness.

Postoperative thrombocytosis and leukocytosis are relatively common after splenectomy. The counts tend to peak between 1 to 2 weeks postsplenectomy. Treatment is rarely required in children.

EDITOR'S NOTES

In most centers, laparoscopic splenectomy is the standard of care for splenectomy in children. It can be performed safely even in small children, is associated with low morbidity and rapid recovery, and the cosmetic results are far superior to that of open splenectomy. Although open splenectomy can (and should, when necessary) be performed through a relatively small "flank" incision, the results cannot approach those of a procedure that uses three or four 5-mm incisions and one 1.5-cm incision, which is typical for most laparoscopic splenectomies.

There are few contraindications to a minimally invasive approach to splenectomy, and all are relative, depending on the experience and comfort level of the surgeon. Severe, uncorrectable coagulopathy, multiple prior laparotomies, a massively enlarged spleen, or a spleen that is suspected of being infiltrated by tumor are all considered contraindications to a laparoscopic approach.

The procedure itself is well described and outlined nicely in the chapter. It should be considered an advanced laparoscopic procedure and performed only by experienced laparoscopists. In most patients, four trocars are sufficient: three 3- or 5-mm incisions in the umbilicus and upper midline and one 12-mm port on the left side of the abdomen. In some cases, a fifth trocar is necessary. The harmonic scalpel can be used for most of the dissection, although a clip applier should be available in case of unexpected bleeding. Although many surgeons describe leaving some of the attachments of the spleen intact until after the hilum is divided, I find that complete mobilization of the spleen simplifies the hilar dissection and shortens the procedure. The mobilized spleen is easily lifted with two long instruments used as levers, one at the upper pole and one at the lower pole, while the stapling device is applied across the hilum. The spleen should always be placed in a plastic bag and removed by morcelation. The 15-mm stem of a large endoscopic bag device will usually fit easily through the incision made for the 12-mm trocar. The device is placed directly into the abdomen, without the use of a trocar and without having to enlarge the incision. Rupture of the bag can result in splenosis if the spleen is morcelated first and then aspirated. It may be preferable to remove the spleen by tearing off one piece at a time so that in case of bag rupture, the relatively intact spleen can be retrieved more easily.

Recovery is typically rapid, with most patients able to go home on the first postoperative day. Most patients can resume normal activities within a few days, unless persistent thrombocytopenia is a concern. Conversion to an open procedure should be uncommon; however, because the most common indication for conversion is bleeding, it is considered in most cases to be a mark of good judgment.

–P.M.

SUGGESTED READINGS

Curran TJ, Foley MI, Swanstrom LL, et al. Laparoscopy improves outcomes for pediatric splenectomy. *J Pediatr Surg* 1998;33:1498–1500.

Jugenburg M, Haddock G, Freedman MH, et al. The morbidity and mortality of pediatric splenectomy: does prophylaxis make a difference? *J Pediatr Surg* 1999;34:1064–1067.

Park A, Heniford BT, Hebra A, et al. Pediatric laparoscopic splenectomy. *Surg Endosc* 2000;14:527–531.

Rothenberg SS. Laparoscopic splenectomy in children. *Semin Laparosc Surg* 1998;5:19–24.

Schiller M. The spleen. In: O'Neill JA Jr, et al., eds. *Pediatric surgery, 5th ed. Vol. 2.* St. Louis: CV Mosby, 1998:1545–1554.

SECTION XI

TRANSPLANTATION

107

RENAL TRANSPLANTATION

PAUL M. COLOMBANI

Approximately 3 million children in the United States have end-stage renal disease (ESRD). There are many causes of ESRD in the pediatric age group. The majority of patients have one of the various forms of obstructive uropathy as the cause of their renal failure. Other common causes include hypoplastic/dysplastic kidney disease, hemolytic uremic syndrome, various glomerulonephritides, and variations of nephrotic syndrome. A more complete list of causes of renal failure in the pediatric age group is given in Table 107.1.

End-stage renal disease is defined as a glomerular filtration rate of less than 10 mL/min per 1.37 m^2 body surface area. The sequelae of ESRD in children are profound and include decreasing cognitive function, poor growth and development, and intractable electrolyte abnormalities. In the past, hemodialysis was the only available method for medically treating a patient with ESRD. Over the past 25 years, peritoneal dialysis has been used with success, even in small infants and others with a contraindication for hemodialysis. In addition, pediatric patients of any age are also now candidates for renal transplantation to treat their end-stage renal disease. Over the past 30 years, renal transplantation in the pediatric age group has gone from an experimental procedure, with a high risk for mortality and poor results, to the treatment of choice for pediatric patients with renal failure.

DIAGNOSTIC APPROACH

Most infants and children with end-stage renal disease are managed with peritoneal dialysis. Growth and development are monitored carefully and patients are observed frequently for the onset of complications related to their disease. The younger child who has failing growth may require a gastrostomy tube placement for nutritional support. In addition to growth failure, poor neurologic development, renal osteodystrophy, and delayed sexual maturation also may be indications for early transplantation. Pediatric patients who are referred for renal transplantation must undergo a vigorous evaluation process to determine suitability for transplantation. Table 107.2 summarizes the workup for a prospective transplant recipient. Patients should optimally reach a size greater than 10 kg in body weight, which usually means that the patients will be 2 to 3 years of age prior to transplantation, although patients who are failing peritoneal dialysis in early infancy also may undergo successful transplantation at a weight of less than 10 kg. The etiology of the renal failure must be identified and the risk of recurrence for certain diagnoses needs to be made known to the parents. Careful evaluation for systemic diseases and an assessment of cardiac and pulmonary function also should be performed.

Given the fact that the sequelae of urologic diseases account for approximately 60% of the pediatric age group with chronic renal failure, a careful genitourinary evaluation must be undertaken. This evaluation includes assessment of infection status, complete records of previous reconstructive surgeries, voiding cystourethrography to determine adequacy of the bladder, and cystometrics for patients who may have a neurogenic bladder. In addition, cystoscopy might be required to complete the urologic evaluation.

Patients who have untreated genitourinary abnormalities should undergo elective urinary reconstruction procedures as needed prior to transplantation. Patients with chronic infection should have aggressive medical management to treat and prevent ongoing urosepsis. Less than 1% of patients require bilateral native nephrectomy prior to transplantation. The most common indications for bilateral native nephrectomy are massive proteinuria from chronic nephrotic syndrome, persistent infection despite urinary reconstruction and urinary bacterial prophylaxis, and sustained and uncontrolled hypertension despite medical management. Finally, a complete psychosocial evaluation of the

P. M. Colombani: Department of Surgery, Johns Hopkins University School of Medicine; and Department of Pediatric Surgery, Johns Hopkins Hospital, Baltimore, Maryland.

TABLE 107.1. ETIOLOGIES OF PEDIATRIC END-STAGE RENAL DISEASE

Genitourinary system anomalies
Aplastic/hypoplastic dysplastic kidney
Obstructive uropathy
Reflux nephropathy
Obstructive uropathy
Medullary cystic disease
Polycystic kidney disease
Agenesis of abdominal musculature syndrome
Focal segmental glomerulosclerosis[a]
Systemic immunologic disease[a]
Chronic glomerulonephritis
Congenital nephrotic syndrome
Hemolytic uremic syndrome[a]
Cystinosis/oxalosis[a]
Pyelonephritis/interstitial nephritis
Familial nephritis[a]
Glomerulonephritis
Membranoproliferative types I and II[a]
Idiopathic crescentic[a]
Diabetic[a]
Renal infarct/cortical necrosis
Wilms tumor
DRASH syndrome
Nephropathy
Membranous[a]
Sickle cell[b]
AIDS[b]

[a]Risk of recurrence in the transplant kidney.
[b]Unknown recurrence risk.

patient and caregivers needs to be performed to determine if the family will be able to cope with the postoperative medical needs of the patient.

Following evaluation and suitable candidacy, patients are placed on the waiting list for cadaveric renal transplantation. Given the long waiting times for cadaveric renal transplantation, many patients have a parental related or nonrelated donor identified for transplantation. With the availability of laparoscopic live donor nephrectomy, an increasing number of donors are now willing to be evaluated for living donation. The marked decrease in postoperative pain, morbidity, and work loss has made significant changes in donor expectations and their willingness to donate.

TABLE 107.2. SELECTION CRITERIA: RECIPIENT EVALUATION

Complete history/physical
Age, weight
Etiology of end-stage renal disease (recurrence risk)
ABO blood group
HLA type/cross-match
Systemic illnesses/sepsis risk
Genitourinary tract evaluation
Psychosocial evaluation (compliance)

OPERATIVE APPROACH

At the time of transplantation, the patients are prepared for surgery with rapid intravenous hydration. A central venous catheter is placed and is used to monitor hydration status. A Foley catheter is placed in the bladder for drainage and, after 50 to 100 mL of antibiotic solution is instilled into the bladder, and the catheter is clamped. A "hockey stick" incision beginning in the midline just above the pubic ramus is made transversely and extended up superiorly along the edge of the rectus abdominis (Fig. 107.1A). In most cases, the common iliac artery and vein are used for the vascular anastomoses for the kidney. Because the left kidney is the most commonly donated live donor kidney (longer renal vein), a left-sided approach is preferable in most cases. The size of the recipient ultimately determines the site of the vascular anastomoses. The smaller the recipient, the more proximal the anastomoses are made. The vena cava and aorta may be used in the very small infant receiving an adult kidney.

In virtually all patients, an extraperitoneal approach can be made even for high vascular anastomoses using the vena cava and aorta. Following creation of the extraperitoneal pocket, the iliac vessels or distal vena cava and aorta are identified and dissected free from the surrounding lymphatic tissue, taking care to prevent injury to the femoral nerve (Fig. 107.1B). After adequate mobilization of the vessels at the appropriate level, the bladder is then identified for the ureteroneocystostomy. The patient is given intravenous heparin, and the vascular anastomoses are performed first. My preference is to perform the renal vein to iliac vein anastomosis first in an end-to-side fashion using a running 5-0 or 6-0 polypropylene suture. Following this, the renal artery is anastomosed end to side to the iliac artery using a 6-0 polypropylene suture. The kidney is then reperfused with release of the clamps and should begin to make urine within 5 minutes. It is important to have placed a central venous line at the time of transplantation to ensure adequate filling pressures. Prior to reperfusion, crystalloid (normal saline) and colloid (5% salt-poor albumin) should be used to raise central venous pressure above 10 to 12 cm H_2O and to maintain systolic blood pressure above 100 mm Hg. Pressors such as dopamine may be necessary.

Following adequate reperfusion and urine production, the ureteroneocystostomy is then performed (Fig. 107.1C). The typical scenario for many of these pediatric recipients is a history of multiple bladder surgeries and possibly reimplanted ureters or augmentation for an inadequate or neurogenic bladder. There are many variations of urinary reconstruction. The most common are the modified Leadbetter-Politano and modified Lich procedure. I prefer a modification of the Lich procedure, creating a nipple valve at the end of the ureter and placing it directly into the bladder through a stab wound in the muscle and mucosa. The nipple valve is anastomosed to the bladder mucosa, and the

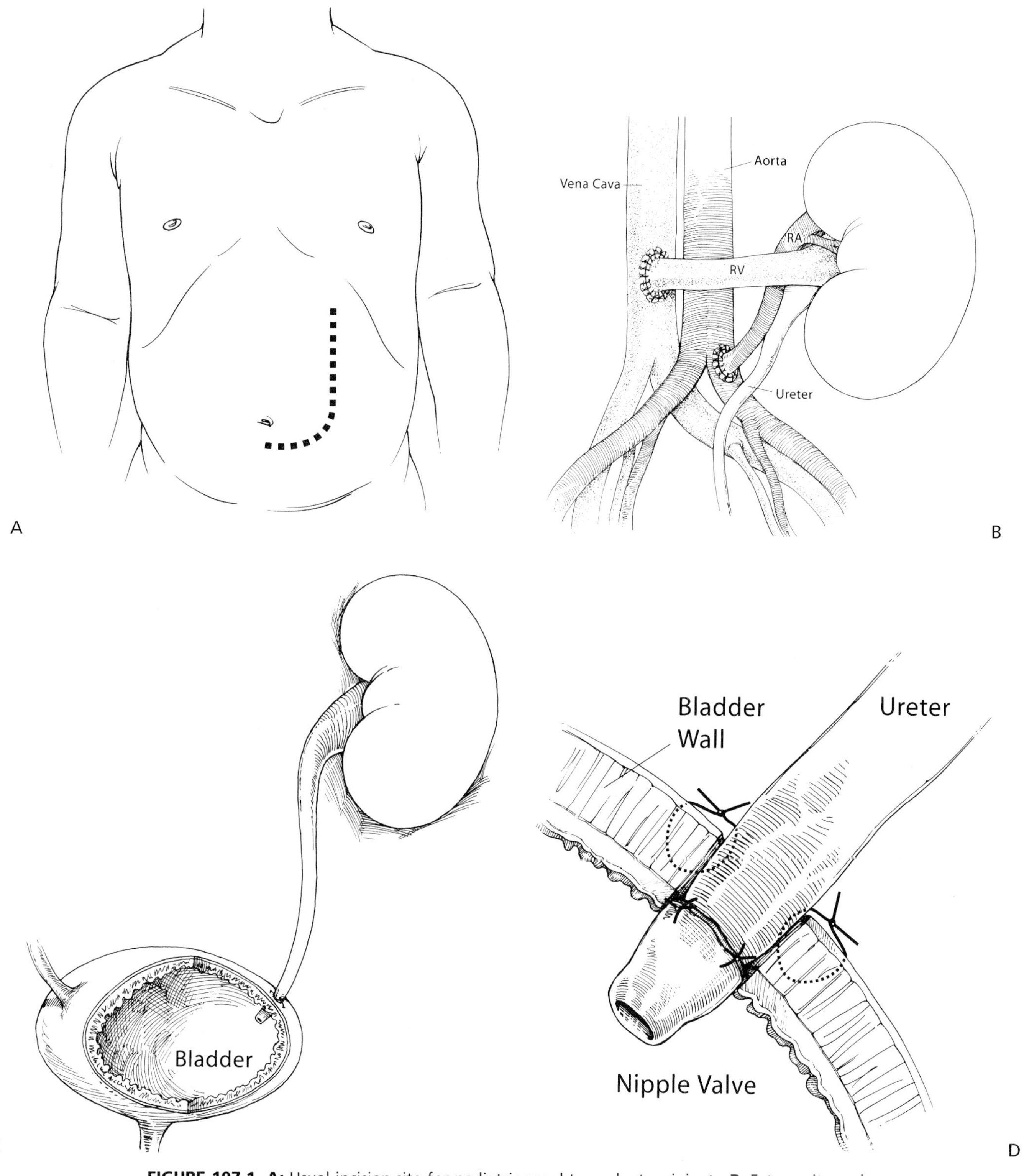

FIGURE 107.1. A: Usual incision site for pediatric renal transplant recipients. **B:** Extraperitoneal exposure of iliac vessels, distal aorta, and vena cava to facilitate vasular occlusion and anastomoses. **C:** Ureteroneocystostomy using modified Lich approach with incision down to bladder mucosa through detrusor muscle. **D:** Creation of nipple valve essentially eliminates vesicoureteral reflux and potential for pyelonephritis.

bladder muscle is closed around the ureter. The nipple valve provides for a nonrefluxing ureteroneocystostomy (Fig. 107.1D).

Following creation of the ureteroneocystostomy, hemostasis is achieved and the wound is closed in layers. If there is significant ooze secondary to the heparinization of the patient, then a drain may be placed to closed continuous suction.

POSTOPERATIVE COURSE

Postoperatively, the patients are taken to the intensive care unit, where their urine output is monitored hourly and central venous filling pressures and blood pressure are monitored continuously. Initial urine output is isosthenuric, presumably due to ischemia-reperfusion injury, and may be quite high. The urine output is initially replaced with intravenous fluids on a milliliter-per-milliliter basis plus insensible losses on an hourly basis. As renal function improves and the urine output comes down over the first few postoperative days, this replacement schedule is gradually tapered down to "maintenance" fluid requirements. Antibiotics are continued for several days, and a diet is started when the patient's ileus has resolved. The Foley catheter is removed when hourly urine output measurements are no longer required and the patient is sufficiently mobile, typically between the 3rd and 5th day. The remainder of the postoperative course is highly protocol driven and varies from program to program.

Immunosuppression regimens vary from institution to institution. Our routine is to use anti–interleukin 2 (IL-2) receptor antibody in the operating room along with a pulse of intravenous methylprednisolone. Postoperatively patients should have mycophenolate mofetil added to their regimen. Tacrolimus is withheld until good renal function is assured and the creatinine has decreased to less than 2.0 mg/dL. This quadruple therapy is continued with a short postoperative course of the anti–IL-2 receptor antibody and a tapering oral dose of methylprednisolone, as well as prednisone, tacrolimus, and mycophenolate mofetil (Table 107.3).

TABLE 107.3. IMMUNOSUPPRESSIVE DRUG PROTOCOLS

Initial and maintenance therapy
- Anti–IL-2 receptor antibody (diclazumab): 1 mg/kg i.v. on days 0, 14, 28
- Methylprednisolone: 10 mg/kg i.v. daily for 2 days, then taper 2 mg/kg every other day until 1 mg/kg/day; convert to oral methylprednisolone when feasible, slow taper down to 0.2–0.3 mg/day by 12 mo
- Mycophenolate mofetil: 600 mg/m^2 orally every 12 hours beginning on day 0
- Tacrolimus: 0.15 mg/kg orally every 12 hours when serum creatinine falls to <2.0 mg%; adjust dosage to maintain initial trough blood levels of 10 ng/kg/day

Rejection treatment
- Methylprednisolone pulse and taper (10 mg/kg/day i.v. and taper to 1 mg/kg/day)
- Steroid-resistant rejection
  - Rabbit antithymocyte globulin (thymoglobulin)
  - Horse antithymocyte globulin (ATGAM)
  - Anti-CD3 monoclonal antibody (orthoclone)

Alternative agents
- Azathioprine (Imuran): 1–2 mg/kg/day orally
- Cyclosporine (Neoral): 5 mg/kg orally every 12 hours; titrate to whole blood trough levels of 150–250 ng/mL
- Rapamycin (Rapamune): 3 mg/m^2 oral loading dose followed by 1 mg/m^2 daily

IL-2, interleukin 2; i.v., intravenously.

COMPLICATIONS

Postoperatively the patients are followed for complications and renal function is monitored. Very commonly in small infants and children, there may be a period of poor graft function attributable to acute tubular necrosis (ATN). This usually resolves over a number of days, and the kidney will begin to make urine and then clear creatinine. Rarely is there a permanent nonfunction of the kidney. This can occur after a very long cold ischemia time in a cadaveric transplant, or if a large kidney is placed into a small infant. Fortunately, this occurs in less than 1% of patients. ATN rates vary between 5% and 15% of patients.

Allograft rejection occurs in 10% and 20% of patients with the use of the anti–IL-2 receptor antibody and quadruple therapy. Most episodes of graft rejection are treated with a pulse and taper of corticosteroids as well as by increasing tacrolimus levels. Occasionally patients may require an antithymocyte preparation to treat steroid-resistant rejection. Graft thrombosis may occur in up to 10% of patients depending on their age and the etiology of their renal failure. There are some patients, for example, those with lupus nephritis or nephrotic syndrome, who may have a hypercoagulable state that makes them prone to vascular occlusion. Urologic complications also may occur. The major urologic complications include ureteral obstruction and stenosis, ureteral necrosis and extraperitoneal urine leak, or bladder fistula. These complications are usually treated with antegrade nephrostomy tube ureteral stenting. Stents are left in place for approximately 6 weeks to allow for healing of the collecting system. Rarely, necrosis of a significant portion of the ureter occurs, which would require reoperation and reconstruction. Minor urologic complications include recurrent urinary tract infections and recurrent pyelonephritis. With the use of a nonrefluxing ureteral anastomosis, the incidence of these complications is less than 1%. Table 107.4 summarizes these complications.

Pediatric patients are at significant risk for postoperative viral infections as well as posttransplant lymphoproliferative

TABLE 107.4. EARLY COMPLICATIONS OF RENAL TRANSPLANTATION

Acute tubular necrosis
Acute rejection
Vascular thrombosis
Hematoma
Wound infection
Urologic complications
  Urine leak
  Ureteral necrosis/stenosis
Lymphocele
Infection
  Bacterial
  Viral
  Protozoal
Hypertension
Metabolic disturbances
Recurrent disease

disorders. Viral prophylaxis regimens and prophylaxis for *Pneumocystis carinii* pneumonia are used in these patients for approximately 6 months. A cytomegalovirus (CMV) infection is particularly problematic and requires prophylaxis for CMV mismatch of patients (CMV-positive donor organ and CMV-negative recipient). Despite prophylaxis, CMV infection may occur and requires treatment with intravenous gancyclovir (Table 107.5). Posttransplantation lymphoproliferative disease can occur in patients who have a reactivation of Epstein-Barr virus (EBV) or a new EBV infection. Patients are initially treated with acyclovir therapy and γ-globulin but may also require withdrawal of immunosuppression. Patients who progress to a lymphoma-like process are treated with chemotherapy.

Patients also have a significant risk for recurrent disease with certain causes of their renal failure. These include Wilms' tumor, focal segmental glomerulosclerosis, nephrotic syndrome, lupus nephritis, hemolytic uremic syndrome, oxalosis, and cystinosis (Table 107.1).

TABLE 107.5. PROPHYLAXIS AND TREATMENT FOR OPPORTUNISTIC INFECTION

Prophylaxis
  CMV
    Cytogam (CMV immune globulin) 30–60 mg/kg/dose; begin 15 mg/kg/h, increase to 60 mg; maximum dose 150 mg/kg
  EBV
    Herpesvirus/varicella zoster virus
    Pneumocystis carinii
Treatment
  CMV
  EBV

CMV, cytomegalovirus; EBV, Epstein-Barr virus.

TABLE 107.6. LATE COMPLICATIONS OF RENAL TRANSPLANTATION

Allograft dysfunction
Chronic rejection
Recurrent disease
Malignancy
  Secondary malignancy (skin, colon, leukemia, lymphoma)
  Epstein-Barr virus–associated posttransplantation lymphoproliferative disease
Opportunistic infection (viral)

Over the long term, most patients should resume normal growth and development and maintain normal renal function. There are significant risks for graft loss over time. The most common reason for late graft loss or rejection is poor compliance. Patients also may develop chronic graft dysfunction or chronic rejection despite adequate immunosuppression. Table 107.6 outlines a number of late complications of renal transplantation and long-term immunosuppression. Patient and graft survival is lower than for adults, with the youngest patients having an approximately 5% lower graft survival rate. Overall, we expect 1-year graft survival to be approximately 85% to 90% in the pediatric age groups (<18 years of age), with patient survival approaching 100%. Five-year graft survival ranges from 45% to 70%, with some age and racial variation. Graft half-life in this age group is 10.1 years.

In summary, pediatric renal transplantation is the universally accepted treatment of choice for pediatric patients with end-stage renal disease. The new kidney should restore normal renal function and prevent the harmful effects of uremia on growth and development as well as neurologic and metabolic function. Overall, long term patient and graft survival is excellent in this age group

SUGGESTED READINGS

Cecka JM, Terasaki PI, eds. *Clinical transplants 2000.* Los Angeles: UCLA Immunogenetics Center, 2001.

Fernando Oswald N. Renal transplantation. In: Oldham KT, Mouriquand Pierre DE, Howard ER, eds. *Pediatric surgery and urology: long term outcomes.* London: WB Saunders, 1998:735–744.

Fine RN. Renal transplantation in children: current practices. In: Ginns LC, Cosimi AB, Morris PJ, eds. *Transplantation.* Malden, MA: Blackwell Science, 1998:312–323.

Ratner LE, Mongomery RA, Maley WR, et al. Laparoscopic live donor nephrectomy: the recipient. *Transplantation* 1998;69: 2319–2323.

Tejani AH, Fine RN, eds. *Pediatric renal transplantation.* New York: Wiley-Liss, 1994.

108

LIVER TRANSPLANTATION

ADELA T. CASAS-MELLEY
STEPHEN P. DUNN

Pediatric liver transplantation has made great strides in the past two decades and is now considered standard therapy for children with end-stage liver disease. We have come a long way from the first pediatric liver transplant performed by Starzl in 1963. With the introduction of cyclosporine in 1984, pediatric liver transplantation became a procedure with an acceptable survival rate. In fact, the survival rate increased from 19% to 65%. Improvements in immunosuppressive therapy as well as improvements in surgical techniques—including reduced-size, split-liver, and living related transplantation—have decreased the number of deaths while patients await transplantation, and the 1-year survival rate has increased to greater than 90%.

Despite these advances, we are still hampered by increasing organ shortages. The number of patients on transplant waiting lists, both pediatric and adult, is increasing at a rate faster than we are able to perform transplantations. The waiting time is increasing, and the number of patients dying while waiting is again increasing. This has led to the development of adult-to-adult living related transplants as well as the use of nonrelated donor transplants.

PATIENT SELECTION

The indications for liver transplantation have expanded as the success of liver transplantation has improved. Advanced liver disease is diagnosed in 1 of 20,000 pediatric patients. One thousand pediatric patients are listed and 500 pediatric transplants are performed each year. The diagnoses leading to liver transplantation in the pediatric population have not changed. Children with biliary atresia account for more than half of the patients undergoing transplantation. The other diagnoses can be separated into the following categories: neonatal cholestasis, metabolic, fulminant hepatic failure, hepatitis, cirrhosis, and tumor (Table 108.1).

Indications

The complications and its prognosis of the liver disease establish the timing for liver transplantation. Complications of portal hypertension leading to bleeding from esophageal or gastric varices is a common occurrence in pediatric patients, and can sometimes tip the balance between stable liver disease and acute deterioration necessitating emergent liver transplantation. Children with complications of portal hypertension are immediately considered for transplantation. Attempts are made to manage bleeding medically with obliterative techniques, such as sclerosant injections and banding, and, in some instances, emergent shunting with a transjugular intrahepatic portosystemic shunt. Transplantation is performed when a suitable donor can be identified. Ascites is managed medically with salt restriction and diuretics. When ascites leads to spontaneous bacterial peritonitis, poor feeding, failure to thrive, or respiratory compromise, transplantation is indicated. Persistent cholestasis (bilirubin level >10 mg/dL), decreased synthetic function leading to falling serum albumin level or elevated prothrombin time, uncontrollable pruritis, and recurrent episodes of cholangitis are all indications for transplantation. One indication for transplantation that cannot be forgotten in the pediatric population is growth failure. If a patient fails to respond to an aggressive feeding program, or develops severe vitamin deficiencies, he or she should be considered for early transplantation. Hepatic malignancies, confined to the liver, also may be treated successfully with hepatic transplantation in certain cases.

Contraindications

Few contraindications to liver transplantation still remain. Extrahepatic malignancy or malignancy metastatic to the liver are absolute contraindications to transplantation. We still consider human immunodeficiency virus (HIV)-posi-

A. T. Casas-Melley: Department of Surgery, Thomas Jefferson University, Philadelphia, Pennsylvania; and Department of Surgery, Division of Solid Organ Transplantation, Alfred I. duPont Hospital for Children, Wilmington, Delaware.

S. P. Dunn: Departments of Surgery and Pediatrics, Thomas Jefferson University, Philadelphia, Pennsylvania; and Department of Surgery, Alfred I. duPont Hospital for Children, Wilmington, Delaware.

TABLE 108.1. INDICATIONS FOR LIVER TRANSPLANTATION

Cholestatic
Biliary atresia
Alagille syndrome
Nonsyndromic biliary hypoplasia
Byler syndrome
Metabolic
α_1-Antitrypsin deficiency
Tyrosinemia
Wilson disease
Hemochromatosis
Cystic fibrosis
Glycogen storage disease
Familial hypercholesterolemia
Hyperoxyluria
Fulminant hepatic failure
Wilson disease
Drug induced
Viral hepatitis
Hepatitis
Neonatal hepatitis
Chronic active hepatitis
Autoimmune
Cirrhosis
Cryptogenic
Tumor
Hepatoblastoma
Hemangioendothelioma

TABLE 108.2. RECIPIENT EVALUATION

History and physical examination
Laboratory test
ABO type
Comprehensive panel
Complete blood cell count
Clotting studies
Urinalysis
Epstein-Barr virus titer
Cytomegalovirus titer
Human immunodeficiency virus
Hepatitis panel
Tissue typing
Purified protein derivative (of tuberculin)
Chest radiograph
Electrocardiogram
Hepatic ultrasonography (to include Doppler flow of vessels)
Dental examination
Immunization update
Consultations
Renal
Cardiology
Social work
Neurology
Pulmonary
Ophthalmology
Audiology
Liver biopsy

tive status to be a contraindication, although several centers in the United States are performing transplantations in adult patients with HIV. Irreversible encephalopathy from advanced liver disease is an absolute contraindication, and determination of the neurologic status of the patient is necessary prior to proceeding with transplantation. Uncontrolled extrahepatic sepsis has been previously used as a contraindication to transplantation; however, we have found that if the patient's source of sepsis is identified and treatment is begun prior to transplantation, the placement of a functioning graft actually improves his or her outcome. This does not seem to extend to fungal sepsis, and we have not been willing to perform transplantation on patients until their fungal disease has been controlled.

EVALUATION

Recipient

The evaluation of potential liver transplant recipients includes a multidisciplinary approach and thorough physical and laboratory evaluations (Table 108.2). The evaluation is used to confirm primary liver disease as well as to establish the presence of extrahepatic manifestations of disease such as portal hypertension and growth failure. Once contraindications to transplantation are excluded, the patient's medical management should be maximized. The medical team should optimize caloric intake, add fat-soluble vitamins, and accelerate their immunization schedule. Recipients are placed on the liver transplant list as soon as they are determined to be candidates. Patients are listed according to ABO blood group, body weight, and acuity of disease. At evaluation, information regarding living related donation is provided to the family. If the family members wish to proceed with evaluation, the appropriate referrals are made.

Living Related Donor

Living related donor evaluations are performed on an outpatient basis. Initially, a family conference is convened to discuss risks and benefits of the procedure with the transplant team. Issues related to postoperative recovery and return to work are discussed. If the donor wishes to proceed, ABO blood typing is performed to identify blood type–compatible donors. The evaluation includes a history and physical examination with an adult hepatologist, psychiatric evaluation, laboratory evaluation, volumetric computed tomography (CT) to determine size of the potential donor segment, and hepatic arteriogram to determine vascular anatomy. Some centers are now substituting magnetic resonance arteriography for the more invasive arteriographic procedure. This evaluation is performed in a stepwise fashion from least invasive to most invasive. The potential donor would have to pass blood tests and physical

TABLE 108.3. DONOR EVALUATION

History and physical by adult hepatologist
Psychiatry evaluation
Laboratory evaluation (same as recipient)
Chest radiograph
Electrocardiogram
Computed tomography scan to determine graft volume
Hepatic arteriogram

examination requirements prior to proceeding with CT and arteriography. In the case of a patient with acute liver failure, this donor evaluation could be completed in 6 to 8 hours, and donation could potentially occur on the same day. At this point we are not accepting organs from living donors over 50 years of age (Table 108.3).

Cadaveric Donor

Assessment of the donor organ is performed by evaluating patient history and laboratory data. Factors such as donor age, length of hospitalization, cause of death, hemodynamic stability, serology results, electrolyte data, and liver functions are evaluated. There are several factors that make a donor high risk. These include past medical history suggestive of alcohol or drug abuse, especially intravenous drug abuse. The longer the donor has been in the hospital, the more likely he or she is to develop infectious complications. Hemodynamic instability requiring pressor support or anemia leading to hypotension and massive blood transfusion make the donor organ more susceptible to injury and to the possibility of organ primary nonfunction or dysfunction. Hypernatremia is a marker for donor instability and correlates with primary liver nonfunction. We do not use organs from donors over 55 years of age unless the recipient is likely not to survive until another donor becomes available. We evaluate electrolytes and liver functions carefully. If the hypernatremia is corrected and liver functions improve with resuscitation, we will consider the donor and evaluate the organ. Liver biopsy performed at recovery to evaluate for fatty infiltration has been useful in excluding donor organs with a high risk for primary nonfunction. If the fatty infiltration is less than 30%, we would recover and use the organ. We do not accept organs with positive hepatitis serology.

OPERATIVE MANAGEMENT

In pediatric patients there are several options for transplantation. All of our patients receive orthotopic transplants. Depending on the recipient size, we either use a whole-organ transplant or split the liver to accommodate patient size. We do our liver splitting *in situ*. We cut down the liver into a left lateral segment for a small child and use the remaining liver for a larger size child. *In situ* splitting decreases cold ischemic time and is associated with good graft function. Of course, a living related donor is always an option for a smaller child and even for a larger child using the right lobe of the donor. We regularly reevaluate the risk of waiting for a cadaveric donor. If a donor does not become available, or the chances of a donor becoming available before the child develops complications is unlikely, we meet with the family to review the possibility of living donation. We have performed over 40 living related donor transplants using the left lateral segment or right lobe with minimal morbidity and no mortality in our donors.

Donor Operation

All cadaveric organ retrieval operations begin in a similar fashion. In most instances, a midline incision is made from the sternal notch to the pubic bone. The chest is opened with a sternotomy. The abdomen is opened, and visualization of the liver is made. If there is concern regarding fatty infiltration, a biopsy is performed. Both triangular ligaments are mobilized. The porta hepatis is dissected to visualize the common bile duct, hepatic artery, and portal vein. The common bile duct is divided near the head of the pancreas. The gallbladder is opened and the biliary tree is flushed free of bile with saline. If the liver is to be split, the left hepatic vein is dissected to allow division at its branch point. The left branches of the hepatic artery and portal vein are identified and looped. Collateral vessels to the portal vein are identified, ligated, and divided. The parenchyma is then divided along the falciform ligament. Several methods can be used to accomplish the parenchymal dissection. We have recently been using the harmonic scalpel with good success. Care is taken to divide the bile duct to segments II and III. The duct, or in some cases two ducts, are found posterior and superior to the portal vein. The ducts are divided with a scalpel to minimize ductal injury.

Once the parenchyma is divided and the only connections remaining are the vessels, the donor is prepared for organ perfusion. The superior mesenteric vein is dissected and a cannula is inserted for portal perfusion. Heparin is administered systemically. The distal aorta is dissected and a cannula is inserted for the aortic flush. If the heart is harvested, the blood is vented into the abdomen via the distal vena cava and the aorta is clamped in the suprahepatic region. If there is no cardiac harvest, the aorta is clamped in the chest and the atrium is used to vent the blood into the thoracic cavity. The organs are flushed with University of Wisconsin solution, which gives us an 18- to 24-hour cold preservation time. Once the flushing is finished, the liver dissection is completed and the organ is retrieved.

If the liver is being split, the left lateral segment is removed by transecting the already dissected vessels at the takeoff of the left hepatic artery and left portal vein. The left hepatic vein is taken at the suprahepatic cava junction. Repair of the remaining vessels can be performed on the back table. The previously transected bile duct on the right lobe is repaired at the time of transection *in situ* to prevent a postoperative bile leak. The remaining liver is then removed, transecting the portal vein at the pancreas, dissecting the hepatic artery, dividing the splenic and gastroduodenal arteries and recovering the celiac axis down to the aorta, transecting the inferior vena cava above the renal veins, and taking a patch of diaphragm around the suprahepatic cava. The procedure for removal of a whole organ is similar to that done for the remaining liver after removal of the left lateral segment graft.

Living Related Donor

The donors are given the choice of epidural placement for postoperative pain. Compression stockings are placed immediately after induction of anesthesia. Large-bore peripheral venous access is established. The procedure is performed via a transverse incision with a midline extension. The left triangular ligament is mobilized and the left hepatic vein is identified. The procedure is the same as described above for *in situ* organ splitting. However, after the vessels have been dissected and the parenchyma has been divided, the donor is given 50 U/kg of heparin. The vessels are then clamped and the left lateral segment is removed. The segment is then perfused with cold University of Wisconsin solution on the back table until the flush return is clear of blood. During this time a second surgeon is repairing the vessels of the donor. The hepatic vein, the hepatic artery, and portal vein orifice are closed and the clamps removed. The bile duct opening is repaired at the time of the bile duct transection. Once there is no evidence of bleeding, a drain is placed at the site of the parenchymal dissection and the abdomen is closed. Patients are extubated postoperatively and monitored overnight in the intensive care unit. They are transferred to the ward on the first postoperative day. They are usually tolerating a regular diet by the third postoperative day and are discharged by postoperative day 6.

Recipient Operation

Hepatectomy

There is a great deal of preparation of the recipient prior to the beginning of surgery. Central venous access must be obtained. We use two arterial lines: one for continuous monitoring and a second for multiple intraoperative blood sampling. Two large-bore peripheral venous catheters are placed. The patient is then prepared and draped and the hepatectomy is begun. This portion of the procedure can be very active. There is usually significant blood loss due to portal hypertension and adhesions from previous abdominal surgery. The abdomen is entered via a bilateral subcostal incision. A midline extension may be added to increase exposure. The triangular ligaments are mobilized. The hepatic veins are identified. The porta is then dissected, identifying the old Roux-en-Y from a previous Kasai procedure or the common bile duct. The common bile duct is ligated close to the liver and transected. If an old Roux-en-Y is present, it is transected with a GIA stapler and salvaged for later use. The hepatic artery and portal vein are dissected and looped. The cava is then dissected. If a whole organ is going to be used, the retrohepatic cava can usually be sacrificed. We have found that most children tolerate caval clamping if they have significant portal hypertension. Therefore, we have not needed to use venous bypass in our children. However, for those children who do not tolerate clamping, we have been able to spare the cava by dividing the small tributaries to the liver, keeping the retrohepatic cava intact and only partially clamping the cava. In some patients, it is necessary to place a temporary portocaval shunt to prevent mesenteric congestion due to the acute portal hypertension caused by portal occlusion in the anhepatic state. These children are usually identified by immediate swelling of the pancreas and small bowel and hemodynamic instability. A temporary shunt can be placed quickly and alleviates the need for venous bypass. If a left lateral segment is being used, the vena cava has to be salvaged as previously described.

Anhepatic Phase

During this time the new graft is sewn into place. The graft is prepared on the back table prior to or during the hepatectomy. If a whole graft is used, the suprahepatic anastomosis is completed first. We do the anastomosis in a running fashion using prolene suture. We prepare the cava in a triangular fashion, with a stitch at each end and one in the middle of the lower edge of the cava. This keeps the anastomosis open and easy to visualize. The infrahepatic caval anastomosis is then performed in a similar fashion. Prior to completion of the anastomosis, the graft is flushed with cold 5% albumin via the portal vein with the flush vented through the infrahepatic caval anastomosis. We use 500 mL for whole grafts and 250 mL for left lateral segments. The infrahepatic anastomosis is then completed. The portal vein anastomosis is then performed, setting up the anastomosis in a triangular fashion and completing it with running suture. Care is taken not to purse-string the anastomosis. Prior to completing the anastomosis, a "growth factor" is left in the portal vein suture. This loop of loose suture is undersewn with a single suture to prevent excess bleeding. The anesthesia personnel is informed that we are ready to remove the clamps so they may prepare the patient with volume, calcium, and bicarbonate solution.

Reperfusion Phase

The suprahepatic, infrahepatic, and portal vein clamps are then removed and the organ is reperfused. Warm saline is used to warm the liver. The anastomosis are then visualized for areas of bleeding, and these are repaired as needed. Once bleeding is controlled, the hepatic artery anastomosis is begun. The donor hepatic artery is flushed with heparinized saline (10 U/mL) and clamped with a small plastic bulldog clamp to prevent back bleeding. We use the donor common hepatic artery to the recipient proper hepatic artery when feasible. If this vessel is less than 3 mm, we dissect the hepatic artery to its junction with the splenic artery and use the confluence of the two vessels for the anastomosis. The anastomosis is performed under a magnification of 2.5 or higher. We use a running suture of polypropylene. Generally, this anastomosis is 3 or 4 mm in diameter. When the anastomosis is completed, the graft is completely vascularized. We then proceed with the bowel preparation for the biliary anastomosis. We rarely use a duct-to-duct anastomosis. We have found that they are usually a high-resistance anastomosis postoperatively and tend to have slower clearance of cholestasis. In children with a short bowel length, a duct-to-duct anastomosis is preferred. In these cases a small silicone elastomer stent is passed through the recipient bile duct into the duodenum to allow for continuous biliary drainage. This is then removed endoscopically a few weeks after transplantation. A Roux-en-Y is performed in the usual way and the bile duct is sewn to the jejunum in an end-to-side fashion. We use a stent during execution of the anastomosis but remove it prior to the completion of the operation. We use interrupted absorbable suture (PDS). The abdomen is then irrigated with copious amounts of saline irrigation. Closed-suction drains are placed in the region of the suprahepatic anastomosis, the biliary anastomosis, and the retrohepatic space, and the abdomen is closed.

Left Lateral Segment

When a left lateral segment is used, the left hepatic vein is sewn to the opening of the recipient hepatic veins in a "piggy-back" fashion. The hepatic veins are triangulated, as previously described, and a running suture is used. Prior to completion of the anastomosis, the graft is flushed via the portal vein with 250 mL of cold 5% albumin. The anastomosis is completed. The procedure then continues similarly with completion of the portal vein anastomosis, reperfusion of the graft, completion of the arterial anastomosis, and Roux-en-Y biliary reconstruction (Fig. 108.1). We have not found it necessary to use vein graft for our anastomosis. We rotate the graft 180 degrees around the long axis of the body from its normal anatomic position and find that it makes the anastomosis easier to perform. The graft fits into the right upper quadrant with minimal mobility postoperatively.

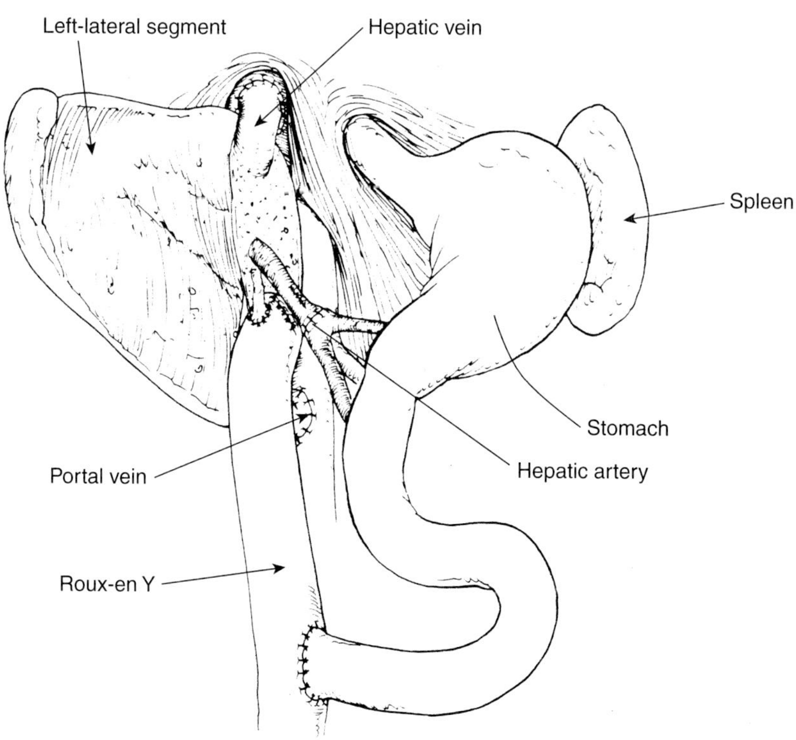

FIGURE 108.1. Left lateral segment in "the flop" position.

IMMUNOSUPPRESSION

We use cyclosporine-based therapy for younger children who are Epstein-Barr virus (EBV) negative at the time of transplantation. In older children, particularly teenagers, we tend to use tacrolimus-based therapy. Our protocol uses a combination of drugs that includes basiliximab, prednisone, and a calcineurin inhibitor. In patients using cyclosporine, we tend to add azathioprine. Immunosuppressive treatment is individualized to the patient, and we change from cyclosporine to tacrolimus if the patient has a significant acute rejection episode, a steroid-resistant rejection episode, or difficulty with attaining an adequate level of cyclosporine due to absorption complications (Table 108.4). Conversion from tacrolimus to cyclosporine is indicated for those children developing hyperglycemia.

COMPLICATIONS

Graft Dysfunction

Graft dysfunction is the most life-threatening complication of liver transplantation. Laboratory values are measured at 12-hour intervals postoperatively. The liver functions can increase for the first 24 hours after surgery from reperfusion injury; however, they should not be increasing exponentially. If the liver functions are doubling every 12 hours, primary nonfunction or dysfunction of the graft should immediately be considered. Graft nonfunction requires emergent retransplantation for patient survival. These patients usually develop severe metabolic derangements and renal failure and are at risk for developing cerebral edema and neurologic damage if transplantation is not performed quickly.

TABLE 108.4. IMMUNOSUPPRESSION THERAPY

Medication	Dosage
Cyclosporine (Neoral)	12–20 mg/kg/day given twice daily Peak levels 2 h postdose 0–3 mo 1,000–1,200 ng/mL 3–6 mo 800–1,000 ng/mL >6 mo 600 ng/mL
Tacrolimus (FK506)	0.2–0.3 mg/kg/day given twice daily Trough levels 0–1 mo 15–20 ng/mL 2–12 mo 10–15 ng/mL >12 mo 5–10 ng/mL
Basiliximab (Simulect)	Patient weight <40 kg, 10 mg i.v. given on days 1 and 4 Patient weight >40 kg, 20 mg i.v. given on days 1 and 4
Azathioprine (Imuran)	1–2 mg/kg/day for 1 yr Hold for WBC count of <5
Methylprednisolone	In operating room 10 mg/kg Day 1, 5 mg/kg Day 2, 4 mg/kg Day 3, 3 mg/kg Day 4, 2 mg/kg Day 5, 1 mg/kg of oral prednisone Wean at 0.2 mg/kg every month until dose 0.2 mg/kg Go to 0.2 mg/kg every other day for 2 mo Discontinue steroids

i.v., intravenously.

Vascular Occlusion

Within the first 24 hours the patient should undergo Doppler ultrasonography to evaluate the patency of the vascular anastomoses. The hepatic artery and portal vein can both develop occlusion immediately postoperatively. Both of these complications require immediate return to the operating room for repair. They usually require declotting and reanastomosis at a more proximal site. Vascular occlusion can lead to early or late biliary complication due to ischemic necrosis of the biliary tree. Patients who develop vascular thrombosis have a higher incidence of bile leaks as well as biliary strictures that require stenting or surgical repair.

Biliary Tract

Bile leaks can occur early after transplantation. They are more common in cut-down livers or living related liver transplants, and are usually from the cut edge of the liver or from missed accessory ducts not seen at the time of surgery. Small leaks in a single drain may be safely watched. Confirmation by hepatobiliary nuclear scanning may be useful and can also evaluate the extent of the leak. Bile leaks can usually require a return to surgery but are usually repaired easily. Bile leaks can become infected and lead to sepsis. Observation of a bile leak must be based on evidence that it is small and well drained.

Rejection

Acute rejection episodes are relatively common early after transplantation, occurring in nearly half of cases. Most episodes are easily managed with increased immunosuppression. Since the addition of interleukin-2 receptor antibody preparations such as daclizumab or basiliximab, the need for the use of OKT3 antibody therapy has decreased significantly. Most episodes are managed with pulse steroids. Early rejection is usually identified by elevation of liver enzymes. Low-grade temperature is not unusual. Because of the similarity in symptoms between rejection and infection, both bacterial and viral, in the early postoperative period, we do not treat the patients until the results of a biopsy are available (Table 108.5).

TABLE 108.5. REJECTION THERAPY

Medication	Dosage
Methylprednisolone pulse	10 mg/kg i.v. for 2 days 5 mg/kg i.v. on day 3 Wean to 1 mg/kg oral prednisone Wean off over 2 wk
Anti-CD3 monoclonal antibody (OKT3)	2.5–5 mg i.v. every day for 7–14 days
Cyclosporine (Neoral)	Adjust to therapeutic range
Tacrolimus (FK506)	Adjust to therapeutic range

i.v., intravenously.

LONG-TERM COMPLICATIONS

Chronic Rejection

A small percentage of patients develop evidence of chronic rejection. These patients develop chronically elevated liver enzymes and on biopsy have evidence of bridging fibrosis and loss of bile ducts. Recent pharmakokinetic studies suggest that inadequate absorption of cyclosporine has contributed to this problem. Children or parents of children who are chronically noncompliant with their immunosuppressant medications are also of significant concern. Chronic rejection usually requires retransplantation.

Biliary Strictures

Cholangitis from biliary strictures and stone formation can occur late after transplantation. This can sometimes develop due to a rejection episode or from a history of hepatic artery thrombosis. Some centers have had success with biliary stenting. We have had better results with surgical repair of the stricture, if the stricture is amenable to surgery. For those that are intrahepatic, we have used transhepatic stent placement. We avoid Palmerez stenting of biliary strictures. Some patients with repeating episodes of cholangitis from intrahepatic strictures require retransplantation.

Posttransplantation Lymphoproliferative Disease

Posttransplantation lymphoproliferative disease (PTLD) is a potentially fatal complication of long-term immunosuppression. Patients present with fever, lymphadenopathy, and hepatosplenomegaly. It seems to correlate with the total exposure to immunosuppression. Patients who have required multiple pulses of steroids, treatment with monoclonal antibodies, or high-dose cyclosporine or tacrolimus tend to have a higher incidence of PTLD. PTLD is almost always associated with EBV infection. Patients develop abnormal proliferation of B-cell lymphocytes that may lead to monomorphic, monoclonal lymphomas. Treatment consists of decreased immunosuppression and supportive measures. Recently there have been attempts at treatment with antibodies directed toward markers on the cell surface of the B cells with some success. EBV polymerase chain reaction (PCR) titers can be measured in patients to determine when they might be exposed or have active EBV infections; however, PTLD may develop in patients irrespective of EBV PCR titers.

SUMMARY

Pediatric liver transplantation has made great strides in the past two decades. The development of better immunosuppressive medications, better monitoring, and better surgical technique have all come together to improve survival. We still have many areas of research left in order to improve medications and attempt to diminish long-term complications of immunosuppression. However, if we progress at the rate of the past decade, we have much to look forward to in the next few years.

SUGGESTED READINGS

Colombani PM, Cigarroa FG, Schwartz K, et al. Liver transplantation in infants younger than 1 year of age. *Ann Surg* 1996; 223:658.

Malatack J, Schaid DJ, Urbach AH, et al. Choosing a pediatric recipient for orthotopic liver transplantation. *J Pediatr* 1987;111:479.

Marcos A, Fisher RA, Ham JM, et al. Right lobe living donor liver transplantation. *Transplantation* 1999;68:798.

Sokal EM, Caragiozoglou T, Lamy M, et al. Epstein-Barr virus serology and Epstein-Barr virus–associated lymphoproliferative disorder in pediatric liver transplant recipients. *Transplantation* 1993; 56:1294.

Starzl TE, et al. Evolution of liver transplantation. *Hepatology* 1982;2: 614.

Starzl TE, Iwatsuki S, Malatack JJ, et al. Liver and kidney transplantation in children under cyclosporine A and steroids. *J Pediatr* 1982;100:681–686.

Starzl TE, Marchioro TL, Von Kaulla KN, et al. Homotransplantation of the liver in humans. *Surg Gynecol Obstet* 1963;117: 659–676.

Tanaka K, Uemoto S, Tokunaga Y, et al. Surgical techniques and innovations in living related liver transplantation. *Ann Surg* 1993; 217:82.

UNOS Update. 1995;2:54.

SECTION

XII

SURGICAL ONCOLOGY

109

NEUROBLASTOMA

EDWARD M. BARKSDALE, JR.
ALA STANFORD

Neuroblastoma is the most common abdominal malignancy in children. These tumors arise from the aberrant migration and differentiation of neural crest cells destined to form the sympathetic ganglia. During their cranial to caudal embryonic descent along the paravertebral ganglia, these primitive neuroblastic cells may become arrested in an immature or incomplete stage of development. Subsequently, they fail to undergo terminal differentiation, giving rise to a variety of neuroblastic tumors ranging from the highly malignant neuroblastoma to the intermediate ganglioneuroblastoma and the benign ganglioneuroma variant. Although these tumors may occur at any site from brain to pelvis, including the neck, posterior mediastinum, retroperitoneal paraspinal ganglia, or the pelvic organ of Zuckerkandl, nearly 60% of neuroblastomas arise in or near the adrenal gland. These tumors can cause symptoms from a mass effect while some are hormonally active and can lead to paraneoplastic symptoms.

Neuroblastoma accounts for 6% to 10% of all childhood cancers and 15% of all pediatric cancer deaths in the United States. Approximately 7 to 12 new cases per million children are diagnosed annually. Of these, 80% present before the age of 4 years, with the greatest incidence in children under 2. Boys are more commonly affected than girls, with a ratio of 1.3 to 1. The vast majority of patients have extensive locoregional (stage 3) or metastatic (stage 4) disease at the time of presentation. Consequently, the prognosis is generally poor, with an overall survival of less than 30%. However, a special category of patients with disseminated disease exists (stage 4s) in which the prognosis is surprisingly favorable. These patients are under 1 year of age and have a primary mass as well as metastases to the bone marrow, liver, and skin. Despite the presence of metastatic disease, these infants paradoxically have an improved prognosis due to the propensity of this disease to undergo spontaneous regression or maturation.

E. M. Barksdale, Jr.: Department of Surgery, University of Pittsburgh; and Division of Pediatric Surgery and Fetal Diagnosis Treatment, Children's Hospital of Pittsburgh, Pittsburgh, Pennsylvania.

A. Stanford: Department of Pediatric Surgery, Children's Hospital of Pittsburgh, Pittsburgh, Pennsylvania.

CLINICAL PRESENTATION

Neuroblastoma has protean clinical manifestations. The signs and symptoms of this disease reflect its biologic diversity and are principally dependent on the location of the primary tumor and metastases, the age of the patient, and metabolic activity of the tumor. Up to 75% of children develop a palpable abdominal mass that usually originates in the flank and extends across the midline. Symptoms of malaise, fever, abdominal distension, anorexia, weight loss, or abdominal pain may be present concurrently. Nearly two thirds of all patients have extensive locoregional disease or widespread metastases at diagnosis. The most frequent sites of early hematogenous spread are to the bone marrow, cortical bone, liver, and skin. Late stage metastases may involve the brain or lung.

Clinical symptoms vary with the primary site of presentation. Abdominal masses may present with progressive distension or more acutely with abdominal pain secondary to intratumor hemorrhage. Bowel or bladder dysfunction can occur as a result of direct compression by a large intra-abdominal or pelvic masses. Cervical masses usually present as firm lesions that may cause dysphagia or stridor. Wheezing, dyspnea, pneumonia, or Horner's syndrome can occur in patients with thoracic tumors. Posterior mediastinal masses with intraspinal extension, or dumbbell tumors, can cause neurologic symptoms of spinal cord compression.

The findings on physical examination parallel the biology of the disease. Nearly 75% of children present with a palpable abdominal mass. The propensity to metastasize to the pelvic and long bones can result in gait disturbances and extremity pain. Intracranial metastases can result in periorbital ecchymoses and proptosis, also known as panda eyes or raccoon eyes. Metastatic lesions to the skin can produce a characteristic "blueberry muffin" appearance in the skin. Severe acute respiratory distress may develop secondary to massive hepatomegaly from liver metastases.

Numerous paraneoplastic syndromes can occur in conjunction with neuroblastoma. Cerebellar ataxia, involuntary movements, and nystagmus are the hallmark of the opsoclonus-myoclonus syndrome, or the "dancing eyes and dancing feet" syndrome, which is felt to be mediated by immunologic cross-reactivity between the tumor and the myelin sheaths of the central nervous system. Excess secretion of vasoactive intestinal peptide may stimulate an intractable electrolyte-losing watery diarrhea. Significant hypertension also may occur due to catecholamine production by these tumors. Neuroblastoma may be associated with other disorders of neural crest cells, including neurofibromatosis, Hirschsprung's disease, Beckwith-Wiedemann syndrome, central hypoventilation syndrome (Ondine's curse), DiGeorge syndrome, and congenital heart disease.

DIAGNOSTIC APPROACH

Although definitive diagnosis requires histologic evaluation of tissue, a high level of clinical suspicion may arise from the history and physical examination. In the child suspected of having neuroblastoma, the serologic and radiologic studies should proceed concurrently. Initial blood studies required include a complete blood count (CBC), serum electrolytes, blood urea nitrogen, creatinine, and liver function studies. Other serologic studies such as lactate dehydrogenase, ferritin, and neuron-specific enolase should be obtained because they have prognostic significance. The urinary catecholamine metabolites vanillymandelic acid and homovanillic acid also should be measured as spot determinations (Table 109.1).

Although ultrasonography is the most frequent radiographic tool for evaluating abdominal masses, there is no characteristic diagnostic appearance of neuroblastoma using this technique. Computed tomography (CT) and magnetic resonance imaging (MRI) are the preferred diagnostic tools for evaluating the primary tumor site in the child suspected of having neuroblastoma. The greater anatomic detail afforded by CT, the ability to stage disease extent, and the presence of metastases make this method our preferred choice for the initial imaging and staging of neuroblastoma.

TABLE 109.1. NEUROBLASTOMA BIOLOGIC MARKERS (SEROLOGIC/MOLECULAR)

Marker	Poor Prognosis
Neuron-specific enolase (NSE)	>15 ng/mL
Lactate dehydrogenase (LDH)	>1,500 IU/mL
Ferritin	>142 ng/mL
Vanillymandelic acid (VMA)/ homovanillic acid (HVA) ratio	<1
N-myc amplification	>10 copies
Chromosome 1	Short arm (p) deletion
DNA ploidy	1
CD44 expression	Decreased
Tyrosine kinase A (TRKA) expression	Increased
Multidrug-resistance–associated protein (MDRP)	Increased

We favor MRI to evaluate patients with thoracic or other tumors that may have intraspinal extension. This modality may provide critical information for the planning of the surgical approach. MRI also may be useful in distinguishing between malignant and benign neuroblastoma variants.

Prior to surgical intervention the patient must be adequately staged. The staging workup is designed to identify the extent of disease and location of metastases. CT evaluation of the lung should be performed in conjunction with the abdominal CT scan. Bone marrow disease should be evaluated with bilateral posterior iliac crest marrow aspirates and biopsies. Children with neuroblastoma should be evaluated for evidence of cortical bone metastases with plain radiography of areas of bony tenderness, and technetium 99m scanning to assess occult areas of metastasis.

Radiolabeled metaiodobenzyl guanidine (MIBG) scintigraphy recognizes receptors for the peptide somatostatin that are present in high abundance in more than 80% of neuroblastomas. Although not universally available, this modality can provide critical information regarding tumor viability, disease extent, recurrence, and prognosis. MIBG is probably the single best study to assess for metastatic disease. Following a complete staging evaluation, adequate tissue must be obtained to both secure the diagnosis and assess the behavior by biologic studies.

Needle, incisional, or excisional biopsy of the primary or metastatic lesions is critical to establish the diagnosis prior to the institution of therapy. Most primary tumors are not amenable to complete surgical excision; however, a determination should be made based on the initial imaging studies as to the resectability of these tumors. Primary excision offers a small incremental improvement in overall prognosis. This should be pursued only in those patients in whom it can be achieved without sacrificing or injuring critical organs such as the kidney. Reported studies suggest that nearly 40% of tumors will be downstaged at surgery.

PATHOLOGY

Macroscopically, neuroblastomas are typically bulky, multilobular, poorly encapsulated, and highly vascular masses. They may have areas of microcalcifications. In contrast, the benign ganglioneuroma variant is usually well circumscribed, with a smooth, dense capsule. Microscopically, the appearance of neuroblastoma is not dissimilar to that of other common pediatric solid tumors such as rhabdomyosarcoma, peripheral neuroectodermal tumor, and extraosseous Ewing's sarcoma. Neuroblastomas are composed of small uniform round blue cells with hyperchromatic nuclei and scant cytoplasm. The cells may form pseudorosettes with eosinophilic fibrinous material in the interstitial space. Some tumors are composed of a mixture of cells that have more differentiated ganglion cells, whereas others are composed exclusively of ganglion cells (gan-

TABLE 109.2. SHIMADA PATHOLOGIC CLASSIFICATION

	Favorable Histology	Unfavorable Histology
Stroma rich	Well differentiated, intermixed	Nodular
Stroma poor		
Age <18 mo	MKI <200/5,000	MKI <100/5,000
Age 18–60 mo	MKI >100/5,000 Differentiated	MKI >100/5,000 Undifferentiated
Age >5 yr	None	All

MKI, Mitosis karyorrhexis index.

glioneuroblastoma or ganglioneuromas). Therefore, other immunohistochemical, cytogenetic, and molecular biologic studies are frequently necessary to make a definitive diagnosis. The amplification of the *N-myc* oncogene, the loss of the short arm of chromosome 1 (1p deletion), and the expression of the *TRK* protooncogene have diagnostic and prognostic implications. A histologic classification system devised by Shimada and colleagues combines the degree of differentiation, the mitotic–karyorhexis index, and the presence or absence of schwannian stroma to determine favorable versus unfavorable outcome (Table 109.2).

Following complete radiographic staging, analysis of the bone marrow, and histologic confirmation, a thorough evaluation of tissue from the primary tumor site with immunohistochemistry, molecular biology, and cytogenetics determinations is performed. Staging is critical for prognostic stratification, therapeutic planning, and comparative analysis of outcome. Although numerous staging modalities have been used in the past, the International Neuroblastoma Staging System (INSS) has nearly supplanted all other schema. The INSS stratifies tumors based on the initial extent of disease (unilateral vs. crossing the midline), resectability (complete vs. incomplete), and the presence of histologically positive lymph nodes. The criteria are summarized in Table 109.3.

TREATMENT

Preoperative Preparation

The management of neuroblastoma relies on the coordinated efforts of several disciplines. Current treatment uses surgery, chemotherapy, radiotherapy, and occasionally myeloablation or immunotherapy. The sequence of therapeutic interventions is protocol driven and guided by the stage of disease at presentation. Although complete eradication of all tumor burden is the goal, this is often not possible at the time of initial diagnosis. In many cases chemotherapy must precede definitive surgical therapy. Therefore, the surgeon's initial role is to critically assess the resectability of the primary tumor and either perform an adequate biopsy for late-stage disease or a safe complete surgical resection of the primary lesion in localized disease. The general principle for the surgical management of neuroblastoma parallels that of other pediatric malignancies: localized, resectable, early-stage (stage 1 or 2) tumors should undergo therapeutic laparotomy and complete resection; locally advanced (stage 2b or 3) or distantly metastatic lesions (stage 4) should receive neoadjuvant chemotherapy followed by surgical resection.

Neuroblastoma resections are often major surgical procedures; therefore, prior to surgery, attention should be focused on the details of care that may have an impact on recovery. Patients should be typed and cross-matched for blood and appropriate blood products. Acquired and inherited coagulopathies should be corrected preoperatively. Preoperative assessment of organ function (e.g., kidney, liver, and heart) should be performed to identify other risk factors or contraindications to surgery. Patients who have received doxorubicin or other cardiotoxic chemotherapeutic agents should receive an echocardiogram prior to general anesthesia. Prophylactic antibiotics should be administered prior to surgical incisions. Finally, a detailed discussion with the family regarding the risks of surgery including major organ loss or dysfunction, vascu-

TABLE 109.3. INTERNATIONAL NEUROBLASTOMA STAGING SYSTEM

Stage	Definition
1	Localized tumor with complete gross excision, with or without microscopic residual disease; representative ipsilateral lymph nodes negative for tumor microscopically (nodes attached to and removed with the primary tumor may be positive)
2A	Localized tumor with incomplete gross excision; representative ipsilateral nonadherent lymph nodes negative for tumor microscopically
2B	Localized tumor with or without complete gross excision, with ipsilateral nonadherent lymph nodes positive for tumor; enlarged contralateral lymph nodes must be negative microscopically
3	Unresectable unilateral tumor infiltrating across the midline, with or without regional lymph node involvement; or localized unilateral tumor with contralateral regional lymph node involvement; or midline tumor with bilateral extension by infiltration (unresectable) or by lymph node involvement
4	Any primary tumor with dissemination to distant lymph nodes, bone, bone marrow, liver, skin, and/or other organs (except as defined for stage 4S)
4S	Localized primary tumor (as defined for stage 1, 2A, or 2B), with dissemination limited to skin, liver, and/or bone marrow (limited to infant <1 yr of age)

lar or neurological injury, and permanent disability or death is mandated prior to surgery.

OPERATIVE MANAGEMENT

The goal of surgical therapy is total or near total tumor resection. Formal, methodical, and planned exposure of the important structures prior to resection and the avoidance of sacrifice of major structures are the guiding principles of operative management. In this context a variety of special considerations arise when approaching neuroblastoma in various body cavities. Major surgical considerations for these sites are summarized below.

CERVICAL AND THORACIC TUMORS

Cervical tumors are usually approached via a low transverse collar incision. Neck lesions that extend into the mediastinum or thoracic masses that extend into the neck should be approached by combined thoracic and supraclavicular incisions. "Trap door" incisions are usually unnecessary and increase perioperative morbidity and long-term disability. Most thoracic tumors require resection via an open thoracotomy, although some may be amenable to a thoracoscopic approach. These tumors usually do not present serious technical obstacles. Most arise in the sympathetic chain and lie in the costovertebral angle. Unlike abdominal tumors, major vessels are typically not encased. The stellate ganglion may be involved in upper thoracic lesions, resulting in a postoperative Horner's syndrome (ptosis, miosis, enophthalmos). This possibility should always be discussed with the patient's family prior to surgery.

SPINAL TUMORS

The dumbbell tumor refers to the extradural extension of an intrathoracic paraspinal tumor. Neurologic symptoms may be absent but can include major impairment. Their clinical presentation significantly impacts the surgical management of these lesions. A great deal of controversy exists as to whether the thoracic or spinal component should be removed first. If the spinal component provides a considerable challenge, some surgeons prefer preoperative chemotherapy or radiotherapy prior to resection. Proponents of this approach feel that these tumors are much less friable, and the risk for intraspinal bleeding and perioperative neurologic complications are significantly decreased. Although this is not unreasonable, we take a somewhat different approach to the management of these lesions. In the absence of clinical symptoms of paralysis, we favor primary surgical excision via thoracotomy with careful teasing of the tumor from the paravertebral space using bipolar cautery to diminish bleeding risks. Most of these lesions are of favorable histology and respond to surgery and adjuvant chemotherapy. In those patients with acute paralysis or cord compressive symptoms, we favor decompressive laminectomy to be performed by a neurosurgeon prior to excision of the thoracic tumor. We recommend neurosurgical excision of the spinal tumor first because of the attendant risk for inducing distal swelling of the spinal cord and worsening symptoms of cord compression by thoracic excision. In our opinion, patients with chronic weakness or fixed neurologic injury should undergo thoracic excision.

ABDOMINAL TUMORS

Most abdominal tumors arise in the upper abdomen. Some of these may be adherent to the liver or diaphragm or extend into the thorax. Following review of the imaging studies, a decision is made whether an abdominal or thoracoabdominal incision is appropriate. Stage 1 and 2 abdominal tumors are usually localized to the adrenal gland without significant extension and are excised without much difficulty. A few surgeons have reported successful laparoscopic resections for localized lesions. Stage 3 and 4 neuroblastomas often encase the major abdominal vessels, including the vena cava, aorta, renal vessels, and mesenteric arteries. These tumors require meticulous technique to avoid vascular injury. Consequently, en bloc resections are impossible, and cutting into the tumor capsule must be accepted. Although some data suggest that patients with complete resections have an improved prognosis, there is clearly a role for surgical debulking and near complete resections. The surgical axioms that guide our operative management of neuroblastoma include (a) gaining generous exposure of the operative field first; (b) recognizing that tumor does not typically invade the tunica media of the major blood vessels; (c) meticulously resecting all tumor; (d) avoiding sacrificing major blood vessels or organs.

For most abdominal tumors we favor a generous chevron or transverse supraumbilical incision, depending on the body habitus. A thoracoabdominal incision is used for large right-sided tumors adherent to the diaphragm or liver, or any tumor that has both intraabdominal and thoracic components. Our next step is to gain full exposure of the retroperitoneum. Exposure of the right retroperitoneum is performed via extensive mobilization and medial reflection of the duodenum and right colon (Catell maneuver). Alternatively, mobilization and medial reflection of the left colon, spleen, stomach, and pancreas facilitate visualization of the abdominal aorta and its branches

(Mattox maneuver). These maneuvers allow for thorough assessment of the extent of intraabdominal disease and evaluation of the technical challenges to complete tumor resection.

At this juncture we focus on a three-step approach to tumor resection: (a) complete vascular exposure, (b) vessel dissection, and (c) tumor resection. The first phase of the operation involves the identification of the major blood vessels and their relationship to the tumor. Proximal and distal vascular exposure is critical. Occasionally vascular control may be necessary if there appears to be a risk of major bleeding. The next step is to perform circumferential subadventitial dissection of the vessel outside of the tumor. This facilitates the final step of safe division and removal of the tumor overlying the vessel down to this layer. The use of bipolar cautery and the Cavitron ultrasonic aspirator (Valleylab, Boulder, Colorado) facilitates the dissection with the minimization of blood loss and significantly decreases the incidence of vessel injury. These maneuvers are then sequentially performed in a caudal to cranial fashion, identifying and exposing all involved major blood vessels along the way and resecting the tumor as described.

The dissections are often lengthy and tedious operations in which tumor is removed in a piecemeal fashion from around the vessels. The major sites for problems occur in the region of the mesenteric and renal arteries, where inadvertent injury is not uncommon. Even in the absence of obvious vascular injury, postoperative vasospasm may lead to organ atrophy or disappearance, especially in infants. Some surgeons propose division and ligation of the renal vein or even nephrectomy. In general, nephrectomy should be avoided, particularly in the setting of previous high-dose chemotherapy or impending bone marrow transplantation. We support the use of near-total perinephric tumor resection. Nephrectomy should be avoided unless a substantial tumor burden will be left behind.

PELVIC TUMORS

Typically these tumors lie deep in the pelvis in the presacral region in close juxtaposition to the pelvic nerves and hypogastric vessels. Although access may be achieved by several approaches, we favor a modified Pfannenstiel incision with bilateral extension to the anterior superior iliac spines as needed. Full exposure of the rectus sheath is performed, and the tendinous attachments of the rectus abdominus muscles to the pubic symphisis are divided and reflected cranially. Lateral muscles of the abdominal wall are divided as needed. Care is taken to avoid disruption of the inguinal canal or its contents. This maneuver facilitates the extensive exposure of the pelvis. As with abdominal tumors, the approach of determining the relationship of the tumor to major vessels, nerves, and viscera is our first maneuver prior to any attempt at resection. Particular focus on the location of the iliac artery, sciatic nerve, pelvic autonomic nerves, ureters, and major visceral structures should be identified before resection.

SPECIAL CONSIDERATIONS

Rarely, stage 4s tumors may present with acute respiratory embarrassment secondary to massive hepatomegaly. The emergency placement of a prosthetic or biosynthetic patch allows abdominal decompression and improved ventilation and visceral perfusion.

POSTOPERATIVE CARE

In general, patients who have undergone major resections should be initially monitored in an acute or intermediate care setting. Although variations exist among institutions, patients may have an epidural catheter for pain management, arterial lines for monitoring, and central venous lines for fluid and nutritional supplementation. Significant third space fluid sequestration is common. This requires close monitoring of volume status and adequacy of resuscitation. A postoperative ileus is anticipated for a minimum of 3 to 5 days. Strong consideration should be given to postoperative parenteral nutrition support because many patients arrive for surgery after chemotherapy with preexisting nutritional deficits. Postoperative intussusception can occur and requires a high index of suspicion. This condition is often heralded by the development of a recurrent ileus after the return of normal bowel function in the postoperative period.

COMPLICATIONS

The most common causes of increased morbidity and mortality include uncontrollable hemorrhage, diarrhea, late presentation peritonitis, and chylous ascites. The diarrhea is permanent and appears to be secondary to tumor dissection adjacent to the superior mesenteric and celiac arteries. It is usually not amenable to the use of loperamide or other antidiarrheal agents and is probably ischemic in nature. The late presentation of abdominal pain, colic, or peritoneal signs following surgery should alert the surgeon to impending intestinal obstruction or ischemia of the intestinal tract. Major organ injury has occurred with these extensive resections in patients with stage 3 or 4 disease who have been treated with chemotherapy; therefore, great care should be taken in the surgical approach to these patients. It is unclear from the current data if 100% tumor resection is necessary. Future studies should elucidate this further.

SUGGESTED READINGS

Brodeur GM, Seeger RC, Barrett A, et al. International criteria for diagnosis, staging and response to treatment with neuroblastoma. *J Clin Oncol* 1988;6:1874–1881.

Chamberlain RS, Quinones R, Dinndorf P, et al. Complete surgical resection combined with aggressive adjuvant chemotherapy and bone marrow transplantation. Survival in children with advanced neuroblastoma. *Ann Surg Oncol* 1996;2:93–100.

Haase GM, Perez C, Atkinson, JB. Current aspects of biology, risk assessment and treatment of neuroblastoma. *Semin Surg Oncol* 1999;16:91–104.

Kiely EM. The surgical challenge of neuroblastoma. *J Pediatr Surg* 1994;29:128–133.

Maris JM, Matthay KK. Biology of neoplasia: molecular biology of neuroblastoma. *J Clin Oncol* 1999;17:2264–2279.

Shimada H, Chatten J, Newton WA Jr, et al. Histopathologic prognostic factors in neuroblastic tumors: definition of subtypes of ganglioneuroblastoma and an age-linked classification of neuroblastomas. *J Natl Cancer Inst* 1984;73:405–416.

Shorter NA, Davidoff AM, Evans AE, et al. The role of surgery in the management of stage IV neuroblastoma: a single institution study. *Med Pediatr Oncol* 1995;24:287–291.

Smith EL, Haase GM, Seeger RC, et al. A surgical perspective on the current staging in neuroblastoma (International Neuroblastoma Staging System) *J Pediatr Surg* 1995;30:289–295.

110

WILMS TUMOR

RICHARD G. AZIZKHAN

The treatment of Wilms tumor (WT, or nephroblastoma) is considered one of the greatest successes of modern pediatric oncology. We now have a cure rate that exceeds 90%—a remarkable contrast to what was once a lethal malignancy. Surgical removal of the primary tumor remains the cornerstone of WT therapy in North America, and the importance of contralateral renal exploration at the time of operation cannot be overstated. Prognosis is related not only to the stage of disease at diagnosis and the histopathologic features of the tumor, but also to the collaborative efforts of pediatric surgeons, pediatric oncologists, and radiation oncologists in carrying out appropriate treatment regimens. The dramatic improvement in prognosis for most affected children can be attributed to the multimodal therapeutic regimens that have developed as a result of several decades of research by the National Wilms Tumor Study (NWTS) Group and the International Society of Pediatric Oncology (SIOP). In addition, there have been important breakthroughs in understanding the genetic and molecular biologic factors involved in Wilms tumorigenesis and normal kidney development. These have had a significant impact on clinical management.

Wilms tumor is the most common primary malignant renal tumor of childhood. Approximately 500 new cases are diagnosed annually in the United States. Seventy-eight percent of these cases are diagnosed at 1 to 5 years of age, with the peak incidence occurring at age 3. The tumor usually develops in otherwise healthy children, but 12% to 15% of cases occur in children with other congenital disorders (Table 110.1). Despite the number of genes that appear to be involved in the development of WT, hereditary WT is uncommon. Estimates of cases of hereditary origin range from 15% to 20%. Only 5% of patients have bilateral involvement, and this may arise from renal dysplasia or nodular or diffuse nephroblastomatosis.

Although exceptional cases may occasionally require approaches to management that extend beyond standard protocols, all children in North America should be treated by multispecialty teams that participate in cooperative groups that adhere to the NWTS protocols. This not only offers the best chance of cure, but also contributes to the overall knowledge that will ultimately lead to the identification of additional markers of prognosis and further advancements and modifications in treatment.

In light of these facts, I present a concise review of genetic and molecular biology findings, but focus primarily on principal aspects of diagnosis and key precepts of management as recommended by the NWTS-5. Emphasis is on surgical principles and considerations.

GENETIC ASPECTS OF WILMS TUMOR

Both hereditary and sporadic WT have been shown to result from changes in one or more of several genes. Specific germline mutations in one of these genes (*WT1*) located on the short arm of chromosome 11 (band 11p13) are associated with WT, and cause a range of genitourinary abnormalities such as cryptorchidism and hypospadias, as well as Denys-Drash syndrome (WT, intersex disorders, and progressive nephropathy). A gene causing aniridia is located near the *WT1* gene on chromosome 11p13, and deletions encompassing the *WT1* and aniridia genes may explain the association between aniridia and WT seen in the WAGR syndrome (WT, aniridia, genitourinary abnormalities, mental retardation). A second WT gene locus, referred to as *WT2*, is thought to reside at chromosome 11p15. Abnormalities of the distal portion of 11p15 have been linked to Beckwith-Wiedemann syndrome (an overgrowth syndrome with omphalocele, visceromegaly, macroglossia, and gigantism).

R.G. Azizkhan: Departments of Surgery and Pediatrics, University of Cincinnati; and Department of Pediatric Surgery, Cincinnati Children's Hospital Medical Center, Cincinnati, Ohio.

TABLE 110.1. CONGENITAL DISORDERS IN PATIENTS WITH WILMS TUMOR

	Incidence (%)
Hamartomas: hemangiomas, "birthmarks," multiple nevi, café-au-lait spots	7.9
Genitourinary anomalies: horseshoe kidney, dysplasia of kidney, cystic disease of kidney, hypospadias, cryptorchidism, duplication of collecting system	4.4
Congenital hemihypertrophy	2.9
Musculoskeletal anomalies: clubfoot, rib fusion, distal phocomelia, hip dislocation	2.9
Congenital aniridia	1.1

DIAGNOSTIC EVALUATION

Clinical Signs and Symptoms

Initial signs and symptoms of WT are presented in Table 110.2. Most patients (60%) present with a palpable, asymptomatic abdominal mass, and parents frequently discover this mass when bathing or dressing the child. Hypertension due to elaboration of renin by tumor cells or from compression of renal vasculature is seen in approximately 25% of patients; hematuria is seen in 15% of patients. Polycythemia is occasionally present from increased erythropoietin production. Bleeding diathesis may be seen as a result of acquired von Willebrand disease (reduced von Willebrand factor antigen level, prolonged bleeding time, and decreased factor VIII and factor VIII:ristocetin cofactor activity).

It is important for surgeons to be aware of the associated clinical phenotypes. Children with WAGR syndrome, Beckwith-Wiedemann syndrome, or Denys-Drash syndrome, or those with sporadic aniridia, isolated hemihypertrophy, and nephropathy with a female genotype/phenotype, are at increased risk for WT. As such, they should undergo abdominal ultrasonography every 3 months until they reach age 6 and yearly thereafter until they attain full growth. Surgeons also must be aware of the possibility that WT can arise in a multicystic dysplastic kidney. Hence, serial ultrasonographic examinations are needed for early detection.

TABLE 110.2. INITIAL SIGNS AND SYMPTOMS OF WILMS TUMOR

	Frequency (%)
Palpable mass in abdomen	60
Hypertension	25
Hematuria	15
Obstipation	4
Weight loss	4
Urinary tract infection	3
Diarrhea	3
Previous trauma	3
Other: bleeding diathesis, polycythemia, nausea, vomiting, abdominal pain, inguinal hernia, cardiac insufficiency, acute surgical abdomen, pleural effusion	8

Differential Diagnosis

Differential diagnosis entails distinguishing WT from neuroblastoma. This is generally not difficult, because most neuroblastomas arise from the adrenal gland or the paravertebral sympathetic ganglia, whereas WT is intrarenal. However, benign processes, as well as other malignant intrarenal neoplasms, can produce clinical and radiographic findings similar to those of WT. Although clear cell sarcoma and rhabdoid tumor of the kidney were historically classified as WT variants, today they are considered distinct and highly malignant tumor types. Another common renal neoplasm to be differentiated from WT is congenital mesoblastic nephroma, which occurs usually in infants under 3 to 4 months of age. This tumor is usually benign but may have perirenal extension. These lesions require complete resection for cure. Recurrence and metastases are extremely rare and require chemotherapy and radiation.

Workup

Preoperative workup comprises medical history, physical examination, laboratory tests, a number of radiographic imaging studies, and a baseline cardiac assessment in patients to receive cardiotoxic chemotherapy. Medical history typically includes information pertaining to family history of cancer, congenital defects, and benign tumors. Because an acquired von Willebrand–type bleeding diathesis has been reported, a careful history of bleeding episodes also should be obtained. Physical examination may reveal congenital anomalies, high blood pressure, or liver enlargement. Laboratory testing should include a differential white blood cell count, urinalysis, and a coagulation profile. Chromosomal analysis should be performed in cases in which congenital disorders are present, especially aniridia, Beckwith-Wiedemann syndrome, and hemihypertrophy. An echocardiogram is useful in detecting the presence of tumor in the right atrium when thrombus is identified in the inferior vena cava (IVC).

Imaging Studies

Imaging studies provide important information for the surgeon, as well as for the radiation oncologist, should postoperative radiation therapy be indicated. Data crucial to surgeons includes the presence and function of the contralateral kidney, whether it is involved with the tumor, and the presence and extent of an intravascular tumor thrombus. The initial radiographic study generally selected is abdominal ultrasonography. This demonstrates whether the abdominal mass is solid or cystic, and may allow identification of the origin of the mass, in addition to measurement of the maximum diameter of the mass. It also allows evaluation of the IVC for flow and for the presence of tumor thrombus. Contrast-enhanced computed tomography (CT) of the abdomen outlines the tumor, but cannot adequately differentiate between compression and invasion of the liver (Fig. 110.1). It may suggest evidence of bilateral involvement or involvement of blood vessels and lymph nodes, or apparent extension of the tumor into adjacent structures such as the liver, spleen, or colon.

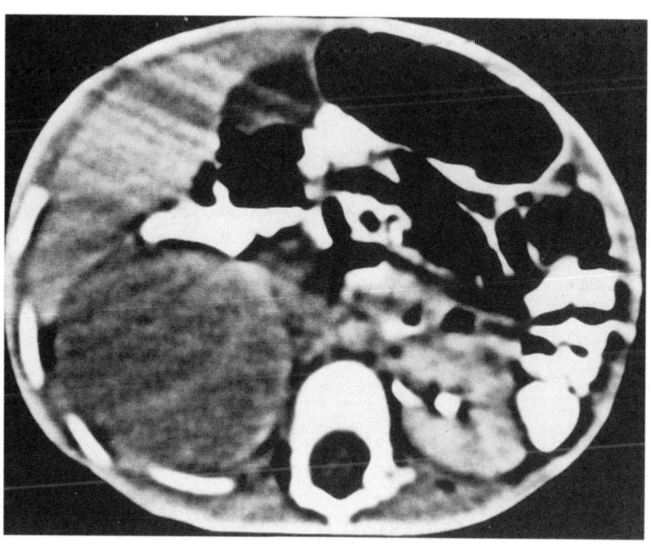

FIGURE 110.1. Computed tomography scan demonstrating a large unilateral Wilms tumor in a 14-month-old boy.

Nephrogenic Rests

Computed tomography also may identify small lesions that could be nephrogenic rests or WT in the contralateral kidney (Fig. 110.2). Nephrogenic rests, which are considered precursor lesions to WT, are seen in 30% to 40% of WT patients; the risk that they will become malignant ranges from 1% to 3%. Ninety percent of synchronous bilateral WTs and 94% of metachronous bilateral tumors contain areas of nephrogenic rests. These rests are not only of theoretical interest in the pathogenesis of WT, but also of practical importance. When multifocal precursor lesions are found in both kidneys at initial exploration or in a kidney removed for WT, there is an increased likelihood of subsequent tumor formation in the remaining parenchyma. This finding indicates the need for close long-term follow-up of the remaining kidney.

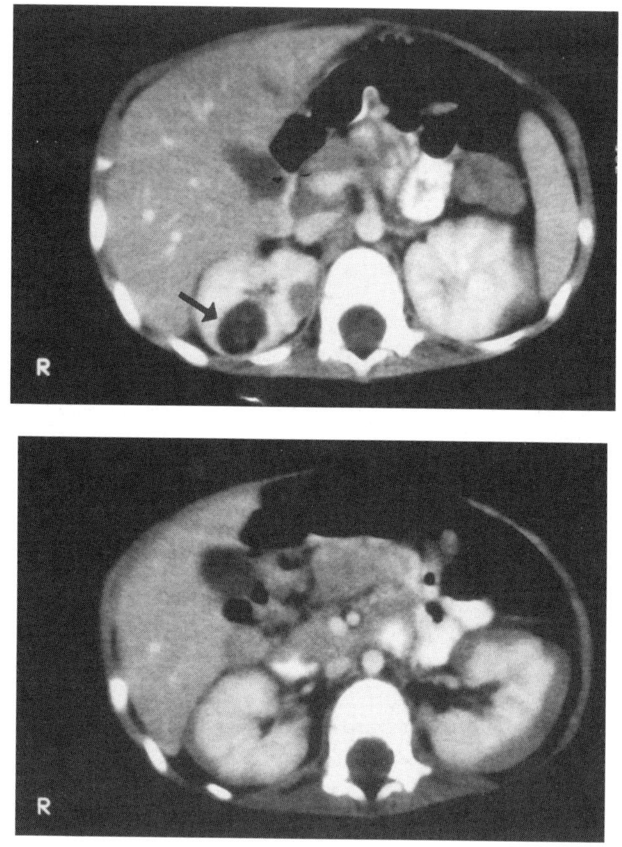

FIGURE 110.2. Computed tomography images demonstrating bilateral nephroblastomatosis (nephrogenic rests) situated in the periphery of the renal parenchyma in a child with a right-sided Wilms tumor (*arrow upper panel*).

Although results of radiographic and ultrasonographic studies generally provide sufficient information on which to base the decision for laparotomy, it is important to keep in mind that no imaging study can unequivocally establish the histologic diagnosis of WT. Results of studies undertaken by both the NWTS and SIOP indicate that 7.6% to 9.9% of patients with the prenephrectomy diagnosis of WT have a condition other than WT. Treatment on the basis of diagnostic imaging findings alone may thus be inappropriate.

Plain chest radiography or CT of the chest may reveal pulmonary metastases. The latter helps recognize small

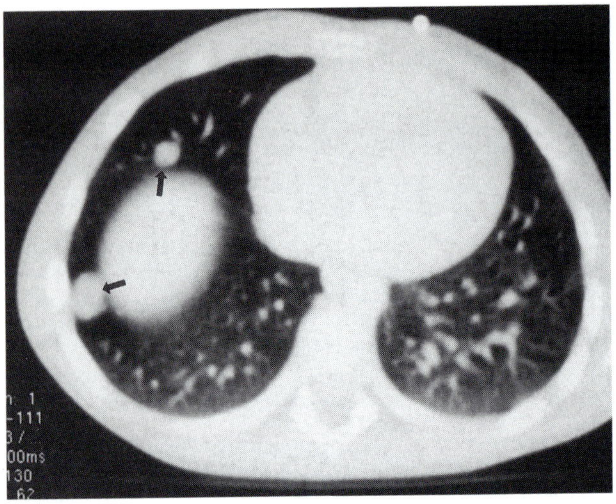

FIGURE 110.3. Computed tomography image demonstrating two large pulmonary metastases located in the right lower lobe.

metastases hidden behind the ribs, diaphragm, and heart, and that may be missed on a chest radiograph (Fig. 110.3). Patients with small pulmonary lesions identified only on chest CT should have biopsies of one or more lesions to confirm that they are due to metastatic tumor, especially if treatment with whole-lung irradiation or doxorubicin is planned.

STAGING

Accurate staging is essential for the determination of the need for radiation therapy and the administration of the appropriate chemotherapy regimen subsequent to surgery. Staging is determined by (a) extent of disease; (b) resectability of the primary tumor; (c) status of perirenal, capsular, and lymph node involvement; (d) local invasion of adjacent organs and structures; (e) presence of metastases; and (f) contralateral kidney involvement. Table 110.3 describes the clinicopathologic staging system as recommended by the NWTS. Staging is defined at the time of celiotomy. It is then confirmed by the pathologist after evaluation of tumor margins and histology.

The NWTS grading system recognizes quantitative (blastemal, epithelial, and stromal predominant) deviations of triphasic WT as having favorable histology (FH). WT with focal or diffuse anaplasia is considered to have unfavorable histology (UH). Staging, which is based on the degree of gross and microscopic tumor extension, is the same for tumors with favorable or unfavorable histologic features. Patients should thus be characterized by a statement of both criteria (e.g., "stage II, FH" or "stage II, UH").

TABLE 110.3. NATIONAL WILMS TUMOR STUDY GROUP STAGING SYSTEM FOR WILMS TUMOR

Stage I	The tumor, limited to the kidney, is completely excised. The renal capsule has an intact outer surface. The tumor is not ruptured or sampled for biopsy before its removal (fine-needle aspiration biopsy is excluded from this restriction). The vessels of the renal sinus are not involved. No evidence of tumor at or beyond the margins of resection is visible.
Stage II	The tumor extends beyond the kidney, but is completely excised. One may see regional extension of tumor (i.e., penetration of the renal capsule or extensive invasion of the renal sinus). The blood vessels outside the renal parenchyma, including those of the renal sinus, may contain tumor. Biopsy was performed (except fine-needle aspiration), or tumor spillage before or during surgery was confined to the flank and did not involve the peritoneal surface. No evidence of tumor at or beyond the margins of resection is present.
Stage III	Residual nonhematogenous tumor is present, confined to the abdomen. Any one of the following may occur: (a) lymph nodes within the abdomen or pelvis are found to be involved by tumor (renal hilar, paraaortic, or beyond; lymph node involvement in the thorax or other extra-abdominal sites is a criterion for stage IV); (b) the tumor has penetrated the peritoneal surface; (c) tumor implants are found on the peritoneal surface; (d) gross or microscopic tumor remains postoperatively (e.g., tumor cells are found at the margin of surgical resection on microscopic examination); (e) the tumor is not completely resectable because of local infiltration into vital structures; or (f) tumor spillage not confined to the flank occurred either before or during surgery.
Stage IV	Hematogenous metastases (lung, liver, bone, brain, etc.) or lymph node metastases outside the abdominopelvic region are present.
Stage V	Bilateral renal involvement is present at diagnosis. An attempt should be made to stage each side according to the foregoing criteria on the basis of the extent of disease before biopsy or treatment.
Stage I–V, anaplasia (UH)	Children with stage I anaplastic tumors have an excellent prognosis. They can be managed with the same regimen as FH patients. Children with stage II–IV diffuse anaplasia, however, represent a higher risk group. These tumors are more resistant to the chemotherapy traditionally used in children with Wilms tumor (FH).

UH, unfavorable histology; FH, favorable histology.

PATTERNS OF DISEASE PROGRESSION

The first signs of spread beyond the tumor pseudocapsule are usually found in the renal sinus or the intrarenal blood and lymphatic vessels. Unless tumor cells are incorporated into a thrombus, are attached to vessel walls, or distend the vessel lumen, there can be no certainty as to whether they were displaced into vessels during manipulation of the tumor specimen. Penetration through the renal capsule is the next most common site of extrarenal spread of WT. The most common sites of metastases are the lungs, regional lymph nodes, and liver. Other metastatic sites are uncommon.

PROGNOSTIC CONSIDERATIONS

Tumor size (<550 g), age of the patient (<24 months), histologic tumor features (FH vs. UH), lymph node metastases, and local features of the tumor (e.g., capsular or vascular invasion) have been used to predict the risk of tumor recurrence or progression. However, the prognostic significance of factors such as age and tumor size has become less important as treatment efficacy has improved. The NWTS has identified histologic features of WT as the key determinant of prognosis. Lymph node involvement remains an important predictor of treatment failure. Chromosomal markers also have been shown to impact prognosis. Findings from NWTS-3 and -4 have shown that loss of heterozygosity of 16q markers, which was present in tumor tissue from 17.2% of patients with FH or anaplastic WT, was associated with poorer 2-year relapse-free and overall survival rates. This difference remained when the analysis was adjusted for stage or histologic features. Loss of heterozygosity of chromosome 1p markers, present in tumor tissue from 11% of children with WT, was also associated with poorer relapse-free and overall survival, although this difference was not statistically significant.

Patients with FH stage IV WT have an excellent prognosis, whereas those who relapse with metastatic disease and especially those with UH have a grave prognosis. Except for patients with diffuse anaplastic stage I tumors, the presence of UH indicates a poorer prognosis in each clinical stage when compared with FH.

PREOPERATIVE THERAPY

Although the NWTS recommends primary surgical treatment, preoperative chemotherapy is beneficial in some children. These patients include those with bilateral involvement, or IVC extension above the hepatic veins, and those declared inoperable at surgical exploration. (Each of these clinical situations is discussed later in this chapter.) Studies conducted by both the SIOP and NWTS have shown that pretreatment with chemotherapy almost always reduces the bulk of the tumor. Pretreatment chemotherapy is also recommended by some as a strategy to decrease the number of patients who have rupture of their renal tumor at the time of nephrectomy. Although this indisputably makes tumor removal easier and reduces the frequency of surgical complications, it does not improve survival rates.

The major concern regarding the management of children who receive prenephrectomy chemotherapy is the potential for loss of important staging information. Clearly, some children may be overtreated or undertreated, as in the case of patients with rhabdoid tumor or clear cell sarcoma. Prenephrectomy chemotherapy does not modify tumor histology to such an extent that the diagnostic features of anaplasia cannot be identified, but it can induce other significant cytologic changes.

If acquired von Willebrand disease is identified either clinically or in the laboratory, desmopressin (DDAVP) should be administered as the initial therapy. If no response is observed, cryoprecipitate or fresh frozen plasma is given. This disease disappears once treatment of WT is initiated. For patients in whom bleeding is resistant to this regimen, dactinomycin and vincristine have been used successfully to correct clotting abnormality before nephrectomy is performed.

GOALS OF THE OPERATIVE PROCEDURE

The goals of the initial operative procedure are threefold. First, the diagnosis must be confirmed. Second, an assessment of the involvement of the contralateral kidney and other organs (e.g., lymph nodes, liver) must be made. Grossly visible regional lymph nodes must be sampled, regardless of whether they appear abnormal or not. If no suspicious lymph nodes are encountered, blind biopsies of the adjacent paraaortic or paracaval lymph nodes should be obtained. Third, a complete resection of the primary tumor must be performed. This includes removal of the involved adrenal gland and sympathetic ganglia or lymph nodes, taking care not to damage other structures. Accurate staging is essential for the subsequent determination of treatment protocol.

Should a mass be present in the contralateral kidney, biopsy of both kidneys for purposes of staging and histology is required. However, biopsy of a unilateral tumor should be avoided prior to removal in order to minimize the risk of local tumor spillage. Most tumors compress and adhere to adjacent organs without actual invasion, but tumors that involve contiguous structures should be sampled for biopsy and assigned a surgical stage. Tumors must be submitted fresh for molecular biology studies.

OPERATIVE PROTOCOL GUIDELINES

Surgical Technique

The transperitoneal approach to the tumor using a generous transverse incision has been the standard surgical technique. In contrast to the flank approach, which should not be used, it allows for both inspection of the regional lymph nodes and for mobilization of the contralateral kidney, which must be inspected on all surfaces for evidence of a synchronous bilateral tumor or evidence of nephrogenic rests. These lesions may not have been identified on preoperative imaging studies.

Radical or modified radical nephrectomy is used to remove the affected kidney (Fig. 110.4), but en bloc resection of nonessential structures (colon, spleen, tail of pancreas, etc.) should be considered only if the surgeon is sure all invasive disease can be removed. These procedures are associated with an increased risk for surgical complications. Moreover, in most cases, small amounts of residual tumor have not been associated with major decreases in survival rates. Colectomy or partial pancreatectomy should not be performed, but wedge resection of an infiltrated portion of the liver is advisable if the lesion can be removed in toto.

Once the peritoneal cavity is entered, the extent of tumor should be assessed and the liver, periaortic area, and vena cava palpated to determine whether primary excision is advisable. Prior to dissection of the tumor, the contralateral kidney should be explored. The Gerota's fascia of the contralateral kidney is opened, and the kidney is mobilized from its perirenal fat and fascia to allow thorough inspection and palpation of both anterior and posterior surfaces. Because the presence of bilateral WT alters the surgical approach significantly, it is essential to determine its status prior to nephrectomy. The importance of making this determination must be emphasized.

The colon is mobilized and reflected medially, with care taken to preserve the colonic blood supply. The renal vein, often splayed over the tumor, must be handled with extreme caution. Although early ligation of the renal vein does not appear to have an appreciable effect on survival, it is preferable (although not always possible) to ligate the renal artery and vein separately before tumor manipulation. With upper pole tumors, complete surgical removal usually includes removal of the perirenal fascia and adrenal gland without opening the Gerota's fascia. The ureter is ligated and divided as low as conveniently possible.

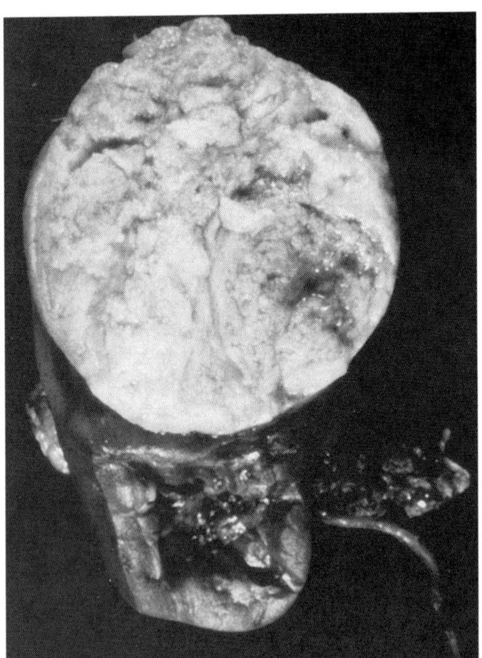

FIGURE 110.4. Cut nephrectomy specimen demonstrating the tumor relationship to the normal renal parenchyma from the same patient as in Fig. 110.1.

Gentle operative technique is essential to avoid spread or spill by inadvertently violating the tumor capsule—a well-documented and important complication in the management of WT. Patients with tumor spill are upstaged and require more aggressive adjuvant therapy.

Lymph Node Involvement

The presence or absence of lymph node metastases is important in determining treatment and long-term relapse-free survival. Positive lymph node involvement assigns patients to stage III disease, which adversely affects the incidence of recurrence and survival. It is important for surgeons to keep in mind that their impressions alone of nodal involvement have been shown to have only a 57% positive predictive value, with a false-negative rate of 31% and a false-positive rate of 18%. Selective sampling of suspicious lymph nodes is thus necessary for accurate staging, and should be performed with a high index of suspicion. Interestingly, however, there is no evidence indicating that extensive lymph node removal alters the outcome. Formal retroperitoneal lymph node dissection is therefore not recommended.

The operative report should clearly identify the site from which lymph nodes are removed and also must differentiate nodes that are contiguous and attached to the primary tumor from those that are not.

Gross Tumor in the Ureter or Renal Pelvis

If the patient has gross hematuria or has documented tumor involvement of the renal pelvis or ureter, a cystoscopy is warranted. Occasionally these patients may have a tumor nodule that has broken free from the main tumor mass and has implanted in the wall of the bladder. These tumor fragments are usually easily removed using the cystocope.

Inferior Vena Caval Extension

Wilms tumor extends into the IVC in approximately 6% of cases, and this involvement may be clinically asymptomatic in more than 50% of cases. Survival does not appear to be affected, and prognosis is comparable stage by stage to patients without caval extension.

If possible, the tumor thrombus should be removed en bloc with the kidney prior to ligation of the renal vein. For

IVC involvement below the level of the hepatic veins, the caval thrombus can be extracted through a cavotomy after proximal and distal vascular control has been obtained. If tumor extension is at or above the hepatic vein level, a biopsy is sufficient initially and a delayed nephrectomy is planned. Attempts at primary surgical excision of the tumor and caval extension are associated with increased surgical morbidity.

Patients with extension of IVC thrombus above the hepatic veins or into the right atrium should undergo preoperative chemotherapy. This usually results in tumor shrinkage, making the standard transabdominal approach feasible and significantly decreasing morbidity. Thoracoabdominal incisions, cardiac bypass, and other maneuvers necessary to extract the tumor from the heart can generally be avoided. In patients with intracardiac extension of tumor that has not responded to prenephrectomy combination chemotherapy, a median sternotomy and midline abdominal incision provide excellent exposure of the right atrium and the intrapericardial portion of the IVC. Extracorporeal bypass is necessary in this situation.

Second-Look Operations

Patients that may require elective surgical reexploration include those with bilateral WT, inoperable tumors pretreated with chemotherapy, abdominal tumor recurrence, and tumors explored through a flank incision.

MANAGEMENT OF BILATERAL WILMS TUMOR

Synchronous or metachronous bilateral WT accounts for approximately 5% of WT patients. Diagnosis made before 2 years of age carries a better prognosis (70%–75% survival) than if made after 2 years of age (20%–45% survival). Survival is better for patients with stage I or II disease (85%) compared with stage III or IV disease (60%). Also, synchronous tumors have a better prognosis than metachronous tumors.

Most cases are not diagnosed on the basis of physical examination. Although advances in imaging techniques have led to an increase in the preoperative diagnosis of bilateral lesions, a review of patients with synchronous bilateral WT who were enrolled in NWTS-4 indicated that 7% of bilateral lesions were not identified by the preoperative imaging studies. Such data emphasize the importance of thorough examination of the contralateral kidney at the time of laparotomy before nephrectomy is undertaken.

The goal of therapy is to eradicate all tumor and to preserve as much normal renal tissue as possible, with the hope of avoiding chronic renal failure. Recommended management is thus initial bilateral renal biopsy with staging of each kidney. This is followed by preoperative chemotherapy. Partial nephrectomy is performed at the initial operation only if the tumor can be removed with preservation of sufficient renal parenchyma on one or both sides for normal renal function. As shown in Table 110.4, which summarizes multimodal treatment regimens, the chemotherapy regimen received depends on stage and histology. Children with stage I or II FH WT receive an 18-week regimen consisting of dactinomycin and vincristine. Those with stage III or IV FH receive a 24-week regimen consisting of dactinomycin, vincristine, and doxorubicin. Children with anaplasia in all stages undergo a 24-week regimen consisting of cyclophosphamide and etoposide, in addition to vincristine and doxorubicin. Following completion of the initial three cycles of chemotherapy, tumor reduction, and the feasibility of partial resection are reassessed by CT. If this evaluation indicates persistent but resectable tumor, or if the tumor has responded completely to chemotherapy, excision of residual tumor mass or biopsy of the former tumor site is indicated. If there is a viable and functioning kidney on one side and the other kidney is extensively involved with tumor, it should be removed. If second-look surgery demonstrates no gross or pathologic evidence of persistent tumor, the chemotherapy regimen

TABLE 110.4. NWTS-5 TREATMENT RECOMMENDATIONS FOR WILMS TUMOR

Stage I (FH): surgery, no radiotherapy, dactinomycin + vincristine for 18 wk
Stage I focal anaplasia: surgery, no radiotherapy, dactinomycin + vincristine for 18 wk
Stage II (FH): surgery, no radiotherapy, dactinomycin + vincristine for 18 wk
Stage II focal anaplasia: surgery, 1,080 cGy to tumor bed, dactinomycin + vincristine + doxorubicin for 24 wk
Stage III (FH): surgery, 1,080 cGy to tumor bed, dactinomycin + vincristine + doxorubicin for 24 wk
Stage III focal anaplasia: surgery, 1,080 cGy to tumor bed, dactinomycin + vincristine + doxorubicin for 24 wk
Stage IV (FH) focal anaplasia: surgery, 1,080 cGy to tumor bed according to local tumor stage, 1,200 cGy to lung and/or other metastatic sites, dactinomycin + vincristine + doxorubicin for 24 wk
Stage II–IV diffuse anaplasia: surgery, radiotherapy (whole lung; abdominal 1,080 cGy), cyclophosphamide + etoposide + vincristine + doxorubicin + mesna for 24 wk
Stage I–IV (clear cell sarcoma): surgery, radiotherapy (abdominal 1,080 cGy; whole lung, stage IV only), cyclophosphamide + etoposide + vincristine + doxorubicin + mesna for 24 wk
Stage I–IV (rhabdoid tumor): surgery, radiotherapy, carboplatinum + etoposide + cyclophosphamide + mesna for 24 wk

Babies 11 months of age or younger should receive half the recommended dose of all drugs. Full doses lead to prohibitive hematologic toxicity in this age group. Full doses of chemotherapeutic agents should be administered to those >12 months of age.
NWTS, National Wilms' Tumor Study.

should be continued for the duration of the treatment regimen. If, on the other hand, surgery demonstrates gross or pathologic evidence of persistent disease, the patient should receive postoperative radiation therapy as well as chemotherapy. Up to 75% of children with bilateral lesions have residual tumor in the remaining kidney, despite repeated surgical procedures. Nevertheless, their survival rate has been extremely high (87%).

SPECIAL SURGICAL CONSIDERATIONS

Parenchymal Sparing Surgery

Although rarely seen in patients with unilateral WT, the occurrence of renal failure as a result of hyperfiltration injury has led European investigators to evaluate the potential for surgery that spares the renal parenchyma in patients with unilateral or bilateral WT. Its possible benefits must be weighed against its potential risks. Surgical complications unique to partial nephrectomy include urine leak and ischemic injury if cross-clamping of the vessels is required. Perilobar or intralobar nephrogenic rests have been identified in 28.8% of unilateral WT specimens. As discussed earlier, these rests are associated with metachronous bilateral WT. Failure to include such microscopic lesions in the surgical specimen could increase the risk of intraabdominal tumor recurrence in patients who have an excellent prognosis with current treatment approaches. Stage I patients are "upstaged" to stage II; they require more chemotherapy and are at risk for both short- and long-term complications related to this therapy.

Using stringent diagnostic imaging criteria, investigators have determined that only 4.6% of unilateral WT patients would have been eligible for partial nephrectomy at the time of diagnosis. These criteria include (a) tumor confined to one pole and occupying less than one third of the renal mass; (b) preserved renal function in the involved kidney; (c) no vascular or collecting system invasion; and (d) clear margins between the tumor, kidney, and surrounding structures.

Partial Nephrectomy

Partial nephrectomy is routinely used in patients with solitary kidneys, synchronous or metachronous bilateral disease, and children known to be at increased risk for multiple neoplasms, such as those with Beckwith-Wiedemann syndrome.

MANAGEMENT OF UNRESECTABLE TUMORS

Tumor size, as well as extension into the suprahepatic IVC, may render the tumor initially inoperable. Because an approximate error rate of 10% has been found in preoperative assessment of resectability by radiographic evaluation, all children with WT should undergo initial exploration to assess operability and to perform a biopsy of the tumor and lymph nodes as previously described. Percutaneous needle biopsy of lesions presumed to be inoperable should be avoided for a several reasons. First, operability cannot generally be accurately assessed without abdominal exploration. Second, the histologic diagnosis based on material obtained from a needle biopsy has an error rate of up to 7.4%. Third, tumor recurrence along the percutaneous biopsy needle tract has been reported.

Patients with FH or focal anaplasia are treated with the 24-week chemotherapy regimen consisting of dactinomycin, doxorubicin, and vincristine (Table 110.4). Those with diffuse anaplasia are treated with the 24-week regimen comprising cyclophosphamide and etoposide, in addition to vincristine and doxorubicin. After 5 weeks of therapy, reevaluation with abdominal CT should be undertaken. If there is no reduction in size of the tumor, radiation therapy is administered. Using the suggested radiation therapy dosage of 1,080 cGy (180 cGy/day for 6 days) with vincristine at weekly intervals during this therapy, shrinkage generally occurs in 6 weeks. Surgery is planned when radiologic assessment indicates that the tumor can be totally excised.

NEONATAL AND EXTRARENAL WILMS TUMOR

Neonatal WT is extremely rare and can be successfully managed with primary nephrectomy alone. Extrarenal WT, found in the pelvis and even the thorax, is also extremely rare. The same therapeutic guidelines are followed as for the affected kidney. Considering the unusual circumstances, it is prudent to use stage III guidelines for chemotherapy and radiation therapy.

FOLLOW-UP

Standard follow-up procedure includes both chest radiography and abdominal ultrasonography. Chest radiographs are taken every 3 months during the second year postsurgery. After this time, they are taken every 6 months for a period of 5 years. Abdominal ultrasonography is performed every 3 months for 2 years posttherapy and then every 6 months until 5 years posttherapy. As demonstrated by a 5- to 10-year follow-up of patients in NWTS-1 and -2, 7% of WT patients developed a benign tumor and 1% developed a second malignancy. The incidence of scoliosis was increased in those patients who received radiation.

METASTATIC TUMOR AND RELAPSE

Disease progression to the lungs, liver, and brain are the main complications of WT. Additionally, the removal of bilateral tumor may leave patients with marginal kidney function. Approximately 12% of patients present with hematogenous metastases at diagnosis and 20% of patients with FH relapse. Over 80% of stage IV patients have pulmonary metastases, and the majority of relapses are also pulmonary in origin. These patients can usually be managed by combined chemotherapy and radiation therapy.

The treatment of metastatic WT depends on the time at which the metastases are diagnosed in relation to the type of therapeutic regimen initially received and the histology of the primary tumor. Patients with FH and stage IV disease have an excellent prognosis, with a 90% survival rate. By contrast, those who relapse with metastatic disease, especially patients with UH, have a grave prognosis. Only 60% of such patients survive.

RADIATION THERAPY

Radiation therapy is usually begun within 10 days after surgery in order to eradicate tumor cells that may have spilled during surgery. As indicated in Table 110.4, stage II (UH), III (FH and UH), and IV (FH and UH) disease require irradiation to the tumor bed. Whole abdominal radiation therapy is unnecessary for patients with tumor spills confined to the flank or for those who have prior biopsy of the neoplasm.

SUGGESTED READING

Beckwith JB. Nephrogenic rests and the pathogenesis of Wilms tumor: developmental and clinical considerations. *Am J Med Genet* 1998;79:268–273.

Breslow NE, Takashima JR, Whitton JA, et al. Second malignant neoplasms following treatment for Wilms tumor: a report from the National Wilms Tumor Study Group. *J Clin Oncol* 1995;13: 1851–1859.

Coppes MJ, Arnold M, Beckwith JB, et al. Factors affecting the risk of contralateral Wilms tumor development: a report from the National Wilms Tumor Study Group. *Cancer* 1999;85: 1616–1625.

Green DM, Breslow NE, Beckwith JB, et al. Comparison between single-dose and divided-dose administration of dactinomycin and doxorubicin for patients with Wilms tumor: a report from the National Wilms Tumor Study Group. *J Clin Oncol* 1998;16: 237–245.

Ritchey ML. Primary nephrectomy for Wilms tumor: approach of the National Wilms Tumor Study Group. *Urology* 1996;47: 787–791.

Ritchey ML, Green DM, Thomas PR, et al. Renal failure in Wilms tumor patients: a report from the National Wilms Tumor Study Group. *Med Pediatr Oncol* 1996;26:75–80.

Ritchey ML, Kelalis PP, Haase GM, et al. Preoperative therapy for intracaval and atrial extension of Wilms tumor. *Cancer* 1993;71: 4104–4110.

Shamberger RC, Guthrie KA, Ritchey ML, et al. Surgery-related factors and local recurrence of Wilms tumor in National Wilms Study 4. *Ann Surg* 1999;229:292–297.

Thomas PR. Wilms tumor: changing role of radiation therapy. *Semin Radiat Oncol* 1997;7:204–211.

Wilimas JA, Kaste SC, Kauffman WM, et al. Use of chest computed tomography in the staging of pediatric Wilms tumor: interobserver variability and prognostic significance. *J Clin Oncol* 1997; 15:2631–2635.

111

RHABDOMYOSARCOMA

HOLLY L. NEVILLE
RICHARD J. ANDRASSY

Approximately 50% of soft tissue sarcomas in children are rhabdomyosarcomas. A rhabdomyosarcoma is one of the small, blue, round cell tumors (neuroblastoma, lymphoma, primitive neuroectodermal tumor, Ewing's sarcoma, rhabdomyosarcoma) of childhood and arises from embryonic mesenchyme, which has the potential to develop into skeletal muscle. Nevertheless, rhabdomyosarcomas may occur anywhere in the body, even where skeletal muscle is generally not present. In the Intergroup Rhabdomyosarcoma Study (IRS) IV, the distribution of primary sites was genitourinary in 29%, head and neck in 28%, extremities in 15%, pelvis in 12%, trunk and thorax in 7%, orbit in 6.5%, and gastrointestinal in 1%. When developing a treatment plan, it is important to recognize several factors, including stage, group, site, and histologic subtype.

There are five subtypes of rhabdomyosarcoma, but most fall into one of two major subtypes: embryonal and alveolar. Other subtypes include botryoid, spindle cell, and pleomorphic rhabdomyosarcomas. Embryonal histology is the most common subtype and is commonly found to arise in the head and neck, genitourinary tract, and orbit. Alveolar rhabdomyosarcoma is most frequently seen in the extremities, trunk, or perineum. Most likely, this occurrence in unfavorable sites associates alveolar histology with a poor prognosis. A recent review did not distinguish the alveolar subtype as a significant independent prognostic indicator in extremity rhabdomyosarcoma. The botryoid variant, named because of its resemblance to a cluster of grapes, arises in cavitary structures such as the vagina and bladder, and is most commonly seen in infants. Spindle cell rhabdomyosarcoma, another variant of the embryonal histology, is most commonly found in the paratesticular area.

R. J. Andrassy: Department of Surgery, University of Texas-Houston Medical School; and Department of Pediatric Surgical Oncology, Memorial-Hermann Hospital, M.D. Anderson Cancer Center, Houston, Texas.

H. L. Neville: Department of Surgery, University of Texas-Houston Medical School, Houston, Texas.

Rhabdomyosarcoma is associated with a p53 mutation and the Li Fraumeni syndrome, a familial cancer syndrome. Therefore, physicians and patients should have a heightened awareness of the potential for second malignancies, including soft tissue or bony sarcomas, leukemia, brain or adrenal neoplasms, and maternal premenopausal breast cancer.

DIAGNOSTIC APPROACH

The evaluation of a patient with a suspected rhabdomyosarcoma should seek to define local extent of tumor, lymph node involvement, and distant metastasis. The patient should initially undergo a thorough physical examination with palpation of the lymph node basins, followed by radiographic evaluation. In most cases, computed tomography or magnetic resonance imaging of the primary tumor is necessary to assess the size of the tumor and its extension into adjacent structures. Magnetic resonance imaging (MRI) is preferred for tumors located in the head and neck or extremity because the resolution allows visualization of tumor proximity to adjacent structures. Magnetic resonance angiography may be added if there is concern about proximity to or invasion of major vascular structures. A bone scan and computed tomography of the chest are also recommended to rule out metastatic disease to the skeletal structures or pulmonary parenchyma. The diagnosis should then be confirmed with a tissue specimen, which may be attained via fine-needle, core biopsy, or incisional biopsy.

Once the histologic diagnosis has been made, the tumor should be staged. In the most recent series by the Intergroup Rhabdomyosarcoma Study Group, patients were prospectively classified for the first time using a pretreatment staging system based on prognostic factors identified in IRS II. The staging system currently used for rhabdomyosarcoma is the Lawrence/Gehan Staging System coupled with the postresection group. The staging system and operative grouping are shown in Tables 111.1 and 111.2. A patient's postsurgical group is multifactorial. Complete resection is necessary to be grouped in group 1.

TABLE 111.1. PREOPERATIVE LAWRENCE/GEHAN STAGING SYSTEM AS DEVISED BY THE INTERGROUP RHABDOMYOSARCOMA STUDY GROUP

Stage	Primary Tumor Site	Size	N	M
I	Orbit/eyelid, Head and Neck (excluding parameningeal [PM]),GU (excluding bladder/prostate)	Any	Nx or N0 or N1	M0
II	Bladder/prostate, Extremity, PM, Other (trunk, retroperitoneum, etc)	<5 cm	Nx or N0	M0
III	Bladder/prostate, Extremity, PM,	<5 cm	N1	M0
	Other	≥5 cm	Nx or N1 or N0	
IV	All			M1

N0, regional nodes not clinically involved; N1, regional nodes clinically involved; Nx, regional nodes not assessed; M0, no distant metastases; M1, distant metastases.
Data from Lawrence W Jr, Gehan EA, Hayes DM, et al. Prognostic significance of staging factors of the UICC staging system in childhood rhabdomyosarcomas: a report from the Intergroup Rhabdomyosarcoma Study. *J Clin Oncol* 1987;5:46–54; with permission.

Primary site, tumor size or invasiveness, and node status separate nonmetastatic patients into distinct prognostic groups. The IRS Group currently uses both pretreatment stage and operative group to stratify patients to therapeutic regimens.

During the diagnostic phase, the patient should be evaluated by both the surgeon and oncologist to provide optimal timing of all therapeutic interventions. Surgery remains a key component in the treatment strategy of pediatric rhabdomyosarcoma, providing both necessary information for histologic diagnosis and staging as well as therapy in many cases. Surgical staging involves excisional or incisional biopsy, and the evaluation of lymphatics through either lymph node sampling or sentinel lymph node biopsy with the use of lymphatic mapping. Primary resection is undertaken only when complete excision can be performed without causing disability or mutilation. Frequently, this is not possible and chemotherapy is given as primary therapy, followed by delayed resection after assessing tumor response. Radiation therapy is reserved for those patients with recurrent, persistent, or locally advanced disease and is most frequently given by external beam. B rachytherapy administered through the use of implants placed at the time of tumor resection is a helpful adjuvant to surgery and chemotherapy in cases with unresectable microscopic disease. This technique allows aggressive treatment of the tumor bed while sparing the growing pediatric patient the morbidity of bone and soft tissue exposure to radiation. Multimodal therapy has allowed for continued improvement in survival as well as cosmetic and functional results in pediatric rhabdomyosarcomas.

TABLE 111.2. POSTOPERATIVE GROUPING SYSTEM BY THE INTERGROUP RHABDOMYOSARCOMA GROUP

Group I	Localized disease, completely resection, N0
Group II	Microscopic residual disease, N0 or N1
Group III	Gross residual disease or biopsy only
Group IV	M1

N0, negative lymph nodes; N1, regional lymph nodes containing tumor; M1, metastatic disease.
Data from Lawrence W Jr, Gehan EA, Hayes DM, et al. Prognostic significance of staging factors of the UICC staging system in childhood rhabdomyosarcomas: a report from the Intergroup Rhabdomyosarcoma Study. *J Clin Oncol* 1987;5:46–54; with permission.

PREOPERATIVE PREPARATION

Preoperative preparation in the patient with rhabdomyosarcoma varies greatly by primary tumor site as well as tumor stage. The extent of surgical resection currently recommended for rhabdomyosarcoma varies by primary tumor site, although initial complete resection is generally recommended if it is thought to be feasible without loss of organ function. Initial surgical resection is not recommended in patients with tumors arising in the orbit, vagina, or bladder because chemotherapy, with or without radiation therapy, or limited surgery performed after multiagent chemotherapy, offers an excellent chance of cure with no decrease in survival when compared with aggressive initial resection.

The surgeon must determine whether complete resection is feasible or recommended at the time of diagnosis. When initial complete resection is not deemed feasible at diagnosis, contemporary therapy for patients with rhabdomyosarcoma includes intensive chemotherapy and radiation therapy after initial biopsy. The biopsy should be carefully planned to ensure that later resection is not hindered. Either a fine needle biopsy, core needle biopsy, or incisional biopsy should be performed. Orientation of the biopsy incision is crucial to allow later surgical intervention with minimal disfiguration. Surgical evaluation of the draining lymph node basins should be performed at the time of biopsy if initial resection is not planned. Delayed resection of gross residual disease should then be performed after optimal response to adjuvant therapy has been achieved.

Such therapy may render a previously unresectable tumor resectable without disability or mutilation.

Primary tumor resection should be considered in patients with localized disease that is amenable to complete resection. Exceptions to this again are primary tumors of the orbit, bladder, or vagina. The preoperative plan should take into account surgical evaluation of lymphatics, which should be done at the time of initial resection. Consideration is currently being given to treating resectable patients with preoperative adjuvant therapy. IRS-V will evaluate the role of tumor resection after neoadjuvant chemotherapy for responding patients. Radiation therapy will be given in all of these cases, but the dose will be reduced according to the extent of the surgical resection.

Reexcision should be considered for patients who are referred with gross, microscopic residual or unknown residual disease status. In our recent study, six patients underwent primary reexcision, and all were alive at the time of the analysis. Surprisingly, several patients referred with complete resection were found to have residual disease at the time of operation. Hays et al. reported that patients with truncal or extremity sarcomas who underwent primary reexcision experienced a survival benefit when compared with patients who received adjuvant therapy prior to complete resection.

The IRS-IV experience with extremity rhabdomyosarcoma emphasized the importance of evaluating regional lymph nodes. Seventeen percent of extremity rhabdomyosarcoma patients with clinically negative regional nodes had microscopic tumor on histologic evaluation. Thirty-eight (50%) of the surgically evaluated lymph nodes contained disease. The true incidence of node positivity in pediatric rhabdomyosarcoma is likely to be underestimated, and does not seem to shadow the behavior of rhabdomyosarcoma in adults.

Lymph node status has important implications for staging and grouping, and thus determines the need for chemotherapy or radiation therapy planning. Although lymph node dissection, even in the face of nodal disease, has not been shown to improve survival, the surgeon may choose from several options to assess the lymph node status. Preoperative lymphoscintigraphy continues to play an important role in sites that have varied drainage, such as the trunk or head and neck. Through the identification of the draining basin, this study aids in performing a focused examination of the lymphatics. Although there has been limited experience with lymph node mapping for rhabdomyosarcoma, our experience to date has demonstrated a good reliability in locating the sentinel node. However, the long-term accuracy of this technique for rhabdomyosarcoma requires further study. Lymphatic mapping with sentinel lymph node biopsy is a technically straightforward, standardized method with minimal morbidity that could be used by pediatric surgeons to enhance the evaluation of lymphatics.

Currently, we use lymphazurin blue in combination with technetium-labeled sulfur colloid. Similar to previous reports, our one failure occurred in a patient who was injected with only lymphazurin. Although more time consuming, and requiring the cooperation of the radiology and nuclear medicine departments, use of technetium-labeled sulfur colloid facilitates the identification of the sentinel node and has been shown to increase the sensitivity of the technique.

TECHNIQUE

All patients with a truncal tumor should undergo preoperative lymphoscintigraphy to identify the draining nodal basin. If lymphatic mapping with sentinel node mapping is being considered, it should be performed at the same time as the biopsy or primary excision. This prevents disruption of the lymphatics, which could obscure or misidentify the sentinel node. Ideally, if a reliable pathologist is available, once the tumor is identified as a malignancy on frozen section analysis, the surgeon should proceed with evaluation of the lymphatics by either sentinel node biopsy or aggressive lymph node sampling. The procedure is performed as follows. The day prior to surgery, or the morning prior to surgery in the event of an afternoon surgery date, lymphoscintigraphy is performed. This allows both the localization of the draining basin and provides the radiolabeling to be used for intraoperative localization.

The patient is then brought to the operating room where the tumor is injected with lymphazurin blue. Routine preparation and draping of both the primary tumor as well as the draining lymphatic basin is then performed, thereby giving adequate time for the dye to stain the lymphatics. The draining basin is then examined using a gamma probe in a sterile sheath. A mark is made with a sterile pen over the areas of high counts. A biopsy of the tumor is then performed to allow for frozen section confirmation of malignancy. Once obtained, the surgeon may proceed with evaluation of the lymphatics, obtain further tissue for permanent sectioning, or perform a complete resection if feasible. Gloves and instruments are then exchanged and the surgeon proceeds with the sentinel node biopsy. Once the areas of high counts are transcutaneously localized, the incisions are planned such that future lymph node dissection, if warranted, would incorporate the planned incisions. A small incision is then made overlying the area of high counts and the underlying tissue examined for the presence of blue dye. Dissection is then undertaken, carefully isolating the blue dye, and ligating any blue lymphatic channels that were traversed, thus decreasing the chance of a chyloma. The gamma probe is again used to assist in localization of the sentinel nodes. The blue nodes with the highest counts are then removed and data recorded regarding their color and count.

We send our nodes for permanent sectioning, because lymph node dissection is not recommended even if positive nodes are identified. For the surgeon's initial cases with lymph node mapping, he or she may consider aggressive lymph node sampling after submitting the sentinel node to confirm accuracy of their technique.

POSTOPERATIVE CARE

Postoperative care varies depending on the site of the primary tumor. Patients with extremity site tumors should be treated with restriction of limb movement, usually aided by a splint placed at the time of surgery or in the recovery room, followed by physical therapy once the incision is healed. Patients are then followed closely by the oncologist and surgeon for local recurrence, distant metastases, and second malignancies. This usually entails visits every 3 to 6 months with physical examination and chest radiography. Pelvic, intraabdominal, and genitourinary tumors may be followed with computed tomography to evaluate for local recurrence.

SUGGESTED READINGS

Alazraki NP, Eshima D, Eshima LA, et al. Lymphoscintigraphy, the sentinel node concept, and the intraoperative gamma probe in melanoma, breast cancer, and other potential cancers. *Semin Nucl Med* 1997;27:55–67.

Andrassy RJ, Hays DM, Raney RM, et al. Conservative surgical management of vaginal and vulvar pediatric rhabdomyosarcoma: a report from the Intergroup Rhabdomyosarcoma Study III. *J Pediatr Surg* 1995;30:1034–1037.

Hays DM, Lawrence W Jr, Wharam M, et al. Primary reexcision for patients with "microscopic residual" tumor following initial excision of sarcomas of trunk and extremity sites. *J Pediatr Surg* 1989;24:5–10.

James J, Andrassy RJ. Rhabdomyosarcoma in children. *Contemp Surg* 1987;30:58–65.

Lawrence W Jr, Hays DM, Heyn R, et al. Surgical lessons from the Intergroup Rhabdomyosarcoma Study (IRS) pertaining to extremity tumors. *World J Surg* 1988;12:676–684.

Neville H, Andrassy RJ, Wiener E, et al. Extremity rhabdomyosarcoma: an analysis of preoperative staging, prognostic factors and outcome from the Intergroup Rhabdomyosarcoma Study IV. *J Pediatr Surg* 2000;35:317–321.

Neville HL, Andrassy RJ. Pediatric rhabdomyosarcoma. In: Hunt K, Ross MI, eds. *Mastery of lymphatic mapping.* New York: Springer-Verlag (in press).

Neville HL, Raney RB, Andrassy RJ, et al. Multidisciplinary management of pediatric soft-tissue sarcoma. *Oncology* 2000;14:1471-1490.

Surgical Directives: Pediatric Surgery, edited by Peter Mattei. Lippincott Williams & Wilkins, Philadelphia © 2002

112

HEPATIC MALIGNANCIES

NICHOLAS A. SHORTER
MICHAEL P. LA QUAGLIA

Worldwide, in all age groups, primary hepatic malignancy, specifically hepatocellular carcinoma, is one of the most common human malignancies. In the West, the frequency of hepatic malignancy is much lower, and in children, malignant tumors of the liver are rare, with only 100 to 150 cases occurring each year in the United States in individuals under 20 years of age, an annual incidence of 1.6 per million children. Of these, about 60% are hepatoblastomas, an embryonal tumor, 33% are hepatocellular carcinomas, seemingly identical to the disease seen in adults, and the rest are various unusual sarcomas. The liver is a common site for metastatic disease, but this topic is beyond the scope of this discussion.

Essentially all cases of hepatoblastoma occur in children under 3 years of age, with the average age being 1 year. Boys are affected more commonly than girls. In contrast, hepatocellular carcinoma usually affects children between the ages of 12 and 15 years. Hepatocellular carcinoma may occur in younger children, however, with a second peak of incidence in children under 4. There is a similar male predominance. Five histologic subtypes of hepatoblastoma exist: fetal, embryonal, mixed mesenchymal, macrotubular, and anaplastic or small cell. The fetal type may have a better prognosis. In general, small cell tumors do poorly. Extramedullary hematopoiesis is typical of hepatoblastoma, and calcification may be present. Vascular invasion and multicentricity are hallmarks of hepatocellular carcinoma. The fibrolamellar variant of hepatocellular carcinoma may be associated with a better prognosis, although recent studies indicate that when patients are controlled for stage, this may not be the case.

Both tumor types can be associated with specific syndromes or diseases. Hepatoblastoma may occur in children with Beckwith-Wiedemann syndrome, Gardner's syndrome, hemihypertrophy, and the familial adenomatous polyposis syndrome. Recently, an important but as yet unexplained association has been noted with very low birth weight. The risk of hepatocellular carcinoma is elevated in the setting of cirrhosis, but the risk differs depending on the etiology. It is high with tyrosinemia and hemochromatosis, moderate with α_1-antitrypsin deficiency, autoimmune hepatitis and alcoholic cirrhosis, and low with Wilson's disease, primary biliary cirrhosis, and primary sclerosing cholangitis. In parts of Africa and Asia, hepatocellular carcinoma often occurs as a result of exposure to aflatoxin B, a natural product of the *Aspergillus* fungus, which often contaminates the food supply. Most significant worldwide is the high incidence of hepatocellular carcinoma in individuals chronically infected with either the hepatitis B or C virus. The mechanisms of viral transformation are often unknown. Studies from Taiwan have demonstrated that the incidence of childhood hepatocellular carcinoma can be reduced with a nationwide program of hepatitis B immunization. In the United States most cases of childhood hepatocellular carcinoma are not virally related and do not occur in the setting of cirrhosis.

The molecular mechanisms of hepatocarcinogenesis are poorly understood. Mutations in the p53 tumor suppressor protein appear to be important in some cases of hepatocellular carcinoma. Abnormalities also have been noted in other cell cycle–related proteins, such as the retinoblastoma protein, p16, p21, and p27, but the significance of these findings is unknown. Loss of heterozygosity at chromosomes 11p15.5 and 1p36 have been described in cases of hepatoblastoma, as have trisomies 20, 2, and 18. The risk of hepatoblastoma is elevated in families with familial adenomatous polyposis, the gene for which is located on the long arm of chromosome 5. Mutations of this gene appear to be common in hepatoblastomas from patients without the syndrome as well, indicating that it is likely to play an important role in tumorigenesis.

In infants and young children, most liver tumors present with an asymptomatic right upper quadrant mass that is detected incidentally by a parent or the family physician. Pain and other symptoms, such as nausea, vomiting,

N. A. Shorter and M. P. La Quaglia: Department of Surgery, Weill-Cornell University Medical School; and Department of Pediatric Surgery, Memorial Sloan-Kettering Cancer Center, New York, New York.

anorexia, and weight loss, are more commonly seen in older children or adolescents with hepatocellular carcinoma. Jaundice is rare. An important point to remember is that some patients with hepatic malignancy present to the trauma service with a liver fracture through the tumor mass, which, unfortunately, can result in misinterpretation of the diagnostic studies. A clue in such cases is that the degree of liver injury usually is disproportionate to the severity of the traumatic event.

The finding of a liver tumor in a child does not necessarily mean that a malignancy is present. In fact, benign masses, such as hemangiomas, account for almost half of all cases. After identifying the liver as the site of origin, evaluation is first directed toward differentiating clearly benign lesions from those that are potentially malignant. Initial diagnostic evaluation depends in part on the capabilities and experience of the institution and on the preferences of the evaluating physicians and surgeons. Plain films are of little value, although calcifications may be present in some hepatoblastomas. Ultrasonography, computed tomography (CT), and magnetic resonance imaging all provide useful, although not identical, information with regard to both diagnosis and resectability, and some combination of these studies is applicable in every case. Angiography is now rarely, if ever, necessary, because vascular structures can be adequately visualized using the other techniques. When malignancy is suspected or confirmed, a metastatic evaluation should include a CT scan of the chest. Lung metastases are present in about 10% of patients at diagnosis.

Results of laboratory evaluation are normal in most children with benign masses. Anemia is common in patients with malignancy, and thrombocytosis (greater than a million platelets per mm3) and sometimes, is a frequent finding in association with hepatoblastoma. Liver function studies are usually normal. Serum alpha-fetoprotein levels should be measured in all patients. They are elevated in up to 90% of patients with hepatoblastoma and at least half of those with hepatocellular carcinoma. Alpha-fetoprotein is a particularly valuable marker when following a child for evidence of recurrence or persistent disease. The values may be difficult to interpret in infants, because alpha-fetoprotein levels are normally elevated at birth and slowly decline to "normal" over the first months of life. Human chorionic gonadotropin levels are elevated in a small subset of hepatoblastoma patients, who may present with precocious puberty. Serum ferritin levels may be elevated with either tumor type.

Once a malignant lesion is suspected, biopsy is necessary, both to confirm the malignant diagnosis and to determine the specific tumor type. Open biopsy is most commonly used. Laparoscopy also may be employed. A determination must be made regarding resectability. Usually this is possible to determine from the radiologic studies, but in some cases the decision can only be made at the time of exploration. If resection is clearly not possible from the radiologic studies, percutaneous needle biopsy can be used to obtain a diagnosis, although this may not be definitive in some cases of hepatocellular carcinoma, which may resemble normal liver tissue in limited samples.

Although the overall approach to hepatoblastoma and hepatocellular carcinoma is similar in that complete resection of the primary tumor is necessary for cure, discrimination between the two has significant prognostic implications. In short, children with hepatoblastoma usually respond well to treatment and have a good chance of cure, whereas hepatocellular carcinoma is typically advanced at diagnosis, responds poorly to treatment, and is usually fatal, except in rare cases that are found incidentally or as a result of screening. Even if unresectable at diagnosis, most hepatoblastomas are unifocal and chemosensitive, and the majority are resectable after therapy. Even some patients with metastatic disease, particularly to the lung, are curable with a combination of chemotherapy, hepatic resection, and, sometimes, surgical excision of the pulmonary lesions. In contrast, hepatocellular carcinoma is frequently multifocal at diagnosis, only resectable in about 30% of patients, responds poorly, if at all, to chemotherapy or radiation, and frequently recurs within the residual liver mass even in cases in which a total resection is performed and felt to be adequate.

Overall survival of about 70% is now achievable in nonmetastatic hepatoblastoma. Survival may be as high as 50% in patients who present with pulmonary metastases. In contrast, long-term survival for children with hepatocellular carcinoma is 10% at best, and, in our experience, it approaches zero.

In both tumor types, initial complete resection is desirable, if it can be accomplished safely. Wedge resections are occasionally possible with small lesions. The possible anatomic resections, based on the segmental anatomy of the liver, are right hepatic lobectomy, left hepatic lobectomy, extended right hepatic lobectomy (right trisegmentectomy), left lateral segmentectomy, and extended left lobectomy (left trisegmentectomy). These are discussed in Chapter 102. On occasion, we have also successfully used a central hepatic resection, removing segments IV, V, and VIII, which has allowed complete resection in several patients, while preserving more normal liver than would have been possible with the more conventional but more extensive procedures that would otherwise have been necessary.

Several staging systems now exist, which are used for both tumor types. None is ideal. In the United States, staging is usually based on the initial extent of disease and the outcome of the initial surgical procedure with regard to the completeness of the resection (Tables 112.1 and 112.2). In Japan, a TNM system is used. In Europe, the most common system is based largely on the initial preoperative extent of disease, the liver being divided into four sectors.

About 50% of hepatoblastomas are resectable at diagnosis. One current area of debate is whether initial resection is always the best approach, or whether with large but still anatomically resectable tumors, chemotherapy should be

TABLE 112.1. HEPATOBLASTOMA STAGING (U.S. SYSTEM)

Stage	Criteria
I	Localized tumor, completely resected
II	Localized tumor, microscopic residual disease
III	Unresectable tumor, gross residual disease
IV	Metastatic disease

TABLE 112.2. HEPATOBLASTOMA STAGING (CHILDREN'S CANCER STUDY GROUP SYSTEM)

Stage	Criteria
I	Complete resection as initial treatment
IIA	Complete resection after chemotherapy or radiotherapy
IIB	Incomplete resection, residual disease localized to one lobe
IIIA	Tumor involves both lobes of liver
IIIB	Regional lymph node involvement
IV	Distant metastases

given first to shrink the lesion, potentially making the resection easier and safer and decreasing the amount of liver tissue that must be removed. At this time opinions are mixed. Theoretical objections to delayed resection are the toxicity of the preoperative therapy, which can delay subsequent operation, a possible adverse effect of chemotherapy on postoperative liver regeneration, the risk for metastases occurring during the period of treatment, and the potential risk for developing drug resistance. Despite these concerns, equivalent cure rates result from both approaches. On the other hand, operative mortality does not appear to have been reduced by preoperative chemotherapy; in fact, reported morbidity rates are higher in those children undergoing delayed resection. These findings are based on small series and anecdotal reports, rather than randomized studies, and therefore should be interpreted cautiously.

Chemotherapy is active against hepatoblastoma. Most regimens are cisplatinum based, usually in combination with vincristine and 5-fluorouracil. Doxorubicin is also active against these tumors, but has much greater toxicity. Chemotherapy can convert up to 75% of previously unresectable hepatoblastomas to a resectable situation, and if a complete resection is eventually achieved, cure rates in the range of 60% can now be expected. Chemotherapy also can cure a significant portion of those with pulmonary metastases, which is sometimes combined with pulmonary resection. In early-stage disease, chemotherapy is of proven benefit following resection, resulting in a survival rate of over 90%. It is not yet clear whether a subset of early-stage patients, perhaps the group with pure fetal histology, can be managed with surgery alone. As previously mentioned, response rates of hepatocellular carcinoma to chemotherapy are minimal. If resection is feasible, it should always be undertaken at presentation. There is little role in the management of either tumor for radiation therapy, except for palliation.

A number of other treatment modalities have been used for malignant liver tumors, usually in adults with hepatocellular carcinoma or metastatic colon cancer. These include such techniques as percutaneous ethanol injection, cryotherapy, radiofrequency ablation, hepatic artery infusion, and transcatheter arterial chemoembolization. Some are only applicable to small lesions, and are rarely useful in childhood tumors. Transcatheter arterial chemoembolization has been tried in children with unresectable hepatocellular carcinoma, but with little success. Hormonal therapy and immunotherapy have thus far been ineffective. The only therapeutic option that has been shown to have some potential value in unresectable patients is liver transplantation, but this is only an option if the disease is completely confined to the liver, and the long-term recurrence rate following transplantation is not yet known, and is likely to be substantial. The initial results appear to be better with hepatoblastoma than they are with hepatocellular carcinoma. This approach is severely limited by the shortage of organs for transplantation, and the use of living related donors in this setting raises significant ethical issues.

SUGGESTED READINGS

Bowman LC, Riely CA. Management of pediatric liver tumors. *Surg Oncol Clin North Am* 1996;5:451–459.

Newman KD. Hepatic tumors in children. *Semin Pediatr Surgery* 1997;6:38–41.

Weinberg AG, Finegold MJ. Primary hepatic tumors of childhood. *Hum Pathol* 1983;14:512–537.

Wheatley JM, LaQuaglia MP. Management of hepatic epithelial malignancy in childhood and adolescence. *Semin Surg Oncol* 1993;9:532–540.

113

TESTICULAR TUMORS

JONATHAN H. ROSS

Tumors occur rarely in the prepubertal testis. The incidence of testis tumors is 0.5 to 2.0 per 100,000 children, accounting for only 1% to 2% of all pediatric tumors. Prepubertal testis tumors are classified by the putative cell of origin. Those arising from germ cells include yolk sac tumor, teratoma, and epidermoid cyst. Stromal tumors include juvenile granulosa cell tumor, Leydig cell tumor, Sertoli cell tumor, and mixed or undifferentiated stromal tumor. Gonadoblastomas contain both germ cell and stromal elements. Secondary tumors rarely affect the testis, although testicular involvement with acute lymphoblastic leukemia is an important exception. Although yolk sac tumors, which are malignant, account for the majority of prepubertal testis tumors, a higher proportion of pediatric testis tumors are benign (compared with testis tumors in adults). Furthermore, the natural history of yolk sac tumors differs significantly from that of postpubertal tumors. For these reasons, the initial surgical management and subsequent treatment of prepubertal testis tumors are quite different.

PRESENTATION AND EVALUATION

Testis tumors most commonly present as a testicular mass that may be noted by the patient or detected on a routine physical examination. A hydrocele is sometimes present, which may be secondary to the tumor or coincidental. The presence of a hydrocele may delay the diagnosis of a testis tumor, and ultrasonography should be considered for any boy with a hydrocele and a testis that cannot be palpated. Occasionally patients present with pain, presumably from an acute bleed into the tumor. Physical examination usually reveals a hard mass in the testicular parenchyma. These masses must be distinguished from benign extratesticular lesions such as epididymal cysts.

J. H. Ross: Section of Pediatric Urology, The Urological Institute, Cleveland Clinic Foundation, Cleveland, Ohio.

Once a testis tumor is suspected, a thorough physical examination is undertaken. Signs of androgenization or feminization should be sought. Metastatic disease is uncommon, and the most common sites—the retroperitoneum and lungs—are unlikely to display symptoms or physical findings. In rare cases, metastases to the bone or central nervous system may produce symptoms.

The initial radiographic evaluation of children with a suspected testis tumor is limited. Because many prepubertal testis tumors are benign, any metastatic evaluation is deferred until tissue confirmation of the tumor's histology is obtained. However, ultrasonography of the primary tumor is helpful. It can be used to distinguish testicular tumors from benign extratesticular lesions. The extent of testicular involvement also can be determined, which is helpful if testis-sparing surgery is being considered. The ultrasonographic appearance of specific testis tumors has been described, but is too inconsistent to allow a definitive diagnosis in most cases.

Tumor markers play an important role in the evaluation and follow-up of childhood testis tumors. Alpha-fetoprotein (AFP) is the most important tumor marker. It is an albumin precursor synthesized by the yolk sac and fetal liver and gut. Levels are elevated in 80% to 90% of children with a yolk sac tumor. Elevated levels of AFP preclude consideration of a testis-sparing approach. An important caveat is that AFP levels are normally quite high in infancy. An "elevated" level in a boy under 1 year of age does not rule out the possibility of a benign tumor, such as teratoma. The β subunit of human chorionic gonadotropin (HCG) is an important marker in adult testis tumors, but is rarely elevated in children because the histologic types that lead to elevated HCG levels are rarely encountered in pediatric testis tumors.

SURGICAL APPROACH

The standard approach to a testis tumor is inguinal orchiectomy. Through an inguinal incision, the spermatic cord is isolated and clamped with a noncrushing clamp. The testis is then delivered into the inguinal incision with the tunica vaginalis intact. Once a testis tumor is confirmed by direct palpation, the cord is ligated and divided at the internal ring.

Testis-sparing surgery is appropriate for benign testicular tumors. This is particularly attractive in prepubertal patients because more than one third of tumors are benign in this population. The preoperative evaluation plays a significant role in patient selection for testis-sparing surgery. An elevated AFP level in a child over 1 year of age virtually always reflects the presence of a yolk sac tumor and precludes a testis-sparing approach. Similarly, diffuse involvement of the testis on preoperative ultrasonography makes the issue moot because there is unlikely to be significant testicular tissue worth preserving. However, in infants, and older children with a normal AFP level, the likelihood of a benign tumor is considerable. This is also true in boys presenting with androgenization. For these patients, if there is salvageable normal testicular parenchyma evident, an inguinal exploration should be undertaken so that testis-sparing surgery may be performed if a benign histology is confirmed (Fig. 113.1). The initial approach is the same as for an inguinal orchiectomy. Once the testis is delivered into the inguinal incision (the cord having been clamped with a noncrushing clamp), the field is draped off with towels and the tunica vaginalis is opened. The tumor is excised with a margin of normal parenchyma and sent for frozen section analysis. If a benign histology is confirmed, then the testicular defect is closed with chromic suture and the testis is returned to the scrotum. If a malignancy is detected, or the frozen section is nondiagnostic, then an orchiectomy is performed.

Following orchiectomy, some children with testicular tumors require additional therapy. The type of adjunctive therapy selected depends on the histology of the primary tumor and the results of radiographic and biochemical studies. The intensity of follow-up also depends on the malignant potential of the primary tumor.

YOLK SAC TUMOR

Yolk sac tumor is the most common prepubertal testis tumor. Yolk sac tumors have gone by a number of other names, including endodermal sinus tumor, orchioblastoma, juvenile embryonal carcinoma, mesoblastoma vitellinum, clear cell adenocarcinoma, extraembryonal mesoblastoma, and archenteronoma. Metastatic evaluation of yolk sac tumors includes computed tomography (CT) of the abdomen and pelvis to rule out retroperitoneal lymph node or hepatic metastases and chest radiography or chest CT to rule out pulmonary metastases. Bone and brain metastases are rare. Therefore, bone scans and head CT scans are obtained only when there is clinical suspicion of metastases at these sites. The serum AFP level is also measured postoperatively. Its half-life is approximately 5 days, and a persistent elevation of AFP following orchiectomy suggests the presence of metastatic disease. However, AFP levels as high as 50,000 ng/mL can occur in normal infants, as can levels greater than 50 ng/mL in children up to 6 months of age.

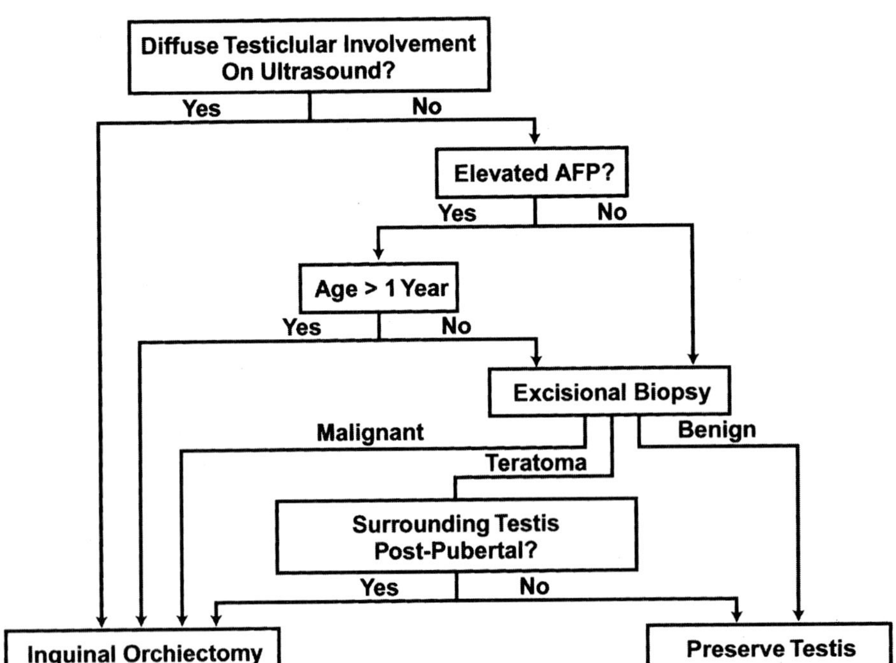

FIGURE 113.1. Surgical management of prepubertal testis tumors.

Therefore, serial measurements are particularly important in small children.

A TNM staging system exists for testis tumors, but its applicability to pediatric tumors is limited due to the infrequent practice of retroperitoneal lymph node dissection (RPLND) in these patients. Several other systems have been proposed. The simplest has been suggested by Boden and Gibb and segregates patients into three stages. Stage I patients have tumor confined to the testis with a negative metastatic evaluation and normalization of AFP postoperatively. Stage II patients have retroperitoneal disease detected by radiographic studies or RPLND, and/or a persistent elevation of AFP postoperatively. Stage III patients have metastatic disease beyond the retroperitoneum. Approximately 80% of children with yolk sac tumors have stage I tumors.

Historically, RPLND was the most common form of adjunctive therapy for the treatment of yolk sac tumors. A standard RPLND is accomplished through a midline or transverse abdominal incision. Complete excision of all lymphatic tissue from the renal hila to 2 cm beyond the bifurcation of the common iliac arteries is accomplished. The lateral margins of dissection are the ureters, and the great vessels are completely skeletonized throughout.

Modified protocols limiting the contralateral dissection and nerve-sparing techniques have been described in adults in an attempt to minimize the morbidity of the dissection, particularly anejaculation. For right-sided tumors, a modified dissection is limited medially by the anterior surface of the aorta. Below the inferior mesenteric artery (IMA), dissection is limited medially by the right common iliac artery, preserving the hypogastric plexus. The modified template for a left-sided tumor is limited medially by the anterior surface of the inferior vena cava. Below the IMA, dissection is again limited medially by the left common iliac artery. The efficacy of these modified techniques has not been clarified in children.

With the widespread use of AFP to detect occult metastases, and improvements in multiagent chemotherapy, the reliance on RPLND to diagnose and treat metastatic disease has faded. Although some series suggested improved survival with RPLND, the studies were uncontrolled and the majority of patients who "benefited" had no histopathologic evidence of disease in the resected nodes. In theory, RPLND is less beneficial for children than for adults because yolk sac tumors in children have a predilection for hematogenous spread. Metastases are limited to the retroperitoneum in only one third of patients with metastatic disease, whereas approximately half of these patients have metastases at hematogenous sites without retroperitoneal involvement. The operative morbidity of RPLND in children is significant, including wound complications, bowel obstruction, chylous ascites, and anejaculation as adults due to injury to the sympathetic nerves.

Chemotherapy is effective in treating metastatic yolk sac tumor. The most commonly used regimens include cisplatin in combination with other agents such as etoposide and bleomycin. Because children with metastatic disease often have multiple sites of spread, chemotherapy is particularly appropriate for these patients.

Radiation is not a standard form of treatment for metastatic yolk sac tumor. Although yolk sac tumor is radiosensitive, the doses required when radiation is used as a primary therapy are prohibitively toxic. Lower doses of radiation may play a role in combination with surgery and chemotherapy for high-risk patients.

The selection of adjuvant therapy for yolk sac tumor depends on the stage of the tumor. The trend in managing stage I tumors is toward observation. Most series reported in the past decade have found no survival advantage to adjuvant therapy in this group. The recurrence rate for patients with stage I tumor managed by observation is approximately 20%, and virtually all of these patients can be salvaged with chemotherapy. Chemotherapy may be considered in high-risk patients, such as those with a normal AFP prior to orchiectomy who cannot be reliably followed biochemically. Patients with stage I tumor are therefore generally observed closely without adjuvant therapy. Patients are evaluated 1 month after orchiectomy with CT of the abdomen and pelvis, chest radiography, and measurement of serum AFP. For 2 years measurement of serum AFP and chest radiography are repeated every 6 weeks, and CT every 3 months. Recurrent disease is usually treated with chemotherapy, even if it appears to be limited to the retroperitoneum. If the patient remains free of disease for 2 years, then he is almost certainly cured, and minimal follow-up is required beyond that point.

Patients with a negative metastatic evaluation, but a failure of the AFP to normalize, are generally treated with chemotherapy. Patients with positive lymph nodes on CT are also treated with chemotherapy, although consideration may be given to performing a modified RPLND in the presence of minimal retroperitoneal disease and a normal AFP level. RPLND should also be considered when retroperitoneal disease is not responding to chemotherapy or for a persistent mass following chemotherapy when the AFP level has normalized. Some of these residual masses contain only necrotic tumor and calcifications.

Chemotherapy is the mainstay of treatment for stage III disease. Chemotherapy with second-line agents should be used for patients failing to respond to standard agents. Surgical excision and radiation should also be considered for those with limited sites of metastatic disease who fail to respond to chemotherapy.

The overall survival rate for patients with yolk sac tumor approaches 90%, with deaths usually occurring within 30 months of presentation. This high survival rate is largely due to the high proportion of patients presenting with stage I disease.

TERATOMA AND EPIDERMOID CYST

Teratoma is the second most common prepubertal testis tumor. The median age of presentation is 13 months, with several patients presenting in the neonatal period. Histologically, teratomas consist of tissues representing the three germinal layers: endoderm, mesoderm, and ectoderm. The presence of cysts on ultrasonography suggests the diagnosis but is neither sensitive nor specific.

Epidermoid cysts are benign tumors composed entirely of keratin-producing epithelium. They are distinguished from dermoid cysts, which contain skin and skin appendages, and from teratomas, which contain derivatives of other germ cell layers. Epidermoid cysts probably represent monophasic teratomas, although development from squamous metaplasia of the rete testis or seminiferous tubules also has been suggested. On ultrasonography, most epidermoid cysts appear as discrete intratesticular masses with areas of increased echogenicity corresponding to the keratin debris or peripheral calcification. Other areas of decreased echogenicity may be present corresponding to regions of the cyst not filled with debris. However, these findings are variable, and an epidermoid cyst may appear as a fairly homogenous solid mass. The primary value of ultrasonography is in characterizing the mass as intratesticular and in excluding abnormalities elsewhere in the testis that would necessitate total orchiectomy.

Teratomas and epidermoid cysts are universally benign in prepubertal children. Testis-sparing surgery is appropriate for these patients. A margin of normal testicular tissue should be included, and frozen sections should be obtained to confirm the diagnosis. In older children with teratoma the normal testicular parenchyma must be carefully evaluated. If there is histologic evidence of pubertal changes, then an orchiectomy should be performed because teratomas are potentially malignant in postpubertal boys. Although epidermoid cysts are benign in children and adults, there have been reports of teratoma being present on the final pathologic evaluation when an epidermoid cyst was the frozen section diagnosis. Therefore, consideration should be given to orchiectomy in patients with presumed epidermoid cyst in a postpubertal testis. Whether biopsies of surrounding testicular parenchyma are necessary is unclear. Although 88% of testes removed for adult teratoma contain areas of intratubular germ cell neoplasia, this has generally not been the case for epidermoid cysts or for pediatric teratoma.

For patients with epidermoid cysts and prepubertal patients with teratoma, no radiographic studies or follow-up for the development of metastatic disease are required. Because of the potential for malignancy, postpubertal patients with teratoma should be evaluated and followed on the same protocol as adults with other malignant germ cell tumors.

MIXED GERM CELL TUMORS

Nonseminomatous mixed germ cell tumors (NSMGCTs) are exceedingly rare in prepubertal patients, but relatively common in adolescents and adults. Adolescents with NSMGCTs should be treated using adult testicular tumor protocols. Stage I patients may be managed with close observation or modified nerve-sparing RPLND. RPLND should definitely be undertaken for tumors with any unfavorable characteristics such as a predominance of embryonal cell histology or lymphatic/vascular invasion. If surveillance is elected, monthly office visits with chest radiography and tumor markers (AFP, human chorionic gonadotropin, and lactate dehydrogenase) are obtained. CT of the abdomen and pelvis is performed every 2 to 3 months. Most relapses in this group occur in the first 8 months, so surveillance studies are obtained every other month in the second year and at increasing intervals thereafter. Stage II patients with minimal retroperitoneal disease undergo RPLND followed by chemotherapy if the lymph nodes are histologically positive. Patients with stage III or bulky stage II disease are treated with primary platinum-based chemotherapy.

GONADAL STROMAL TUMORS

Stromal testis tumors are rare in children, and there are no large series to guide their management. However, anecdotal reports and small series in the literature offer some experience on which to base therapy.

Leydig Cell Tumor

Leydig cell tumors are universally benign in children. They usually present between 5 and 10 years of age with precocious puberty. Presenting symptoms include an early growth spurt, prominent external genitalia, erections, pubic and axillary hair, facial hair, acne, and deepening of the voice. Although feminization (particularly gynecomastia) is common in adults, it is rare in children and, when present, is usually superimposed on the virilizing signs. Other causes of precocious puberty include central nervous system lesions, adrenocortical carcinoma, and congenital adrenal hyperplasia. In the presence of a testicular mass, a Leydig cell tumor is the most likely diagnosis. An elevated testosterone level with low or normal follicle-stimulating hormone and luteinizing hormone levels is consistent with a Leydig cell tumor. Normal levels of 17-hydroxyprogesterone exclude the diagnosis of congenital adrenal hyperplasia. Because virilization may present before a tumor is palpable, all boys with precocious puberty and no obvious cause should undergo ultrasonography of the testicles to rule out a small tumor.

When possible, Leydig cell tumors should be treated by testis-sparing excision. Persistence of androgenic effects may be due to a contralateral tumor, but this is rare in children. Because Leydig cell tumors are sometimes difficult to detect on physical examination, ultrasonography may be necessary to rule out a contralateral tumor. However, even after successful removal of a solitary tumor, androgenic changes are not completely reversible, and some children may proceed through premature puberty due to activation of the hypothalamic–pituitary–gonadal axis.

Sertoli Cell Tumor

Sertoli cell tumors account for only 2% of primary prepubertal testis tumors. A review of 60 cases of Sertoli cell tumors reported only 4 cases in patients under 20 years of age, the youngest being 15 years old. Approximately 10% of adult Sertoli cell tumors are malignant. These malignant tumors are usually characterized by large tumor size, areas of necrosis, vascular invasion, cellular atypia, and increased mitotic activity. In contrast to general series dominated by adult patients, the median age of patients in the Prepubertal Testis Tumor Registry was 6 months, with a range of 4 months to 10 years. There were no reports of metastatic disease. Sertoli cell tumors are usually hormonally inactive in children, although they may occasionally cause gynecomastia or isosexual precocious puberty. While all reported cases to date have been benign in children under 5 years of age, there have been a few cases of malignant Sertoli cell tumors in older children. Orchiectomy is sufficient treatment in infants, though a metastatic evaluation could be considered in infants with worrisome histologic findings. Older children should undergo abdominal CT and chest radiography to rule out metastases. When metastatic disease is present, aggressive combination treatment, including RPLND, chemotherapy, and radiation therapy, should be considered.

The large-cell calcifying Sertoli cell tumor is a clinically and histologically distinct entity with a higher incidence of multifocality and hormonal activity. Although standard Sertoli cell tumors are more common in adults, large-cell calcifying Sertoli cell tumors are found predominantly in children and adolescents. Most present with a testicular mass. Approximately 25% of patients have bilateral and multifocal tumors. The presence of calcifications results in a characteristic ultrasonographic appearance, including multiple hyperechoic areas.

Approximately one third of patients with large-cell calcifying Sertoli cell tumors have an associated genetic syndrome or endocrine abnormality. Although occasionally malignant in adults, large-cell calcifying Sertoli cell tumors have been universally benign in patients under 25 years of age. Orchiectomy is sufficient treatment for children.

Juvenile Granulosa Cell Tumor

Juvenile granulosa cell tumor is a stromal tumor bearing a light microscopic resemblance to ovarian juvenile granulosa cell tumor. Granulosa cell tumors occur almost exclusively in the first year of life, most in the first 6 months. Structural abnormalities of the Y chromosome and mosaicism are common in boys with juvenile granulosa cell tumor. Several cases have been described in association with ambiguous genitalia. These tumors are hormonally inactive and benign. Although these children should undergo chromosomal analysis, no treatment or metastatic evaluation is required beyond orchiectomy.

Mixed or Undifferentiated Stromal Tumors

Histologically, mixed or undifferentiated stromal tumors consist of areas of gonadal stromal neoplasia and undifferentiated regions of spindle cells that may exhibit a high mitotic rate. These stromal tumors have an epidemiology similar to that of granulosa cell tumors. Although some of these tumors have histologic characteristics commonly associated with malignancy, most are benign. There are inadequate data in the literature to formulate rigid guidelines for managing these tumors. Histologic features do not appear to correlate with invasive or metastatic potential. Although aggressive behavior has not occurred in infants, there are reports of such behavior in older children. Because orchiectomy cures most of these patients, RPLND and adjuvant therapy are probably not appropriate in the absence of radiographic evidence of metastatic disease. However, given the uncertainty, postoperative evaluation and follow-up for the development of metastatic disease seems prudent.

GONADOBLASTOMA

Gonadoblastomas contain both germ cells and stromal cells. Usually three distinct elements are present: large germ cells resembling seminoma, sex cord nongerminal elements such as Sertoli or granulosa cells, and stromal elements such as Leydig cells. Gonadoblastomas occur more frequently in postpubertal patients, but may be seen in childhood. Gonadoblastoma occurs almost exclusively in dysgenetic gonads, usually in association with an intersex disorder. Dysgenetic gonads are gonads that have failed to develop normally and are composed of gonadal-type fibrous tissue. They are also termed "streak gonads." Although the nomenclature is inconsistent, dysgenetic gonads may contain some primitive ovarian structures. On the other hand, when partial differentiation along testicular lines is present, the gonad is referred to as a dysgenetic testis. Gonadoblastoma is more likely to occur in dysgenetic gonads or dysgenetic testes in patients with a Y chromosome or evidence of some Y chromatin. Gonadoblastomas occur in 3% of patients with true hermaphroditism, and 10% to 30% of patients with mixed gonadal dysgenesis or pure gonadal dysgenesis and an XY karyotype. They also occur commonly in the dysgenetic testis syndrome.

Gonadoblastomas are usually asymptomatic, often detected incidentally when dysgenetic gonads are removed. However, virilization has been associated with some of these tumors. Forty percent of gonadoblastomas are bilateral. Although gonadoblastomas are benign, overgrowth of the germinal components leading to a dysgerminoma (i.e., seminoma) occurs in as many as 50% of cases. Approximately 10% develop overtly malignant tumors. Although most invasive tumors associated with intersex occur in young adulthood, there are several reports in children as well. Intraepithelial germ cell neoplasia may be identified in many of these gonads and is associated with germ cell tumors.

Gonadoblastomas are treated by orchiectomy. Indeed, any dysgenetic gonad in a child with a Y chromosome should be removed prophylactically in infancy or early childhood. Tumors are much less likely in patients who lack a Y chromosome, such as those with Turner syndrome or XX patients with pure gonadal dysgenesis. When malignant degeneration is present, a metastatic evaluation and appropriate follow-up are indicated. Fortunately, these tumors are radiosensitive and have a favorable prognosis. However, if unfavorable elements such as choriocarcinoma or embryonal carcinoma are present, the outlook is poor.

Five percent to 10% of patients with androgen insensitivity syndrome (AIS) develop germ cell tumors. Patients with AIS do not have dysgenetic gonads, and are not prone to gonadoblastoma. Rather, like otherwise normal males with undescended testicles, the tumors associated with AIS are most often seminomas occurring post-pubertally. However, all standard types of postpubertal germ cell tumors may occur. Patients with AIS also may develop Sertoli cell adenomas, which are benign hamartomatous nodules composed of multiple small tubules lined by prepubertal-type Sertoli cells.

HYPERPLASTIC NODULES IN CONGENITAL ADRENAL HYPERPLASIA

Adrenal rest tissue can be found along the spermatic cord and in the testicular hilum of newborns. This tissue generally regresses in infancy, but may persist in boys with congenital adrenal hyperplasia (CAH). Stimulation of the tissue by high levels of adrenocorticotropic hormone can lead to multiple, usually bilateral nodular growths in the testes. Some patients with milder unrecognized forms of CAH may present with testicular masses. In such patients who present with precocious puberty, the testicular masses could be misinterpreted as Leydig cell tumors. The nodules of CAH are similar histologically to Leydig cell tumors, potentially perpetuating the error even after excision. Therefore, any child presenting with precocious puberty and a testicular mass should undergo an endocrinologic evaluation, including measurement of serum 17-hydroxyprogesterone, to distinguish these two entities.

The hyperplastic nodules of CAH are benign. Most of these nodules resolve or significantly reduce in size in response to steroid replacement. If this occurs, the patient may safely be followed with serial examinations or ultrasonography. Because any testicle may develop a true testicular tumor, nodules that fail to respond to steroid replacement should be sampled for biopsy. Orchiectomy should be avoided unless the biopsy reveals some lesion other than an adrenal rest nodule. Large tumors that fail to regress may be enucleated.

LEUKEMIA

Secondary malignancies of the testicle are rare. The most important is acute lymphoblastic/lymphocytic leukemia (ALL). Only 2% of boys with ALL have overt clinical evidence of testicular involvement at diagnosis. This is usually reflected in firm diffuse enlargement of one or both testicles and portends a poorer prognosis. Subclinical (i.e., microscopic) involvement of the testes is present in approximately 20% of patients with ALL at the time of diagnosis. However, most patients with microscopic testicular involvement achieve a complete remission following modern standard chemotherapy. Conversely, some patients without evidence of testicular involvement at diagnosis ultimately relapse in the testicles. Therefore, pretreatment testicular biopsy is unnecessary because it does not predict those patients who are prone to have persistent or relapsing disease at that site.

Relapse in the testicles following chemotherapy used to occur in approximately 10% of patients. The testis may represent a protected site from chemotherapy, more prone to relapse. However, with modern ALL, chemotherapy testicular relapse occurs in less than 1% of cases. Postchemotherapy biopsy in the absence of physical findings (to rule out occult persistence of tumor in the testes) is therefore no longer routine. Those few patients with testicular enlargement persisting or occurring after chemotherapy should undergo biopsy to confirm testicular ALL. Most of these patients are found to have relapsed at other sites as well and require additional intensive systemic chemotherapy to prevent ultimate clinical hematologic relapse. Radiation to the testicles is also required. In the rare case of unilateral testicular relapse, consideration should be given to orchiectomy. This could allow lower doses of radiation to the remaining testicle, and ultimately better endocrine function than would occur with higher doses of radiation to both testicles if the affected testicle were left in place. In any case, testicular salvage can be achieved in most patients with testicular relapse following chemotherapy, and they can attain long-term survival. Relapse during chemotherapy portends a more dire outcome.

SUGGESTED READINGS

Connolly JA, Gearhart JP. Management of yolk sac tumors in children. *Urol Clin North Am* 1993;20:7.

Grady R, Ross JH, Kay R. Epidemiologic features of teratomas of the testis in a prepubertal population. *J Urol* 1997;158:1191.

Kay R. Prepubertal testicular tumor registry. *J Urol* 1993;150:671.

Pui C-H, Crist WM. Acute lymphoblastic leukemia. In: Pui C-H, ed. *Childhood leukemias.* New York: Cambridge University Press, 1999:288–312.

Rushton HG, Belman AB, Sesterhenn I, et al. Testicular sparing surgery for prepubertal teratoma of the testis: a clinical and pathological study. *J Urol* 1990;144:726.

114

OVARIAN TUMORS

DANIEL VON ALLMEN

Ovarian masses in children represent a heterogeneous group of lesions that may be benign or malignant. The presentation, workup, and management vary greatly depending on the patient's age and the underlying risk for malignancy. Simple cysts in newborns that are small and asymptomatic can be observed for spontaneous resolution, whereas larger cysts may require aspiration or excision to prevent torsion or confirm the diagnosis, but the risk of malignancy is low and ovarian tissue should be preserved on the ipsilateral side. Conversely, complex cysts in the premenarchal child have a significant malignant potential and must be treated as such. Although the malignant potential of cystic masses in the postmenarchal teenager decreases, both "pediatric" and "adult" type tumors may be present. In this chapter, I will focus on the workup and management of the potentially malignant lesions in prepubertal and teenage patients. Germ cell tumors are the most common ovarian neoplasm in children and account for 60% to 70% of cases. Epithelial tumors and sex cord tumors each account for 10% to 15% of cases, and the remainder are rare primary tumors and ovarian manifestations of lymphomas and leukemias (Table 114.1).

PRESENTATION

Most ovarian lesions present with either pain or an abdominal mass. Others report pain as the most common presenting symptom, but in my experience, many girls present with abdominal masses that are frequently quite large but relatively asymptomatic. The patient and parents are often oblivious to the presence of these huge lesions that can fill the abdomen and are ultimately noted by relatives or health care personnel.

Patients who present with acute abdominal or pelvic pain require a prompt workup to identify the source of the pain. On physical examination a mass may or may not be palpable. The differential diagnosis includes appendicitis, cystitis, ovarian torsion, and constipation. Pregnancy and pelvic inflammatory disease should always be considered in postmenarchal patients who are sexually active. Routine laboratory studies are usually unrevealing, but abdominal and pelvic ultrasonography will show a mass in the pelvis.

Identification of a solid or complex cystic ovarian mass should prompt additional diagnostic studies. Laboratory studies should include measurement of tumor markers, including α-fetoprotein (AFP), quantitative β-human chorionic gonadotropin (β-HCG), and CA-125. In cases of acute abdominal pain with a question of ovarian torsion, the patient should undergo early operation for evaluation of the mass. In cases that do not require immediate operation for pain and possible torsion, a CT scan of the abdomen and pelvis is useful to characterize the mass itself as well as its relationship to surrounding structures. This can provide some indication of the etiology of the mass prior to surgery. Germ cell tumors are often asymptomatic large and heterogeneous lesions with both cystic and solid components. Large calcifications are characteristic of benign teratomas. Conversely, the presence of ascites and a poorly circumscribed lesion in the setting of significant abdominal pain in a postmenarchal patient should raise suspicion for an epithelial neoplasm. The differentiation is important given the different staging systems (Tables 114.2 and 114.3) and operative guidelines for the various tumor types. Obviously, identification of metastatic disease confirms the presence of a malignant lesion. Unfortunately, the absence of metastatic lesions does not rule out the possibility of a malignant process, and any complex ovarian mass must be treated as a malignancy.

TUMOR TYPES

Germ cell tumors are the most common type of tumor in children. They are further divided into five subgroups based on the degree of differentiation and the cellular components involved. Dysgerminomas are the least differentiated

D. von Allmen: Department of Surgery, Division of Pediatric Surgery, University of Pennsylvania School of Medicine; and Department of Pediatric General and Thoracic Surgery, Children's Hospital of Philadelphia, Philadelphia, Pennsylvania.

TABLE 114.1. OVARIAN TUMORS

Germ cell tumors
- Undifferentiated
  - Dysgerminoma
- Embryonic
  - Teratoma
  - Embryonal carcinoma
- Extraembryonal
  - Endodermal sinus tumor
  - Choriocarcinoma

Sex cord-stromal tumors
- Granulosa-thecal cell
- Sertoli-Leydig cell

Epithelial tumors
- Serous cystadenoma
- Mucinous cystadenoma

Miscellaneous
- Lymphoma
- Leukemia
- Polyembryoma
- Ovarian myxoma
- Mesothelioma
- Gonadoblastoma

TABLE 114.2. FIGO STAGING SYSTEM FOR PRIMARY CARCINOMA OF THE OVARY

Stage I: Growth limited to the ovaries
- IA: Growth limited to one ovary; no ascites; no tumor on the external surface; capsule intact
- IB: Growth limited to both ovaries; no ascites; no tumor on the external surface; capsule intact
- IC: Tumor either stage IA or IB, but with ascites or peritoneal washings containing malignant cells; tumor on the surface or capsule ruptured

Stage II: Growth involving one or both ovaries with pelvic extension
- IIA. Extension to the uterus or tubes
- IIB. Extension to other pelvic tissues
- IIC. Tumor either IIA or IIB, but with ascites or peritoneal washings containing malignant cells; tumor on the surface or capsule ruptured

Stage III: Tumor involving one or both ovaries with peritoneal implants outside the pelvis or positive retroperitoneal or inguinal lymph nodes; superficial liver metastasis equals stage III; tumor is limited to the true pelvis but with histologically proven malignant extension to small bowel or omentum
- IIIA. Tumor grossly limited to the true pelvis with negative nodes but histologically proven microscopic seeding of the peritoneal surfaces
- IIIB. Tumor of one or both ovaries with histologically confirmed implants of abdominal peritoneal surfaces, none exceeding 2 cm in diameter; nodes are negative
- IIIC. Abdominal implants greater than 2 cm in diameter or positive retroperitoneal or inguinal lymph nodes

Stage IV: Growth involving one or both ovaries with distant metastases; if pleural effusion present, there must be positive cytology to allot a case to stage IV; parenchymal liver metastasis equals stage IV

TABLE 114.3. PEDIATRIC GERM CELL STAGING: PEDIATRIC ONCOLOGY GROUP

Stage I: Limited to ovary (ovaries) peritoneal washings negative; tumor markers normal after appropriate half-life decline (α-fetoprotein, 5 days; β-human chorionic gonadotropin, 16 h)

Stage II: Microscopic residual disease or disease in lymph nodes <2 cm; peritoneal washings normal; tumor markers positive or negative

Stage III: Gross residual disease or biopsy only; lymph nodes >2 cm; contiguous spread to other organs (omentum, intestine, bladder); peritoneal washings positive for malignant cells; markers negative or positive

Stage IV: Metastatic disease, including liver

tumors and are comparable with the seminoma in males. Some degree of differentiation yields the embryonic tumors, embryonal carcinoma or teratoma or the extraembryonic tumors, endodermal sinus tumors (yolk sac tumors), or choriocarcinoma. Although each of the tumor types arises from the primordial germ cell, they express different tumor markers and have different malignant potential (Table 114.4).

Teratomas are the most common lesions and may be mature, immature, or malignant. Immature tumors are graded from I to III based on the degree of differentiation of the neural elements of the mass. The more immature the neural tissue, the higher the grade and more malignant the behavior of the neoplasm in adults. In children, however, surgery alone is thought to be adequate therapy for immature lesions. Careful pathologic evaluation is important to avoid missing malignant elements in heterogenous lesions.

Pure dysgerminomas are malignant but highly responsive to chemotherapy and radiation. Unlike other germ cell tumors, dysgerminomas are bilateral in 10% to 15% of cases. Serum lactic dehydrogenase (LDH-1) is frequently elevated in dysgerminoma. Standard tumor markers are negative except in cases of mixed tumors, which may have components of endodermal sinus tumor or choriocarcinoma that account for elevation of the AFP and/or β-HCG. Endodermal sinus tumor is nearly always associated with elevations of AFP and is a more aggressive tumor that

TABLE 114.4. TUMOR MARKERS AND INCIDENCE OF BILATERALITY

Tumor	Markers	Bilaterality
Teratoma	+/– AFP	10%
Dysgerminoma	LDH-1	15%
Endodermal sinus tumor	AFP	LOW
Choriocarcinoma	β-HCG	LOW
Epithelial tumors	CA-125	15%

AFP, α-fetoprotein; LDH, lactate dehydrogenase; β-HCG, β-human chorionic gonadotropin.

can metastasize within the peritoneum and to liver, lung, and brain. Choriocarcinoma is associated with elevation of β-HCG and has aggressive malignant potential when it is not associated with pregnancy.

The sex cord tumors, granulosa-thecal cell tumors and Sertoli-Leydig cell tumors, arise from stromal components of the ovary and frequently produce hormones that may result in clinically apparent changes in the patient. The granulosa-thecal cell tumors may be associated with isosexual precocious puberty, and the malignant potential is based on the granulosa cell component. Sertoli-Leydig cell tumors (arrhenoblastomas) produce androgenizing hormones and may present with hirsutism and other signs of virilization.

Epithelial tumors present a particular problem in management for pediatric surgeons. Serous and mucinous cystadenomas are frequently characterized as being of low malignant potential histologically. These are indolent tumors that have a high incidence of bilaterality and local spread within the pelvis. Cystadenocarcinoma is much less common. Adult epithelial tumor markers (e.g., CA-125) must be obtained for follow-up and after appropriate surgical staging has been done. These tumors may be locally invasive, requiring extensive resections that can leave the patient infertile. In many institutions, the adult gynecologic oncologists manage these patients, and it is my practice to refer them prior to surgery if there is a suspicion for this type of tumor preoperatively. However, the diagnosis is not always apparent preoperatively, and the pediatric surgeon must be aware of the appropriate laboratory workup and operative management.

SURGICAL PRINCIPLES

Ovarian lesions can be approached from either a midline incision or a Pfannensteil approach depending on the size of the lesion and the likelihood of malignancy. Regardless of the approach, one must be prepared to perform a cancer operation because it is frequently impossible to know at the time of surgery whether the lesion is benign or malignant. For this reason, the use of laparoscopy is controversial. Although I occasionally use laparoscopy diagnostically in cases of suspected torsion, I do not decompress cystic lesions to facilitate removal. The recommendations of the Germ Cell Committee of the Children's Oncology Group specifically discourage this approach and stress the importance of removing the tumor intact. Violating the capsule laparoscopically or rupturing the tumor intraoperativly can result in upstaging of malignant lesions. If the mass is large, I prefer a midline incision that can be extended sufficiently to remove the tumor without rupture.

Once the incision is made and the peritoneal cavity entered, it is important to proceed through the necessary steps to adequately stage a patient in the event a malignancy is present. First, any ascites should be aspirated and sent for cytology. In the absence of ascites, peritoneal washings should be performed in suspicious cases. The omentum should be carefully inspected and removed if any evidence of a mass lesion is present. For germ cell tumors, omentectomy is no longer mandatory if the omentum is grossly negative for tumor. However, I have a low threshold for proceeding with omentectomy if the tumor is adherent to the omentum or there is any possibility of a non–germ cell malignancy. The peritoneal surfaces, including the surface of the diaphragm, should be carefully examined for signs of peritoneal implants. Some benign teratomas are associated with diffuse implants of benign glial tissue (gliomatosis peritonei), which do not require therapy other than adequate biopsies to assure the proper diagnosis. Iliac and retroperitoneal lymph nodes should be sought and sampled for biopsy if present. Although a formal lymph node dissection is not necessary in most cases of germ cell tumors, lymph node metastasis will alter staging and treatment in both germ cell and epithelial tumors. The contralateral ovary should be carefully inspected and any suspicious areas sampled for biopsy. Dysgerminomas and epithelial tumors are bilateral in 10% to 15% of cases.

Resection of the actual tumor is usually straightforward. The tumors are often large and amenable to a salpingo-oophorectomy. Occasionally, if the tumor is an encapsulated teratoma, the ipsilateral fallopian tube can be preserved. In the case of bilateral teratomas, it is frequently possible to enucleate the lesions on at least one ovary to preserve fertility. Extensive germ cell tumors should be sampled for diagnostic biopsy without resecting vital structures. Current chemotherapy regimens are effective in treating these tumors, and a second-look procedure may be indicated to achieve a complete response in patients treated with biopsy alone at the initial operation. Once the tumor is removed and appropriate staging complete, the abdomen is closed. A nasogastric tube is typically not necessary. A Foley catheter may be required if an epidural catheter is used for postoperative pain control.

POSTOPERATIVE CARE

Postoperatively, the patient's diet is advanced as tolerated and the patient is discharged home once she is able to eat and maintain adequate pain control with oral medications.

The key aspect of the postoperative care is the pathologic diagnosis of the specimens removed during the operation. Patients found to have malignant tumors may require chemotherapy. The current treatment protocols for germ cell tumors from the Children's Oncology Group are based on regimens that include bleomycin, platinum, and etoposide. These regimens have proven to be very effective and have resulted in significant improvements in survival, even for advanced-stage tumors. Current studies in the Children's Oncology Group are aimed at reducing therapy for low-stage procedures and decreasing toxicity of high-stage regimens.

SUGGESTED READINGS

Castleberry RP, Cushing B, Perlman E, et al. Germ cell tumors. In: Pizzo PA, Poplack DG, eds. *Principles and practice of pediatric oncology, 3rd ed.* Philadelphia: Lippincott-Raven, 1997:921–945.

Cushing B, Giller R, Ablin A, et al. Surgical resection alone is effective treatment for ovarian immature teratoma in children and adolescents: a report of the Pediatric Oncology Group and the Children's Cancer Group. *Am J Obstet Gynecol* 1999;181:353–358.

Gribbon M, Ein SH, Mancer K. Pediatric malignant ovarian tumors: a 43-year review. *J Pediatr Surg* 1992;27:480–484.

Helmrath MA, Shin CE, Warner BW. Ovarian cysts in the pediatric population. *Semin Pediatr Surg* 1998;7:19–28.

Lazar EL, Stolar CJ. Evaluation and management of pediatric solid ovarian tumors. *Semin Pediatr Surg* 1998;7:29–34.

Lovvorn HN, Tucci LA, Stafford PW. Ovarian masses in the pediatric patient. *AORN J* 1901;67:568–576.

Rescorla F. Pediatric germ-cell tumors. In: Andrassy R, ed. *Pediatric surgical oncology.* Philadelphia: WB Saunders, 1998:239–266.

Skinner MA, Schlatter MG, Heifetz SA, et al. Ovarian neoplasms in children. *Arch Surg* 1993;128:849–853.

115

SURGICAL CONSIDERATIONS IN PEDIATRIC METASTATIC DISEASE

MARY BRINDLE
R. LAWRENCE MOSS

Pediatric tumors generally arise within germinal tissues. Most primary pediatric tumors grow rapidly but are sensitive to chemotherapy. An aggressive effort to diagnose and treat these tumors early in their course is necessary because pediatric tumors generally have a great potential for metastasis.

New chemotherapeutic agents are extremely successful at controlling primary tumors and micrometastases. Chemotherapy is less successful at treating gross metastatic disease. The poor results of chemotherapy in the treatment of metastases may be due to poor tissue penetration in bulky tumors as well as a smaller population of dividing cells. It is also possible that metastases that develop in the presence of chemotherapy may represent a selected population of drug-resistant tumor cells. Management strategies for select metastatic pediatric cancers involve aggressive tumor resection and high-dose chemotherapy.

The pattern of metastatic spread in most pediatric tumors is hematogenous. The lung seems to act as a filter, receiving the metastatic cells from the tumor's venous drainage. Examples include tumors of the head, neck, kidney, and testes, as well as bone and soft tissue sarcomas, melanoma, and endocrine tumors. The major solid pediatric tumors, with the exception of neuroblastoma, metastasize most commonly to the lungs. Less common sites of metastasis include the bone marrow, liver, and central nervous system.

Site-specific cellular interactions play an important role in determining the location of metastatic deposits. These factors explain why cancers such as melanoma metastasize to the lungs to a greater degree than would be explained simply by the pattern of venous drainage.

M. Brindle: Department of General Surgery, Department of Pediatrics, Stanford University Medical School; and Division of Pediatric Surgery, Lucile Packard Children's Hospital, Palo Alto, California.

R. L. Moss: Department of Surgery, Yale University School of Medicine; and Department of Surgery, Yale-New Haven Children's Hospital, New Haven, Connecticut.

PULMONARY METASTASES

Pulmonary metastases are by far the most common and the most amenable to surgical therapy. Pulmonary metastases are almost always asymptomatic and are usually discovered through radiologic imaging. The presence of symptoms usually indicates an ominous prognosis. Dyspnea may indicate a large tumor compressing the airway or replacement of lung parenchyma by multiple lesions. Chest pain may signify development of parietal pleura metastases or chest wall invasion.

Even in the setting of a known primary tumor, new radiographically detected pulmonary nodules in a pediatric patient cannot be presumed to be cancer. There are numerous benign causes of pulmonary nodules in patients with cancer. Infectious infiltrates, which are common in immunosuppressed children, may be radiographically indistinguishable from metastatic lesions. Bacteria are responsible for the majority of these infections; however, patients with prolonged neutropenia also may develop fungal lung disease. Noninfectious causes of pulmonary lesions include drug-induced pneumonitis and radiation pneumonitis. Even small regions of atelectasis may be indistinguishable from malignant lesions. Computed tomography (CT) can be used to detect pulmonary lesions as small as 2 to 3 mm. It is difficult to differentiate benign from malignant lesions on the basis of CT findings alone. Most studies have found that the correlation between radiologic diagnosis and pathologic findings is poor.

The treatment of pulmonary metastatic disease is dependent on the biology and natural history of the primary tumor and tumor response to combined therapy. The therapeutic approach also differs depending on whether pulmonary metastases appear at the same time as the primary tumor, or develop at a later stage. Prior to considering pulmonary metastasectomy, there must be complete eradication of the primary tumor, and the patient must undergo thorough screening for other metastatic sites. Pulmonary metastasectomy is most often performed for osteosarcoma. It is also sometimes performed in select soft tissue sarcomas, Wilms tumors, and primary hepatic tumors.

OSTEOSARCOMA

Historically, osteosarcoma has been associated with a poor chance for survival. Thirty years ago, a patient who underwent successful resection of a nonmetastatic osteosarcoma had an 80% risk for developing metastases within the next 6 months. Few patients survived beyond a year. The natural history of this disease and its poor response to simple surgical resection are indicative of early micrometastatic spread. With the development of multiagent chemotherapy, the survival of patients with osteosarcoma has improved dramatically. Today, 60% to 75% of these patients attain long-term disease-free survival.

The prognosis for patients with metastatic osteosarcoma at initial presentation remains poor, with only 10% to 30% of patients achieving long-term disease-free survival. The lung is the first site of osteosarcoma metastasis in 90% of children; most often this is the only metastatic focus. Chemotherapy is the most effective method of preventing pulmonary metastatic spread. Trials that have explored the use of prophylactic whole-lung irradiation demonstrate little benefit. On the other hand, numerous studies have demonstrated the value of aggressive resection of established pulmonary metastases, including repeat resection for recurrent pulmonary disease.

Generally, patients who present with a primary osteosarcoma are treated with aggressive, multiagent chemotherapy. Therefore, metastatic deposits that appear later in the patient's course are likely to contain drug-resistant tumor cells, whereas pulmonary metastases detected at the same time as the primary tumor are more likely to be chemosensitive.

At the time of diagnosis of a primary osteosarcoma, the evaluation should include (a) CT or magnetic resonance imaging (MRI) of the primary site, (b) radiography and CT of the chest to determine the presence or absence of pulmonary metastases, and (c) 99m-technetium bone scan to determine the presence or absence of "skip lesions" or distant bony metastases. If pulmonary metastases are suspected from CT imaging, biopsy confirmation of tumor is necessary.

Patients treated for primary osteosarcoma undergo an aggressive screening regimen to detect subsequent metastases. This regimen includes chest radiography every 2 months, as well as a chest CT and a bone scan every 4 to 6 months for the first 2 years. The frequency of screening procedures is gradually decreased. Rarely will patients present with metastatic disease after 5 years of disease-free survival.

Pulmonary metastases are considered unresectable in the presence of (a) extrathoracic metastases, (b) hilar involvement, (c) malignant pleural effusion, (d) massive disease, and (e) more than 16 pulmonary nodules (debatable).

At the time of diagnosis of osteosarcoma, a thorough workup is performed, evaluating the primary tumor site and screening for bony and pulmonary metastases. Management of pulmonary metastatic disease is dependent on the timing of metastatic diagnosis in relation to the diagnosis of the primary cancer.

Synchronous Metastases

If the metastatic deposit is discovered at the same time as the primary disease, the primary tumor is first treated with surgical resection and systemic chemotherapy, followed later by pulmonary metastatic resection. The chemotherapeutic regimen given to patients with metastases before and after resection of the primary tumor is considerably more aggressive than chemotherapy given to patients with nonmetastatic disease. The majority of chemotherapeutic regimens for osteosarcoma involve doxorubicin and cisplatin as well as the use of high-dose methotrexate. Isofosfamide has been found to be tolerable and effective in these patients. However, its role is still being defined.

Chemotherapy is generally given prior to resection of the primary tumor, after resection of the primary tumor, and after resection of pulmonary metastases. Resection of pulmonary metastases is undertaken only if complete resection can be performed while maintaining adequate pulmonary parenchyma.

Metachronous Metastases

Metastases that develop after the patient has already received chemotherapy tend to be very aggressive. Once pulmonary metastases are detected, the primary site is reevaluated and a bone scan is performed to ensure that there are no extrathoracic metastases. The extent of the pulmonary metastases is determined, and resection is performed. There is no role for preoperative chemotherapy in patients who present with resectable pulmonary metastases. Preoperative pulmonary function tests are only rarely necessary when an anatomic resection is considered and in some cases of repeat metastasectomy, to ensure that there will be adequate functional tissue after resection.

The surgical approach should provide adequate exposure in order to thoroughly examine the lung and allow for resection of all detectable metastatic disease. Identifying metastatic deposits not evident on preoperative CT is not unusual. Patients are intubated with a double-lumen endotracheal tube, allowing for the affected lung to be deflated and more easily manipulated. Most surgeons perform pulmonary metastasectomy through a thoracotomy. The presence of bilateral disease may necessitate a staged procedure, with the second thoracotomy being performed 1 to 2 weeks after the first operation. This also may be accomplished through a median sternotomy, which is a method preferred by some surgeons. This approach, however, provides poor exposure to retrocardiac lesions and lesions located in the left lower lobe.

Complete metastatic resection with lung conservation is the rule in the management of metastatic lesions. Whenever possible, wedge resections are used to remove all metastatic foci. Repeat resection may be necessary in the case of disease recurrence. Anatomic resections, such as those performed for primary bronchogenic carcinomas, are not necessary, because there is no need to resect the lymphatic drainage from hematogenously spread osteosarcoma metastases. It is therefore only in rare instances that segmentectomy, lobectomy, or pneumonectomy are performed. Survival is diminished with pulmonary recurrences, but a significant increase in survival has been demonstrated with repeat resections up to a total of four times.

Postoperative Adjuvant Therapy

There are no controlled studies examining the use of post-thoracotomy adjuvant chemotherapy. Metastases developing after intensive, multiagent chemotherapy are less likely to respond to salvage chemotherapy. Nonetheless, chemotherapy is often instituted in these patients and is certainly recommended for the following patients: those with multiple lesions (three or more), patients who present with metastases within 6 months to 1 year of resection of the primary tumor, and patients who have not had complete resection of the pulmonary lesions or were noted to have visceral pleural disruption at the time of surgery.

Unresectable Tumors

Osteosarcoma is poorly radiosensitive. However, when a tumor arises that is not resectable, it is appropriate to consider radiation therapy for local control. There is support for the use of chemotherapy in these patients. Although a complete response is rare, chemotherapy may cause enough tumor regression to allow resection.

Results

After metastasectomy, patients undergo chest CT every 3 months to evaluate for recurrence. Imaging of the primary site is performed on a yearly basis accompanied by a bone scan to determine the presence of distant bony metastases.

A number of factors influence patient survival. Factors that indicate a poor prognosis at the time of treatment of the primary tumor in the pediatric patient include young age (<10 years), poor response of tumor to preoperative chemotherapy, axial skeleton involvement, skip lesions, rapid progression of disease, and the presence of certain oncogenes. The oncogenes that are felt to play the greatest role in osteosarcoma tumorigenesis are the retinoblastoma (RB) oncogene and the p53 oncogene. Patients with hereditary retinoblastoma have the highest genetic predisposition for osteosarcoma of any patient population. Several studies have demonstrated that the genetic locus implicated in the development of retinoblastoma (band q14 of chromosome 13) is also implicated in the development of osteosarcoma. Mutation of the p53 gene has been implicated in a number of tumors and is present in 25% of the cases of osteosarcoma. Other factors that have been associated with a worse prognosis include hyperdiploid, high-grade tumors, an incompletely treated primary cancer, and the presence of extrapulmonary metastases.

In the case of a fully treated primary tumor with pulmonary metastases, the following factors also contribute to a poor outcome:

1. Incomplete resection of pulmonary metastases or unresectable metastases.
2. Disruption of visceral pleura by metastases.
3. Large number of metastatic deposits. Numerous studies have examined the relationship between the number of metastases and patient survival. Many studies demonstrate a worse prognosis with the development of more than three pulmonary nodules within 6 months of the primary surgery. There is disagreement, however, on the number of metastases associated with a worse outcome. With greater than 16 nodules, complete resection is unlikely.
4. Bilateral metastases or left-sided metastases are shown, in some studies, to have a decreased rate of survival.
5. A short disease-free interval from the time of resection of the primary tumor until appearance of metastases.

RHABDOMYOSARCOMA

Rhabdomyosarcoma and other soft tissue sarcomas frequently metastasize to the lungs. These tumors are generally chemoresponsive. Tumors treated at stages I to III with primary resection, chemotherapy, and radiation therapy, have a good prognosis. Metastatic disease is associated with a poor long-term prognosis. Five-year survival decreases precipitously in the presence of stage IV disease. Metastases are often widespread and unresectable. Metastatic resections for soft-tissue sarcomas are reserved for isolated pulmonary lesions that are unresponsive to chemotherapy and radiation.

WILMS TUMOR

Initial screening tests in the presence of a Wilms tumor include CT of the abdomen and chest to determine the nature of the primary tumor as well as metastatic spread. Suspicious pulmonary lesions require biopsy to confirm the presence of metastatic disease. Although pulmonary metastases are associated with a worse outcome, survival is still much greater than for other metastatic pediatric cancers. This is due to the responsiveness of these tumors to whole-lung irradiation and chemotherapy.

There is little evidence to support pulmonary resection in the presence of metastatic disease. Trials of pulmonary metastasectomy have not shown superior results to those achieved with chemotherapy and radiation. For this reason, metastasectomy is reserved for patients who do not respond to conventional therapy.

HEPATIC TUMORS

Hepatoblastoma and hepatocellular carcinoma comprise the majority of pediatric hepatic tumors. In one third of all cases of pediatric hepatic tumors, there is radiologic evidence of either regional or distant metastatic spread at the time of diagnosis. Pulmonary metastases also may be detected through an increasing alpha-fetoprotein level after initial hepatic resection. Resection of the primary tumor is essential in order to provide the best chance for long-term disease-free survival. This may be accomplished through hepatic lobectomy or trisegmentectomy. A number of small studies have supported aggressive resection of pulmonary metastases after successful resection of the primary tumor. As in the case of metastatic osteosarcoma, repeat resections conserving lung tissue may result in improved survival.

HEPATIC METASTASES

Hepatic metastases are uncommon in pediatric tumors and generally represent extensive, unresectable disease. In the case of a Wilms tumor, however, resection of liver affected by direct extension of the primary tumor results in improved long-term survival. In this situation, there may be invasion of the primary tumor into the liver or hematogenous spread of tumor involving the liver. Resection may be performed at the time of the initial surgery. But in most instances, hepatic resection is delayed. Factors that must be considered by the surgeon include the magnitude of the original operation, the anticipated extent of hepatic resection, and the general status of the patient. Chemotherapy and radiation significantly decrease the extent of the tumor; therefore, bulky tumors and tumors involving crucial anatomic structures may be more easily resected at a second laparotomy.

NEUROBLASTOMA

Neuroblastoma represents a unique example of metastatic hepatic disease that warrants discussion. Infants with stage IV-S neuroblastoma present with hepatomegaly, subcutaneous nodules, and a positive bone marrow. The massive tumor-filled liver in these infants may cause respiratory insufficiency, coagulopathy, gastrointestinal dysfunction (frequent vomiting), and renal compromise. The liver mass resolves without therapy in most affected patients, and long-term survival is comparable with that of stage I and II disease. Complications of massive hepatomegaly, however, may be fatal. Therapeutic intervention includes low-dose radiation therapy or low-dose cyclophosphamide. Some surgeons have recommended surgical enlargement of the abdominal wall with placement of either an external Silastic patch or internal polytetrafluoroethylene patch. The efficacy of this technique is questionable, and septic complications have been observed. Palliative resection does not play a role in stage IV-S disease.

CENTRAL NERVOUS SYSTEM METASTASES

Brain metastases are rare in children with solid tumors. Improvements in survival resulting from the evolution of a multidisciplinary approach to pediatric cancers have increased the period of time during which children are at risk for developing brain metastases. There is a high incidence of relapsing brain metastases in patients on systemic chemotherapy, which suggests that the brain is a pharmacologically protected site in patients initially diagnosed with metastatic disease.

Ewing's sarcoma and rhabdomyosarcoma are among the most likely cancers to metastasize to the brain. Roughly 3% of all patients with Ewing's sarcoma have central nervous system (CNS) metastases at the time of primary diagnosis. Almost all affected patients have clinical signs of CNS involvement, including headache (most common), morning vomiting, and lethargy. Metastatic CNS lesions may produce increased intracranial pressure, which can present as the Cushing's triad (hypertension, bradycardia, and apnea). In extreme cases, brain herniation may occur with changes in responsiveness, respiratory pattern, pupil size and reactivity, extraocular movements, and motor function. Treatment of increased intracranial pressure secondary to metastatic disease includes decreasing intravenous fluids to 75% of maintenance and administering dexamethasone (1 mg/kg loading dose followed by 0.5 mg/kg four times a day). Other supplemental therapies include diuretics, acetazolamide (to decrease CSF production), and hyperventilation (which should be used with caution because excessive hyperventilation may lead to cerebral ischemia). Intracranial pressure monitoring and antiseizure prophylaxis may be considered.

Even in the absence of increased intracranial pressure, the outcome of patients with metastatic CNS lesions is dismal. The median duration of survival after diagnosis of brain metastasis, irrespective of histology, is less than 3 months. Aggressive chemotherapy is the mainstay of treatment and offers the best chance of long-term survival. Although there are isolated reports of pediatric patients achieving long-term survival after resection of CNS metastases, there is not enough evidence to support surgical resection of these lesions.

SPINAL METASTASES

Metastases to bone rarely require surgical treatment. Spinal metastatic disease with cord compromise does, however, demand prompt evaluation and treatment and may require surgical intervention. Neuroblastoma is the most common non-CNS pediatric tumor to metastasize to the spine. Spinal involvement may be secondary to tumor extension, lymphatic spread into the vertebral foramina, or hematogenous deposit in the bone marrow. Although the lumbar spine is the most frequently involved site, it is thoracic spine involvement that tends to compromise the spinal cord and necessitate surgical intervention.

The most common presenting symptoms of spinal metastases are back pain and a change in gait. Neurologic sequelae that may develop include radicular pain, sensory loss, bowel and bladder dysfunction, and, eventually, paraplegia. The development of these findings in the first 24 hours after the onset of symptoms denotes a poor prognosis. MRI is the best method for determining the extent of metastatic disease in the spine.

In the absence of extensive neurologic involvement, a multiagent regimen of chemotherapy should be initiated. High-dose steroids play a role primarily in pain relief. Radiation therapy is initiated in tumors that are associated with neurologic impairment but where the bony structures remain intact. Failure of radiation therapy necessitates surgical intervention.

Surgical decompression is generally reserved for older children and in those who have significant bone destruction. Decompression may be accomplished through an anterior or posterior approach. The anterior approach allows resection of an anterior tumor and correction of kyphosis. The posterior approach is suitable for multilevel vertebral decompression. Removal of posterior bony elements necessitates the use of fixation devices such as Luque rods. Both surgical options provide excellent pain relief to the patient.

SUGGESTED READINGS

Bergen GA, Shelhamer JH. Pulmonary infiltrates in the cancer patient. *Infect Dis Clin North Am* 1996;10:297–325.

Black CT, Luck SR, Musemeche CA, et al. Aggressive excision of pulmonary metastases is warranted in the management of childhood hepatic tumors. *J Pediatr Surg* 1991;26:1082–1086.

Bouffet E, Doumni N, Thiesse P, et al. Brain metastases in children with solid tumors. *Cancer* 1997;5;403–410.

Harris MB, Gieser P, Goorin AM, et al. Treatment of metastatic osteosarcoma at diagnosis: a Pediatric Oncology Group study. *J Clin Oncol* 1998;16:3641–3648.

Pogrebniak HW, Pass HI. Initial and reoperative pulmonary metastasectomy: indications, technique and results. *Semin Surg Oncol* 1993;9:142–149.

Sinha AK, Seki JT, Moreau G, et al. The management of spinal metastasis in children. *Can J Surg* 1997;40:218–226.

Temeck BK, Wexler LH, Steinberg SM, et al. Metastasectomy for sarcomatous pediatric histologies: results and prognostic factors. *Ann Thorac Surg* 1995;59:1385–1390.

Temeck BK, Wexler LH, Steinberg SM, et al. Reoperative pulmonary metastasectomy for sarcomatous pediatric histologies. *Ann Thorac Surg* 1998;66:908–913.

116

MUSCULOSKELETAL SURGICAL ONCOLOGY

ROBERT P. STANTON

Malignant neoplasms of the musculoskeletal system are rare in children: osteogenic sarcoma occurs in 1 per million population and Ewing's sarcoma 1 per 1.5 million population. It is not surprising that young patients with malignant musculoskeletal neoplasms often do not receive an optimal preoperative workup. In most cases the patient's complaints are attributed to traumatic events, and proper management is delayed for weeks or even months. If an abnormal mass is appreciated, the cause is often ascribed to an infection or other more common etiology. Unfortunately, ill-advised surgical procedures are often recommended, which can have severe adverse implications for future management of the patient. In this chapter I review the basic management principles that should be used to evaluate a child presenting with a suspected musculoskeletal neoplasm.

CLINICAL EVALUATION

One of my professors once told me, "Every child falls every day." It is almost inevitable that the child presenting with a tumor will have a history of some form of injury to the area. Those of us practicing oncologic surgery do not really believe that trauma is a factor in the development of malignant tumors, but it is logical to believe that the minor trauma brings attention to the area affected by the tumor. In other instances, incidental trauma such as a sprained knee or ankle lead to the ordering of a radiograph of the area, and a bone tumor may be identified as an incidental finding, initiating tumor workup. It is important to determine the real history for the problem being evaluated. Clinicians should try to talk to the patient when taking a history. The parents often try to answer questions that the clinician asks the child. If possible, the child should be encouraged to respond to the questions. It is surprising how much accurate information can be obtained from a child as young as 8 years. One thing children are not very good at is assessing the timing of their problems. For this, the parents are a better source of information. How long has this been present? What is the type of pain (if any) and how is it affecting the normal activity of the child? Altered activity is the "pain meter" for the child. Is the pain related to activity or is the pain independent of activity? What fun or favorite activities have been curtailed as a result of the pain? Does the pain wake the child from sleep? What has been done for the pain so far? What medications (including over-the-counter preparations) have been used, and what was the response?

The physical examination is the most important part of the evaluation. The examination begins by having the child undress down to the underclothing. An experienced clinician never attempts to evaluate a patient who is not undressed. The gait is evaluated by having the child walk in the room. This is more easily done if the floor is carpeted, because small children do not walk normally on cold floors if they are barefoot, and the gait cannot be evaluated if the child is in shoes. Small children are often fearful of physicians, and one is wise to begin the examination of the child by evaluating a portion of the anatomy that is as far away from the area of concern as possible. Children are fascinated by counting, and I prefer to start the examination by counting the fingers or toes of an uninvolved extremity. Gradually moving carefully to the involved extremity is less likely to result in a hysterical child whose examination is unrewarding. The skin should be evaluated carefully, because changes in superficial skin temperature and the distribution of superficial blood vessels is often seen in musculoskeletal neoplasms. The physician should do a complete check of the range of motion of each joint and a careful palpation of each portion of the extremity between joints. Masses can usually be appreciated and characterized by careful palpation. Is the lesion bony? Does it have a soft mushy feel (lipoma) or is it more firm and rubbery (fibroma)? Most sarcomas have a discrete border on palpation. Inflammatory masses are less discrete and more likely to be painful to the touch. Muscle her-

R. P. Stanton: Musculoskeletal Tumor Program, Department of Surgery, Alfred I. duPont Hospital for Children, Wilmington, Delaware.

nias are nearly invisible when the muscle is relaxed, yet with contraction, a worrisome mass becomes visible and palpable. Does the mass move with the normal motion of the tendons? For an underlying bony mass, what is the relationship of the overlying structures? Is there a painful soft tissue bursa over the protuberant mass? A careful evaluation of the regional lymph nodes is indicated, although a general principle of musculoskeletal malignancies is that they generally show widespread metastatic spread to the lungs without regional lymph node metastasis.

STAGING

All definitive surgery for malignant lesions of the extremities is predicated on staging the lesion in accordance with the Musculoskeletal Tumor Society (MSTS) staging system. This system was developed and adopted in the early 1970s and is sufficiently different from the tumor staging systems commonly in use in general surgical oncology that a review is in order.

Musculoskeletal Tumor Society Staging System

I. Low-grade malignancy
   a. Intracompartmental
   b. Extracompartmental
II. High-grade malignancy
   a. Intracompartmental
   b. Extracompartmental
III. Metastatic disease

When considering surgical resection to control local disease, the concept of anatomic compartment localization is one of the most important factors. Examples of anatomic compartments would be one muscle, joint, or bone. A malignant rhabdomyosarcoma that is contained within the fascial envelope of the vastus medialis muscle would be staged as IIa, because the tumor is histologically high grade, but only involves one discrete anatomic compartment. A typical osteogenic sarcoma of the distal femur that started within the medullary canal of the bone but has now broken through the cortex and has a 7 × 15 cm, soft tissue extension into the quadriceps muscle would be a IIb, because it is high grade, but now involves more than one compartment. The bone itself is considered one compartment. If the tumor were involving the entire femur from one end to the other, but was confined to the bone with no evidence of extension through the cortex to the soft tissues, the stage would be Ia or IIa, depending on the histologic grade. Certain areas of the body do not have discrete compartments; therefore, tumors in these areas are arbitrarily designated to be extracompartmental. Examples of these areas include the palm of the hand and the popliteal fossa. This staging system allows the surgeon to plan for a definitive resection and allows the prediction of long-term survival.

General surgeons and orthopaedic surgeons use different terms to describe their surgical margins. Even when the same term is used by both specialties, it is not uncommon to find that the definition of the term is not the same for both specialties. A review of these terms will be helpful in allowing more accurate discussion of tumor margins across specialties. Sarcomas grow by local cell division and pressure on the surrounding normal soft tissues. This is in distinction to carcinomas, which more typically show a tendency to infiltrate between cell layers of the surrounding normal tissues. As the sarcoma grows, its outermost cells are compressed and form a pseudocapsule. This capsule is composed of compressed tumor cells, not normal cells, and thus does not represent a viable surgical margin. In addition, there is a reactive zone surrounding the pseudocapsule of a malignant sarcoma. This represents an area of normal tissue within which can be found lymphocytes, monocytes, and histiocytes as a result of local inflammatory changes caused by the nearby presence of the tumor. Exactly how this response is elicited is unknown. In the reactive zone one may find microscopic foci of tumor cells not in contact with the main tumor. These are known as satellite lesions.

Staging Studies

The staging of a musculoskeletal lesion always begins with ordinary radiographs. Even soft tissue neoplasms may have an effect on the underlying skeletal structures. For bone tumors, radiographs give an excellent picture of the biologic behavior of the tumor. Aggressive lesions are ill defined and demonstrate aggressive destruction of the adjacent normal cortex. In some instances the tumor matrix produces neoplastic bone, and the pattern of this "bone" may be diagnostic for the particular histologic tumor type. In virtually every case, the radiographs allow the development of an accurate differential diagnosis. Additional studies are often needed to develop a detailed assessment of the extent of the tumor. Computed tomography (CT) is especially useful in musculoskeletal tumors. Subtle changes in the quality of the bone cortex are easily demonstrated by adjusting the "windows" of the scan and give a level of detail not available with other imaging techniques. In addition, if malignancy is extremely likely, one should remember that most musculoskeletal sarcomas are prone to metastasize to the lungs. Whole-lung CT is the most specific and sensitive test for early metastatic disease. One should consider the radiation dose to the chest when deciding whether to proceed with lung CT before receiving histologic confirmation of the diagnosis. Magnetic resonance imaging (MRI) is of immense help in imaging soft tissue tumors of the extremities, and also gives much useful information concerning marrow cavity involvement in bone tumors. The cortex is poorly visualized by MRI; therefore CT and MRI are complementary. Whole-body nuclear imaging is often useful to exclude unexpected multifocal disease and occult metastatic spread to the skeleton. The activity in the lesion being evaluated is sometimes of use to the surgeon, but this biologic information is usually already apparent from the radiographs. The skeleton is the second most common location for metastatic spread of musculoskeletal neoplasms. Therefore, the bone scan should be obtained to complete the staging studies of most patients. Invasive studies such as arteriography and lymphangiography are almost never indicated.

SURGICAL MARGINS

Surgical margins may be differentiated as intralesional, marginal, wide, or radical. Intralesional surgery includes any surgical procedure during which the pseudocapsule of the tumor is exposed or entered. By definition, the capsule is considered to be tumor tissue; therefore, the tumor resection bed contains at the very least, microscopic tumor cells. In addition, the reactive zone has not been removed, and therefore must be considered to contain satellite lesions. This type of surgery cannot be considered adequate for a malignant musculoskeletal neoplasm.

A marginal excision removes the tumor by dissection through the reactive zone. The pseudocapsule is not exposed at any time during the procedure. The tumor is enclosed entirely by "normal" tissue, although the reactive zone may contain satellite lesions. For this reason, local recurrence may be expected in a high number of cases of marginal excision unless some form of adjuvant therapy (i.e., local radiation therapy) is used to extend the effective margin.

A wide margin is the first margin that is considered to be adequate for a high-grade malignancy of the musculoskeletal system. In this type of resection the tumor is excised by dissection around the tumor through the normal tissue outside the reactive zone. The amount of normal tissue that must be sacrificed to ensure that the surgeon does not leave any reactive zone material behind is variable and depends on the exact histology of the tumor and whether neoadjuvants (preoperative chemotherapy or radiation therapy) have been used. In general, one would need several millimeters of soft tissue margin, and several (7–10) centimeters of bone to achieve such a margin. In this type of resection, the entire compartment is not removed. One may expect local recurrence rates of 2% to 3% with a wide margin, regardless of whether it is achieved by limb salvage procedures or amputation.

A *radical margin* is obtained by removing the entire contents of the anatomic compartment in which the tumor is found. The resection is performed en bloc so that the compartment itself is not entered, therefore ensuring that microscopic spread of tumor cells is not possible. A radical margin provides a nearly zero local recurrence rate, but of course, the patient may have already developed microscopic metastatic disease. In some anatomic locations, a radical margin is not possible without performing an amputation of the limb. In other cases, a radical margin may be obtained at the expense of vital structures (i.e., sciatic nerve) that make the retained limb less functional than a prosthetic replacement. In such cases, there is no reason to retain a functionless limb at the risk of a higher local recurrence rate.

BIOPSY CONSIDERATIONS

In most cases of suspected malignancy, an incisional biopsy should be performed. Ideally the surgeon performing the biopsy should be the same surgeon that will be performing the definitive resection of the tumor. This ensures that the biopsy incision is placed in such a fashion as to be resectable with the definitive specimen resection. All incisions must be placed to allow subsequent extensive exposure; thus, transverse incisions would almost never be appropriate. Transverse incisions do not allow sufficient exposure to allow an extensive resection. The removal of transverse incisions en bloc with the underlying specimen often require the use of flaps to close the surgical site. These techniques are inappropriate for patients who need to start or continue chemotherapy shortly after a resection. In many cases, a transverse biopsy incision leads to an amputation in a patient who would otherwise have been a candidate for limb salvage.

The approach to the tumor should be direct, and through a muscle whenever possible. Dissection between muscles is inappropriate, because it encourages spread of the biopsy hematoma to more than one compartment. Dissection through a muscle belly allows the muscle fascia to control the hematoma, thereby limiting the extent of subsequent surgery.

A generous incisional biopsy sample should be obtained and sent for frozen section analysis. Musculoskeletal tumors are often composed of many cell types; therefore, small specimens may only contain reactive bone or portions of the tumor that are not diagnostic for the entire neoplasm. Some sarcomas grow so rapidly that they outgrow their blood supply and are prone to necrosis. If the specimen contains only "ghost" cells of the original tumor, a specific histologic diagnosis may not be possible. These factors mandate frozen section review of the specimen to be sure that it is representative and likely to be diagnostic. In addition, frozen section review often gives a preliminary diagnosis and thus guides the pathologist to order the appropriate special stains and cytogenetic tests that are often crucial in developing an exact diagnosis in a timely fashion. In rare cases, a potential malignancy turns out to be an unusual presentation of an infection, and the frozen section results are often the first indication that the material will need to be cultured to determine the causative organism.

If the preliminary diagnosis from the frozen section analysis confirms the probable malignant nature of the lesion, the biopsy defect must be managed to control the hematoma. Meticulous hemostasis is mandatory, using a combination of electrocautery and hemostatic agents. The pseudocapsule should be closed watertight using a running interlocking stitch. Each layer of tissue should receive a meticulous closure and the skin should be closed using a nonabsorbable and nonreactive suture, because often the patient is started on chemotherapy several weeks before a definitive resection is performed. Biopsy wounds may open once chemotherapy is started if they are not adequately closed. Drains are rarely necessary. If drains are necessary, they should be placed in line with the skin incision, and their location should be clearly documented in the dictated operative note. If a hole has been created in the bone cortex to obtain a specimen, and the frozen section results confirm the probable malignant nature of the process, one should consider plugging the bone hole with a substance such as polymethylmethacrylate (orthopedic bone cement) to contain the hematoma of bone.

EXCISIONAL BIOPSY

Excisional biopsy is seldom appropriate in a malignant musculoskeletal tumor. If the frozen section diagnosis reveals that a previously suspected malignancy is in fact entirely benign, and the surgeon is sufficiently familiar with the management of that particular benign tumor, the procedure may be converted to an excisional biopsy. Many benign musculoskeletal neoplasms are aggressive and have high recurrence rates. In many instances, more aggressive surgery is indicated than what might be expected for a totally benign process. In these cases the surgeon may be advised to conclude the incisional biopsy and defer the definitive resection to a surgeon familiar with the particular characteristics of that tumor. By leaving the peripheral aspects of the tumor in place, the definitive resection may be more easily planned.

The majority of children with malignant musculoskeletal neoplasms are eligible for management in accordance with standardized treatment protocols developed by national cooperative study groups (e.g., Children's Oncology Group). Increasingly, these protocols use neoadjuvant chemotherapy. Following the incisional biopsy, the patient receives several weeks of "up-front" chemotherapy, and then is restaged prior to the definitive resection of the remaining tumor. Following the resection, the histologic response of the tumor to the chemotherapy is assessed, and in some instances, alterations to the remaining chemotherapy regimen are made in an attempt to customize the chemotherapy to the specific response of the tumor. For these reasons, definitive resection of the tumor as the initial procedure is a rare event.

DEFINITIVE RESECTION OF MALIGNANT BONE TUMORS

In all instances, the goals of the surgeon should be to entirely remove the entire tumor and any potentially contaminated tissues in an en bloc fashion to prevent local recurrence and to maximize the survival of the patient. A variety of innovative surgical resections are available to provide reconstruction of the limb following tumor resection. The use of limb-sparing techniques has increased dramatically without any compromise in long-term patient survival. Modular endoprosthetic replacements are commercially available that allow the surgeon to reconstruct massive lengths of missing skeleton and to replace resected joints.

These devices are similar to the endoprotheses used in adult joint reconstructions and thus are subject to the limitations of host bone–prosthesis fixation and are also likely to have limited functional life spans when used in young, active patients. Experience has shown that these prosthetic replacements have functioned well beyond the initial expected life span of a similar prosthesis implanted in a young patient as a result of injury rather than neoplasm. This is likely due to the fact that the bone and substantial muscle is often removed in cancer surgery, thus placing some constraints on the subsequent physical activity of the patient. Human allografts are often used in limb reconstructions if the joints do not have to be sacrificed. Human tissue banks can usually supply appropriately sized allograft replacements for nearly any skeletal segment.

With both endoprosthetic and allograft reconstructions, no human growth can be expected in the reconstructed segment, and for immature patients, limb length inequality may be expected at skeletal maturity. Several innovative endoprosthetic devices have been produced that allow incremental elongation of the prosthesis to keep pace with the natural growth of the opposite limb; however, reliability and durability of the devices have continued to be a problem. None of these devices are generally available outside of investigational protocols.

In all cases, the soft tissue reconstructions require salvage of the neurovascular structures. If vessels are involved with tumor, reconstruction requires vascular grafts. Due to loss of graft patency and high postoperative infection rates, vascular reconstructions are not appropriate if postoperative chemotherapy or radiation therapy will be required. Surgical resection of major motor nerves is almost always an indication to consider an amputation. Paralyzed and insensate limbs almost certainly have worse function than the appropriate corresponding prosthesis, and there is no reason to subject the patient to the potential of contaminated resection margins for inferior postoperative function. Although the techniques of surgical limb salvage allow the retention of virtually any limb, these techniques must not be used indiscriminately.

SUMMARY

The evaluation and management of musculoskeletal neoplasms requires a working knowledge of the radiographic and clinical aspects of a wide variety of both benign and malignant neoplasms. To avoid iatrogenic complications, the surgeon should be familiar with the principles discussed above and should have the experience, training, and ancillary support to provide optimum care for the patient. Ideally, a coordinated team approach including the surgeon, medical oncologist, radiologist, and pathologist should be used throughout the patient's care to optimize the chances for an excellent long-term outcome.

SUGGESTED READINGS

Enneking WF. *Musculoskeletal tumor surgery.* New York: Churchill Livingstone, 1983.

Simon MA. Biopsy of musculoskeletal tumors. *J Bone Joint Surg [Am]* 1982;64:1253–1257.

Stanton RP. Complications associated with the treatment of benign tumors and tumor-like conditions. In: Epps CH Jr, Bowen JR, eds. *Complications in pediatric orthopaedic surgery.* Philadelphia: JB Lippincott, 1995:685–714.

SECTION XIII

SKIN AND SOFT TISSUES

117

BENIGN SKIN LESIONS

PETER MATTEI

Skin lesions are a frequent indication for pediatric surgical consultation. Some patients are asking the opinion of the surgeon as to whether the lesion needs to be removed or sampled for biopsy, whereas others come to the office having already decided, usually with the help of their primary care physician or a dermatologist, that they desire to have the lesion removed and they are asking the surgeon's help in facilitating that decision. It is important to know the mindset of the patient and the referring physician beforehand, because this can change the tenor of the recommendation and can help prevent an awkward encounter.

NEVI

Melanoma occurs infrequently in children, although the incidence may be increasing. Nevertheless, a common indication for pediatric surgical evaluation is the child with a worrisome pigmented mole or freckle. It is at times a difficult balance to strike: we want to respect the concerns of the parents without being overly aggressive, while maintaining a rational approach without being too cavalier. Fortunately, the vast majority of suspicious nevi are benign and few are malignant or even premalignant.

Most would agree that giant nevi and those that are symptomatic (itchy, painful, bleeding) should be removed, regardless of age or location. There is less agreement about the much more common small, asymptomatic lesions. We are all familiar with the characteristics of moles that are considered grounds for concern in adults: an irregular border, heterogeneous coloration, size greater than 5 mm, changes in the surrounding normal skin, any change over time, and location in certain sites, such as the palms, soles, and areas of the skin that are protected from sunlight. Patients who are fair-skinned or who have a family history of melanoma are also considered at higher risk. Unfortunately, most nevi in children seem to have at least one of these worrisome features, and nevi that are followed from infancy go through changes in color and size as the patient grows, especially during adolescence. To add to the confusion, childhood melanoma sometimes occurs in nevi that are rather benign in appearance.

Although occasionally a child presents for the surgeon's opinion regarding a particular lesion and whether it should be removed, the majority of patients present already having decided that the mole is worrisome to them and that they would like to have it removed. I think we place the patient in a potentially dangerous position when we try to dissuade a parent from having a particular lesion removed, unless we can be absolutely certain that the lesion is benign and is unlikely to undergo malignant transformation in the future. Because this is so difficult to determine by visual inspection alone, it is usually advisable to recommend excisional biopsy in these cases. Although there would seem to be the potential for abuse and multiple unnecessary operations, this seems to occur only rarely.

Once the decision is made to proceed with biopsy, the setting and type of anesthesia need to be planned. For most infants and small children, the biopsy procedure should be performed under general anesthesia. For older children, the procedure can be performed safely and comfortably under local anesthesia, depending on the maturity and temperament of the child. In most cases, a single oral dose of an anxiolytic such as midazolam is quite useful. In some centers, it is routine to perform "minor" procedures with the patient under sedation administered intravenously or by inhalation.

All suspicious nevi should be excised completely with a full-thickness excision down to and including a few millimeters of underlying subcutaneous fat. Shave biopsies and incisional biopsies are inadequate for pigmented nevi, and can compromise the ability to accurately stage a malignant lesion. A margin of at least 1 mm of normal skin is considered acceptable for all but the most worrisome lesions. Elliptical incisions oriented along skin lines are cosmetically superior to circular incisions and punch biopsies. Of course, lesions that are irregular and whose long axis is not parallel

P. Mattei: Department of Surgery, Thomas Jefferson University, Philadelphia, Pennsylvania; and Department of Pediatric Surgery, Alfred I. duPont Hospital for Children, Wilmington, Delaware to the skin lines may require more creative excisional techniques to minimize scarring. Fortunately, the elastic nature of the skin in childhood allows most incisions to be closed with little tension and excellent cosmetic results.

Almost all incisions can be closed with absorbable suture, avoiding the distress of suture removal and the cosmetically unacceptable cross-hatching that occurs with other closure techniques involving permanent suture. My preference is interrupted, buried, deep-dermal sutures using 4-0 or 5-0 braided absorbable suture on a small tapered needle and sterile strips applied longitudinally with a skin adhesive. These are strong stitches that are useful even when the skin is under significant tension. The parents are instructed to keep the wound dry for 48 hours, unless a waterproof dressing is applied, in which case they can get wet immediately.

Giant nevi pose a technical challenge because of the resulting large skin defect that needs to be closed. Some are so large that advanced plastic surgical techniques need to be applied, including the use of tissue expanders, cutaneous flaps, or skin grafting. Alternatively, a large lesion can be excised in stages. Removing the first specimen from the center of the lesion, thus leaving the scar to be completely excised later, leaves the surrounding normal skin intact for a more cosmetically acceptable closure at the final stage.

Nevus sebaceum is a lesion that appears on the scalp in young children. These lesions have a waxy plaque-like appearance and are usually yellowish, nonpigmented, and hairless. They usually have an irregular shape and can be quite a bit longer than they are wide. Because they have a propensity to undergo neoplastic change in adulthood, they should be excised at some point during childhood. If a young child with a sebaceous nevus is to undergo general anesthesia for another reason, the nevus can be removed simultaneously. Otherwise, they can be removed when the child is a teenager.

CUTANEOUS HEMANGIOMAS

These are raised red dermal lesions that begin in infancy and continue to grow during the first year of life. They have a characteristic appearance and growth history, so that further studies are rarely necessary to confirm the diagnosis. Some have a significant subcutaneous component and can occur anywhere on the skin. If left alone, these generally have a predictable clinical course that includes gradual spontaneous involution beginning after the first year and continuing for several years thereafter.

Because of the natural history and the difficulty with achieving acceptable cosmesis after primary excision, most of these lesions are simply observed. Excision is recommended only if the location of the lesion poses significant health concerns, for example, lesions near the eye that obstruct vision. Lesions that pose significant cosmetic concerns are troublesome because the resulting scar is rarely an improvement in the patient's appearance. For large lesions and those that cannot be safely excised, systemic corticosteroids sometimes result in early involution. More recently, antiangiogenesis drugs have been proposed as an alternative to steroids, but α-interferon, the most commonly recommended agent in the past, has been associated with troubling adverse affects on the spinal cord and lower extremity function. Lesions of the head and face appear to be more sensitive to the effects of corticosteroids, which can be administered by local injection, avoiding systemic effects.

CYSTS

Epidermal inclusion cysts result from the accumulation of shed skin cells and keratin produced by epidermal skin elements that become trapped beneath the skin. This is presumably due to a minor traumatic event that causes these cells to be pushed below the dermis, although the actual mechanism is not known. They are usually slow growing and asymptomatic, unless they are infected or ruptured. Infected cysts present as an abscess, which when drained produces the characteristic white, cheesy keratin deposits (formerly described as "sebaceous" material) in addition to pus. Infected cysts eventually require excision, although it is generally best to delay excision until the acute infection has resolved. Cysts that rupture beneath the skin produce a foreign body reaction that can simulate infection. These are also best excised when signs of local inflammation have resolved.

The cysts are located in the subcutaneous fat just below the dermis. They are typically well encapsulated, nontender and vaguely fluctuant. They are classically described as having an umbilicated center or a punctum at their attachment to the skin, but this is often difficult to identify. Further studies are rarely necessary except for the rare lesion that mimics a neoplasm. Cysts that develop on the scalp or behind the ear are often indistinguishable from hyperplastic lymph nodes.

Epidermal inclusion cysts can be excised under general or local anesthesia, depending on the age and maturity of the patient. A narrow elliptical incision is made parallel to the skin lines and should incorporate the punctum to minimize recurrence. The entire cyst wall should be excised to prevent recurrence. Keeping the cyst wall intact during removal is preferable but rupture is sometimes inevitable. The presence of cyst contents in the wound can cause a minor local foreign body reaction and may increase the risk for a wound infection, but probably does not in and of itself lead to an increased risk of recurrence. However, cyst rupture may make it more difficult to achieve a complete excision of the wall itself. The wound is irrigated and closed primarily with absorbable sutures.

Dermoid cysts are grossly indistinguishable from epidermal inclusion cysts, and the keratinous material contained within them is essentially the same. They differ in their origin, in that dermoid cysts are presumably congenital, not acquired, and occur in characteristic locations of the head and chest where embryonic fusion planes occur. They typically occur on the scalp, at the lateral eyebrow, or on the anterior chest near the midline. They can be distinguished histologically by the presence of accessory skin elements that are lacking in epidermal inclusion cysts, which consist of pure epidermal tissue. The natural history and the approach to treatment are the same. Lesions of the scalp in infants occasionally have an intracranial component and therefore should be evaluated first by plain radiography of the skull, looking for an area of radiolucency, or by computed tomography (CT), especially for midline lesions. Cysts on the scalp and lateral brow are typically densely adherent to the periostium of the skull and are usually cupped by a saucer-shaped area of adjacent bone. Frequently, the periostium itself needs to be excised in order to completely remove the cyst wall. Incisions on the scalp should follow lines of tension, whereas brow lesions should be excised through an incision placed within or slightly above and parallel to the eyebrow. The eyebrow should not be shaved, and incisions below the eyebrow should be avoided because of the risk of local bleeding with ecchymosis and an inferior cosmetic result.

SUBCUTANEOUS MASSES

Subcutaneous soft tissue masses are usually asymptomatic. They are soft, somewhat mobile, and nontender. Although the specific diagnosis can be suggested by the clinical appearance, the differential diagnosis generally includes lipoma, lymphangioma, and hemangioma. Treatment is excision for all three, so that an extensive workup to make an absolute diagnosis is unnecessary. A possible exception is a hemangioma in an infant in whom it may be elected to observe the lesion with the hope that it may spontaneously resolve. Large lesions of the neck should be evaluated with imaging studies for possible involvement of deeper structures. Ultrasonography offers a noninvasive and accurate method of screening for deeper involvement, with CT or magnetic resonance imaging reserved for cases that are shown by ultrasonography to be more complex.

Most of these lesions should be excised under general anesthesia. The incision is oriented parallel to lines of tension and does not always need to be as large as the diameter of the lesion. The incision should be continued carefully through the deeper tissues so that a subtle change in the appearance of the fat could be appreciated immediately, avoiding violation of the capsule of the lesion. Eventually, the mass can be distinguished from surrounding normal fat, and a plane can be established between the two.

At operation, hemangiomas have the unmistakable appearance of purplish red cystic structures in a cluster-of-grapes configuration. They are usually well encapsulated, and the plane between the lesion and the surrounding fat is usually easy to define with blunt dissection. The dissection should stay close to the wall with control of small feeding vessels with cautery or suture where appropriate. The mass occasionally involves the underlying fascia, which may need to be excised with the lesion. An attempt to excise a perceived intramuscular component is usually fraught with bleeding and an inability to identify the true extent of the lesion. In these rare cases, it is usually best to close the wound after hemostasis is achieved and plan to image the area postoperatively to better assess the deeper component. When the subcutaneous component has been completely excised, hemostasis is achieved and the wound closed in layers with absorbable sutures. Closed-suction drains are occasionally necessary for large defects. Postoperative recovery is typically uneventful and recurrence is unusual.

Lymphangiomas are usually identified by the presence of multiple tiny cysts, but can grossly resemble a lipoma. The limits of the dissection are not always clear, because the mass is often fatty and can blend in with the surrounding adipose tissue. Feeding vessels at the periphery include tiny lymphatics that are difficult to visualize and may contribute to a postoperative seroma or recurrence if not controlled. The skin is closed in the usual fashion. A closed-suction drain is used only if the defect is large. The parents should be warned that a postoperative seroma is likely. A small seroma can be safely observed. A large seroma can be drained painlessly with a needle placed directly through the incision. This may need to be repeated every week or two for two or three aspirations, but it will eventually resolve. Recurrence is uncommon, but patients should be followed for up to a year.

Lipomas and lipoblastomas are asymptomatic, benign fatty tumors that occur in the subcutaneous space. On examination, they are similar to lymphangiomas and hemangiomas, although they are not always as well encapsulated. The surgical approach is the same. An incision smaller than the diameter of the lesion is usually adequate. The dissection should proceed carefully so that the capsule of the mass can be identified and preserved. The tumors frequently lie deep to Scarpa's fascia. Once the proper plane of dissection is identified, the majority of the dissection can be performed bluntly, with small feeding vessels controlled with cautery. Some lipomas blend in well with the surrounding fat, but they usually have a firmer consistency that can be appreciated by careful palpation. Complete excision is the goal. The defect that remains is rarely large or vacuous, and the wound can usually be closed in layers without a drain.

SKIN NODULES

A small, hard nodule in the subcutaneous fat just below the dermis is usually a pilomatrixoma (calcifying epithelioma of

Malherbe). This is a benign cystic tumor derived from the hair follicle that begins in the dermis and extends into the subcutaneous space. These nodules occur almost exclusively in children and young adults. They are usually asymptomatic, although they can be mildly tender to the touch. They rarely become infected and do not have premalignant potential. Excision is straightforward and should include the small area of dermis to which the lesion is attached. They are usually well encapsulated and can be delivered by blunt dissection.

Neurofibromas can occur in any child and usually present as firm, irregular nodules with a cartilaginous feel. They are sometimes associated with a small superficial nerve branch, which can usually be sacrificed without sequelae. Although sporadic and not usually associated with neurofibromatosis, every child with a neurofibroma should be evaluated carefully for café au lait spots (the presence of more than six is diagnostic of neurofibromatosis) or, if multiple nodules are present, by a medical geneticist.

Various other fibromas, nodules, and cysts arise frequently in children and are usually best removed to allay parental anxiety and avoid diagnostic uncertainty. Lesions that are tender or show signs of infection or inflammation should be evaluated for the possibility of a foreign body. The history might be suggestive, but in most cases it is prudent to perform plain radiography or ultrasonography specifically to rule out the possibility of a foreign body despite a negative history. This is particularly true if the family decides not to proceed with surgical excision right away.

Warts are viral lesions that are sometimes referred to a surgeon for consideration of excision. Small warts can be treated with liquid nitrogen, although larger ones may require primary excision. This should be approached with caution, because the resulting skin defect can be difficult to cover and recurrence rates are high. Shaving warts allows retention of the intradermal component and guarantees recurrence. It should be noted that nearly all warts have a natural history of spontaneous involution, although this can take 2 to 3 years. Plantar warts are painful nodules that develop on the sole of the foot. These are also likely to eventually spontaneously resolve, but because of the length of time involved and the pain they cause with walking, most are excised. Small lesions are treated with liquid nitrogen, whereas larger ones may require surgical excision. The wound is usually best left to heal by secondary intention, because wound dehiscence is common after primary closure. Condyloma acuminata are large warty growths that develop around the anus, genitalia, or mouth. Although the possibility of sexual abuse must be considered in any child with anal warts, some reports suggest that the association with abuse may not be as high as once thought, especially in infants. Condylomata can be excised sharply or fulgurated with various energy sources. Recurrence is high, and repeated attempts are usually required.

LYMPH NODES

Few clinical signs are more anxiety provoking to parents than an enlarged lymph node in a child. Although statistically it is almost always more likely to be infectious or otherwise nonspecific, the assumption on their part is that it represents a malignancy. A careful workup and close follow-up usually allow the parents to be reassured without unnecessary surgery, although in some cases excisional biopsy is needed.

Small, tense lymph nodes are frequently palpable on the scalp or over the mastoid process, where they can be difficult to distinguish from dermoid cysts. In general, these can be observed rather than excised, unless they are seen to increase in size over time. More commonly, the node in question is on the neck, in the axilla, or in the inguinal region. The family should be asked about when they first noticed the mass, how much it has increased in size over time, and whether it is causing any symptoms. Masses that have been present for many months without significant change are less likely to be significant, although other factors may prompt concern. Nodes present for less than a few weeks may warrant a period of observation, with or without a trial of empiric antibiotics, before proceeding with excision. A family history of lymphoma or blood dyscrasias should be sought. A history of travel and of exposure to a cat may be significant. Specific questions should be asked about constitutional symptoms such as weight loss, fevers, chills, and night sweats. Orthopnea or new-onset dyspnea can be a sign of a mediastinal component compressing the airway. Specific questions regarding behaviors that place the patient at risk for exposure to human immunodeficiency virus (HIV) need to be asked, although the answers should be interpreted with caution.

While it is impossible to distinguish a benign lymph node from one involved with malignancy purely on the basis of physical examination, certain characteristics are more worrisome than others. Supraclavicular lymph nodes are felt to carry a higher risk for malignancy than other cervical nodes. Lymph nodes that are larger than 2 cm in diameter, hard, or fixed are also more worrisome, although suppurative lymph nodes in young children can be quite tense (rather than fluctuant) and fixed, but are usually very tender and have local skin changes or a history that suggests an infectious cause. Needle aspiration may be diagnostic and therapeutic in these cases.

In an asymptomatic child, most nodes smaller than 1 cm, especially on the face or scalp, can be safely observed. Any lesion larger than 1 cm that is symptomatic, located in the supraclavicular region, or getting progressively larger should be excised. Prior to excision, the workup should include a complete blood count, chest x-ray, cat scratch titers, and Monospot (Meridian Diagnostics, Cincinnati, Ohio) or Epstein-Barr virus titers. In most patients, a purified protein derivative (of tuberculin) and HIV test also should be performed. Most patients can be observed for a period of about 2 weeks, during which time I usually recommend a trial of empiric antibiotics (broad-spectrum cephalosporin or ampicillin with a β-lactamase inhibitor). The final decision about whether to operate should always include the views and opinions of the family and the primary care physician.

Excision of a lymph node is generally a straightforward procedure, but the risks should not be underestimated. Although the likelihood of wound infection and bleeding is low, the risk for injury to adjacent structures, especially peripheral nerves, is high. This is why the decision to operate should be a thoughtful one, the incision needs to be planned with care, and the surgical technique must be meticulous. Lymph nodes are located below the platysma in the neck and below the Scarpa's fascia in the axilla and groin. The incision should be placed parallel to skin lines of tension and rarely needs to be larger than the diameter of the largest node being removed. In the neck, the typical course of important superficial nerves should be reviewed and the incision placed accordingly. This is especially true for the spinal accessory nerve and the great auricular nerve (which runs close to and parallel with the external jugular vein) and to a lesser degree for the transverse cervical and lesser occipital nerves. The incision is continued carefully through the platysma, parallel to the course of its fibers. Once the subplatysmal plane is reached, the remainder of the dissection should be performed with gentle blunt dissection using a fine curved hemostat. When the characteristic faint purplish color of the lymph node is reached, further dissection immediately adjacent to the capsule allows the node to practically rise out of the incision. The narrow vascular pedicle of the node should then be cauterized close to the capsule and the node removed. Further sampling can be undertaken if the remaining nodes are a source of continued anxiety for the patient or family, but only if they can be removed safely. Nodes in the internal jugular, axillary, and inguinal regions are typically multiple and matted together, although it is usually only necessary to remove just enough of the mass to provide a pathologic diagnosis and not to remove the entire chain.

Lymph nodes that are excised to rule out lymphoma should be sent to the pathologist fresh so that a touch preparation and immunohistochemical studies can be performed, if necessary. Similarly, cultures can be performed if an infectious process is suspected.

FOREIGN BODIES

Foreign bodies that penetrate the skin and become embedded in the subcutaneous tissues can be made of wood, plastic, metal, glass, or stone. The history is often suggestive, but the presence of an occult foreign body should be considered during the evaluation of any patient with a localized skin infection of unclear etiology or a nodule with an atypical history or appearance. The presence of a wooden foreign body is nearly always accompanied by local inflammation and intense pain, whereas most other foreign body materials are well tolerated unless infection has occurred.

Although nonradiopaque foreign bodies such as wood and plastic are better visualized with ultrasonography, plain radiography should be performed in every case for documentation purposes. It is occasionally possible to retrieve a superficial foreign body at the bedside or in the emergency department, but prolonged attempts that involve restraining the child and painful probing of the wound are usually futile and inhumane. This is especially true for metallic foreign bodies in the foot, where the plantar tissue planes are complex and allow the fragment to be concealed effectively. It is almost always best to perform the procedure in the operating room, preferably under general anesthesia, and with fluoroscopic guidance. Nonradiopaque foreign bodies are also usually best removed by examination under anesthesia in a controlled setting such as the operating room, and it may be necessary to use ultrasonographic guidance for particularly stubborn fragments. Depending on the nature of the laceration, most small wounds can be left open to granulate or closed loosely with fine sutures. After removal, it is imperative that radiography (or ultrasonography) be performed to verify complete removal of every fragment and to provide documentation as well.

FOLLOW-UP

After surgery, routine follow-up is essential to evaluate wound healing, address parental concerns, and discuss the pathology results in person. Suture removal can almost always be avoided by the routine use of absorbable suture for skin closure. Seromas can be addressed, as described above, with needle aspiration and observation.

Most lesions that are not excised after the initial visit should be evaluated on serial office visits by the same examiner, unless it can be declared with absolute certainty that the lesion is benign and will not progress to something more serious. This may be every 2 or 3 weeks for lymph nodes or up to 6 months or a year for nevi. It is important to ensure proper follow-up because patients frequently forget that you might have expressed concern about the lesion or they remember only that you said it was "nothing to worry about."

In summary, skin lesions and various lumps and bumps are a significant component of most pediatric surgical practices. Parents are often anxious about these seemingly minor problems, which requires that the surgeon approach them thoughtfully and with sensitivity. A systematic approach that avoids unnecessary surgery but maintains the safety of the patient is important. Proper handling to ensure accurate pathologic assessment is also important. Lastly, some lesions that do not require immediate surgery may nonetheless require close follow-up, which is the responsibility of the surgeon to provide.

SUGGESTED READINGS

Bartlett SP, Lin KY, Grossman R, et al. The surgical management of orbitofacial dermoids in the pediatric patient. *Plast Reconstr Surg* 1993;91:1208–1215.

Cohen BA, Honig P, Androphy E. Anogenital warts in children: clinical and virological evaluation for sexual abuse. *Arch Dermatol* 1990;126:1575–1580.

Dunkin CS, Abouzeid M, Sarangapani K. Malignant transformation in congenital sebaceous naevi in childhood. *J R Coll Surg Edinb* 2001;46:303–306.

Lammers RL, Magill T. Detection and management of foreign bodies in soft tissue. *Emerg Med Clin North Am* 1992;10:767–781.

Nason RW, Abdulrauf BM, Stranc MF. The anatomy of the accessory nerve and cervical lymph node biopsy. *Am J Surg* 2000;180: 241–243.

118

MALIGNANT MELANOMA

MICHAEL B. ISHITANI

Malignant melanoma in children is rare but appears to be increasing in frequency. In the United States, the annual incidence of melanoma in adults has been estimated to be 1 in 90, and in children, 0.8 per million and 6.3 per million in the first and second decades of life, respectively. Older reports of melanoma in children concentrated on its presentation in congenital lesions of the skin or passage of metastases across the placenta. More recent reports have noted an increased incidence in children exposed to intense sunlight and concomitant exposure to high levels of ultraviolet radiation, especially those in racial and ethnic groups predisposed to the development of melanoma. Children in Sweden and Queensland, Australia, in the second decade of life have a high incidence of melanoma of between 30 and 50 cases per million; however, children in these areas in the first decade of life do not have an increased risk of melanoma. As in adults, melanoma in children is a disease of white individuals, with very few cases reported in African Americans. The incidence of melanoma is similar in girls and boys.

Factors that increase the risk of melanoma in children have been reported. Melanomas can present as a congenital lesion or a malignancy arising in preexisting childhood skin lesions. Other known risk factors include certain genetic mutations and diseases and certain phenotypes with a known predisposition to the development of melanoma. In some children, an acquired or innate alteration in immune competence contributes to the development of disease. Also, it is highly probable that exposure to ultraviolet radiation is important in the pathogenesis of melanoma (Table 118.1).

Congenital melanoma is extremely rare but should be considered in children born with a rapidly growing pigmented nodule. Although melanomas arising in preexisting skin lesions are also unusual, they must be sought in children with a giant congenital nevus that is larger than 20 cm or involves more than 5% of the body surface area. In these children, the risk of melanoma may be up to 1,000 times higher than usual. Whether prophylactic resection of a giant congenital nevus should be performed is debated because major reconstructive surgery may be required to achieve complete removal. Smaller congenital nevi are of less concern, although there is an increased risk of melanoma as these children become adults.

Children with known genetic mutations or diseases such as xeroderma pigmentosum that increase the risk of melanoma should be followed carefully, and excisional biopsy should be performed promptly at the first sign of a worrisome lesion. To decrease the overall risk for the development of melanoma and other skin cancers, all children should be protected from excessive exposure to strong ultraviolet radiation. Children with a phenotype that increases the risk for melanoma or those with altered immune systems should be especially careful to avoid sunburns and prolonged exposure to the sun.

DIAGNOSTIC APPROACH

Making the diagnosis of malignant melanoma in a child can be difficult. Several ominous looking but ultimately benign lesions, such as Spitz nevus, can mimic the gross appearance and behavior of malignant melanoma. About 20% of melanomas in children occur in the head and neck region, 20% on the upper extremities, 20% on the lower extremities, and 40% on the trunk.

The classic clinical signs and symptoms of malignant melanoma are the same in children as in adults. These include the "ABCDEs" of *a*symmetry; tan irregular, scalloped or poorly circumscribed *b*orders; variable *c*olors with shades of brown, black, white, red, or blue; large *d*iameter (>6 mm); or *e*xpanding size. Skin lesions that bleed, rapidly increase in size, change color, or ulcerate should be evaluated. In general, an excisional biopsy should be performed on any suspicious pigmented lesion whenever possible. This permits microscopic evaluation of the entire lesion, including the depth and level of tissue invasion. Punch or inci-

M. B. Ishitani: Department of Surgery, Divisions of Pediatric Surgery and Transplantation, Mayo Clinic, Rochester, Minnesota.

TABLE 118.1. RISK FACTORS FOR CHILDHOOD MALIGNANT MELANOMA

Congenital
De novo melanoma
Transplacental transmission
Arising in a preexisting lesion
Giant congenital nevus
Small congenital nevi
Dysplastic nevi/dysplastic nevus syndrome
Other nevi (blue nevus, nevus spilus)
Neurocutaneous melanosis
Genetic predisposition
Family history
Phenotype (red or blonde hair, propensity to sunburn or inability to tan)
p16 gene (CDKN2A, CDK4 and MTS1 mutations
Xeroderma pigmentosum
Acquired
Immunosuppression?
HIV infection?
Ultraviolet radiation exposure

HIV, human immunodeficiency virus.

sional biopsy should be performed on the most suspicious areas of lesions that cannot be excised completely because of adjacent critical structures or for cosmetic reasons.

The lesion should be examined microscopically by a pathologist experienced in differentiating malignant melanoma from other benign forms of pediatric skin disease. If there is any question, the biopsy sample should be referred to an established center for additional confirmation of the diagnosis.

PREOPERATIVE EVALUATION

After the diagnosis of malignant melanoma has been confirmed, preoperative evaluation for lymphatic spread should be performed. The physical examination should be repeated, with particular attention to potential sites of lymphatic and metastatic spread. Areas of concern include contiguous lymph nodes, the liver, the central nervous system, and the lungs. Physical examination findings or laboratory abnormalities should lead to further diagnostic evaluation of the potential problem area.

Recently, lymphatic mapping with sentinel lymph node biopsy using technetium-labeled sulfur colloid or lymphazurin blue stain (or both) has been successful in determining if metastatic spread of tumor has occurred and, at the same time, limiting morbidity associated with a full superficial or deep lymph node dissection. This technique has been widely used to determine lymph node status in adults after the diagnosis of melanoma, breast cancer, and other tumors; a limited but encouraging experience in children with melanoma also has been reported.

TECHNICAL APPROACH

For melanomas thinner than 1.0 mm, current recommendations are to perform wide excision of the malignant melanoma or to reexcise the area of biopsy to leave a 1-cm margin of clear tissue. Wider resection has not been shown to be of benefit. Melanomas thicker than 1.0 mm should be excised with wider margins, ranging from 1.5 to 3.0 cm depending on lesional depth. Primary closure should be performed if possible. Use of tissue expanders and modern plastic surgical techniques usually allow primary closure of the wound even in small children. Skin grafts are seldom necessary.

Lymph node dissection should be performed on the basis of the findings at physical examination or lymphatic mapping. A formal lymph node dissection should be performed if metastatic nodal disease is present, because in adults a limited but measurable survival benefit is gained. Aggressive resection of metastases to other organs may prolong survival, occasionally with long-term benefit.

POSTOPERATIVE COMPLICATIONS

The main postoperative complication of resection of malignant melanoma is recurrence of disease at the site of resection, in local or regional lymph nodes, or as distant metastases. Recurrent disease can appear years after resection of the initial tumor; therefore, routine surveillance for metastatic disease must be performed indefinitely. This should consist of a history and physical examination with the physician looking for suspicious new skin lesions and evidence of lymphatic spread. Laboratory studies should be performed to evaluate for potential spread to the liver, and chest radiography should be performed to look for metastases to the lung. Signs or symptoms suggestive of involvement of other organ systems or locations should prompt investigation of those areas as indicated.

Patients who have had more extensive resection of lymph nodes for metastatic disease may have lymphedema and swelling. Compression stockings and physical therapy can help control these conditions.

In children, as in adults, survival appears to be correlated with the depth of invasion. Eighty percent of children present with stage I/II disease and have a 5-year disease-free survival rate of 77% to 84%. However, children with stage II disease with deeply invasive melanomas (Clark's level IV/V) or lesions more than 1.5 mm thick have a nearly two-thirds chance of having nodal metastases. In this case, survival decreases to 50% at 5 years. Children with metastatic disease have a 5-year survival rate of 34%.

Adjuvant chemotherapy in children has had limited usefulness. Experimental treatments with α-interferon, interleukin-2, melanoma vaccines, and advanced immunotherapy techniques are being evaluated.

SUGGESTED READINGS

Ceballos PI, Ruiz-Maldonado R, Mihm MC Jr. Melanoma in children. *N Engl J Med* 1995;332:656–662.

Chamlin SL, Williams ML. Moles and melanoma. *Curr Opin Pediatr* 1998;10:398–404.

Neville HL, Andrassy RJ, Lally KP, et al. Lymphatic mapping with sentinel node biopsy in pediatric patients. *J Pediatr Surg* 2000;35: 961–964.

Saenz NC, Saenz-Badillos J, Busam K, et al. Childhood melanoma survival. *Cancer* 1999;85:750–754.

Sander B, Karlsson P, Rosdahl I, et al. Cutaneous malignant melanoma in Swedish children and teenagers 1973–1992: a clinico-pathological study of 130 cases. *Int J Cancer* 1999;80:646–651.

Spatz A, Avril M. Melanoma in childhood: review and perspectives. *Pediatr Dev Pathol* 1998;1:463–474.

Whiteman DC, Valery P, McWhirter W, et al. Risk factors for childhood melanoma in Queensland, Australia. *Int J Cancer* 1997;70: 26–31.

119

NECROTIZING SOFT TISSUE INFECTIONS

SHAWN J. RANGEL
R. LAWRENCE MOSS

Necrotizing infections of the skin and soft tissues encompass a variety of conditions that can be rapidly fatal if not treated in a timely fashion. Many classification schemes have been proposed for these infections, with the most straightforward separating the entities into those involving the skin (necrotizing cellulitis), those involving the superficial fascia (necrotizing fasciitis), and deeper infections characterized by necrosis of underlying muscle and its investing fascia (myonecrosis). The specific classification of these infections is somewhat arbitrary to the surgeon, because the principles of aggressive resuscitation and extensive debridement remain the same for all necrotizing processes.

A variety of conditions have been associated with the development of necrotizing infections in the pediatric population. Long-term invasive monitoring, omphalitis, and circumcision are recognized risk factors in neonates, whereas trauma, diabetes, and various immunocompromised states have been found to predispose older children. It is important to note that greater than 90% of pediatric patients who develop invasive soft tissue infections do not have identifiable risk factors. This is in stark contrast to data from the adult literature, where over 75% of patients with necrotizing fasciitis were found to have compromised immune function secondary to diabetes, chronic renal insufficiency, and other systemic illnesses. There is increasing evidence to suggest that varicella infection and the use of nonsteroidal antiinflammatory drugs (NSAIDs) may directly impact the clinical course of necrotizing soft tissue infections. Observational data have repeatedly demonstrated an increased risk for developing invasive group A streptococcal (GAS) infections following primary varicella infection. Proposed mechanisms include increased bacterial ingress through superficial skin lesions, novel entry portals via mucosal and respiratory lesions, and an immune-modulating effect of the virus on the developing immune system. Retrospective data also suggest a trend of increased severity of necrotizing soft tissue infections with NSAID use, but this is confounded by varicella infection in a number of studies. Until the role of NSAIDs is further clarified, it is generally recommended that these agents be avoided in pediatric patients during known varicella infection.

Culture data from necrotizing soft tissue infections has demonstrated a variety of offending organisms, including gram-positive cocci, enteric gram-negative rods, anaerobes, and fungal pathogens. Necrotizing cellulitis is most often caused by polymicrobial infections, although isolated cases of GAS and *Clostridia* species are not uncommon. Nearly all cases of necrotizing fasciitis are caused by mixed flora, with gram-negative enteric bacteria (*Escherichia coli, Klebsiella, Pseudomonas,* and *Citrobacter*) and anaerobes (*Bacteroides, Peptostreptococcus,* and *Clostridia*) most frequently isolated. Pseudomonal species are often found in cases of necrotizing fasciitis associated with neutropenia and leukemic conditions. Similar to necrotizing cellulitis, cases of isolated GAS-associated necrotizing fasciitis are not infrequent in the pediatric population. In the past few decades, there have been an increasing number of reports of necrotizing fasciitis attributed to mucormycosis. Predominately seen in severely immunocompromised patients, these infections result in massive gangrenous soft tissue lesions and carry a particularly high risk for mortality. Myonecrosis can result from a variety of anaerobic organisms, although *Clostridium perfringens* is isolated from most cases.

The devastating nature of necrotizing soft tissue infections is a function of the particularly virulent organisms. Collagenases, proteases, and a host of other enzymatic compounds are secreted to facilitate rapid necrosis and invasion along tissue planes. Progressive edema and thrombosis of feeding vessels lead to further ischemia and accelerated tissue necrosis. In addition to progressive and devastating local infection, pathogens such as *Clostridia* and GAS may pro-

R. L. Moss: Department of Surgery, Yale University School of Medicine; and Department of Surgery, Yale-New Haven Children's Hospital, New Haven, Connecticut.

S. J. Rangel: Division of Pediatric Surgery, Stanford University School of Medicine, Stanford, California.

duce exotoxins, resulting in highly lethal toxemia syndromes (e.g., streptococcal toxic shock syndrome with *Streptococcus pyogenes*). Necrotizing soft-tissue infections with associated toxemia syndromes are among the most fulminant infections known.

It is essential to recognize the earliest clinical signs of necrotizing infections because prompt diagnosis and treatment offer the best chances for survival. This is evidenced by the stark contrast in mortality between patients undergoing early debridement and those treated conservatively in both adult and pediatric series. In a retrospective review of 20 pediatric patients with necrotizing fasciitis, all patients who underwent debridement within 3 hours of admission survived, whereas a mortality rate of 100% was associated with delayed intervention. A recent large review of 68 patients that included both adults and children further supports the strategy of early operative management. Thirty-eight percent of patients who underwent delayed exploration eventually died from their infection, compared with only 4.2% treated with early debridement.

The clinical presentation of pediatric patients with necrotizing soft tissue infections can be variable. About three quarters of patients were found to be tachycardic, whereas less than 50% were febrile at initial presentation. In retrospective studies, virtually 100% of children with necrotizing infections were described as "ill" or "toxic appearing" by the admitting physician. Almost all patients had an altered sensorium, with infants appearing lethargic and older children either listless or agitated. Given that necrotizing soft tissue infections typically occur in previously healthy children, the physician must have a high index of suspicion when soft tissue infections present in association with mental status changes.

Cutaneous manifestations of necrotizing soft tissue infections can be variable and even absent early in the course of disease. Some degree of tissue edema is almost always present, but this finding is not specific to necrotizing infections. Edema secondary to dermal lymphatic obstruction, commonly described as peau d'orange, is seen in up to 90% of reported cases and is very suggestive of an underlying necrotizing process. Violaceous skin changes also are quite suggestive of necrotizing soft tissue infections, with a predictive value of 100% in many reported series (Table 119.1). With progressive necrosis, crepitus and bullous lesions develop in the overlying skin and frank cutaneous necrosis may become evident. These are late findings and often herald an unsalvageable situation. Sepsis and multisystem organ dysfunction are other signs of advanced infection that portend a particularly poor prognosis. Virtually all patients presenting with shock or respiratory failure died in most pediatric series.

Laboratory data including white blood cell count, differential analysis, and blood cultures have been found to be neither sensitive nor specific in the diagnosis of necrotizing infections. However, some reported series have shown predictive value with markedly elevated white blood cell counts and the presence of significant bandemia (Table 119.1). Blood cultures are frequently negative and rarely impact the course of antibiotic therapy. Attempts at gram-staining exudates from bullous lesions have little utility in the management of these infections. With progressive infection, laboratory data may suggest an underlying septic picture characterized by progressively increasing white blood cell count and bandemia, elevated C-reactive protein, refractory metabolic acidosis, and disseminated intravascular coagulation. Severe electrolyte disturbances also can be seen, including hypocalcemia. Rapid depletion of serum calcium may occur in cases of massive soft tissue necrosis secondary to saponification of subcutaneous fat.

Once necrotizing infection is suspected, antibiotic therapy and aggressive resuscitation efforts should be implemented immediately in preparation for surgery. Wide-spectrum antibiotic coverage with a penicillin, clindamycin, and aminoglycoside should be used until culture results dictate otherwise. Double-coverage of pseudomonal species should be considered in cases of necrotizing soft tissue infections associated with neutropenia or other immunocompromised conditions. Hyperbaric oxygen therapy has been used as an adjunctive therapy, but no study to date has demonstrated a clear benefit in cases of necrotizing infections. The use of pooled gamma globulin to attenuate associated toxemia syndromes also has been reported, although the efficacy of this therapy remains in question. Both of these therapies should be considered adjunctive at best, because neither adequately addresses the underlying infectious process.

Operative exploration should begin immediately following adequate resuscitation. If intraoperative findings are not consistent with a necrotizing process, the wound is closed and antibiotics are continued. In cases of necrotizing fasciitis, the wound is characterized by watery drainage and grossly devitalized subcutaneous tissue. Use of a probe or gentle pressure from the surgeon's finger readily dissects the necrotic plane between subcutaneous tissues and the underlying fascia. Careful examination of deep muscle groups and their associated fascia is required to rule out myonecrosis and the need for further debridement. Extensive resection of all involved tissue to grossly viable margins regardless of tissue loss or aesthetic consideration is essential to control local infection. The initial debridement may be the most critical, and the surgeon should therefore err on the side of removing any tissue where viability is in question. The practice of raising tissue flaps to debride areas of significant functional or cosmetic importance has been advocated in an effort to conserve tissue. This approach may be appropriate in areas such as the head and neck, but only if the overlying tissue is clearly viable. Others have reported the use of intraoperative frozen-section biopsy to determine the extent of resection margin. There appears to be little or no benefit with this approach compared with simple gross debridement, and delays in obtaining biopsy results may

TABLE 119.1. SYNOPSIS OF THE SEVEN LARGEST CASE-SERIES OF NECROTIZING FASCIITIS (NF) IN CHILDREN

Study	No. of Patients	Clinical Presentation	Anatomic Region	Associated Conditions	Outcome
Moss/Kosloske et al. *J Pediatr Surg* 1996;31:1142–1146 (Case-series)	20	95% previously healthy (1 with ALL) Peau d' Orange in 90% of NF Altered sensorium in 100% NF	12/20 (60%) trunk 6/20 (30%) extremity 2/20 (10%) head/neck	5/20 (25%) trauma 5/20 (25%) varicella 4/20 (20%) oomphalitis 3/20 (15%) postoperative 3/20 (15%) other	5/20 (25%) total mortality 100% survival with early debridement 100% mortality with debridement >3 h Mortality associated with positive blood cultures, renal failure, DIC, ARDS Mean 3.8 debridements per patient
Waldhausen et al. *J Pediatr Surg* 1996; 31:1138–1141 (Case-series: cellulitis vs. NF in active varicella)	18	Violaceous or bullous skin changes 100% predictive of NF 94% sensitivity, 62% specificity for NF with bands >5%	12/18 (67%) extremities 9/18 (50%) trunk 5/18 (22%) head/neck (patients with multiple sites)	18/18 (100%) varicella	0% total mortality (0/18) Mean time from diagnosis to debridement 1.4 days Delay from diagnosis to operation >2 days associated with more extensive debridement, need for STSG and increased duration of hospital stay Mean 1.2 debridements per patient
Samuel et al. *J Pediatr Surg* 1994; 29:1414–1416 (Case-series: NF in setting of oomphalitis)	14	All cases healthy full-term infants 100% with retained umbilical stump 86% of patients with NF had WBC >22,000	14/14 (100%) trunk	All cases preceded by gastroenteritis or broncho-pneumonia	86% total mortality (12/14) 100% mortality with conservative therapy 67% mortality with early operation
Wilson et al. *Am J Dis Child* 1973;125:591–595 (Case-series)	11	91% previously healthy (1 with aplastic anemia, 1 debilitated from gastroschisis)	9/11 (82%) trunk 2/11 (18%) extremities	7/11 (64%) trauma or postoperative 3/11 (27%) other infection 1/11 (9%) unknown	36% total mortality (4/11)
Lally et al. *Ann Surg* 1984;199:101–103 (Case-series)	8	Mean WBC 33,000 83% presenting with hypothermia 100% of NF associated with oomphalitis admitted from home NF found in 10% of community acquired oomphalitis	N/A	N/A	83% total mortality (7/8) All operations performed between 12 h and 3 days after admission
Sawin et al. *Am J Surg* 1994;167: 481–484 (Case-series)	7	Violaceous or peau d'orange appearance 100% predictive of NF Mean WBC 23.1 in NF vs. 13.1 for cellulitis ($p < 0.02$) HR 186 for NF vs. 142 for cellulitis ($p < 0.02$) 100% of NF associated with oomphalitis admitted from home NF found in 16% of community acquired oomphalitis	(7/7) 100% trunk	6/7 (86%) oomphalitis 1/7 (14%) postoperative	71% total mortality (5/7) 100% survival for debridement <18 h from onset of symptoms 100% mortality if debridement >18 h
Murphy et al. *J Pediatr Surg* 1995;30:1131–1134	5		4/5 (80%) trunk 1/5 (20%) extremities	3/5 (60%) neutropenic from chemotherapy	20% total mortality (1/5)

ALL, acute lymphocytic leukemia; DIC, disseminated intravascular coagulation; ARDS, adult respiratory distress syndrome; STSG, split-thickness skin graft; WBC, white blood cell count; N/A, not applicable.

significantly lengthen operative time. In all cases, thorough debridement should be performed as quickly as possible with immediate transfer of the patient back to the critical care environment.

For necrotizing soft tissue infections of the perineal region, we advocate performing a diverting colostomy because the majority of infections demonstrate enteric organisms on culture. Necrotizing infections arising from complicated omphalitis also deserve special mention. Simple excision of the necrotic umbilicus is rarely sufficient. Extensive debridement of all involved tissue to grossly viable margins is essential, including complete resection of umbilical structures back to their site of origin if necessary (Fig. 119.1).

Tissue defects resulting from adequate debridement can be considerable, but the need for frank amputation is rare. Cosmetic and functional defects resulting from extensive debridement can present daunting reconstructive challenges, and may require the work of a plastic surgeon. Less extensive defects can be adequately covered with split-thickness skin grafts or delayed primary closure when appropriate.

Although the diagnosis of necrotizing soft tissue infections remains primarily clinical, the utility of various imaging modalities including computed tomography (CT), magnetic resonance imaging (MRI), and ultrasonography has recently been described in the literature. Inflammatory changes in subcutaneous tissues such as fascial thickening are readily demonstrated on CT, and perhaps even more so

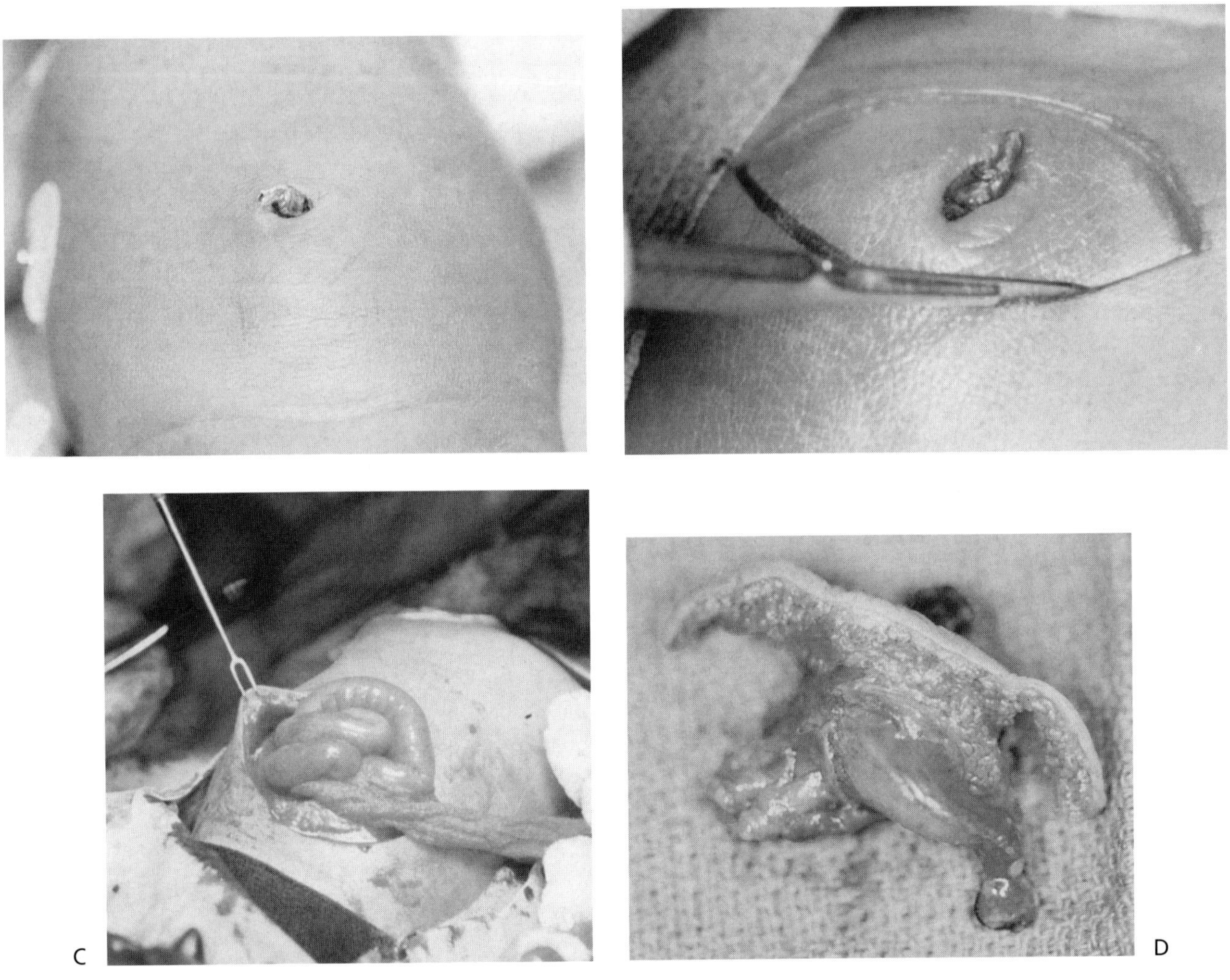

A B C D

FIGURE 119.1. A: Necrotizing fasciitis arising from complicated omphalitis. The necrotic base of the umbilical stump is seen in association with grossly edematous and cellulitic skin changes. **B:** Incision in preparation to excise all involved periumbilical tissues. **C:** Tissue defect following complete excision of all nonviable tissue, including the rectus muscles and fascia. **D:** Excised specimen with attached urachal remnant and umbilical vessels. The wound was subsequently closed with a synthetic absorbable mesh and a split-thickness skin graft.

on MRI. MRI may be particularly useful in delineating anatomic structures in areas of significant cosmetic or functional importance where extensive debridement may be necessary (e.g., the head and neck region). Ultrasonography is somewhat more practical than other imaging studies in its ability to perform rapid bedside examinations and identify subcutaneous fluid collections. False-negative examinations and delays in interpretation of results have limited their utility, however, and there is no evidence that outcomes are improved when these modalities are used. Once there is adequate clinical suspicion for a necrotizing process, definitive diagnosis and treatment by operative exploration should never be delayed by imaging studies.

The technique of bedside frozen section biopsy using local anesthesia also has been reported in an attempt to facilitate early diagnosis. The ability to obtain an adequate sample using this technique in pediatric patients can be challenging, and false-negative samples due to technical limitations are a significant concern. Most pediatric surgeons would prefer a more thorough exploration under general anesthesia to facilitate any required debridement. As with imaging modalities, there appears to be no clear role for frozen-section biopsy when clinical suspicion suggests a necrotizing process.

Following effective debridement, survival depends on the ability of intensive critical care to minimize progression of the inflammatory response and associated multiorgan dysfunction. Aggressive wound care and maintaining a low threshold for repeat debridement is paramount. The prognosis for necrotizing soft tissue infections is primarily determined by the time to intervention, with treatment delays of greater than 24 hours associated with a doubling of mortality risk. Even in the era of wide-spectrum antibiotics and aggressive surgical management, the mortality rate exceeds 64% in some series secondary to progressive sepsis and multiorgan dysfunction. The mortality rate is particularly high when there are frank necrotizing changes in the overlying skin and signs of organ dysfunction prior to operative management. As with all cases of soft tissue sepsis, the best chance for survival hinges on prompt recognition of the septic source and early, thorough debridement. As our understanding of multiorgan dysfunction and critical care practice continue to improve, we will undoubtedly see a decrease in the mortality associated with necrotizing infections. However, at the present time the most important factor for survival remains prompt recognition of necrotizing infections by the treating clinician, such that life-saving interventions can be implemented at the earliest possible time.

SUGGESTED READINGS

AAP Committee on Infectious Diseases. Severe invasive group A streptococcal infections: a subject review. *Pediatrics* 1998;101: 136–140.

Beltran J. Magnetic resonance imaging of soft-tissue infection. *Magn Reson Imag Clin North Am* 1995;3:743.

Bilton BD, Zibari GB, McMillan RW, et al. Aggressive surgical management of necrotizing fasciitis serves to decrease mortality: a retrospective study. *Am Surg* 1998;64:397–400.

Brook I, Frazier EH. Clinical and microbiological features of necrotizing fasciitis. *J Clin Microbiol*1995;33:2382.

Freischlag JA, Ajalat G, Busuttil RW. Treatment of necrotizing soft-tissue infections: the need for a new approach. *Am J Surg* 1985; 149:751–755.

Kosloske AM, Bartow SA. Debridement of peri-umbilical necrotizing fasciitis: importance of excision of the umbilical vessels and urachal remnant. *J Pediatr Surg* 1991;26:808.

Meleney FL. Hemolytic streptococcus gangrene. *Arch Surg* 1924;9: 317–364.

Moss RL, Musemeche CA, Kosloske AM. Necrotizing fasciitis in children: prompt recognition and aggressive therapy improve survival. *J Pediatr Surg* 1996; 31:1142–1146.

Wilson B. Necrotizing fasciitis. *Am Surg* 1952;18:416–431.

Zerr DM, Alexander ER, Duchin JS, et al. A case-control study of necrotizing fasciitis during primary varicella. *Pediatrics* 1999;103: 783–790.

120

VASCULAR ANOMALIES

STEVEN J. FISHMAN

There is probably no area in pediatric surgery more poorly understood by most practitioners than vascular anomalies. This results from the widespread propagation of improper terminology to describe the various vascular lesions. Unfortunately, this field has fallen between the cracks of all the traditional disciplines of medicine. It is not well studied, taught, or practiced in dermatology, radiology, pathology, hematology, or any of the various surgical specialty training programs. Thus, the medical literature and textbooks are riddled with an extensive cross-fertilization of misinformation. Given the limited scope of this chapter, I will attempt to provide a broad outline for understanding the various types of vascular anomalies, including their classification and natural history. An overview of treatment options is also presented.

CLASSIFICATION

Vascular anomalies can be broadly grouped into two general types: vascular tumors and vascular malformations (Table 120.1). The vascular tumors are neoplasms of endothelium, which are almost always histologically benign. Nevertheless, they can be threatening to vital function or life. The vast majority are hemangiomas. Vascular malformations result from errors of vascular morphogenesis. Like other congenital malformations, they occur during embryogenesis and are relatively stable in postnatal life. Vascular malformations are most simply classified and termed by their aberrant channel types. These can include capillaries, veins, lymphatics, arteries, and almost any combination thereof. Unfortunately many antiquated terms continue to be applied to these lesions. These terms often confuse the nature of the lesion. In general medical parlance, terms ending in the suffix *-oma* imply a proliferative process. Thus, use of terms such as *cystic hygroma* and *lymphangioma* should be abandoned. These lesions refer to microcystic and macrocystic lymphatic malformations. They are not proliferative processes and do not respond to antiproliferative or antiangiogenic therapies as their improper names might suggest. Similarly, it is common to see fictitious admixtures of terms referring to tumors and malformations. There is no such lesion as a "lymphohemangioma." More likely this refers to a lymphaticovenous malformation. The most frequently misused term is *cavernous hemangioma.* True proliferative hemangiomas have narrow endothelial-lined channels. Red lesions with blood filled large spaces or "caverns" are venous malformations. Again, the term *cavernous hemangioma* is misleading, of no value, and should be abandoned. Venous malformations have a completely different natural history than hemangiomas and do not respond to any of the pharmacologic agents used to enhance involution of true hemangiomas.

VASCULAR TUMORS

Hemangiomas

Hemangioma is the most common tumor of infancy, occurring in 4% to 11% of white babies. It is less common in other races and extremely rare in patients of African descent. Girls are affected approximately four times more commonly than boys. Hemangiomas are most commonly seen about the head and neck, followed by the trunk and extremities, and much more rarely the visceral organs. Typically, a hemangioma is first noted at 1 or 2 weeks of age, having been either undetectable or a very faint pink stain at the time of birth. A hemangioma proliferates, sometimes dramatically and horrifically, for the first year of life. The proliferative phase is followed by stabilization and then slow gradual involution over the ensuing 4 to 6 years. Superficial

S. J. Fishman: Department of Surgery, Harvard University Medical School; and Department of Surgery, Children's Hospital, Boston, Massachusetts.

TABLE 120.1. BIOLOGIC CLASSIFICATION OF VASCULAR ANOMALIES

Tumors	Malformations
Hemangioma	Capillary
Congenital hemangioma	Venous
Kaposiform hemangioendothelioma	Lymphatic
Angiosarcoma	Arterial Combinations (AVM, CLVM, CAVM, LVM, etc.)

AVM, arteriovenous malformation; CLVM, capillary-lymphatico-venous malformations; CAVM, capillary arteriovenous malformations; LVM, lymphatico-venous malformations.

hemangiomas of the skin have a classic strawberry-like appearance (Fig. 120.1). A deeper lesion may have normal overlying skin with either no discoloration or a bluish hue under the skin. Lesions may range from several millimeters to many centimeters in size. Most lesions are singular, but multiple lesions may occur in 20% of cases. Multifocal cutaneous lesions enhance the likelihood of visceral lesions being present.

Most hemangiomas are of cosmetic significance only. However, some lesions, such as those involving the eyes, ears, airway, liver and gastrointestinal tract, may be threatening to life, vision, or hearing. Large lesions in other areas may cause significant tissue destruction or high-output cardiac failure due to massive flow through the tumor. Small non-threatening lesions of minimal significance are generally observed. Parents are provided reassurance that the lesions will involute with time. However, lesions threatening life, vital function, or critical tissues may require therapeutic intervention. Some lesions that are not of enormous medical risk but potentially significantly disfiguring may be treated as well. Corticosteroids are the mainstay of therapy.

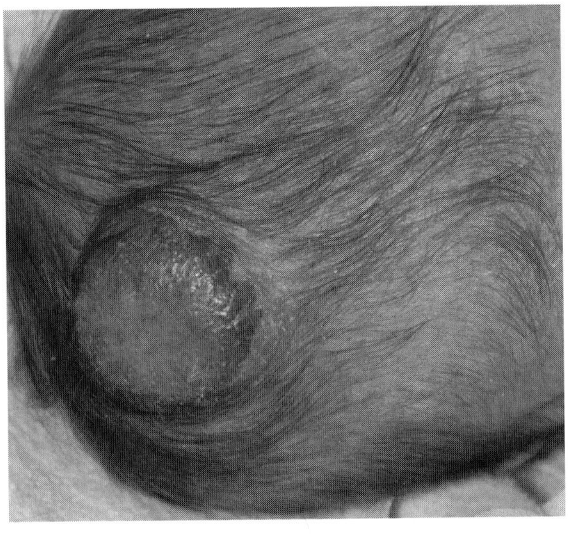

FIGURE 120.1. Typical hemangioma.

Likely acting by an antiangiogenic mechanism, corticosteroids generally accelerate the natural history of a lesion, aborting proliferation and enhancing involution. We generally administer prednisone equivalent at 2 mg/kg/day for 1 month, then halve and slowly taper this dose over the ensuing 6 months or so. Those lesions that do not respond at this dose will likely respond to 4 or 5 mg/kg/day, although we prefer to reserve these doses for refractory cases. Small lesions in facial locations may be treated with intralesional injections of triamcinolone rather than long-term daily administration of systemic steroids. Alarming hemangiomas, which do not respond to steroids, almost always involute with administration of α-interferon. However, there is a significant risk of spastic diplegia with this agent. It should be used cautiously and only in refractory cases and with careful and frequent neurologic assessment.

Surgical intervention is only occasionally warranted in proliferative phase hemangiomas. Certainly, endotracheal laser application is useful in many cases of subglottic airway hemangiomas. Much more frequently, surgical excision plays a role in the treatment of involuting and involuted hemangiomas. Although the tumors regress, large hemangiomas often leave a bulky fibrofatty residuum requiring excision. The overlying skin is often atrophic, thin, and scarred if there had been prior ulceration.

Hemangiomas of the liver require special attention. Many are small and asymptomatic and require only serial evaluation. Larger lesions may have intralesional macrovascular shunting causing cardiac failure. These should be treated pharmacologically. If drug therapy is unsuccessful or too slow in a life-threatening case, subselective hepatic arteriography with embolization of the shunts may be indicated. This should be performed only by an experienced pediatric interventional radiologist. Embolization or surgical ligation of the proximal hepatic arteries is not as effective, and the benefits may be of short duration, because collateral flow is quickly recruited. Still more complex are the enormous hepatic hemangiomas, which encompass the entire abdominal cavity, leading to abdominal compartment syndrome, impaired vena caval return, and compromise of diaphragmatic excursion. This situation is frequently fatal and should be prevented by pharmacologic intervention before this stage is reached. Surgical intervention is almost never necessary in the diagnosis or management of liver hemangiomas. Properly interpreted imaging studies can usually differentiate a hemangioma from other hepatic lesions of infancy. I believe that surgical excision of a liver hemangioma is almost never necessary. However, massive lesions compromising ventilation and perfusion may justify liver transplantation due to their high risk for mortality.

Large hemangiomas, particularly those in the liver, have recently been demonstrated to cause profound hypothyroidism. This results from the expression of a deiodinase by the hemangioma, which cleaves iodine from active thyroid hormones. If the hemangioma is large enough, it can inactive thyroid hormone more rapidly than the thyroid gland can replenish it. In this unusual circumstance, massive doses of thyroid hormone replacement are necessary. The hypothyroidism resolves when the hemangioma involutes.

Congenital Hemangiomas

A congenital hemangioma appears quite similar to a typical hemangioma of infancy. However, its life cycle is vastly accelerated. A congenital hemangioma is fully grown at birth and begins its spontaneous involution early in infancy. It is generally completely involuted before 1 year of age. Congenital hemangiomas have a characteristic appearance. They are generally bulbous hemispherical lesions. They are often somewhat dark purple in coloration with a pale halo of skin around the base. Histologically, congenital hemangiomas are not entirely identical to standard hemangiomas and likely have a different cause. Generally, congenital hemangiomas require no treatment, because they involute so quickly. Interestingly, review of some of the literature reporting seemingly miraculous responses to various therapies for hemangioma suggests that these lesions were actually congenital hemangiomas. Thus, these lesions would have involuted just as quickly with no therapy at all.

Kaposiform Hemangioendotheliomas

Kaposiform hemangioendotheliomas are relatively rare, benign, but often aggressive vascular neoplasms. Only recently has it been recognized that this lesion is a separate entity and is not just an "aggressive hemangioma." There can be similarities in life cycle, with appearance shortly after birth followed by aggressive proliferation and then slow involution. A kaposiform hemangioendothelioma never completely involutes; at least a pale residual stain persists. These lesions are diffuse in their cutaneous pattern and permeate the subcutaneous tissues and underlying vasculature (Fig. 120.2). They most commonly involve a proximal extremity and adjacent areas of the trunk. The tissues in the regions are often thickened and edematous and have a deep purple ecchymotic appearance. There are not usually distinct borders, as would typically be seen with true hemangiomas. Most kaposiform hemangioendotheliomas manifest the Kasabach-Merritt phenomenon. This consists of a profound consumptive thrombocytopenia in which the platelet count generally decreases to between 2,000 and 10,000 platelets/mm^3. This thrombocytopenia is not correctable by platelet transfusion, because the exogenous platelets also become trapped in the lesion. Indeed, during the transfusion the lesion often swells massively. Contrary to popular belief, the Kasabach-Merritt phenomenon does not occur in typical hemangiomas of infancy or in any of the vascular malformations. Mild anemia and thrombocytopenia may be seen with hemangiomas, typically those of

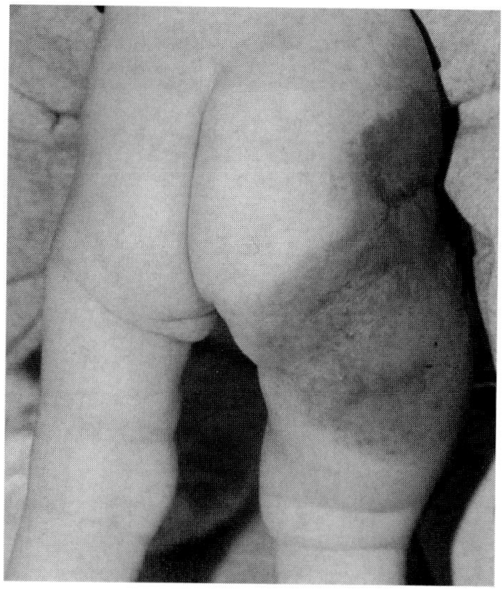

FIGURE 120.2. Kaposiform hemangioendothelioma.

the liver, especially if there has been intralesional hemorrhage and clotting. The coagulopathy most typically seen with vascular malformations is that of clotting factor consumption rather than platelet consumption. Kaposiform lesions can be responsive to steroids. Steroid-resistant lesions often respond to α–interferon. This lesion continues to be associated with a mortality rate approaching 50%. Intracranial hemorrhage is a significant risk in these young infants with often uncorrectable thrombocytopenia.

VASCULAR MALFORMATIONS

Capillary Malformations

The most typical type of capillary malformation is that commonly referred to as a port-wine stain. These are flat, light purple geographic stains of cosmetic significance only. If such a lesion appears over the V1 and V2 distribution of the face, there must be suspicion for Sturge-Weber syndrome, which includes vascular lesions of the leptomeniges and glaucoma. Magnetic resonance imaging should be performed in these situations. Capillary malformations often can be significantly improved cosmetically with pulsed dye laser treatment.

Lymphatic Malformations

Lymphatic malformations are common. They may contain groupings of large cysts up to several centimeters in diameter, tiny microcysts not visible to the naked eye, or a combination of the two. Lymphatic malformations are most commonly seen in the supraclavicular, axillary, and cervicofacial regions (Fig. 120.3). They also can be seen in the mediastinum, groin, retroperitoneum, pelvis, and extremi-

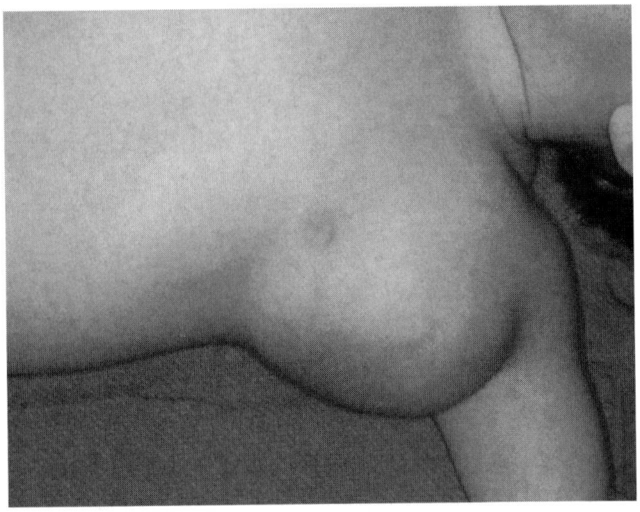

FIGURE 120.3. Lymphatic malformation of axilla.

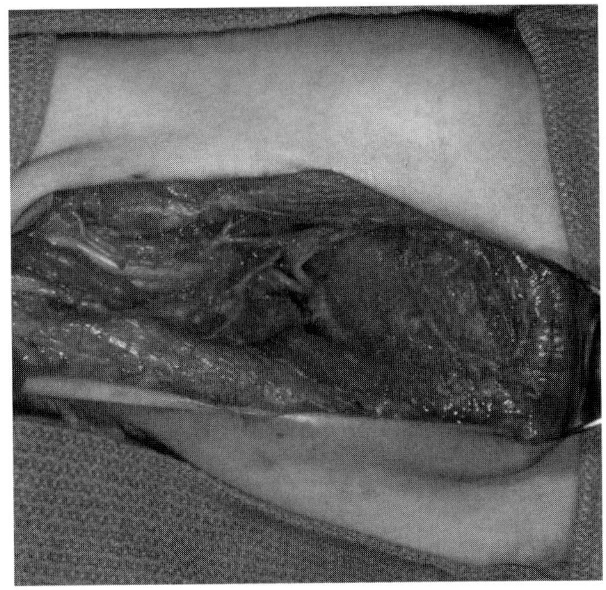

FIGURE 120.4. Brachial plexus dissection for excision of lymphatic malformation.

ties. Large lymphatic malformations can be extremely disfiguring. Bony overgrowth, especially in the mandible and facial bones, is not uncommon. Lymphatic malformations, especially those that permeate through the skin manifesting as groupings of vesicular lesions, may develop repetitive cellulitic infections. Streptococcal organisms are the most common offending agents. However, regions of the buttock and thigh region may demonstrate gram-negative enteric infections. These may result from translocation of organisms from the rectum when pelvic tissues are densely involved.

Lymphatic malformations may be treated by excision or sclerotherapy. Microcystic lesions do not respond to sclerotherapy. Surgical excision often can be extremely tedious. Although these lesions are benign, they generally do not respect normal tissue planes. I approach these procedures with the intent to remove as much of the malformation as possible without damaging normal structures, regardless of the necessary time commitment. Meticulous dissection is often required, because these lesions frequently envelop neurovascular structures such as the brachial plexus (Fig. 120.4). With a large lesion, an anatomic region should be chosen to perform complete dissection in a given sitting. Other defined anatomic regions can be resected in a staged fashion if necessary. One should not attempt these procedures unless prepared to remove as much of the lesion as possible. An incomplete dissection near delicate vital structures is likely to result in re-expansion of the lesion in this region. A second operation in the face of scarring from the prior dissection is more difficult and of greater risk. When only a portion of a large malformation can be resected in a single sitting, expansion of the remaining portion of the lesion should be expected and the family warned so that they will not be alarmed. Prolonged drainage from surgical drains is the rule. It is not uncommon for drains to be required for several months postoperatively. There is also a relatively high incidence of postoperative infection. These infections should be treated aggressively with antibiotics. Ironically, an infection often leads to sclerosis of the remaining leaking lymphatics, allowing the drains to be removed shortly after the infection begins.

Some of the most difficult lymphatic lesions involve congenital anomalies of the thoracic duct and cisterna chyli. These often manifest with chylous ascites, chylothorax, or occasionally chylous pericardial effusion. Some of these anomalies are associated with a mass lesion in the mediastinum or retroperitoneum. Cross-sectional imaging is not successful at demonstrating the anatomic and physiologic aberration in these situations. Rather, dynamic contrast lymphangiography may be required. Some of these lesions may be improved by thoracic duct ligation. Others are seemingly insoluble.

Venous Malformations

Venous malformations are the most prevalent of the vascular malformations. They are all too frequently confused with hemangiomas. A venous malformation, if involving the skin, is generally visible at birth. They generally grow proportionate with the patient and persist throughout life. They may become proportionately larger during puberty and pregnancies. Venous malformations are less rubbery in consistency than hemangiomas. Compression may evacuate a large percentage of the blood from the lesion, with refilling occurring within several seconds after releasing pressure. These lesions can range from minute cosmetic lesions to extensive lesions involving large portions of the body (Fig. 120.5). Patients with venous malformations often complain of pain in the lesion, most typically upon awakening in the morning or after vigorous activity. Swelling and discomfort can be minimized with elastic compression garments, especially for extremity lesions. Low-dose aspirin, beyond early childhood, is also often helpful in preventing discomfort. Aspirin is used not for its analgesic properties but rather for its antithrombotic properties. These lesions have nonlaminar venous flow through spongelike channels, which can induce chronic low-grade thrombosis, especially with stagnation.

Venous malformations are often amenable to treatment with intralesional sclerotherapy. Successful sclerotherapy may reduce the bulk of lesions and eliminate the painful episodes. Many venous malformations are best addressed with surgical excision. Preoperative sclerotherapy is often useful to reduce intraoperative hemorrhage with large lesions. Operative tourniquets are extremely useful while dissecting extremity lesions. Close collaboration with the anesthesia team is necessary to safely resect large lesions of the face, neck, torso, or genitalia, because profound uncontrollable bleeding is not uncommon. In many cases, complete excision is not possible due to extensive infiltration of adjacent or vital tissues. Hemorrhage can be controlled by simply closing the skin and soft tissues. Postoperative hematoma and wound breakdown are not uncommon, but generally heal without difficulty. Incomplete resection of a venous malformation in a body cavity where skin closure cannot be used to tamponade bleeding should be avoided at virtually all costs.

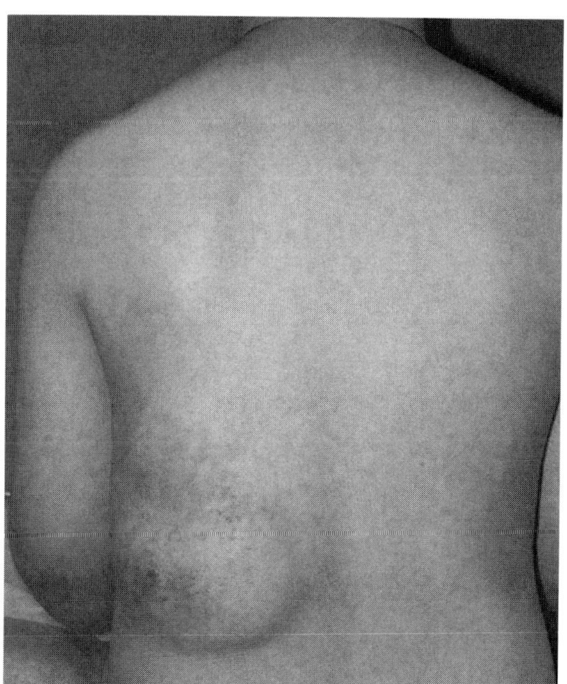

FIGURE 120.5. Venous malformation.

Although rare in comparison with lesions of the skin and soft tissues, venous malformations of the gastrointestinal tract may be of interest to pediatric surgeons. Gastrointestinal bleeding is the most common manifestation of such lesions. Focal lesions often can be resected or sclerosed if small and superficial. Multifocal polyp-like lesions are typical of the blue rubber bleb nevus syndrome. These patients have multifocal lesions affecting the skin and gastrointestinal tract. They are typically distributed throughout the gut. Like other venous malformations, these lesions do not respond significantly to pharmacologic therapy. Endoscopic banding or sclerotherapy of accessible lesions in the esophagus, stomach, and colon can be undertaken, but many lesions are transmural, and there is a significant risk for perforation. In general, the majority of lesions are in the small bowel and are therefore not easily accessible by endoscopy. I have taken an approach of intraoperative total enteroscopy and excision of every visible lesion. Although extremely tedious, this can eradicate the need for repetitive blood transfusion. Diffuse venous malformations may involve the anorectum and variable lengths of the colon. If bleeding is significant, requiring transfusion, partial colectomy, anorectal mucosectomy, and coloanal pull-through can be performed successfully.

Arteriovenous Malformations

Arteriovenous malformations range from small pink stains to massive lesions of an entire extremity, which may cause high-output cardiac failure. Although it is difficult to predict which lesions will progress and to what extent, arteriovenous malformations can exacerbate dramatically. A small asymptomatic lesion can go on to cause local pain, ulceration, progressive tissue destruction, and even pathologic fractures (Fig. 120.6). The most extreme cases can cause death due to enormous cardiac overload. Treatment must be individualized. Even in the care of experienced clinicians, it can be difficult to counsel whether or when to treat a particular lesion. Cure of an arteriovenous malformation is only possible by complete excision or rarely by complete eradication of the nidus by embolization. Ligation of proximal feeding vessels should never be performed. In such cases, the malformation will always parasitize flow from surrounding tissues. All that is accomplished by proximal vessel ligation is the elimination of appropriate access channels for embolization. Similarly, if embolization is undertaken, it should be performed in the nidus portion of the lesion rather than in the feeding vessels. Embolization should only be undertaken by an interventional radiologist with significant expertise and experience in treating these lesions, because improper embolization techniques can make future therapy much more difficult or impossible. Operative excision of arteriovenous malformations can be

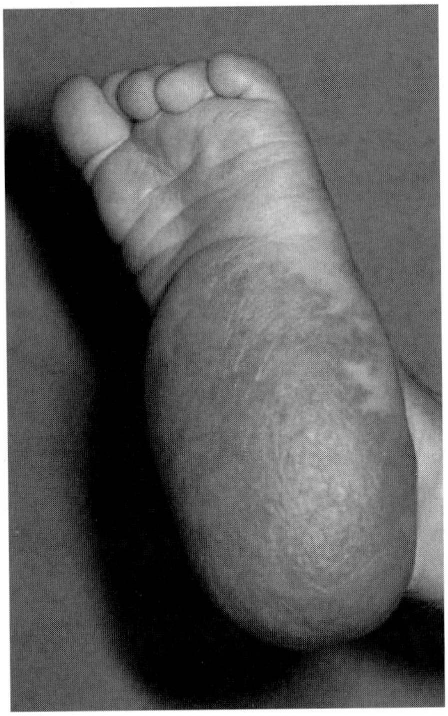

FIGURE 120.6. Arteriovenous malformation.

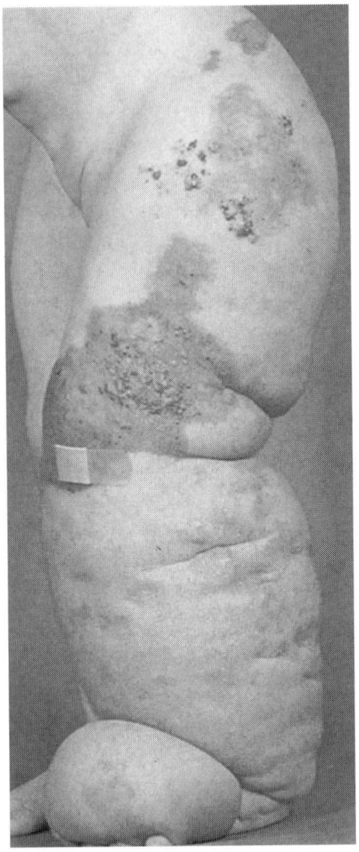

FIGURE 120.7. Combined capillary lymphaticovenous malformation (Klippel-Trenaunay syndrome).

made significantly less hemorrhagic by preoperative embolization, being careful not to render surrounding tissues ischemic, because this can impair healing of the surgical wound.

Complex Combined Vascular Malformations

Vascular malformations can encompass almost any combination of abnormal channel types. The most common example is the combined capillary lymphaticovenous malformation of the Klippel-Trenaunay syndrome. Patients with Klippel-Trenaunay typically have involvement of a lower extremity and hemipelvis (Fig. 120.7). The affected extremity is often overgrown in both length and girth. There are typically geographic areas of purplish capillary malformations with small black lymphatic vesicles within them. These often ooze serosanguineous fluid and serve as a portal of entry for bacteria to cause cellulitic infections. Leg length discrepancy should be carefully monitored by an orthopedic surgeon experienced in this regard. Shoe lifts are often helpful during childhood. When the overgrown extremity reaches the anticipated mature length of the opposite normal leg, an epiphysiodesis can be performed to prevent further growth, leading to nearly symmetric lengths of the two legs in adulthood. The venous component of the malformation can lead to discomfort and is often best treated with elastic compression stockings. Patients often seek surgical excision and contouring of the bulky components of their extremity or buttock. Great care should be taken to establish the presence and patency of the deep venous system before contemplating any surgical procedure. Many patients have a prominent lateral embryonic vein ascending up the leg or torso. In the absence of a deep venous system, this vein should not be resected or interrupted. Significant pelvic involvement of the malformation can lead to rectal bleeding, hematuria, or mass compression on the bladder or rectum.

CONCLUSION

Although not commonly appreciated, vascular anomalies often present in recognizable patterns with predictable natural histories and outcomes. It is crucial to differentiate whether a lesion represents a tumor or a vascular malformation, because the classification of the lesion dictates whether the lesion will undergo spontaneous involution or will persist and progress. Pharmacologic therapy is usually successful for hemangiomas when indicated. Pharmacologic therapy is not yet available for vascular malformations. However, appropriate use of interventional radiologic and surgical techniques can significantly benefit many patients.

Interdisciplinary evaluation and care by a team dedicated to the understanding and management of vascular anomalies is often appropriate and helpful.

SUGGESTED READINGS

Barlow CF, Priebe CJ, Mulliken JB, et al. Spastic diplegia as a complication of interferon alfa-2a treatment of hemangiomas of infancy. *J Pediatr* 1998;132:527–530.

Boon LM, Enjolras O, Mulliken JB. Congenital hemangioma: evidence of accelerated involution. *J Pediatr* 1996;128:329–335.

Drolet BA, Esterly NB, Frieden IJ. Hemangiomas in children. *N Engl J Med* 1999;341:173–181.

Ezekowitz RA, Mulliken JB, Folkman J. Interferon alfa-2a therapy for life-threatening hemangiomas of infancy. *N Engl J Med* 1992;326: 1456–1463.

Fishman SJ, Burrows PE, Leichtner AM, et al. Gastrointestinal manifestations of vascular anomalies in childhood: varied etiologies require multiple therapeutic modalities. *J Pediatr Surg*1998;33: 1163–1167.

Fishman SJ, Burrows PE, Upton J, et al. Life-threatening anomalies of the thoracic duct: anatomic delineation dictates management. *J Pediatr Surg* 2001;36:1269–1272.

Fishman SJ, Fox VL. Visceral vascular anomalies. *Gastrointest Endosc Clin North Am* 2001;11:813–834.

Fishman SJ, Mulliken JB. Vasular anomalies. A primer for pediatricians. *Pediatr Clin North Am*1998;45:1455–1477.

Fishman SJ, Shamberger RC, Fox VL, et al. Endorectal pull-through abates gastrointestinal hemorrhage from colorectal venous malformation. *J Pediatr Surg* 2000;35:982–984.

Huang SA, Tu HM, Harney JW, et al. Severe hypothyroidism caused by type 3 iodothyronine deiodinase in infantile hemangiomas. *N Engl J Med* 2000;343:185–189.

Mulliken JB, Fishman SJ, Burrows PE. Vascular anomalies. *Curr Prob Surg* 2000;37:517–584.

Mulliken JB, Young AE. *Vascular birthmarks: hemangiomas and malformations.* Philadelphia: WB Saunders, 1988.

Sarkar M, Mulliken JB, Kozakewich HP, et al. Thrombocytopenic coagulopathy (Kasabach-Merritt phenomenon) is associated with kaposiform hemangioendothelioma and not with common infantile hemangioma. *Plast Reconstr Surg* 1997;100:1377–1386.

Vikkula MB, Boon LM, Mulliken JB. Molecular genetics of vascular malformations. *Matrix Biol* 2001;20:327–335.

121

LYMPHEDEMA

NEIL R. FEINS
KONSTANTINOS PAPADAKIS

Lymphedema is a swelling caused by an abnormal collection of lymph fluid in the interstitial tissues, resulting from anomalies or functional overload. There are two types of lymphedema: idiopathic (primary) and acquired (secondary).

Primary lymphedema is divided into three categories: congenital, praecox, and tarda. Congenital lymphedema, which is present at birth, is the rarest form of primary lymphedema, comprising only 11% of the cases. It is commonly believed that congenital lymphedema carries the poorest prognosis. Because the disease is caused mainly by a decreased number of functioning lymphatics, the symptoms that are present at birth are more severe than those that appear later in life.

Lymphedema praecox, the most common form of primary lymphedema, presents before the age of 35 years. The usual age of onset is during the teens or early twenties. The edema usually begins concurrently with a growth spurt. It is thought that with increased growth, there is increased tissue hydrostatic pressure. Therefore, the decreased or abnormal lymphatics are overwhelmed, and the resultant edema becomes clinically manifest and eventually permanent. The history may reveal the onset of edema after trauma or an infectious process. In these cases, the decreased number of lymphatics decompensate with the additional insult or there is further damage to the already compromised lymph channels.

Of patients with primary lymphedema, 85% present with symptoms before the age of 35 years. The remaining 15% develop symptoms after the age of 35 and are referred to as having primary lymphedema tarda.

In 1957, Kinmonth and associates established that primary lymphedema was due to a structural, developmental fault of the regional lymphatics, resulting in functional derangement of lymphostasis. If formed subcutaneous lymph trunks are not found, the disease is classified as aplasia. The classification of hypoplasia is used for patients with smaller lymph vessels and fewer than normal lymph vessels. Eighty-seven percent of patients with primary lymphedema are considered to be in this group.

The surgical management of lymphedema in children and young adults remains a challenge. Because lymphedema is a rare problem, few surgeons have been able to acquire extensive experience.

PATIENT SELECTION

Patients with lymphedema commonly present with a painless swelling of an extremity. The swelling decreases with bed rest but does not disappear. Fifteen percent of patients exhibit accompanying vascular or lymphatic malformations, double rows of eyelashes, or yellow toenails and fingernails. Patients do not complain of pain. A lymphangiogram is rarely required to make a clinical diagnosis of lymphedema. Sometimes lymphangioscintography or magnetic resonance imaging may be necessary.

Experience at our institution involved 324 patients during a span of 24 years. The patients ranged in age from 8 months to 60 years. The predominant group consisted of patients 22 years of age and younger when surgery was performed initially. Almost all patients had primary lymphedema. The most common cause was paucity or hypoplasia of the lymphatics in the subcutaneous tissue.

Most clinicians believe that the lymphatic system is divided into a valveless superficial and a valved deep system. In cases of lymphedema, the fluid lies in the superficial system, the subcutaneous tissue. The deep system beneath the fascia, the muscle component, is separate and unaffected. The universal observation that the deep muscles and their lymph systems seem competent in all cases of lymphedema has been the key factor in procedures that attempt to deliver lymph into valved deep systems to move the fluid in a cephalad direction.

N.R. Feins and K. Papadakis: Department of Surgery, The Children's Hospital, Harvard Medical School, Boston, Massachusetts.

Lymphedema occurs in the subcutaneous tissues when the system is abnormal or overloaded. Protein-rich fluid collects, and increases the oncotic pressure, perpetuating the edema and leading to stasis, infection, and fibrosis. If the skin over an extremity has been stretched for a long time, the elastic fibers lose considerable tensile strength. These fibers can no longer confine minimal edema to normal contours without the aid of external support.

Surgery is indicated when conservative measures fail, including elastic stockings and pneumatic compression devices for an extremity that is too heavy and cumbersome to manipulate during daily activities. These patients may not be able to wear normal clothing or shoes. Recurrent cellulitis and lymphangitis can be relieved by surgery and are further indications for operative intervention.

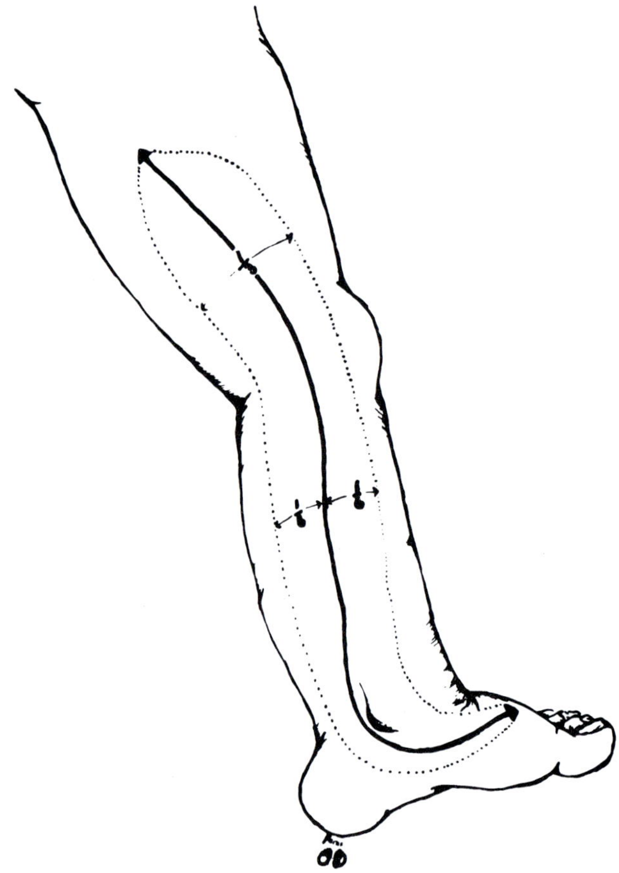

FIGURE 121.1. An incision is made on the medial aspect of the foot. Each flap is developed for one-sixth the circumference of the leg for a total exposure of one-third the extremity.

METHODS AND SURGICAL TECHNIQUES

Attempts at surgical correction of lymphedema date back to 1841. Methods are divided into physiologic and excisional procedures. Physiologic surgery is based on the goal of reconnecting, reconstructing, or stimulating the growth of lymphatic pathways. These procedures rarely work in cases of primary lymphedema, unless a large amount of subcutaneous tissue is excised during the procedure or the edema is actually secondary lymphedema with local blockage.

Because the lymph of lymphedema is generated and collects in the subcutaneous tissue, excision of this tissue would seem to be the logical operative choice. Charles reported success by removing edematous tissue down to the muscle and covering the denuded surface with split-thickness grafts that have been obtained from other areas. This procedure and its modifications are the most successful for permanently reducing the size of a leg with lymphedema. The drawbacks include resultant bizarre limb disfigurement, breakdown of the grafts, and chronic infections. In 1936, Homans excised the subcutaneous tissue and deep fascia and created thin skin flaps, which were used to cover the excised area. After an evaluation of the various procedures, we developed a method modified from that performed by Homans.

THE FIRST PROCEDURE

The first operation is begun on the medial aspect of the leg because this incision is less visible (Fig. 121.1). With proper use of a pneumatic tourniquet, transfusions are rarely necessary. The skin flaps are developed one-sixth medially and one-sixth laterally for a total of one-third the circumference of the entire leg. The flaps are full thickness but as thin as possible (Fig. 121.2). The total size of the skin flaps must not be larger than one-third the circumference of the leg to decrease the chance of necrosis. Removal of most of the edematous subcutaneous tissue is performed by blunt finger dissection. The greater saphenous venous system is removed or interrupted during the excisional procedure. It is imperative that a functioning deep venous system be present. The fascia aponeurosis is removed from the muscle with sharp dissection (Fig. 121.3).

In the case of bilateral disease, it is preferable to operate on one extremity at a time. If the original procedure is without problems, we operate on the opposite leg in 7 to 10 days.

Approximately 21% of patients have a satisfactory result from the original operation. They are pleased with the reduction in size and the contour of the extremity, and the result is stable. However, some results do not remain stable and may require further surgery.

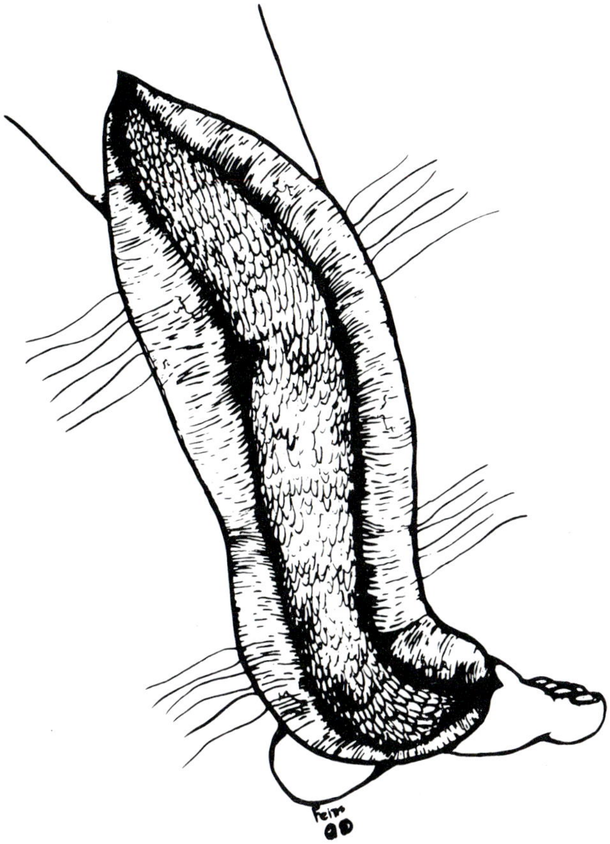

FIGURE 121.2. The flaps are very thin, but full thickness. The exposed subcutaneous tissue and underlying fascia are removed entirely.

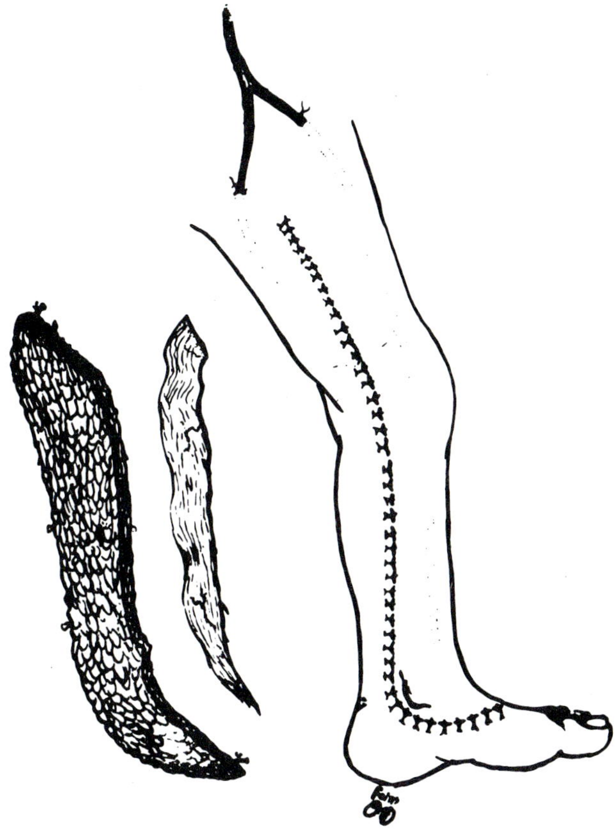

FIGURE 121.3. The subcutaneous tissue is removed in one piece. The deep fascia is removed as a separate specimen.

THE SECOND PROCEDURE

Because of continued enlargement of the extremity, some patients return for staged or serial excision. The second procedure is performed on the lateral aspect of the extremity. After surgery, lymphatic function increases with time and improves for up to 1 year. Because of these findings, we usually do not perform the second stage procedure during the first postoperative year. Approximately 31% of patients require three excisional procedures.

THE THIRD PROCEDURE

The third operation, if necessary, is performed on the posterior aspect of the extremity. Postoperatively, the patient must wear support hose indefinitely to help minimize swelling. Excisional techniques, similar to those described, can be used in the surgical management of lymphedema of the upper extremities. Some patients have chyle reflux into their legs and can develop chyle fistulas of their lower extremities or genitalia. If dilated incompetent retroperitoneal lymphatics are found on computed tomography, these can be ligated and result in decreased drainage and fistula formation.

PROCEDURE FOR INVOLVEMENT OF THE PENIS OR SCROTUM

Some patients in our series had lymphedema of the genitalia. Female patients responded to straightforward labial resection. In the course of managing lymphedema of the penis, scrotum, or both, a safe and uncomplicated operation was developed.

The procedure is performed as outlined in Figures 121.4 through 121.6. The cosmetic and functional results of this operation are generally good or excellent. Using this technique, the penile skin is never separated from the glans, and suture lines on the penis are prevented. The only contraindication is chronically damaged skin that will necessi-

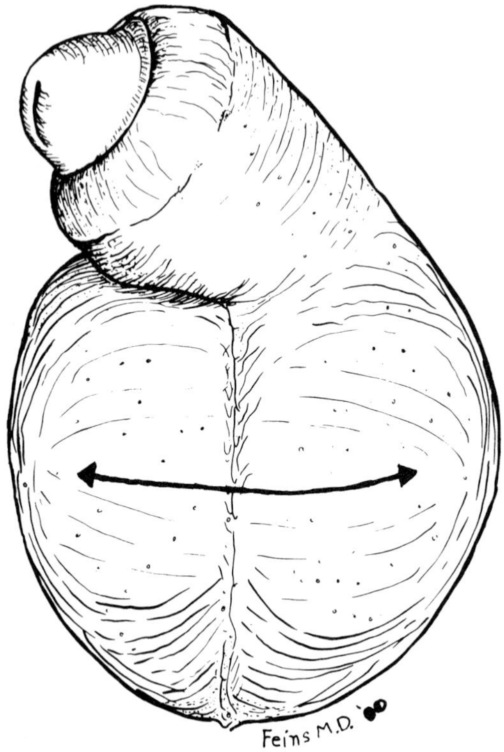

FIGURE 121.4. The incision (*arrows*) is made transverse in the scrotum at the base of the penile shaft. The same incision is made whether the penis and/or the scrotum is involved.

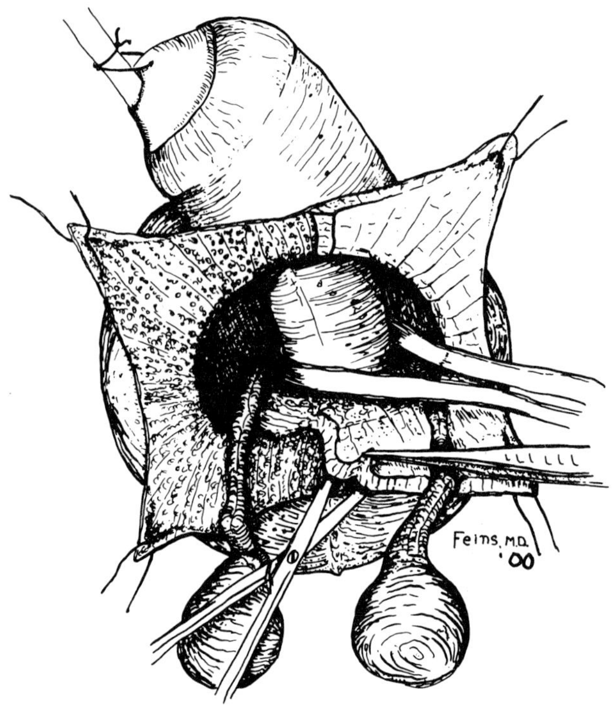

FIGURE 121.5. The skin flaps of the scrotum are developed. The subcutaneous tissue is partially excised, and the testes and cord structures are secured. The dissection on Buck's fascia begins. The base of the penis is surrounded by a drain.

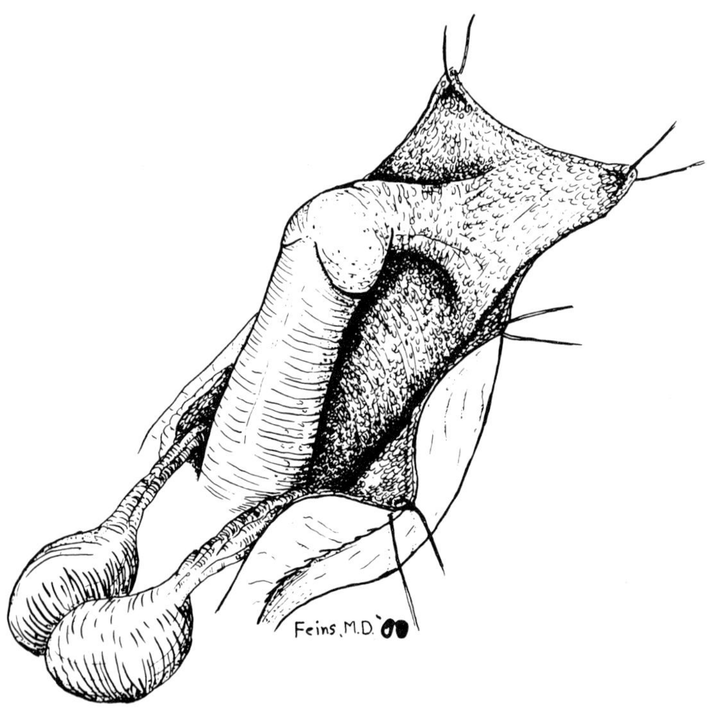

FIGURE 121.6. The penis is inverted into the wound and dissected circumferentially up to the coronal sulcus. Thin penile and scrotal flaps are constructed, and the subcutaneous tissues excised. The skin is redraped over the penis and sutured to the base from the inside.

tate grafting. If enough subcutaneous tissue is removed, reoperation is not necessary, but some swelling recurs and remains. A narrow bandage wrapped around the penis helps prevent recurrent edema, and patients are encouraged to wear an athletic supporter. If a large amount of edema remains or recurs, additional excision is necessary.

RESULTS

In our series of 324 patients, 208 underwent excisional surgery for lymphedema. In this group, 371 operative procedures were performed: the sex ratio was five females to every three males. The lymphedema was primary in 320 patients. The majority of the patients had surgery on their lower extremities, and 23 had procedures related to their genitalia. Ninety-five percent of the patients are being followed and treated with elastic stockings, air splints, weight control, elevation, hygiene, and antibiotics.

The longest follow-up is 23 years. Some patients have marked improvement after one procedure. Other patients are only moderately improved after three excisional operations; however, the cycle of increasing edema has been controlled in most of these patients. The severe attacks of lymphangitis that were present preoperatively in 31 patients have not recurred. Isolated attacks of lymphangitis seen after surgery were due to delayed wound healing in one patient, furuncles in three patients, and trauma in four patients. It appears that excisional therapy (i.e., total superficial lymphangiectomy and debulking) enhances drainage, or at least inhibits stasis, explaining the marked decrease in inflammatory episodes.

Of the patients, 92% were pleased with the results or surgery; 8% were not satisfied. Early in our experience, we found that patients with mild to moderate lymphedema who desired cosmetic improvement were rarely pleased with the resultant scarring and contour.

DISCUSSION

All patients require support hose specifically designed for them. Liberal use of the air splint at home enhances control of swelling. Any injury to the involved area should be treated vigorously to prevent infection. No limitations on activities are necessary.

Presently, 48% of patients require two-stage serial excisional procedures, 31% require three procedures, and 21% require one procedure. Some younger patients can be managed without surgery. However, the number of patients who can be controlled without surgical intervention is difficult to estimate. Attempts at nonoperative control should be exhausted before surgery is contemplated because surgery is not curative.

Due to the uncertainty regarding the optimal procedure for lymphedema, we chose a variation of the serial subcutaneous excisions described by Homans in 1936. This operation was appealing due to its ease, safety, and relatively good cosmetic result.

The anatomy of the lymphatics in the extremities remains unclear. However, the deep muscle has never been involved with the lymphedematous process. Therefore, it seems logical to resect the subcutaneous tissue and attempt total lymphangiectomy, removing the large amounts of the tissue that were producing lymph fluid. The skin flaps are attached to the underlying muscle, eliminating the space where the fluid can collect.

CONCLUSION

All of the patients in this series who had undergone excisional surgery have improved and have a more normal appearance. The morbidity of this simple procedure is negligible. At this time, staged subcutaneous excision appears to be the procedure of choice for treating moderate to severe lymphedema, regardless of the cause or classification. The procedure is not a cure. Hopefully, a true physiologic method will be developed.

SUGGESTED READINGS

Charles RH. In: Latham A, English TC, eds. *A system of treatment.* Vol. 3. London: Churchill, 1912.

Feins NR. A new surgical technique for lymphedema of the penis and scrotum. *J Pediatr Surg* 1980;15:787–789.

Feins NR. Lymphatic disorders. In: O'Neill JH, et al., eds. *Pediatric surgery, 5th ed.* St. Louis: CV Mosby, 1998:1973–1981.

Homans J. The treatment of elephantiasis of the legs: preliminary report. *N Engl J Med* 1936;215:1099–1104.

Kinmonth JB, Tracy GD, Marsh JK. Primary lymphedema: clinical and lymphangiographic studies of a series of 107 patients in which the lower limbs were affected. *Br J Surg* 1957;45:1–9.

Serville M. Surgical treatment of lymphedema: a report of 652 cases. *Surgery* 1987;101:485–495.

122

BREAST DISORDERS

M. ANN KUHN
GAIL E. BESNER

Breast tissue development begins in the 20-day embryo as a mammary ridge that extends from the forelimb to the hind limb. In the 6th week of gestation the nipple and areola form over a bud of breast tissue. Initially this tissue is composed of primary mammary ducts and loose fibrous stroma. The duct system forms from the development of 15 to 20 secondary buds that bifurcate into tubules. Normal development occurs at 8 to 15 years of age.

DEVELOPMENTAL ANOMALIES

Premature Thelarche

Premature thelarche is defined as breast growth in girls under 8 years of age with the absence of other signs of precocious puberty. This condition is most often seen in infants and toddlers. The typical finding on physical examination is a smooth, firm 3- to 4-cm subareolar swelling that is nontender with no associated nipple or areolar development. This finding may be unilateral or bilateral and often recedes after a few months. In 30% to 50% of girls it may persist until puberty, at which time breast development occurs normally. The underlying breast bud can be palpated on physical examination. These patients should have continued follow-up and parental reassurance. We feel comfortable observing this type of premature breast development as long as other signs of precocious puberty are not present. It is important not to misdiagnose premature thelarche as a breast mass because biopsy or excision can lead to loss of or injury to the breast bud with subsequent amastia or breast distortion.

If signs of precocious puberty are present, then evaluation should include examination for other signs of sexual maturation, including darkening of the areola, appearance of pubic and axillary hair, or vaginal bleeding. A height curve should be plotted to look for evidence of accelerated growth, and a wrist radiograph should be obtained to determine bone age. If the results of these evaluations are normal, then no further workup is needed. If other signs of sexual maturation are present, the diagnosis of precocious puberty is made. A complete endocrine evaluation should be performed, including a gonadotropin-releasing hormone stimulation test, as well as ultrasonographic studies of the adrenal glands and ovaries. In most cases, no specific cause is identified, and the precocious puberty is assumed to have a central origin. Computed tomography or magnetic resonance imaging of the brain can sometimes demonstrate hamartomas and other hypothalamic lesions in idiopathic precocious puberty. In cases where surgical correction of the underlying cause of precocious puberty is not possible, medical management is instituted. Leuprolide acetate, a gonadotropin-releasing hormone analogue, can be given to suppress the release of luteinizing hormone and follicle-stimulating hormone, in turn decreasing estrogen production. Leuprolide acetate at 0.15 to 0.3 mg/kg/dose is administered intramuscularly every 28 days.

Asynchronous Thelarche

Breast development may begin on one side and progress at a faster rate than on the other side. This usually is a self-limited condition and both sides become equal by the end of puberty. The patient requires reassurance. If significant asymmetric breast development persists, then augmentation or reduction mammoplasty can be performed to correct the disparity in size between the breasts.

Tuberous Breast Deformity

Tuberous breast deformity is breast hypoplasia with a protuberant and overdeveloped areola. There is usually inadequate skin in the infraareolar area with decreased tissue at

M. A. Kuhn and G. E. Besner: Departments of Surgery and Pediatrics, The Ohio State University, and Children's Hospital, Columbus, Ohio.

the breast base. Surgical management has included the use of tissue expansion, breast augmentation, Z-plasty, and flap creation.

Juvenile Hypertrophy and Macromastia

Juvenile hypertrophy and macromastia refer to breast overgrowth in adolescent girls. All children with diffuse breast enlargement should have a detailed history, physical examination, and periodic follow-up examinations. All sources of exogenous estrogen should be excluded, including drugs, tumors, neurologic disorders, pulmonary disease, and chronic liver disease.

Females with macromastia have large but histologically normal breasts. This is a subjective diagnosis and should be made with caution. Girls usually complain of chronic backache and shoulder irritation from bra straps. Many of these teenagers desire reduction mammoplasty, but this should be deferred until skeletal growth and breast maturation is complete. At this time, the patient should undergo careful evaluation and counseling.

Juvenile hypertrophy is an uncommon condition characterized by massive breast hypertrophy. The breasts are firm and nodular with a histologic increase in fibrous connective tissue of the breast and only moderate ductal proliferation. There are no associated hormonal abnormalities or remote tumors, and this is not a premalignant lesion. Modes of treatment that have been recommended are reduction mammoplasty, mastectomy with implantation of a prosthesis, hormonal manipulation, and a combination of surgical and medical management. The large size of the breasts makes reduction mammoplasty technically difficult, and the condition has a tendency to recur after surgery. In severe cases the preferred treatment may be subcutaneous mastectomy with free nipple transplant and insertion of a prosthesis.

Polymastia and Polythelia

Accessory breast tissue is the most common developmental anomaly that occurs in the breast. Polymastia refers to any accessory breast tissue and polythelia refers to supernumerary nipples. The usual location of this accessory breast tissue is from the midclavicular or axillary area to the inguinal ligament along the embryonic milk line. It is rare to find this tissue below the umbilicus. Patients usually have no clinical symptoms, but the accessory breast tissue may become swollen and painful postpartum. This tissue is also at risk for breast disease, as is the normal breast tissue. Surgical intervention is usually undertaken for cosmetic reasons.

Amastia and Athelia

Amastia refers to absence of one breast; athelia refers to absence of the nipple. Amastia can be associated with absence of the pectoralis major muscle. Poland syndrome is characterized by amastia, ipsilateral rib deformity, webbed fingers, and radial nerve palsy. In the teenage population, amastia can be disturbing. Surgical correction involves implant placement with serial injection of saline to match breast growth on the opposite side. After puberty is complete, a permanent implant is placed. Patients with Poland syndrome may require a latissimus dorsi flap to reconstruct the missing pectoralis major muscle.

BREAST MASSES

Masses in the prepubertal breast are uncommon and usually benign when found. Biopsy is rarely needed for diagnosis. In particular, we avoid biopsy or surgical excision in the developing breast because the breast bud can be partially or completely destroyed, causing significant hypoplasia at puberty. Although most breast masses in children can be evaluated with a careful physical examination and managed conservatively, the rapidly enlarging lesion or painful lesion should be examined by excisional biopsy. Also, children with a history of malignancy who have a suspicious breast mass should undergo biopsy. Patients with breast masses need appropriate long-term follow-up and parental reassurance for both operative and nonoperative cases.

A localized breast mass in boys and postpubertal girls usually requires surgical excision. We use ultrasonography as the initial imaging tool in adolescent girls to differentiate solid from cystic breast masses. Mammography is not useful in evaluating masses in the adolescent breast because of the predominantly fibroglandular composition of the breast. Sonography does not help to determine whether a breast mass is benign or malignant. To help with this determination, fine needle aspiration (FNA) can be used to determine whether a surgical biopsy is necessary. Excision should not be deferred until the lesion is large and bulky because reconstruction of normal breast contour may be more difficult. When possible, we prefer to excise breast masses through a circumareolar incision, which leads to an excellent cosmetic result. We find that the best cosmetic result is obtained by avoiding approximation of the breast tissue itself once the mass is removed. We prefer to approximate the skin with a layer of absorbable subcutaneous sutures followed by a running subcuticular skin closure.

Non-Neoplastic Breast Masses

Gynecomastia

Gynecomastia refers to palpable breast enlargement that occurs in boys. It can occur in the neonatal period from excess placental estrogen from the fetal circulation, which induces enlargement of the breast tissue. Breast enlargement in adolescent boys is not uncommon and can be found in up to 30% to 60% of boys. Gynecomastia is uncommon in prepubertal boys, and can be associated with adrenal or testicular tumors or endocrine disorders. Therefore, referral to a pediatric endocrinologist for a complete evaluation is warranted in a prepubertal boy with gynecomastia.

Simple pubertal gynecomastia begins about a year after the onset of puberty. The breast tissue enlarges for 1 to 2 years and then gradually recedes. This frequently occurs bilaterally, either simultaneously or sequentially. Patients typically present complaining of unilateral breast pain, asymmetry, or both. On physical examination a smooth, fine discoid mass can be seen and felt beneath the nipple–areolar complex. Most cases of pubertal gynecomastia are idiopathic, and extensive evaluation is not necessary unless the history or physical examination reveals other abnormalities such as lack of secondary sexual characteristics or the presence of a testicular mass. If the testes are small, Klinefelter's syndrome should be considered. Adolescents should be given strong reassurance and frequent follow-up until the gynecomastia has completely resolved.

Breast diameter greater than 4 cm rarely undergoes spontaneous regression. A complete drug history is important in the evaluation of these patients because drugs such as anabolic steroids, digitalis, isoniazid, tricyclic antidepressants, spironolactone, and marijuana can cause gynecomastia. Patients with gynecomastia may have persistent pain as well as poor self-esteem. In these cases a simple mastectomy is performed with all the breast tissue excised down to the pectoralis fascia, including the axillary tail. We perform the operation through a circumareolar incision that extends for 180 degrees around the lower areolar margin. The majority of the breast tissue and subcutaneous tissue is removed, but some subcutaneous tissue under the areola should be preserved to prevent adhesions to the underlying fascia with depression of the nipple–areolar complex. In patients with a large amount of subcutaneous fat in addition to gynecomastia, liposuction can be added to the subcutaneous mastectomy procedure. We tend to avoid the use of closed-suction catheter drainage in most cases, but we do use a circumferential compressive gauze dressing and elastic tape. The skin is closed with a running subcuticular absorbable suture. Preoperatively, we advise the patient that postoperative seromas may develop requiring needle aspiration in the office. The medical management of gynecomastia with climiphene, danazol, or tamoxifen has not been effective and is not used in our institution as an alternative to surgical therapy. Obesity is a common cause of pseudogynecomastia. A careful examination should make the distinction clear. These patients are better treated with counseling for weight loss than with surgery.

Abscess

Infection of the breast is uncommon in children except in neonates, but may also follow trauma or occur during lactation. An abscess usually presents as a tender, indurated or fluctuant erythematous mass. It may result from obstruction of a mammary duct, irritation or abrasion of the nipple, or from cellulitis of the surrounding chest wall. *Staphylococcus aureus* is the major etiologic agent. Treatment is usually with oral antibiotics and either needle aspiration for smaller lesions or incision and drainage for larger lesions.

Mastitis neonatorum presents as an abscess in the second or third week of life. The incidence does not correlate with the degree of physiologic breast enlargement, but the disorder may be more likely to occur if the engorged breasts are manipulated excessively. Significant fever and other systemic reactions do not frequently occur. Antibiotic therapy is used if there is significant cellulitis. We prefer needle aspiration of the abscess, which may need to be repeated. We reserve formal incision and drainage for failure of needle aspiration, because severe reduction in adult breast size following neonatal abscess drainage has been reported.

Breast Tumors

Fibroadenomas

This benign encapsulated tumor is the most common pathologic diagnosis in the adolescent breast. It usually develops in the upper outer quadrants of the breast and is more common in African Americans. Physical examination reveals a firm, smooth, mobile mass. Enlargement is seen during the menstrual cycle, and 10% of such masses regress spontaneously. They tend to enlarge slowly but may grow rapidly and become giant fibroadenomas. Giant fibroadenomas are benign but distort the normal breast architecture and can actually erode through the skin or the areola. There is no link between fibroadenoma and carcinoma.

Excision of fibroadenomas is often indicated and is usually technically easy because the tumor is so well encapsulated. Children who present with this breast mass can be observed over one or two menstrual cycles prior to excision. Mammography is not helpful in assessing masses in the adolescent breast because of the large amount of fibroglandular tissue compared with fatty tissue. Histologically the tumor is composed of abundant fibrous tissue and a network of branching ducts without significant tuboalveolar development. These lesions cannot be distinguished from phyllodes tumor until histologic examination is performed. Local recurrence is rare, but other fibroadenomas may develop in either breast and can often be followed nonoperatively.

Fibrocystic Disease

Fibrocystic disease is the next most common lesion of the breast after fibroadenoma. It may affect one or both breasts at the same or different times. Physical examination usually reveals a localized or diffuse area of cordlike thickening.

One or more cysts are usually palpable and at times may be difficult to distinguish from solid masses. Pain and tenderness usually increase just before each menstrual period. Examination at different times in the menstrual cycle may help to confirm the diagnosis. FNA may lead to resolution of cystic masses that persist after several menstrual cycles. Excisional biopsy may be necessary if a mass remains present though two or three menstrual cycles and does not resolve with aspiration. Adolescents, especially those with this condition, should learn the technique of self-breast examination.

Phyllodes Tumor

This tumor develops from breast tissue and is closely related to the fibroadenoma but lacks a true capsule. It is distinguishable from fibroadenoma histologically by increased hypertrophy and greater cellularity of the fibrous tissue stroma. It is the most common malignant breast mass in adolescents. Phyllodes tumor is classified into three groups: benign, intermediate (borderline), and malignant. The stromal cellularity, atypia, anaplasia, and degree of mitotic activity determine the classification of the tumor. The behavior of the tumor cannot be predicted by the classification because even the benign lesions can metastasize. Management is controversial, but we prefer simple wide excision. These tumors have a tendency to recur locally, which can be treated by repeat excision. Mastectomy is reserved for recurrent tumors not amenable to local excision, and possibly for high-grade malignant lesions. Prognosis is poor in the case of malignant disease even with the use of multimodal therapy.

Primary Carcinoma

Malignant tumors of the breast in women under 20 are rare. They account for only 1% of all neoplasia in girls and adolescents. Malignant pathology, including lymphoma, fibrosarcoma, and reticulum sarcoma, is extremely rare. As many as 30% of adolescents with breast carcinoma have a positive family history. Breast cancer commonly presents as an asymptomatic mass that is hard, subareolar, and usually fixed to deep tissue. Axillary lymphadenopathy is not common.

Primary carcinoma of the breast is usually due to juvenile secretory carcinoma. This carcinoma is characterized by abundant secretion of mucin and mucopolysaccharide-containing materials with rare metastatic spread. Wide local excision is adequate for treatment in young children, but careful follow-up is needed because these tumors may recur locally or present with axillary node metastases. At this time, reexcision with or without simple mastectomy is appropriate.

Adolescent girls presenting with carcinoma of the breast should be managed as adults. As yet, the option of breast-conserving procedures for early-stage carcinoma has not been addressed but should be dependent on the patient's age and breast size.

Primary rhabdomyosarcoma of the breast is extremely rare. Treatment of this lesion includes wide local excision of the primary lesion and use of multiagent chemotherapy. Non-Hodgkin's lymphoma can occur as a primary malignancy in the breast, and surgical therapy is limited to an adequate biopsy for diagnostic purposes followed by chemotherapy.

Metastatic Disease

Metastatic disease is rare but can occur following hematogenous or lymphatic spread. The most frequent primary tumors that metastasize to the breast are rhabdomyosarcoma, non-Hodgkin's lymphoma, and leukemia. Rarely histiocytosis, medulloblastoma, and neuroblastoma can result in breast metastasis. There also has been one case of renal carcinoma metastasizing to the breast. Therefore, a thorough breast examination should be part of the surveillance program for patients with a history of cancer, and a biopsy of any enlarging suspicious mass should be performed. FNA should be performed before the patient undergoes incisional or excisional biopsy. A complete metastatic workup also should be performed. Further surgical therapy in patients with metastatic disease to the breast is limited.

Other Breast Masses

Cystic lesions such as simple cysts, blue-domed cysts, and galactoceles can occur at any age. Pain, tenderness, nipple discharge, infection, and progressive enlargement are common. Excision is usually indicated. Fibrous mastopathy, lobular hyperplasia, sclerosing adenosis, fat necrosis, and other mastopathies present as discrete, firm, often irregular masses. On palpation these lesions may be mobile or fixed, and it is difficult to distinguish them from neoplastic masses. Excision is indicated. Juvenile papillomatosis presents as a mass similar to fibroadenoma but has a distinct histologic appearance. It has an unknown potential for subsequent malignancy. Hemangiomas may occur in infants but usually resolve. If the underlying breast bud is involved in the lesion, associated mammary hypoplasia can occur. MRI may be useful to distinguish the breast bud from the vascular lesion. Steroid therapy may be used to promote involution of the hemangioma while sparing the breast bud. Surgical intervention is reserved for lesions causing life-threatening symptoms. Cystic hygromas also can occur in young children. Excision may be necessary but should be limited to avoid injury to the breast bud.

NIPPLE DISCHARGE

Nipple discharge in the pediatric patient is usually not the result of malignancy. The discharge can be unilateral or bilateral, milky, green, gray, black, or bloody. Causes can include galactorrhea, Montgomery's tubercles, intraductal papillomatosis, and duct ectasia. The character of the discharge can help with the diagnosis. Milky discharge is suggestive of galactorrhea, whereas purulent discharge suggests infection. Serous or serosanguinous discharge can be seen with intraductal papilloma, proliferative breast changes, duct ectasia, or cancer. Watery nipple discharge implies papilloma or cancer.

Galactorrhea results from an increase in prolactin levels. Increased prolactin may be secondary to pregnancy, postabortion or postpartum states, pituitary adenomas, chronic renal failure, and hypothyroidism. The presence of pituitary adenoma is evaluated with a serum prolactin level and a CT or MRI of the pituitary gland. Treatment consists of medical management with bromocriptine or surgical removal. Drugs that affect the hypothalamic–pituitary axis such as birth control pills, phenothiazines, spironolactone, estrogens, opiates, prochlorperazine, metoclopramide, tricyclic antidepressants, cimetidine, verapamil, and methyldopa also may induce galactorrhea.

Intraductal papillomas may present with a bloody nipple discharge and are rare in adolescents. These lesions form from an abnormal proliferation of cells in mammary ducts supported by a vascular stalk. Trauma may rupture the stalk, leading to a bloody discharge. Montgomery's tubercles are small, soft papules around the areola. They enlarge with pregnancy and are involved with lactation. Adolescents with this condition may have a lump under the areola and complain of a thin, clear to brown discharge. The discharge usually disappears in 3 to 5 weeks and the lump within 4 months.

All patients with persistent discharge from a single duct require surgical excision of the duct to obtain a diagnosis. The extent of excision should be limited to the involved duct and its adjacent breast tissue. Preoperatively, the location of the offending duct should be determined on physical examination by palpating all four quadrants of the areolar complex to see which area leads to nipple discharge. Ultrasonography can be used to confirm localization, or in cases where physical examination is inconclusive. If this still does not allow localization, collodion can be applied to the nipple and covered with Tegaderm (3M Health Care, St. Paul, Minnesota) for 48 hours, followed by repeat ultrasonography and physical examination to again attempt to locate the involved duct.

SUGGESTED READINGS

Neinstein LS. Breast disease in adolescents and young women. *Pediatr Clin North Am* 1999;46:607–629.

Rogers DA, Lobe TE, Rao BN, et al. Breast malignancy in children. *J Pediatr Surg* 1994;29:48–51.

West KW, Rescorla FJ, Scherer LR, et al. Diagnosis and treatment of symptomatic breast masses in the pediatric population. *J Pediatr Surg* 1995;30:182–187.

SECTION XIV

GENITOURINARY SYSTEM

123

CIRCUMCISION

T. ERNESTO FIGUEROA
PAT CASALE

Few topics have generated such passionate and polarizing debate as circumcision. Every pediatric surgeon and urologist is likely to confront this issue on a daily occurrence, from parents seeking advice, to parents wishing a different appearance of their son's genitalia, to pediatricians arguing about the pros and cons of this historic and oldest type of surgery. In the past 30 years, the American Academy of Pediatric's Task Force on Circumcision has outlined three different proposals for the management of the foreskin. The most recent recommendations by this task force, published in 1999, expressed that neonatal circumcisions may offer some potential medical benefits, but the present medical evidence is not sufficient to recommend routine neonatal circumcisions. The use of procedural analgesia was advocated in this report. This is a significant change from the initial policy statement, published in 1971, which expressed that there was no absolute medical indication for routine circumcisions. Attitudes about circumcision are colored by medical knowledge, cultural beliefs, and personal experiences, and, as we approach different patients, we must be cautious that our own bias does not have a bearing on the recommendations offered to a given family. Neonatal circumcision is still widely practiced in the United States. Obstetricians perform most of these circumcisions, although pediatricians, family medicine physicians, and pediatric surgical specialists are also often asked to perform this procedure.

NEONATAL CIRCUMCISION

Indications and Contraindications

The major indication for a neonatal circumcision is the parental decision to have their son circumcised. The parent should be informed of the potential medical benefits of the circumcision as well as the risks associated with the procedure. We make the point that this is not meant to be a cosmetic procedure, and specifically tell the parents that the appearance of the penis will change as the child grows. The purpose of the procedure is to remove the most apical constricting portion of the prepuce, so that the residual prepuce can be retracted without difficulty. Most of the problems that we see in our practice following neonatal circumcisions are related to misinformation and the expectations that the glans will always be visible in every child following the circumcision. We tell the parents that most boys develop a hidden penis in infancy due to the rapid weight gain, which in turn produces the appearance of "excess" or "residual" prepuce. When confronted with this situation, we always reassure the families and discourage the quest for a revision of the circumcision. A second indication for a neonatal or infant circumcision is the potential benefit to prevent urinary tract infections in boys predisposed to these infections (urinary tract anomalies or a documented episode of pyelonephritis).

There are several contraindications to a neonatal circumcision. A neonatal circumcision should be reserved for healthy and stable infants. Any history of bleeding disorders in the family should prompt a thorough investigation of the patient's hematologic status prior to proceeding with a circumcision. This usually entails determining the prothrombin time, partial thromboplastin time, bleeding time, and platelet count. Finally, any abnormalities of the penis, no matter how minor, should deter the physician from performing the procedure. Some of these anomalies include penile torsion, incomplete formation of the prepuce, chordee, hypospadias, penoscrotal fusion, micropenis, or any other evidence of an intersex state (including bilateral nonpalpable testes).

Analgesia

The first step in performing a neonatal circumcision is the use of a procedural analgesic. Penile blocks using 1 to 2 mL

T. E. Figueroa: Department of Urology, Thomas Jefferson University, Philadelphia, Pennsylvania; and Division of Pediatric Urology, Alfred I. duPont Hospital for Children, Wilmington, Delaware.

P. Casale: Department of Urology, Thomas Jefferson University, Philadelphia, Pennsylvania.

of lidocaine 1% solution are effective. Penile blocks have been described as dorsal penile blocks or circumferential "ring" blocks. We prefer to use a combination of the two to maximize the analgesic effect. Using a 27-gauge needle, we like to inject 0.5 mL into the penopubic angle as a dorsal penile block, and then 1 to 1.5 mL around the base of the penis as a subcutaneous ring block. We also inject 0.3 mL to the dorsal distal prepuce, in the area where the dorsal slit will be made. We have found this step to minimize the reaction of the neonate to the procedure. After injecting the area, we compress the tissues for 2 minutes with a small gauze pad to minimize edema and allow for satisfactory effect of the block. Some clinicians have advocated the use of a distal ring block at the level of the corona, although we do not have experience with this approach.

Eutectic mixture lidocaine-prilocaine topical anesthetic (EMLA) cream also has been used with reported safety and effectiveness. The dose is 1 to 2 g of EMLA cream applied 60 to 90 minutes prior to the procedure. Although there is a theoretical concern about the potential for neonates to develop methemoglobinemia, this dosage produces levels well below the toxic range. In our experience, the combination of a dorsal penile block and subcutaneous ring block has been more effective than EMLA in providing consistent analgesia.

The use of acetaminophen after the procedure and allowing the baby to suck on dextrose water during the procedure are also helpful maneuvers to minimize discomfort associated with the procedure. We always ask the parents if they wish to be present during the procedure, because their presence may be of comfort to the child undergoing the procedure.

Procedures and Complications

Neonatal circumcisions are performed by using a variety of clamping devices that crush the prepuce to minimize bleeding and the need for suturing the skin edges. Currently, the most commonly used devices include the Gomco clamp (Allied Health Care Products, St. Louis, Missouri), the Plastibell (Hollister Inc., Libertyville, Illinois), and the Mogen clamp. Each device has positive as well as potentially negative characteristics. Which device to use is a matter of personal preference, but the surgeon should be familiar with all of these devices because occasionally only one of them is available.

Once the penile block has been administered, we like to place two small hemostat clamps to the distal dorsal prepuce. Placing these clamps on slight traction allows the surgeon to develop the plane between the glans and the inner prepuce with a third small clamp. This should be done with gentle, incremental advances toward the corona of the glans, always pointing the tips of the dissecting clamp dorsally against the inner prepuce to avoid directing the clamp into the urethral meatus. The dissected dorsal prepuce between the two holding clamps is crushed and divided, completing the dorsal slit. The prepuce is separated from the glans until the corona sulcus is visualized. Dissection is always avoided ventrally, leaving the frenulum intact to minimize bleeding.

The Gomco clamp comes in various sizes (1.1, 1.3, 1.45, and 1.6 cm) depending on the diameter of the crown that fits over the glans. This device consists of four pieces: the crown, base, hinge, and nut. The device has to be put together at the time of the circumcision, which requires some dexterity. Once a dorsal slit is preformed to midglans, the crown is fitted over the glans. The right fit should be a crown that reaches the corona of the glans. Selecting too small of a crown produces a poor cosmetic result (too much residual prepuce), and too big of a crown can result in a degloving injury to the penis by removing too much skin, or possibly, a urethral injury and a subsequent urethrocutaneous fistula. Once the device is assembled, it is maintained in place for 3 to 5 minutes, during which time the prepuce distal to the clamp is amputated. After releasing the clamp, it is important to retract the fused cut edges proximal to the corona. Failure to do so results in a secondary phimosis. Other complications associated with this device include bleeding and separation of the fused edges. When this occurs, fine sutures (5-0, 6-0 chromic catgut) may be used to approximate the edges. An asymmetrical (oblique) circumcision can result if the device is not placed correctly. Recently, there have been some reports of inadequate fusion of the skin edges, which may be related to the use of an old or worn device.

The Plastibell is a simple device that is readily available. It is simpler to apply than the Gomco, and like the Gomco, it protects the glans during the circumcision. The device is left in place with a coarse suture tied at the sulcus of the device to crush the prepuce. Most of these devices fall off 4 to 7 days after being placed. The crowns come in various sizes: 1.1, 1.2, 1.3, 1.4, 1.5, and 1.7 cm. The most common sizes are 1.3 and 1.5 cm. Selection of the correct size is similar as with the Gomco. Postoperative problems are rare. Occasionally, a portion of the prepuce remains attached after the Plastibell has separated from most of the wound, causing a hinging effect. When this occurs it will be necessary to cut the band of tissue with scissors to remove the Plastibell. An unusual complication of this device is proximal migration of the device, which occurs when the crown is too large for the glans. This is a potentially serious complication because it produces a constricting band or tourniquet action around the penis, which can result in urinary retention and necrosis of the skin or organ. Cellulitis also can occur with this type of device, and there have been a handful of case reports of necrotizing fasciitis (Fournier's gangrene) following a Plastibell circumcision. Bleeding seems to be less of a problem with this device.

Those who prefer the Mogen clamp state that it is a fast and effective method, with minimal complications. It is a light clamp, which is applied to the prepuce on traction. There is a small bevel or indentation on the clamp to accommodate the glans. The skin is cut distal to the crushing effect. Unlike the other devices described previously, it does not have a crown or protective portion for the glans. The clamp is applied to the intact prepuce without visualizing the glans. The glans should be pulled away from the clamp as the clamp is positioned in place. Once the circumcision is performed, the fused, cut edges must be retracted proximal to the corona sulcus, or a secondary phimosis will occur. Degloving injuries can occur if too much foreskin is pulled distal to the clamp. The most devastating complication associated with the use of this device is partial amputation of the glans. This occurs when the glans is trapped in the clamp and amputated with the cut foreskin. When this occurs, there is usually profuse bleeding from the cut surface of the glans. Applying pressure with gauze around the glans can help control bleeding. The amputated portion of the glans should be retrieved and preserved in saline on ice until it can be reattached to the glans using microsurgical techniques in the operating room. If the transection has occurred proximal to the urethral meatus, a urethral anastomosis will be necessary as well. In those instances, we have placed a small feeding tube as a urethral stent, and approximated the urethra with 8-0 Vicryl sutures. The glans epithelium is approximated with 7-0 PDS sutures (Ethicon Inc.). The stent is left in place for 7 days. Partial loss of the glans and meatal stenosis can occur after glans reattachment.

Bleeding can occur following any of the techniques described above. This is always an emergency. The first approach is to apply gentle and constant pressure around the anastomosis of the skin and the prepuce to control bleeding. Application of a small amount of lidocaine with epinephrine topically also can aid in controlling the bleeding. If a specific bleeding point is identified, then this area can be touched with the tip of a silver nitrate stick or a fine suture can be placed. Any more extensive use of these techniques should be done in the operating room under controlled circumstances. A circumferential compressive dressing can be used to control bleeding in the neonate. In those cases, placing a small urethral catheter prevents difficulty with urination or urinary retention. Rarely does the bleeding require a formal surgical exploration. All of these patients should undergo a hematologic assessment to determine if there is a bleeding disorder. In the rare event that urgent exploration may be necessary to control bleeding acutely, fresh frozen plasma can be given prophylactically until the hematologic evaluation is completed.

The care of the circumcision wound is often ignored. Many of the problems leading to a poor circumcision result can be prevented with simple, but definitive, wound care. Following the circumcision, we recommend applying an antibiotic ointment to the wound, three to four times a day, for a week. At this point, we recommend switching to a nonantibiotic ointment, such as A&D (Fougera, Melville, New York), and gently retracting the penile skin and mucosal apron away from the corona as the ointment is applied. This maneuver is performed for 3 months once or twice a day. This simple maneuver prevents some of the common problems that continue to plague this procedure, such as mucosal adhesions, formation of penoglandular epithelial bridges, and secondary phimoses. Maintaining a protective skin barrier such as A&D ointment on the glans also may prevent the formation of urethral meatal stenosis, thought to result from the chronic irritation of the meatus as it rubs against the urine-soaked diaper.

When a secondary phimosis occurs, prompt action is essential. If the parents report that they can no longer see the glans, the infant should be evaluated for the possibility of a secondary phimosis. In this instance, the healing wound moves distal to the glans. The combination of healing and the presence of urine can produce rapidly contracting cicatrix. This cicatrix can be so dramatic as to produce urinary retention. If the child is having difficulty urinating, then a dorsal slit incision should be performed. If the child is urinating well, we now routinely use a topical agent to try to arrest the progressive contraction of the wound. Our choice is hydrocortisone cream 2.5% applied to the cicatrix, while the penile skin is pulled back on stretch. We have seen many of these phimoses resolve in 4 to 6 weeks. If the cicatrix does not respond to this type of therapy, then a secondary operation, or revision of the circumcision, is necessary. Some of these patients develop a concealed penis, and it is important to limit the amount of skin removed in these revisions, because frequently there is a real paucity of penile shaft skin in these patients.

PEDIATRIC CIRCUMCISION

Technique

When the infant is over 3 months of age, or if there is a penile abnormality that would prevent the use of a neonatal circumcision, a surgical circumcision is then performed after the age of 6 months. The popular techniques to do a freehanded circumcision include a sleeve technique and a guillotine technique. The guillotine technique is not well suited for infants and children, leaving a less than ideal cosmetic result. We prefer approaching the circumcision as we approach hypospadias surgery. A traction glans stitch of 4-0 silk is placed on the dorsum of the glans, the frenulum is divided, the mucosal apron is marked with the surgical pen to 6 to 8 mm, and then incised. The penile skin overlying the corona is marked and incised with the scalpel. We have found that bipolar cautery, or fine-point forceps and electrocautery, is helpful in achieving accurate hemostasis. If there is a penile torsion or chordee, the penile skin is completely degloved, which usually corrects the cutaneous abnormality. Closure of the wound is achieved with fine absorbable suture, such as 6-0 chromic catgut, either with interrupted or running suturing. As in hypospadias surgery, optical magnification with surgical loupes and the use of fine ophthalmic instruments are invaluable assets to this type of surgery.

Dressings

Dressings after a circumcision are used mostly to aid in hemostasis. A tight dressing may be difficult to remove postoperatively, and a very loose dressing rarely makes it to the recovery room after the patient is awakened from the general anesthesia. In non–toilet-trained patients, we prefer the use of an unraveled cotton ball soaked in benzoin. This dressing stays on for 3 to 4 days and is easily removed by the parents. If the patient is toilet trained, we do not recommend this type of dressing, because it is very difficult to remove. In those instances, it may be simpler just to apply a coating of antibacterial ointment over the wound, without a specific dressing. In the past we were enthusiastic about the use of occlusive and circumferential dressings such as Tegaderm (3M Health Care, St. Paul, Minnesota), but over time found too many instances in which the dressing was difficult to remove, or that it prompted bleeding by sliding back and forth on the wound.

Complications and Their Management

Bleeding is the most common complication reported after a circumcision, and it may occur in 0.1% to 1% of cases. If bleeding develops after surgery, it can be managed in two ways, depending on whether the bleeding is from the anastomosis or from a penile vessel. Mucosal bleeding that occurs after the circumcision can be readily managed with gentle compression and application of a vasoconstricting agent, such as epinephrine. Many emergency rooms stock solutions such as lidocaine-epinephrine-tetracaine (LET), which are used as topical anesthetics for lacerations. This is a highly effective agent in inducing hemostasis when the bleeding is from the mucosal edge. Patients who develop bleeding from a penile vessel usually present with bleeding and a penile hematoma. These patients require reexploration to correct this problem.

Urinary retention can occur in young boys, particularly in those who recently have completed toilet training (2–4 years of age). Retention occurs because of fear to urinate, because the child anticipates pain during urination. When notified that a young boy has not urinated, we encourage the parents to give pain medication and allow the boy to go to sleep. These boys will often wet during sleep (nocturnal enuresis). If the child wakes up still apprehensive about urinating, or if the child appears to be in distress from a full bladder, we ask the family to bring the child back to the hospital, where the child receives a dose of midazolam. This medication calms the child and relaxes the external sphincter, allowing him to void. We try to avoid catheterizing these boys, because this action may perpetuate the child's apprehension to urinate.

Penile wound infections are extremely rare. Fever, wound pain, erythema of the wound, and crepitus are all serious findings. Any indication of a wound infection requires immediate and aggressive antimicrobial coverage and wound care.

SUGGESTED READINGS

AAP Task Force on Circumcision. Circumcision policy statement. *Pediatrics* 1999;103:686–693.

Duckett JW. A temperate approach to neonatal circumcision. *Urology* 1995;46:771–772.

Gollaher DL. From ritual to science: the medical transformation of circumcision in America. *J Social History* 1994;28:5–36.

Kunin SA. Circumcision in newborns: not why, but how. *Dialogues Pediatr Urol* 1994;17:1–8.

Wallerstein E. Circumcision: the uniquely American medical enigma. *Urol Clin North Am* 1985;12:123–132.

Williams N, Kapila L. Complications of circumcision. *Br J Urol* 1993;80:1231–1236.

124

HYPOSPADIAS

NEIL R. FEINS
KONSTANTINOS PAPADAKIS

Hypospadias is a congenital defect associated with proximal placement of the urethral meatus. The meatus can be located from the glans to the perineum. A chordee, a ventral curvature, may accompany this anomaly. Repair is focused on attaining normal voiding and sexual function.

The incidence of hypospadias is reported at 4.7 to 8 per 1,000 males. Associated anomalies are inguinal hernias and undescended testes. The more proximal the defect, the more numerous are the accompanying abnormalities. Ninety percent of cases present with the meatus on the distal shaft or glans. Most classification systems are based on the location of the meatus and if a chordee is present. Over 300 different procedures have been described for repair. Many of these procedures are similar, and all of them stress meticulous surgical technique and adequate skin coverage. Most surgeons have a few favorite repairs, but one must remember that no one procedure will work for the variety of presentations.

The repairs, methods, and suture material are ones that have worked well for us, but with experience, continuous evolution is apparent.

TECHNIQUE

Glanular hypospadias is amenable to a modified meatal advancement glanoplasty repair. Following general anesthesia, a penile block of 0.5% marcaine and 0.5% lidocaine with 1/200,000 epinephrine is given. The block is given at the beginning of the operation and at the end.

Most hypospadias repair surgery is performed at about 6 months of age, and one dose of a broad-spectrum antibiotic is given intravenously prior to making the incision. A 5-0 silk holding suture is placed vertically in the glans, and a round 7 French Silastic catheter (Allegiance Jackson Pratt, McGaw Park, Illinois) is placed into the urethra and bladder followed by a rubber band tourniquet to decrease blood loss and allow visualization of the delicate tissues.

N. R. Feins and K. Papadakis: Department of Surgery, The Children's Hospital, Harvard Medical School, Boston, Massachusetts.

A triangle of dorsal tissue is removed to advance the dorsal meatus, and the meatus is sutured to the new apex with 7-0 ophthalmic chromic sutures. A horseshoe incision is made with a sharp ophthalmic knife proximal to the meatus, the incision in the glans is deepened and a ventral flap is raised with sharp tenotomy scissors. A ventral flap helps release the ventral meatus. The flap is used for traction distally, and the glans is now approximated with horizontal mattress sutures of 6-0 Vicryl (Ethicon Inc.). The glans is further closed with a second more superficial layer of interrupted 6-0 chromic sutures. The ventral meatus is matured with 7-0 ophthalmic chromic sutures, and the excess ventral flap can be excised. The tourniquet can be removed and a mucosal collar formed. The excess foreskin is removed, and the penile incisions closed with 5-0 or 6-0 chromic. There is rarely a need for the catheter to remain in place, and the wound is covered with Betadine ointment (The Purdue Frederick Co., Norwalk, Connecticut) every six hours (Fig. 124.1).

Mid- to distal shaft hypospadias with minimal chordee is best managed using the Snodgrass tubularized incised plate urethroplasty technique. The operation is begun as in the previous procedure. The two longitudinal perpendicular incisions are made in the glans and joined 1 or 2 mm proximal to the meatus. A circumferential skin incision is made proximal to the coronal sulcus, and the shaft skin is degloved. An artificial erection is performed to evaluate any penile curvature (see Fig. 124.4C). If present and not corrected by resection of ventral fibrotic tissue, a dorsal tunica albuginea plication will be needed (see Fig. 124.4D).

A longitudinal midline incision is made in the urethral plate from the dorsal aspect of the urethral meatus to the tip of the glans. A tube is then fashioned over a 7 French Silastic catheter using a 7-0 PDS running subcuticular technique. The neourethra should fit loosely around the catheter and is covered with a thin layer of dorsal subcutaneous tissue. The glans wings are closed with deep mattress sutures of 6-0 Vicryl and a superficial layer of 6-0 chromic. The meatus is matured with interrupted 7-0 ophthalmic chromic sutures. The 7 French Silastic catheter is left in the bladder and sutured to the glans with a 6-0 Prolene suture

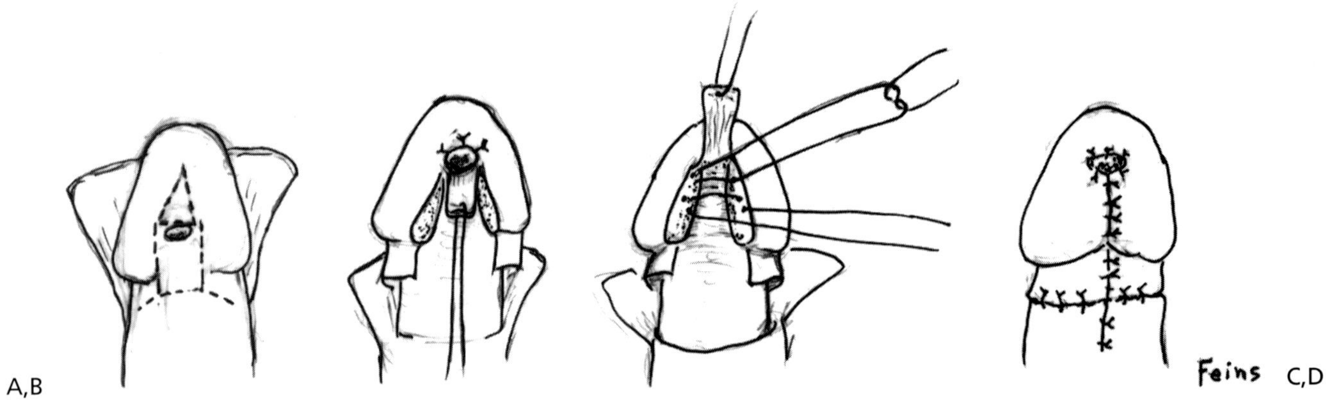

FIGURE 124.1. Modified meatal advancement glanoplasty repair. **A:** The dotted lines represent the proposed incisions. **B:** The triangle of tissue distal to the meatus has been removed and the distal meatus advanced toward the tip. The glanular incisions have been executed and the ventral flap freed. **C:** The ventral flap has been drawn distally and the glanoplasty begun. **D:** The meatus has been matured, and the excess flap and hooded prepuce excised. The glans has been closed in two layers and the mucosal collar has been sutured to the shaft skin.

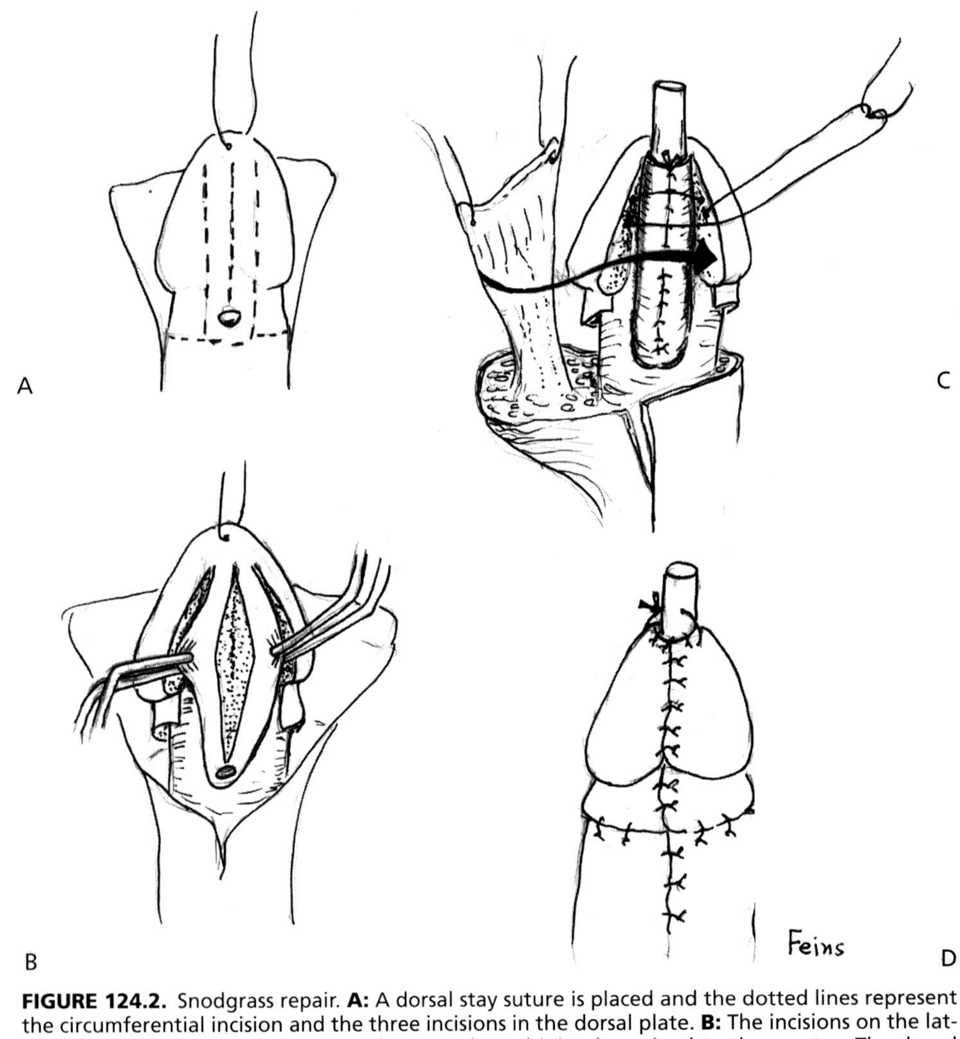

FIGURE 124.2. Snodgrass repair. **A:** A dorsal stay suture is placed and the dotted lines represent the circumferential incision and the three incisions in the dorsal plate. **B:** The incisions on the lateral aspect of the dorsal plate have been made and joined proximal to the meatus. The dorsal plate in the midline has been incised deeply. **C:** The urethral plate has been tubularized over a 7 French Silastic catheter, and a subcutaneous tissue flap has been developed and will be rotated over the neourethra prior to closing the glans. **D:** The skin closure has been accomplished and the catheter sutured in place with a 6-0 Prolene suture.

(Ethicon, Inc.). The shaft is covered with dorsal Byars flaps or available ventral skin. A Tegaderm dressing (3M Health Care, St. Paul, Minnesota) is fashioned and the patient is kept supine with three corner restraints or in a car seat for 48 hours. The dressing is removed in 4 days, and the catheter is removed in 7 days (Fig. 124.2).

For the more proximal hypospadias that cannot be corrected by the Snodgrass repair, we usually perform the transverse preputial island flap repair. The procedure is started as the Snodgrass, and then a ventral midline longitudinal incision is made from around the urethral meatus to the distal circumcising incision. The skin is incised circumferentially, and the shaft is degloved. The fibrotic corpus spongiosum is excised and an artificial erection established. If a curvature is present, it is managed by dorsal plication as described previously in the text (Fig. 124.4D). A transverse rectangle of preputial skin is marked to match the distance from the meatus to the tip of the glans and made 15 mm wide. After the tissue is dissected, it is tubularized loosely using a subcuticular suture of 7-0 PDS over a 7 French or larger Silastic catheter to form a neourethra.

The neourethra is brought to the ventral surface of the penis on a tension-free pedicle. The dorsal aspect of the proximal meatus is fixed to the corpora with a few fine absorbable sutures. The ventral surface of the glans is split in the midline. The neourethra is sutured to the native meatus with two separate sutures of 7-0 PDS joined in a running locking full-thickness technique. The distal neourethra is placed in the bed of the glans. The distal meatus is matured with 7-0 chromic sutures and the glans is closed. The pedicle can be brought over the neourethra or a second layer of viable tunica vaginalis can be placed over the repair and the skin closed in a routine fashion. The Silastic catheter should be sutured in place and removed in 7 to 10 days (Fig. 124.3).

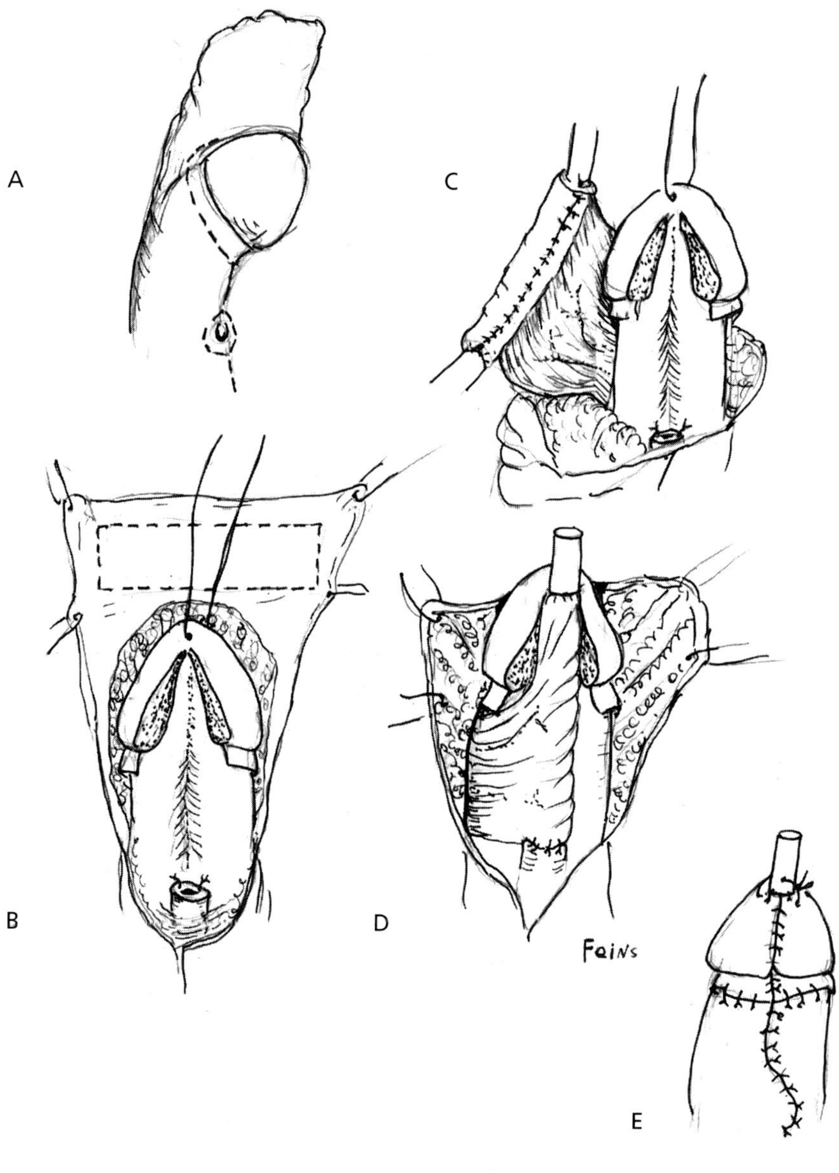

FIGURE 124.3. The transverse preputial island flap repair. **A:** The incision is made on dotted lines around the distal shaft and in the ventral midline to eventually go around the meatus. **B:** The glans has been opened, chordee tissue resected, the native meatus fixed to the corpora cavernosa. The dashed lines represent the measured width and length of the proposed neourethra. **C:** Tubularization of the transverse preputial island flap is performed over a 7 French or larger Silastic catheter using a 7-0 PDS running subcuticular suture. **D:** The neourethra has been joined to the proximal urethra after having been rotated on a tension-free pedicle. **E:** The catheter has been sutured in place and the skin closed with the remaining preputial skin that has been divided in the dorsal midline.

TWO-STAGE HYPOSPADIAS REPAIR

Hypospadias in most patients can be corrected with one operation. In severe cases of perineal hypospadias, we usually prefer a two-stage repair.

The first stage is to correct the curvature with a dermal graft placed following a transverse incision in the tunica albuginea beneath the maximal penile bend. A midline longitudinal incision is made in the preputial and dorsal penile skin. Each half is brought to the ventral surface and closed

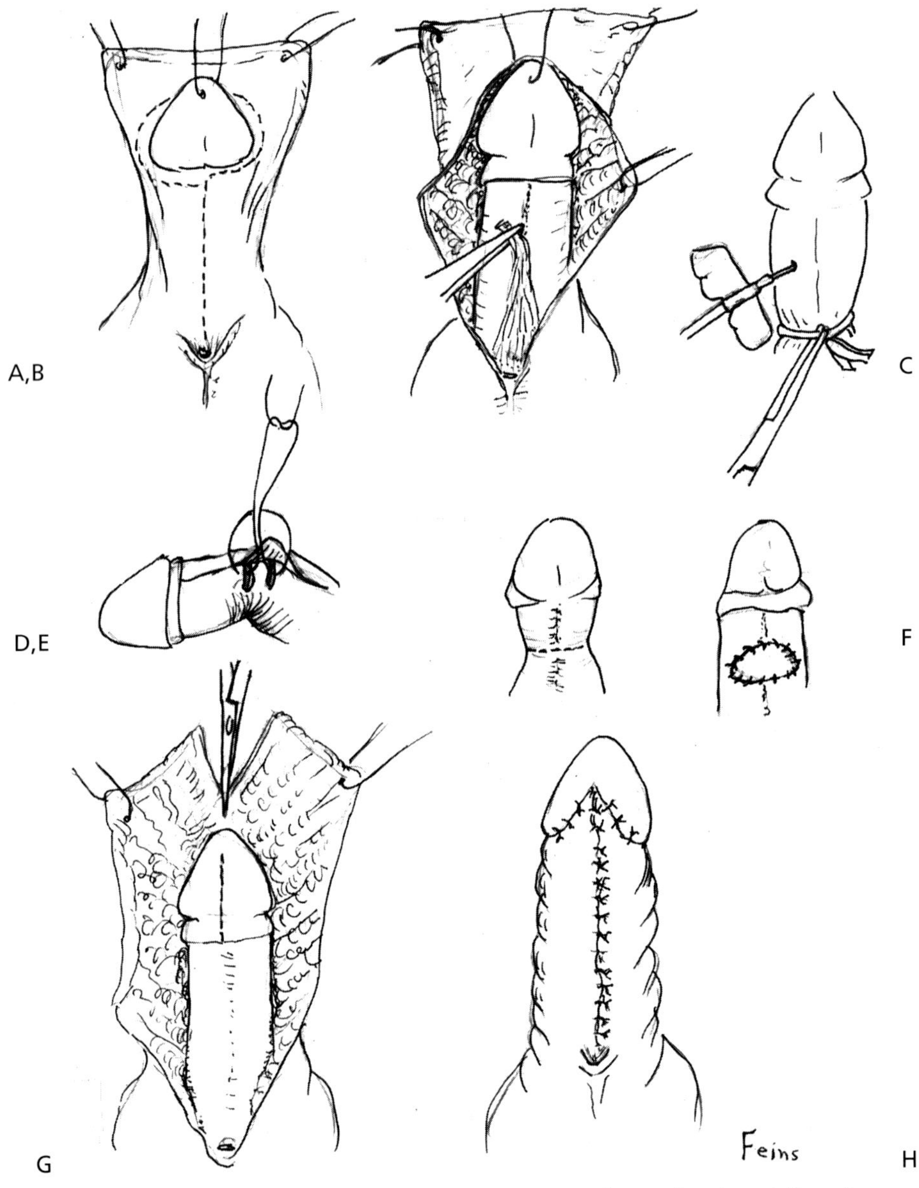

FIGURE 124.4. The two-stage repair. **A:** An incision is made on the dotted lines for scrotal hypospadias. **B:** Removal of fibrotic corpus spongiosum. **C:** Artificial erection is induced to evaluate the presence of chordee. **D:** The neurovascular bundle is elevated and incisions are made in the tunica albuginea opposite the point of maximal curvature. An inverting suture of PDS is used to close the gap, burying the knot and correcting the ventral curvature. **E:** Another method for severe chordee correction is to make an incision along the dotted line across the maximum ventral curvature. **F:** The defect in the tunica albuginea of corpora cavernosum is closed with an ellipse of defatted dermis, usually harvested from the groin, and sewn into the created defect. **G:** The glans is opened along the dotted line, the penis degloved, and Byars flaps developed with a dorsal incision in the preputial skin. **H:** The preputial skin is transferred to the ventral surface and sewn in place.

with chromic sutures. This step yields healthy skin that eventually will be used to form the neourethra. The second stage is performed about 6 months later. The ventral skin is tubularized over a Silastic catheter (7 French or larger) to form a neourethra. The incisions are 15 mm apart, and the edges are not elevated excessively. The neourethra is closed with a subcuticular 7-0 PDS suture. The second layer over the neourethra is local subcutaneous tissue or tunica vaginalis, and the skin is closed with interrupted 5-0 chromic sutures. A urethral stent is left in place for 10 days (Fig. 124.4).

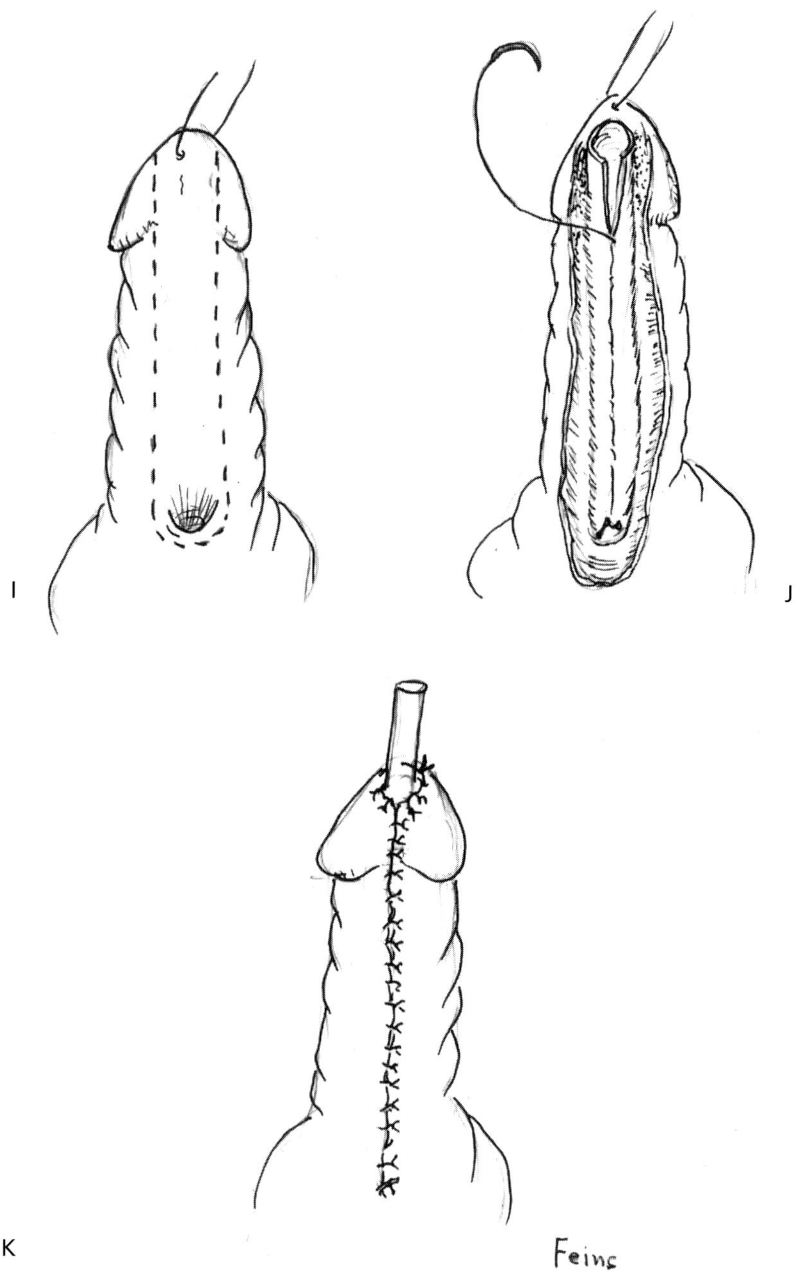

FIGURE 124.4. *Continued.* **I:** Six months later the second stage is begun with incisions 15 mm wide for tubularization. **J:** The neourethra is closed with a running subcuticular suture. **K:** The neourethra is covered by a layer of subcutaneous tissue and skin. A 7 French Silastic catheter is left in place.

SUGGESTED READINGS

Baskin LS, Duckett JW. Dorsal tunica albuginea plication (TAP) for hypospadias curvature. *J Urol* 1994;151:1668.

Devine CJ, Horton CE. Use of dermal graft to correct chordee. *J Urol* 1975;113:56.

Duckett JW. Transverse preputial island flap: technique for repair of severe hypospadias. *Urol Clin North Am* 1980;7:423.

Duckett JW, Snyder HM II. The MAGPI hypospadias repair after 1000 cases: avoidance of meatal stenosis and regression. *J Urol* 1992;147:665.

Gittes RF, McLaughlin AP III. Injection techniques to induce penile erection. *Urology* 1974;4:473.

Retik AB, Bauer SB, Mandell J, et al. Management of severe hypospadias with a two-stage repair. *J Urol* 1994;152:749.

Snodgrass W. Tubularized incised plate urethroplasty for distal hypospadias. *J Urol* 1994;151:464.

Snow BW. Use of tunica vaginalis to prevent fistulas in hypospadias surgery. *J Urol* 1986;136:861.

125

HYDROCELES AND VARICOCELES

T. ERNESTO FIGUEROA
PAT CASALE

HYDROCELES

Hydroceles can occur in infancy or childhood as the clinical manifestation of a patent processus vaginalis (communicating hydrocele), or later in life as accumulation of fluid between the visceral and parietal layers of the tunica vaginalis (noncommunicating hydrocele). The fluid content of the patent processus is peritoneal fluid, and the fluid content of the noncommunicating type is lymph fluid. In infancy, the peritoneal fluid gains free access through the patent sac. The build-up of fluid in the noncommunicating hydrocele is felt to occur because of an imbalance between the secretory and absorptive capacities of the tunica vaginalis, resulting in an accumulation of fluid. This imbalance may be primary or idiopathic, or secondary to a testicular process, such as a tumor, inflammation, infection, or trauma.

Infant hydroceles are estimated to occur in approximately 6% of healthy full-term boys. By the first birthday, the majority of these boys have shown resolution of the hydroceles, probably because of closure of the patent processus. In the absence of a hernia, surgical ligation of the patent processus is usually delayed until after the first birthday.

Diagnostic Approach

The approach to infant hydroceles is straightforward, and rarely does it require imaging studies. Demonstration of a fully decompressible or partially decompressible hydrocele is sufficient to confirm the diagnosis. A nondecompressible hydrocele in infancy is also the product of a patent processus, which may be compressed by the large hydrocele or act as a one-way valve. This latter condition usually creates the tense, large hydroceles of infancy. An extreme form of this condition is what has been labeled abdominoscrotal hydroceles. It is always intriguing to find these enormous hydroceles with a barely patent processus.

Adolescents who present with a hydrocele always pose a diagnostic concern. If the hydrocele is large, the anatomic landmarks of the testis and epididymis will not be evident. In these situations it is advisable to perform ultrasonography to assure that the testis is benign. Most of these hydroceles are primary or idiopathic.

Preoperative Preparation

Laboratory studies are not necessary for either condition. Sonographic evaluation, as indicated above, should be performed in the postpubertal boy with a large hydrocele. In infancy, if the testis is not palpable due to the large size of the hydrocele, it may be prudent to assess the area sonographically.

Fully decompressible hydroceles pose the problem that they may not be clinically evident (fully decompressed) at the time of surgery. This is critical, because most hydroceles are clinically unilateral; consequently, only one side is typically explored. It is imperative that the expected surgical site be marked in the presence of the family just prior to taking the child to the operating room to avoid the embarrassing mistake of operating on the incorrect side. Occasionally we encounter patients with a presumed hydrocele that is not evident on the clinic visit. Our approach to these patients is to inform the family of why the hydrocele is apparent only occasionally, and have them monitor the child for scrotal enlargement. Once this occurs, they call us to confirm the side of involvement. Because the majority of these cases are unilateral, we always inform the families of the 10% to 15% chance of appearance of clinically evident contralateral hydrocele.

Technical Approach

Hydroceles in infancy and childhood, as well as those that demonstrate variation in size, are always explored

T. E. Figueroa: Department of Urology, Thomas Jefferson University, Philadelphia, Pennsylvania; and Division of Pediatric Urology, Alfred I. duPont Hospital for Children, Wilmington, Delaware.

P. Casale: Department of Urology, Thomas Jefferson University, Philadelphia, Pennsylvania.

inguinally. A preincision injection of bupivicaine as an ilioinguinal nerve block is advantageous. A small, cosmetic, transverse inguinal incision over a skin crease is ideal. In infants and children, we perform the dissection distal to the external ring, after spreading the cremasteric fascia. In older boys and adolescents, the aponeurosis of the external oblique muscle is opened. Some surgeons have argued about the need to get completely around the cord, although we feel that a limited dissection is preferable. The sac is identified and gently separated from the adjacent cord structures. A high ligation is performed with much care to separate the sac from the vas deferens. A limited dissection is sufficient in the majority of cases. Occasionally, however, the testis may need to be brought into the wound to identify key structures. This maneuver carries the risk of everting the tunical space, which may preclude satisfactory scrotal placement of the testis at the end of the procedure. If there is difficulty returning the testis into the scrotum, an orchiopexy may be necessary. It is critical to pull down on the testis at the completion of the procedure to assure that the testis is in a dependent portion of the scrotum. We always tell the mothers to carry out the same maneuver daily for 7 days by lubricating their fingers with soap and gently pulling down on the testis to prevent secondary entrapment.

In postpubertal boys with the noncommunicating type of hydroceles, the approach is transscrotal. A transverse scrotal incision is made over the affected side. We usually make the skin incision and all subsequent dissection with needle tip electrocautery using the pure cut mode. This limits bleeding, one of the common complications of this type of repair. Once the dartos is incised, the bulging tunica is identified and carefully separated bluntly from the dartos muscle. After incising the tunica, the fluid is drained. This allows for evisceration of the testis. The excess sac is divided with the electrocautery, and the edges oversewn with 4-0 chromic sutures, with the tunica near the testis wrapped behind the testis and epididymis in a bottleneck fashion. The dartos and skin are closed with running layers of 4-0 chromic sutures. We do not routinely leave a drain.

Postoperative Care

The care of the infant who has undergone a hydrocele repair is straightforward. We recommend no bathing for 3 days, then slow return to usual activities. As stated previously, we instruct the mothers to pull down gently on the testis to assure that entrapment does not occur.

Postpubertal boys who have undergone a scrotal hydrocelectomy must be on restricted activity for at least 10 days. Rapid return to athletic activity may prompt the development of significant hematomas. Many of these scrota take several months to achieve a symmetric appearance, because the enlarged, thickened tunics require several weeks to months to resolve.

VARICOCELE

Abnormal dilatation of the internal spermatic vein plexus, or varicocele, is one of the most common conditions in adolescence. This condition is estimated to occur in 15% of the population, and they first become evident near the time of puberty. Ninety-five percent of varicoceles are left-sided, with the remaining 5% being bilateral. Right-sided varicoceles are rare, and should always prompt evaluation for an abdominal tumor. Varicoceles are mostly asymptomatic, usually discovered by the pediatrician during a yearly physical examination. Occasionally, the varicoceles may present with dull, heavy pain at the end of a day of standing. We have seen a handful of young men present with a large scrotal hematoma secondary to bleeding from the dilated veins after a direct injury to the scrotal area. The greatest concern about varicoceles is that they may produce testicular injury and eventually infertility. It is estimated that 50% of men attending infertility clinics are found to have a varicocele. Varicocele also represents the most common cause of correctable infertility in the male. When all of the patients with varicocele are grouped, only 20% to 30% may experience infertility. So the majority of patients with varicoceles do not go on to develop infertility. The challenge for the physician caring for the adolescent with a varicocele is to identify those patients who may be exhibiting evidence of testicular growth compromise, or testicular size asymmetry. As a general rule, if there is a difference of 30% or greater between the affected, smaller left testis and the normal-sized right testis, those patients should undergo surgical repair.

Diagnostic Approach

Examination is performed with the patient in the supine and then erect positions to document the presence and grade (I, II, III) of the varicocele. Testicular size assessment can be performed with calipers, orchidometers, or with sonography. Testicular volume can be calculated using the following formula: length $\times$ width $\times$ thickness $\times$ 0.65. If the testes are symmetric, then yearly reexaminations are performed until the patient completes puberty.

Preoperative Preparation

Once the decision is made to proceed with surgery, it is important to remind the family why this operation is being performed. We do not routinely assess sperm parameters in adolescents. The family is reminded that varicocele can recur in up to 15% of cases. Other potential complications include hydrocele formation (from ligation of lymphatic channels), injury to the vas deferens, and injury to the testicular artery.

Technical Approach

The surgical approach to the varicocele can be divided into three general categories:

- Subinguinal with or without microscopy
- Suprainguinal (open or laparoscopic) with mass ligation of the spermatic vessels including artery, or excluding the artery
- Venous embolization using radiographic techniques

Each method has ardent supporters and advocates, as well as critics. There is little consensus in the literature about the preferred approach. It appears that the most accurate and complete dissection is accomplished with a subinguinal approach under microscopic magnification. Using this technique, the testicular artery and lymphatic channels can be identified and preserved. Avoiding damage to the lymphatic channels reduces the risk for hydrocele (noncommunicating) formation. The operative table is placed in a 15 degree reversed Trendelenberg position to maximize the distention of the veins. It is useful to have a sterile Doppler probe that can be placed over a given vessel to determine if there is pulsatile, or arterial, flow. The large veins in the pampiniform plexus and the cremasteric vessels are individually ligated and divided.

Suprainguinal or Palomo procedures are simpler in that the vessels are approached prior to their branching, and can be ligated easily. Proponents of this operation cite high success rates. Division of the testicular artery potentially places the testis at risk. Hydrocele formation is also common. This procedure can be accomplished laparoscopically. Embolization techniques are not widely available and require expertise in invasive radiology.

Postoperative Care

Rest and limited activity are essential after this type of operation. Bleeding can occur initially with exertion. We routinely perform sonography on the scrotum at about 3 and 6 months after the operation to assess for testicular growth. These patients must be followed for at least 2 years after the operation to assure that they do not develop a recurrence or one of the complications of the operation.

SUGGESTED READINGS

Bloom DA, Wan J, Key D. Disorders of the male external genitalia and inguinal canal. In: Kelalis PP, King L, Belman AB, eds. *Clinical pediatric urology, 3rd ed.* New York: Harcourt, 1992:1015–1049.

Hirsch IH, Abdel-Meguid TA, Gomella LG. Postsurgical outcomes assessment following varicocele ligation: laparoscopic versus subinguinal approach. *Urology* 1985;51:810–815.

Jarrow JP, Cobur M, Sigman M. Incidence of varicoceles in men with primary and secondary infertility. *Urology* 1996;47:73–76.

Skoog SJ, Roberts KP, Goldstein M, et al. The adolescent varicocele: what's new with an old problem in young patients? *Pediatrics* 1997;100:112–122.

Turek PJ, Lipshultz LI. The varicocele controversy. *AUA Update Series* Volume XIV, Lessons 13, 14, 1995.

126

UNDESCENDED TESTIS

JULIA S. BARTHOLD

Cryptorchidism or undescended testis (UDT) is present if a testis does not reside in a normal scrotal location. In the vast majority of boys with isolated cryptorchidism, a completely developed testis is located somewhere along the normal line of descent between the internal inguinal ring and scrotum. Occasionally, the testis has "vanished" or atrophied completely due to antenatal testicular torsion; true testicular agenesis is extremely rare.

EPIDEMIOLOGY AND NATURAL HISTORY

Two percent to 5% of all newborn boys have UDT, while up to 25% of premature and small-for-gestational-age neonates are affected. Occurrence is unilateral in 65% to 75% and slightly more frequent on the right side. UDT is a heterogeneous disease whose pathogenesis is poorly understood. When occurring as an isolated entity, it may be hereditary (likely polygenic) or due to environmental or maternal hormonal influences. UDT is commonly found in combination with myelomeningocele, mental retardation, abdominal wall defects such as gastroschisis, omphalocele, and prune belly syndrome, and in association with many known syndromes. UDT is often present in combination with endocrine diseases associated with failure of testicular hormone secretion and action, such as hypogonadotrophic hypogonadism, androgen insensitivity, and deficiency of enzymes required for androgen biosynthesis. This review focuses primarily on isolated, nonsyndromic cryptorchidism.

Spontaneous descent of a testis that is undescended at birth may occur in as many as one third of cases, although secondary ascent also may occur, necessitating close follow-up during the first year of life. When testes descend, they usually do so in the first 6 months of life; any testis that remains undescended at age 1 will not attain a scrotal position without treatment. The cause of spontaneous descent is thought to be activation of the hypothalamic–pituitary–gonadal axis in the first 2 to 3 months of life with a dramatic surge in the levels of serum testosterone, luteinizing hormone (LH), and follicle-stimulating hormone (FSH). Mean levels of these hormones are lower in cryptorchid infants whose testes fail to descend as compared with levels in boys with spontaneous descent in the first year of life.

In many reported series, more than half of patients who undergo orchidopexy are of school age, despite long-standing recommendations that orchidopexy be performed prior to at least age 2. Overall, the incidence of surgery is 2 to 3 times the 1% incidence of UDT present at age 1. The reason for this discrepancy is not fully understood. In the past, it was theorized that boys with retractile testes were inappropriately undergoing orchidopexy. However, well-documented cases of testicular "ascent" have been reported in recent years in boys known to have descended testes on at least one previous examination. Some of these boys were followed closely because of marked testicular retractility by experienced examiners and eventually diagnosed with true UDT. The true incidence and etiology of this phenomenon are unclear. Ascended testes are sometimes found in the superficial inguinal pouch at the time of surgery, suggesting that their increased mobility may have allowed scrotal positioning in infancy that was no longer possible with continued linear growth. Some investigators theorize that ascent is due in some cases to abnormalities of the processus vaginalis. These include abnormal closure resulting in a tethering fibrous band or lack of closure allowing proximal migration of the testis. Limited data suggest that germ cell development may be as impaired in ascended testes as is found in primary cryptorchidism.

Clear histologic changes are evident in the UDT as early as the second year of life; these are characterized primarily by failure of transformation of gonocytes to differentiated spermatogonia with reduction in total germ cell counts. Some studies suggest that germ cell development may even be impaired prior to birth. In later childhood, further premeiotic maturation of the germinal epithelium is impaired. Leydig cell atrophy in infancy and Sertoli cell abnormalities

J. S. Barthold: Department of Urology, Thomas Jefferson University, Philadelphia, Pennsylvania; and Division of Urology, Alfred I. duPont Hospital for Children, Wilmington, Delaware.

are also reported. Abnormal germ cell development is also reported frequently in the contralateral scrotal testis of boys with unilateral UDT, suggesting that a global developmental or endocrine defect may be present. Another finding that supports this is the high frequency of epididymal anomalies in boys with UDT. In order of occurrence, these include failure of normal suspension, incomplete fusion with the testis, atresia, and agenesis. Inguinal hernia is present ipsilaterally in up to 90% of infants with UDT but is less common in older boys and is rarely clinically evident. Hypospadias is seen in up to 10% of boys with nonsyndromic UDT.

Left untreated, about one third of cryptorchid testes lack germ cells by age 2. By puberty, Sertoli cell–only histology is expected. The risk for germ cell tumor is greater in the UDT, and may not be substantially reduced by orchidopexy. These tumors are thought to originate in untransformed gonocytes that remain dormant until after puberty. Other problems that occur more frequently in boys with untreated UDT include spermatic cord torsion (Fig. 126.1) and incarcerated inguinal hernia. It is therefore critical to identify the position of the testis in infants presenting with a tender inguinal mass. A cryptorchid testis not placed in the scrotum at the time of inguinal hernia repair will require subsequent, often tedious, orchidopexy associated with a higher risk for testicular injury. Conversely, testes may become secondarily cryptorchid after routine inguinal surgery, even if care is taken to palpate the testis in the scrotum at the conclusion of the case. These testes do not appear to have the same risk for germ cell maldevelopment, at least in the short term, or malignancy, as does the primary UDT.

DIAGNOSIS

Identification of testicular position can be notoriously difficult. In newborns, a large hydrocele may be present, which limits palpation of the hemiscrotum. In boys between 6 months of age and puberty, the normal testis is typically retractile, with brisk contraction of the cremaster muscle occurring in response to a variety of stimuli.

Examination should begin with careful inspection of the genitalia. Scrotal asymmetry is highly suggestive of unilateral UDT. Other abnormalities of genital development suggesting a possible endocrine disorder, such as micropenis or hypospadias, should be identified if present. If one testis is not palpable, contralateral testicular hypertrophy characterized by a volume of 2 mL or greater is suggestive but not diagnostic of monorchia.

If possible, the patient should be examined initially in an upright, cross-legged position to inhibit the cremaster reflex. Retractile testes usually descend spontaneously if the patient is relaxed in this position. If the testis is not in the scrotum during this initial maneuver, the patient should be examined in the supine position with legs

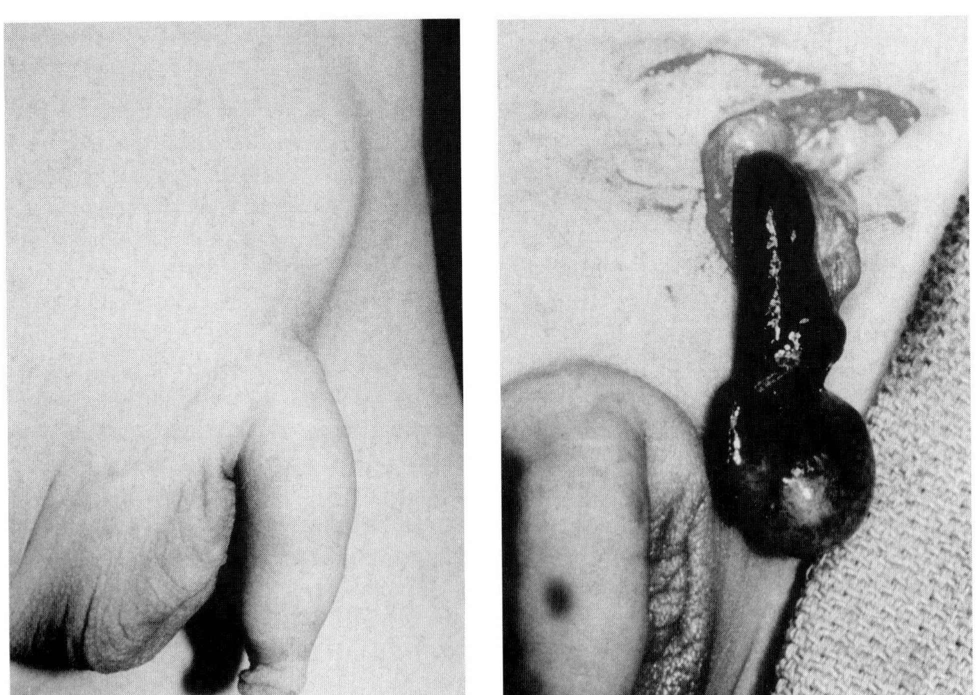

A B

FIGURE 126.1. Torsion of an undescended testis. **A:** Inguinal mass visible. **B:** Nonviable testis found at the time of inguinal exploration.

abducted. Other methods to reduce cremaster muscle hyperactivity include a warm room, warm examining hands, and distraction of the patient. If the testis is palpable, transfer to a dependent scrotal position should be attempted. When the testis does not remain in the scrotum for any length of time, particularly after stretching of the cremaster muscle or if the cord feels tight, it is undescended. If the examination is difficult or equivocal, a subsequent examination should be scheduled.

If the testis is not palpable, it may become so with gentle milking along the inguinal canal or with application of soap to the examiner's hands. Care should be taken to examine possible ectopic sites, such as the prepenile, femoral, and perineal (Fig. 126.2) areas. Despite careful examination, 10% to 20% of UDTs are nonpalpable. However, other structures may be palpable that should not confuse the examiner. These include ductal structures within the canal or a small, 1- to 2-mm nubbin of firm tissue in the scrotum. Palpation of the epididymis does not confirm that the testis is extraabdominal, because complete separation of the two structures may occur. A nubbin palpable in the scrotum is suggestive of a "vanishing" testis, particularly if contralateral testicular hypertrophy is present. Findings at surgery for nonpalpable testes indicate that vanishing testes are most common (43%), followed by intraabdominal testes (36%) and extra-abdominal viable testes (21%). Bilaterally nonpalpable testes are found in the abdomen or inguinal canal in over 90% of cases.

Imaging studies are rarely useful for preoperative localization of testes. Ultrasonography does not identify testes proximal to the internal inguinal ring, and often identify testes as being inguinal in normal boys whose testes retract in response to the examination. It is useful only for documenting testicular size after secondary or recurrent cryptorchidism and for identifying inguinal testes in obese older boys with nonpalpable testes. Magnetic resonance imaging with gadolinium injection also may occasionally be useful in obese boys or after failure to identify a testis during inguinal or abdominal exploration. However, the most effective method for localizing and potentially treating the nonpalpable testis is laparoscopy.

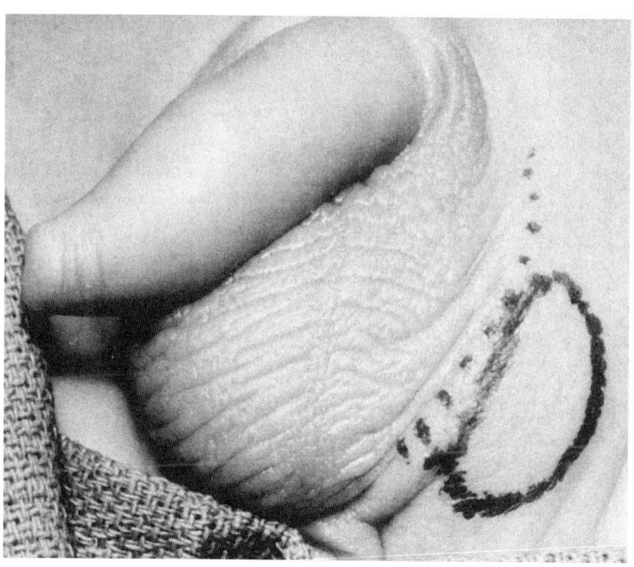

FIGURE 126.2. Patient with a left perineal testis and underdevelopment of the ipsilateral hemiscrotum.

TREATMENT

Intervention is indicated if the testis fails to descend spontaneously or if cryptorchidism is initially diagnosed after the first year of life. Orchidopexy prevents torsion and clinical hernia, minimizes psychologic concerns, reduces the risk of infertility, and allows reliable self-examination to identify tumor. Treatment options include surgery or hormonal therapy with either LH-releasing hormone (LHRH) or human chorionic gonadotropin (HCG).

In the United States, intranasal LHRH is not available, so intramuscular HCG is used. Regimens vary widely, with duration of treatment ranging from 1 day to 1 year, although HCG is usually given in a series of 3 or 10 doses given over 1 to 2 weeks. Careful review of the results of hormone therapy suggests that this approach is only occasionally effective. Randomized studies indicate poorer results than nonrandomized studies or studies in which retractile testes were specifically excluded. These results show success rates of 12% to 20% at the conclusion of therapy, although recurrence may occur in 25% to 50% of patients after long-term follow-up. Testes closer to the scrotum are more likely to respond to hormonal therapy. However, some data suggest that hormonal therapy is not only less effective in infants than in older boys but may inhibit germ cell development in the younger age group. The most important use of HCG may be differentiation of retractile from truly undescended testes in selected cases because hormone therapy inhibits testicular retractility.

Surgery is the standard treatment for UDT at any age. In recent years, the timing of recommended orchidopexy has progressively decreased, because spontaneous descent is rare after 6 months and histologic deterioration of the testis likely begins within the first year of life. No data are available to suggest that surgical risk is greater in infants. In fact, orchidopexy may be easier in a small infant after recent exposure to the endogenous hormone production that occurs at 2 to 3 months of age. Orchidopexy is usually performed as an outpatient. The first step should always be reexamination of the patient under anesthesia, because almost one fifth of testes that were nonpalpable during the office examination may become palpable, changing the surgical approach. Rarely, UDT may descend into normal scrotal position under anesthesia. The procedure should not be aborted unless the testis is in a truly dependent position under no tension, because continued concerns about UDT being present and eventual return to the operating room are likely. A special category is the patient with UDT who is already pubertal or postpubertal. Orchiectomy is reasonable in many of these cases if the UDT is unilateral. If orchidopexy is performed, the testis should be sampled by biopsy to rule out carcinoma *in situ.*

The optimal approach to orchidopexy depends primarily on whether the testis is palpable or nonpalpable.

Palpable Testes

A standard low inguinal incision beginning superolateral to the pubic tubercle is appropriate for routine orchidopexy. Isolation of the spermatic cord and testis from within the cremaster muscle and fascia as described by Redman is useful, particularly in reoperative cases. After the testis is delivered, the internal spermatic fascia is incised and the hernia sac isolated and ligated at the level of the internal inguinal ring. Often these maneuvers provide sufficient length for easy placement of the testis in the scrotum. If not, lateral retroperitoneal bands can be identified along the cord and incised to provide additional length. Other options include further mobilization of the cord by incising the transversalis fascia at the level of the internal ring. This allows higher retroperitoneal dissection and transposition of the cord medial to the epigastric vessels, if needed, to allow a more direct route for the testis into the scrotum. If the spermatic vessels are unusually short, the incision may be extended cephalad through the internal oblique muscle or a counterincision made and the vessels mobilized trans- or retroperitoneally.

Prior to scrotal placement of the testis, it should be measured, the epididymal anatomy documented, and any appendiceal structures removed. Testicular volume can be calculated by the formula 0.7(length)(width)(depth) or 0.7(length)(width^2). A scrotal pouch is created, usually between the skin and the dartos layer, and hemostasis assured. Tension on the testis should be minimized and the cord straightened prior to transfer of the testis into the scrotum. The tunica vaginalis should be opened completely. The testis should be immobilized in the scrotal pouch by closure of the neck of the pouch enough to prevent retraction out of the scrotum. Fixation of the testis itself using transparenchymal sutures is not recommended because of the risk of vascular injury and the demonstrated association with lower fertility potential. Instead, absorbable sutures are placed between the tunica vaginalis and dartos layers to provide fixation. Fixation of the testis extravaginally provides enough inflammatory reaction to maintain the testis within the scrotum in the vast majority of cases. In fact, testicular torsion has been reported after orchidopexy only when the testis is left within an intact tunica vaginalis, and can occur in this circumstance even when permanent suture fixation through the parenchyma is used.

Nonpalpable Testes

When both testes are nonpalpable, additional workup is useful, particularly to rule out congenital adrenal hyperplasia with severe masculinization of the phallus in a genotypic female. In genotypic males with bilateral nonpalpable testes, the combination of high serum FSH and absent testosterone response to HCG stimulation is diagnostic of anorchia. However, even in these cases and most cases of unilateral nonpalpable testes, laparoscopy is a reliable and useful adjunct. When used appropriately, laparoscopy can confirm the presence and position or absence of a testis in essentially every patient. It may be especially useful in boys who have had a previous surgical exploration that failed to identify spermatic vessels or testis. In addition, laparoscopic surgery can be used to either remove or mobilize an abdominal testis into the scrotum.

Many pediatric urologists and surgeons use an open Hasson technique for placement of the umbilical trocar unless 2-mm instrumentation is used, because the risk of injury to abdominal contents is lower. The inguinal anatomy on the side of the descended testis, if present, is viewed first to provide a reference (Fig. 126.3A). The spermatic vessels, extending caudally, and the vas deferens, coursing laterally, should be easily visualized at their confluence at the internal inguinal ring, which should be closed. If the vas deferens and vessels end abruptly prior to reaching the internal ring (Fig. 126.3B), the diagnosis of abdominal vanishing testis is made, and the procedure is terminated. If the vas deferens and vessels are atretic (i.e., substantially reduced in diameter) but course through a closed inguinal ring, a high likelihood of scrotal or, less commonly, inguinal vanishing testis is present. Management of this entity is controversial. Many surgeons advocate making a low inguinal incision over the external ring and excising the distal testicular remnant, which contains testicular tissue in 0 to 10% of cases. Other surgeons advocate no additional surgery if the cord is atretic, because vanishing testes contain viable tubules so rarely and the risk of malignant degeneration is negligible because antenatal torsion is the likely etiology. Despite the low risk of torsion of the remaining scrotal testis, many surgeons perform scrotal orchidopexy on that side to reduce the risk of catastrophic subsequent loss due to trauma or torsion.

When a normal spermatic cord traverses the internal ring, particularly if a hernia is present (Fig. 126.4A), a testis is likely present within the inguinal canal and inguinal exploration is necessary. Up to half of the testes that are found in these cases may be atrophic, however. Certainly, if an inguinal hernia is identified ipsilateral to a scrotal testis during diagnostic laparoscopy, repair is indicated.

If an abdominal testis is visualized by laparoscopy (Fig. 126.4B and C), several options exist. If the vas deferens takes a long, looping course, extending caudally within the inguinal canal and then cranially to the testis, a one- or two-

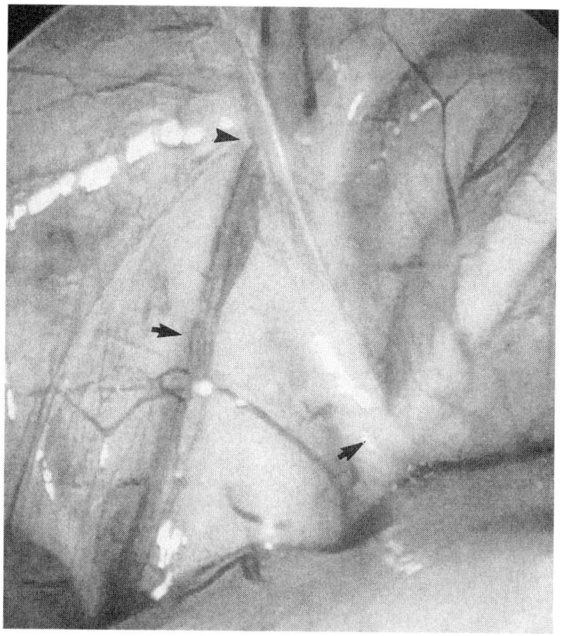

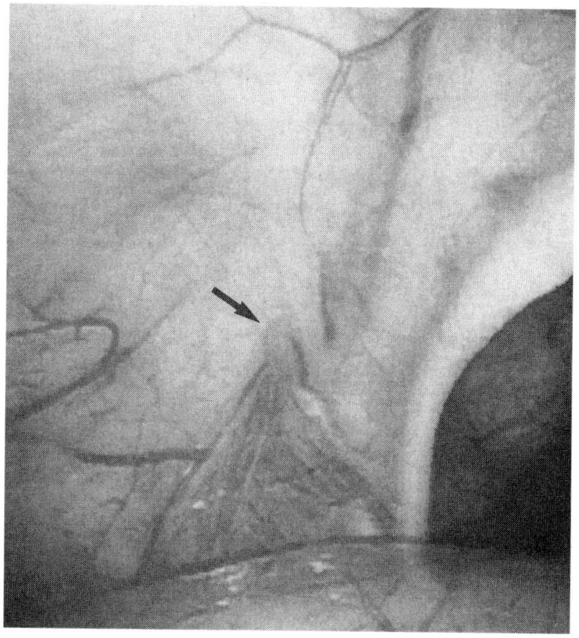

FIGURE 126.3. Laparoscopy for diagnosis of vanishing testis. **A:** Normal left inguinal anatomy. Note normal vas deferens and spermatic vessels (*arrows*) exiting the closed internal inguinal ring (*arrowhead*). **B:** Intraabdominal vanishing testis. Note abrupt termination of spermatic cord (*arrow*) proximal to a closed internal inguinal ring.

stage Fowler-Stephens orchidopexy with transection of the spermatic vessels may be considered. A decision to proceed with this approach must be made prior to mobilization of the testis, because viability of the testis is dependent on preservation of the collateral vessels between the distal remnant of the spermatic vessels and the vas deferens. The single-stage Fowler-Stephens orchidopexy is usually performed as an open procedure but can be performed laparoscopically. The two-stage Fowler-Stephens procedure involves laparoscopic clipping of the vessels with completion of the orchidopexy surgically or laparoscopically 6 months later.

If the testis is within a few centimeters of the internal inguinal ring, preservation of the spermatic vessels is preferable. The orchidopexy can be performed laparoscopically or via an open preperitoneal (Jones) approach. The laparoscopic approach requires placement of two additional trocars in the lower abdominal quadrants. Mobilization of the spermatic vessels all the way to the renal hilum with release of the peritoneal attachments is possible with good visualization under magnification. Percutaneous techniques can be used to create a neoexternal ring medial to the medial umbilical ligament and bring the testis directly into the scrotum. Formal closure of a patent processus vaginalis does not appear to be necessary in these cases. Alternatively, the Jones approach may be used to achieve the same result. By using laparoscopy first, the surgeon can choose a standard orchidopexy incision or the higher Jones incision located medial to the anterior superior iliac spine depending on the position of the testis. Both the Jones approach and laparoscopic orchidopexy reduce the need for transection of the spermatic vessels, orchiectomy, or the outdated and risky two-stage open surgical orchidopexy.

Special consideration is required if both testes are abdominal or a solitary abdominal testis is present. For bilateral abdominal testes, the procedures should be staged with an interval of 6 months between procedures. If atrophy of one testis occurs, testicular autotransplantation by an experienced team should be considered because it may provide the most reliable method for bringing a solitary abdominal testis into the scrotum, particularly one in a high abdominal position. This procedure can be performed successfully even in very young boys, but should be performed by a specialized team with experience in performing the procedure. At the very least, an abdominal testis should be brought into a palpable position so that endocrine function can be maintained and surveillance for malignancy is possible.

If no spermatic vessels are seen by laparoscopic endoscopy via the umbilical port, a second trocar may be placed in the ipsilateral lower quadrant to facilitate visualization of the anterior aspect of the psoas up to the renal hilum. Using two established ports, excision of a very high testis or a testis in a pubertal boy can be expedited.

Other unusual findings may be encountered at the time of orchidopexy, particularly when testes are nonpalpable. Boys with persistent müllerian duct syndrome have normal external genitalia but development of uterus, tubes, and vasa internally. Unilateral or bilateral UDT, transverse testicular ectopy (both testes on the same side), and hernias are common. Excision of at least some portions of the tubes and uterus is usually necessary to allow orchidopexy, but

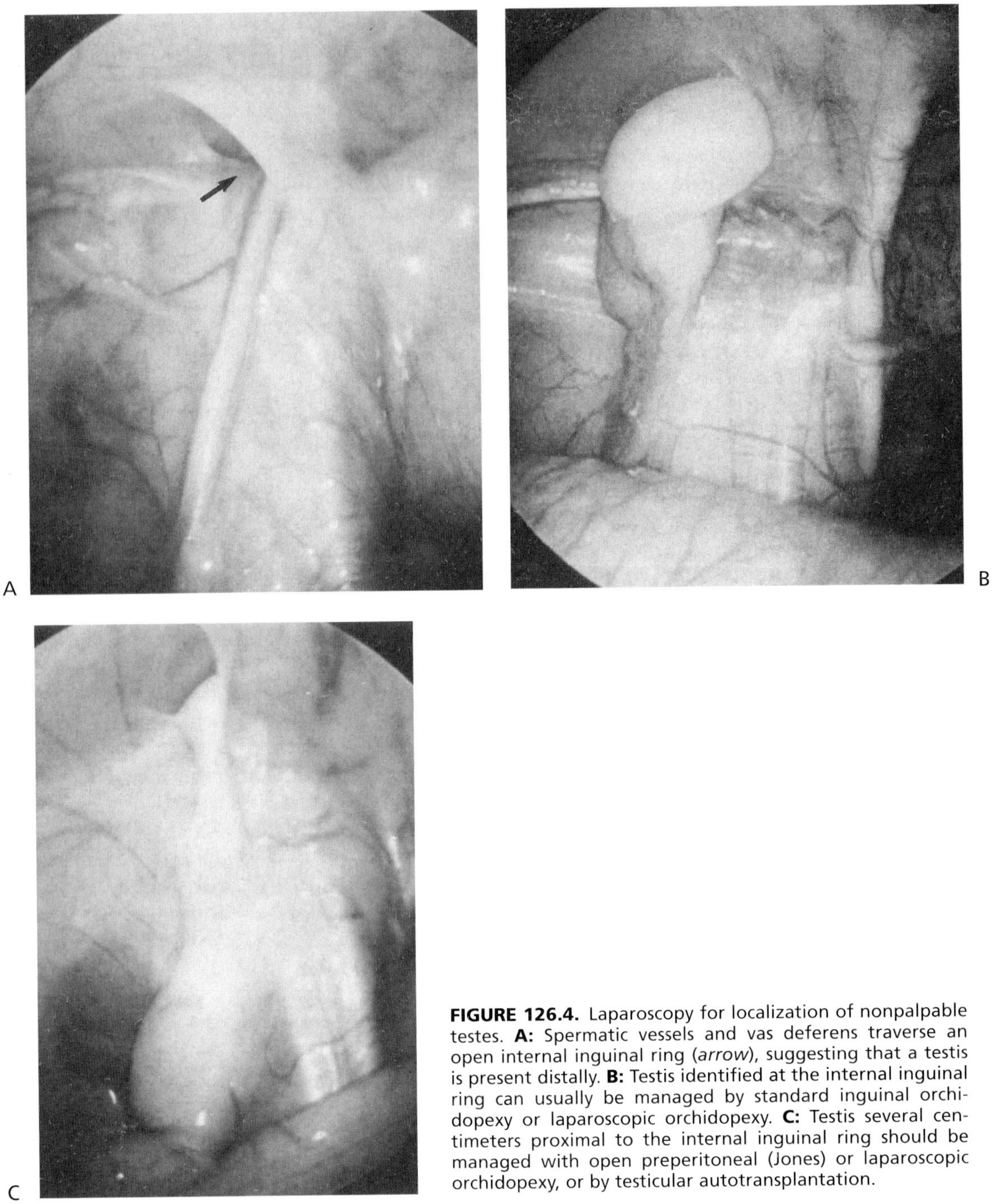

FIGURE 126.4. Laparoscopy for localization of nonpalpable testes. **A:** Spermatic vessels and vas deferens traverse an open internal inguinal ring (*arrow*), suggesting that a testis is present distally. **B:** Testis identified at the internal inguinal ring can usually be managed by standard inguinal orchidopexy or laparoscopic orchidopexy. **C:** Testis several centimeters proximal to the internal inguinal ring should be managed with open preperitoneal (Jones) or laparoscopic orchidopexy, or by testicular autotransplantation.

care must be taken to avoid injury to the vasa. Another form of intersex that may occasionally be associated with nonambiguous genitalia is partial gonadal dysgenesis. This entity includes a spectrum of abnormal gonadal development, including true hermaphroditism (ovarian and testicular tissue both present) and testicular or mixed gonadal dysgenesis. These patients also have some degree of müllerian ductal development. Although the testicular portion of ovotestes may be retained and placed in the scrotum, abdominal streak or dysgenetic gonads should be removed because of a substantial risk for malignancy.

POSTOPERATIVE RESULTS AND COMPLICATIONS

The results and complication rates of the various types of orchidopexy depend on the severity of the cryptorchidism and the surgical technique. Success should be determined by observing an intrascrotal testis without atrophy at least 6 months postoperatively. For testes that are originally abdominal, canalicular, and distal to the external ring, success rates are 75% to 77%, 84% to 96%, and 92% to 100%, respectively. Two-stage orchidopexy and the single-stage Fowler-Stephens procedure fail in approximately one third of cases. Staged transection of the spermatic vessels appears to be more successful, particularly if both stages are performed laparoscopically, and transabdominal mobilization without vessel transection is successful in 80% to 95% of cases. Success rates for laparoscopic orchidopexy are over 90% in recent series. Microvascular orchidopexy is successful in 84% to 95% and standard inguinal orchidopexy in over 88% of cases. In general, success rates are higher in boys undergoing surgery prior to 6 years of age. Preservation of blood flow through the spermatic vessels should be achieved whenever possible.

Complications of orchidopexy include bleeding, infection, testicular retraction or atrophy, and injury to the vas deferens or epididymis. Laparoscopy introduces risk of bleeding or injury of intraabdominal contents. If atrophy of an intrascrotal testis is documented, no further intervention is necessary. However, if retraction out of the scrotum occurs, repeat orchidopexy or orchiectomy, depending on the size of the testis and age of the patient, should be performed. The surgeon may consider the use of HCG in some cases of redo orchidopexy to stimulate spermatic cord lengthening. Some surgeons recommend its use preoperatively in patients with abdominal testes in an attempt to stimulate extraabdominal migration of the testis and facilitate primary orchidopexy.

PROGNOSIS

Impaired spermatogenesis is common in men with a history of UDT. Oligospermia or azoospermia is present in up to 50% and 100% of men with a history of unilateral and bilateral cryptorchidism, respectively. These data support the biopsy data showing that germ cell development is also impaired in the scrotal testis of boys with unilateral UDT. Although testicular biopsies at the time of orchidopexy correlate overall with long-term fertility potential, their predictive value in individual cases is questionable. Furthermore, early data, not yet independently confirmed, suggest that the risk for malignancy may be higher when testicular biopsy is performed at the time of orchidopexy.

Although semen analysis data suggest that the risk for infertility is high in previously cryptorchid men, careful paternity studies suggest that the conception rate in those with only one testis affected is not significantly different from that of normal men. About 50% of men with a history of bilateral UDT report paternity. Although paternity data are not always reliable, it is well known that sperm counts alone are not always indicative of fertility potential. Nevertheless, some clinicians recommend that low, stimulatory doses of an LHRH analogue be used after orchidopexy to maximize germ cell counts and, hopefully, future sperm production. The effectiveness of this approach has not been confirmed in rigorous studies, but it may be most useful in bilateral cases of UDT in which the risk of infertility is significant.

Testicular germ cell tumors are more common in men with a history of UDT, and may even occur in the contralateral scrotal testis. These tumors occur after puberty in 1% or less of patients. The presence of carcinoma *in situ* indicates a high (at least 50%) chance of subsequent malignancy. Although orchidopexy does not appear to reduce the risk for malignancy, the biology of the tumor appears to be affected by surgery. Tumors occurring in testes after previous successful orchidopexy are more frequently nonseminomatous germ cell tumors, whereas seminomas are more common in untreated abdominal testes.

SUMMARY

Nonsyndromic cryptorchidism is one of the most common congenital anomalies. The cause is unknown, but is likely multifactorial. The risk is higher in boys born prematurely or who are small for gestational age. About one third of undescended testes descend in the first year of life, usually within 6 months. After 6 months of age, testicular retractility is common, and accurate examination may be difficult. Evaluation by an experienced examiner is mandatory in questionable cases.

Treatment should begin by 6 to 12 months of age to reduce the long-term risks to the testis. Surgical treatment is much more effective than hormonal therapy, but the success of each is dependent on many factors, particularly the position of the testis. If the testis is nonpalpable, laparoscopy is the most reliable technique for localization; imaging studies are rarely used. Abdominal testes appear to survive best when spermatic artery–sparing techniques are used for orchidopexy. Final results of any therapy used should be determined at least 6 months after treatment is completed. Although spermatogenesis is impaired in many men with previous UDT, earlier surgery may minimize this effect and the likelihood of paternity in unilateral cases is high. Malignancy is rare, but patients should be educated about the risk and taught testicular self-examination after puberty.

Some cases of UDT present initially at older ages. At present, it is unclear if these are true examples of testicular ascent or are due to failure or inability to diagnose the problem in infancy. Nevertheless, it is clearly imperative that serial examination of the testes continue until puberty, particularly when the testes are markedly retractile.

SUGGESTED READINGS

Baker LA, Docimo SG, Surer I, et al. A multi-institutional analysis of laparoscopic orchidopexy. *BJU Int* 2001;87:484–489.

Cendron M, Huff DS, Keating MA, et al. Anatomical, morphological and volumetric analysis: a review of 759 cases of testicular maldescent. *J Urol* 1993;149:570–573.

Cisek LJ, Peters CA, Atala A, et al. Current findings in diagnostic laparoscopic evaluation of the nonpalpable testis. *J Urol* 1998; 160:1145–1149.

Docimo SG. The results of surgical therapy for cryptorchidism: a literature review and analysis. *J Urol* 1995;154:1148–1152.

Gheiler EL, Barthold JS, González R. Benefits of laparoscopy and the Jones technique for the nonpalpable testis. *J Urol* 1997;158: 1948–1951.

Gill B, Kogan S. Cryptorchidism: current concepts. *Pediatr Clin North Am* 1997;44:1211–1227.

Lee PA. Consequence of cryptorchidism: relationship to etiology and treatment. *Curr Probl Pediatr* 1995;5:232–236.

Mayr JM, Lawrenz K, Berghold A. Undescended testicles: an epidemiological review. *Acta Paediatr* 1999;88:1089–1093.

Pyorala S, Huttennen N-P, Uhari M. A review and meta-analysis of hormonal treatment of cryptorchidism. *J Clin Endocrinol Metab* 1995;80:2795–2799.

Redman JF. Inguinal reoperation for undescended testis and hernia: approach to the spermatic cord through the cremaster fascia. *J Urol* 2000;164:1705–1707.

Toppari J, Kaleva M. Maldescendus testis. *Horm Res* 1999;51: 261–269.

127

THE ACUTE SCROTUM

T. ERNESTO FIGUEROA
PAT CASALE

The acute scrotum refers to the clinical presentation characterized by the hallmarks of *pain and swelling* of the scrotum. This presentation is always considered an emergency, because the potential for testicular loss is real. Delay in the recognition and management of this presentation can result in loss of the testis, infertility, and possibly subsequent legal action against the managing physicians and hospital. The accurate diagnosis of the condition producing the acute scrotum is often limited by the similarity in presentation and physical findings of the different causes of acute painful scrotal swelling. Radiographic techniques, although helpful, do not have absolute sensitivity and specificity, and obtaining a study may cause a delay in the management of the problem. Surgical intervention might be required for diagnostic and therapeutic reasons, but many patients do not require surgical intervention. The old axiom "when in doubt, operate" is always the correct approach in patients presenting with an acute scrotal condition.

Painless swelling of the scrotum, although it can occur acutely, is not addressed in this chapter. Some of the conditions that may produce painless swelling of the scrotum include hydroceles and hernias, testicular masses, lymphedema, and postsurgical scrotal wall edema.

DIFFERENTIAL DIAGNOSIS

Four conditions account for the majority of the cases of acute scrotum: spermatic cord torsion (testicular torsion), which includes extravaginal and intravaginal torsion; torsion of a testicular appendage; acute epididymitis; and testicular injury due to trauma. Each of these conditions is discussed individually in relation to history, physical findings, laboratory findings, radiographic tools, and surgical approaches.

T. E. Figueroa: Department of Urology, Thomas Jefferson University, Philadelphia, Pennsylvania; and Division of Pediatric Urology, Alfred I. duPont Hospital for Children, Wilmington, Delaware.

P. Casale: Department of Urology, Thomas Jefferson University, Philadelphia, Pennsylvania.

THE AGE FACTOR

These conditions can occur in any age group, and the conditions should not be excluded based on the age of the patient. However, there is a relationship between the age of the patient and the likely etiology of the acute presentation. In general terms, neonates present with an extravaginal torsion of the spermatic cord. In childhood and preadolescent years, the most common presentation is torsion of the testicular or epididymal appendages. As the testes increase in size during adolescence, particularly at the onset of puberty, the most likely presentation is intravaginal torsion of the spermatic cord. If the patient is sexually active, then epididymitis is a strong consideration. In non–sexually active males, epididymitis is exceptionally rare. Based on these generalizations, a pubertal, non–sexually active boy presenting with an acute scrotal condition should be considered to have testicular torsion until proven otherwise, and urgent surgical exploration is always indicated. If the boy is sexually active, the history and laboratory findings, as well as radiographic studies, should allow the physician to differentiate epididymitis from spermatic cord torsion. In prepubertal boys, the diagnosis of torsion of a testicular appendage can usually be made with certainty based on history and physical findings, unless the inflammatory process is advanced and the physical landmarks are obscured by the inflammatory mass. In that scenario, surgical exploration is the most definitive management because it accurately confirms the diagnosis.

DIAGNOSTIC APPROACH

Spermatic Cord Torsion

The most serious of these conditions is spermatic cord torsion. Two types of torsion have been described: extravaginal and intravaginal torsions.

Extravaginal torsions involve all of the elements of the cord. This type of torsion has traditionally been described to occur in the neonate, although some recent studies have questioned this long-standing belief. The torsion occurs due to poor attachments of the tunica vaginalis to the adjacent dartos muscle. This allows the cord to twist, resulting in severe ischemia, necrosis, and loss to the gonad. These events invariably occur prenatally, and always lead to loss of the affected testis. Depending on when in pregnancy the torsion occurs, the presentation can range from edematous and fixed scrotal skin with an indurated intrascrotal mass (closer to the time of delivery), to a marble-like testis without any associated scrotal skin changes, to a vanished testis (early in pregnancy). The skin may be discolored or appear bruised. Torsion that occurs in the immediate postnatal time has been reported, but it is extremely rare. It is not unusual to receive a call from the nursery to see a neonate with an indurated hemiscrotum after an initial "normal" examination of the scrotum. Laboratory findings are usually not helpful in this condition. Differential diagnoses include incarcerated hernia, tense hydrocele, or a neonatal testicular tumor. We have found that scrotal ultrasonography in this scenario is often useful to distinguish an acute event from a chronic torsion, based on the sonographic appearance of the testicular parenchyma (echo-texture). Ultrasonography in the acute event will show normal testicular parenchyma, whereas the appearance of a chronic torsion is a nonhomogeneous parenchyma, with areas of fluid echoes, representing liquefied necrosis, and a calcified rim around the testis, representing secondary atrophic changes and resolving inflammation. The presence or absence of blood flow by Doppler techniques is not a reliable finding in neonates in whom the testicular vessels are extremely small. We have seen good pulsatile Doppler flow in testes later found to be necrotic at exploration, and also we have failed to see flow in perfectly normal testes.

The decision to operate or not in a neonate with a suspected testicular torsion rests on the availability of competent and experienced pediatric anesthesia. In a general hospital, where the majority of these babies are delivered, around-the-clock pediatric anesthesia is not always available. In that case, the decision to be made is whether to transfer the baby to a facility with pediatric anesthesia services or not. Transferring the newborn entails separation from the family, significant parental anxiety, and the risks associated with the anesthesia of a newborn. These are important considerations, because these testes are rarely salvageable. The family should never be given the impression that surgery is likely to save these testes. The main reason to operate, however, is to perform a prophylactic orchiopexy on the normal testis to minimize the low risk of subsequent torsion. Asynchronous testicular torsion has been reported, prompting many pediatric urologists and surgeons to offer exploration in the neonatal period.

Bilateral prenatal torsion also can occur. Using the diagnostic capabilities of ultrasonography, the findings of chronic changes in the testes make immediate surgical exploration an exercise in futility, because neither testis is likely to be salvageable.

The surgical approach can be either transscrotal or inguinal, although we tend to prefer the inguinal approach to explore the affected side. We usually approach the benign side through a scrotal approach, open the tunica vaginalis, and probe the processus. If the processus is patent, a small inguinal incision is necessary to perform a high ligation. If the processus is not patent, the tunica vaginalis is everted and its edges attached to the adjacent dartos muscle with absorbable sutures. The most important step is to evert the tunica vaginalis and expose the tunica albuginea of the testis to the dartos. The affected testis is removed. When the decision is made not to operate in the newborn period, we advise the parents to be vigilant about the appearance of the scrotum and to notify us immediately if there is any change. We continue to advocate prophylactic orchiopexy of the remaining testis, although we recognize that the incidence of torsion in the untreated testis is small.

Intravaginal torsions are believed to occur after infancy due to the so-called bell-clapper deformity, or narrow attachment of the testis within the tunica vaginalis. The testis can swing within the tunical space, like a bell-clapper, and torsion can result. As indicated previously, these are more likely to occur in the pubertal young man, because the testes grow rapidly during puberty. These torsions occur predominantly from lateral to medial, and may be 180 to 720 degrees, or more, in severity. The result is vascular compromise and ischemic changes in the testis. Traditionally, the timing from torsion to salvage by detorsion has been said to be 6 to 8 hours. However, this is highly variable, because the more severe the torsion, the more complete the vascular compromise, and the shorter the likelihood of survival.

These events produce intense immediate pain. The pain may occur at any time, and it may or may not be related to physical activity. Sometimes the patient is awakened by the pain. Examination early on shows a retracted testis with unusual landmarks, because the epididymis may be anterior, superior, or even inferior depending on the number of twists of the cord. The testis is diffusely tender. The cremasteric reflex should be absent in these patients, but this is not a reliable sign. Later presentation is usually clouded by the associated hydrocele formation and scrotal wall edema. Radiographic studies, although interesting, have no role in the management of suspected spermatic cord torsion. The management of these events is urgent surgical exploration, keeping in mind that this is a race against time. When the patient presents early on (within 6 hours of onset), it is worthwhile to try to detorse the cord manually. We follow the metaphor of "opening the book" to approach manual detorsion. The testis is untwisted medially to laterally. When this results in resolution of the event, there is immediate relief of the pain and elongation of the cord. This is a useful guideline, but it is important to be aware that torsions can also occur in the opposite direction.

If manual detorsion cannot be accomplished, or if there is too much edema and inflammation, then immediate surgical exploration is mandatory. At surgery, a midline scrotal raphe incision works well. The affected side is approached first, untwisted, and placed in warm saline-soaked pads. The benign side is exposed, and the tunica vaginalis is opened and everted. The traditional approach has been to place nonabsorbable sutures in three fixing points between the tunica albuginea and the adjacent dartos. Others have advocated creating a dartos pouch, as is done with a standard orchiopexy, and fixing the edges of the everted tunica vaginalis to the dartos with absorbable suture. This approach avoids placing sutures directly into the testis. Once the benign side is fixed, attention is directed to the involved testis. If the testis appears viable, then fixation is performed. If the testis does not appear viable, then it is removed. If untreated, the torsed testis will undergo progressive ischemic damage, seminiferous tubular cell death, necrosis, and atrophy.

A special condition deserves mentioning: *intermittent (subacute) spermatic cord torsion*. These patients experience intermittent episodes of severe testicular pain, which resolve spontaneously within a short period of time. Most of these cases are in young pubertal boys. When witnessed, these are easily recognized, because these boys are in excruciating pain with the physical findings of a retracted or elevated, tender testis. Then suddenly it resolves. Testicular technetium scanning shortly after the resolution of the pain shows a classic "hyperemia response." The management of choice is elective surgical fixation as soon as possible. A problem occurs, however, when the history is not diagnostic, and the episodes are unwitnessed. Some of these patients may be experiencing orchialgia unrelated to torsion, which would not warrant surgical exploration. This is a difficult dilemma, and we often elect to monitor these patients and tell them to contact us as soon as the pain episode occurs.

Torsion of the Testicular Appendages

One of the most common urologic presentations to the emergency room is torsion of the testicular appendages. These appendages represent vestigial remnants of the wolffian duct (appendix epididymis) or müllerian duct (appendix testis). Both of these are located in the apical portion of the testis, near the head of the epididymis; thus they produce identical symptoms. Unlike torsions of the spermatic cord, torsions of the appendages do not pose any risk to the testes. The natural history is for these events to resolve spontaneously without sequelae.

These patients are typically prepubertal, 7 to 11 years of age. The pain comes acutely and may be mild or severe. The pain tends to improve after a few hours. Its onset is not associated with any specific activity, although many patients indicate anecdotally that they were hit in the scrotum with an object when they first developed pain. When examined early on, prior to any inflammatory changes of the skin, the elusive "blue dot sign" may be identified, representing the congested, torsed appendage. When asked to point to the area of pain, these boys can pinpoint the area with the tip of their index finger. With time, inflammatory changes may become evident: erythema of the superior portion of the involved hemiscrotum, hydrocele formation, thickening of the tunica vaginalis, and lastly, reactive epididymitis. It is this latter associated event that can create a diagnostic quandary. The initial torsion is a limited event, localized to the uppermost aspect of the testis. However, when secondary reactive epididymitis occurs, the pain becomes more diffuse, the inflammatory changes more widespread, and the evaluation more difficult. When the inflammatory changes are advanced, it may be impossible to distinguish this condition from torsion of the spermatic cord.

Sonographic assessment at this stage shows a hyperemic appearance with an enlarged epididymis. One of the shortcomings of testicular sonography in the evaluation of these patients is the impression that the acute event is secondary to epididymitis. This is an important distinction, because the reactive epididymitis associated with torsion of the appendages does not require any further investigation, whereas the diagnosis of epididymitis in a non–sexually active male (without torsion) requires further investigation. If the urinalysis is negative, it is unlikely that these patients are experiencing acute epididymitis. Testicular technetium scanning is not a good study when there are significant inflammatory changes of the skin and dartos muscle. These changes may lead to a missed testicular torsion, obscured by the increased vascularity of the dartos muscle and skin. Surgical exploration may be necessary for diagnostic purposes when the diagnosis is uncertain, because the reactive epididymitis will take several days to resolve and will not improve from the surgical exploration.

The management of these boys is expectant and supportive. Limited activity until the discomfort completely disappears (5–7 days) is paramount. Most of the cases that advance to the more severe inflammatory stages are seen in boys who, after experiencing the initial pain from the torsion event, go out and play actively. Progressively, these boys develop worsening pain, erythema, and scrotal enlargement. We routinely recommend using nonsteroidal antiinflammatory agents, like ibuprofen, to control the pain and minimize the inflammatory phase.

Acute Epididymitis

Acute epididymitis is extremely rare in childhood, and it occurs in association with a urinary tract infection. The diagnosis of epididymitis in childhood carries the burden to demonstrate a possible urogenital tract anomaly, for example, a rare ectopic ureter. Consequently, these patients should undergo extensive radiographic and cystoscopic evaluation. In the absence of urinary tract infections, epididymitis has been thought to occur in some boys with severe voiding dysfunction, who void at very high pressures against a nonrelaxed external urinary sphincter. In our practice, this entity is extremely rare.

The most common presentation of acute epididymitis is the postpubertal, sexually active male. The symptoms are gradual in nature, and can have the associated findings of dysuria, flank pain, fever, and pyuria. The physical findings are variable depending on the severity of the process. Initially, the epididymis is tender, mostly at its base. Eventually, the testis may become involved in what is referred to as epididymoorchiitis. This is a diffusely tender, enlarged mass with loss of the anatomic landmarks. Rectal examination may reveal a tender prostate. Laboratory findings may show pyuria, bacteriuria, and leukocytosis. Sonographic assessment is often useful to confirm this diagnosis, and to exclude testicular torsion. The study should reveal intratesticular Doppler flow. Management of this condition is antibiotic coverage and supportive care. The choice of antibiotics should provide coverage for *Chlamydia trachomatis, Ureaplasma urealyticum,* and gonococcal infections, as is done for the treatment of sexually transmitted diseases. A common protocol is a 1-g dose of ceftriaxone given intramuscularly followed by a week-long course of 100 mg doxycycline taken twice daily. It is important to treat the sexual partners as well. All of these young men should receive counseling on the risks of unprotected sexual intercourse.

Testicular Trauma

Trauma to the testes is an infrequent presentation. The history of a direct injury to the scrotal area is always present. The findings vary from a completely normal-appearing scrotum with minor tenderness to a diffusely enlarged scrotum with ecchymoses and loss of the anatomic landmarks. If the physical findings prevent accurate assessment of the testis, then one should proceed rapidly with a sonographic evaluation. There are two conditions that require identification acutely: testicular rupture and torsion of the spermatic cord. Many patients present with torsion after a direct injury to the testis. Testicular rupture is not always simple to identify, but loss of the normally well-defined rim of the tunica vaginalis by ultrasonography is the telltale sign. This condition requires scrotal exploration and closure of the defect. Scrotal hematomas are managed expectantly.

SUGGESTED READINGS

Das S, Singer A. Controversies of perinatal torsion of the spermatic cord: a review, survey and recommendations. *J Urol* 1990;143: 231–233.

Jones DJ. Recurrent subacute torsion: prospective study of effects on testicular morphology and function. *J Urol* 1990;145:297–299.

Rajfer J. Congenital anomalies of the testis and scrotum. In: Walsh PC, Retik AB, Vaughan ED, et al., eds. *Campbell's urology, 7th ed.* Philadelphia: WB Saunders Co., 1997:2172–2192.

Redman JF, Barthold JS. Technique for atraumatic scrotal pouch orchiopexy in management of testicular torsion. *J Urol* 1995;154: 1511–1512.

Stone KT, Kass EJ, Cacciarelli AA, et al. Management of suspected antenatal torsion: what is the best strategy? *J Urol* 1995;153: 782–784.

128

VESICOURETERAL REFLUX

MICHAEL A. KEATING
MARK A. RICH

Vesicoureteral reflux, the retrograde flow of urine from the bladder to the upper urinary tract, is one of the most common problems in pediatric urology. The surgical solutions for the anomaly have withstood the test of time. In contrast, the recommendations for its management seem to continually change. New insight offered by perinatal detection, an evolving understanding of the influence of urinary tract infections (UTIs), and prospective randomized clinical studies often raise more questions than they answer. Reflux is the focus of over 150 manuscripts in the literature each year. As a consequence, physicians are cautioned to keep abreast of this expanding body of knowledge and, when necessary, search beyond the distillation presented here.

ANATOMIC CONSIDERATIONS AND FUNCTIONAL CORRELATES

The normal ureter actively propels urine into the bladder and prevents reflux by occluding with bladder filling and contraction. Active and passive components are required of the ureterovesical junction (UVJ) to achieve a flap-valve effect. The intravesical ureter must have an oblique course as it enters the bladder, proper muscular fixation, and posterior support to enable occlusion and adequate submucosal length. Effective peristalsis and low pressures within the bladder are also required for normal urine flow.

The factor most critical to a competent UVJ is the length of submucosal ureter relative to its diameter. *Primary reflux* results from large-caliber ureters or those having short intravesical segments that cannot be effectively shut by the junction. Ureters that cannot coapt because of chronic scarring from urinary infections (UTIs) are also a problem. A 5:1 tunnel length:ureteral diameter ratio is found in normal children and sets the standard for surgical correction.

Secondary reflux results from the elevated pressures of bladder obstruction. The maximum pressure ureters can generate is 40 cm H_2O. When bladder pressures exceed this, ureteral dilatation begins. Gradual breakdown of the junction is followed by reflux. Such obstructions can be anatomic (urethral valves in boys and ureteroceles in girls being most frequent) or functional. The latter are far more common and include neurogenic bladder, non-neurogenic neurogenic bladder, and bladder dysfunction. Any bladder with altered dynamics causing increased intravesical pressures poses a threat. Children with spina bifida are the classic example, but bladder dysfunction is intimately related to reflux in many cases.

IMPORTANCE OF BLADDER DYSFUNCTION

During toilet training, children demonstrate infantile-type uninhibited contractions in response to bladder filling. In an attempt to become continent, the child responds by contracting the external sphincter. Continence is ultimately achieved but sometimes at the expense of abnormally elevated bladder pressures. Problems arise when incomplete emptying results from what is essentially learned sphincter dyssynergy. This, in turn, leads to frequency, incontinence, and recurrent UTIs. A history of premature toilet training accompanies many children evaluated for reflux. Simply put, it is easier for toddlers to "hold on" to please parents and caregivers than to "let go." Families are cautioned to go slowly with toilet training to avoid these problems.

It is no coincidence that most children with reflux present soon after the onset of toilet training. Reflux and bladder dysfunction both peak between 3 and 5 years of age. Reflux occurs in nearly half of children with bladder dysfunction and, conversely, the most common urodynamic abnormality seen with reflux is uninhibited bladder contractions. Most children outgrow these tendencies, although identifying bladder dysfunction is key to the management of many chil-

M. A. Keating: Department of Surgery, Division of Urology, University of South Florida, Tampa; and Department of Children's Surgery, Arnold Palmer Hospital for Children, Orlando, Florida.

M. A. Rich: Department of Urology, University of South Florida, Tampa; and Division of Pediatric Urology, Nemours Children's Clinic, Orlando, Florida.

dren with reflux. Overlooking the diagnosis also might decrease the effectiveness of a surgical approach.

Signs or symptoms of voiding dysfunction include dribbling, urgency, and incontinence. Little girls may curtsey and boys squeeze the penis in an attempt to suppress bladder contractions. Encopresis and constipation also suggest abnormal toilet behavior and present a significant risk to recurrent UTIs. A careful examination rules out occult spina bifida as a cause of such symptoms. When spinal dysraphism is suspected, magnetic resonance imaging is the study of choice. Incomplete evacuation with residual urine on diagnostic studies and a thickened bladder wall or multiple diverticula are other suggestive findings.

Treatment of bladder dysfunction is directed at dampening bladder contractions and lowering pressures. Anticholinergics make a difference. Refluxers whose uninhibited contractions are treated with medication show better rates of resolution when compared to controls with normal bladder dynamics and refluxers whose bladder instability is not treated. Timed voids (every 2–3 hours), double voiding, and relaxation are also used to facilitate emptying. In severe cases such as non-neurogenic neurogenic bladder, which mimics spina bifida, myogenic failure and residual urine cause resting pressures of greater than 40 cm H_2O. Hydronephrosis can be quickly followed by the appearance of reflux, and intermittent catheterization becomes necessary. Regardless of the neuropathic bladder's cause, unless the UVJ has been irreparably damaged, even severe reflux can resolve by lowering bladder pressures. When medical management is unsuccessful in correcting secondary reflux, enterocystoplasty, vesicostomy, or some other form of urinary diversion becomes necessary.

WHO HAS REFLUX

The overall incidence of reflux in healthy children is perhaps 1%. The older the child, the less likely he or she is to have reflux. Reflux is present in more than half of infants with UTIs, emphasizing the need to evaluate these children. It is less common in older children who are similarly evaluated, presumably because of the spontaneous resolution that occurs with development in many cases. The vast majority (85%) of reflux occurs in girls, but boys who present with UTIs have a higher likelihood of having the anomaly. Reflux is also the most common cause of antenatally diagnosed hydronephrosis. A male predominance exists, perhaps because of a temporary urethral obstruction causing the transiently abnormal bladder dynamics seen in newborns.

Reflux has a multifactorial etiology, including a genetic component. It is the most common inherited anomaly of the urinary tract. The progeny of refluxers are at risk (66% in one series) and up to 45% of siblings are affected, depending on age at screening. Notably, the large majority (75%) are asymptomatic, and many already have renal scars. Most will spontaneously resolve, but awareness is key because of its innocuous nature. Although some prefer to evaluate siblings using voiding cystourethrography (VCUG), we find urinary ultrasonography (UUS) alone a reasonable screen. If the kidneys are normal and the sibling never has a UTI, the bladder study is deferred. Sterile reflux, if present, does not pose a threat to the child, although cautions are given of signs and symptoms of UTIs that should prompt further evaluation.

Reflux commonly occurs in children with the VACTERL (vertebral, anal, tracheoesophageal, renal, radial, cardiac, and limb) and CHARGE (coloboma of the eye, heart defects, atresia of the choanae, renal anomalies and retardation of growth or development, genital anomalies, and ear abnormalities or deafness) associations. Reflux is also a common finding with imperforate anus, whether neurogenic bladder dysfunction is present or not. Patients with a rectovesical or rectourethral fistula should be managed with a completely diverting colostomy to avoid problems with urinary tract infections. Voiding studies are indicated in any child with one of these problems.

Reflux also commonly occurs with other urologic anomalies. Vesicoureteral reflux is the most common abnormality associated with complete ureteral duplication. Although urine may reflux into either ureter, it more commonly involves that from the lower pole because of its lateral position and shorter submucosal tunnel. Contrary to earlier teaching, the frequency of resolution of reflux appears to be the same whether the patient has a single ureter or a double ureter, although resolution may take longer in patients with duplications. Reflux also occurs commonly in patients with bladder diverticula. The most common location for bladder diverticula is lateral and cephalad to the ureteral orifice. Here they can alter the anatomy of the UVJ and cause reflux. Reflux associated with small diverticula resolves at rates similar to that of primary reflux and can be managed accordingly. In contrast, reflux found with large paraureteral diverticula is less likely to resolve and usually requires correction. In cases where the ureter enters the diverticulum, regardless of size, surgery is recommended. Reflux is a common finding with renal agenesis and usually involves the contralateral ureter, although involvement of a blind-ending ipsilateral ureter also occurs. The incidence of reflux is also increased with multicystic dysplastic kidneys, where the contralateral ureter is involved in 15% to 20% of cases.

CLASSIFICATION AND GRADING

The severity of reflux is graded to better predict its likelihood of resolution and the risks of developing associated complications. The International Classification provides the standard based on the appearance of the ureter and collecting system during VCUG. Because reflux occurs in a continuum, any system suffers from being somewhat arbitrary. Other inconsistencies also exist. In cases where lower ureteral dilatation exceeds that of the calices, the prognosis may differ from those having uniform ureteral caliber throughout. Accurate grading is also difficult if ipsilateral obstruction, nonobstructive dilatation, or postinfectious scarring causes pelvocaliceal distortion. Overestimation of grade is fairly common. Classifying reflux with radionuclide cystography (RNC) does not assess ureteral and pelvocaliceal anatomy. Although grading systems exist for the modality, when management decisions depend on comparisons of grade and trends in the degree of reflux, standard VCUG provides the best standard.

DIAGNOSIS

Most patients present with symptoms that suggest a UTI. High fevers are uncommon in newborns, who instead present with failure to thrive and lethargy. Infants and toddlers present with fever, malodorous urine, dysuria, and frequency. Pyelonephritis often causes vague abdominal discomfort rather than localized flank pain. Fever may not be a reliable sign of upper tract involvement. When reflux has gone undetected and renal scarring has occurred, children of any age can present with renal insufficiency, hypertension, and impaired growth.

A urine culture is performed in any child who presents with fever or malaise or is suspected of having a UTI. Unfortunately, UTIs are often mistaken for otitis, gastroenteritis, or respiratory infections. Microscopy is notoriously inaccurate, although dipsticks can be suggestive. Method of collection becomes an important issue. In toilet-trained children, a midstream-voided specimen is adequate. Any growth greater than 100,000 colonies warrants further evaluation. Intermediate yields (10,000 to 50,000 colonies) have no correlation with actual infections. Adhesive bags are widely used in infants but are the least reliable. Specimens with no growth are valid. Those specimens with multiple organisms are typically contaminated. Catheterization is a better way to minimize contamination and is the preferred method in infants or children whose specimens may be contaminated. Bacterial counts of greater than 1,000 colony-forming units/mL are considered significant. Suprapubic aspiration is rarely necessary.

Reflux is found in 30% to 50% of children with UTIs. Approximately 30% of these children already have renal scarring that is usually proportional to the severity of reflux. Notably, scarring can occur after a single UTI, even in the absence of fever, and there are no reliable signs that differentiate children with reflux who are at risk for upper tract changes from those without. These realizations amplify the need for thorough evaluations of any child suspected of having a UTI.

We modify the workup according to age, sex, and clinical history. Complete evaluations that include VCUG and UUS are required of three groups: any child under 5 years of age with a true UTI; children with a febrile UTI, regardless of age; and any boy with a UTI unless he is sexually active or has a past urologic history. Children who have had one UTI are highly prone (80%–85%) to have another, whether an anomaly like reflux or voiding dysfunction is the cause. As many as half are asymptomatic. It seems reasonable, then, to work up the first UTI to lay this issue to rest. If reflux or other anomalies are absent, parents can be reassured that the urinary tract is normal and that further UTIs generally remain confined to the lower urinary tract where they do not pose a serious health threat. Therapeutic efforts are then directed at improving toilet behavior.

Older children with asymptomatic bacteriuria or UTIs causing only lower tract symptoms are screened initially with UUS alone. Cystography is reserved for those with abnormal ultrasonographic results or recalcitrant infections. Finally, because reflux is the cause of antenatal hydronephrosis in many cases, newborns with moderate to severe degrees of hydronephrosis are fully evaluated with VCUG. Cystography is also indicated in babies who had intermittent hydronephrosis *in utero*. Ultrasonography is a notoriously poor screen for reflux in newborns where a significant number (25%) are normal despite having reflux on VCUG. Although most reflux is low-grade and resolves, it is reasonable to empirically treat these children at an age when they are most susceptible to pyelonephritis and renal scarring.

LOWER URINARY TRACT ASSESSMENT

Fluoroscopic VCUG is the initial study of choice. This allows standard grading, provides anatomic details that could alter management (bladder diverticulum or urethral valves), and offers insight into function by assessing postvoid residual and bladder capacity. Static cystograms that miss the voiding phase or studies performed with Foley catheters are not valid. Studies performed under anesthesia, where the detrusor is affected, are also of equivocal value.

In the past, the VCUG was completed a few weeks after a UTI to allow for inflammation to resolve and to prevent patient discomfort. This approach may overlook reflux that occurs with infection, when cystitis can weaken the UVJ. To avoid such false-negative findings, we often obtain the study early after a UTI, because cystography poses no increased risk to the child. We commonly see children whose history suggests a UTI with upper tract involvement, yet the infection is treated and the VCUG is negative. These children are treated medically for a few months as low-grade refluxers while efforts are directed at improving toilet behavior, which, by default, may be the only risk factor.

Nuclear cystography (RNC) does not provide the anatomic detail of fluoroscopy, but is an accurate method for detecting reflux. We find it helpful for following reflux after initial grading and anatomic detail is obtained by standard VCUG. The study also can be used to document resolution after corrective surgery.

UPPER TRACT ASSESSMENT

Ultrasonography is the diagnostic study of choice to initially evaluate the upper urinary tracts of patients suspected of having reflux. Although the study cannot rule out reflux, especially because lower grades do not cause hydronephrosis, it can be used to assess renal size, the presence of scars, hydronephrosis, postvoid residual volume, bladder wall thickness, and other renal anomalies. The noninvasive study is also used for follow-up of renal growth.

Functional studies are required of the scarred kidney when the question of salvageability is raised. A baseline study is also obtained before reimplantation surgery but is probably unnecessary with a normal UUS. Excretory urography, intravenous pyelogram (IVP), has been displaced by the more sophisticated data provided by renal scintigraphy using technetium 99m–labeled dimercaptosuccinic acid. Scans are the best study for detecting pyelonephritis and cortical scarring. Their role in the management of reflux, however, remains unclear.

Cystoscopy has no role in evaluating reflux. There is little information gained from viewing the anatomy not provided by VCUG and UUS. Although terms such as "golf-hole orifice" linger, they do not predict the presence of reflux. Instead, progressive bladder filling gives an orifice a more abnormal appearance and shortens its tunnel. Although some surgeons routinely cystoscope prior to reimplantation, deferring surgery on the basis of its findings is rare, especially if a recent urine culture is negative. Urodynamics help direct therapy in any child suspected of having a secondary cause for reflux, although when massive reflux is present, a valid assessment of bladder dynamics is difficult.

COMPLICATIONS

Reflux by itself does not pose a threat, unless elevated bladder pressures are chronically transmitted to the upper urinary tract with a severely neuropathic bladder. The anomaly does offer bacteria easy access to the kidneys, where their effects can be devastating. Reflux nephropathy describes changes associated with focal thinning of the parenchyma, caliceal dilatation, and impaired renal growth. Although the majority of renal scars never pose a problem, progression can result in proteinuria, hypertension, eclampsia, and renal failure.

There is a direct relationship between the grade of reflux and nephropathy (5% with grade I and 50% with grade V). Studies of antenatally diagnosed reflux, in which one third of kidneys are scarred yet UTIs have not occurred, suggest a congenital basis in some. In theory, the interplay between the ureteral bud and renal blastema determines renal development as well as that of the UVJ. Male infants are particularly prone because of their tendency to have high grades of reflux, and boys are much less likely to acquire scarring because they rarely have recurrent UTIs.

Most studies underscore the importance of UTIs in the evolution of nephropathy. Reflux appears to amplify the effects of pathogens and predispose the kidney to scarring. Most scars occur in patients who have had recurrent UTIs, especially with higher grades of reflux. Other than grade, other factors that determine the severity of renal injury include age, bacterial virulence, host susceptibility and renal inflammatory response.

The development of scars is an age-related phenomenon. The infant kidney is more vulnerable to damage by infection. Just as the highest incidence of reflux is found in younger children, the risk of scarring is greatest in newborns and infants. Immaturity of the immune system probably plays a role. Reflux nephropathy is less uncommon after 5 years of age. Despite these observations, we treat older children with significant UTIs no differently, because scars can develop in children of any age who are not properly treated.

A variety of bacterial virulence factors and host receptor differences help explain differences in the predisposition to pyelonephritis. Their description exceeds the scope of this discussion. It is more important to remember that bacteria ascend in retrograde fashion and that the bladder is infected before the kidneys. Any patient's most important defense mechanism is effective bladder emptying on a regular basis. Normal bladders empty completely, leaving no culture medium for bacteria. In contrast, patients with bladder dysfunction void infrequently and empty incompletely.

Reflux nephropathy is the most common cause of severe hypertension in children and young adults. Arterial damage presumably leads to segmental ischemia and renin-driven hypertension. Importantly, most patients who develop hypertension have nearly normal renal function. Hypertension is related to the grade of reflux and severity of scarring, especially in patients with bilateral involvement. The elimination of reflux or its spontaneous resolution does not reverse the risks of hypertension once scarring is present. This emphasizes the need for periodic checks of the blood pressure in any patient with a history of reflux nephropathy.

With the exception of kidneys that are developmentally arrested, most studies implicate UTI as the cause for altered renal growth. Acceptable growth occurs if UTIs are controlled with medication. Successful antireflux surgery can also accelerate growth but may not allow affected kidneys to return to normal size, especially if they already have significant nephropathy. In contrast, kidneys without scarring usually show rebound growth with the correction of reflux or its spontaneous resolution with medical management.

Chronic pyelonephritis was reported as the cause of end-stage renal disease in 25% of children and young adults in earlier studies, although the disease now accounts for less than 3% of transplantations performed in North America. Preventive treatment aimed at delaying the onset of hyperfiltration and segmental glomerulosclerosis using angiotensin-converting enzyme (captopril) shows promise.

Women with a history of reflux have increased morbidity during pregnancy because of infection-related complications, whether their reflux has been corrected or not. Women with renal scars, hypertension, and an element of renal failure are at increased risk. Women with renal scars whose reflux is uncorrected appear to be at particular risk and should have their reflux corrected before pregnancy to minimize maternal and fetal morbidity. The morbidity during pregnancy of women with persistent reflux without renal scarring remains poorly defined, but the tendency toward developing UTIs seems increased.

MEDICAL MANAGEMENT

Reflux resolves spontaneously in many children. In theory, two mechanisms contribute. The first is elongation of the submucosal tunnel that occurs with interval growth of the bladder and ureter. The second is a beneficial change in bladder dynamics from an infantile hyperreflexic pattern to one having larger capacity and lower pressures. The likelihood of resolution depends on initial grade and age at presentation. Weighing these factors allows clinicians to prognosticate, with some degree of accuracy, which child is a candidate for medical therapy and who is best served by surgical correction.

Most low grades (I–II) of reflux spontaneously resolve (80%–85%). Intermediate grade (III) reflux resolves in approximately 50% of patients. High grades are less likely to resolve (grade IV, perhaps 25%; grade V, <10%). Patient age is an equally important factor. Younger children, especially newborns, are more likely to have reflux and are more likely to have it resolve, regardless of grade. Later childhood sees more slowly cumulative rates of resolution, perhaps 15% per year. The likelihood of resolution presumably ends with puberty and the cessation of longitudinal growth. Recent studies suggest that if resolution is to occur, it usually does so within the first 2 to 3 years after diagnosis. How long one should wait is unclear, although 5 years seems long enough if families are willing to wait, but many are not. In fact, what may be more important are trends in follow-up. The absence of improvement in the grade of reflux on serial cystograms after a few years is a sign that resolution may not occur.

The procedures designed to correct reflux set a high standard for comparison with medical management. Nevertheless, the latter becomes the choice for most children with reflux as long as they remain free of infection. Both modalities have risks and benefits that must be discussed with parents in light of the natural history of the anomaly. The treatment plan should be individualized and must consider parental compliance and socioeconomic concerns. Nevertheless, some generalized recommendations can be made.

Medical management is recommended for prepubertal children with grade I, II, or III reflux because most cases will resolve. A period of observation is also warranted for most grade IV reflux, especially in younger children and those with unilateral disease. Some improvement should become evident within 2 to 3 years. If not, surgery should be considered. Newborns with grade V reflux, who can be maintained on prophylaxis, also should be managed medically at first. Grade V reflux that persists or is discovered in older children is unlikely to spontaneously resolve and should be corrected surgically.

The onset of puberty alters the recommendations for adolescents whose reflux is being medically managed. Surgery is recommended for girls with reflux that persists, especially if they have nephropathy or have shown a tendency toward urinary infections, because they seem prone to problems during pregnancy. In girls with normal kidneys, antibiotics are discontinued as puberty approaches. If UTIs appear and reflux persists, it is corrected. There is little doubt that ureteral reimplantation in girls is more challenging after puberty. Maturation of the pelvic adnexa makes ureteral mobilization difficult and increases bleeding. Because older boys are less prone to UTIs, prophylaxis can be discontinued and most reflux observed, unless infections or other symptoms arise. Using this approach, only about 15% of adolescents (usually girls) require surgery, and new renal scars are uncommon.

Medical management assumes that sterile reflux does not pose a health risk. To achieve this, low-dose prophylaxis is continued until reflux resolves. Medications are usually given once daily at half the standard therapeutic dose. Nighttime dosing is most effective because it precedes the longest period of urinary retention in toilet-trained children. Amoxacillin is recommended for children up to 6 weeks of age. After 6 weeks the biliary system is able to handle trimethoprim-sulfamethoxazole, which usually becomes the prophylaxis of choice. Potential side effects (leukopenia, Stevens-Johnson syndrome) are discussed with parents. Nitrofurantoin is another acceptable option. Best at minimizing fecal resistance, its long-term application can pose problems (pulmonary fibrosis and interstitial pneumonia are occasional side effects). Alternating the medications every other day or taking one in the morning and the other at night is effective for children who develop infections resistant to single-agent therapy but where surgery should be deferred, especially in children with bladder dysfunction.

Improving toilet hygiene and eliminating constipation all help achieve the goals of medical management. Bladder dysfunction is treated with anticholinergics. Urine cultures are obtained every 3 months to screen for UTIs. Negative cultures are usually reliable, regardless of collection technique. When questions of culture validity arise, confirmation with catheterization becomes necessary. In rare cases, pyelonephritis recurs despite these efforts and reimplantation becomes necessary to protect the kidneys. Parents should be warned that UTIs typically continue after surgery when bladder dysfunction is an issue. These remain confined to the bladder where they do not present a threat, although their symptoms can be a nuisance.

We have gone to periodic radiologic studies at 18-month intervals. The latter allows more time for interval growth, is cost effective and requires only two catheterizations for VCUG in a 3-year period. Prophylaxis is discontinued when cystography documents resolution. A repeat confirmatory cystogram is unnecessary in the asymptomatic child. Complete reevaluations are required in children who develop pyelonephritis.

The expectations required of families must be frankly discussed. Approximately one third of children treated medically for reflux are lost to follow-up, many after the first year. Intermittently treating UTIs associated with reflux is ineffective. Children who are only treated when symptomatic demonstrate progressive nephropathy compared with those maintained on chronic suppression. If compliance is an issue, some children are best served by correcting their reflux surgically rather than embarking on a futile course of medical management or suboptimal follow-up.

SURGICAL MANAGEMENT

The expectations of surgery must be understood beforehand. Successful ureteral reimplantation may not completely eliminate the incidence of pyelonephritis in children where other host factors exist. Bacteriuria is still fairly common (found in as many as 40% of patients), especially if there are problems with toilet dysfunction, but pyelonephritis is less common (found in about 10%) once reflux has been corrected.

A variety of techniques have been described for the correction of reflux. Technical descriptions and illustrations may be found in standard texts of urology and pediatric surgery. We will limit our discussion to indications, technical nuances, and complications. Common to each technique is the creation of a valvular mechanism that recreates normal anatomy, providing a submucosal tunnel for the ureter having sufficient length and muscular backing. Reflux that persists is usually caused by inadequate length to the reimplant or unrecognized bladder dysfunction.

Cross-Trigonal (Cohen) Technique

This versatile reimplantation is probably the most popular technique used today and is our preference for most patients. Creating a submucosal tunnel along the posterior aspect of the bladder is possible in most patients, and the repair is probably the easiest to complete and to teach. The cross-trigonal approach is especially useful for small or neuropathic bladders, because a gentler curve is given to the ureter than with other repairs. We cite a 98% to 99% success rate to parents. The technique's one drawback is difficulty with retrograde, although the introduction of flexible cystoscopes and retrograde catheters has lessened the significance of this concern.

Skeletalization of the ureter must be avoided during its mobilization with this or any technique. Dissection is performed with minimal tissue handling. A 5-0 silk suture is placed within the future perimeatal cuff and through a fine (3.5 or 5 French) feeding tube placed in the ureter to facilitate handling. A generous mucosal cuff is outlined around the meatus using a needle-tip cautery. This helps with later suturing of the ureter and identification of its lumen. After incising the mucosa and taking down the superficial detrusor, the plane for ureteral dissection is found inferiorly by spreading with a fine hemostat. Excessive dissection of the detrusor is unnecessary and causes bleeding. Sharp dissection parallel to the ureter with tenotomy scissors establishes the correct plane, and hemostasis is accomplished with selective cautery on periureteral attachments. Angulations should be corrected. If the distal ureter is narrow or unhealthy after being mobilized, it is excised back to healthy viable tissue and spatulated to avoid stenosis.

Closure of the original hiatus is performed if the opening is patulous. Inadequate closure can lead to diverticulum formation, the most common complication of this repair. The hiatus should allow a hemostat to lie next to the ureter to avoid obstruction. A groove is created in the detrusor medially to avoid a shelf at the entrance to the new tunnel. For some small bladders it helps to change the position of the ureteral entrance by incising the superolateral margin of the hiatus and mobilizing the peritoneum off the back of the bladder, giving the ureter a more lateral position and creating a longer tunnel. Once the ureters are brought beneath their tunnels and anastomosed into position, a fine infant feeding tube should pass easily to assure patency. A Penrose drain is left in the perivesical space, but ureteral stents and bladder catheters are unnecessary in most cases.

Advancement (Glenn-Anderson) Technique

The advantage of the advancement technique is similar to that of the cross-trigonal method. Because the ureter remains in its original hiatus, obstruction or kinking is highly unusual. Success rates as high as 97% to 98% have been cited, although this technique is implicated in many patients referred to us for persistent postreimplantation reflux. Adequate tunnel length can be a problem. Like most operations, selection is the key to success. The best candidates for advancements are ureters that are laterally positioned and a generous (3–4 cm) distance to the bladder neck. This is ideal for unilateral repairs, because the contralateral ureter is not potentially disrupted. If the bladder is small or the ureters are medially positioned, a suprahiatal detrusor "cut-back" modification and more extensive transvesical dissection can be used to gain additional tunnel length, although we would generally recommend switching to the cross-trigonal technique.

Politano-Leadbetter Technique

The popularity of Politano-Leadbetter is waning. Reluctance to use the repair stems from the somewhat "blind" nature of its transfer of the ureter behind the bladder, especially when compared with the simpler methods described above. This drawback can be overcome and we still prefer the technique for unilateral reimplantations to avoid disruption of the valvular mechanism of the contralateral ureter. Success rates are similar to those of other repairs.

After mobilizing the ureter, a dissector is used to sweep the peritoneum from the posterior bladder and proposed new hiatus. This helps prevent placing the ureter through the peritoneum or viscera. A right-angle clamp hugs the posterior bladder wall and indents the proposed new hiatus from without. This location is superior, medial, and, in most instances, 2 to 2.5 cm from the old hiatus. Excessive lateral placement can lead to ureteral obstruction as the bladder fills. The mucosa and muscle are then sharply incised and the right angle spread generously upon entering the bladder. Incomplete separation of the detrusor can cause obstruction at the new hiatus. Incising a few millimeters of its medial lip helps prevent kinking. A second right angle is passed outside the bladder by the initial clamp and guides the ureter through the new hiatus. An unobstructed route into the bladder can be confirmed. A fine feeding tube is passed to rule out obstruction. Wide mucosal mobilization is needed to avoid ureteral obstruction when the new submucosal tunnel is created. When the bladder is trabeculated, it is sometimes easier to raise mucosal flaps with cautery to form the ureteral bed.

Extravesical (Lich-Gregoir) Technique

Extravesical reimplantation is becoming increasingly popular. Extended follow-up in large series, especially when combined with the ureteral advancement (detrusorrhaphy), finds the procedure as effective as any. Because the bladder is left intact, bladder spasms and hematuria are minimized. The technique is also less invasive than other repairs, and hospitalization may be shortened. There are some drawbacks, however. Concerns about disrupting the nerves to the bladder cause some surgeons to defer the technique with bilateral reimplants for fear of causing urinary retention. Transient retention requiring as long as 4 weeks of intermittent catheterization occurred in 16% of patients in one series. Long-term voiding efficacy is unaffected.

The obliterated hypogastric artery is identified and ligated and the ureter gently mobilized after isolating it with a vessel loop. The peritoneum is also cleared from the posterior aspect of the bladder intended for implantation. Major blood vessels are preserved during the perivesical dissection. The serosal and muscular layers of the detrusor are opened along a straight course cephalad and lateral from the UVJ, freeing up the ureter during the dissection. Four or 5 cm of detrusor is cleared along this route from the underlying musoca to create the antirefluxing trough. Additional dissection is performed circumferentially to the bladder mucosa so that the ureter is attached only at its juncture with the bladder mucosa. Ureterotrigonal continuity is not disrupted. A pair of "vest-type" sutures (4-0 polyglycolic acid) approximate, in succession, detrusor at the distal limit of the dissected trigone, proximal ureter, and detrusor (inside/out) to advance the ureter into the bladder. Any mucosal rents are closed with fine interrupted chromic sutures. The ureter is placed in the trough and the detrusor closed over it. A Penrose drain is left in the perivesical space.

Endoscopic Treatment

The concept of treating reflux endoscopically is a valid one. In theory, an object or injectable material positioned behind the ureter provides the backing necessary to cause coaptation during bladder filling and contraction. Such an approach is particularly appealing because of its simplicity, lessened morbidity, and potential cost effectiveness. The decision making in the management of reflux often balances the uncertainty of spontaneous resolution against surgical morbidity. A significant reduction in the latter might shift management decisions in favor of correction in selected patients.

Any endoscopically injected substance for treating reflux should be easily delivered, biocompatible, nonantigenic, and non-migratory. A number of materials have been offered to meet these criteria, including silicone, collagen, bioglass, and autologous cartilage and fat. Success rates, especially in short-term follow-up, have been encouraging. Unfortunately, longer follow-up is either unavailable or cite lower rates of resolution, suggesting reabsorption with loss in efficacy. Currently, the concept of the endoscopic approach is reasonable but an ideal substance is unavailable. The permanency of open surgical techniques seems preferable to offering what might be a transient response that subjects patients to an undefined length of follow-up and the possibility of future urologic problems.

Duplicated Ureters

Approximately 10% of children undergoing surgery have a variant of ureteral duplication. The most common configuration is a complete duplication that results in two separate orifices. This is best managed by preserving a cuff of bladder mucosa that encompasses both orifices. Because the pair typically share blood supply along their adjoining wall, mobilization as one unit with a "common sheath" preserves vascularity and minimizes trauma. Reimplantation then follows in a sequence similar to that used in any of the techniques described above. In instances of a Y or V configuration, a single orifice refluxes into both systems. If the common stem is long enough to be reimplanted alone, standard techniques are used. Otherwise, to avoid obstruction at the union, the stem is excised and the ureters converted to a complete duplication.

FOLLOW-UP

Radiologic studies are used to assess initial and long-term surgical results and to follow parameters of renal growth. Successful reimplants usually control ascending infections, although pyelonephritis sometimes reappears. UUS is performed 6 to 8 weeks after surgery and should show minimal ureteral dilatation. VCUG 6 months later checks the quality of the repair. If the results of both studies are satisfactory, further studies are unnecessary unless the patient develops upper tract changes or significant UTIs. Periodic visits with UUS at 18 months, 3 years, and 5 years are also recommended. The reappearance of hydronephrosis, new renal scars, retarded renal growth, or recurrent UTIs may warrant a complete reevaluation. Children with minimally symptomatic bacteriuria are evaluated for dysfunctional voiding and treated accordingly.

COMPLICATIONS

Reflux during the postoperative period can occur in either the repaired ureter or the contralateral ureter. Presumably, these changes are secondary to trigonal edema. Exacerbations of bladder dysfunction during the perioperative period are also implicated. Fortunately, the vast majority of postoperative reflux is low grade and transient. Most resolves within 1 year. Parents should be reassured that conservative management is all that is usually required.

Early after surgery, various degrees of hydronephrosis can be expected of the reimplanted ureter. Edema, subtrigonal bleeding, and bladder spasms all contribute. Mucus plugs or blood clots are other causes. Most obstructions are mild, asymptomatic, and resolve spontaneously. Significant obstructions are usually symptomatic. Affected children typically present 1 to 2 weeks after surgery with abdominal pain, nausea, and vomiting. Fever is less common. Renal scans usually show marked delay in excretion, whereas severe hydroureteronephrosis is present on UUS. The large majority subside spontaneously, but placement of a nephrostomy tube or ureteral stent sometimes becomes necessary. Treatment is otherwise supportive and includes parenteral antibiotics and hydration.

True failures of ureteroneocystostomy are rare. Before reoperation, the cause of the complication should be fully defined so that any error of earlier surgery is not repeated. Standard radiologic studies (VCUG and IVP) and cystoscopy with retrograde ureterography provide anatomic detail, but additional diagnostics including urodynamics and renal pressure perfusion studies are also sometimes helpful, especially when a functional cause is suspected.

Reflux that persists after surgery usually results from failure to achieve sufficient submucosal length or provide adequate backing for the ureter within its new tunnel. Advancement techniques are particularly prone in this regard. Another common error occurs when reimplanting the dilated ureter. Reluctance to perform appropriate tapering makes attainment of a proper diameter-to-tunnel ratio impossible.

Other than technical errors, failure to identify and treat secondary causes of reflux is a common cause of its reappearance. Foremost among these are unrecognized neuropathic bladder and severe voiding dysfunction. Performing reimplantations in bladders that exhibit abnormal dynamics significantly lessens the likelihood of success. In severe cases, the reappearance of hydroureteronephrosis followed by reflux is a predictable scenario. Urodynamic studies are indicated in any child who has a failed reimplantation. Aggressive treatment of the underlying disorder resolve some cases and must be effective to assure the success of any secondary surgery that might be indicated.

Significant ureteral obstructions vary in location and degree depending on etiology. Most can be avoided by adhering to the principles cited above. Complete obstructions usually result from ischemia and typically involve the implanted segment. Other causes of ureteral occlusion include angulation at the new hiatus, inadvertent passage through the peritoneum or viscera, or compromise at the hiatus or within a poorly developed submucosal tunnel. Intermittent obstructions also occur. Ureters reimplanted in abnormally lateral positions become increasingly angulated with progressive bladder filling. Ureterectasis with J hooking of the distal ureter is seen by IVP. Bladder emptying results in alleviation of angulation with decompression. Revision is necessary if the obstruction becomes chronic.

After thoroughly defining a complication of reimplantation, the surgical approach to its correction is dictated by the type of failure, degree of ureteral dilatation, and whether one or both ureters are affected.

An intravesical approach is used for ureters that continue to reflux. The technique of mobilization differs from that in standard reimplantation by incising the mucosa of the old submucosal tunnel and sharply removing scarred ureteral attachments. As much mobilization as possible is done within the bladder, but it is often necessary to move outside to gain adequate length for repair.

Intravesical mobilization is futile with obstructed ureters because they are usually irreparably damaged within the bladder wall. Instead, the bladder is opened to assess its interior and to plan the site for the new ureteral hiatus and tunnel.

After entering the peritoneum and packing away the bowel, virgin ureter is identified at the bifurcation of the iliac vessels. It is then freed as distally as possible and transected outside the bladder. With any type of ureter, mobilization is made to healthy tissue and scarred or fibrotic tissue excised. Any necessary tailoring of the dilated ureter is also completed. The amount of viable ureter and the quality of the recipient bladder help determine the surgical approach.

Refluxing ureters can be repaired in a manner similar to that described for primary reimplantations. Any method can be used to complete the repair intravesically, provided sufficient ureteral length is obtained from within. When the mobilization must be extended extravesically, selection of a neohiatus and reimplantation using the Politano-Leadbetter repair is a good choice.

Obstructed ureters present the additional dilemma of obtaining adequate length for reimplantation. Careful proximal mobilization is the first maneuver used to obtain length. When this alone is inadequate, a psoas hitch is used to bridge significant ureteral defects that remain. The bladder can be tacked to the psoas tendon above the iliac vessels and still maintain normal function. The technique provides as much as 8 to 10 cm and effective immobile muscular backing along the bladder base.

Ureters with defects that cannot be bridged by a psoas hitch or those that continue to reflux despite repeated efforts at reimplantation are ideal candidates for transureteroureterostomy (TUU), in effect bypassing the problem. Historically, hesitation to use a TUU stemmed from potentially affecting the recipient ureter. This is not a problem if the recipient ureter is minimally mobilized, there is no angulation of the donor ureter under the sigmoid, and a tension-free, spatulated anastomosis is created. The combination of a psoas hitch and TUU is especially useful in cases of bilateral failure where the feasibility of creating two adequately long tunnels might be limited by the anatomy of the bladder. After both ureters are freed, the healthiest and longest ureter can be reimplanted into a long submucosal tunnel using a psoas hitch. The second ureter is then joined to the reimplanted ureter as a TUU.

SUGGESTED READINGS

Belman AB. A perspective on vesicoureteral reflux. *Urol Clin North Am* 1995;22:139–149.

Burbige K. Ureteral reimplantation: a comparison of results with the cross-trigonal and Politano-Leadbetter techniques in 120 patients. *J Urol* 1991;146:1352–1353.

Cooper CS, Chung BI, Kirsch AJ, et al. The outcome of stopping prophylactic antibiotics in older children with vesicoureteral reflux. *J Urol* 2000;163:269–272.

Elder JS, Peters CA, Arant BS, et al. Pediatric Vesicoureteral Reflux Guidelines Panel summary report on the management of primary vesicoureteral reflux in children. *J Urol* 1997;157:1846–1851.

Koff SA, Wagner YY, Jayanthi VR. The relationship among dysfunctional elimination syndromes, primary vesicoureteral reflux and urinary tract infections in children. *J Urol* 1998;160:1019–1022.

Mansfield JT, Snow BW, Cartwright PC, et al. Complications of pregnancy in women after childhood reimplantation for vesicoureteral reflux: an update with 25 years followup. *H Urol* 1995; 154:787–790.

O'Donnell B, Puri P. Treatment of vesicoureteral reflux by endoscopic injection of Teflon. *BMJ* 1984;289:7–9.

Paltiel HJ, Lebowitz RL. Neonatal hydronephrosis due to primary vesicoureteral reflux: trends in diagnosis and treatment. *Radiology* 1989;170:787–789.

129

BLADDER AUGMENTATION

UZAY YASAR
CURTIS A. SHELDON

Bladder augmentation is a complex yet highly successful option in the field of surgical reconstruction of the pediatric bladder. Refinements of surgical technique, the application of clean intermittent catheterization (CIC), advances in urodynamics, and review of our experience in urinary diversion and undiversion have led to major advances in this dynamic field. Despite these successes, there remain adverse sequelae and long-term complications that must be considered before undertaking augmentation cystoplasty.

There are several goals in the surgical restoration of bladder function. First and foremost is the protection of the upper urinary tracts with the creation of a large-capacity, low-pressure reservoir for urine storage. Patients should be able to go 4 hours between catheterizations while maintaining a low intravesical storage pressure. When bladder pressure is greater than 40 cm H_2O, patients are at high risk for upper tract deterioration. Urinary continence is another important goal of reconstruction. This is often a difficult problem to diagnose and treat because of its multiple causes, ranging from bladder neck incompetence to uninhibited detrusor contractions to an areflexic detrusor muscle, resulting in overflow incontinence. If possible, the preservation of spontaneous voiding should be attempted. When spontaneous voiding is not feasible, access for easy catheterization becomes a necessity, whether by the native urethra or by the creation of a continent, catheterizable conduit. Keeping these fundamentals of bladder reconstruction in mind, augmentation may be applied for the correction of many urinary tract anomalies with good expectation for success.

U. Yasar and C. A. Sheldon: Department of Surgery, Division of Urology, University of Cincinnati; and Division of Pediatric Urology, Cincinnati Children's Hospital Medical Center, Cincinnati, Ohio.

WORKUP

Before surgical reconstruction on the bladder is pursued, more conservative measures must be attempted. Initial treatment for any patient with a dysfunctional bladder being considered for augmentation should first consist of pharmacologic therapy, often in combination with CIC. Anticholinergics can be used to increase the capacity and compliance of the bladder to an acceptable degree. Behavioral modifications also may play a part in conservative therapy. If these measures fail, surgical therapy might be warranted.

Meticulous preoperative evaluation of the patient is critical to determine if the patient is a candidate for bladder augmentation. A careful history and physical examination are performed. Preoperative evaluation of the patient should assess renal function, a 24-hour urine collection for volume measurement, and glomerular filtration rate if renal function is in question. Determining urine output is essential for creating an augmented bladder with a large enough capacity to store at least 4 hours of urine output. This is especially true for children in high-output renal failure who may produce up to 4 L of urine in 1 day. *Nuclear renography* is indicated if elements of obstruction or renal scarring are present. *Voiding cystourethrography* is an important study to determine the presence of vesicoureteral reflux, whereas formal *urodynamics* provide crucial information on leak point pressure, bladder capacity, bladder compliance, and the presence of uninhibited detrusor contractions. Lastly, *upright cystography* can be performed to evaluate the competency of the bladder neck.

PREOPERATIVE PREPARATION

Once the decision for augmentation is made, the patient must be properly prepared. The full nature of the operation and its inherent risks and potential complications must be discussed. The patient must understand that he or she may lose the ability for spontaneous voiding and that intermittent catheterization may become a permanent part of life postoperatively. Because postoperative compliance with management is critical to the success of any bladder reconstruction, a careful assessment of the child's willingness and ability to comply is important. A full bowel preparation must be performed preoperatively. This must be done regardless of the reconstructive procedure planned, for the surgeon must have the ability to tailor the case intraoperatively for any eventuality. The preparation can be performed in an outpatient setting with less complicated patients, but often requires a full 2 days of in-hospital mechanical preparation for those children with a neuropathic bladder and bowel. Performing an adequate bowel preparation in this patient population can be a challenge.

Cystoscopy should be performed immediately before the augmentation to assess native anatomy such as bladder size and morphology, location of ureteral orifices, and competency of the bladder neck. This can provide important anatomic insight and aid the surgeon in determining which reconstruction to perform. Additionally, a urine culture should be sent a few days before the operation and a positive culture should be treated preoperatively to prevent seeding of the peritoneal cavity with infected urine.

TECHNICAL CONSIDERATIONS

Several important concepts are pertinent to bladder reconstruction. Detubularization of an intestinal segment consists of opening an isolated bowel segment along its antimesenteric border. Detubularization of a bowel segment results in an interruption of its circular muscle fibers, causing an interruption of its basic electrical rhythm. This interruption results in blunting of bowel contractions and an increased compliance of the reconfigured bowel segment. This isolated segment is then reconfigured into a more spherical shape to fit the bladder. This is done by folding the intestinal segment upon itself in the shape of a U, S, or W and anastomosing the bowel wall together. In addition, reconfiguring the segment into a spherical shape maximizes the volume achievable for any given length of bowel segment. This results in a dramatic increase in effective bladder capacity when used to augment the bladder.

Another concept important in bladder reconstruction is management of the native bladder. If the detrusor muscle of the native bladder is left intact, it generates high pressures that can cause the augmented bowel segment to act as a diverticulum. There are two ways to avoid this problem. The first involves excision of the supertrigonal detrusor originally described by Gil-Vernet, leaving just a cuff of bladder to be anastomosed to the reconfigured intestinal segment. The second involves preserving the native bladder and opening it with a wide sagittal incision starting just cephalad to the bladder neck anteriorly. This incision is carried posteriorly to the trigone of the bladder. The augmenting segment is then anastomosed to this "clam-shell" bladder. This seems to be a more advantageous technique for management of the native bladder. It is technically easier to anastomose the reconfigured bowel segment to the remaining bladder, and the supertrigonal bladder adds to the overall capacity of the augmentation. Additionally, both appendicovesicostomy (Mitrofanoff principle) and ureteral reimplantation are more easily performed into the detrusor muscle than into a bowel segment. This becomes especially important if vesicoureteral reflux exists preoperatively, necessitating ureteral reimplantation.

The Mitrofanoff principle was introduced in 1980 and is currently an important option for the surgeon performing augmentation cystoplasty in the pediatric population. It involves the creation of a continent, catheterizable conduit that allows easy catheter access to the bladder. This involves the implantation of a tubularized visceral segment using a one-way flap valve mechanism into the urinary bladder with the exteriorization of the other end to the skin. This exteriorization is usually to the abdominal wall, but also may be to the umbilicus or the perineum. The conduit is commonly fashioned from appendix but also can be created using a segment of ureter or tapered ileum. It is the one-way flap valve mechanism that provides continence, and effective implantation of the valve has been demonstrated not only into native bladder but also into colonic and gastric augmented segments of the reconstructed bladder. Antegrade passage of a catheter is easily accomplished, making this technique particularly well suited to the patient who has difficulty catheterizing the native urethra. This is a frequent finding in this population and includes children bound to a wheelchair, those who have a tortuous urethra from congenital deformity or reconstruction, and children who have only marginal control of their upper extremities. In addition, catheterizing the conduit is less uncomfortable than catheterizing the native urethra and may enhance patient compliance.

Various donor tissue can be used to augment the bladder, including ileum, an ileocecal segment, stomach, sigmoid colon, and ureter (Table 129.1). Recently, autoaugmentation, either alone or with the use of an intestinal seromuscular patch overlying denuded bladder epithelium, has been used. However these newer techniques have not replaced the gold standard of augmenting bladder with a segment of the intestinal tract.

The most common segment of bowel to be used in bladder augmentation is ileum. In the ileocystoplasty, a segment of ileum approximately 20 to 40 cm long is isolated and detubularized (Fig. 129.1). It is important that the mesentery of the isolated segment is long enough to reach the bladder. An ileoileostomy is performed and the

TABLE 129.1. SIGNIFICANT CHARACTERISTICS OF AUGMENTATION MODALITIES

Technique	Pros	Cons
Ileocystoplasty	Technically simple	Acidosis, infection, mucus Antirefluxing implantation unreliable
Sigmoid colocystoplasty	Technically simple Allows implantation of ureter or Mitrofanoff into tenia	Risks interruption of blood supply to rectum after reconstruction for imperforate anus Acidosis, infection, mucus
Ileocecocystoplasty	Technically simple Allows antirefluxing implantation of dilated ureters with intussusception technique	Intussusception antireflux mechanism inherently unstable Risks devastating fecal incontinence in patients with marginal continence mechanism (e.g., myelomeningocele or VATER)
Gastrocystoplasty	Reduced risk of infection and mucus production Allows easy implantation of ureter or Mitrofanoff No risk of acidosis	Hematuria-dysuria
Ureterocystoplasty	Metabolically inert No mucus May be performed extraperitoneally	Antirefluxing implantation not possible Dilated ureter only occasionally available Risk of failure to attain adequate compliance and capacity
Autoaugmentation	Technically simple Metabolically inert No mucus May be performed extraperitoneally	Antirefluxing implantation not possible Risk of failure to attain adequate compliance and capacity

From Sheldon CA. Urinary reconstruction (rather than diversion) for continence in difficult pediatric urologic disorders. *Semin Pediatr Surg* 1996;5:11.

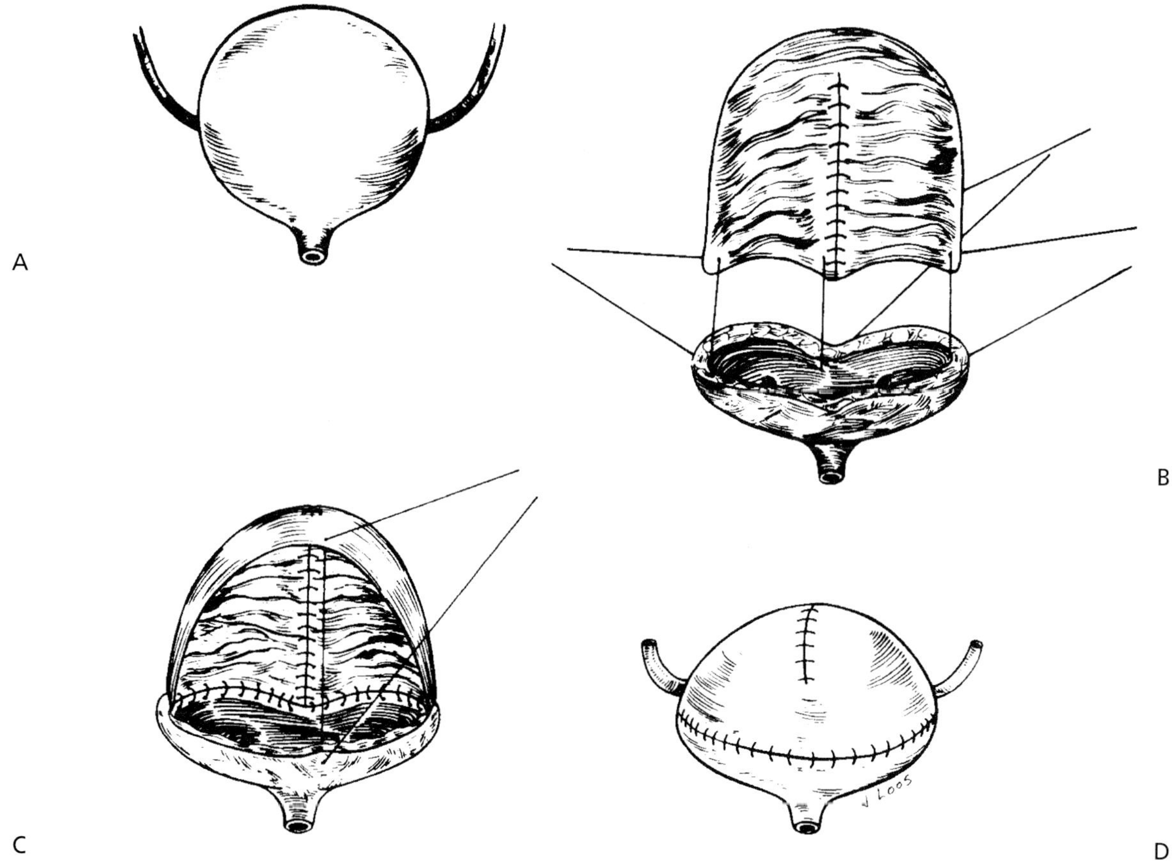

FIGURE 129.1. Bladder augmentation using an intestinal segment. **A:** The bladder is opened like a clam shell. **B:** The intestinal segment is detubularized by longitudinal incision along the antimesenteric border. A cup patch is fashioned by suturing one edge of the resultant rectangle to itself. **C:** The cup patch is sutured to the remnant bladder plate. **D:** Final appearance. (Reprinted from Sheldon CA, Bukowski T. Bladder function. In: Rowe MI, O'Neill JA, Grosfeld JL, et al., eds. *Essentials of pediatric surgery.* St. Louis: Mosby Year Book, 1995:731–747; with permission.)

mesenteric window closed to prevent internal herniation. Once the segment of ileum is reconfigured for maximum capacity, it is anastomosed to the clam-shelled bladder. The closure is started at the posterior aspect of the native bladder, and I prefer to close with two separate layers of running absorbable suture, the first layer interlocking. Before the closure is complete, a Malecot suprapubic tube (SPT) is brought out through a separate incision in the native bladder. Drains are left in place, and the urethral catheter placed preoperatively is left as a secondary means for postoperative bladder drainage.

The ileocecocystoplasty is performed in much the same manner as the ileocystoplasty. The right colon is mobilized, and an ileocecal segment is isolated. Approximately 20 to 30 cm of terminal ileum is isolated. The segment is opened in its entirety along the antimesenteric border and reconfigured for anastomosis to the bladder. The advantage of the ileocecocystoplasty is that it allows construction of an ileal antirefluxing nipple to which dilated ureters can be attached, thus preventing the transmission of pressure and refluxing urine to the upper tracts. If necessary, the ureters also can be tunneled through the cecal segment, creating an antirefluxing mechanism. When the ureters are too short for reanastomosis to the bladder, a limb of ileum can be left intact to reach the shortened ureters. The ileocecocystoplasty is rarely performed in the pediatric population, however, because removal of the ileocecal valve in children can result in intractable diarrhea. This is especially true in children with marginal continence mechanisms (myelomeningocele and imperforate anus patients), the very population most likely to need the bladder augmentation procedure.

Gastrocystoplasty involves the augmentation of the bladder using a segment of stomach, usually from the body. The segment is isolated by taking a wedge of stomach along the greater curvature, being careful to avoid the lesser curvature and thus injury to the vagus nerve (Fig. 129.2). This segment is brought down on a right gas-

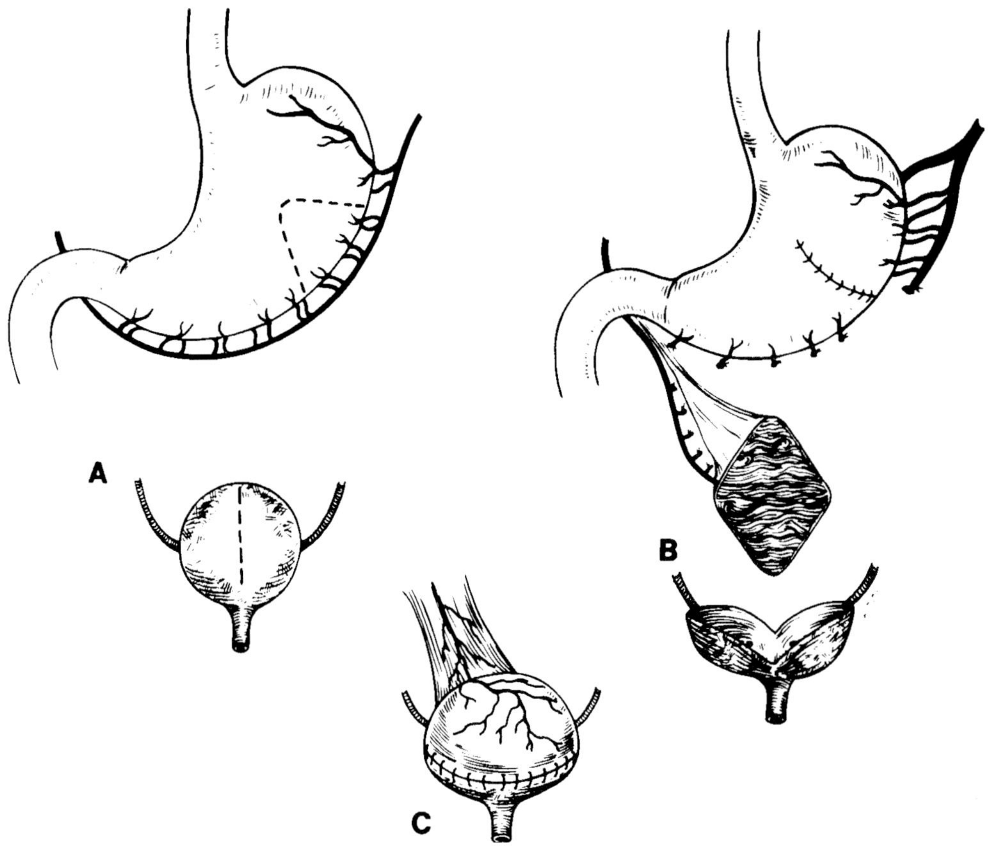

FIGURE 129.2. Bladder augmentation using a gastric segment: gastrocystoplasty. **A:** A wedge of nonantral stomach is isolated, based on the right gastroepiploic vessels. **B:** The bladder is prepared to open like a clam shell. **C:** The anastomosis is completed with a running double layer of absorbable suture. (Reprinted from Sheldon CA, Bukowski T. Bladder function. In: Rowe MI, O'Neill JA, Grosfeld JL, et al., eds. *Essentials of pediatric surgery.* St. Louis: Mosby Year Book, 1995: 731–747; with permission.)

troepiploic vascular pedicle, although infrequently the left gastroepiploic artery is used. This segment is then anastomosed to the opened bladder with a running double layer of absorbable suture. Using a segment of stomach has some distinct advantages over using small or large bowel. Compared with intestinal segments, it is less permeable to urinary solutes, specifically chloride, and presents no risk for causing acidosis, which is better suited for patients with renal insufficiency. Because the stomach segment secretes acid, children with renal insufficiency may see a reversal of their baseline acidotic state. In addition, gastrocystoplasties are less prone to mucus production, have a reduced risk for infection, and allow easy implantation of ureters or Mitrofanoff neourethras.

Colocystoplasty using sigmoid colon is a common option for pediatric bladder augmentation. A 20-cm segment of sigmoid colon is selected and isolated. A colocolostomy is performed and the mesenteric window closed. In order to disrupt the strong contractions that the sigmoid colon tends to have, the segment of sigmoid is detubularized and reconfigured to provide maximal compliance and capacity. Anastomosis to the bivalved bladder is performed in a similar fashion as other intestinal segments, and a suprapubic tube and drains are left in place before closing. The advantage of the colocystoplasty lies in the fact that ureters can easily be reimplanted by an antirefluxing manner by tunneling the ureters through the teniae.

Ureterocystoplasty and autoaugmentation are alternatives to using a gastrointestinal segment for bladder augmentation. These two options are well suited for children with renal insufficiency. In both cases the tissue used to augment the bladder is urothelium, a metabolically inert tissue that consists of transitional epithelium. This epithelium is relatively impermeable and does not lead to electrolyte changes or acidosis secondary to urinary solute absorption, and it does not produce mucus. Additionally, both procedures can be performed retroperitoneally. This avoids the complications associated with entering the peritoneal cavity and is advantageous for the patient who has a ventriculoperitoneal shunt or is dependent on peritoneal dialysis.

In the ureterocystoplasty, dilated ureter is used to augment the bladder. Massively dilated ureters are often seen in the pediatric population. Not uncommonly, such ureters may be associated with kidneys that have minimal or no function. When this is the case, the dilated ureter is mobilized and detubularized. Often the entire renal pelvis of the nonfunctioning kidney can be carefully mobilized along with the ureter. Because the blood supply to the ureter approaches medially above the true pelvis and laterally in the true pelvis, care must be taken not to devascularize it during its mobilization. After it is detubularized, the ureter is reconfigured into a "U-shaped" patch. This patch is then anastomosed to the bivalved bladder with a double-layer of running absorbable suture, the first layer interlocking. The bladder is opened in a similar manner as the ileocystoplasty. The difference is that the sagittal incision is extended posteriorly to the ureteral orifice of the dilated ureter. In this manner, the ureter is never detached from the bladder, helping to preserve its blood supply. When the kidney of the dilated ureter still functions, the distal segment of the ureter can be used to augment the bladder while the proximal ureter is either reimplanted into the bladder or anastomosed to the contralateral ureter. A major disadvantage to this technique is the small number of children requiring a bladder augmentation that fit the criteria for this procedure.

Autoaugmentation involves the excision of the detrusor muscle overlying the bladder dome, leaving the underlying bladder mucosa intact (Fig. 129.3). With time, this bladder mucosa bulges like a wide-mouthed bladder diverticulum, increasing bladder capacity and compliance. A thick, fibrous layer replaces the excised detrusor. There are two variations in the surgical technique, both with equally good results. The first involves simple excision of the detrusor muscle to create the diverticulum. With the second technique, the detrusor muscle is incised to allow the mucosa to bulge. In both cases, the detrusor edges are secured to the psoas muscle bilaterally to prevent reapproximation of the muscle. The advantages of the autoaugmentation are those of maintaining a native urothelial surface. Additionally, it is an extraperitoneal procedure with complete maintenance of bowel integrity. Complications from this operation are few, and reoperative bladder reconstruction does not seem to be hindered. However, there are concerns over the limited improvement in bladder capacity and compliance, and it is generally not recommended for children with low-capacity, high-pressure bladders.

Because of concerns over minimal improvements in bladder volume and compliance secondary to fibrosis after the autoaugmentation procedure, some surgeons have been covering the exposed bladder mucosal surface with a demucosalized enteric segment in an attempt to decrease the amount of scarring. Different enteric segments have been tried with varying success. Demucosalized stomach and sigmoid colon placed over the bladder mucosa after autoaugmentation seem to offer some promise, but further investigation is needed.

POSTOPERATIVE CARE

As with any patient that undergoes major abdominal surgery, postoperative care of the bladder-augmented patient can be complex. Immediately after surgery, elec-

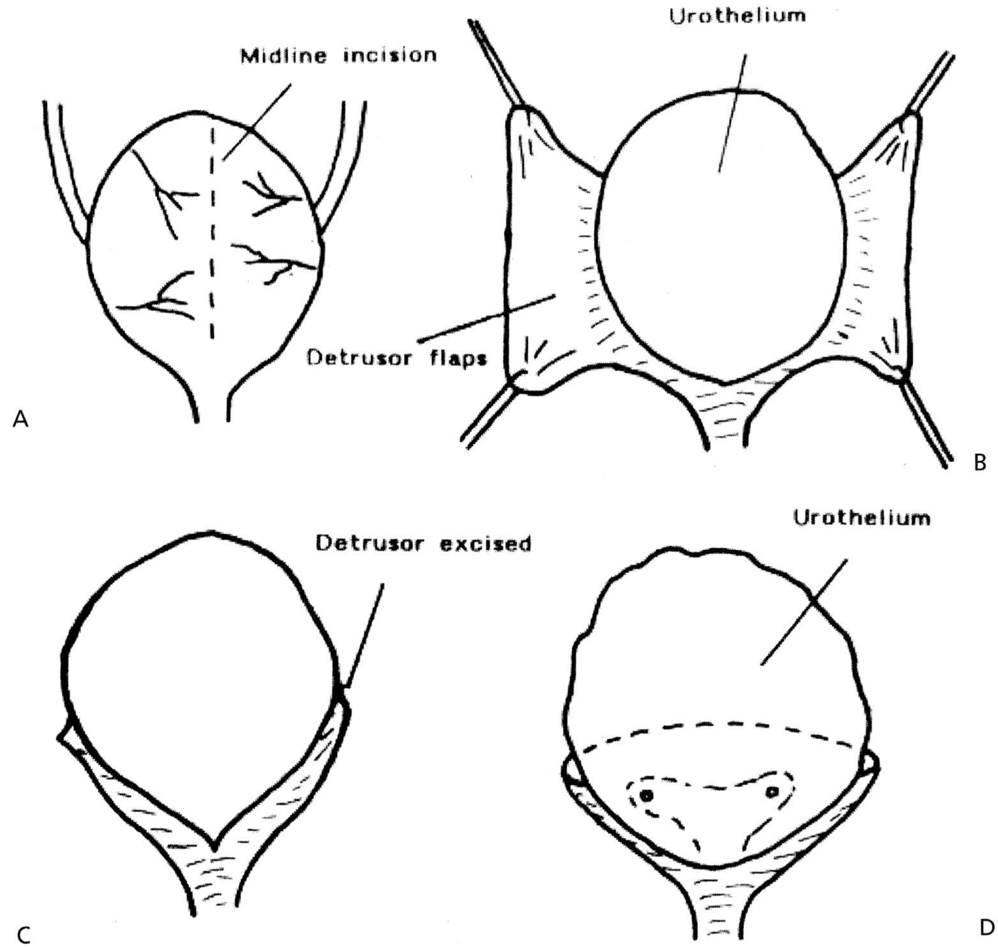

FIGURE 129.3. Autoaugmentation. **A:** Midline incision in the detrusor muscle, leaving bladder mucosa intact. **B:** The detrusor muscle is dissected away from underlying urothelium. **C:** The mobilized detrusor muscle is excised. **D:** Final appearance. Only a rim of detrusor muscle surrounding the trigone remains. The remainder of the urothelium is devoid of its original muscular support. (Reprinted from Sheldon CA, Bukowski T. Bladder function. In: Rowe MI, O'Neill JA, Grosfeld JL, et al., eds. *Essentials of pediatric surgery.* St. Louis: Mosby Year Book, 1995:731–747; with permission.)

trolyte and blood counts must be followed carefully, especially in the face of bleeding and third-space fluid shifts. Intravenous fluids should be sufficient to compensate for intravascular deficits. The patient should be maintained on bowel rest, with nasogastric tube (NGT) decompression and broad-spectrum antibiotic coverage. Urine output from the urethral catheter, SPT, and Mitrofanoff catheter (if present), as well as drain and NGT output, should be monitored carefully. Parenteral nutrition should be considered, because some of these children are often without oral nutrition for 5 days or more. Depending on which augmentation technique is used, it may be necessary to gently irrigate the bladder free of mucus several times each day. The NGT is removed after the resolution of ileus, and the diet is slowly advanced. The patient can be discharged from the hospital only after being without fever, tolerating a regular diet, and receiving the supplies and teaching needed for proper tube care. They go home on oral antibiotics, with their SPT, urethral catheter, and Mitrofanoff catheter to drainage. Typically, our patients are followed carefully postoperatively by telephone, and ultrasonography and a panel of renal tests are performed at the 2-week follow-up visit. Approximately 4 weeks postoperatively, indwelling catheters are removed and intermittent catheterization is resumed. The time between catheterizations is gradually increased from every 3 hours to four times a day.

COMPLICATIONS

Augmentation cystoplasty can be a highly rewarding undertaking for both patient and surgeon. However, it can be challenging and is fraught with many potential complications. These include metabolic derangements, alterations in gastrointestinal function, urinary tract infection (UTI), urolithiasis, malignancy, bone demineralization, and spontaneous bladder rupture. These complications are specific to bladder augmentation, and are in addition to those normally encountered with major abdominal surgery. The risk of a complication varies according to the type of augmentation performed and is outlined in Table 129.1.

Metabolic derangements are commonly encountered after bladder augmentation with a gastrointestinal segment. The determinants of the character and severity of these metabolic derangements are a consequence of the nature of the segment used, the absorptive surface area, the dwell time, and the metabolic reserve of the patient. Intestinal segments tend to absorb many urinary solutes that can lead to alterations in acid-base status, electrolyte abnormalities, hyperammonemia, and eventually bone demineralization. The major solutes absorbed by ileum and colon are ammonium and chloride. Patients with normal renal function compensate by excreting this additional acid load. However, in patients with compromised renal function, this absorption can quickly lead to an acidotic state, marked by hyponatremia and hyperchloremia. Buffering of even a slightly acidotic state is provided by bone, which can lead to demineralization and secondary hyperparathyroidism. Jejunum is rarely used for augmentation cystoplasty. This is because it often leads to the unique metabolic state of a hyponatremic, hypochloremic, hyperkalemic, and metabolic acidosis. Patients with such metabolic derangements present with fatigue, weakness, anorexia, and polydipsia. However, perhaps the most worrisome effect seen in children is the retardation of growth and development, especially in those children with compromised renal function.

Gastrocystoplasty leads to a distinct metabolic state. The stomach segment secretes chloride ions and acid into the augmented bladder, occasionally leading to a hypochloremic metabolic alkalosis. This often has the beneficial effect of improving the acidotic state seen in children with renal insufficiency. However, there are consequences to using stomach. These children seem to be vulnerable to dehydration during episodes of viral gastroenteritis. This is especially true in children with renal insufficiency. Additionally, gastrocystoplasty can result in the hematuria-dysuria syndrome, a syndrome marked by pain and urinary bleeding due to erosion of urothelium by acidic urine. It is more commonly seen in children who are incontinent and have exposure of the urethra to acidic urine. It is also seen in children with renal insufficiency who do not produce enough urine to dilute the acid load secreted by the stomach segment. This syndrome is usually mild and is treatable with histamine blockers or proton pump blockade. Infrequently, the symptoms can be intractable, and may require consideration of another augmentation modality.

Many of the complications brought on by augmentation cystoplasty are secondary to resection of the bowel. Bowel obstruction is uncommon after augmentation cystoplasty, occurring in approximately 3% of patients. The incidence of obstruction is the same regardless of which bowel segment is used. In addition, vitamin B_{12} deficiency can occur with bladder augmentation in two separate ways. Intrinsic factor (IF) is responsible for binding vitamin B_{12} in the gut and its eventual absorption in the terminal ileum. Because IF is produced by the parietal cells in the fundus of the stomach, gastrocystoplasty can in theory cause a shortage of IF production and thus vitamin B_{12} deficiency. Because distal ileum is the sole site of vitamin B_{12} absorption, its resection during an ileocystoplasty also can result in a malabsorption of vitamin B_{12}. A deficiency of vitamin B_{12} can lead to megaloblastic anemia, although this may take years to occur.

Diarrhea can become a significant problem in children after bladder augmentation using a segment of intestine. Resection of the ileocecal valve is most often implicated. Resection of the valve can do this in two ways. First, it causes a decreased transit time from the ileum to the cecum. Second, it allows backflow of bacteria from cecum to ileum, causing bacterial overgrowth and malabsorption of fat and vitamin B_{12}. This is especially true in children with neurogenic dysfunction of bladder and bowel who typically rely on chronic constipation for fecal continence. It is estimated that up to 10% of children undergoing resection of the valve will have problems with chronic diarrhea. Resection of large segments of ileum also can result in diarrhea as a consequence of decreased bile acid reabsorption. This overflow of bile acid into the colon results in both a secretory diarrhea as well as steatorrhea. It would seem prudent not to resect large segments of ileum or the ileocecal valve for augmentation cystoplasty in children, especially those with preexisting risk factors.

Another risk of augmentation cystoplasty is that of tumor formation. Most of our experience comes from studying the ureterosigmoidostomy model, where the risk of malignancy near the site of ureterocolonic anastomosis is increased several hundred times above normal. These tumors are usually adenocarcinomas, although benign tumors, and rarely a transitional cell carcinoma, have been documented. This is believed to be a result of urinary nitrosamines, known to have a carcinogenic influence on the colon, which originate from the mixing of feces and urine. Tumor development has been seen in the augmented bladder as well. The exact incidence is unknown at this point, but it is clearly much greater than in the general population, and may not be influenced by which gastrointestinal segment is used to augment the bladder. Because of the long latency period of these tumors (>20 years), periodic endoscopy is warranted for the lifetime of the patient.

Patients have a higher incidence of both upper tract and reservoir bladder calculi after augmentation. Although varied in composition, struvite stones are most commonly seen. There are several reasons for this increased incidence. Stasis of urine in a dependent reservoir is a contributing factor, and the presence of mucus in the reservoir can further act toward stone propagation. Mucus also can serve as a nidus for infection, often by urea-splitting bacteria such as *Proteus* or *Klebsiella.* Metabolic changes in these patients and periods of dehydration also contribute to stone formation. Another causative agent is a foreign body, such as nonabsorbable sutures or staples used during the reconstruction. Care should be taken to avoid as many of these factors as possible, and the patient should be instructed to completely empty their bladder with CIC. UTIs caused by stone-forming organisms should be treated aggressively with antibiotics. Metabolic abnormalities and bouts of dehydration should be addressed and treated appropriately.

One of the most treacherous complications of bladder reconstruction is perforation of the augmented bladder. It is one of the most common causes of an acute abdomen in these patients, and suspicion should be high when a child with an augmented bladder presents with abdominal pain, distension, fever, decreased urine output, and sepsis. The etiology of perforation often goes undiscovered, and no single bowel segment seems to be at greater risk than another. Cystography can be diagnostic, demonstrating extravasation of contrast from the augmented bladder. However, there is a significant incidence of false-negative results with cystography, and if suspicion remains high, computed tomography with bladder contrast can be more definitive. Surgical exploration and repair are the standard course for bladder rupture management after augmentation cystoplasty.

SUGGESTED READINGS

Churchill BM, Aliabadi H, Landau EH, et al. Ureteral bladder augmentation. *J Urol* 1993;150:716–720.

Duckett JW, Snyder HM. Continent urinary diversion: variations on the Mitrofanoff principle. *J Urol* 1986;135:58–62.

Gearhart JP, Albertsen PC, Marshall FF, et al. Pediatric applications of augmentation cystoplasty: the Johns Hopkins experience. *J Urol* 1986;136:430.

Gil-Vernet JM Jr. The ileocolic segment in urologic surgery. *J Urol* 1965;94:418–426.

King LR. Protection of upper tracts in undiversion. In: King LR, Stone AR, Webster GD, eds. *Bladder reconstruction and continent urinary diversion.* Chicago: Year-Book Medical, 1987:127–153.

Kulb TB, Rink RC, Mitchell ME. Gastrocystoplasty in azotemic canines. Presented at the American Urological Association, North Central Section Meeting, Palm Springs, Florida, 1986.

McGuire EJ, Woodside JR, Borden TA, et al. Prognostic value of urodynamic testing in myelodysplastic patients. *J Urol* 1981;126:205–209.

Mitrofanoff P. Cystostomie continente trans-appendiculaire dans le traitement des vessies neurologiques. *Chir Pediatr* 1980;21:297–305.

Rink RC, Adams MC. Augmentation cystoplasty. In: Walsh PC, ed. *Campbell's urology, 7th ed.* Philadelphia: WB Saunders, 1998:3167–3189.

Sheldon CA, Snyder HM. Principles of urinary tract reconstruction. In: Gillenwater JY, ed. *Adult and pediatric urology, 3rd ed.* St. Louis: CV Mosby, 1996:2317–2410.

130

INTERSEX

RUPA V. KOTHANDAPANI
CURTIS A. SHELDON

Although a relatively complex field, the subject of intersex states is a fascinating one and a true challenge to the pediatric surgical specialist in terms of diagnosis, surgical reconstruction, and various controversial issues that relate to these disorders. However fascinating it is to the surgeon, it has the potential to be physiologically devastating and socially detrimental to the patient and his or her family if not treated and recognized quickly and accurately. The very first question pondered by the new parents is regarding the sex of the child. When this is not readily apparent, it can create much confusion and anxiety, prompting the surgeon and others, such as endocrinologists and geneticists, to be available for guidance, reassurance, and compassion.

Potential sequelae also need to be addressed after the initial diagnosis is made. These include such issues as risk of malignancy, electrolyte abnormalities, recurrence of abnormalities in future children, and psychologic complications. The intersex patient also may be affected by infertility, delayed puberty, or primary amenorrhea.

A detailed discussion of pertinent embryology and reconstruction is beyond the scope of this chapter but is available in several published reviews.

DIAGNOSIS

The differential diagnosis of ambiguous genitalia includes four prominent entities: female pseudohermaphroditism, male pseudohermaphroditism, true hermaphroditism, and primary gonadal disorders (Table 130.1).

Female pseudohermaphroditism is a condition in which the patient has two ovaries, bilateral müllerian structures, and a 46,XX karyotype. The most common condition is congenital adrenal hyperplasia (CAH), primarily in the form of 21α-hydroxylase deficiency (90%), 11β-hydroxylase deficiency, or 3β-hydroxysteroid dehydrogenase deficiency. These enzymatic defects result in deficiencies of glucocorticoids and lead to an excess of androgens, causing virilization. It is important to realize that CAH in boys may present with excessive masculinization. Additionally, less common forms of CAH may cause diminished virilization of boys. Mineralocorticoid activity may be diminished or increased depending on the particular enzymatic deficiency, resulting in either salt-wasting dehydration or hypertension. This disorder also may be due to transfer of exogenous maternal medications to the developing fetus or to maternal androgen-producing neoplasms.

In male pseudohermaphroditism, the majority of patients have two testes, bilateral wolffian structures, and a 46,XY karyotype. These disorders are primarily due to end-organ resistance to androgens, various defects in androgen synthesis, and disorders of testicular development. Several other etiologies are shown in Table 130.1.

True hermaphroditism is a less common condition and is characterized by harboring both ovarian and testicular tissue. Müllerian and wolffian ductal structures may be evident, and the karyotype is variable, with 46,XX being the most common. The most important piece of evidence needed to make this diagnosis is the gonad, of which the most characteristic is the ovotestis. Müllerian structures are generally associated with the presence of an ipsilateral ovary or ovotestis, and wolffian structures are seen with the presence of an ipsilateral testis.

Primary gonadal disorders are a significant source of ambiguous genitalia. The most common type is mixed gonadal dysgenesis, which is commonly associated with the presence of a streak gonad and a testis. The karyotype is 45,X/46,XY. If the testis is dysgenetic, one can expect to see müllerian structures ipsilaterally. If the testis is viable, then the resulting ductal structures on the ipsilateral side are likely wolffian. Phenotype is tremendously variable, ranging from a phenotypic female with clitoral hypertrophy to a phenotypic male with cryptorchidism and hypospadias. One important issue not to overlook in this patient popu-

R.V. Kothandapani and C.A. Sheldon: Department of Surgery, Division of Urology, University of Cincinnati; and Division of Pediatric Urology, Cincinnati Children's Hospital Medical Center, Cincinnati, Ohio.

TABLE 130.1. CONCEPTUAL CLASSIFICATION OF COMMON CAUSES OF AMBIGUOUS GENITALIA

Category	Gonad	Internal Ducts	Karyotype	Diagnosis
Female pseudohermaphrodite	Ovary/ovary	Müllerian/müllerian	46,XX	Congenital adrenal hyperplasia Transfer of maternal androgens
True hermaphrodite	Ovary/testis Ovotestis/testis Ovotestis/ovary Ovotestis/ovotestis	Müllerian/wolffian Variable/wolffian Variable/müllerian Variable/variable	46,XX 46,XX/46,XY 46,XY	True hermaphroditism
Male pseudohermaphrodite	Testis/testis	Wolffian/wolffian	46,XY	Incomplete androgen insensitivity 5α-reductase deficiency Defects in androgen synthesis
Primary gonadal disorders	Testis/streak Absent/absent Dysgenetic/dysgenetic	Wolffian/müllerian Variable Variable	45,X/46,XY 46,XY 46,XY	Mixed gonadal dysgenesis Embryonic testicular regression Dysgenetic male pseudohermaphroditism

lation is the high incidence of gonadoblastoma, or dysgerminoma. Removal of the dysgenetic gonad, therefore, is important in the management of these patients.

Diagnostic Evaluation

All neonates need to have their external genitalia evaluated in detail during their initial newborn physical examination. Any neonate with ambiguous genitalia must have a full diagnostic workup. Evaluation is also required for patients with hypospadias associated with undescended testes, patients with micropenis, boys with excessive masculinization, and girls with palpable hernias, as well as for those with a salt-wasting or salt retention presentation.

As with any other medical evaluation, a good history should be obtained from the patient's family. One should inquire about maternal exogenous hormone exposure and evidence of maternal virilization during the gestational period. Questioning also should involve a history of the patient's siblings for evidence of intersex states. It is helpful to find out if there has been a family history of unexpected early deaths, infertility, or delayed puberty, each of which can suggest the possibility of an intersex state.

A detailed physical examination should then follow. Vital signs are evaluated, especially the blood pressure, because it may be high if 11β-hydroxylase deficiency is the underlying disorder. Signs of dehydration should be noted if there is a salt-wasting deficiency. The number of orifices in the perineal and genital regions should be recognized. If the patient is a phenotypic male, the position of the meatus is addressed. The length of the shaft of the phallus, the size of the glans, and the presence or absence and location of the testes also are noted. For a phenotypic female, inguinal and labial masses should be carefully examined, because they may represent herniated or partially descended gonads.

After the initial history and physical examination, attention is then focused on laboratory testing. Testing ensues based on the physical examination. For example, if gonads are palpable in an undervirilized male, a β-human chorionic gonadotropin (β-HCG) stimulation test may be performed, and 48 hours later the testosterone to dihydrotestosterone ratio is measured. Testosterone and other metabolites in the pathway (Fig. 130.1) also may be assayed in selected cases. Adrenocorticotropic hormone may be administered to enhance the levels of the metabolites and help discern the level of enzyme deficiency as well as the level of serum cortisol. On the other hand, a patient with nonpalpable gonads, such as a virilized phenotypic female, must be evaluated for CAH. A serum 17-hydroxyprogesterone level is ordered, which is the biochemical marker for 21α-hydroxylase deficiency. A standard panel of electrolytes also may be evaluated, especially to rule out hyponatremia and hyperkalemia, which are both seen in 21α-hydroxylase deficiency secondary to glucocorticoid and mineralocorticoid deficiencies (Fig. 130.1). Finally, all patients with ambiguous genitalia should undergo karyotype determination. Of historical significance, the buccal smear was a modality used in the past to determine the presence and frequency of Barr bodies. Today, however, karyotypes can be determined in less than 72 hours, are more accurate, and have replaced buccal smears.

Females presenting with hernias, especially if bilateral, should have an attempt made at identifying Fallopian structures during hernia repair. If none are noted, vaginoscopy or laparascopy should be performed. If the cervix and other müllerian elements are absent, the karyotype is determined to exclude testicular feminization (complete androgen insufficiency).

Imaging modalities can be useful in some types of ambiguous genitalia. For example, one form of congenital adrenal hyperplasia, side-chain cleavage deficiency, has the appearance on imaging of markedly enlarged adrenals with evidence of lipid density. For other types of adrenal hyperplasia, a cerebriform pattern has been seen on ultrasonography. Ultrasonography also may be used to differentiate between an irreducible inguinal mass in a phenotypic female that is suspicious for an incarcerated ovary versus testis or lymph node. Ultrasonography will help delineate a lymph node by a characteristic central echolucency. The

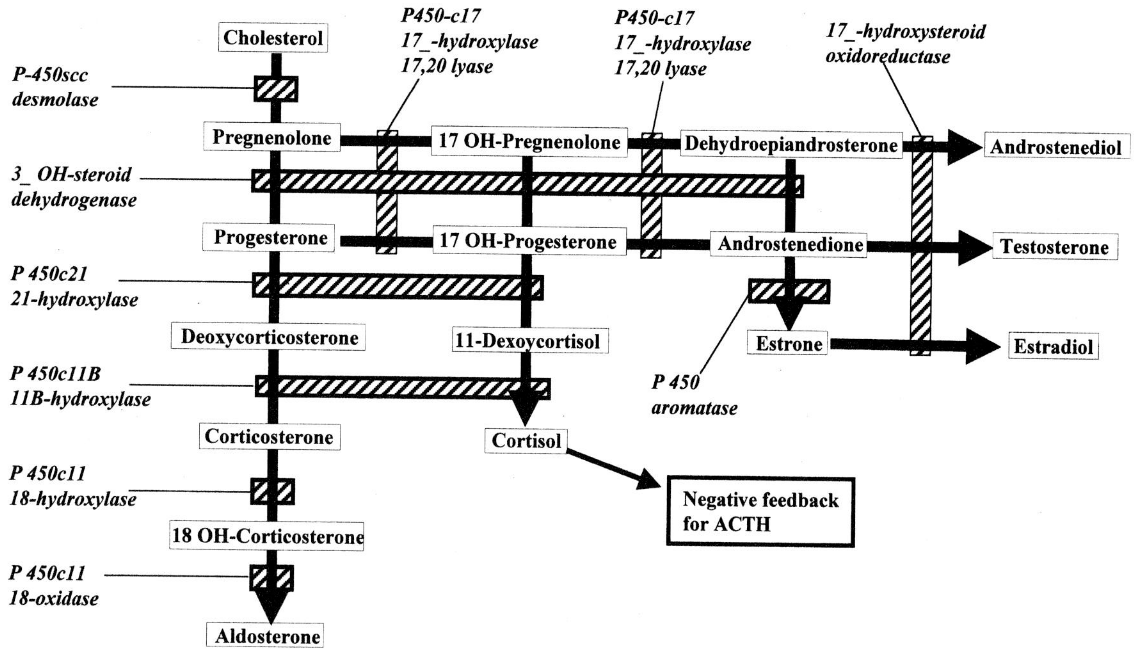

FIGURE 130.1. Biochemical pathways by which steroid hormones are synthesized from cholesterol. An enzyme deficiency at any level results in the absence of detectable levels of the final product and elevated levels of precursor substrates.

presence or absence of müllerian structures and ovaries in the pelvis also may be delineated. Additionally, ultrasonography is helpful in the search for müllerian remnants in a patient with hypospadias and cryptorchidism.

Endoscopy is a critical tool for evaluation of the patient's anatomy when reconstruction is being considered. In patients in whom vaginal reconstruction is required, vaginoscopy must be performed to identify the level of entry of the vagina into the urogenital sinus relative to the striated sphincter, determining the surgical approach. Diagnostic laparascopy is indicated to evaluate gonads and pelvic ductal structures in selected cases.

MEDICAL TREATMENT

If the underlying disorder is congenital adrenal hyperplasia, attention needs to be focused on correction of electrolyte imbalances and volume resuscitation, especially if the enzymatic defect is 21α-hydroxylase deficiency, which occurs in 90% of cases. Cortisol deficiency should be remedied, and androgen overproduction should be suppressed. Close clinical and biochemical monitoring of glucocorticoid replacement therapy (usually hydrocortisone) is necessary to avoid the side effects of either excessive or insufficient therapy. Steroid levels are monitored by obtaining serum 17-hydroxyprogesterone, androstenedione, and urinary pregnanetriol levels every 3 to 4 months. In addition, those with the salt-wasting form of congenital adrenal hyperplasia will need mineralocorticoid replacements in the form of fluorocortisone. Intravenous normal saline may be required for volume resuscitation. Fluorocortisone levels may be monitored by routine blood pressure monitoring, or less commonly, by plasma renin activity.

If undescended testicles are noted in an otherwise phenotypic male, an HCG stimulation test may promote descent into a more correct anatomic position. Some true hermaphrodites as well as selected individuals with male pseudohermaphroditism and primary gonadal disorders who are raised as males need hormone replacement therapy. Similarly, those patients with inadequate ovarian tissue who are raised as females, such as those with testicular feminization syndrome, should have hormone replacement therapy started at puberty. Consultation with an experienced endocrinologist is recommended in the management of all patients with an intersex diagnosis.

SURGICAL TREATMENT

In the case of female pseudohermaphroditism, a female gender assignment is made and feminizing reconstruction is planned. Feminizing genitoplasty is undertaken at 6 to 12 months of age and includes clitoroplasty, vaginoplasty, and labioplasty. Feminizing genitoplasty is a common operation used in the management of those patients with ambiguous genitalia. It can range from a straightforward procedure to one that is enormously complex and difficult.

If the patient is steroid deficient, preoperative preparation includes a steroid preparation in the form of cortisone acetate or hydrocortisone, which is given starting 2 days prior to surgery so that adequate levels of glucocorticoids are present in the bloodstream in the perioperative period. If the patient is volume contracted with abnormal electrolytes, aggressive volume resuscitation and sodium repletion is critical. Prophylactic intravenous antibiotics are also administered.

The low type of urogenital sinus malformation is the most common type of malformation. It is defined by the entry of the vagina into the urogenital sinus distal to the striated muscle sphincter. The urethra and vagina are obscured by midline fusion of the labioscrotal folds. These are managed by single-stage procedures using urogenital sinus mobilization with advancement and either an inverted "U" inlay flap or an "M" inlay flap from the labioscrotal folds. An incision is made along the coronal sulcus of the glans and along the lateral edges of the urethral plate to join beneath the urogenital sinus introitus. The dorsal prepuce is then mobilized. The corpora cavernosa are excised and oversewn with preservation of the dorsal neurovascular complex. The clitoroplasty is then performed to reduce the size of the phallus to a size typical of a clitoris while preserving sensation to the clitoris. The clitoris is approximated to the prepubic fascia. The urogenital sinus is circumferentially mobilized and advanced. If needed, the urogenital sinus is incised in the midline and an M flap is developed, reapproximated in the midline, and inserted to facilitate exteriorization of the vagina. The dorsal prepuce is divided in the midline and brought down bilaterally to reconstruct the labia minora (labioplasty). The goals of vaginoplasty are to create good cosmesis, as well as a vaginal vault that is of adequate size to potentiate successful intercourse later in life. It also must be of satisfactory dimensions to easily allow efflux of uterine secretions. Results of reconstruction can be seen in Fig. 130.2.

High urogenital sinus malformations, defined by the entry of the vagina into the urogenital sinus proximal to the striated sphincter, are more complex. For these types of vaginal reconstructions, a routine bowel preparation is used preoperatively along with intravenous antibiotics. In addition, detailed preoperative counseling is required so that the parents of the patient understand the need for long-term follow-up, the risk for vaginal stenosis, and the potential need for vaginal dilatation until sexual maturity is reached.

The vaginal insertion can rarely occur as high as the trigone of the bladder. Inlay flaps are not appropriate in this setting because of poor cosmesis and subsequent urinary incontinence. Initially, an M-shaped incision is made and the pelvic floor musculature is divided in the midline. Clitoroplasty is performed. The vagina is divided from its insertion and the defect is oversewn. The vagina is spatulated and the labioscrotal flap is tubularized. These two structures are then sewn together. The musculature is then reapproximated. For those patients in whom the vagina enters above the bladder neck, the vagina may be mobilized transperitoneally or transvesically. Final results are shown in Fig. 130.3. Patients whose vagina cannot be adequately mobilized to reach the perineum may require an interposition of small or large bowel. Similarly, patients requiring feminizing genitoplasty who have no vaginal tissue are reconstructed with the creation of a neovagina, usually from a colonic segment.

Masculinizing genitoplasty often can be successfully performed in a single-stage procedure. Attention is focused to urethral reconstruction, chordee release, and scrotoplasty.

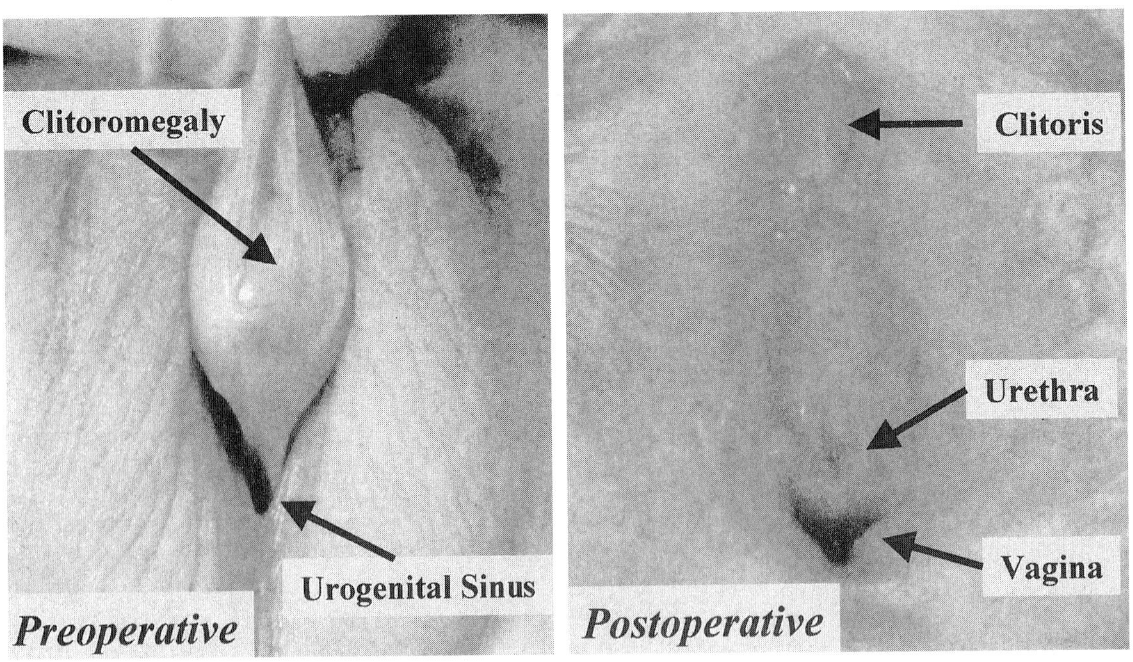

FIGURE 130.2. Feminizing genitoplasty of a patient with a low type of urogenital sinus malformation.

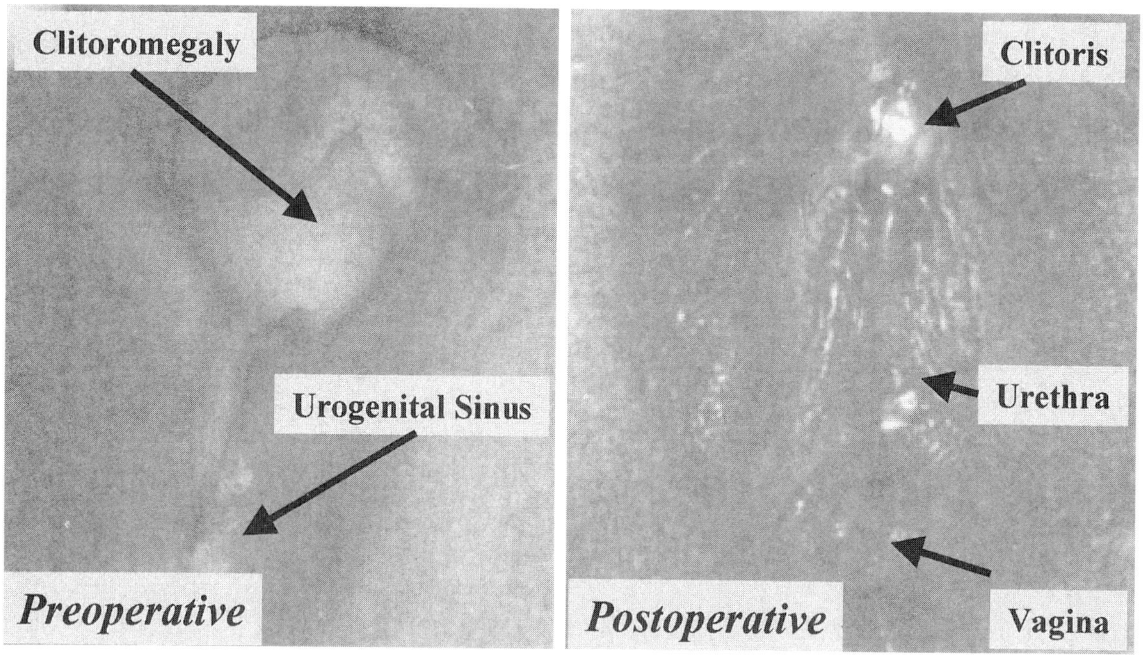

FIGURE 130.3. Feminizing genitoplasty of a patient with a high urogenital sinus malformation.

The optimal time for surgical intervention is prior to 12 months of age. Urethral reconstruction for hypospadias is accomplished by using a vascular pedicle flap, a free-graft technique, or a combination of the two. Chordee release is fairly routine, unless there is a degree of corporal disproportion, in which case ventral corporoplasty techniques need to be used. The defective corporal tissue is removed, and resurfacing is performed using a dermal graft or a pedicle flap of tunica vaginalis.

Staged reconstructions can be performed in severe malformations. Chordee release is performed, and glanular flaps are developed. An incision is made through the dorsal foreskin, and this is used to resurface the ventral shaft and the exposed areas of the glans. The second part of the procedure is undertaken 3 to 6 months later. An extended U-shaped incision is made ventrally, and a neourethra is created by tubularization of the underlying tissue. Preoperative and postoperative results are shown in Fig. 130.4.

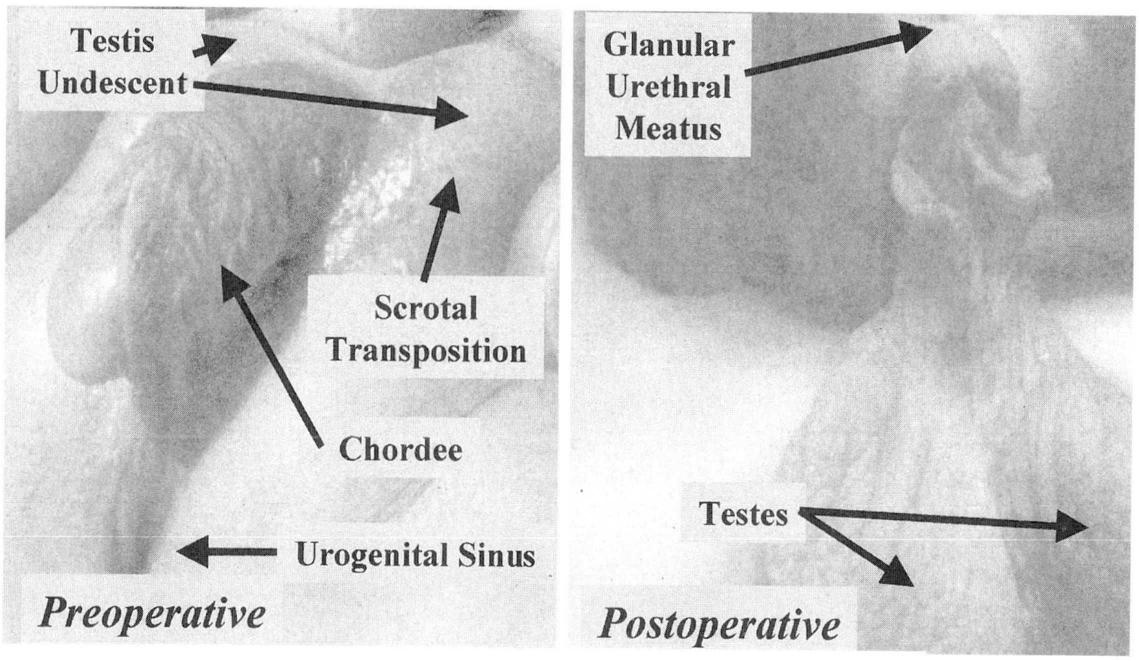

FIGURE 130.4. Preoperative and postoperative results of a masculinizing genitoplasty.

SPECIAL ISSUES

Internal Ductal Structures

In addition to feminizing and masculinizing genitoplasties, the surgical management of ductal structures also needs to be addressed. Patients diagnosed with true hermaphroditism or gonadal diagnosis and raised as males should have müllerian remnant tissues removed. If testes can reach a scrotal position, they should be sampled for biopsy to rule out any degree of dysgenesis. If the testicle is viable, then penile reconstruction, gonadectomy, and testicular prosthesis placement is appropriate.

Gonadectomy

There are two primary reasons for gonadectomy: avoidance of inappropriate secondary sexual changes during puberty and avoidance of malignancy. In general, any gonadal tissue not appropriate for gender is removed. This is most critical with respect to testis removal due to the risk of inappropriate masculinization. Patients with true hermaphroditism may have gender-appropriate ovaries or testes retained provided that biopsy excludes ovatestis or dysgenesis and for males, it can be positioned within the scrotum. The gender appropriate component of ovotestis can occasionally be retained if it meets biopsy criteria. This is relatively rare for the testicular component, however.

In mixed gonadal dysgenesis, there is a high risk of developing gonadoblastoma, which is composed of germ cells with malignant potential. Because of a high incidence of bilaterality, some surgeons have recommended bilateral gonadectomy. Streak gonads and dysgenetic testes are removed unconditionally.

In male pseudohermaphroditism with testicular feminization, most patients are raised as females unless there is a marked response to androgen exposure. Patients should undergo bilateral orchiectomy because of the potential for malignant degeneration, although there remains some controversy regarding the timing for gonadectomy. Gonadectomy in infancy eliminates the risk of malignant degeneration, which has been reported in children less than 1 year of age, and avoids the physical and emotional consequences of having a girl undergo orchiectomy around the time of puberty. Leaving the testes throughout childhood has the theoretical advantage of providing some hormonal support during development.

Gender Assignment Controversies

Presently, there is an ongoing debate regarding the role of definitive gender assignment for patients with ambiguous genitalia. There are many investigators who believe that anatomy and endocrine studies are not reliable enough to assign a particular gender. Reiner suggests fusing these practical data with the overall picture of gender identity, giving more credence to psychosocial and psychosexual outcomes, and doing more research on long-term outcomes of identity and sexuality. Some argue that pre- and postnatal hormones have a significant influence on future gender role behavior, leading to the potential for deviant behavior and psychopathology. Others advocate delayed surgical reconstruction until the patient is old enough to give informed consent. However, it is unknown if outcomes would be better based on reconstruction as an adult; delayed repair may actually endanger a previously healthy psychosocial status.

It also has been observed that psychosocial adaptation has been affected by the results of surgical reconstruction. With a functional reconstruction as an infant, many patients go on to do well with adequate family and peer support. Surgical reconstruction is performed with the consideration of karyotype and gonadal findings, and should be performed by surgeons who are well versed in both masculine and feminine reconstructions to eliminate any bias.

Indeed, the long-standing nurture versus nature controversy remains, and there is evidence at this point that both contribute to gender identity. A multidisciplinary team of physicians, child psychiatrists, and social workers is clearly indicated. Longitudinal studies are needed to further address problems with gender identity.

SUGGESTED READINGS

Glassberg KI. Editorial: gender assignment and the pediatric urologist. *J Urol* 1999;161:1308–1310.

Parrott TS, Woodward JR. Abdominoperitoneal approach to management of the high short vagina in the adrenogenital syndrome. *J Urol* 1991;146:647.

Passarini-Glazel G. A new 1-stage procedure for clitorovaginoplasty in severely masculinized female pseudohermaphrodites. *J Urol* 1989;142:55.

Reiner WG. Assignment of sex in neonates with ambiguous genitalia. *Curr Opin Pediatr* 1999;11:363–365.

Sheldon CA, Gilbert A, Lewis AG. Vaginal reconstruction: critical technical principles. *J Urol* 1994;152:190.

Sheldon CA. Intersex States. In: Oldham KT, Colombani PM, Foglia RP, eds. *Surgery of infants and children: scientific principles and practice.* Philadelphia: Lippincott-Raven, 1997:1577–1616.

Sheldon CA. Editorial: functional social and psychosexual adjustment after vaginal reconstruction. *J Urol* 1999;162:188–189.

Slijper FM, Drop SL, Molenaar JC, et al. Long-term psychological evaluation of intersex children. *Arch Sex Behav* 1998;27:125–144.

Snyder MH, Retik AB, Bauer SB, et al. Feminizing genitoplasty: a synthesis. *J Urol* 1983;129:1024.

Van Niekerk WA, Retief AE. The gonads of human true hermaphrodites. *Hum Genet* 1981;58:117.

131

CLOACAL EXSTROPHY

DENNIS P. LUND

Cloacal exstrophy is one of the most complex anomalies compatible with survival. Although there is a wide spectrum of complexity of the anomaly, it basically consists of five parts: omphalocele, imperforate anus, exstrophy of two small hemibladders that are separated by a lateral cecal fissure, and ambiguous genitalia (Fig. 131.1). As in all bladder exstrophy patients, the symphysis pubis is widely separated. Newborns frequently have prolapse of the terminal ileum through the lateral cecal fissure, and this appears as an elephant's trunk deformity. Almost all of the children have anomalies of their spinal cord ranging from simple tethering to more complex lesions such as terminal myelocystocele or lipomeningocele. There are frequent anomalies of the upper urinary tracts such as pelvic kidneys, and all children have vesicoureteral reflux.

The incidence of this anomaly is approximately 1 in 300,000 live births. Embryologically, this is thought to occur due to premature rupture of the cloacal membrane before descent of the urorectal septum in the embryo at 5 weeks' gestation. However, recent ultrasonographic evidence has suggested that there might be something going on later in gestation because some patients have been seen with an intact cloacal membrane on prenatal ultrasonography as late as 22 weeks' gestation but are then subsequently born with cloacal exstrophy.

This lesion was first described in 1709 by Littre. The first survivor was reported in 1960 by Rickham. Survival now is nearly 100%, and the challenge for the pediatric surgeon is functional reconstruction of these children.

TREATMENT OF THE NEWBORN CHILD

Frequently, this lesion can be diagnosed antenatally. If this is the case, it is ideal for the parents to meet with a pediatric surgeon capable of reconstructing these cases so that they can begin to have some understanding of the complexity of the problem and what will be involved in reconstruction. All of the anomalies associated with cloacal exstrophy are reconstructable if they are not too severe and if there is an adequate amount of tissue with which to work. However, this may not be the case. For example, the male baby with a microphallus or more commonly two tiny hemi-phalluses may be best raised as a female. Although great progress has been made in penile reconstruction, it is still extremely difficult to create a functional phallus when there is simply no tissue with which

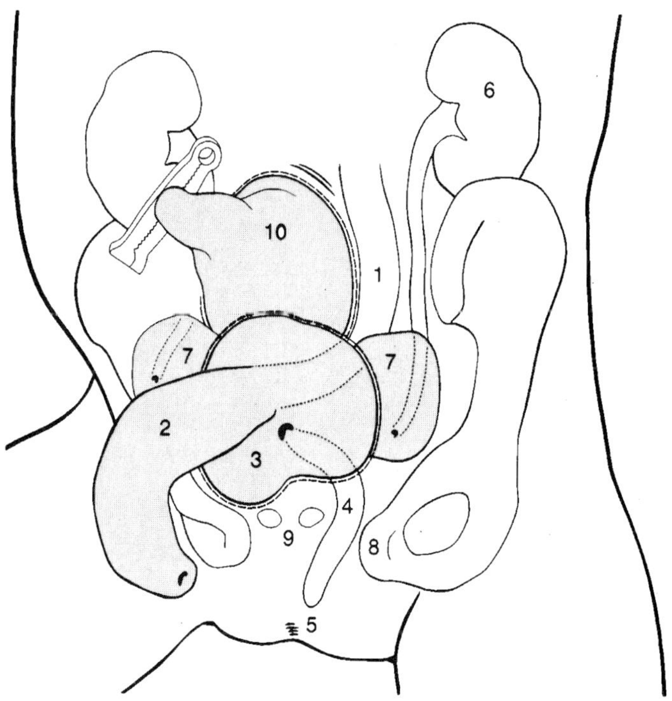

FIGURE 131.1. Typical characteristics of a newborn cloacal exstrophy patient. The females usually have two vaginas attached to the open hemibladders (*7*), each with a hemiuterus, fallopian tube, and ovary. The males have an absent or extremely deficient hemiphallus on each side near the symphisis bones (*8*), with labioscrotal tissue that is sometimes widely separated. Frequently the testes are undescended. (1) Proximal ileum, (2) prolapsed ileum, (3) open cecum, (4) microcolon, (5) imperforate anus, (6) kidney, (7) hemibladder, (8) wide symphysis, (9) ambiguous genitalia, (10) omphalocele.

D. P. Lund: Department of Surgery, University of Wisconsin; and Department of Surgery, University of Wisconsin Children's Hospital, Madison, Wisconsin.

to work. This kind of dilemma is best addressed very early after birth and may require the involvement of a gender identity team, including a pediatric surgeon, a urologist, an endocrinologist, and someone capable of providing psychologic and psychiatric support for the family.

The steps in reconstruction of the newborn are demonstrated in Fig. 131.2. This should be undertaken soon after birth since this makes bladder and pelvic closure easier and the bladder does not have a chance to become heavily colonized with bacteria. Newborn evaluation should include sonography of the kidneys and spinal cord.

The cecum should be separated from the two hemibladders. The cecum is then tubularized and left in continuity with the intestine. This is very important so that the maximum amount of bowel is available for nutritional purposes in these babies, who frequently have less than the normal length of intestine. Depending on the quality of the gluteal cleft and the severity of the spinal cord anomaly, it may be possible to perform a primary rectal pull-through operation by bringing the hindgut down through the center of the perineal sphincter. If this is done, it is probably wise to protect the cecal closure with an ileostomy. An alternative is to create a terminal colostomy from the end of the hindgut. The hindgut should be functionalized as soon as possible because there is significant growth of this short piece of large intestine when it is used, and it is helpful in controlling fluid and electrolyte loss.

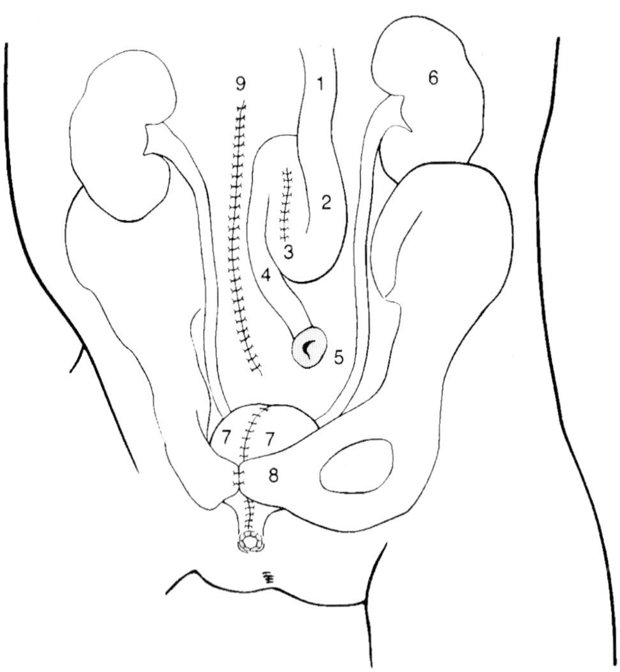

FIGURE 131.2. Postoperative neonate after separation and closure of bowel and bladder. Pull-through of the rectum can be performed at this stage, but may be deferred until definitive reconstruction. (1) Proximal ileum, (2) inverted distal ileum, (3) closed cecum, (4) microcolon, (5) colostomy, (6) kidney, (7) hemibladder, conduit, (8) closed symphysis, (9) abdomenal wall closure.

The two small hemibladders are then joined together. No effort is made to correct vesicoureteral reflux in the newborn. A urinary introitus that drains freely must be created so that there is no obstruction to the drainage of urine, which can set the baby up for urinary tract infections and renal damage. It is wise to leave ureteral stents and a urinary drainage tube so that postoperative edema does not lead to urinary obstruction. The symphysis pubis should be brought together with heavy absorbable sutures in front of the urinary opening. This can usually be done without pelvic osteotomies in the newborn. In order to promote healing of the symphysis, the baby is placed in a modified Bryant's traction for 3 weeks postoperatively.

In the genetic female, there are typically two small hemivaginas that empty into the urethral plate area. These are left to freely drain as part of the urinary introitus. They should both be preserved for future reconstruction. In the case of the genetic male for whom the decision has been made to raise the child in the female gender, the author recommends gonadectomies at the first operation to try to minimize imprinting due to testosterone.

Finally, the omphalocele should be closed as part of the abdominal closure. This is frequently possible to do in a single stage, but if not, a piece of temporary prosthetic material may be placed as a silo, which can then be removed in a staged manner analogous to closure of a large omphalocele or gastroschisis case.

As previously stated, the baby is placed in a modified Bryant's traction for 3 weeks while the symphysis heals. Feeding may be started as soon as the ileostomy or colostomy begins to function, but these babies frequently require a period of total parenteral nutrition until bowel function becomes adequate. After 3 weeks, the baby is taken down from traction and allowed to function normally.

Some of the technical aspects of treatment of the newborn child include placement of a temporary central venous line for use intraoperatively and also for parenteral nutrition postoperatively. The baby should be positioned and prepared for surgery so that he or she is circumferentially prepared and draped from the nipples downward. This allows access to the perineum as well as the ability to bring the legs together for the symphysis closure. In the past, some surgeons have removed the small hemibladders. This practice should be avoided because even the small hemibladders can be used for ultimate reconstruction of the urinary conduit. Also, as mentioned above, it is essential to separate the cecum from the hemibladders and incorporate it into the gastrointestinal tract for nutritional purposes.

Management in the first few years of life includes correction of the neurologic defects involving the spine. Thereafter, continuous support for the patient and the family is necessary so that the child can grow and develop as normally as possible. Urinary tract infections may be a problem, and it is essential to make sure that there is good, unobstructed urinary drainage. The kidneys should be followed for growth and to watch for development of significant hydronephrosis. This can be done with regular renal ultrasonography examinations. If there is good urinary drainage, it is not necessary to use suppressive antibiotics. If urinary tract infections are a problem, however, it may be necessary to use suppression.

DEFINITIVE RECONSTRUCTION

Definitive reconstruction needs to be undertaken when the child is a bit older. Because these cases are exceedingly rare, with about 15 new cases per year in the United States, it may be wisest to refer these cases to a reconstructive center that has experience in this type of reconstruction. The goals of reconstruction include urinary continence without recurrent urinary tract infections, genital reconstruction, and, if possible, rectal reconstruction. Every effort is made to try to rid the patient of colostomy and urostomy appliances and to make the child appear and function as normally as possible. There is no "right" age for reconstruction, but I prefer to try to have the child trained out of diapers prior to the commencement of regular schooling. Because almost all of these children will require clean intermittent catheterization to empty their bladders, having children a bit older so that they can participate in this activity themselves may be helpful. However, even children 3 to 5 years of age can learn to perform clean intermittent catheterization themselves. Therefore, it seems reasonable to plan for the commencement of reconstructive activity in the child's third or fourth year. By this age, the child's growth will have slowed and the nutritional problems and the caloric demands of early childhood growth will have lessened. Furthermore, because these reconstructions are extensive undertakings, this allows time to achieve a good functional result prior to the start of school.

URINARY TRACT RECONSTRUCTION

Reconstruction of the urinary tract requires that the child have a conduit that is compliant so that it does not generate excessive pressure as it fills and that the child has a mechanism for outlet resistance. All of these children will require clean intermittent catheterization to empty their bladders. In addition, urinary tract reconstruction needs to address the upper tract anomalies if they require surgical correction, such as megaureters and vesicoureteral reflux.

In order to make a compliant conduit, the bladder will have to be augmented. This is done using either a piece of stomach (a gastrocystoplasty) or a piece of small bowel. I favor the use of stomach, if possible, because this reconstruction does not borrow too extensively from the small bowel, which is already in short supply. The advantages of gastrocystoplasty include creation of an acid environment in the bladder, making urinary tract infection and stone formation less likely, and less mucus formation. However, some children develop bladder discomfort or even hemorrhagic cystitis from the acid, especially in cases where the patient is not completely dry. Acid blockade or bicarbonate irrigations are necessary in some of these children. If stomach is not suitable, however, one may use a detubularized piece of small intestine and attach this to the two small hemibladders that had been closed previously. Sometimes it is necessary to use both stomach and small bowel. During the urinary tract reconstruction, the ureters must be reimplanted using either the Cohen or the Politano-Leadbetter technique. The ureters can be reimplanted into the augmented section of bladder, and this is somewhat more easily done into a gastric augmentation than into small bowel. Again, the use of ureteral stents is recommended during healing.

After reimplantation of the ureters and creation of the bladder augmentation, a continence mechanism must be devised. The possible mechanisms for this include creation of a bladder neck at the previously constructed urinary introitus or creation of a Mitrofanoff catheterizable conduit (Fig. 131.3). The Young-Dees bladder neck procedure can be used to create a bladder neck if local tissues allow. It is

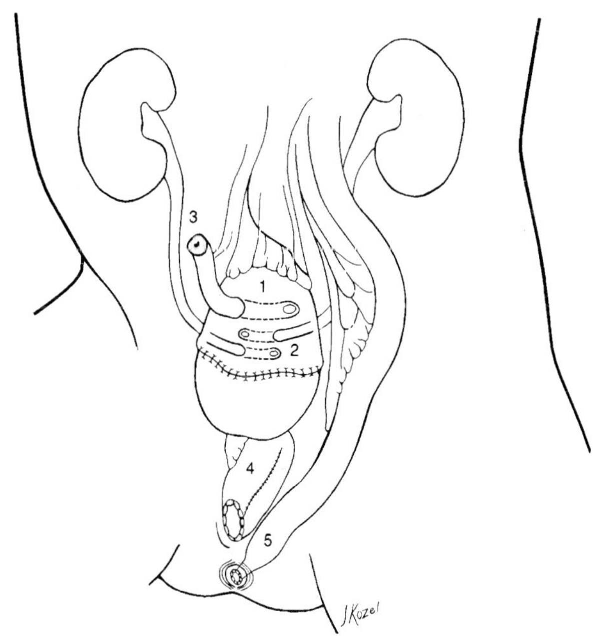

FIGURE 131.3. An idealized reconstruction in a patient who required a bowel vagina and underwent rectal pull-through. Each case must be individualized depending on the available local tissues. In this case, after the bladder augmentation, the ureters were reimplanted and a Mitrofanoff conduit was constructed out of small bowel for urinary continence. (1) Bladder augmentation (stomach or small bowel), (2) ureteral reimplants, (3) microfanoff conduit, (4) small bowel vagina, (5) colon pull through.

also possible to do this with a nipple valve created from small bowel and placed in the bladder neck. However, I now prefer the Mitrofanoff principle and most often create a conduit out of small bowel using the technique of Monti, which is then implanted into the gastrocystoplasty and brought out low in the abdomen. This technique requires surgical closure of the previously created urinary introitus. This small Mitrofanoff stoma is cosmetically satisfactory and does not require any appliance or pad to cover it. It is usually easy to catheterize because the patient can easily see it. The major disadvantage of this technique is that it makes subsequent endoscopic visualization of the bladder and ureters more difficult.

As the urinary tract is reconstructed, it is necessary to leave a catheter sutured into the continence mechanism and to place a suprapubic tube. The suprapubic tube should be left in place until it is established that the patient can be easily catheterized.

In some cases, it may be necessary to perform two augmentations to the bladder in order to have a large enough, compliant conduit. In this case both small bowel and stomach can be applied. Use of colon or hindgut for this purpose is strongly discouraged. Because the hindgut is so essential for fluid removal from the fecal stream, either colostomy or rectal management are considerably easier if the stools are more formed.

GASTROINTESTINAL RECONSTRUCTION

Some patients with cloacal exstrophy will be candidates for a rectal pull-through. The factors that influence the choice of a rectal pull-through include the following:

1. Good strength of sphincter muscles when they are electrically stimulated must be established.
2. The sphincter must be appropriately positioned.
3. The spinal cord tethering should be minimal and not accompanied by any complexities such as a large lipomeningocele or myelomeningocele.
4. The presence of a good gluteal cleft is a much better anatomic situation for rectal pull-through than the classic "rocker bottom."
5. Parents' wishes must be acknowledged and they must be made aware that a bowel regimen will be necessary for acceptable fecal continence.

If, during the years leading up to reconstruction, the patient is able to produce fairly formed stool through the colostomy, this makes continence more likely in the setting of a good bowel regimen. However, dietary manipulation, as well as an enema program and pharmacologic agents, may well be necessary in order to produce acceptable social continence.

The pull-through procedure itself is usually performed at the time of the urinary tract and genital reconstruction. The technique used is a combined abdominal perineal pull-through. It may be advantageous to use a posterior sagittal approach in combination with the abdominal approach and this requires that the child be prepared circumferentially should intraoperative turning of the patient be necessary. The patient should not be paralyzed intraoperatively, and the electrical nerve stimulator should be used to map out the rectal sphincter so that the pull-through can be placed exactly centered in the sphincter muscles. With proper bowel preparation, it is not necessary to protect the pulled-through bowel with a diverting enterostomy.

Hendren and Lund reported on 25 patients who underwent rectal pull-through procedures for cloacal exstrophy. Of these, 77% claimed to have acceptable fecal continence with the bowel program. However, 16% of patients who underwent rectal pull-through procedures were ultimately reversed to permanent colostomies. Clearly, it is important that the family be aware of the implications of pull-through of the rectum.

GENITAL RECONSTRUCTION

Vaginal reconstruction in the genetic female requires separation of the vaginas from the bladder neck. Typically there are two separate vaginas with a hemiuterus, fallopian tube, and ovary associated with each. If one vagina is very diminutive, as is often the case, then this vagina and uterus should be discarded while saving the ovary. If both are of suitable caliber and they can be anastomosed side to side and brought to the perineum, this will allow for a larger vaginal vault. More often, however, only one vagina is suitable and this can be mobilized and brought to the perineum. If neither vagina is suitable to bring to the perineum, a vagina may be created using a segment of small bowel and anastomosed to the uterus or vagina to create a vaginal introitus on the perineum.

Genetic males who are being raised in the female gender may undergo vaginal reconstruction at the time of urinary tract reconstruction or this may be deferred until adolescence. The technique preferred by the author is to utilize small bowel. The small bowel should be detubularized and fashioned so that it has a large enough capacity and brought down on its vascular pedicle behind the bladder to the perineum. This is demonstrated in Fig. 131.3.

The most difficult reconstructive problem is in the genetic male who has been raised as a male and has no phallic tissue. Even the smallest amount of sensory tissue should be maintained in both boys and girls. These patients should be referred to one of the few centers around the country that are attempting phallic reconstruction using techniques such as a vascularized, sensate forearm flap. This is clearly an area of intense research, and it may well be that tissue-engineering approaches to solving this problem will offer the best hope for these patients in the future.

DISCUSSION

Cloacal exstrophy is no longer the hopeless entity it was once thought to be. Nearly all children now survive and furthermore can undergo reconstruction to achieve a satisfactory state of function and appearance. These children are almost always neurologically normal from the waist up and are frequently very bright. Some of this sophistication may be the result of extensive hospitalization in the early years of life. My experience, however, is that most of these children have above-average intelligence.

Many of these children can now be diagnosed antenatally and are referred to surgeons for antenatal counseling. It is necessary to make parents aware of the complexity of the problem, but it is also important to reassure them that the majority of these problems can be solved surgically. From the surgeon's perspective, there must be the realization that these children are perpetual works in progress. The surgeon must be patient and, above all, persistent. Many times more than one operation is necessary to solve a particular reconstructive problem.

The large number and complexity of anomalies in these patients requires a thoughtful and systematic approach. As a baby develops and grows, his or her requirements begin to differ. Early in life, nutrition and growth are of paramount importance and every effort needs to be made to optimize gastrointestinal tract function. As the child grows, the surgeon can then begin to address the individual reconstructive problems.

The goal of reconstruction should be to try to rid the patient of stomas and particularly of appliances. The use of a urinary stoma that requires an appliance is now mostly unnecessary. A functional bladder neck or Mitrofanoff conduit can almost always be created, but it requires persistence. All of these patients need to empty their bladders by clean intermittent catheterization. Therefore, urinary continence requires both a compliant conduit and a compliant patient, who is willing to catheterize regularly.

In my experience, about 50% of patients will be candidates for pull-through of the rectum. If the patient is a good candidate for pull-through, the patient and family need to recognize that fecal continence will be achieved only with the use of a good bowel program that may involve use of medications as well as enema washouts. Use of all large bowel in the gastrointestinal tract maximizes the chances for a successful pull-through. Even in cases where a pull-through is not possible, an intact hindgut makes colostomy management much simpler.

Despite the complex array of anomalies in patients with cloacal exstrophy, the most difficult psychosocial problem is often related to gender assignment of those genetic male patients who have absent phallic tissue. Although tremendous progress has been made in phallic reconstruction, there are no good long-term functional data on these techniques. Tissue engineering clearly holds promise in this area. If gender reassignment is chosen, it is recommended that this choice be made as early as possible and that testosterone-producing tissue be removed as early as possible. Even so, in these cases, patients may sometimes exhibit male-type behavior. The converse situation, where male patients without phallic tissue are raised as boys, can lead to situations of intense frustration when those boys become men. I have seen both situations occur. Clearly there is no easy answer to this problem, and gender assignment decisions must be individualized. This decision should be made as early as possible, however, and the use of a gender assignment team may be beneficial. If techniques of phallic reconstruction continue to improve, this subset of cloacal exstrophy patients will be less problematic.

Cloacal exstrophy is clearly one of the most complex reconstructive problems for the pediatric surgeon. With a thoughtful approach, however, these patients can undergo satisfactory reconstruction and live healthy and functional lives. The interaction between the surgeon and the patient with this disease must be unique. Patients and surgeons need to realize that they are involved "for the long haul" in the care of these children. However, the satisfaction that can be derived for the surgeon in seeing successful reconstruction in one of these children is without parallel.

SUGGESTED READINGS

Hendren WH, Atala A. Use of bowel for vaginal reconstruction. *J Urol* 1994;152:752–755.

Jordan GH. Penile reconstruction, phallic construction and urethral reconstruction. *Urol Clin North Am* 1999;26:1–13.

Lund DP, Hendren WH. Cloacal exstrophy: a twenty-five year experience with 50 cases. *J Pediatr Surg* 2001;36:68–75.

Lund DP, Hendren WH. Cloacal exstrophy: experience with twenty cases. *J Pediatr Surg* 1993;28:1360–1369.

Matthews R, Jeffs RD, Reiner WG, et al. Cloacal exstrophy—improving the quality of life: the Johns Hopkins experience. *J Urol* 1998;160:2452–2456.

Monti PR, Lara RC, Dutra MA, et al. New techniques for construction of efferent conduits based on the Mitrofanoff principle. *Urology* 1997;49:112–115.

Ricketts RR, Woodward JR, Zwiren GT, et al. Modern treatment of cloacal exstrophy. *J Pediatr Surg* 1991;26:444–448.

132

BENIGN GYNECOLOGIC DISORDERS

AVIVA L. KATZ

Pediatric surgeons are frequently responsible for the diagnosis and management of gynecologic processes that affect children and adolescents. In addition to the various ovarian neoplasms that occur in these age groups, we need to be familiar with many benign gynecologic disorders. Ovarian and paraovarian processes also should be considered in the differential diagnosis of any girl who presents with abdominal pain, because the symptoms are often nonspecific and can mimic those of appendicitis and other gastrointestinal processes.

VAGINAL BLEEDING

The likely etiology of vaginal bleeding is related to the age of the patient; this knowledge helps direct an age-appropriate and concise evaluation. These changes are in part related to the changing hormonal milieu as development proceeds. Vaginal bleeding in the newborn period is most often physiologic and secondary to the influence of maternal estrogen. The fetal endometrium and external genitalia may be stimulated *in utero* by maternal estrogens and gonadotropins that cross the placenta. This can result in thickening and enlargement of the labia minora and the clitoris and stimulation of growth of the endometrium. Endometrial shedding, with vaginal discharge or vaginal bleeding, may result from the relatively abrupt estrogen withdrawal that occurs after birth. This bleeding is generally self-limited.

Bleeding that persists beyond 2 weeks should be considered pathologic, not physiologic, and deserves further investigation. Following this period of early infancy there should be no source of endogenous estrogen until the development of premenarchal activity, usually at 7 to 10 years of age. Most gynecologic problems seen during this period are related to a lack of estrogen and its usual protective effect on tissues, rather than estrogen stimulation. Problems related to estrogen stimulation require a search for exogenous (hormone replacement therapy is a common medical therapy) or pathologic endogenous estrogens.

Vaginal foreign bodies are a relatively common cause of vaginal bleeding, especially in the older toddler or school-aged child. The foreign body may produce a local inflammation or vaginitis resulting in discharge that may be serosanguinous or blood stained. The most common foreign body encountered are wads of toilet paper, which usually appear as a grayish mass. Occasionally, with a cooperative and calm parent/child pair, the foreign body can be floated free from the vagina with gentle lavage with a small 8 or 10 French catheter. More commonly, due to anxiety and the sensitivity of the unestrogenized vaginal wall and atrophic mucosa, retrieval of the foreign body requires an examination under a general anesthetic. Other causes of vulvovaginitis are less likely to result in vaginal bleeding.

Urethral prolapse is another source of apparent vaginal bleeding. Redundant urethral mucosa may prolapse through the urethral meatus, encircling the urethral meatus, and with the development of vascular congestion there may be tissue strangulation appearing as a friable polypoid mass. The cause of this lesion is uncertain, but it has been linked to the hypoestrogenic state. Urethral prolapse is an often misdiagnosed cause of genital bleeding in young girls, and more commonly presents with bleeding rather than dysuria. Most often, the prolapse responds to conservative measures, including sitz baths and estrogen cream application. If the prolapsed mucosa has become necrotic, excision with approximation of the mucosal edges may be necessary.

Genital trauma is another relatively common cause of vaginal bleeding. Minor trauma in the premenarchal child may result in significant bleeding. Lack of estrogen stimulation results in atrophic tissues with poor distensibility and exposure of the underlying capillary beds. It is key in this situation to anticipate and address the anxiety that this bleeding will cause the patient and her family. Additional goals are to determine the extent of the injury, especially whether the wound extends above the pelvic floor, and whether the history of the injury matches the type and extent of wound found. An examination under anesthesia may be required to allow determination of the full

A. L. Katz: Departments of Surgery and Pediatrics, Thomas Jefferson University, Philadelphia, Pennsylvania, and Alfred I. duPont Hospital for Children, Wilmington, Delaware.

extent of the injuries and appropriate repair of extensive injuries. Bathtub rims, counter doors, bicycle bars, and gym and playground equipment are frequently the source of straddle injuries and genital trauma in young children. Although there may be urethral injury or vulvar hematoma or laceration, these injuries rarely result in wounds that extend through the vaginal vault and above the pelvic floor. In these situations, blood seen coming from the vaginal orifice does not necessarily originate in the vaginal cavity and does not clearly indicate a true vaginal injury. If a source of bleeding is seen on the external genitalia and the hymen is intact, it is unlikely that the bleeding originates in the vagina.

Although accidental vaginal penetrating injuries may occur, *sexual abuse* must be suspected. Prepubertal children subjected to blunt penetrating forceful trauma may sustain lacerations to the hymen with extension into the vagina, rectum, and peritoneal cavity. Bleeding from these injuries may be extensive and requires operative evaluation and repair. All injuries with damage oriented posteriorly should be considered suspicious and evaluated to avoid missing extensive injuries. Most accidental blunt injuries are oriented anteriorly on the perineum, with involvement of the labia minora and clitoris.

Additional sources of vaginal bleeding include urogenital tumors, including benign hemangiomas and arteriovenous malformations, and malignant tumors, including primarily rhabdomyosarcoma, especially botryoid sarcoma, and ovarian tumors with hormonal production and stimulation of endometrial shedding. These tumors and the various causes of precocious puberty are beyond the scope of this chapter.

VULVOVAGINITIS

Vulvovaginitis is an inflammation of the vulva and vaginal tissues. In most children the vulva is usually inflamed first and the vagina either uninvolved or secondarily affected. Vulvovaginitis is the most common gynecologic disorder in children. The vulva of the young child is relatively unprotected without labial fat pads or pubic hair. Additionally, the vulvar skin and vaginal mucosa are thin and atrophic due to the lack of estrogen and are far less resistant to infectious organisms. The child's vaginal cavity has a neutral pH, with limited native bacterial colonization, again providing limited protection from invading bacteria. Poor perineal hygiene and contamination with stool and other debris are additional elements leading to the development of vulvovaginitis.

The child most commonly presents with complaints of discharge, discomfort, pruritis, and urinary symptoms, chiefly dysuria. Nonspecific vulvovaginitis accounts for 25% to 75% of the cases seen in prepubertal girls. It may be related to chemical or mechanical irritants such as soaps, bubble baths, and laundry detergents. Physical examination reveals irritation with a nonpurulent, nonodorous discharge. Treatment consists of reassurance and attention to hygiene with elimination of the irritating agent. If the inflammation is resistant to these interventions, oral antibiotics directed against *Escherichia coli* and other intestinal pathogens may be used.

A variety of specific causes of vulvovaginitis are seen less commonly in the prepubertal girl. *Candidal infections* are less common in the age group, partly due to an alkaline to neutral vaginal pH that is hostile to yeast. Most candidal infections result from poor hygiene, with contamination of the organism from the gastrointestinal tract. Decreased cellular immunity and broad-spectrum antibiotic use are additional predisposing factors. The presentation in the prepubertal patient less frequently includes the anticipated thick white discharge and more commonly includes minimal discharge, with pruritis, erythema, edema, and satellite lesions. Treatment is with standard antifungal agents.

Bacterial vaginosis results from a mixed flora of predominately anaerobic bacteria, including *Gardnerella vaginalis.* Although this vaginosis is common in adolescents and young women, it is relatively rare in prepubertal girls, although an increased prevalence is noted in sexually abused girls. The diagnosis is made by noting a thin homogenous, malodorous discharge, because cultures are generally not helpful. Bacterial vaginosis is generally responsive to metronidazole. *Chlamydia, Neisseria gonorrhoeae,* and *Trichomonas* may all cause vaginitis in the sexually abused child or sexually active adolescent. These infections may be asymptomatic, requiring thorough evaluation of culture material for appropriate diagnosis, or may present with vaginitis with infection usually confined to the vagina, rather than ascending endocervically to the upper genital tract.

Lichen sclerosis et atrophicus is a genital dermatologic condition that may yield abnormal examination results and may be confused with vulvovaginitis. Lichen sclerosis is thought to be secondary to a testosterone receptor insensitivity on the perineum and may be associated with pigmentation changes and pruritis. There may be secondary changes to the involved tissue due to scratching in easily traumatized areas, occasionally raising the concern of differentiating this lesion from abuse. The skin changes may wax and wane without specific treatment. Treatment may consist of topical corticosteroids to control the pruritis. Specific therapy with topical testosterone is limited due to the concern of virilizing changes and effects on growth.

LABIAL ADHESIONS

Adhesions of the labia minora are common from infancy until puberty. This relatively common gynecologic disorder is another estrogen deficiency disorder, with low estrogen levels in the prepubertal child resulting in thin, relatively atrophic, easily traumatized labial tissue. This thin skin may become easily denuded with minor trauma, followed by adherence of tissue in the midline, with reepithelialization and resultant fusion. These adhesions generally appear as a thin membrane between the labia minora, not covering the clitoris. Labial adhesions are not seen in the neonate, because the tissue at this time is well estrogenized secondary to the transplacental passage of maternal hormones. Fusion of the labia noted in the newborn therefore requires evaluation for ambiguous genitalia. Most labial adhesions demonstrate posterior fusion, which may extend for a variable distance anteriorly. These adhesions may frequently be discovered incidentally, and treatment is only required if they become symptomatic. Fusion may persist until the tissues become estrogenized at puberty, but persistence of this finding alone does not dictate the need for therapy. Most children remain asymptomatic, and the only therapy required is reassurance of the benign nature of this problem and the anticipated spontaneous resolution at or slightly before puberty. Symptoms, when present, are most commonly related to relative obstruction and include vaginitis, urinary tract infection, dysuria, and dribbling of urine with resultant chronic perineal irritation.

Treatment is initiated with topical conjugated estrogens applied twice a day for a period of 2 weeks. This therapy is directed just at the area of the adhesions, anticipating that allowing adequate maturation of the tissues will allow the cycle of tissue fragility, injury, and fusion to resolve. Unfortunately, topical therapy is only successful in approximately half of patients. For those patients who remain symptomatic and fail topical therapy, the next step is manual separation. This requires the use of either a topical analgesic or a brief general anesthetic. Manual separation must still be followed by topical estrogen therapy because the tissue will be raw immediately following separation and may quickly readhere. The use of a simple protecting ointment following a 2- to 4-week course of topical estrogen therapy may help minimize tissue trauma and the recurrence of adhesions. With long-term use of topical estrogen therapy, there is the potential for systemic absorption. This estrogen stimulation may result in changes in other estrogen-responsive tissue, such as early breast development and vulva pigmentation. Families should be cautioned to watch for these potential changes and be reassured that they will regress when the estrogen therapy is completed.

OVARIAN CYSTS

Knowledge regarding the incidence and natural history of ovarian cysts throughout the period of late fetal development through infancy and childhood has developed rapidly over the past decade, in significant part due to the increased use of ultrasonographic imaging.

Antenatal diagnosis of ovarian cysts has become increasingly common. This phenomenon is most likely secondary to transplacental passage of maternal and placental hormones, resulting in ovarian stimulation. This high estrogen state may be responsible for the stimulation and growth of functional ovarian follicular cysts. These cysts can occasionally become a source of autonomous estrogen production. An additional factor stimulating ovarian follicular cyst formation is high fetal gonadotropin secretion. This elevated gonadotropin secretion continues until the 25th to 29th week of gestation, despite a high fetoplacental estrogen level, due to a lack of pituitary steroid receptors at this developmental stage. This physiology also explains the development of large ovarian cysts in extremely premature neonates. Since the initial findings of ovarian cysts on antenatal ultrasonography, there has been ongoing debate regarding how best to manage this fetal finding. Most fetal cysts resolve spontaneously and are first noted after 26 to 28 weeks of gestation. The goal of all proposed therapy is to balance a safe and accessible intervention in the hopes of maximizing salvage of ovarian tissue. Fetal intervention is complicated by the inherent difficulties in antenatal diagnosis. Ovarian cysts may be difficult to differentiate from enteric duplication cysts, mesenteric cysts, and omental cysts. Other cystic structures in the pelvis that may be confused with an ovarian cyst include hydrometrocolpos, urachal cyst, bowel atresia, renal cysts and anterior meningocele.

There are clearly no data to support any intervention for the smaller, uncomplicated ovarian cyst, and there is excellent documentation of resolution over time. The issue of fetal intervention in larger cysts has been raised in the literature, without clear resolution at present. Cysts larger than 5 cm are thought to be at increased risk for complications, most importantly torsion, resulting in the loss of ovarian tissue. The risks of *in utero* aspiration of the cyst, with intervention to the mother, fetus, and pregnancy, must be weighed against an undefined risk of ovarian loss. Cyst aspiration becomes a more pressing concern in those rare fetuses with extremely large cysts causing compression of the thorax, raising the concern of pulmonary hypoplasia, or compressing and obstructing the urinary system. Here, the risks to the fetus would seem clearer and would support the argument for intervention. The aspirated cyst fluid should be assessed for estrogen levels to help confirm the ovarian source of the cyst.

Most ovarian cysts continue to regress throughout the neonatal period and beyond, with complete resolution anticipated by 3 to 4 months of age. This is a result of the abrupt decline in hormonal stimulation and the hyperestrogenized state at the time of birth. Once again, in the neonate, intervention is recommended for the larger simple cysts due to the concern about ovarian loss through torsion, with the size of concern usually 5 cm, although there are limited prospective data to help support this position. Intervention may start with ultrasonography-guided needle aspiration of simple, anechoic cysts, with laparoscopy or laparotomy reserved for recurrences of the simple cyst. Complex cysts, noted on ultrasonography by a fluid-debris level, a retracting clot, septations, or a solid masslike appearance, reflect complications of the cyst, most commonly hemorrhage or torsion. Rarely, these ultrasonographic changes may represent an ovarian tumor. These changes require surgical intervention, either by laparoscopy or limited laparotomy to allow visualization of the gonad, and cystectomy or oophorectomy as needed. These complex cysts do not resolve over time.

Beyond the neonatal period and prior to the onset of puberty is a period of relative hormonal quiescence. The risk of malignancy in a complex ovarian mass is higher during this age period, as compared with infancy, and simple, anechoic cysts are less common. For this reason, a surgical approach is required for all complex cysts, and for all simple cysts that do not show changes of resolution during a short period of observation of 2 to 4 weeks. Again, laparoscopy or laparotomy should allow adequate visualization of the ovary to proceed with appropriate resection, either cystectomy or oophorectomy in the case of tumor.

The hormonal changes accompanying puberty again increase the potential for development of ovarian cysts. Simple, anechoic cysts are most likely functional follicular cysts, demonstrating an exuberant response to hormonal cycling. Many of these cysts resolve over time, and cysts smaller than 7 to 8 cm frequently do not require intervention, unless increasingly symptomatic with pain or fever. Hemorrhagic cysts in this age group also may demonstrate spontaneous resolution over time. Surgical intervention should be limited, and there is significant experience with laparoscopy in the treatment of ovarian cysts. Laparoscopic fenestration or excision of the cyst wall and drainage, with preservation of ovarian tissue, is an excellent approach, with conversion to a laparotomy as needed if the cystic change proves to be a complex ovarian tumor on visualization. Follow-up after ovarian cystectomy is vital to try to minimize the recurrence of follicular ovarian cysts. Combination oral contraceptives, containing both estrogen and progesterone, are a useful adjunct in an attempt to prevent cyst recurrence. These agents may be effective by suppressing gonadotropin stimulation and subsequent ovulation and follicular cyst formation. A number of products are available, each with a slightly different ratio of estrogenic, progestational, and androgenic activity. It may take several cycles to achieve optimum response to the agent chosen, or a different formulation may be required to minimize side effects and achieve cyst suppression. There is no evidence that the use of oral contraceptives will encourage sexual activity in otherwise abstinent teenagers, a commonly held misunderstanding that sometimes interferes with the use of this extremely effective agent.

OVARIAN TORSION

Ovarian torsion may be related to the presence and size of an ovarian cyst, the size of the ovary itself, or the length of the ovarian suspensory ligaments or the fallopian tube. A high level of clinical suspicion is required to make the diagnosis of ovarian torsion in a timely fashion. Most cases of torsion involve otherwise normal ovaries, and an element of urgency in diagnosis and treatment is justified in an attempt to salvage ovarian tissue. Torsion is a relatively common but often unanticipated finding, accounting for nearly 20% of the cases in a series examining ovarian masses in children and teenagers. Most patients with torsion present with abdominal pain; there is often also associated nausea and vomiting. There may be fever and leukocytosis, making the diagnosis difficult on clinical grounds alone.

Transabdominal or transvaginal ultrasonography can be of significant assistance in diagnosing ovarian torsion. Sonographic findings indicative of torsion include ovarian edema, an enlarged ovary with dilated peripherally located cysts, absent ovarian arterial or venous flow on color Doppler imaging, an enlarged dishomogenous ovary, often with associated pelvic ascites, and an echogenic adnexal mass. Although the absence of flow on color Doppler images is suspicious for torsion, the presence of flow, even internal ovarian flow, does not rule out the diagnosis of torsion. There may be some variation based on age in the sonographic findings in torsion. Neonates and young children tend to demonstrate extrapelvic cystic or complex masses, whereas pubertal young women frequently demonstrate a more solid mass. There is some evidence that the combination of Doppler flow imaging with the morphologic assessment improves the diagnostic accuracy of ultrasonography for ovarian torsion. Ovarian edema appears to be a reactive state in response to torsion and may in some patients represent intermittent ovarian torsion. Only limited experience has been reported with the use of magnetic resonance imaging in diagnosing ovarian torsion, although changes seen include thickened ovarian vessels and an absence of enhancement.

There is increasing evidence that rapid surgical intervention upon the diagnosis of torsion helps to preserve ovarian tissue. Although detorsion accomplished within 4 to 6 hours is traditionally considered optimal, ovarian salvage is possible long after the onset of symptoms. Prompt surgical intervention is therefore appropriate regardless of the time of presentation. There are increasing reports of laparoscopic intervention for torsion throughout all age groups. This modality permits excellent visualization and access, usually allowing detorsion of the affected ovary. Because the ovaries involved in torsion are overwhelmingly either normal or affected only with simple cysts or benign teratoma, oophorectomy, if necessary due to ovarian necrosis, also may be completed laparoscopically. There is abundant support in the literature for the safety of detorsing ovarian torsion with no documented risk of embolus or the development of a septic-like state. Additionally, there is increasing evidence that this salvaged ovarian tissue remains functional, as demonstrated by hormonal response and follicle development, even successful oocyte retrieval for *in vitro* fertilization.

There are increasing reports of the advisability of including a procedure at the time of surgery to minimize the risk for future torsion of either the affected or contralateral ovary. This is especially of concern when there has been loss of ovarian tissue secondary to torsion. Two techniques have been suggested: oophoropexy with tacking of the ovaries to the pelvic sidewalls, and plication or shortening of a long ovarian ligament. Theoretical concerns regarding mechanical impairment to fallopian tube function have been raised due to the stretch on the tube in oophoropexy to the pelvic sidewall. Similar to the situation in testicular torsion, it is hoped that fixating the ovary will prevent bilateral ovarian torsion and loss with resultant sterility. There are no data on the true incidence of contralateral ovarian torsion. An additional situation in which the ovary may be at increased risk for torsion is the irreducible ovary trapped in an inguinal hernia sac, again raising the issue of relatively urgent surgical repair.

ENDOMETRIOSIS

Endometriosis is defined as the presence of endometrial glands and stroma outside the normal anatomic location of the uterine endometrium. There is no clear cause of endometriosis, although it is found in a significant minority of menstruating women. Its true incidence in adolescents is not at all defined, in part due to the need for laparoscopy to define the presence of disease. Adolescents with endometriosis most frequently present with pain. The most severe pain typically occurs just before and during menses, tends to increase over time, and does not entirely respond to oral contraceptives and nonsteroidal antiinflammatory drugs.

Most patients have normal physical examination results, with only mild tenderness on abdominal or pelvic examination. In limited studies of adolescents with chronic pelvic and abdominal pain without findings on physical examination or radiologic studies and no response to oral contraceptives or nonsteroidals, as many as 70% of patients prove to have endometriosis on laparoscopy. Endometrial implants in adolescents may present as classic lesions with a blue/brown/gray "powder burn" appearance, or more commonly as atypical implants, including white lesions, clear vesicular lesions, and red flame or petechial lesions. There may be a progression of lesions from atypical sparse lesions in adolescents to the more classic findings in adults, with adolescents rarely having extensive disease. Adolescents with severe obstructing lesions of the genital tract, including imperforate hymen, vaginal septum, and hematocolpos, may have a higher incidence of more severe endometriosis.

The optimal treatment of endometriosis remains unclear. Surgical resection or destruction of the lesions may be successful in relieving pain, but may be associated with a high rate of recurrence, with the risk for postoperative adhesions. Medical therapy is directed at suppressing the ectopic endometrial tissue, and involves hormonal manipulation including oral contraceptives, progestins, and androgens, all of which have associated side effects.

PREGNANCY

Pregnancy can occur in girls as young as 9. Most pediatric centers have strict patient care guidelines that mandate transfer of any pregnant patient to an appropriate obstetric unit for any and all evaluations or interventions, so a detailed discussion of the topic is beyond the scope of this chapter. Nevertheless, pregnancy must be considered in the evaluation of any girl who has started her menses and any girl over 11 years of age who presents with abdominal pain, an abdominal mass, or gastrointestinal symptoms of unclear etiology. It cannot be overemphasized that pregnancy must be excluded with certainty in these patients regardless of the patient's sexual history and physical findings. In addition to a careful physical examination, a urine pregnancy test is usually sufficiently sensitive to rule out both intrauterine and ectopic pregnancy, although in cases where there is a high index of suspicion, a pelvic ultrasonographic examination should be performed. This is especially true of patients with pain localized to the lower abdomen and who are at risk for a tubal pregnancy, a potentially life-threatening process and one that must be assessed emergently. One should keep in mind that an elevated β-human chorionic gonadotropin level can occur with trophoblastic germ cell tumors, such as choriocarcinoma, and rarely with other neoplasms such as hepatoma. The possibility of a false-positive pregnancy test, admittedly an exceedingly rare event, should be considered in the appropriate clinical setting. Clinicians should also be familiar with the laws and policies that apply in the state and institution where they work to avoid an infringement of the pregnant patient's right to privacy.

SUGGESTED READINGS

Baldwin DD, Landa HM. Common problems in pediatric gynecology. *Urol Clin North Am* 1995;22:161–176.

Banerjee R, Laufer MR. Reproductive disorders associated with pelvic pain. *Semin Pediatr Surg* 1998;7:52–61.

Brown MR, Cartwright PC, Snow BW. Common office problems in pediatric urology and gynecology. *Pediatr Clin North Am* 1997;44:1091–1115.

Dodds ML. Vulvar disorders of the infant and young child. *Clin Obstet Gynecol* 1997;40:141–152.

Dolgin SE, Lublin M, Shlasko E. Maximizing ovarian salvage when treating idiopathic adnexal torsion. *J Pediatr Surg* 2000;35: 624–626.

Farrington PF. Pediatric vulvo-vaginitis. *Clin Obstet Gynecol* 1997;40: 135–140.

Helmrath MA, Shin CE, Warner BW. Ovarian cysts in the pediatric population. *Semin Pediatr Surg* 1998;7:19–28.

Pokorny SF. Genital trauma. *Clin Obstet Gynecol* 1997;40:219–225.

Schmahmann S, Haller JO. Neonatal ovarian cysts: pathogenesis, diagnosis and management. *Pediatr Radiol* 1997;27:101–105.

133

CONGENITAL ANOMALIES OF THE VAGINA AND UTERUS

REBECKA L. MEYERS

Vaginal anomalies are most common in the female infant with congenital adrenal hyperplasia and virilization. In endocrinologically normal girls, anomalies of the vagina and uterus may be isolated or associated with persistent urogenital sinus, imperforate anus, or cloacal malformations. All of these anomalies represent a failure of normal embryologic development. Normal embryologic development of these female reproductive structures is the result of pairing, fusion, and recanalization of the müllerian (paramesonephric) ducts. The most proximal müllerian ducts remain unfused and form the fallopian tubes. The middle and distal müllerian ducts fuse to form the uterus and the proximal vagina. The distal vagina and its separation from the urinary tract and rectum result from a complex interaction between the caudal end of the fused müllerian ducts, müllerian tubercle, sinovaginal bulbs, vaginal plate, urogenital sinus, and cloaca. Urogenital sinus and cloacal anomalies are examples of caudal regression syndromes, which can present with various vaginal, bladder, kidney, and rectal anomalies.

IMPERFORATE HYMEN AND TRANSVERSE VAGINAL SEPTUM

These simple vaginal obstruction anomalies manifest either in infancy or puberty. Infant girls may retain mucinous secretions stimulated by maternal estrogens and develop a mucocolpos (vagina distended with mucus). If the proximal vaginal distension is severe, pressure and distortion of the bladder and urethra may lead to secondary hydroureter and hydronephrosis. In a neonate with imperforate hymen, the thin solid or partially fenestrated membrane may be seen bulging between the labia. In some girls the imperforate hymen may not be detected until adolescence, when it presents with recurrent crampy lower abdominal pain and failure of menstruation. Physical examination shows a bulging membrane between the labia. The diagnosis is confirmed with the ultrasonographic finding of hematocolpos (vagina distended with blood). Treatment of neonates and adolescents is the same: a cruciate incision of the hymen and suture reapproximation of the epithelium.

In rare cases, the vaginal obstruction is due to a more proximal transverse vaginal septum, the result of a failure of vaginal canalization. The level of a transverse septum is variable and directly influences the degree of hematocolpos and hematometrocolpos (vagina and uterus distended with blood). Ultrasonography and occasionally magnetic resonance imaging are useful in distinguishing between vaginal obstruction due to a transverse septum, a vaginal duplication (vertical septum), or a proximal vaginal atresia. Low transverse membranes less than 2 cm in thickness can be exposed transvaginally, pulled down with stay sutures, and excised completely to prevent future stenosis. Interdigitating flaps of proximal and distal mucosa are then fashioned with absorbable sutures. A vaginal septum thicker than 2 cm or a septum located high in the vagina may require an abdominovaginal surgical approach and sometimes perineal skin flaps for reconstruction. Whether the surgical approach is simple or complex, postoperative vaginal dilation should be used to prevent formation of a stricture from concentric scar.

VAGINAL AND UTERINE DUPLICATION

Disorders of müllerian duct fusion result in a spectrum of vaginal and uterine duplication anomalies. Double vaginas have multiple variations; they occur side by side, diverge from each other, or are totally separate. Vaginal duplication is almost invariably associated with concomitant uterine duplication. However, isolated uterine anomalies are more common and include the bicornuate (two cervices) and sep-

R. L. Meyers: Division of Pediatric Surgery, Department of Surgery, University of Utah School of Medicine, and Primary Children's Medical Center, Salt Lake City, Utah.

tate (one cervix) uterus. The wide variation in uterine anomalies is commonly classified into six subgroups according to Buttram: (a) agenesis; (b) unicornuate uterus; (c) uterus didelphys; (d) bicornuate uterus; (e) septate uterus; and (f) diethylstilbesterol-related T-shaped defects. Longitudinal septa may be asymptomatic, or present with leukorrhea or pain during intercourse. In some cases one side of the vagina is obstructed, forming a cystic structure that may become sufficiently distended to cause secondary obstruction of the second vaginal lumen (Fig. 133.1). There is an increased frequency of endometriosis in those with functioning endometrium and vaginal obstruction. Hypomenorrhea is common in anomalies that involve a lack of functioning uterine tissue such as a unicornuate uterus or a rudimentary horn of a bicornuate uterus. Approximately 25% of women with uterine anomalies have fertility and obstetric problems, including spontaneous abortion, abnormal fetal presentation, premature birth, dystocia, stillbirth, and ectopic pregnancy.

In patients with longitudinal vaginal septum without obstruction, a vaginal septectomy will suffice. In double vagina with unilateral obstruction the septum is resected completely or marsupialized into the patent vagina. If the obstructed vagina and uterus are rudimentary, or if there is no response to the septectomy or marsupialization, a hysterovaginectomy of the obstructed side will be necessary. In its most severe form, there may be proximal atresia of both vaginas, which necessitates a combined marsupialization of the more rudimentary vagina (or tubularization of the double vagina) and vaginal abdominoperineal pull-through.

VAGINAL ATRESIA

Vaginal atresia with persistent urogenital sinus is most often seen in girls with congenital adrenal hyperplasia. In its most common form the genitalia are virilized by excess adrenal precursor androgen production due to the absence of the enzyme 21-hydroxylase. Sporadic vaginal atresia may be complete agenesis (vaginal agenesis is discussed below), proximal, or distal and may or may not be associated with urinary tract fusion and persistent urogenital sinus. As in the case with imperforate hymen and transverse vaginal septum, the symptoms of cyclic abdominal pain and sciatic-like pelvic pain are secondary to vaginal obstruction and retained menses causing vaginal (hematocolpos) or vaginal and uterine (hematometrocolpos) distension. Vaginal atresia with urogenital sinus can be "low," with vaginal entry into the urogenital sinus below the external sphincter, or "high," with vaginal entry into the urogenital sinus above the external urethral sphincter.

The timing of neonatal or early adolescent surgery depends on surgeon and parental preference and upon the individual child's symptoms. Ultrasonography, voiding cystourethrography, cystoscopy, and occasionally magnetic resonance imaging should be used to absolutely define the anatomy before any surgical intervention is contemplated.

Repair of Vaginal Atresia without Urogenital Sinus

Distal vaginal atresia without urogenital sinus can be treated with perineal flap vaginoplasty alone. Proximal vagi-

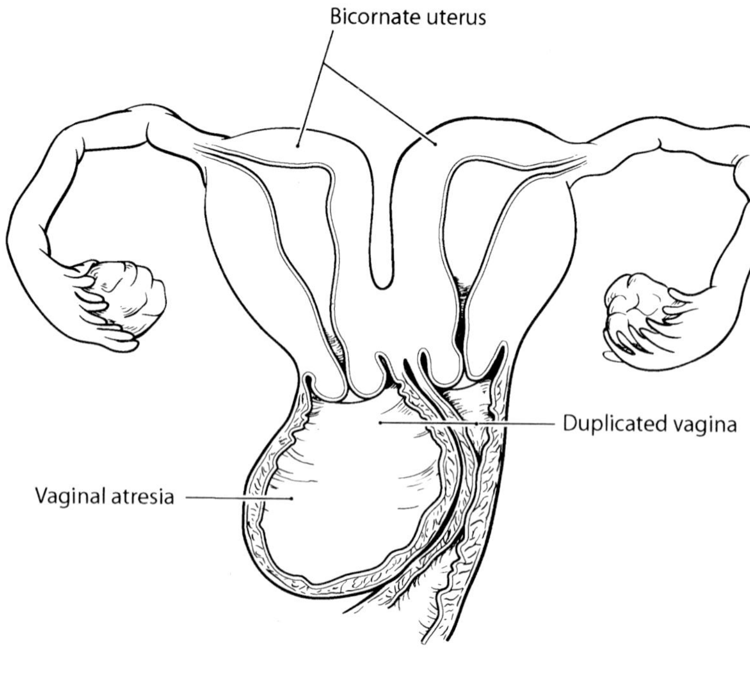

FIGURE 133.1. Duplication of the vagina. Atresia of one lumen and obstruction of the adjacent lumen caused by retained secretions and distension of the atretic lumen. Associated bicornuate uterus is typical.

nal atresia without urogenital sinus requires abdominoperineal vaginal pull-through with abdominal mobilization of the obstructed proximal vagina from the bladder anteriorly and the rectum posteriorly and pull-through to meet perineal flaps that form the introitus and lower vagina. A variety of perineal flaps have been advocated in the literature, including bilateral labial flaps combined with an inverted posterior U-flap, bilateral buttock flaps, bilateral pudendal thigh flaps, and a perineal artery-based axial flap. If the atresia is very high, many pediatric surgeons prefer the use of a vascularized graft of sigmoid colon. In extreme cases, some treatment failures may prefer hysterectomy for definitive management of their retained menses.

Repair of Vaginal Atresia with Urogenital Sinus

In its lowest form, persistent urogenital sinus presents as a simple fusion of the labia minora that conceals an otherwise normal vestibule; it is easily repaired with cutback vaginoplasty (Fig. 133.2). When the vagina enters the urogenital sinus low, below the level of the external urethral sphincter, the vaginal opening is exteriorized with a perineal flap vaginoplasty (Fig. 133.3). When the vagina enters the urogenital sinus high, above the level of the external urethral sphincter, the infant may present with massive vaginal dilation (hydrocolpos) secondary to retrograde urination into the vagina. Ultrasonography will show a huge abdominal mass with a thin, almost imperceptible wall (the hydrocolpos) capped by a displaced and minimally distended uterus. The bladder frequently cannot be identified on sonography, presumably because of compression by the distended vagina or because the vagina is more distensible than the bladder and fills preferentially. Neonatal surgical decompression of the bladder (vesicostomy) or vagina (vaginostomy) is often necessary.

Definitive surgical repair of high urogenital sinus is with a vaginal pull-through procedure. The perineal flap vaginoplasty used for low lesions is inappropriate for two reasons. First, the external urethral sphincter would be cut and predispose to postoperative urinary incontinence. Second, the resulting extreme degree of female hypospadias would predispose to frequent urinary tract infection and entrapment of urine in the vagina. Therefore, with a high urogenital

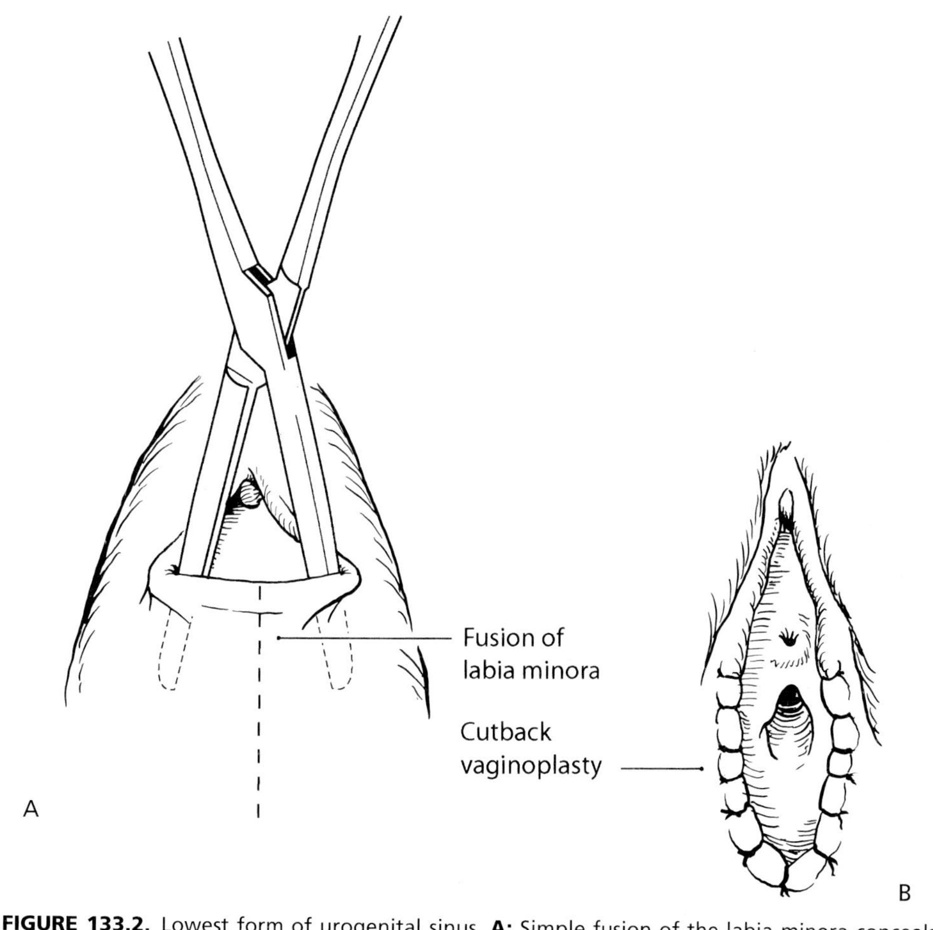

FIGURE 133.2. Lowest form of urogenital sinus. **A:** Simple fusion of the labia minora conceals an otherwise normal vestibule. **B:** Easily repaired by cutback division of the fused labia minora.

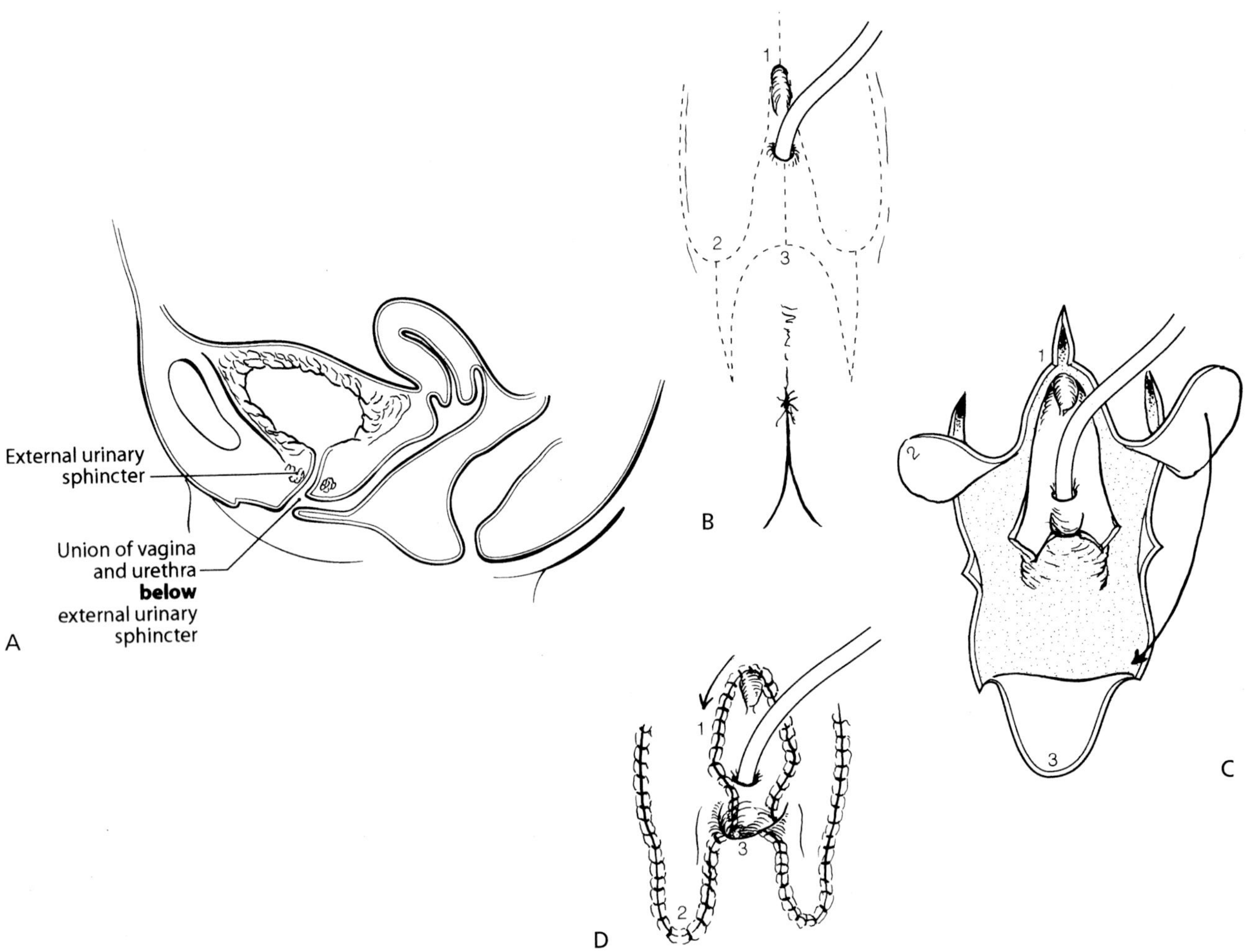

FIGURE 133.3. A: Low vaginal atresia with urogenital sinus. Union of vagina and urogenital sinus is below the external urinary sphincter. **B–D:** Surgical repair is commonly accomplished with perineal flap vaginoplasty using two anterolateral labial flaps and a posterior U-flap.

sinus, the urogenital sinus below the confluence is preserved as the distal urethra, and the vagina is disconnected above the external urethral sphincter and brought down to the perineum as a perineal pull-through vaginoplasty. In girls with a proximal vagina too short to reach the perineum, the sigmoid colon may be used as an interposition graft (Fig. 133.4). For patients with a very high confluence, Hendren has described urethral lengthening using a portion of the vagina to create a neourethra and a buttock flap to reconstruct the lower vagina. Peña has advocated surgical reconstruction of the very high confluence by mobilization and distal transposition of the urogenital sinus as a unit. He uses a posterior saggital, transanorectal exposure protected by a temporary colostomy and justifies this approach, which requires bivalving an otherwise normal anus and rectum, by excellent surgical exposure and ability to mobilize the high union of the vagina and urogenital sinus and bring them down toward the perineum as a unit.

If the procedure is performed in infancy, it is often combined with clitoral reduction surgery. Others prefer a two-stage correction with clitoroplasty in infancy and definitive vaginoplasty just before the onset of menses. In girls without complete obstruction of menses, some surgeons advocate delay until sexual maturity. In girls with severe forms of virilization not well controlled by steroid suppression medical management, we have used a two-stage approach with clitoroplasty in infancy and vaginoplasty prior to puberty. Whatever the timing of surgery, long-term follow-up is mandatory. Numerous reports have documented postoperative stricture formation and the need for redo vaginal reconstructive surgery to achieve a normal vaginal outlet. Whether the vaginal reconstruction is performed in infancy or in the prepubescent girl, details such as placement of the perineal flap well into the vagina without tension, attempts to avoid future hair-bearing skin for flaps where possible, and careful follow-

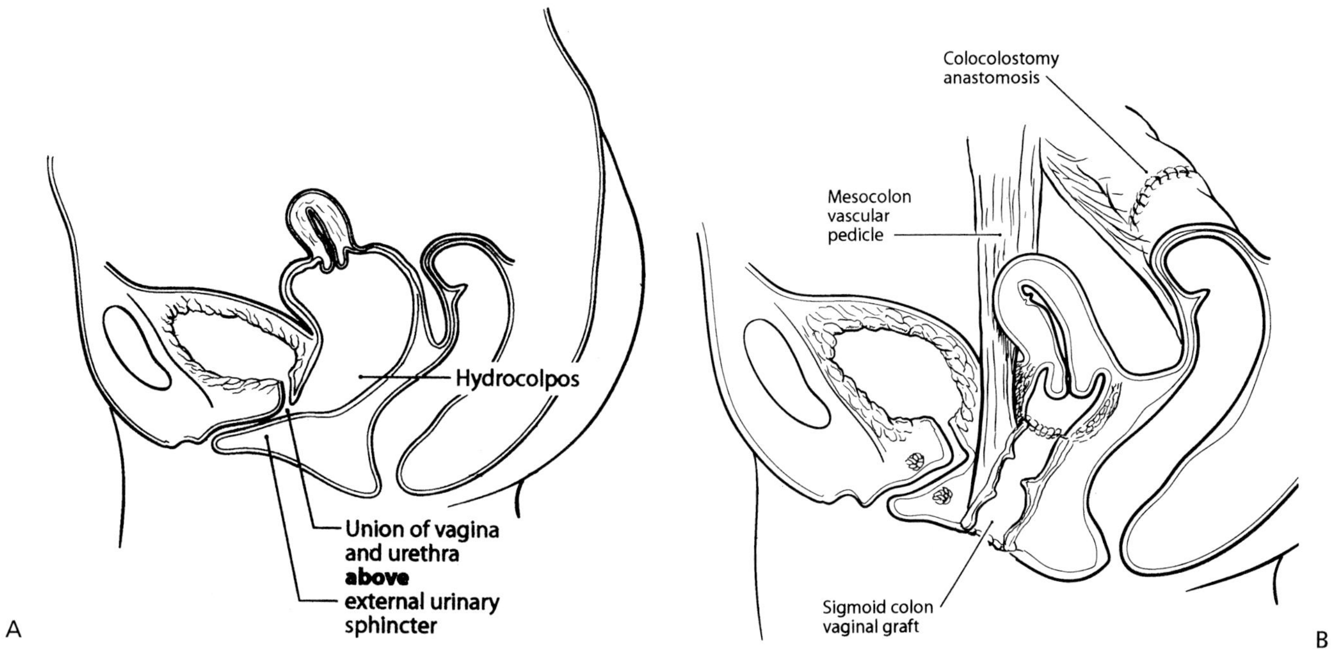

FIGURE 133.4. A: High vaginal atresia with urogenital sinus. Union of vagina and urogenital sinus is above the external urinary sphincter. Hydrocolpos may be seen secondary to retrograde urination. **B:** Definitive surgical repair is with a vaginal pull-through procedure. Several variations of repair have been described. Shown here is a sigmoid colon interposition graft.

up and vaginal dilation regimens are mandatory to reduce the need for secondary surgery.

VAGINAL AGENESIS, AND CONGENITAL ABSENCE OF THE VAGINA AND UTERUS

Congenital absence of the vagina in the presence of a normal uterus has been described in association with imperforate anus. Congenital absence of both the vagina and uterus, an anomaly known as the Mayer-Rokitansky-Küster-Hauser (MRKH) syndrome, is second only to gonadal dysgenesis as a cause of primary amenorrhea. The patients have a 46,XX karyotype, with normal endocrine and ovarian function. Urinary tract anomalies are common, and many girls have associated musculoskeletal (usually spinal) anomalies. The typical form of the syndrome is characterized by the absence of both the vagina and the uterus with persistent symmetric uterine remnants (muscular buds), normal fallopian tubes, and normal ovaries. An atypical form of the MRKH syndrome includes asymmetric uterine remnants and abnormal fallopian tubes, urinary anomalies, and cystic or malpositioned ovaries. Because the surgical management of complete vaginal agenesis requires creation of a new vagina, rather than drainage of a rudimentary vagina, these anomalies have been discussed separately.

If any functional uterine tissue is present, menstrual secretions are retained in the uterus and, as with vaginal obstruction anomalies, these girls present with cyclic abdominal pain and a pelvic or abdominal mass. When there are associated urinary tract abnormalities, frequent urinary tract infection may lead to an earlier diagnosis. Ultrasonography, voiding cystourethrography, magnetic resonance imaging, cystoscopy, and sometimes laparoscopy are useful in precisely defining the anatomy. Because the vaginal introitus derives from the urogenital sinus, not the müllerian ducts, it is usually present and can be incorporated into the vaginal reconstruction. To prepare the patient for vaginal reconstruction, dilation of the introitus can be instituted after menarche when the introitus has started to be toughened by endogenous estrogens (Fig. 133.5). In some cases, with a generous introitus and a motivated patient, the historical method of Frank, which involves prolonged daily vigorous dilation of the introitus on a specially designed seat, may prove adequate. Although it is occasionally useful, the Frank technique has a high long-term failure rate.

The most common surgical approach is the McIndoe procedure in which a neovagina is created by split-thickness skin grafts implanted over a semirigid mold placed into a surgically created potential vaginal space. After initial postoperative healing is complete, the surgically implanted mold is removed and replaced by the patient each night. A modification of the McIndoe technique was described by Serra and uses gradual inflation of a chronically placed tissue expander, rather than a semirigid mold to promote graft adherence and to prevent vaginal retrac-

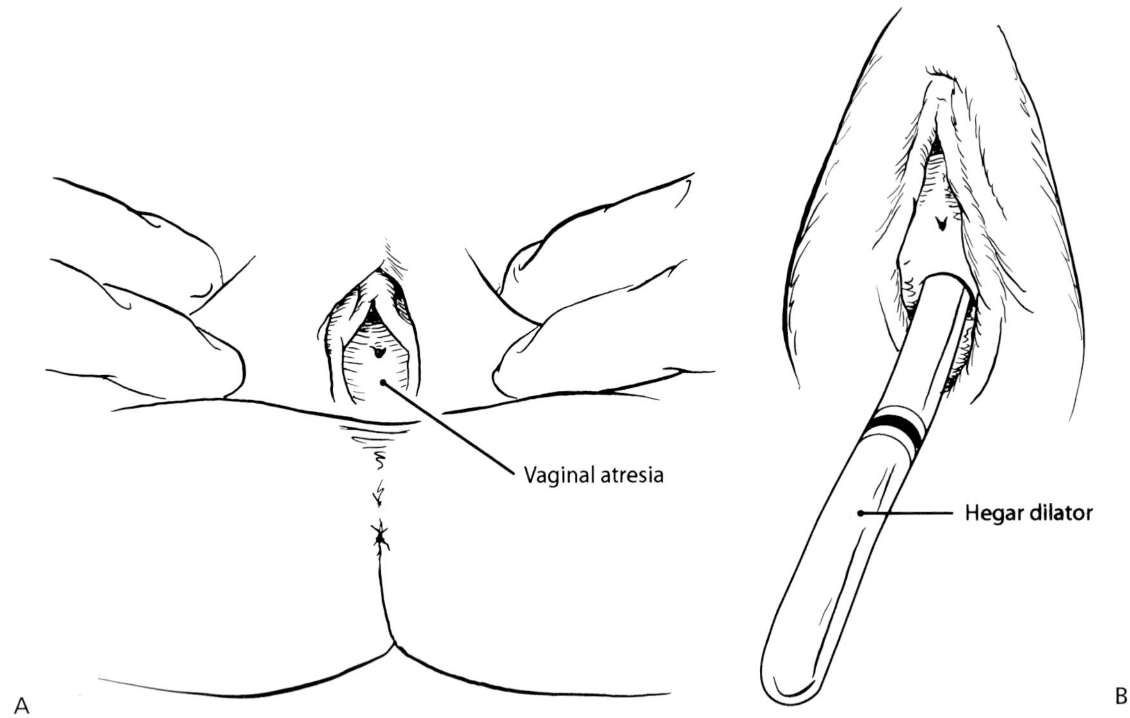

FIGURE 133.5. A: Vaginal atresia. **B:** Dilation of the introitus for 6 to 12 months with a Hegar dilator may deepen the introitus and toughen the skin prior to surgical vaginal reconstruction.

tion. The expander is left in place for several months, with inflation at weekly intervals.

VAGINAL ATRESIA WITH CLOACAL ANOMALIES

Cloacal anomalies are characterized by a confluence of rectum, vagina, and urinary tract into a single channel, the persistent cloaca. Persistent cloacal anomalies result from the failure of the urorectal septum to reach the perineum and secondary failure of development of the müllerian tubercle, sinovaginal bulbs and plate, and urogenital sinus. Cloacal anomalies virtually always present with distal vaginal atresia, usually present with varying degrees of retrograde urination and urinary distention of the vagina and uterus (hydrometrocolpos), and may present with vaginal and uterine duplication (Fig. 133.6). The surgical recon-

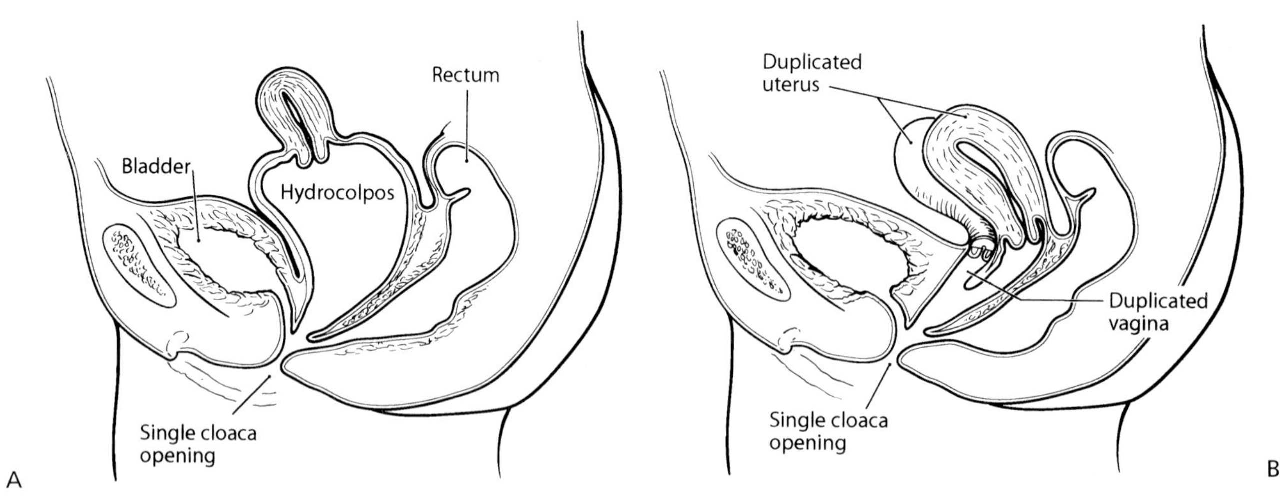

FIGURE 133.6. Examples of vaginal atresia with persistent cloaca. **A:** Single cloaca opening with hydrocolpos. **B:** Single cloaca opening with vaginal duplication.

struction of cloacal anomalies is discussed in detail in Chapter 73.

SUGGESTED READINGS

Donahoe P, Gustafson M. Early one-stage reconstruction of the extremely high vagina in patients with congenital adrenal hyperplasia. *J Pediatr Surg* 1994;29:352–358.

Hendren W, Atala A. Repair of the high vagina in girls with severely masculinized anatomy from the adrenogenital syndrome. *J Pediatr Surg* 1995;30:91–94.

Kim H, Laufer M. Developmental abnormalities of the female reproductive tract. *Curr Opin Obstet Gynecol* 1994;6:518–525.

Meyers, R. Congenital anomalies of the vagina and their reconstruction. *Clin Obstet Gynecol* 1997;40:168–180.

Peña A, Filmer B, Bonilla E, et al. Transanorectal approach for the treatment of urogenital sinus. *J Pediatr Surg* 1992;27:681–685.

Powell D, Newman K, Randolph J. A proposed classification of vaginal anomalies and their surgical correction. *J Pediatr Surg* 1995; 30:271–276.

SECTION XV

MISCELLANEOUS

134

ABDOMINAL PAIN

PETER MATTEI

Few clinical problems are more humbling, even for experienced senior clinicians, than the child with abdominal pain. Despite recent and dramatic advances in medical imaging, the diagnosis and clinical approach to children with abdominal pain is based principally on the history and physical examination. Although this results in a high degree of diagnostic accuracy, there is also an unsettling potential for bias and often a great deal of anxiety on the part of both the family and the surgeon.

The purpose of this chapter is to compile useful clinical pearls, dispel some common myths, and, it is hoped, help in the formulation of a diagnostic approach to the child with acute abdominal pain. I believe it is impossible to create a one-size-fits-all algorithm that will allow the correct diagnosis and treatment of every child with absolute certainty. It is helpful to remember that our goal should not be to be right every time, but to do the right thing every time—timely intervention while avoiding unnecessary surgery, when possible. It is also a good practice to involve the parents in the decision-making process, within reason, and to remind them that the "right answer" is frequently hard to pin down in these cases.

PERCEPTION OF ABDOMINAL PAIN

Conventional teaching about the neural pathways and conscious interpretation of abdominal pain proposes that there are three general "types" of abdominal pain: visceral, somatic, and referred. Visceral pain is caused by stretching of any hollow viscus, and is classically described as a dull or cramping ache that is poorly localized to the midline. Pain originating in foregut structures (stomach, duodenum, biliary tree) vaguely localizes to the epigastrium, whereas pain originating in the midgut (small bowel, appendix) and hindgut (colon) are perceived in the periumbilical region and hypogastrium, respectively. Somatic abdominal pain is caused by stimulation of sensory nerves in the peritoneum itself and is described as sharp, steady, and well localized to the site of the injury or inflammation. Referred pain is perceived in a site that is some distance from the location of the organ involved. Examples include shoulder pain that is caused by diaphragmatic irritation and scapular pain seen in some cases of cholecystitis.

This paradigm helps us understand the clinical pattern associated with certain common inflammatory processes such as appendicitis. The classic presentation of acute appendicitis is that of vague periumbilical pain, due to stretching of the obstructed appendix, followed by localized right lower quadrant pain when the inflammatory process begins to affect the peritoneum. It also can be useful when we are faced with an unusual presentation of a common condition or with an uncommon process, such as bowel ischemia in the setting of a bowel obstruction. However, it is important to recognize that variations and exceptions occur frequently. For example, retroperitoneal processes, such as a retrocecal appendix, do not necessarily follow the accepted pattern. Similarly, conditions such as biliary and appendiceal colic, which would be expected to produce classic visceral symptoms, frequently result in well-localized pain and tenderness in the absence of peritoneal inflammation. Clearly the neural pathways that mediate sensations of the viscera are poorly understood and probably quite variable, making the practice of trying to force a given set of clinical observations to fit the conventional doctrine somewhat dangerous.

HISTORY AND PHYSICAL EXAMINATION

A careful history includes the time of onset, the location, the quality and progression of the pain, and associated complaints such as nausea, vomiting, fever, and a change in bowel habits. Time course is important, especially when considering the possibility of appendicitis. Although rare cases of acute appendicitis can be identified within a few hours of the onset of pain, the diagnosis should be made with great caution when the pain has been present for less

P. Mattei: Department of Surgery, Thomas Jefferson University, Philadelphia, Pennsylvania; and Department of Pediatric Surgery, Alfred I. duPont Hospital for Children, Wilmington, Delaware.

than 12 hours and almost never when it has been present for less than 6 hours. Early acute appendicitis is clinically indistinguishable from the more common causes of abdominal pain such as gastroenteritis. It is precisely the more prolonged time course that makes one begin to consider a surgical process such as appendicitis. The location of the pain can suggest the organ of involvement, but the most important cause of localized abdominal pain anywhere on the abdomen in children is acute appendicitis. Unfortunately, it also seems that any abdominal process can cause localized right lower quadrant pain in any given patient, thus mimicking appendicitis. It is important to always consider all possibilities, regardless of the location of pain. Recurrent pain that is made worse with eating suggests gallbladder pain, but appendiceal colic and other intestinal processes can produce a similar pattern. Acute appendicitis is nearly always accompanied by gastrointestinal complaints and at least a low-grade fever, so the lack of such symptoms makes the diagnosis much less likely. Nevertheless, these are nonspecific symptoms that can be caused by any number of processes

Other historical points are sometimes helpful, but generally not to the degree that we would hope. It seems clear, for example, that most children do not really understand the concepts of hunger and appetite, so trying to decide about anorexia is probably a futile and potentially misleading exercise. Similarly, any answer related to a question about sexual activity is suspect, so it is always best to assume that a child over 11 years of age is at risk for pregnancy and sexually transmitted disease, regardless of the history obtained. A favorite question is about the car ride to the hospital and whether the pain was exacerbated by going over bumps in the road. Although taught to medical students as a reliable indicator of peritonitis, I have found this finding to lack any worthwhile degree of sensitivity or specificity. Lastly, the history related to bowel movements and their pattern are frequently unreliable. Moreover, parents are sometimes disbelieving or deeply offended by the suggestion that their child is constipated, especially when there is a history of daily bowel movements without hard stool or straining. This situation should be handled with great care, because there is a danger of unintentionally coming across as condescending or arrogant when discussing such a sensitive subject.

One should perform a methodical abdominal examination with warm hands and a gentle, unhurried demeanor. Auscultation for bowel sounds is a pointless exercise, because the findings rarely add anything to the workup. Sequential palpation of the entire abdomen with a flat hand (as opposed to poking with the fingertips) and avoiding sudden movements that can startle the patient will allow an accurate assessment in all but the most uncooperative patient. Light palpation should be followed by deep palpation. Gentle percussion is useful to determine the degree of tympany as well as a sensitive (but not perfectly specific) test for peritonitis. Costovertebral angle tenderness should be assessed by gentle palpation. Rectal examination should not be performed routinely, unless there is a specific question to be answered, such as a low pelvic abscess. The diagnostic yield is low and, in most cases, does not justify the time and trauma that is typically involved. Similarly, unless the patient is an experienced adolescent in whom pelvic inflammatory disease or pregnancy is being considered as a likely diagnosis, the pelvic examination should probably be deferred in favor of less invasive imaging studies such as ultrasonography. Obviously, exceptions occur, and it is up to the examining physician to weigh the options carefully. I have never found tests for obturator or psoas tenderness useful, and when reported by residents or primary care physicians, it is often falsely positive and misleading.

It is important to avoid making a definitive decision on any patient with abdominal pain on the basis of a single examination. Examination findings vary not only between examiners but also over time for the same examiner. Serial examinations are therefore critical and, I believe, obligatory before a decision to operate or to discharge is made. This is especially true in the patient who has been given narcotic analgesics, although it is unlikely that the peritoneal signs of acute appendicitis will be masked with a standard dose of morphine, for example. In equivocal cases, admission to the hospital for observation and serial examinations is useful and probably more accurate than current imaging modalities.

Urinalysis should be performed in all patients, although some red blood cells and lymphocytes may be seen in cases of appendicitis due to the presence of an inflamed appendix adjacent to the ureter or bladder. A urine pregnancy test is mandatory in all girls who are beyond menarche or over 11 years of age. An elevated white blood cell count is suggestive of appendicitis, but it must be kept in mind that the sensitivity of this test for acute appendicitis is no better than 90% and the specificity is probably around 50%. Abdominal radiographs are rarely useful unless another diagnosis such as obstruction is being considered. I have found ultrasonography only useful in girls to rule out adnexal pathology but not particularly helpful in ruling out or confirming the diagnosis of acute appendicitis. Computed tomography (CT) is being used frequently in adults, but I use it only in exceptional cases, for example, in children who are difficult to examine or when another diagnosis is being considered. In a child with a history and physical examination suggestive of appendicitis, one is obligated to recommend appendectomy regardless of the CT findings. However, it may occasionally be useful in truly borderline cases.

PERITONITIS

The concept of peritonitis is sometimes hazy, especially when dealing with children less than 5 years of age. Although the classic picture of the frightened, immobile patient with a rigid abdomen is immediately recognizable, it is the more subtle picture that is more common and difficult to identify. Many young children lack the ability to produce rigidity, making the presence of guarding a much more useful finding. The distinction between voluntary and involuntary guarding, however, is difficult and probably of little value—*any* guarding should suggest the possibility of peritonitis. Similarly, the patient with severe tenderness to light palpation or gentle percussion may be suspected of having peritonitis, even in the absence of true guarding.

Abdominal examination in a child should be approached carefully and with a gentle manner, so as not to induce findings that can falsely suggest peritonitis. This includes testing for rebound tenderness. I feel that, with the exception of testing for the Rovsing's sign, the rebound test should never be performed. It is not specific for peritonitis and, in cases of true peritonitis, it is painful and cruel. Similarly, there is nothing pathognomonic about motion tenderness (cough, heel strike, shaking the bed), regardless of the results, and, as mentioned above, a history of pain when going over bumps in the car ride to the hospital is notoriously misleading.

Young children with abdominal pain are especially problematic. Although the usual rules related to historical and physical findings apply, it is often difficult to elicit an accurate history from children less than 6 years of age, and they are often also difficult to examine. It is in these situations that the principles of serial, gentle, and careful examinations are most important. Young children with right lower lobe pneumonia frequently present with right-sided abdominal pain and tenderness, so it is extremely important to auscultate the lung fields and consider obtaining a chest radiograph. Unfortunately, the majority of young children with acute appendicitis will have perforated prior to operation.

Children under 6 years of age with diffuse peritonitis tend to lie perfectly still and to not want to be moved. They frequently have a breathing pattern characterized by panting or grunting, which minimizes excursion of the diaphragm. The abdomen is typically distended and very tender to light palpation, but actual guarding and rigidity may be absent. With this clinical picture, the diagnosis is perforated acute appendicitis with diffuse peritonitis until proven otherwise, although pneumonia (as well as pericarditis and meningitis) can cause a nearly identical presentation in this age group.

SPECIFIC DIAGNOSES

Appendicitis is the most common cause of abdominal pain that is treated surgically and is covered in depth elsewhere. It can be extremely difficult to diagnose with certainty, especially in very young children. Any child with abdominal pain of more than 6 hours duration has acute appendicitis until proven otherwise. A history of vague pain that begins in the epigastrium or periumbilical region and then progresses to become steady and localized to the right lower quadrant is a reliable finding that strongly suggests the diagnosis of acute appendicitis. The diagnosis is more likely if there is associated nausea, vomiting, or fever. Anorexia is an inconstant and unreliable finding. Diarrhea is sometimes present but is not useful. Physical examination is the single most important diagnostic tool in children with a history compatible with acute appendicitis. Localized tenderness with guarding confirms the need for appendectomy, although subtle findings warrant either further testing or serial examinations. The Rovsing's sign is reliable but not pathognomonic. A history longer than 3 days or frank peritonitis suggest the likelihood of perforated appendicitis.

Intussusception is a cause of abdominal pain in children between the ages of 3 months and 3 years, although it can occur at any age. The classic presentation is that of children who appear well but have intermittent episodes of severe, cramping abdominal pain that causes them to cry and double over or draw up their legs. However, in some children with intussusception, the pain is atypical or is a much less prominent symptom. Some children present with lethargy as the chief complaint and have minimal abdominal pain or heme-positive stools as the only clue that intussusception is the cause. Results of the physical examination are nearly always benign, except in the rare case of bowel ischemia or perforation, and can never be used to rule out intussusception with certainty. Because of this inherent uncertainty, all patients with even a suggestion of intussusception require a contrast study.

Abdominal pain due to *constipation* can be severe, and the physical findings are variable. The diagnosis is seldom made on the basis of history, and results of the physical examination are variable. Rectal examination may be helpful, but it is often necessary to obtain an abdominal radiograph to demonstrate to the family that the child is actually constipated. It remains a diagnosis of exclusion and one must be careful not to dismiss the family's concerns as "just constipation."

The ovaries are a relatively common cause of abdominal pain. The most important diagnosis to consider and rule out early (besides tubal pregnancy) is *ovarian torsion*. The pattern of onset and physical patterns are extremely variable and nonspecific. The onset can be abrupt or gradual. Some patients are nauseated while others lack gastrointestinal complaints. Results of the physical examination can be normal or may suggest peritonitis. The diagnosis needs to be considered in any girl with lower abdominal pain in whom another diagnosis cannot be made with certainty. Those with peritoneal findings should undergo laparotomy, whereas all others should undergo urgent Doppler ultrasonographic imaging. If the diagnosis remains equivocal, laparoscopy or laparotomy is mandatory to rule it out with certainty. This applies even to patients with a history of greater than 24 hours, because the ovary may still be viable due to intermittent or partial torsion. *Ovarian cysts* can be symptomatic due to hemorrhage or rupture. Pain is caused by acute stretching of the ovarian capsule or by the presence of blood or cyst fluid in the pelvis. The pain is usually deep and difficult to localize, although it may be worse on one side or the other, adding to the confusion. Ovarian cysts can usually be confirmed with ultrasonography, although follicular cysts are common and can be coincidental, whereas large cysts that have ruptured may reveal only free fluid in the pelvis. A small amount of free fluid in the pelvis is considered a normal finding in girls (there should be none in boys), and a moderate or large amount is abnormal but nonspecific. Even in cases in which a benign ovarian process has been confirmed, surgical intervention may still be required for persistent, debilitating symptoms or if neoplasm remains a concern.

Pelvic inflammatory disease and tuboovarian abscess can cause severe abdominal pain that can be confused with appendicitis or ovarian pain. Abdominal examination findings can be confusing, because the tenderness may seem severe (wincing, patient pushes examiner's hand away), but true peritoneal signs are usually absent. A careful gynecologic examination by an experienced examiner should be performed with appropriate cultures and smears obtained. In all adolescents with a sexually transmitted disease, a history of sexual abuse should be sought and sexual contacts should be treated.

A urinary tract infection (UTI) can cause abdominal pain, but usually only after it has progressed to cystitis or pyelonephritis. A more typical UTI should not result in significant abdominal pain or tenderness. The pain of cystitis is localized to the suprapubic region and is nearly always associated with significant dysuria and mucus on urinalysis. These clinical findings also can be induced by acute appendicitis when the appendix is located in the pelvis. Pyelonephritis can cause surprisingly localized anterior abdominal pain but is usually accompanied by flank tenderness and pyuria. Many children with ascending infection of the urinary tract have a history of urinary tract anomalies, vesicoureteral reflux, or neurogenic bladder. Therefore, all children with a UTI should undergo anatomic ultrasonography of the urinary tract and, in most cases, a formal urologic evaluation. Establishing an ascending UTI as a cause of abdominal pain can be quite difficult and requires a great deal of experience and good judgment, especially because pelvic acute appendicitis can mimic many of the same findings.

Renal colic due to nephrolithiasis classically presents with excruciating flank or abdominal pain, but in children frequently presents in an atypical and less dramatic fashion. Hematuria is usually present, but its absence does not rule out stone disease with certainty. Appendicitis adjacent to the ureter also can result in mild hematuria. Workup should include ultrasonography of the kidneys and complete urologic evaluation.

Mesenteric adenitis is a diagnosis that is often invoked when all other causes of abdominal pain have been excluded or when appendectomy reveals a normal appendix. It also seems to be a much more common diagnosis in the emergency department and primary physician's office, especially in children with streptococcal pharyngitis and right lower quadrant pain. It remains a somewhat mysterious disease process that nevertheless helps to provide a more tangible, albeit dubious, explanation for otherwise inexplicable abdominal pain. It seems unlikely that mesenteric adenitis should cause pain for more than 12 hours or so, and it should probably never cause true peritonitis. In equivocal cases, these patients should be observed carefully with serial examinations, imaging studies, or even diagnostic laparoscopy to prevent the delayed diagnosis of acute appendicitis.

Acute ileitis, whether due to infection or Crohn's disease, should be suspected in patients with right lower quadrant pain that has developed gradually over the course of several days. It is usually accompanied by fever and gastrointestinal complaints. On physical examination, there is tenderness and guarding in the right lower quadrant that may mimic acute appendicitis. It is usually the time course (if it has been more than 48 hours), the absence of peritonitis on physical examination, or the presence of a sausage-shaped mass that suggests the diagnosis. Although sometimes made at the time of appendectomy, the diagnosis is usually confirmed by CT and treated nonoperatively.

Biliary tract disease is a relatively uncommon cause of abdominal pain in young children but becomes more prevalent in adolescents. Children with gallstones seem to rarely develop acute cholecystitis, although biliary colic occurs much more frequently. The symptoms and signs are generally the same as those that occur in adults, although the pain may be less well localized or worse in the epigastrium. Patients with biliary dyskinesia present with progressive right upper quadrant or epigastric pain and nausea after meals but have no evidence of gallstones by ultrasonography. The diagnosis is confirmed by biliary nuclear medicine scan with administration of cholecystokinin, which reveals poor gallbladder emptying. Abdominal examination is usually unremarkable.

Pancreatitis can occur in children, but the classic picture of epigastric pain radiating through to the back is frequently lacking. The symptoms are often vague or nonspecific. Any child with abdominal pain or nausea of unclear origin should have serum amylase and lipase levels checked. Imaging of the pancreas is difficult because of the lack of natural contrast provided by retroperitoneal fat present in adults. In general, CT and ultrasonography are unreliable in making the diagnosis or quantifying the degree of inflammation of pancreatitis, but may be useful if a pseudocyst is suspected.

Volvulus is a rare but potentially catastrophic cause of abdominal pain. The clinical picture is usually dominated by signs of a bowel obstruction (bilious emesis) but we have seen patients with intermittent volvulus who complain only of pain. These can be difficult to sort out, but most patients with chronic or recurrent abdominal pain eventually undergo a barium upper gastrointestinal study, which will demonstrate malrotation. Patients with vitelline duct remnant bands to the umbilicus or with a Meckel's diverticulum sometimes have recurrent cramping abdominal pain due to partial or intermittent volvulus, but these patients are often not discovered to have an abnormality until they undergo laparoscopy or laparotomy. Meckel's diverticulitis can mimic appendicitis, although the pain and tenderness may not be localized to the right lower quadrant. In patients with a normal appendix at appendectomy for presumed appendicitis, the ileum needs to be evaluated fully for Meckel's diverticulitis.

Gastritis is a viral illness that can cause epigastric or left upper quadrant pain in children. Vomiting and brown hematemesis can occur as well. On examination, there is tenderness in the epigastrium but no peritoneal findings. Treatment is conservative with histamine blockers and a bland diet. *Peptic ulcer disease* is uncommon but typically follows the same pattern as in adults. Perforated ulcer disease with peritonitis or bleeding is exceedingly rare and should prompt a workup for gastrinoma. Patients who are immunocompromised, for example, after bone marrow transplantation, can develop bleeding or perforation from cytomegalovirus infection. Patients with an absolute neutrophil count of less than 1,000 are at risk for *typhlitis*. This inflammatory and presumably infectious disease of the right colon and terminal ileum can clinically resemble appendicitis. CT will confirm the diagnosis, thus preventing an unnecessary operation. The treatment is bowel rest and broad-spectrum antibiotics. Serial examinations and judicious reimaging are important to rule out perforation, because most of these patients are on corticosteroids and therefore may lack the typical signs of peritonitis.

Henoch-Schoenlein purpura can cause severe cramping and diffuse or wandering abdominal pain. There may be some guarding on examination, but true peritoneal findings are uncommon. The diagnosis is confirmed by the presence of the characteristic palpable purpura. Treatment is with systemic corticosteroids. Operative intervention is rarely necessary except in the event of bowel obstruction (usually due to intussusception) or life-threatening hemorrhage. *Hemolytic uremic syndrome* can cause abdominal pain and is associated with thrombocytopenia and renal dysfunction. These patients should be observed carefully for signs of colonic ischemia, which can occasionally be severe enough to require bowel resection.

Primary peritonitis is a condition in which young children, typically between 2 and 6 years of age and almost always female, develop severe abdominal pain and fever, with or without nausea and vomiting, and have diffuse peritonitis on physical examination. The findings are almost always attributed to perforated appendicitis. At operation, there is purulent ascites but a normal appendix. An extensive search for a bowel perforation should be performed but is nearly always negative. Cultures typically grow *Streptococcus*. Treatment is by saline irrigation of the abdominal cavity at the time of laparotomy and systemic broad-spectrum antibiotics for 7 to 10 days. Patients typically recover quickly after a brief postoperative ileus, and sequelae are unusual. The cause of this unusual condition is unknown, although several theories have been proposed, including hematogenous seeding of the peritoneal cavity, microperforation of the bowel, and retrograde contamination of the peritoneum via the fallopian tubes.

OPERATIVE APPROACH

The concept of the "surgical abdomen" is difficult to define, because it is more of a clinical judgment than a diagnosis. It may refer to the patient with diffuse peritonitis or localized peritonitis, or a patient who is severely systemically ill or "septic" who happens also to have abdominal pain. The implication is that although the origin or extent of disease may be unclear, the judgment has been made that the patient requires an operation.

Regardless of the cause or severity of the abdominal complaints, it is almost always advisable to prepare the patient properly for surgery. This may include fluid resuscitation, antibiotics, and analgesics. A detailed plan of action should be decided upon, and all possibilities should be discussed with the family. Further imaging should be considered only if the patient is stable and if the results of the study are likely to lead to a significant alteration in the approach or prevent an unnecessary operation. Although in adults it is customary to perform a midline incision that can be extended up or down depending on the operative findings ("incision of indecision"), nearly all pediatric laparotomies can be safely performed using a transverse incision. Upper abdominal causes of acute surgical disease, such as perforated peptic ulcer disease, gastric emergencies, and necrotizing pancreatitis, are extraordinarily rare in the pediatric population. The vast majority of patients have had some complication of acute appendicitis as the cause of their pain and most of the other possible disease entities can be adequately addressed through a generous right lower quadrant incision with or without extension across the midline. Midline incisions are painful and disfiguring and are rarely necessary. In some cases, it may be reasonable to perform a diagnostic laparoscopy first so that the problem can be identified and the incision placed in the best location. This approach is especially useful in the management of ovarian processes, in which a Pfannensteil incision may provide the best exposure and optimal cosmesis. Victims of trauma in whom a small bowel injury is suspected can be approached through a small periumbilical incision or by laparoscopy.

Every pediatric surgeon has had the experience of operating on a child with "textbook" acute appendicitis, only to find that the appendix is perfectly normal. Although I do not believe the adage that a surgeon must perform a certain number of negative appendectomies as a quality assurance mechanism, cases like this are inevitable. Parents should always be warned ahead of time that despite a typical presentation and the availability of imaging, there is a risk (less than 5% to 10%) of negative appendectomy. The appendix should be removed even if it appears to be normal and a brief inspection through the same small incision should be performed to rule out acute ileitis, Meckel's diverticulitis, and ovarian pathology. If turbid or purulent ascites is present, the bowel needs to be inspected more completely to rule out bowel perforation. Many of these children have primary peritonitis.

SUMMARY

Abdominal pain is a frequent complaint in children and can test the clinical acumen of even the most careful, experienced, and conscientious clinician. Children often present with atypical patterns of disease, and therefore serial examinations and an approach of systematic exclusion are important. It is important to consider all possible diagnoses and to remember that an unusual presentation of a common problem (acute appendicitis) is much more likely than an unusual diagnosis.

135

LAPAROSCOPIC TECHNIQUES

THOMAS H. INGE
KEITH E. GEORGESON

Minimal-access techniques have revolutionized the practice of pediatric surgery. Patient benefits are many: reduced postoperative discomfort, fewer wound complications, and quicker return to school for patients and return to work for their caregivers. Newer, miniaturized instrumentation specifically engineered for the pediatric patient further decreases the morbidity of peritoneal access, without compromising exposure or performance. This chapter reviews the technical aspects of laparoscopic procedures commonly performed in children. These include Nissen fundoplication, gastrostomy, pyloromyotomy, anorectoplasty, intussusception, and contralateral inguinal exploration.

BASIC TECHNIQUES

The success of a minimal-access procedure first depends on safe establishment of pneumoperitoneum and trocar placement. Prior to making an incision, the skin, abdominal wall, and peritoneum are infiltrated with a large volume of dilute 0.125% lidocaine (or a smaller volume of 0.25% bupivacaine) solution with 1:200,000 epinephrine for local anesthesia. Pneumoperitoneum can be established using a Veress needle or open Hasson technique. The needle method is quicker and creates a tighter seal. It can be performed safely if the fascia is grasped to oppose the entry force of the needle. The added length of the 120-mm Veress needle provides a good handle and superior control. The needle is passed downward at an angle, so that inadvertent penetration of intraabdominal viscera and retroperitoneal structures is avoided. The Veress needle should be passed with an initial rapid but controlled downward motion through the fascia at the umbilicus. In one fluid "J-stroke" motion, the needle is then redirected in a more horizontal plane, usually toward the left upper quadrant, and the peritoneum is penetrated. Once insufflated, trocars can be inserted using the same J-stroke technique to safely access the peritoneal cavity.

NISSEN FUNDOPLICATION AND GASTROSTOMY

Fundoplications for gastroesophageal reflux disease are one of the most common pediatric surgical procedures. Frequently, infants or children have failed to thrive because of a severe underlying medical problem that renders them less able to tolerate oral feeding. Gaseous bowel distension can make any laparoscopic procedure difficult. Therefore, preparation begins the day prior to operation with a single oral dose of castor oil to evacuate the colon. Feedings are stopped 12 hours before the procedure, and a glycerin or dulcolax suppository is administered.

Skillful induction of anesthesia is important, because laparoscopy is more difficult if bowel insufflation occurs during intubation. After intubation, the patient is positioned at the end of the operating table in a frog-leg position (infants and toddlers) or with the legs in stirrups for older children. The bladder is emptied by Credé or bladder catheterization. An orogastric tube is passed to completely evacuate air from the stomach. A Maloney bougie is placed into the stomach to facilitate the esophageal dissection. A steep reverse Trendelenberg position is used with the right side slightly down to allow gravitational "retraction" of the bowel and liver. A Mayo stand is positioned over the patient's head to allow access to the head for the anesthesiologist. The surgeon stands between the patient's legs and the assistant stands on the surgeon's left

T. H. Inge: Department of Surgery, University of Cincinnati; and Department of Pediatric Surgery, Cincinnati Children's Hospital Medical Center, Cincinnati, Ohio.

K. E. Georgeson: Department of Surgery, Division of Pediatric Surgery, University of Alabama School of Medicine; and Department of Pediatric Surgery, Children's Hospital of Alabama, Birmingham, Alabama.

side. The scrub nurse and Mayo stand for instruments are to the surgeon's right.

After the peritoneal cavity is insufflated (12–15 mm Hg), five trocars are placed, beginning with a 5-mm trocar through the umbilicus (Fig. 135.1). The port for the liver retraction should be placed next. This exposes the gastroesophageal junction and allows optimal strategic placement of the other working ports. A 4-mm trocar should be inserted immediately subxyphoid to allow maximal elevation of the left lateral segment, with a grasp of the diaphragm just above the right crus. The surgeon's right-hand port is placed in the far left lateral position, slightly superior to the transverse plane of the umbilicus. The surgeon's left-hand port should be placed to enter the abdomen to the right of the falciform ligament, below the edge of the elevated liver. The fifth (camera) port should be placed in approximately the left midclavicular line, equidistant from the umbilicus and the surgeon's right-hand port, at the level of the greater curvature of the stomach.

The operation begins by opening of the lesser omentum over the caudate lobe of the liver using scissor cautery, aided by the Babcock grasper applied to the lesser curve of the stomach by the assistant. Dissection in a cephalad direction continues, and the phrenoesophageal ligament is completely divided. Complete dissection down to the longitudinal fibers of the esophagus is critical. This ensures that the distal esophagus can be mobilized for fixation in the abdomen. The assistant's caudad retraction on the gastroesophageal fat pad is important for safe dissection of the hiatus. Next, the short gastric vessels are divided using hook electrocautery. Small amounts of tissue must be taken to free the short gastric vessels. These vessels can be readily taken with the hook cautery in all infants and most children. Dissection of the posterior gastric wall from the pancreas and diaphragm is performed to allow adequate mobility of the fundus. Without adequate posterior mobilization, an unsatisfactory (spiral) wrap can result. The superior end point of the posterior dissection is the left crus, behind the gastroesophageal junction. The esophageal bougie is next retracted up into the thoracic esophagus to afford better visualization. A window is created behind the esophagus. The assistant facilitates exposure of the retroesophageal space by placing a grasper from right to left through the window to both lift the gastroesophageal junction and provide caudal retraction. This window must be created superior to the left gastric artery to ensure that the fundus is wrapping the distal esophagus. After all fibers of the posterior phrenoesophageal ligament are divided, there should be at least 2 cm of esophagus visible below the hiatus. A figure-of-eight 2-0 silk stitch is next used to approximate the crura posteriorly. The fundus is grasped and pulled from left to right through the window behind the esophagus. With a grasper on the fundus on either side of the esophagus, the fundus is gently rocked back and forth behind the gastroesophageal junction (like a shoeshine) to visually ensure that no posterior tethering of the fundus is present. The bougie is again passed into the stomach. The first suture is placed in the uppermost edge of the wrap on the left side of the esophagus and then through the edge of fundus that has been pulled through to the right of the esophagus. Next, the superiormost stitch is placed about 1 cm more cephalad than the first. This stitch incorporates fundus on the left, esophageal wall (just to the right of anterior vagus), right anterior crus, and finally a portion of fundus on the right side of the esophagus. The third fundoplication suture is then placed 1 cm below the middle suture, incorporating esophagus at the gastroesophageal junction.

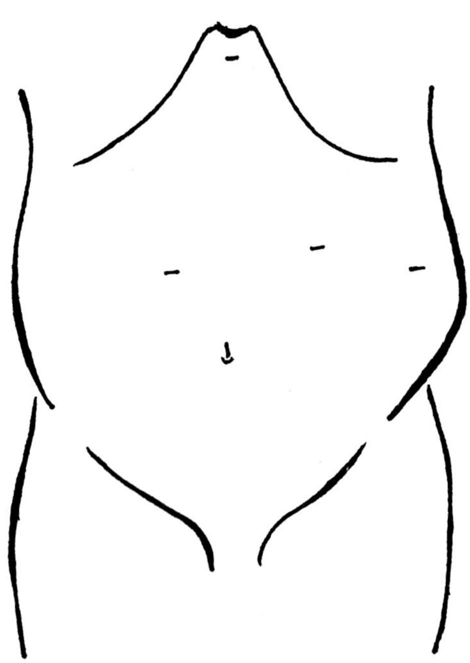

FIGURE 135.1. Trocar placement for laparoscopic Nissen fundoplication.

For gastrostomy placement, the bougie is removed, the stomach is insufflated with air by orogastric tube, and pneumoperitoneum reduced to 6 to 8 mm Hg. The 0 degree telescope is placed into the umbilical port. The anterior wall of greater curvature is grasped through the left midclavicular port and elevated toward the abdominal wall. Transabdominal stay sutures of zero polydioxanon on a large needle are used to incorporate 1 cm of gastric wall on either side of the grasper. Because stay sutures are used to position the stomach during gastrostomy tube placement, they are not tied initially. The grasper and trocar are removed, and the same tract is dilated up to the desired gastrostomy tube size using the Seldinger's technique. The dilator kit is ideal for this purpose because it includes needle, wire, and disposable dilators. The needle is inserted transabdominally (through the trocar site) to puncture the gastric wall between the stay sutures. The wire is then placed into the gastric lumen, and the tract is dilated. If placing a skin level device (button) as the gastrostomy, the thickness of the abdominal wall is measured with the 8 French dilator. This allows accurate choice of the stem length of the button. Once an adequate tract has been dilated, the 8 French dilator can be used within the button to stiffen the stem so that it can be negotiated over the wire into the gastric lumen. A tube gastrostomy can be used through this tract if desired. The zero polydioxanon sutures are gently tied over the button. Only the fascia at the 5-mm port site is closed.

Liquids are offered by postoperative day 1. Full feedings can begin by day 2. Stay sutures are removed by days 2 to 4. Normal gastrostomy care is withheld for 2 weeks, and parents are instructed to leave the button accessed during this time to prevent manipulation of the button during the initial healing phase. The right-angle tube attachment is used during this time and is secured to the skin with adhesive film. This measure prevents inadvertent traction on the button, which can enlarge the tract and cause pain.

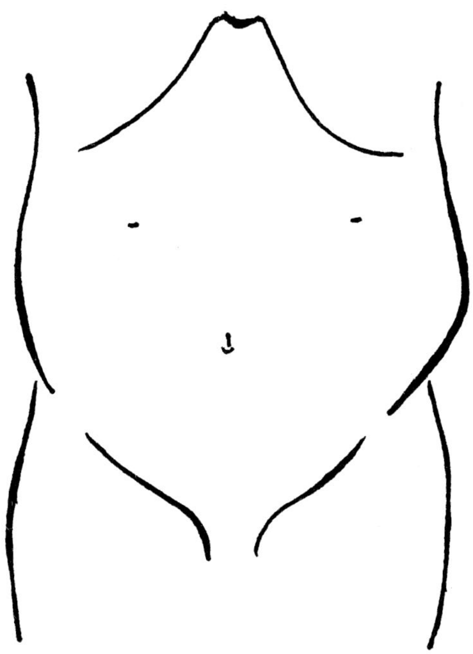

FIGURE 135.2. Instrument placement sites for laparoscopic pyloromyotomy.

LAPAROSCOPIC PYLOROMYOTOMY

Laparoscopic pyloromyotomy is one type of minimal-access technique that is growing in acceptance. In the vast majority of cases, laparoscopic pyloromyotomy is short, well tolerated, minimizes operative trauma, reduces ileus, and improves cosmesis. Preoperative treatment of infants with hypertrophic pyloric stenosis emphasizes correction of electrolyte abnormalities and rehydration as well as assessment of their cardiac and respiratory status. Pulmonary hypertension is a possible consequence of hypercapnia, hypoxia, acidosis, or hypovolemia in the poorly prepared patient, and these problems can be exacerbated by pneumoperitoneum.

After an orogastric tube is placed, the patient is positioned crosswise on the operating room table with the monitor at the head of the patient and the surgeon standing at the foot of the patient. The assistant stands to the left of the surgeon. A generous infiltration of local anesthetic (0.125% lidocaine) is provided at each of the three entry wound sites. After pneumoperitoneum to 8 to 10 mm Hg is established, a 4-mm port is placed through the lower margin of the umbilicus (Fig. 135.2). A 4-mm 30 degree telescope is then inserted into the trocar. The right upper quadrant incision is made using a stab technique with the arthroscopy knife that will be used for the pyloromyotomy. The 3-mm tissue grasper is passed directly through the abdominal wall (no trocar is needed) and is used to grasp the duodenum just beyond the pylorus to rotate the pylorus into view. The same knife is placed through the abdominal wall just to the left of the umbilicus, and is used to score the pylorus in a longitudinal direction. The blade is then retracted and the more blunt end of this instrument is inserted into the pyloromyotomy incision until the surgeon feels a definite "give," indicating penetration through the thickened muscular wall down to the mucosa. Because the sharp blade has been retracted, the instrument does not penetrate the mucosal layer. The blade is rotated back and forth to enlarge the defect in the hypertrophied pyloric muscle. The pyloric spreader is advanced into the abdomen through the left upper quadrant stab wound. It is inserted into the opening in the muscle and the jaws are gently opened to spread the muscle layer and open the pyloric channel. The two edges of the pyloromyotomy should now move independently. Once a satisfactory pyloromyotomy has been achieved, air can be insufflated into the orogastric tube to rule out perforation. Instruments are removed and pneumoperitoneum is evacuated through the umbilical trocar. The umbilical trocar is removed and fascia is closed at the umbilical site. The two stab wounds are closed using only sterile strips.

Acetaminophen is used for pain for 24 hours. Feeding is started according to the surgeon's protocol. We have been uniformly pleased with the outcomes of this procedure. When compared with pyloromyotomy performed using a laparotomy (right upper quadrant or umbilical approach), there are numerous advantages to laparoscopic pyloromyotomy. First, a smaller surgical wound exists, so there is a lower potential for wound complications. Wound closure takes less time, and with the laparoscopic approach one avoids trauma to the stomach and pylorus at the time of delivery of the structures out of the abdomen. Finally, cosmesis is improved when compared with open procedures.

LAPAROSCOPICALLY ASSISTED ANORECTOPLASTY

Laparoscopically assisted anorectoplasty (LAARP) uses minimally invasive techniques to dissect the atretic rectum, to close and divide any associated fistula, and to achieve accurate placement of the rectum within the levator and sphincter muscles using a minimal perineal dissection with laparoscopic guidance.

Although most patients with high imperforate anus first undergo divided sigmoid colostomy at birth, LAARP also can be performed as a primary procedure. When a colostomy has been performed at birth, a distal colostogram is obtained prior to LAARP to define the site of communication of the rectal fistula with genitourinary structures. LAARP is performed at 4 to 6 weeks of age, provided there are no other medical contraindications.

The patient is placed in a transverse orientation at the end of the operating table so that the surgeon and assistant have free access on three sides. A blanket is placed below the trunk and lower extremities, which extends the neck so that the head is safely out of the way after draping. The active stoma is sutured closed, and the mucous fistula is irrigated with saline prior to skin preparation. No lower extremity intravenous catheters can be placed because a full body preparation from the nipples to toes is performed. After stockinettes are placed on each leg, the baby is pulled through an extremity drape so that a snug fit is achieved. The urinary bladder is decompressed by transurethral catheterization, which sometimes requires cystoscopy for placement. Pneumoperitoneum to a pressure of 10 to 12 mm Hg is established using a Veress needle inserted in the right upper quadrant just below the costal margin. Three 4-mm trocars are placed in the right upper and lower quadrants, and left lower quadrant (Fig. 135.3). A 5-mm trocar is placed in the left upper quadrant or umbilicus. Dissection begins at the peritoneal reflection. Using hook cautery, the distal mesorectum is divided. The bipolar scissors (Evershears; Gyrus Medical, Maple Grove, Minnesota) are used more distally near the prostate to prevent collateral damage to the nerves and urethra. As the rectum tapers, the fistula to the urethra or vagina is identified. It is then clipped (using a 5-mm applicator) or ligated with suture at the junction with the posterior urethra and divided sharply. When the distal bowel is retracted out of the pelvis, the pelvic floor can be inspected. The pubococcygeus muscle can usually be visualized, unless it is congenitally hypoplastic. If the muscle is not well visualized, the position of the divided fistula is used to mark the midline. The anal area of the perineum is electrostimulated transcutaneously, and the area of maximal contraction and elevation of the perineum is noted. The anterior, lateral, and posterior limits of this anal area are marked with sutures. Next, a 1-cm vertical midline incision is made and the intrasphincteric plane is bluntly dissected from below to the level of the levator sling. A radially expanding sheath over a Veress needle (Innerdyne Corp., Salt Lake City, Utah) is passed through the intrasphincteric plane and advanced between the two bellies of the pubococcygeus muscle in the midline using laparoscopic guidance, just posterior to the urethra. If the needle is inaccurately passed to either side of the midline, it is readily apparent due to laparoscopic surveillance and corrected prior to dilation of the tract. The 10-mm trocar is then inserted through the sheath to dilate the tract. The divided rectal fistula is grasped and pulled onto the perineum trailing behind the trocar. The anastomosis between rectum and anus is completed with interrupted 3-0 polyglycolic acid suture. The rectum is retracted cephalad laparoscopically and "hitched" to the presacral fascia with 2-0 silk sutures. This fixed retraction lengthens the skin-lined anal canal, with the goal of improving anal sensation in the future.

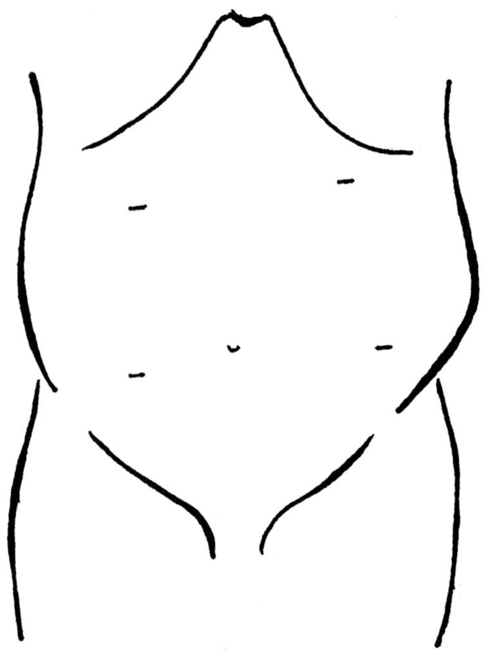

FIGURE 135.3. Trocar placement for laparoscopically assisted anorectoplasty.

LAARP allows the surgeon to treat a high lesion essentially like a low lesion, avoiding potential operative trauma to the sphincter musculature. The basic concept is that of fistula transfer from the urethra or vagina through the levator sling, and external anal sphincter muscle complex to the anal surface. There is no need to divide the sphincter muscle complex from below, because the pubococcygeus muscle can be visualized and targeted laparoscopically, and immediately after the procedure, strong and symmetric contraction of the sphincter around the neoanus can be seen. Although primary colostomy is not absolutely necessary for this procedure, it seems prudent as initial experience is gained. This technique provides a unique opportunity for inspection of the condition of the pelvic musculature of patients with anorectal malformations. In particular, the pubococcygeus muscle, through which the rectum should normally pass, can be visualized with this technique. The center of the two bellies of the pubococcygeus muscle can then be targeted for precise pull-through of the distal rectum, using minimally invasive abdominal and perineal incisions.

LAPAROSCOPIC REDUCTION OF INTUSSUSCEPTION

When satisfactory attempts at hydrostatic or pneumatic reduction of ileocolic intussusception fail, operative intervention is required. Often, laparoscopic reduction can be performed. The limitations to successful laparoscopic reduction are (a) obstructed, dilated small bowel loops that do not permit visualization of the ileocecal region, and (b) a gangrenous intussuscipiens that requires bowel resection.

The key to successful laparoscopic reduction of intussusception is instrumentation, and the graspers chosen must be atraumatic and able to completely grasp the entire diameter of bowel wall, to avoid pressure- and traction-related bowel wall injury. Atraumatic nonaggressive 5-mm bowel graspers (no. 33210LF, Storz Endoscopy, Culver City, CA) and Babcock graspers are used with satisfactory results. After gastric and urinary bladder decompression, induction of pneumoperitoneum is performed through the umbilicus. Three 5-mm trocars are placed in the child's left upper and lower quadrants and right lower quadrant. We have found that using the umbilicus for the camera puts the scope too close to the intussuscepted bowel to be useful. If the patient is an older toddler, the port sites become left lower quadrant, suprapubic midline, and left midabdominal.

The operation begins by first inspecting the colon to assess the distalmost extent of the intussuscipiens. This mass within the colon often can be palpated in the transverse colon, and can sometimes be "walked" back proximally with a hand-over-hand action using two bowel graspers. When this method fails, attention focuses on the ileocecal junction where the intussusception is occurring. With one grasper on the cecum, the other is used to gently rock back and forth on the small bowel, and gentle traction is applied to gradually reduce the intussusception. A fourth trocar for an assistant's grasper can be inserted into the right side of the abdomen to stabilize the cecum and allow the surgeon to use both graspers to manipulate the small bowel. If a complete reduction is not possible using these techniques, a right midabdominal incision is made to deliver the intussusception out of the abdomen for open reduction or bowel resection.

LAPAROSCOPIC INGUINAL EXPLORATION OF THE CONTRALATERAL GROIN DURING INGUINAL HERNIORRHAPHY

The evaluation and management of the contralateral groin in infants and children with an inguinal hernia is controversial. When sufficient suspicion exists for a contralateral hernia (i.e., child <2 years of age, former premature infant, inconclusive physical examination findings), it is reasonable to perform a laparoscopic contralateral exploration to avoid the risks associated with an open inguinal exploration. Once the symptomatic hernia sac has been identified and dissected down to the internal ring, the sac is opened and the 4-mm trocar is gently placed into the sac. It is important to recognize the potential for injury of adjacent structures with this maneuver. With the sharp inner trocar removed, the sheath alone can be passed into the internal ring, and with an anterior torque it is gently advanced into the peritoneal cavity. Pneumoperitoneum to 10 mm Hg is achieved through the trocar sleeve, and the 4-mm 70 degree telescope is inserted. The contralateral internal ring is visualized. In many cases, either the adjacent umbilical ligament or a veil of peritoneum obscures visualization of the ring. In this case a 14-gauge angiocatheter is inserted percutaneously through the abdominal wall just lateral and inferior to the umbilicus. A lacrimal duct probe is used to determine the presence and length of a patent processus vaginalis. If a patent processus is greater than 1 cm in length, an open inguinal herniorrhaphy is performed. The angiocatheter and trocar are then removed, and a high ligation of the symptomatic hernia is performed.

APPENDIX

Although many companies produce high-quality instruments, the following specialty devices have been found useful. With these instruments and a basic 5-mm laparoscopic set, most pediatric minimally invasive procedures can be performed.

1. Telescope, 4 mm × 18 cm, 30 degree (no. 7210AA; Storz Endoscopy, Culver City, CA)
2. Babcock grasper (no. 630-147; Jarit Instruments, Hawthorne, NY)
3. Tissue graspers, 4 mm × 24 cm, two suggested (no. 26180KO; Storz)
4. Scissors, 24 cm (no. 630-202; Jarit)
5. Curved dissector, 24 cm (no. 630-126; Jarit)
6. Hook cautery (no. 630-318; Jarit)
7. Suction irrigator system, 5 mm
8. Nonabsorbable 2-0 suture on SKI needle (Ethicon Corporation, Somerville, NJ)
9. Veress needle (no. UV 120; Ethicon)
10. Radially expandable 5-mm short trocars (Step SL75; Innerdyne Corporation, Salt Lake City, UT)
11. Trocars, 4 mm (no. 30115; Storz)
12. Needle holder (no. 630-251; Jarit)

13. Liver retractor, 3 mm (no. 89-6121) or 5 mm (no. 89-6112) (Snowden-pencer, Tucker, Georgia)
14. Reducers, 5 to 4 mm (no. SR3000003; Innerdyne)
15. Cook dilator set for GT placement (no. C-JCDS-100-CHB; 238974; Cook Corporation, Bloomington, Indiana)
16. Pyloric spreader (no. 26180VT; Storz)
17. Silk suture on SKI needle (no. D8015; Ethicon)

SUGGESTED READINGS

Bax NMA, Georgeson KE, Najmaldin AS, et al., eds. *Endoscopic surgery in children.* Berlin: Springer-Verlag, 1999.

Chung DH, Georgeson KE. Fundoplication and gastrostomy. *Semin Pediatr Surg* 1998;7:213.

Georgeson K, Inge T, Albanese C. Laparoscopically-assisted anorectoplasty for high imperforate anus—a new technique. *J Pediatr Surg* 2000;35:927–930.

136

VENTRICULAR SHUNTS FOR HYDROCEPHALUS: GENERAL SURGICAL ISSUES

JOSEPH QUEENAN
PETER MATTEI

It is increasingly common for pediatric general surgeons to encounter patients with a history of hydrocephalus and who have been treated with a ventricular drainage procedure. These are often former premature infants who can now be chronically treated with ventricular drainage devices into adolescence and adulthood. In the past, children being treated with such a device often presented with mental retardation and significant physical disabilities; however, with current protocols that emphasize early diagnosis and an aggressive approach to management, many patients are now able to achieve developmental milestones, sometimes with few significant limitations.

ANATOMY OF A VENTRICULAR SHUNT

Ventricular drainage shunts are created using long segments of flexible polymer tubing with a fenestrated end placed into a suitable cerebrospinal fluid (CSF)-containing space of the brain and the drainage end placed in a low-pressure body cavity or the intravascular space. The most common sites for drainage are the peritoneal cavity, the pleural space, and the right atrium. The CSF drains passively, driven by the pressure gradient between the ventricle and the drainage site. A reservoir is placed in line with the drainage pathway and serves several functions. The first is to regulate flow from the ventricle to the distal site, via a pressure- or flow-controlled valve. The reservoir also functions as a one-way valve, to prevent reflux of fluid or blood into the brain, especially during transient episodes of increased abdominal or thoracic pressure with reversal of the pressure gradient. They are often designed with a pump mechanism that with direct manual pressure pushes the CSF toward the drainage site. Finally, the reservoir allows percutaneous aspiration of CSF for analysis and culture, "tapping" the shunt. The reservoir is placed in the subgaleal space in an easily accessible location, typically over the mastoid bone or occiput.

The vast majority of ventricular shunts are placed by pediatric neurosurgeons, although occasionally we as pediatric general surgeons are asked to assist in gaining access to a suitable drainage site. The details of the surgical technique used to place the cranial portion of the catheter is beyond the scope of this chapter, but it usually involves a burr hole in either the frontal or the occipital area. The drainage catheter is then tunneled subcutaneously down to the site of drainage. For a peritoneal shunt, a small upper abdominal transverse incision is made. The peritoneum is identified and entered under direct vision. The catheter is placed into the peritoneal space and the incision is closed using standard techniques. Alternatively, a peritoneal trocar can be used under Valsalva to gain access to the peritoneum. A substantial length of catheter is typically used.

OPERATING ON A PATIENT WITH A VENTRICULOPERITONEAL SHUNT

Most patients with a functional ventriculoperitoneal shunt can safely undergo laparotomy despite the presence of a length of catheter within the peritoneal space. However, the surgeon needs to be mindful of several issues. The first is placement of the incision. The subcutaneous portion of the shunt should be carefully palpated, mapped, and marked to avoid accidental injury to the shunt tubing during the opening incision or by the placement of retractors. If the child is obese or if the catheter is otherwise difficult to palpate, a "shunt survey" (plain radiographs of the catheter from top to bottom) should be considered. Once the peri-

J. Queenan: Division of Neurosurgery, Alfred I. duPont Hospital for Children, Wilmington, Delware.

P. Mattei: Department of Surgery, Thomas Jefferson University, Philadelphia, Pennsylvania; and Department of Pediatric Surgery, Alfred I. duPont Hospital for Children, Wilmington, Delaware.

toneum has been entered safely, the intraabdominal portion of the catheter is usually not difficult to manage. Packing it away with a moist sponge can help to keep it out of harm's way. A patient with a history of having had multiple peritoneal shunts might be expected to have multiple adhesions or walled-off collections of CSF, but these are usually easily managed with standard general surgical techniques.

Bacterial contamination of the abdominal portion of the catheter exposes the patient to the risk of meningitis. For clean procedures that do not involve entering contaminated viscera, standard antibiotic prophylaxis should be sufficient to prevent this complication. If a colonized or infected structure needs to be opened, thus directly exposing the catheter to bacteria, consultation with the neurosurgical team should be made. In some cases, they will elect to externalize the shunt, which is to remove the distal catheter from the peritoneum to allow the CSF to be diverted into a drainage bag.

ACCESS TO THE PERITONEAL SPACE

Occasionally, the assistance of a general surgeon is requested to help gain access to the peritoneum. This is usually necessary in patients who have had multiple prior laparotomies, multiple prior shunts, or the need for unique placement of the catheter, for example, over the dome of the liver or in the gallbladder. Although a standard or laparoscopic lysis of adhesions can easily provide adequate space into which the CSF may drain freely, catheters placed under such circumstances often fail. This is due to recurrent adhesions and the fact that the scarified peritoneal surface that remains often provides inadequate absorption. In other cases, the abdomen has been divided by adhesions into separate compartments, one or more of which might be adequate for drainage and absorption. Gaining access to such a compartment might require a lysis of adhesions, although laparoscopy with placement of the catheter under direct visualization also should be considered. A laparoscopy access port can be placed through the small incision used for placement of the shunt to confirm an adequate space and safe placement of the catheter in patients who are at risk for adhesions.

In rare cases, and depending somewhat on institutional preferences, one might be asked to assist with placement of a drainage catheter into the gallbladder. It should be confirmed before surgery that the gallbladder is free of stones or sludge and that there is no history of biliary tract disease or infection. A patient with a biliary tract anomaly or obstruction is always at risk for cholangitis. The gallbladder can usually be accessed through a relatively small right upper quadrant transverse or subcostal incision. The fundus of the gallbladder is all that needs to be free, but enough of the gallbladder should be dissected to be absolutely certain that the catheter is being placed in the proper structure. Bile should be aspirated and sent for immediate analysis by Gram stain and culture. A Gram stain positive for bacteria is a relative contraindication for placement of the shunt. A redundant length of catheter is placed into the lumen of the gallbladder via a tiny incision and secured with concentric purse-string sutures of an absorbable monofilament suture. The gallbladder does not need to be fixed to the abdominal wall. Stone formation is reportedly quite rare despite the presence of a foreign body. Infection with subsequent meningitis is a risk of the procedure.

PSEUDOCYSTS

Drainage of CSF into the peritoneum results in chronic inflammation that leads to the formation of adhesions. These are sometimes in the form of a pseudocyst, or a chronic collection of CSF that forms adjacent to the catheter. Although often of no clinical significance, pseudocysts can be associated with shunt dysfunction or small bowel obstruction due to adhesions. Infected pseudocysts produce signs and symptoms of an intraabdominal infection (abdominal pain, fever, ileus, tender mass) and can result in ascending infection and meningitis. In some cases, a frank abscess may develop.

Patients with a ventriculoperitoneal shunt who present with abdominal pain need to be evaluated for infected pseudocyst in addition to the usual causes of abdominal pain in their age group. Although ultrasonography is sometimes useful, computed tomography (CT) of the abdomen and pelvis is the most useful study. Findings on CT of a fluid collection near the tip of the catheter confirms the diagnosis of a pseudocyst. In the absence of an alternative source of sepsis, the pseudocyst must be presumed to be infected. Image-guided percutaneous drainage provides fluid for analysis and Gram stain. Treatment includes drainage of the infected fluid, removal of the shunt tubing, externalization of the shunt, and appropriate antibiotics. These are usually done in association with or by the neurosurgical team.

VENTRICULOTHORACIC SHUNTS

When the peritoneal space is no longer available as a site of drainage, the pleural space is a reasonable alternative in children over 6 or 7 years of age. The negative pressure of the thorax is conducive to good drainage, and the pleura provides an excellent absorptive surface for the CSF. The ventricular portion of the shunt is constructed in the usual fashion. The catheter is tunneled subcutaneously along the lateral chest wall, and a small stab incision is made in the fourth or fifth intercostal space, as though a small chest tube were being placed. A length of catheter is inserted and allowed to gather in the pleural space. As the incision is closed, a small suction cannula can be inserted and used to remove air that might have accumulated during the procedure. A chest tube is rarely necessary. A small pneumothorax is usually well tolerated and will resolve on its own, unless the lung was injured in the process of making the incision or placing the catheter.

VENTRICULOATRIAL SHUNTS

Drainage catheters also can be placed in the right atrium. The standard principles of central venous access apply. The catheters can be placed with a percutaneous approach into the subclavian vein or the internal jugular vein, using the Seldinger technique and a peelaway sheath system. Alternatively, a cutdown approach to the external jugular vein, the facial vein, or the internal jugular vein can be used. The catheter is fed directly into the vein through a venotomy and secured with ligatures. It is usually best to gain access to the atrium first. The catheter is flushed with heparinized saline, clamped, and then tunneled subcutaneously to the reservoir.

COMPLICATIONS

In addition to the complications related to pseudocysts and adhesions that are described above, ventricular shunts are susceptible to a number of other unique complications. Ventriculoperitoneal drainage catheters can erode into a hollow viscus, most commonly the bowel or the bladder. Catheters have been known to enter the bowel lumen and become visible at the anus. The resultant "perforation" is generally small and self-limited and rarely results in peritonitis or ascites. In the asymptomatic patient, the shunt must be externalized and the distal catheter removed. The catheter should be removed by applying traction on the distal end so that the contaminated portion is not dragged through the peritoneum. Patients are observed for 24 hours but rarely require formal laparotomy. Lastly, some patients with a ventriculoperitoneal shunt can develop large hydroceles or hernias as a result of progressive enlargement of a preexisting patent processus vaginalis. Patients with small hydroceles or hernias should therefore undergo repair before or at the time of their shunt placement. Repair after they have become very large can be technically challenging but is typically well tolerated with a relatively low recurrence rate.

Ventriculopleural shunts are usually well tolerated but can cause a pleural effusion. If the effusion is large or symptomatic, it is exceedingly unlikely that the site will be salvageable. Thoracentesis is typically followed by reaccumulation and increases the risk for infection, as does placement of a pleural tube. In most cases, the catheter should be removed and the shunt placed in a different site. Ventriculoatrial shunts carry the same risk as central venous catheters, including infection, thrombosis, embolization, and atrial perforation with pericardial effusion. Any of these complications mandates removal of the catheter and temporary externalization of the shunt. Atrial and venous perforations due to catheter erosion are usually self-limited and heal spontaneously after removal of the catheter, although pericardiocentesis may be required if symptoms persist. Ventriculoatrial shunts use fixed-length catheters and therefore require lengthening procedures as the child grows. This involves removal of the intravascular portion of the catheter and replacing it with a longer segment that is spliced to the more proximal portion of the catheter or the reservoir itself. Patients with ventriculoatrial shunts for several years also have developed chronic and progressive pulmonary hypertension (cor pulmonale), which in some cases has been fatal. The cause is unknown and the disease tends to be insidious. Other patients have developed shunt-related glomerulonephritis, which appears to be related to shunt infection with coagulase-negative *Staphylococcus*. Renal function usually improves after removal of the shunt, but finding another suitable site for drainage can be a problem.

In summary, although ventricular drainage catheters are placed and maintained by pediatric neurosurgeons, general surgeons are sometimes asked to assist in placement of the drainage portion of the shunt or to manage a complication. In addition, many of these patients require other surgical procedures that could interfere with the function of or be complicated by the presence of the shunt. Pediatric surgeons should therefore be aware of the purpose and function of the shunts as well as the potential for complications unique to these devices. Consultation with a pediatric neurosurgeon also can be very useful.

SUGGESTED READINGS

Beach C, Manthey DE. Tension hydrothorax due to ventriculopleural shunting. *J Emerg Med* 1998;16:33–36.

Drake JM, Iantosca MR. Management of pediatric hydrocephalus with shunts. In: McGlone DG, ed. *Pediatric neurosurgery, surgery of the developing nervous system, 4th ed.* Philadelphia: WB Saunders, 2001.

Drake JM, Kestle JR, Tuli S. Cerebrospinal fluid shunt technology. *Clin Neurosurg* 2000;47:336–345.

Ketoff JA, Klein RL, Maukkassa KF. Ventricular cholecystic shunts in children. *J Pediatr Surg* 1997;32:181–183.

Lundar T, Langmoen IA, Hovind KH. Fatal cardiopulmonary complications in children treated with ventriculoatrial shunts. *Childs Nerv Syst* 1991;7:215–217.

Sathyanarayana S, Wylen EL, Baskaya MK, et al. Spontaneous bowel perforation after ventriculoperitoneal shunt surgery: case report and a review of 45 cases. *Surg Neurol* 2000;54:388–396.

Sleigh G, Dawson A, Penny WJ. Cor pulmonale as a complication of ventriculo-atrial shunts reviewed. *Dev Med Child Neurol* 1993;35:74–78.

Vella J, Carmody M, Campbell E, et al. Glomerulonephritis after ventriculo-atrial shunt. *Q J Med* 1995;88:911–918.

137

PERMANENT DIALYSIS ACCESS

HÉLÈNE FLAGEOLE

Care of the patient with end-stage renal disease (ESRD) is both rewarding and challenging. These are children one comes to know very well because they often require multiple procedures, ranging from their first dialysis access to hopefully a successful transplantation. When instituting dialysis, especially in the pediatric population, it is important to keep in mind that access may be required for many years. Each potential site for access, particularly for hemodialysis (HD), is therefore extremely precious. Dialysis is also occasionally required for patients with potentially reversible conditions such as hemolytic-uremic syndrome, poststreptococcal glomerulonephritis, tumor lysis syndrome, hypovolemic shock, and so forth. A not uncommon indication for dialysis in children is acute poisoning.

Children suffering from renal insufficiency have many medical problems that the surgeon needs to be aware of before performing any procedure, especially if dialysis is required acutely. Those include:

- Abnormalities in acid-base status
- Electrolyte imbalances, especially hyperkalemia, which can cause arrhythmias, but also abnormal calcium/phosphorus and sodium levels
- Fluid overload, which may make ventilatory management difficult
- Anemia, to the extent that pre- or intraoperative transfusions may be necessary
- Abnormal platelet function, which may require treatment with desmopressin acetate.

Even for more elective dialysis access procedures, these children are complicated from a medical point of view. I cannot emphasize enough the importance of a close collaboration between surgeon, nephrologist, and anesthesiologist. This team approach is also essential when the time comes to select a dialysis device. Surgeons who are performing dialysis access operations need to familiarize themselves with the catheters that are available in their institution, both for peritoneal dialysis (PD) and for HD. This will ensure clear communication between concerned parties, and maximize the efficiency of the implanted device.

PERITONEAL DIALYSIS

Preoperative Preparation

The decision to institute PD has often been made when the surgical consultant gets a request by his or her fellow nephrologist. However, it is essential to understand the issues leading to that decision. In infants and children weighing less than 20 kg, vascular access is technically difficult; therefore, PD is the modality of choice.

Other considerations for long-term access include family choice, distance between the home and the hospital, and the parents' willingness and ability to perform dialysis at home. There are also relative contraindications to performing PD—multiple abdominal operations with secondary adhesions and presence of nearby stomas being the most common.

Technical Approach

At our center, we use a catheter with a single cuff. To minimize the risk of leakage around the catheter, it is usually placed in the rectus muscle. I like to use the following technique: a one-inch transverse incision is made over the rectus muscle just below the umbilicus. The anterior rectus sheath is also incised. The muscle fibers are separated, not cut, and the peritoneum identified. A small opening is made in the peritoneum, and all the omentum that can be brought out through it is resected, otherwise it can become entangled around the catheter and cause a blockage.

Using a wire guide, the catheter is guided toward the pelvis. After removal of the guide, the peritoneum is closed around the cuff in a purse-string fashion. I then create a tunnel under the anterior rectus sheath and place the exit site on the skin 2 inches above the first incision. This maneuver permits complete closure of the rectus sheath and decreases the risk for leaks. Next, the catheter is tested with 10 mL/kg of heparinized saline (40 units/mL) to assess ease

H. Flageole: Department of Surgery, McGill University; and Department of Pediatric Surgical Services, Montreal Children's Hospital, Montreal, Quebec, Canada.

of instillation and drainage. The appropriate connections are then made, and the tubing is completely covered with the dressing. Our nephrologists like to obtain a routine postoperative abdominal radiograph to verify the position of the catheter.

Notes of Caution

1. Unless the catheter is manufactured with a curve, it should always be placed straight. If an attempt is made to give it a "gentle bend," it will eventually return to its original straight shape and come out of the pelvis as a result.
2. Depending on the available selection of catheters for patients of different sizes, the placement of the incision may vary.

Postoperative Considerations

After successful placement of a PD catheter, it may be used immediately if the situation is urgent. In these instances, the risk for leakage around the catheter is increased and the dialysis is usually begun with small volume exchanges (e.g., 10 mL/kg). If the catheter is placed electively, it is preferable to allow sufficient time for proper wound healing before using it. Other causes of catheter failure are blockage from omentum wrapping around it, which is minimized by performing partial omentectomy at the time of catheter insertion, and the formation of fibrin clots in the catheter. The incidence of clot formation is decreased with the addition of heparin to the dialysate. If it occurs nonetheless, administration of a fibrinolytic agent often resolves the problem. At our center, we use recombinant tissue plasminogen activator (rTPA).

The most common medical complication seen in patients on PD is peritonitis, which occurs more often in children than in adults. The mainstay of therapy is instillation of intraperitoneal antibiotics, and the response to treatment is usually rapid. When there is no response after 2 to 3 days or if there are frequent relapses with the same organism, the catheter will need to be removed because it is most likely colonized. Moreover, most cases of fungal peritonitis also require catheter removal as part of the treatment.

Another factor that may lead to failure of PD in the pediatric population is parental "burnout." PD is very demanding on families and this should be kept in mind if suddenly a pattern of increased episodes of peritonitis develop, with noncompliance to medications, missed appointments, and so forth.

HEMODIALYSIS

As with PD, HD may be required acutely and temporarily, or chronically. Temporary vascular access for HD is usually obtained by inserting a short rigid hemodialysis catheter in the femoral vein using the Seldinger technique. Chronic vascular access in children remains a much greater challenge than it is in adults. It is important to pay attention early in the course of the disease to preserving vessels that could later be used for access. Despite the likelihood of a successful transplant, many children spend years on HD, and each access procedure has an average life of only 2 years. The choice of a specific type of vascular access is influenced by several factors, including the size of the child, availability of peripheral vessels, and estimated duration of dialysis before transplantation. The choices available include arteriovenous (AV) fistulas, single- or double-lumen catheters, and, less frequently, bridge grafts. Each will be addressed separately in the sections that follow.

As described in the section on PD, the medical status of the patient needs to be examined in detail prior to surgery and anesthesia, and all significant abnormalities corrected before proceeding with an operation.

Catheters

Preoperative Preparation

Catheters are the initial form of vascular access for HD in more than 60% of children and in some centers remain the most frequently used long-term device. In small children, they may be the only method of access available because their small vessels may not support a fistula or a graft. We use surgically implanted soft, flexible silicone catheters that come in a variety of sizes and lengths, and in single or double lumens. Which catheter to use in a given patient depends on his or her size. Again, a clear line of communication with the nephrologist is essential to select the best device for each patient. The choice is made on the principle that the smallest catheter that will allow sufficient flow for efficient dialysis is used, and double-lumen catheters create less recirculation, making them preferable. Generally, single-lumen catheters are only used in small infants.

Technical Approach

The ideal site for insertion of an HD catheter is the internal jugular vein. We generally use the right side first if it is available. However, the left side works equally well, with the difference that a slightly longer catheter is needed. Although frequently used in the past, the subclavian vein has been shown to develop stenosis in a matter of days following catheter insertion. This complication could preclude the creation of an AV fistula later on. At our center, we use a cutdown technique under general anesthesia. A small transverse supraclavicular incision is made overlying the area where the sternomastoid muscle divides in two heads. Between those two heads, the carotid fascia is identified, opened, and proximal and distal control of the internal jugular vein is obtained. A segment of at least 2 cm of vein is dissected. Next, a 6-0 polypropylene purse-string suture is placed on the anterior wall of the vein. Avoiding ligation of the vein distally may allow circulation around the catheter and make the vein reusable. The exit site on the skin is then selected in the infraclavicular fossa, and the two incisions are joined via a subcutaneous tunnel. The catheter is then advanced and great care is exercised to prevent kinking of the catheter. If that were to occur, the flow on the dialysis machine would be insufficient and it would be necessary to replace the catheter. A small venotomy is made in the center of the purse-string suture and the catheter is advanced into the right atrium. This is done under fluoroscopic guidance. It is of paramount importance to then test each lumen for ease of blood return. If the clinician cannot aspirate 10 mL in 2 to 3 seconds, or if there are any "catches," the catheter needs to be slightly repositioned until flow is satisfactory from both lumens. This sometimes requires a lot of patience, but if things do not function properly in the operating room, they surely will not in the dialysis unit. Once the position is optimized, the purse-string suture is gently tied around the catheter to ensure hemostasis and the incision is closed. The catheter is then secured at the skin exit site. The line is heparinized and the entire catheter is covered with a sterile dressing.

Notes of Caution

1. When using a silicone catheter without a built-in curve, the subcutaneous tunnel must be very shallow because this material kinks easily.
2. The skin site should be placed far enough from the initial incision to allow changes in position without risking the cuff coming out of the skin.
3. In children, one cannot secure the catheter at its exit site enough. These patients often exhibit poor wound healing, and insufficient fibrous tissue forms around the cuff. Moreover they are active when not connected to the dialysis machine. These factors make catheter extrusion a common cause of failure in this population.

Postoperative Considerations

There are many possible and frequent complications of HD catheters, and most of them are more frequent in children than in adults. The most common complication reported in the literature is infection, with *Staphylococcus* the usual offending organism. When an infection is suspected, parenteral antibiotics are the first line of treatment. At our center, the infection rate is minimal, which contrasts somewhat with the literature. Other causes of catheter failure, which are far more common in children than adults, are trauma and extrusion. In our institution, this mechanical type of complication is much more common than infections. Even if the catheter comes out only a few centimeters, and the cuff is still subcutaneous, if the tip moves out of the right atrium into the superior vena cava, the flows will be inadequate and the catheter will need to be replaced.

Thrombotic complications also can occur, sometimes with serious consequences. The lumen of the catheter may become obstructed with a clot. In such cases, rTPA may be used successfully to lyse the clot. A more severe occurrence is vascular thrombosis. Some patients have required open-heart surgery to remove intraatrial clots. To minimize the risk of thrombotic complications, our patients are anticoagulated.

Arteriovenous Fistulas

Preoperative Preparation

An AV fistula at the wrist, usually between the radial artery and the cephalic vein (Brescia-Cimino fistula), is probably the most desirable method of long-term vascular access for dialysis. Although not often used in infants and very small children, it is commonly used in older children and adolescents, unless transplantation is planned for the weeks or months following the beginning of dialysis. This scenario is seen more and more frequently in centers with an active living-related renal transplant program. In our institution, transplantation is discussed with families shortly after the diagnosis of ESRD is made. Some patients are not dialyzed at all (preemptive transplantation), whereas others spend only a few months on dialysis if they have a suitable living donor.

Patients who are candidates for AV fistula creation require careful evaluation of their vascular status. Assessment of arterial inflow is done by performing Allen tests on both sides, and if results are normal bilaterally, the nondominant side is usually chosen. This gives patients more freedom during the long hours spent in the dialysis suite. Suitability of the veins is verified by applying a tourniquet and checking the caliber of the veins, the wall elasticity, and the length of the segment available for later cannulation. We routinely perform Doppler studies of the neck veins as well, particularly if central catheters have been used. Subclavian stenosis is common in patients who had catheters placed in this vein, even for short periods of time.

If the radiocephalic site at the wrist is unavailable, alternatives in the upper extremity include the ulnobasilic fistula at the wrist, the radiocephalic site in the upper forearm, and a cubital fistula involving the brachial artery.

Technical Approach

In children, we perform this operation under a combination of general anesthesia and axillary block. The block induces vasodilatation, which is desirable in these cases. We also recommend routine use of magnifying loupes or an operating microscope due to the small caliber of the vessels in pediatric patients.

After a free-arm preparation is done, an incision measuring a few centimeters is made over the radial aspect of the wrist. The vein is usually identified first and gently dissected as far distally as possible. The radial artery is then identified and dissected. The site of anastomosis is chosen. It is important to create a fistula that is long enough to maximize patency rates. The vein is ligated distally, and a side-to-end arteriovenous anastomosis is performed using 7-0 or 8-0 monofilament suture. The umbrella suturing technique allows good visualization at the heel.

Postoperative Considerations

In the immediate postoperative period, occlusion is the main issue. We check patency hourly for the first 12 hours, manually or with Doppler imaging, and every 2 hours for the next 12 hours. In children, we have a splint for the fistula made before discharge, usually the next day, to decrease the risk of trauma. If no complications occur, the fistula is ready for puncture in approximately 8 to 12 weeks, depending on the initial size of the veins and the speed of dilatation.

Arteriovenous fistulas are not immune to long-term complications because of the inevitable changes that take place in the walls of the involved vessels. Thrombosis is by far the most common cause of failure. The usual cause is intimal hyperplasia on the venous side of the anastomosis that develops regardless of all extrinsic factors, including surgical technique. Specific pediatric data on 1-year patency rates are scarce. Across the literature, it is 50% to 70%. The management of the thrombosed fistula is controversial, with some groups advocating balloon dilatation and others claiming that the benefits of dilation are very short term and that these fistulas should be revised surgically. At our center we have limited experience with dilatation. When surgically revising a fistula, it is recommended to create a new anastomosis proximal to the site of occlusion. Thrombosis also can occur as a result of too frequent cannulation of the same vein. Infection in AV fistulas is a rare event and can normally be treated conservatively with antibiotics. It causes sclerosis of the venous wall that can contribute to thrombosis.

Grafts

Preoperative Preparation

For patients who are not candidates for an arteriovenous fistula, a bridge graft can be useful. The material of choice for graft placement is polytetrafluoroethylene (PTFE). Because of the increasing use of transplantation, and consequently less time spent on HD, we seldom need to resort to a graft at our center. However, when necessary, we would favor the forearm loop as the graft of choice. If that is not possible, thigh grafts, between the superficial femoral artery and femoral vein, have been used with success at some centers.

Technical Approach

For the forearm loop, a long-segment conduit with an internal diameter of 6 mm is tunneled subcutaneously in the upper forearm and the arterial anastomosis is fashioned end-to-side with the brachial artery above the elbow. The venous anastomosis is to the cephalic or basilic vein, also above the elbow. In small children with tiny vessels, the anastomoses can be placed just below the axilla.

Postoperative Considerations

A major difference in complications between fistulas and grafts is infection. Infection in a prosthetic conduit can be serious, sometimes requiring removal of the entire graft. Pseudoaneurysms also can develop in grafts, resulting from puncturing the same site too frequently, and if they rupture, life-threatening hemorrhage may occur.

SUGGESTED READINGS

Ash SR, Nichols WK. Placement, repair, and removal of chronic peritoneal catheters. In: Gokal R, Nolph KD, eds. *The textbook of peritoneal dialysis.* The Netherlands: Kluwer Academic, 1994:315–333.

Brittinger WD, Walker G, Twittenhoff WD, et al. Vascular access for hemodialysis in children. *Pediatr Nephrol* 1997;11:87–95.

Dougherty MJ, Calligaro KD, Schinder N, et al. Endovascular versus surgical treatment for thrombosed hemodialysis grafts: a prospective, randomized study. *J Vasc Surg* 1999;30:1016–1023.

Goldstein SL, Macierowski CT, Jabs K. Hemodialysis catheter survival and complications in children and adolescents. *Pediatr Nephrol* 1997;11:74–77.

Hodges TC, Fillinger MF, Zwolak RM, et al. Longitudinal comparison of dialysis access methods: risk factors for failure. *J Vasc Surg* 1997;26:1009–1019.

Lahoche A, Beregi JP, Kherbek K, et al. Percutaneous angioplasty of arteriovenous (Brescia-Cimino) fistulae in children. *Pediatr Nephrol* 1997;11:468–472.

Nissenson AR, Fine RN, Gentile DE. *Clinical dialysis.* Norwalk, CT: Appleton & Lange, 1995.

Twardowski ZJ, Khanna R. Peritoneal dialysis access and exit site care. In: Gokal R, Nolph KD, eds. *The textbook of peritoneal dialysis.* The Netherlands: Kluwer Academic, 1994:271–314.

138

RENOVASCULAR HYPERTENSION

JAMES A. O'NEILL, JR.

Unfortunately, blood pressure is not routinely measured in children, particularly small children, so the diagnosis of hypertension in this age group is often delayed. In many instances, the presence of hypertension is found incidentally when children are being anesthetized for elective surgical procedures. In only rare instances are children obviously symptomatic, with encephalopathy, visual disturbances or headaches, and similar findings. When hypertension occurs in infants under 6 months of age, congestive heart failure may be the presenting sign. However, in the majority of instances patients are overtly asymptomatic.

The studies by Goldblatt and co-workers in the early 1930s demonstrated the relationship between renal ischemia and hypertension based on the renin–angiotensin axis, even though the latter was not described until the 1960s. So-called essential hypertension or hypertension of no known etiology occurs in children, but this cause of hypertension does not predominate until adolescence and adulthood. In most young children, a specific correctable etiology can be demonstrated, and in children under 5 years of age, the incidence of potentially correctable hypertension is close to 80%. Correctable forms of hypertension in children may be thought of as congenital or acquired and include endocrine, neurologic, metabolic, renal infectious, and vascular disorders. Hypertension of renovascular origin also may be thought of as congenital or acquired, and their recognition is important because the most common cause of surgically correctable hypertension in childhood is renovascular disease. The congenital causes include arterial hypoplasia or occlusion, neurofibromatosis involving the renal artery, and William's syndrome, which includes elfin facies, hypercalcemia, supravalvular aortic stenosis, and systolic hypertension associated with a variety of peripheral vascular stenoses including, particularly, subclavian and renal artery stenosis. The acquired forms of renovascular hypertension include anastomotic stenosis, renal artery trauma or thrombosis, Kawasaki's disease, and, most common of all, fibromuscular hyperplasia, either localized to the renal artery or a more generalized form of the disease similar to Takayasu's arteritis and subisthmic coarctation.

Although it is thought that fibromuscular hyperplasia in its various forms is autoimmune in origin, firm proof of this relationship is still lacking. There is no question, however, that the disorder involves an inflammatory arteritis that goes through a phase of active inflammation followed by a quiescent period during which time the lesions do not tend to progress. Lesions may involve both renal arteries or single segments of renal arteries or the entire mid-aortic area and its associated visceral branches. The radiographic pattern of fibromuscular hyperplasia in young adults, when it involves the renal artery, is usually one of multiple stenotic lesions, whereas in children the pattern is one of narrowing of the renal artery origin and sometimes its branch vessels.

Also, although females predominate in the older age group of patients with fibromuscular hyperplasia, in children the gender incidence is equal. With fibromuscular hyperplasia, the lesions are characteristically stenotic, whereas in Kawasaki's disease aneurysms may form, primarily in the branch vessels. Identification of the inflammatory phase of fibromuscular hyperplasia is important. It is preferable not to intervene surgically or with angioplasty during the inflammatory phase because recurrence predictably occurs. However, intervention during the quiescent phase is safe. Patients with renovascular lesions may have multiple lesions, and both kidneys are involved up to 70% of the time. Although in most instances bilateral involvement is evident at the time of diagnosis, some patients have recurrent disease many years later at another site or in the opposite kidney, which mandates long-term follow-up.

DIAGNOSIS

Once hypertension has been documented in a child, a variety of diagnostic studies should be performed, but the primary emphasis is on aortography with selective renal angiog-

J. A. O'Neill, Jr.: Section of Surgical Sciences, Vanderbilt University Medical Center, Nashville, Tennessee.

raphy (Table 138.1). Although a variety of laboratory studies are in order for general evaluation, only a few are of real help in terms of the specific entity involved. Urine catecholamine studies should be performed in all patients to rule out pheochromocytoma. Erythrocyte sedimentation rates should be determined in order to determine whether patients have active arteritis. Electrocardiography may help to determine whether patients have left ventricular strain or cardiac failure, and renal function should be assessed fully before dye studies are performed. Because we have seen a number of patients with oliguric renal failure when they first presented, timing of angiography was carefully coordinated with treatment of renal impairment. Measurements of blood urea nitrogen and serum creatinine are key in this respect.

With regard to radiologic studies, certain screening studies may be helpful. For screening, we have used either 99m-technetium diethylenetriamine pentaacetic acid (DTPA) flow scans or 99mTc-dimercaptosuccinic acid (DMSA) renal scans, which usually indicate delayed flow to the involved kidney if only one is involved. These studies are not as helpful in patients with bilateral lesions, although the time to full uptake is usually delayed as compared with normal. While captopril renography is useful in adults, we have not found this provocative test to be useful in children because it is not usually necessary to determine whether a particular lesion is significant in terms of causing the hypertension or not in the childhood age group. The presence of a renovascular stenotic lesion in a child is virtually always of significance. The most definitive approach is abdominal aortography and selective renal angiography. These procedures have helped us determine the presence of lesions within the kidneys as well as narrowing of the aorta, so called midaortic syndrome, and its visceral branches, particularly the superior mesenteric artery.

Plasma renin is ordinarily elevated in patients with renovascular hypertension, but its use as a screening test in children is limited. The prime use of renal vein renin studies is to distinguish the significance of a branch vessel lesion or aneurysm, in terms of determining whether the lesion is significant or not, but we have not found such determinations necessary in patients who have orificial narrowing of the main renal artery. Renal vein renin studies also may be useful to distinguish the significance of postoperative anastomotic stenoses should they occur.

In addition to making the diagnosis of renal artery stenosis, midaortic syndrome, or other forms of renovascular hypertension, full angiography is essential to planning operative repair. It is our preference to repair all lesions simultaneously rather than to stage operations. Although it was initially felt that staging vascular repairs was safer than performing procedures on both kidneys simultaneously, experience has shown that better results can be obtained when primary repair of all lesions is done at the same time. This is because reoperative surgery is difficult in a field where there is previous arteritis-related inflammatory reaction. The accuracy rate of aortography with selective renal arteriography is close to 100%. Although intravenous digital subtraction angiography may be helpful as a screening study, it does not provide sufficient detail in visualization to be definitive. Although the clarity of detail with magnetic resonance angiography is not currently sufficient for operative planning, emerging improvements in this modality may well obviate the need for aortography in the future.

TABLE 138.1. DIAGNOSIS OF RENOVASCULAR HYPERTENSION

Screening studies
Urinary catecholamines
Erythrocyte sedimentation rate
Complete blood count, serum electrolytes, urea nitrogen, creatinine
99mTc- DTPA flow scan or 99mTc- DMSA renal scan
Electrocardiogram, chest radiograph
Definitive studies
Aortography
Selective renal arteriography

DTPA, diethylenetriamine pentaacetic acid; DMSA, dimercaptosuccinic acid.

PREOPERATIVE PREPARATION

Preoperative preparation and postoperative treatment form a continuum. Patients who present with extreme hypertension should have treatment started immediately, even before all diagnostic studies are obtained. Control of blood pressure is highly desirable prior to performing angiography. For patients with severe hypertension that is symptomatic, intravenous drugs are usually preferable initially, gradually phasing to oral medications (Table 138.2). In extreme cases, nitroprusside is the preferred drug. In lesser degrees of hypertension, propranolol, hydralazine, and diuretics are in order. Once the patient can be transitioned to oral medications, then either long- or short-acting β-blocker agents such as propranolol as well as minoxidil, hydrochlorothiazide, and spironolactone may be used. Several other long-acting drugs are also available. However, it is our preference

TABLE 138.2. USEFUL DRUGS FOR RENOVASCULAR HYPERTENSION

Intravenous drugs for emergencies or postoperatively	
Nitroprusside	0.5–6 μg/kg/min infusion
Labetalol	1–3 mg/kg/h bolus or infusion
Nifedipine	0.25–0.5 mg/kg
Oral drugs for long-term treatment	
Propranolol	1–6 mg/kg/24 h
Atenolol	1–6 mg/kg/24 h
Minoxidil	0.1–1 mg/kg/24 h
Hydrochlorothiazide	1–3 mg/kg/24 h

not to use angiotensin-converting enzyme (ACE) inhibitor drugs such as captopril on patients with renovascular hypertension because of the potential for drug-induced renal ischemia and potentiation of renal failure. Although ACE inhibitor drugs are known to be extremely useful in patients with essential hypertension, they are potentially dangerous in patients with renovascular lesions. The same preoperative drugs are useful postoperatively with a similar transition because hypertension usually worsens immediately following operation because of cross-clamping and the time it takes to perform repairs, although the sequence usually goes rapidly when adequate revascularization has been accomplished. Resolution or improvement in the degree of hypertension may take up to 6 months following operation, so weaning of antihypertensive medicines should be accomplished gradually.

TECHNIQUES OF REPAIR

Because of the wide variation in presentation and distribution of lesions responsible for renovascular hypertension, the surgeon should be familiar with a number of operative approaches that may be needed. The first consideration is the matter of balloon angioplasty. We have found that balloon angioplasty is a definitive solution in instances of branch vessel stenoses or anastomotic stenoses, but it either did not work or was only temporarily successful in patients with ostial lesions. Because of the fact that many children with renovascular hypertension are quite young, we have avoided the use of stents because of the potential for both short- and long-term complications. However, with technical improvements in the future, it may be appropriate to reconsider this policy. Nonetheless, the results have been so satisfactory with definitive repair that the placement of stents has not been attractive in our experience. Balloon dilatation may be very useful in some instances where it is used as a temporalizing procedure while treating emergent hypertension. For example, in two of our three patients with total occlusion of both renal arteries associated with oliguric renal failure, it was possible to normalize renal function and treat the hypertension using balloon dilatation, and although the stenoses recurred, these patients were in much better condition for definitive operation because of angioplasty.

As a matter of philosophy, in very young children, partial and total nephrectomy have only been used when absolutely necessary. For example, in occasional neonates with severe hypertension related to renal hypoplasia and presumed congenital arterial hypoplasia, nephrectomy has been undertaken. In addition, primary partial nephrectomy has been used occasionally because of renal atrophy, extensive vascular damage, or vessels thought to be too small for a successful reconstruction. It is always preferable to perform revascularization whenever possible because partial or total nephrectomy is always available as a last resort. Because recurrent fibromuscular hyperplasia can occur, ablation of renal tissue is undesirable in children.

In the case of ostial lesions of the renal artery, one possibility is patch angioplasty, but this is rarely possible because of the extent of these lesions. Also, in patients with neurofibromatosis lesions of the origin of the renal artery, patch angioplasty is not feasible.

The most desirable approach to ostial lesions of the renal artery is reimplantation, provided that the aorta itself is normal. Unfortunately, fibromuscular hyperplasia frequently involves the wall of the aorta, as evidenced by the frequent occurrence of mid-aortic syndrome or subisthmic coarctation. In our experience, patients who have had successful reimplantation of the renal artery as a method of definitive repair have had lasting relief of their hypertension. Neither patch angioplasty nor direct anastomosis has been applicable in patients with branch vessel lesions. We have treated branch vessel lesions by balloon dilatation whenever possible, partial nephrectomy when the lesions were too distal for revascularization, and bypass with saphenous vein on occasion.

Because involvement of the renal artery with poststenotic dilatation is extensive in many instances, and because the wall of the aorta is often involved, bypass from the distal aorta to the renal artery distal to its point of narrowing is the most commonly applicable procedure. In instances of unilateral stenosis, it is sometimes possible to use hypogastric artery but often it is not long enough. When bypass procedures are performed, arterial grafts are the most theoretically appealing, but they are frequently not long enough. When bilateral renal artery stenosis is present, it is probably preferable not to harvest both hypogastric arteries because of the long-term potential for complications such as impotence or bladder dysfunction. For all of the above reasons and in order to avoid the potential that the hypogastric artery is involved with fibromuscular hyperplasia, which we have documented, we have preferred to use reversed saphenous vein as bypass material. These grafts should be placed end to side to either the distal aorta or to an aortoaortic bypass graft if one is needed because of midaortic narrowing. It is of interest that in our early experience with saphenous vein bypass grafts in the aortorenal location, graft aneurysm formation occurred. If such an aneurysm was going to form, it usually occurred within the first 12 months postoperatively, with an incidence of 20% to 30%. Significant aneurysm in a bypass graft usually results either in thrombosis or partial thrombosis with distal embolization to the kidney. Therefore, beginning in 1980, we modified the procedure.

Specifically, saphenous vein is harvested at the outset of the procedure, making an effort to obtain a segment without side branches if possible. The vein is left *in situ* until ready for use and then removed and gently washed out with heparinized saline. The end-to-side anastomosis to the aorta is completed initially by cross-clamping the aorta and then removing a small button of aortic tissue with a punch. Spatulation of the graft is performed, and the graft is sutured end-to-side with 5-0 or 6-0 polypropylene sutures interrupted at three points to permit future growth. Depending on the size of the vein graft, 4- or 6-mm tubular Dacron mesh (Pilling Surgical Corp., Horsham, Pennsylvania) is placed around the vein graft to prevent aneurysmal dilatation, and this has proven to be effective on follow-up. After completion of the graft-to-aorta anastomosis and placement of the protective tubular mesh, the distal end of the vein is anastomosed end-to-end to the renal artery, again with spatulation of both sides to be anastomosed and using a running technique posteriorly and an interrupted technique anteriorly. The anastomosis distally should be performed in an oblique fashion to produce an anastomotic circumference approximately three times the arterial diameter. When the distal anastomosis is completed, the mesh is fitted to the appropriate size and care is taken to be certain that its placement has not resulted in kinking of the graft.

In patients with combined midaortic syndrome and renal artery stenosis, two approaches are available. The first is lengthy aortoplasty with renal arterioplasty, filling the gap with a piece of Dacron graft or autogenous artery. This approach is preferred by some surgeons. The second approach, which we prefer, has been to bypass the midaortic lesions with woven Dacron grafts of 10 to 14 mm. In the majority of patients, it has been possible to perform the bypass entirely within the abdomen from the retroesophageal aorta to the bifurcation below, but two patients with longer lengths of aortic narrowing have required placement of the proximal aortic anastomosis of the bypass graft in the descending thoracic aorta. Then the saphenous bypass vein grafts have been taken off the Dacron bypass graft instead of the native aorta whenever the distal aorta could not accommodate them. This has proven to be most satisfactory. In young children, sufficient redundancy of the bypass graft has been allowed in placement to compensate for growth.

These techniques have held up for as long as 20 years thus far in follow-up. Some patients with midaortic syndrome also have significant narrowing of the superior mesenteric and celiac arteries. Because all of our patients have demonstrated extensive collateralization from the distal aorta, and because aortoaortic bypass has been anticipated, primary revascularization of these visceral vessels has not been performed by us, and no such patient has become symptomatic to date on long-term follow-up. However, some have taken the position that it is best to perform prophylactic revascularization of the superior mesenteric and celiac arteries, basing this on the thought that these patients would eventually become symptomatic. Only time and long-term follow-up will settle this issue, but allowing collateral circulation to provide for adequate proximal visceral flow has been most satisfactory to date, so whether visceral revascularization is worth the risk remains to be seen. The placement of a mesh protector around saphenous veins has held up and eliminated aneurysm formation. Other methods of renal artery revascularization such as splenorenal anastomosis and other makeshift procedures should probably be reserved for instances where all other approaches have failed.

COMPLICATIONS

Whenever patients can be treated with medications to the point that their vasculature is close to adult size, postoperative complications are less than if early repairs are needed. Because the vasculature of children does not have involvement with atherosclerosis, distal embolization during operative repair is not an issue. If appropriate precautions are taken, intraoperative hemorrhage and delayed bleeding from anastomoses should be rare. Systemic heparinization is used during operation, and it is allowed to dissipate following completion of all the anastomoses. Using this approach, bleeding complications have been nil, but the potential does exist, of course. Graft thrombosis may occur in the postoperative period because of kinking or unevenness of the anastomosis. Immediate reoperation is preferable to the use of thrombolytic agents because anastomotic revision is usually needed in these instances. Late thrombosis may occur because of aneurysm formation or flow changes, in which case a new bypass will be needed. Autogenous tissue should be used whenever possible, but occasionally PTFE or Dacron bypass grafts will be required. They have a much higher incidence of late thrombosis than autogenous grafts, however, so should only be used when absolutely necessary. Although chylous ascites was encountered early in our experience in one patient, it has not occurred subsequently since we have been using broad exposure of the retroperitoneum by means of reflection of the right colon for right-sided lesions, and of the spleen, pancreas, stomach, and left colon for left-sided lesions.

Two patients who had recurrent hypertension 12 to 18 months following bilateral repairs were found to have narrowing of one distal renal graft anastomosis, and each was successfully dilated by percutaneous transluminal angioplasty.

Another potential complication is recurrent hypertension related to recurrent fibromuscular hyperplasia, so long-term follow-up is essential. Patients are followed at 6-month intervals initially and yearly intervals thereafter to be sure that blood pressure remains normal or under good control with minimal medication requirement, including with exercise. It is probably prudent to perform magnetic resonance angiography every 5 years in asymptomatic patients to be sure the repairs are holding up. Aortography with selective renal arteriography or graft arteriography is indicated if hypertension recurs. Although we have not encountered long-term graft complications so far, there is still a potential for it to occur. In the majority of instances, the long-term results will be excellent so an aggressive approach to revascularization is clearly in order.

SUGGESTED READINGS

Dean RH, Robaczewski D. Arteriopathies of childhood. *Semin Pediatr Surg* 1994;3:103–113.

Messina LM, Riley LM, Goldstone J, et al. Middle aortic syndrome. Effectiveness and durability of complex arterial revascularization techniques. *Ann Surg* 1986;204:331–339.

O'Neill JA. Long-term outcome with surgical treatment of renovascular hypertension. *J Pediatr Surg* 1998;33:106–111.

O'Neill JA, Berkowitz H, Fellows KJ, et al. Mid-aortic syndrome and hypertension in childhood. *J Pediatr Surg* 1995;30:164–172.

Stanley JC, Frye WJ. Pediatric renal artery occlusive disease and renovascular hypertension. Etiology, diagnosis and operative treatment. *Arch Surg* 1981;116:669–676.

Surgical Directives: Pediatric Surgery, edited by Peter Mattei. Lippincott Williams & Wilkins, Philadelphia © 2002

139

FETAL SURGERY

ROMAN M. SYDORAK
CRAIG T. ALBANESE

In the past two decades, major advances in fetal imaging and diagnostic techniques have dramatically changed our understanding and management of prenatally diagnosed malformations. Although most of these abnormalities are best managed after birth, a few select diseases have devastating developmental consequences and nearly uniform fatality with standard postnatal care. These defects have prompted efforts for repair with *in utero* operative intervention. Years of research have identified selection criteria for fetuses amenable to intervention, and, at the same time, anesthetic, tocolytic, and, surgical techniques have been developed and refined. Using a team effort that includes pediatric surgeons, perinatologists, and sonographers, fetal surgery has become a reality, with the successful treatment of a number of these malformations.

MATERNOFETAL RISKS

Fetal surgery is primarily predicated on the fact that there are two patients being treated, the mother and fetus. The risk:benefit ratio favors the fetus with a lethal malformation, because without intervention the mortality rate is 100% and with intervention survival is possible. However, initiating such surgery is not that easily justified for the mother, whose physical health is usually not affected by her unborn child's condition. For this reason, it was paramount to prove that any intervention made through the mother could be performed safely. Early experience found that mothers had few complications and that their future fertility was not affected by fetal intervention. Bleeding caused by hysterotomy was diminished by the use of an absorbable stapling device, morbidity related to preterm labor (PTL) controlled by tocolytics, and pulmonary edema associated with use of tocolytics responsive to diuretics.

R. M. Sydorak and C. T. Albanese: Department of Surgery, Division of Pediatric Surgery, The University of California, San Francisco, and The University of California, San Francisco Medical Center, San Francisco, California.

FETAL SURGICAL TECHNIQUES

The development of both open and minimal-access fetal surgical techniques continues to evolve. Anesthesia of the mother and fetus is established with halogenated agents, which also provide profound uterine relaxation, thereby preventing intraoperative contractions. The fetus additionally receives an intramuscular injection of a narcotic and a paralytic agent. An epidural catheter is inserted to enhance postoperative maternal pain control. Tocolytics include a regimen of indomethacin, magnesium sulfate, intravenous nitroglycerin, and β-sympathomimetics. In the operating room, the mother is positioned with the right side elevated to avoid inferior vena caval compression by the gravid uterus and with her legs in lithotomy. Maternal monitoring is accomplished with standard techniques, including pulse oximetry, a blood pressure cuff, large-bore intravenous catheters, measurement of the urine output, and electrocardiography. The two principal routes of access to the fetus are discussed below.

OPEN FETAL SURGERY

The timing of fetal surgery is dependent on the malformation being treated and the pathophysiologic course encompassing the disorder. Commonly, accurate early diagnosis and the fragility of fetal tissue become limiting factors at less than 18 weeks' gestation. After 30 weeks' gestation, manipulations of the uterus are associated with a high risk for premature rupture of membranes (PROM), and PTL. Thus, it is then more reasonable to deliver the fetus and treat the malformation with postnatal care.

The uterus is exposed through a low transverse abdominal incision. The site of the hysterotomy is dictated by placental position. The uterus is opened using an absorbable uterine stapler, which facilitates hemostasis and control of the membranes. Four reverse biting compression clamps are placed at the lateral edges of the uterine incision to prevent venous bleeding at the unstapled edges and to keep the hysterotomy open. The appropriate part of the fetus is then exposed. A pulse oximeter is placed on the fetus because this has proven to be the most promising noninvasive method of monitoring fetal well-being. Warmed lactated Ringer's solution is continuously infused around the fetus to maintain fetal body temperature and uterine volume. Following repair of the defect, the fetus is returned to the amniotic cavity. Amniotic fluid is restored with a combination of the saved amniotic fluid, warmed saline, and an antibiotic. The membranes are closed with a monofilament absorbable suture, and the myometrium with two layers of absorbable sutures. Fibrin glue is applied to help seal the uterine incision. Cesarean delivery is performed when membranes rupture or labor cannot be controlled, usually before 36 weeks' gestation. Future deliveries after open fetal intervention must be by cesarean section to avoid the risk for uterine scar dehiscence during labor, because nearly all hysterotomies are in a nontransverse segment location.

MINIMAL ACCESS FETAL SURGERY

Although techniques for direct optical visualization of the fetus are not new, recent modifications of existing postnatal endoscopic techniques and the development of new fetoscopic instruments have resulted in the development of fetal endoscopic surgery, better known as FETENDO. The FETENDO strategy preserves fetal homeostasis by protecting the intrauterine physiologic milieu and avoiding the morbidity of a uterine incision, resulting in less PTL with less use of tocolytics, decreased maternal hospital stay, and decreased maternal complications related to the tocolytic therapy.

The surgeon stands between the patient's legs with an assistant on either side and the ultrasonographer on the patient's right. Monitors are placed side by side at the head of the table. An anterior placenta often requires a laparotomy to gain access to the posterior wall of the uterus, whereas a posterior placenta allows the procedure to be performed either percutaneously or with a mini-laparotomy. The sonologist is crucial to the case, determining trocar placement in relation to the placenta, guiding insertion of trocars, and monitoring the fetus throughout the operation. Standard 3- and 5-mm radially expanding trocars (InnerDyne, Sunnyvale, CA) are introduced via a diamond-tipped needle. They control bleeding by outward pressure, and membrane separation via a swift insertion technique with the sharp needle.

In contrast to adult laparoscopy performed within a gaseous medium, fetoscopy is performed within a fluid medium, preventing acidosis, hypothermia, and problems with ultrasonic visualization. A continuous pump irrigation system is used that delivers a variable fluid flow at a constant physiologic temperature via the tip of the endoscope. Working in this medium has not precluded the use of the laser or harmonic scalpel. Visualization is augmented by dispelling bleeding and replacing turbid amniotic fluid with saline.

POSTOPERATIVE MANAGEMENT

Tocolysis begins before anesthesia induction and continues after emergence. Fetal sonography, heart rate monitoring, magnetic resonance imaging (MRI), and echocardiography are substitutes for direct fetal physical examination in the postoperative period. Patient-controlled anesthesia pumps or epidural catheters ease maternal stress, provide analgesia, and aid tocolysis. Average length of hospital stay is 2 to 7 days, and outpatient tocolysis continues with an oral calcium channel blocker or a terbutaline pump. Fetal sonography and nonstress testing are performed weekly. Delivery occurs when membranes rupture, labor cannot be controlled, or the fetus is at full term.

FETAL MALFORMATIONS AMENABLE TO SURGICAL CORRECTION

Prenatal diagnosis has defined a "hidden" mortality rate for some lesions, such as congenital diaphragmatic hernia (CDH), urinary tract obstruction (UTO), sacrococcygeal teratoma (SCT), and congenital cystic adenomatoid malformation (CCAM) of the lung. These lesions, when first evaluated and treated postnatally, demonstrate a favorable selection bias because the most severely affected fetuses often die *in utero* or immediately after birth. Although most prenatally diagnosed malformations are best treated by standard postnatal care and planned delivery at a tertiary care center, a growing number of simple anatomic abnormalities with predictable, lethal consequences have been successfully corrected before birth with good outcomes. The development of minimal-access fetal surgical techniques, along with improvements in treatment and prevention of PTL, may enable us to make the transition from treating only life-threatening defects to treating non–life-threatening but substantially morbid malformations, namely myelomeningocele.

URINARY TRACT OBSTRUCTION

Fetal urinary tract abnormalities are the most frequent congenital anomaly diagnosed. Although 90% of fetuses need no treatment, findings of bilateral obstruction, most commonly caused by posterior urethral valves, may produce pulmonary hypoplasia and renal dysplasia. These fatal consequences can be ameliorated in selected patients by urinary tract decompression. Determination of the renal biochemical profile and ultrasonographic appearance of the kidneys and ureters helps determine which fetuses are amenable to operative intervention.

The aim of prenatal intervention is to bypass or directly treat the obstruction, restoring the amniotic fluid to normal levels. Initial intervention involving open fetal surgery is no longer necessary, because vesicoamniotic shunts can now be placed percutaneously and newer endoscopic alternatives have evolved. The most widely used and accepted means of treating bladder outlet obstruction is by percutaneous insertion of a double-J vesicoamniotic shunt. Complications associated with shunting include shunt occlusion, migration,

PTL, urinary ascites, and chorioamnionitis. The overall survival rate is 47%, and shunt-related complications occur in 45% of cases, a marked improvement for what is a nearly uniformly fatal condition. Quintero and colleagues have described a promising experience with *in utero* percutaneous cystoscopy in the management of lower obstructive uropathy.

CONGENITAL DIAPHRAGMATIC HERNIA

Congenital diaphragmatic hernia is a simple defect involving failure of development of the diaphragm, resulting in pulmonary hypoplasia. Despite advances in pre- and postnatal care and the development of extracorporeal membrane oxygenation, there continues to be a high neonatal mortality rate and appreciable long-term morbidity. Initial experience with open fetal surgical diaphragmatic repair was fraught with high mortality rates and prompted alternative approaches designed to reverse lung hypoplasia. After extensive animal research and observation of fetuses with high airway obstruction (see later section on Congenital High Airway Obstruction), fetoscopic tracheal occlusion was performed in human fetuses and was found to increase lung growth and have better outcomes than both open repair and standard postnatal care. This retrospective data is currently being evaluated in a National Institutes of Health–sponsored randomized control trial. Fetuses with a poor prognosis (a lung:head ratio less than 1.4 and the left lateral lobe of the liver in the hemithorax) and in whom the diagnosis is made prior to 25 weeks' gestation are randomized to standard postnatal care or fetal intervention (Fig. 139.1). Outcomes of this randomized control trial are

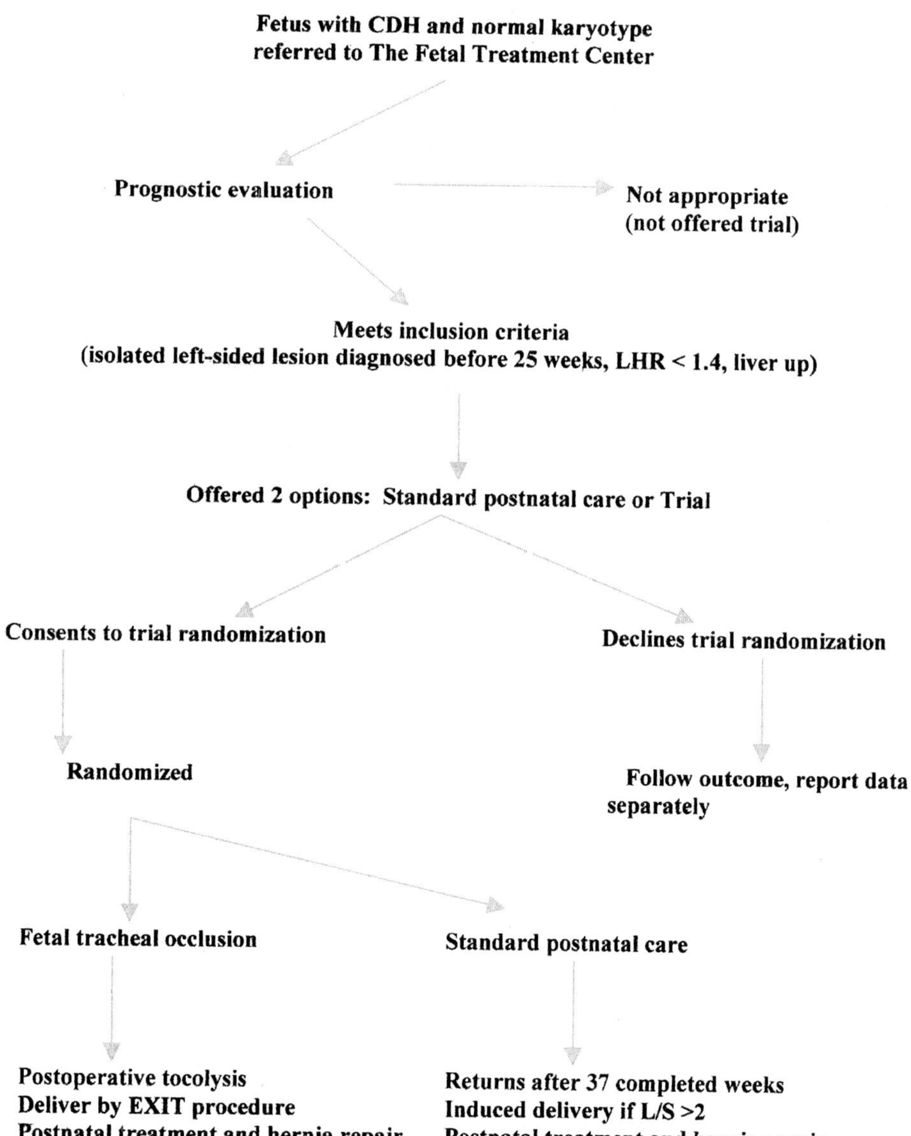

FIGURE 139.1. Algorithm for management of congenital diaphragmatic hernia.

pending, but retrospective results have shown a dramatic reduction in mortality with fetoscopic tracheal occlusion compared with standard postnatal care.

The technical goal of the procedure involves placement of an intratracheal balloon. The fetoscope is used to enter the amniotic cavity using a single 5-mm radially expanding trocar. Once inside, landmarks and ultrasonography are used to guide the surgeon to the mouth. With gentle pressure and hydrodissection, the mouth is opened, the hypopharynx exposed, and the trachea cannulated with the fetoscope. Following adequate visualization of the carina, a detachable occlusive balloon is deployed 2 cm proximal to the carina. Removal of the balloon and delivery of the fetus is performed using the EXIT (*ex utero* intrapartum treatment) strategy. The uterus is opened (avoiding the placenta), the baby's head and shoulders delivered, and the balloon is popped and removed via an endoscope. The child is then intubated, surfactant delivered, and mechanical ventilation begun. Once the oxygen saturation increases, the cord is cut and the child delivered. The diaphragmatic defect is repaired when the baby is stable (usually 3–7 days after delivery).

FETAL CYSTIC LUNG LESIONS

The natural history of prenatally diagnosed cystic lung masses is variable, and associated anomalies are rare. Pulmonary sequestration, defined as nonfunctional lung tissue with systemic arterial supply but not communicating with the tracheobronchial tree, causes minimal morbidity and no mortality. Fetal surgery is rarely needed except in rare cases where large effusions can lead to a tension hydrothorax and hydrops. Treatment then consists of thoracoamniotic shunting or, if no resolution of hydrops occurs, prenatal resection (Fig. 139.2).

Congenital cystic adenomatoid malformation (CCAM), the most common type of fetal thoracic mass, is a space-occupying lobar hamartoma. It may be cystic, solid, or both and is diagnosed by ultrasonography or ultrafast fetal MRI. CCAMs have a broad spectrum of clinical severity. They may enlarge significantly, may remain the same size, or may disappear prenatally. They lead to fetal demise in 100% of cases when cardiac and great vessel compression leads to hydrops. Only the most severely affected fetuses may be candidates for fetal intervention. Careful ultrasonographic

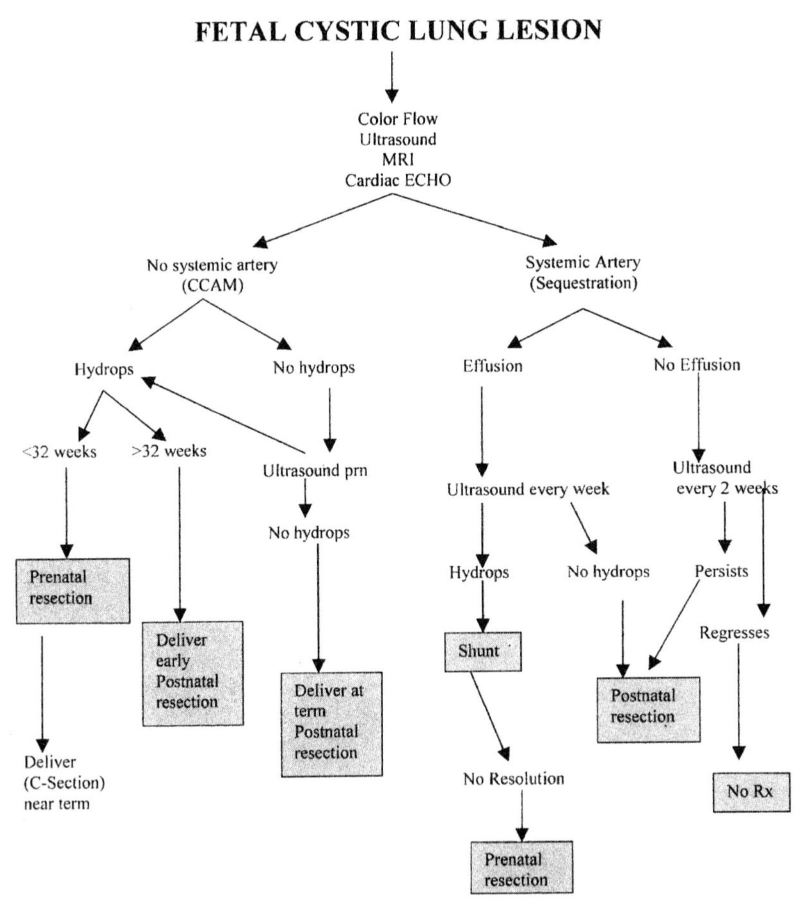

FIGURE 139.2. Algorithm for the evaluation and treatment of a prenatally diagnosed fetal cystic lung mass.

surveillance of large lesions is necessary to detect the first signs of hydrops, because fetuses in whom hydrops develops (<10%) can be saved with resection of the mass, with a 60% survival rate. Open fetal surgical resection of the massively enlarged solid pulmonary lobe (fetal lobectomy) is performed with a posterolateral thoracotomy at the fifth intercostal space. The hilar vessels are isolated and ligated with an endoloop, stapler, or nonabsorbable suture. Alternatively, primarily cystic lesions can be decompressed percutaneously by needle aspiration or a thoracoamniotic shunt.

SACROCOCCYGEAL TERATOMA

Sacrococcygeal teratoma is the most common congenital tumor diagnosed prenatally. Although most fetuses diagnosed with SCT have an uneventful intrauterine course, a small subset (<20%) with large tumors develop hydrops from high-output failure due to the shunting effect of large arteriovenous fistulas at the tumor base, a finding that may rapidly lead to fetal demise. Options for treatment include hysterotomy and removal of the tumor, or minimal-access techniques to stop the blood flow to the tumor via an ultrasonography-guided radiofrequency ablation (RFA) probe or fetoscopically guided laser. Because the need for intervention is rare, determining the approach that provides the best outcome has been difficult.

COMPLICATIONS OF MONOCHORIONIC TWINNING

A variety of abnormalities occur in monochorionic twin pregnancies where shared placental circulation and abnormal vascular connections can lead to twin-twin transfusion syndrome (TTTS), twin reversed arterial perfusion (TRAP), or potential death of a healthy fetus if a co-twin discordant for a lethal anomaly should die. TTTS, the most common of these abnormalities (occurring in up to a third of monochorionic twins), is characterized by abnormal vascular connections between the twins, resulting in a hydropic "recipient" twin with cardiac failure and polyhydramnios and one "stuck" (donor) twin with intrauterine growth retardation and oligohydramnios. Early expectant management results in 80% to 100% mortality primarily due to the high risk of miscarriage and brain damage.

There are differing views about the best treatment strategy to employ for TTTS, but options include serial amniocenteses, laser photocoagulation of abnormal vascular connections, or selective termination of the unhealthy twin in severe cases (Fig. 139.3). Patients are staged sonographically (Fig. 139.3), and patients with stages II to IV receive treatment. The initial treatment is one or more amniocenteses of the recipient sac. For those nonresponders or those recipients with hydrops, laser photocoagulation is performed

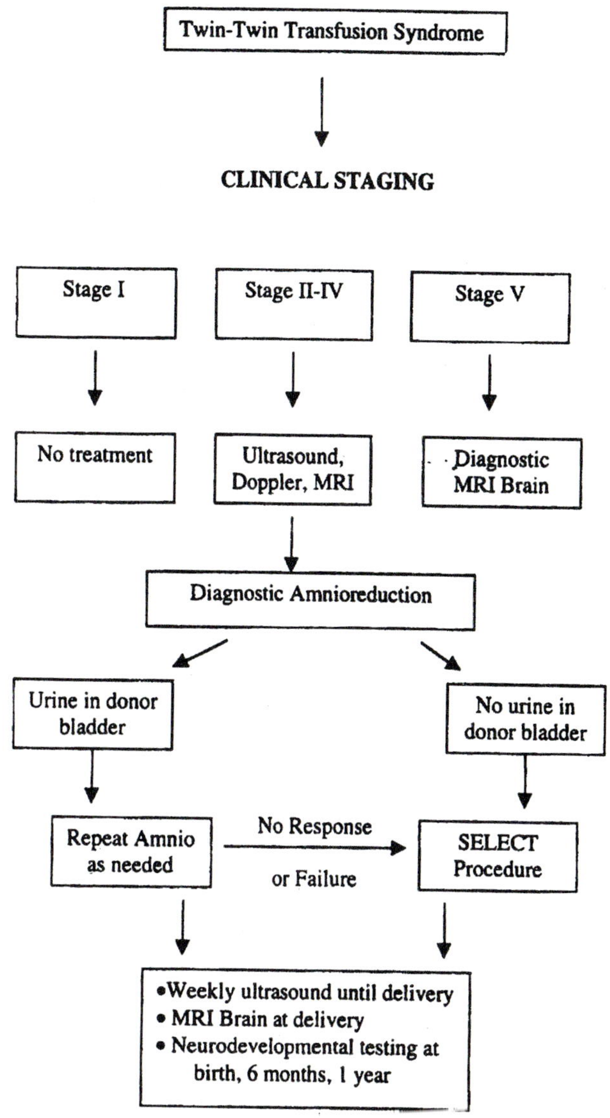

FIGURE 139.3. Algorithm for management of twin-twin transfusion syndrome.

using the neodymium:yttrium-aluminum-garnet (Nd-YAG) laser passed via a fiber through an operating endoscope. The vessels in question are unpaired vessels with flow from the donor to recipient. Spectral Doppler interrogation demonstrates the characteristic pulsatile arterial blood flow on the donor's side, whereas the vessel shows a continuous venous flow on the recipient's side. Some surgeons elect to coagulate all vessels seen crossing the intertwin septum, whereas others selectively divide communicating vessels along the shared meridian intertwin membrane. Laser surgery may be a more effective alternative than serial amniocentesis because there are more pregnancies with greater than one survivor, fewer intrauterine fetal deaths, and a lower incidence of brain abnormalities. Survival statistics with laser treatment show survival of both twins in 69% of cases and at least one twin in 82%. When the disease has progressed so far that the donor twin's life is threatened (hydrops, poor cardiac contractility), the recipient twin can be selectively terminated.

For some discordant monochorionic twins and for an acardiac-acephalic twin with TRAP syndrome, obliteration of the umbilical cord of the abnormal twin is preferable because the demise of one twin threatens the other. Should the compromised twin die, the sequela to the healthy twin is a 25% risk for developing necrotic lesions, usually affecting the cerebral white matter with a comparable risk for co-twin intrauterine death. The therapeutic goal of completely interrupting the vascular communication between the two twins, although simple in concept, has been difficult to accomplish. Initial attempts to remove the abnormal fetus from the uterus (sectio parva) or embolize the umbilical cord were characterized by frequent failures. As a result, umbilical cord ligation became the most commonly used procedure for vascular interruption. A variety of techniques have been used to divide the cord, including extracorporeal knot ligation, laser obliteration, bipolar coagulation, and ultrasonography-guided transection with a harmonic scalpel. All of these techniques have been successful in small series, and the optimal approach has not been determined. The most commonly used methods at our institution use selective ultrasonography-guided RFA termination (unpublished data) at the umbilical cord insertion and the CUT (cord ultrasonic transection) procedure using the harmonic scalpel.

MYELOMENINGOCELE

Myelomeningocele, or spina bifida, is a complex developmental defect involving failure of closure of the neural plate, resulting in a variety of abnormalities, including paraplegia, skeletal deformities, sexual dysfunction, hydrocephalus, and often impaired mental development. Between 1,500 and 2,000 babies are born with myelomeningocele in the United States every year. More than 80% of children with myelomeningocele may be identified before birth with maternal serum α-fetoprotein screening. Direct sonographic visualization of the abnormal fetal spine and brain can usually be accomplished by 16 weeks' gestation.

The rationale for prenatal intervention is based on the observation that lower extremity function present in early pregnancy is progressively lost in later gestation. Animal experiments have demonstrated that intrauterine repair of myelomeningocele may preserve peripheral neurologic function. Furthermore, experimental studies indicate that the Chiari II malformation, which is nearly always associated with myelomeningocele, may be prevented by prenatal repair. Recent clinical experience has demonstrated that open fetal surgery may improve neurologic function and resolve the hindbrain herniation associated with myelomeningocele. These early studies appear promising, but the variable natural history, lack of accurate prenatal indicators of neurologic function, absence of matched controls and long-term follow-up hamper the assessment of benefits of prenatal intervention.

These crucial unanswered questions in the prenatal natural history of myelomeningocele will be evaluated in a three-center randomized control trial beginning in 2002. Following evaluation at a designated fetal treatment center, fetuses at less than 25 weeks' gestation with L1 to S1 lesions will be randomized comparing *in utero* microsurgical three-layered open repair to standard postnatal care (Fig. 139.4).

CONGENITAL HIGH AIRWAY OBSTRUCTION

Congenital high airway obstruction is usually caused by laryngeal or tracheal atresia and rarely by isolated tracheal stenosis. Obstruction prevents the normal egress of fluid from the lungs into amniotic space. Thus, the growth factor–rich fluid builds up under pressure and greatly expands the lungs. The characteristic sonographic findings are large lungs with flattened or inverted diaphragms. Hydrops, secondary to mediastinal compression from the hyperplastic lungs, is common. If no hydrops is present, the fetus is delivered by the EXIT procedure, with tracheostomy and interval laryngotracheal reconstruction. However, for selected fetuses who develop hydrops, early delivery or *in utero* fetoscopic tracheostomy can relieve the obstruction and may reverse the hydrops.

AMNIOTIC BAND SYNDROME

Amniotic band syndrome is a frequent cause of fetal deformations involving the limbs, craniofacial region, and trunk. The spectrum of morbidity ranges from syndactyly to limb amputation. The syndrome may be fatal if umbilical cord constriction is present. Mild forms of the syndrome do not warrant fetoscopic intervention given the potential fetal and maternal morbidity. Fetuses with severe forms of this syndrome are good candidates for early release if it can be accomplished fetoscopically. Quintero treated two such cases, dividing the bands using scissors via a single port with ultrasonographic guidance. This restored adequate blood flow distal to the obstruction, and only mild or minimal limb dysfunction was present at birth.

PLEURAL AND PERICARDIAL EFFUSIONS

Percutaneous thoracoamniotic shunting may be effective in relieving lung compression and any coexistent mediastinal shift caused by pleural effusions from thoracic masses (pulmonary sequestration, CCAM). Similarly, pericardiocentesis may relieve caval compression by large fluid-filled pericardial teratomas. These interventions may prevent pulmonary

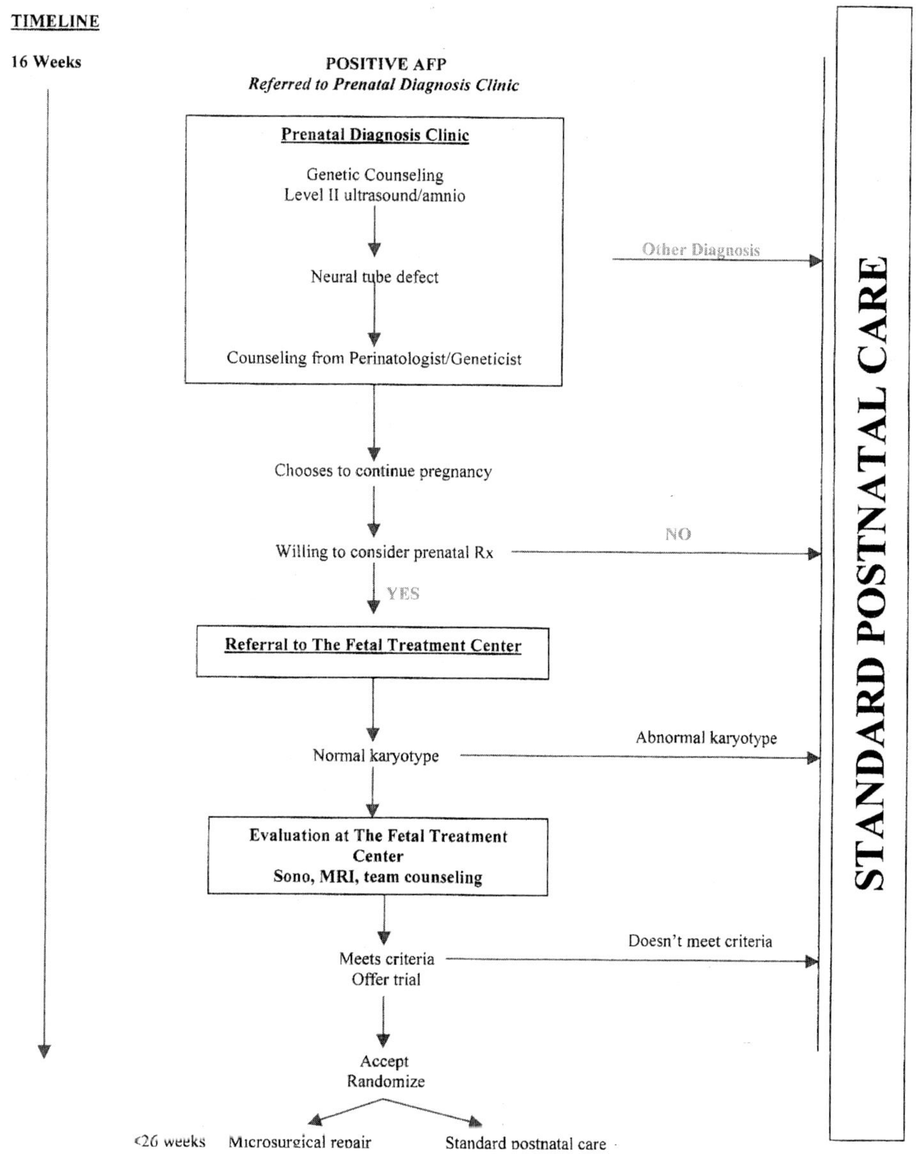

FIGURE 139.4. Algorithm for management of myelomeningocele.

hypoplasia, reverse fetal hydrops, and resolve polyhydramnios, thereby reducing the risk for fetal death or preterm delivery. When shunting or pericardiocentesis prove to be ineffective, prenatal resection may be attempted (Fig. 139.2).

COMPLICATIONS OF FETAL SURGICAL INTERVENTION

Preterm labor and PROM are the predominant limiting factors preventing the broad application of fetal surgery. PTL has been referred to as the Achilles heel of fetal intervention. Although numerous tocolytics and less invasive surgical techniques have been used, little progress has been made in preventing PTL, which occurs, in some degree, to all mothers undergoing fetal surgery. Minimal access techniques have shown trends toward decreasing the incidence of PTL, but conclusive studies showing that fewer and smaller trocars lessen the risk of PTL have not been published.

Perhaps the greatest problem with fetal surgery is PROM, the most common complication associated with fetoscopy. Despite experimentation with a variety of closure techniques, breaching the uterine membranes leads to both a functional weakness and an as yet unknown biochemical change that leads to PROM in 6% to 10% of cases in single-port procedures and up to 40% to 60% in multiport procedures with longer operating times. This can lead to perinatal loss rates as high as 50% in some series, in large part due to sequelae of PROM (e.g., PTL, oligohydramnios, premature delivery, chorioamnionitis, and even fetal demise). Although alternative techniques to close the membranes have been tried, observation of the membranes at delivery has often shown that the rupture occurred at a site distant from trocar insertion. Once the diagnosis of PROM is made, mothers can rarely carry their fetuses for longer than a few weeks, although an innovative approach to seal ruptured membranes has been attempted.

FUTURE OF FETAL THERAPY

Operative fetal intervention is only now approaching the end of its second decade. Minimal-access surgery has largely taken over the field in the past 5 years save for a few diseases that require open operative intervention. Many challenges remain, including devising less invasive operative methods, determining better predictors of fetuses at risk, and reducing the incidence of PTL and PROM, the two nemeses of fetal surgery. The elucidation of the natural history of several fetal disorders has paved the way for the development of fetal surgical intervention. The short but eventful history of fetal surgical intervention offers new hope for the fetus with an isolated congenital malformation. The great promise is that for some diseases, the earliest possible intervention (i.e., before birth) will produce the best possible outcomes. As experience develops and the results of many of the currently running trials become known, the role of fetal surgery will become clearer. Although significant progress has been made in the treatment of nearly fatal fetal diseases such as TTTS, CDH, monochorionic twins, and UTO, the future of fetal surgery will rely on a better understanding of the pathophysiology and treatment of PROM and PTL.

SUGGESTED READINGS

Adzick NS, Harrison MR, Crombleholme TM, et al. Fetal lung lesions: management and outcome. *Am J Obstet Gynecol* 1998;179:884–889.

Adzick NS, Harrison MR, Flake AW, et al. Fetal surgery for cystic adenomatoid malformation of the lung. *J Pediatr Surg* 1993;28:806–812.

Albanese CT, Harrison MR. Surgical treatment for fetal disease. The state of the art. *Ann N Y Acad Sci* 1998;847:74–85.

Farrell JA, Albanese CT, Jennings RW, et al. Maternal fertility is not affected by fetal surgery. *Fetal Diagn Ther* 1999;14:190–192.

Freedman AL, Johnson MP, Smith CA, et al. Long-term outcome in children after antenatal intervention for obstructive uropathies. *Lancet* 1999;354:374–377.

Harrison MR. Fetal surgery. *Am J Obstet Gynecol* 1996;174:1255–1264.

Harrison MR, Evans MI, Adzick NS, et al., eds. *The unborn patient, 3rd ed.* Philadelphia: WB Saunders, 2001:11–18.

Luks FI, Johnson BD, Papadakis K, et al. Predictive value of monitoring parameters in fetal surgery. *J Pediatr Surg* 1998;33:1297–1301.

Machin GA, Keith LG. *An atlas of multiple pregnancy.* New York: Parthenon, 1999.

Mychaliska GB, Bealer JF, Graf JL, et al. Operating on placental support: the ex utero intrapartum treatment procedure. *J Pediatr Surg* 1997;32:227–230; discussion 230–231.

SUBJECT INDEX

Page numbers followed by f indicate figures; page numbers followed by t indicate tables.

C

D

H

I

J

K

L

M

O

P

R